CONTENTS

evolve

ELSEVIER

YOU'VE JUST PURCHASED
MORE THAN
A TEXTBOOK!

Evolve Student Resources for *Gray, Grove, & Sutherland:
Burns and Grove's The Practice of Nursing Research:
Appraisal, Synthesis, and Generation of Evidence, Eighth
Edition,* include the following:

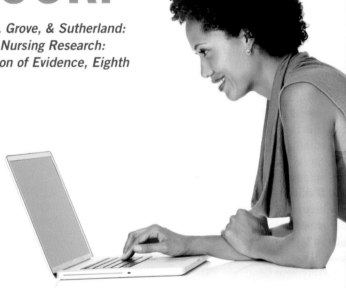

- **Interactive Review Questions**
  More than 400 questions,
  with feedback for both correct
  and incorrect responses.

Activate the complete learning experience that comes with each
textbook purchase by registering at

http://evolve.elsevier.com/Gray/practice

REGISTER TODAY!

2015v1.0

EDITION 8

BURNS AND GROVE'S
THE Practice of Nursing Research

Appraisal, Synthesis, and Generation of Evidence

Jennifer R. Gray, PhD, RN, FAAN
Associate Dean
College of Natural and Health Sciences
Oklahoma Christian University
Edmond, Oklahoma;
Professor Emeritus
College of Nursing and Health Innovation
The University of Texas at Arlington
Arlington, Texas

Susan K. Grove, PhD, RN, ANP-BC, GNP-BC
Professor Emeritus
College of Nursing and Health Innovation
The University of Texas at Arlington
Arlington, Texas;
Adult Nurse Practitioner
Family Practice
Grand Prairie, Texas

Suzanne Sutherland, PhD, RN
Professor Emeritus and Part-Time Lecturer
California State University, Sacramento
Sacramento, California

ELSEVIER

ELSEVIER

3251 Riverport Lane
St. Louis, Missouri 63043

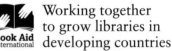

To our readers and researchers, nationally and internationally, who will provide the science to develop an evidence-based practice for nursing. To our family members for their constant input, support, and love, and especially to our husbands
Randy Gray,
Jay Suggs,
and
Jerry Sutherland

Jennifer, Susan, and Suzanne

CONTRIBUTORS

Daisha J. Cipher, PhD
Clinical Associate Professor
College of Nursing and Health Innovation
University of Texas at Arlington
Arlington, Texas

Kathryn M. Daniel, PhD, RN, ANP-BC, GNP-BC, AGSF
Associate Professor
Associate Chair for Nurse Practitioner Programs, Graduate Program
Director, Adult-Gerontology Primary Care Nurse Practitioner Program
Interim Director, Family Nurse Practitioner Program
College of Nursing and Health Innovation
University of Texas at Arlington
Arlington, Texas

REVIEWERS

Sara L. Clutter, PhD, RN
Associate Professor of Nursing
Department of Nursing
Waynesburg University
Waynesburg, Pennsylvania

Betsy Frank, RN, PhD, ANEF
Professor Emerita
Department of Baccalaureate Nursing Completion
Indiana State University
Terre Haute, Indiana

Sharon Kitchie, RN, PhD
Adjunct Instructor
Department of Nursing
Keuka College
Keuka Park, New York

Teresa M. O'Neill, PhD, APRN, RNC
Professor Emerita
Our Lady of Holy Cross College
New Orleans, Louisiana

Jeanne Tucker, RN, MSN, HSAD, PhD, CHES, PCEP
Assistant Professor of Nursing
Patty Hanks Shelton School of Nursing
A Consortium of Hardin Simmons University and
   McMurry University
Abilene, Texas

Angela F. Wood, RN, PhD, NNP
Professor of Nursing, Chair
Department of Nursing
Carson-Newman University
Jefferson City, Tennessee

PREFACE

Research is a major force in the nursing profession that is used to change practice, education, and health policy. Our aim in developing the eighth edition of *The Practice of Nursing Research: Appraisal, Synthesis, and Generation of Evidence* is to increase excitement about research and to facilitate the development of evidence-based practice for nursing. It is critically important that all nurses, especially those in advanced-practice roles (nurse practitioners, clinical nurse specialists, nurse anesthetists, and nurse midwives) and those assuming roles as administrators and educators, have a strong understanding of the research methods conducted to generate evidence-based knowledge for nursing practice. Graduate and undergraduate nursing students and practicing nurses must be actively involved in critically appraising and synthesizing research evidence for the delivery of quality, cost-effective care. This text provides detailed content and guidelines for implementing critical appraisal and synthesis processes. The text also contains extensive coverage of the research methodologies—quantitative, qualitative, mixed methods, and outcomes—commonly employed in nursing. Doctoral students might use this text to facilitate their conduct of quality studies essential for generating nursing knowledge.

The depth and breadth of content presented in this edition reflect the increase in research activities and the growth in research knowledge since the previous edition. Nursing research is introduced at the baccalaureate level and becomes an integral part of graduate education (master's and doctoral) and clinical practice. We hope that this new edition might increase the number of nurses at all levels involved in research activities, so as to improve outcomes for nursing practice.

This eighth edition is written and organized to facilitate ease in reading, understanding, and implementing the research process. The major strengths of this text are as follows:

- State-of-the-art coverage of evidence-based practice (EBP)—a topic of vital and growing importance in a healthcare arena focused on quality, cost-effective patient care.
- Addition of a chapter on mixed methods research, a methodology that is employed today with increasing frequency, reflecting the modern proliferation of multifaceted problems.
- A clear, concise writing style for facilitation of student learning that is consistent throughout all chapters.
- Comprehensive coverage of quantitative, qualitative, mixed methods, and outcomes research strategies, with examples provided from published studies.
- A balanced coverage of qualitative and quantitative research methodologies.
- An introduction to ethical issues related to genomics research.
- Electronic references and websites that direct the student to an extensive array of information that is important for conducting studies and using research findings in practice.
- Rich and frequent illustration of major points and concepts from the most current nursing research literature, emphasizing a variety of clinical practice areas.
- A strong conceptual framework that links nursing research with EBP, theory, knowledge, and philosophy.

Our text provides a comprehensive introduction to nursing research for graduate and practicing nurses. Of particular usefulness at the master's and doctoral level, the text provides not only substantive content related to research but also practical applications based on the authors' experiences in conducting various types of nursing research, familiarity with the research literature, and experience in teaching nursing research at various educational levels.

The eighth edition of this text is organized into 5 units and 29 chapters. Unit One provides an introduction to the general concepts of nursing research. The content and presentation of this unit have been designed to introduce EBP, quantitative research, and qualitative research.

Unit Two provides an in-depth presentation of the research process for quantitative, qualitative, mixed methods, and outcomes research, including two detailed chapters on measurement. As with previous editions, this text provides extensive coverage of study designs and statistical analyses.

Unit Three addresses the implications of research for the discipline and profession of nursing. Content is provided to direct the student in conducting critical appraisals of both quantitative and qualitative research. A detailed discussion of types of research synthesis and strategies for promoting EBP is provided.

Unit Four provides students and practicing nurses the content they require for implementation of actual research studies. This unit includes chapters focused on data collection and management, statistical analysis, interpretation of research outcomes, and dissemination of research findings.

Unit Five addresses proposal development and seeking support for research. Readers are given direction for developing successful research proposals and seeking funding for their proposed research.

The changes in the eighth edition of this text reflect advances in nursing research and also incorporate comments from outside reviewers, colleagues, and students. Our desire to promote the continuing development of the profession of nursing was the incentive for investing the time and energy required to develop this new edition.

NEW CONTENT

The eighth edition provides current comprehensive coverage of nursing research and is focused on the learning needs and styles of today's nursing students and practicing nurses. Several exciting new areas of content based on the changes and expansion in the field of nursing research are included in this edition. Some of the major changes from the previous edition are as follows:

- Chapter 1, "Discovering the World of Nursing Research," provides a stronger introduction to EBP and includes an example of the most current evidence-based guidelines for the management of hypertension.
- Chapter 2, "Evolution of Research in Building Evidence-Based Nursing Practice," has a new figure for demonstrating the levels of research knowledge. In addition, this chapter introduces the most current processes for synthesizing research knowledge, which are systematic reviews, meta-analyses, meta-syntheses, and mixed-method systematic reviews.
- Chapter 3, "Introduction to Quantitative Research," was rewritten to provide a clearer overview of the quantitative research process and the role of iteration in the design process, for the beginning researcher. It also includes the concept of theoretical substruction and the application of this strategy.
- Chapter 5, "Research Problem and Purpose," was rewritten to reflect practical considerations of how to identify a problem area and define the purpose of a study.
- Chapters 6, 7, and 8 have been reordered, reflecting a more logical sequencing.
- Chapter 6, "Objectives, Questions, Variables, and Hypotheses," has been rewritten to guide the student in how to word research questions for various

quantitative and qualitative designs, identify types of variables, write conceptual and operational definitions, and construct various types of hypotheses.

- Chapter 7, "Review of Relevant Literature," provides practical steps in searching the literature, synthesizing the information, and writing the review.
- Chapter 9, "Ethics in Research," features new coverage of genomics research, recent ethical violations, and government regulations. This chapter also details the escalating problem of scientific misconduct in all healthcare disciplines and the actions that have been taken to manage this problem.
- Chapters 10 and 11 have been rewritten and re-organized, presenting noninterventional designs in one chapter and interventional designs in the other.
- Chapter 10 "Quantitative Methodology: Noninterventional Designs and Methods" presents concepts pertinent to noninterventional research, including specifics of design validity. It also describes and provides examples and new illustrations for various descriptive and correlational designs used frequently in nursing research, or potentially useful for healthcare research. Its algorithms for differentiating among the four major quantitative design types, and for selecting specific designs from among both descriptive and correlational methods, have been revised.
- Chapter 11 "Quantitative Methodology: Interventional Designs and Methods" presents concepts pertinent to interventional research, including descriptions of specific threats to validity for interventional studies. It also describes and provides new examples and illustrations for various experimental and quasi-experimental designs used frequently in nursing research, or potentially useful for healthcare research. Its algorithms for selecting specific interventional designs from among both experimental and quasi-experimental methods, have been revised.
- Chapter 12, "Qualitative Research Methods," describes each step of the research process from writing the problem statement to interpreting the findings for qualitative studies. In addition to the data collection methods of observing, interviewing, and conducting focus groups, content was added about web-based research and other electronic means of collecting qualitative data.
- Chapter 13, "Outcomes Research," a unique feature of our text, was rewritten to extend the revisions begun by Dr. Diane Doran, a leading authority in the conduct of outcomes research, for edition 7, and to update content so that it reflects current trends in outcomes research. More detail in content is included

for the foundational concepts described by Donabedian, including his theoretical bases for outcomes research and his own history. The interplay between outcomes research and EBP, from standpoints of quantitative and qualitative research, has been clarified and is displayed in a new diagrammatic model.

- Chapter 14, "Mixed Methods Research," is a new chapter and proposes three broad categories of mixed methods research: exploratory sequential design, explanatory sequential design, and convergent concurrent designs. The often-missing steps of integrating the findings across methods is newly described.
- Chapter 15, "Sampling," was revised to reflect the most current coverage of sampling methods and the processes for determining sample size for quantitative and qualitative studies in nursing. Discussion of sampling methods and settings are supported with examples from current, relevant studies.
- Chapter 16, "Measurement Concepts," features detailed, current information for examining the reliability and validity of measurement methods and the precision and accuracy of physiological measures used in nursing studies. The discussions of sensitivity, specificity, and likelihood ratios are expanded and supported with examples from current studies.
- Chapter 17, "Measurement Methods Used in Developing Evidence-Based Practice," provides more current detail on the use of physiological measurement methods in research. A new diagram is added to promote the use of Q-sort methodology in studies.
- Chapter 18, "Critical Appraisal of Nursing Studies," now includes consistent steps for the critical appraisal of quantitative and qualitative studies: (1) identifying the steps or elements of the research process; (2) determining study strengths and limitations; and (3) evaluating the credibility, trustworthiness, and meaning of study findings for future research, nursing knowledge, and practice.
- Chapter 19, "Evidence Synthesis and Strategies for Implementing Evidence-Based Practice," has

undergone revision to promote the conduct of research syntheses and the use of best research evidence in nursing practice. The chapter contains current, extensive details for conducting systematic reviews, meta-analyses, meta-syntheses, and mixed-method systematic reviews.

- Major revisions have been made in the chapters focused on statistical concepts and analysis techniques (Chapters 21 through 25). The content is presented in a clear, concise manner and supported with examples of analyses conducted on actual clinical data. Dr. Daisha Cipher, a noted statistician and healthcare researcher, provided the revisions of these chapters.
- Chapter 26, "Interpreting Research Outcomes," has been revised, using a design validity-based model as underpinning for identification of limitations, generalizations, and recommendations for further research.

STUDENT ANCILLARIES

An **Evolve Resources website,** which is available at http://evolve.elsevier.com/Gray/practice/, includes the following:

- Interactive Review Questions, which have been revised so that more questions are now at the application, analysis, or synthesis level.

INSTRUCTOR ANCILLARIES

The **Instructor Resources** are available on Evolve, at http://evolve.elsevier.com/Gray/practice/. Instructors also have access to the online student resources. The Instructor Resources feature a revised Test Bank of more than 600 items reflecting eighth edition changes and revisions, PowerPoint presentations totaling more than 700 slides, updated to eighth edition changes and revisions, and an Image Collection consisting of the images from the text.

ACKNOWLEDGMENTS

Writing the eighth edition of this textbook has allowed us the opportunity to examine and revise the content of the previous edition based on input from a number of scholarly colleagues, the literature, and our graduate and undergraduate students. A textbook such as this requires synthesizing the ideas of many people and resources.

We also want to thank the people who contributed to this new edition. Dr. Daisha Cipher provided an excellent revision of Chapters 21 through 25 with her strong statistical expertise and ability to explain data analysis in an understandable way. We also thank Dr. Kathy Daniel for her contribution of a current, quality quasi-experimental research proposal to Chapter 28. Our gratitude is also extended to Dr. Nancy Burns, an original co-creator of *The Practice of Nursing Research*, who has a passion for nursing research.

We also have attempted to extract from the nursing and healthcare literature the essence of knowledge related to the conduct of nursing research. Thus, we would like to thank those scholars who shared their knowledge with the rest of us in nursing and who have made this knowledge accessible for inclusion in this textbook. The ideas from the literature were synthesized and discussed with our colleagues and students to determine the revisions needed for the eighth edition.

We also express our appreciation to the administrators and fellow faculty at our respective universities for their support during the long and time-consuming experience of revising a book of this magnitude. We particularly value the questions raised by our students regarding the content of this text, which allow us a unique view of our learners' perceptions.

We also recognize the excellent reviews of the colleagues who helped us make important revisions in this text. These reviewers are located in large and small universities across the United States and provided a broad range of research expertise.

On a personal level, we acknowledge that such an extensive project has an impact on all aspects of our lives. We are indebted to our families and friends for patient understanding and for their efforts to maintain the status quo of our "real lives."

Finally, we thank the people at Elsevier, who have been extremely helpful to us in producing a scholarly, attractive, appealing text. We extend a special thank-you to the people most instrumental in the development and production of this book: Lee Henderson, Executive Content Strategist; and Laurel Shea, Associate Content Development Specialist. We also want to thank others involved with the production and marketing of this book—Abbie Bradberry, Project Manager; Maggie Reid, Designer; and Kristen Oyirifi, Marketing Manager.

Jennifer R. Gray, PhD, RN, FAAN | **Susan K. Grove**, PhD, RN, ANP-BC, GNP-BC | **Suzanne Sutherland**, PhD, RN

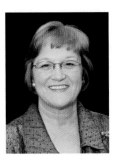
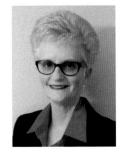
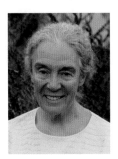

CONTENTS

APPENDICES

Discovering the World of Nursing Research

Susan K. Grove

http://evolve.elsevier.com/Gray/practice/

Welcome to the world of nursing research. You might think it is strange to consider research a *world,* but research is truly a new way of experiencing reality. Entering a new world requires learning a unique language, incorporating new rules, and using new experiences to learn how to interact effectively within that world. As you become a part of this new world, your perceptions and methods of reasoning will be modified and expanded. Understanding the world of nursing research is critical to providing evidence-based care to your patients. Since the 1990s, there has been a growing emphasis for nurses—especially advanced practice nurses (APNs), administrators, educators, and nurse researchers—to promote an evidence-based practice (EBP) in nursing (Brown, 2014; Craig & Smyth, 2012; Melnyk & Fineout-Overholt, 2015). EBP in nursing requires a strong body of research knowledge that nurses must synthesize and use to promote quality care for their patients, families, and communities. We developed this text to facilitate your understanding of nursing research and its contribution to the implementation of evidenced-based nursing practice.

This chapter broadly explains the world of research. A definition of nursing research is provided, followed by the framework for this textbook that connects nursing research to the world of nursing. The chapter concludes with a discussion of the significance of research in developing an EBP for nursing.

DEFINITION OF NURSING RESEARCH

The root meaning of the word research is "search again" or "examine carefully." More specifically, **research** is the diligent, systematic inquiry or investigation to validate and refine existing knowledge and generate new knowledge. The concepts *systematic* and *diligent* are critical to the meaning of research because they imply planning, organization, rigor, and persistence. Many disciplines conduct research, so what distinguishes nursing research from research in other disciplines? In some ways, there are no differences, because the knowledge and skills required to conduct research are similar from one discipline to another. However, when one looks at other dimensions of research within a discipline, it is clear that research in nursing must be unique to address the questions relevant to the profession. Nurse researchers need to implement the most effective research methodologies to develop a unique body of knowledge that is core to the discipline of nursing. This body of knowledge needs to encompass nursing's "unique focus of vision and social mandate" (Thorne, 2014, p. 1).

The American Nurses Association (ANA) developed a definition of nursing that identifies the unique body of knowledge needed by the profession. "Nursing is the protection, promotion, and optimization of health and abilities, prevention of illness and injury, facilitation of healing, alleviation of suffering through the diagnosis and treatment of human response, and advocacy in the care of individuals, families, groups, communities, and populations" (ANA, 2016). On the basis of this definition, nursing research is needed to generate knowledge about human responses and the best interventions to promote health, prevent illness, and manage illness (ANA, 2010b).

Many nurses hold the view that nursing research should focus on acquiring knowledge that can be directly implemented in clinical practice, which is often referred to as applied research or practical research. However, another view is that nursing research should include studies of nursing education, nursing administration, health services, and nurses' characteristics and roles as well as clinical situations (Brown, 2014; Riley, Beal, Levi, & McCausland, 2002). Therefore, the generation of nursing knowledge needs to focus on education, practice, and service. Research is needed to identify teaching-learning strategies to promote excellence in nursing education. Thus, some nurse researchers are involved in advancing a science for nursing education so the teaching-learning strategies used are evidence-based (National League for Nursing [NLN], 2016). Nurse administrators are involved in research to enhance nursing leadership and the delivery of quality, cost-effective patient care. Studies of health services and nursing roles are important to quality outcomes in the nursing profession and the healthcare system (Doran, 2011; Holt, 2014).

Thus, the body of knowledge generated through nursing research provides the scientific foundation essential for all areas of nursing and encompasses the vision and social mandate for the profession. In this text, **nursing research** is defined as a scientific process that validates and refines existing knowledge and generates new knowledge that directly and indirectly influences the delivery of evidence-based nursing.

FRAMEWORK LINKING NURSING RESEARCH TO THE WORLD OF NURSING

To best explore nursing research, we have developed a framework to help establish connections between research and the various aspects of nursing. The framework presented in the following pages links nursing research to the world of nursing and is used as an organizing model for this textbook. Figure 1-1 demonstrates that nursing research is not an entity disconnected from the rest of nursing but rather is influenced by and influences all other nursing aspects. The concepts in this model are pictured on a continuum from concrete to abstract. The discussion introduces this continuum and progresses from the concrete concept of the empirical

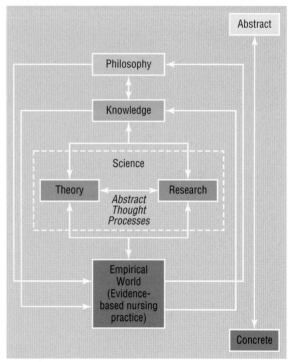

FIGURE 1-1 Framework linking nursing research to the world of nursing.

world of nursing practice to the most abstract concept of nursing philosophy. The use of two-way arrows in the model indicates the dynamic interaction among the concepts.

Concrete-Abstract Continuum

As previously mentioned, Figure 1-1 presents the components of nursing on a concrete-abstract continuum. This continuum demonstrates that nursing thought flows both from concrete to abstract thinking and from abstract to concrete. **Concrete thinking** is oriented toward and limited by tangible things or by events that we observe and experience in reality. Thus, the focus of concrete thinking is immediate events that are limited by time and space. Many nurses believe they are mainly concrete thinkers because they focus on the specific actions in nursing practice. **Abstract thinking** is oriented toward the development of an idea without application to, or association with, a particular instance (Chinn & Kramer, 2015). Abstract thinkers tend to look at the broader situation or system for meaning, patterns, and relationships rather than at a specific behavior or incident. This type of thinking is independent of time and space. Graduate nursing education fosters abstract thinking, because it is an essential skill for developing theory and generating ideas for study. Nurses assuming advanced roles and registered nurses (RNs) need to use both abstract and concrete thinking. For example, a nurse practitioner (NP) must explore the best research evidence about a practice problem (abstract or general thinking) before using his or her clinical expertise to diagnose and manage a particular patient's health problem (concrete thinking) (Thorne & Sawatzky, 2014). RNs review evidence-based agency protocols (abstract thinking) to direct their implementation of a protocol to manage a particular patient problem (concrete thinking).

Nursing research requires skills in both concrete and abstract thinking. Abstract thought is required to identify researchable problems, design studies, and interpret findings. Concrete thought is necessary in both planning and implementing the detailed steps of data collection and analysis. This back-and-forth flow between abstract and concrete thought may be one reason nursing research seems complex and challenging.

Empirical World

The **empirical world** is what we experience through our senses and is the concrete portion of our existence. It is what we often call *reality*, and *doing* kinds of kinetic activities are part of this world. There is a sense of certainty about the empirical or real world; it seems understandable, predictable, and even controllable. Concrete thinking in the empirical world is associated with such words as "practical," "down-to-earth," "solid," and "factual." Concrete thinkers want facts. They want to be able to apply whatever they know to the current situation.

The practice of nursing takes place in the empirical world, as demonstrated in Figure 1-1. The scope of nursing practice varies for the RN and the APN. RNs provide care to and coordinate care for patients, families, and communities in a variety of settings. They initiate interventions as well as carry out treatments authorized by other healthcare providers (ANA, 2010a). APNs, such as NPs, nurse anesthetists (NAs), nurse midwives (NMs), and clinical nurse specialists (CNSs), have an expanded clinical practice. Their knowledge, skills, and expertise promote role autonomy and overlap with medical practice. APNs usually concentrate their clinical practice in a specialty area, such as acute care, neonatal, pediatrics, gerontology, adult or family primary care, psychiatric-mental health, women's health, maternal child, or anesthesia (ANA, 2010b). You can access the most current nursing scope and standards for practice

from ANA (2010a). Within the empirical world of nursing, the goal is to provide EBP to improve the health outcomes of individuals, families, and communities and the outcomes for the nursing profession and healthcare system (Thorne & Sawatzky, 2014). The aspects of EBP and the significance of research in developing EBP are covered later in this chapter. Throughout this text, research examples are provided from the areas of clinical practice, education, and administration.

Reality Testing Using Research

People tend to *validate* or test the reality of their existence through their senses. In everyday activities, they constantly check out the messages received from their senses. For example, they might ask, "Am I really seeing what I think I am seeing?" Sometimes their senses can play tricks on them. This is why instruments have been developed to record sensory experiences accurately. For example, does the patient merely feel hot or actually have a fever? Thermometers were developed to test this sensory perception accurately. Through research, the most accurate and precise measurement devices have been developed to assess the temperatures of patients based on age and health status (Waltz, Strickland, & Lenz, 2010). Thus, research is a way to test reality and generate the best evidence to guide nursing practice.

Nurses use a variety of research methodologies to test their reality and generate nursing knowledge, including quantitative research, qualitative research, mixed methods research, and outcomes research. **Quantitative research**, the most frequently conducted method in nursing, is a formal, objective, systematic methodology that counts or measures to describe variables, test relationships, and examine cause-and-effect interactions (Kerlinger & Lee, 2000; Shadish, Cook, & Campbell, 2002). Since the 1980s, nurses have conducted qualitative research to generate essential theories and knowledge for nursing. **Qualitative research** is a rigorous, scholarly, interactive, holistic, subjective research approach used to describe life experiences, cultures, and social processes from the perspectives of the persons involved (Creswell, 2013; Marshall & Rossman, 2016; Morse, 2012; Munhall, 2012). More recently, nurse researchers have effectively combined quantitative and qualitative methods in implementing **mixed methods research** to address selected nursing problems (Clark & Ivankova, 2016; Creswell, 2014, 2015).

Medicine, healthcare agencies, and now nursing are focusing on the outcomes of patient care and nurses' roles and actions. **Outcomes research** is an important scientific methodology that has evolved to examine the end results of patient care and the outcomes for healthcare providers, such as RNs, APNs, nurse administrators, and physicians, and for healthcare agencies (Doran, 2011). These different types of research are all essential to the development of nursing science, theory, and knowledge (see Figure 1-1). Nurses have varying roles related to research that include conducting research, critically appraising research, synthesizing studies, and using research evidence in practice.

Roles of Nurses in Research

Generating scientific knowledge with real potential for implementation in practice requires the participation of all nurses in a variety of research activities. Some nurses are developers of research and conduct studies to generate and refine the knowledge needed for nursing practice. Others are consumers of research and use research evidence to improve their nursing practice. The American Association of Colleges of Nursing (AACN, 2006) and ANA (2010a, 2010b) have published statements about the roles of nurses in research. Regardless of their education or position, all nurses have roles in research, and some ideas about those roles are presented in Table 1-1. The research role a nurse assumes usually expands with his or her advanced education, expertise, and career path. Nurses with a Bachelor of Science in Nursing (BSN) degree have knowledge of the research process and skills in reading and critically appraising studies (Fawcett & Garity, 2009). They assist with the implementation of evidence-based guidelines, protocols, algorithms, and policies in practice (Brown, 2014). In addition, these nurses might provide valuable assistance in identifying research problems and collecting data for studies.

Nurses with a Master of Science in Nursing (MSN) have undergone the educational preparation to critically appraise and synthesize findings from studies to revise or develop protocols, algorithms, or policies for use in practice. They also have the ability to identify and critically appraise the quality of evidence-based guidelines developed by national organizations. APNs and nurse administrators have the ability to lead healthcare teams in making essential changes in nursing practice and in the healthcare system based on current research evidence. Some MSN-prepared nurses conduct studies but usually do so in collaboration with other nurse scientists (AACN, 2016; ANA, 2010a).

Doctoral degrees in nursing can be practice-focused (Doctor of Nursing Practice [DNP]) or research-focused (Doctor of Philosophy [PhD]). Nurses with DNPs are educated to have the highest level of clinical expertise, with the ability to translate scientific knowledge for use in practice (Smeltzer et al., 2015). These doctorally prepared nurses have advanced research and leadership knowledge to develop, implement, evaluate, and revise evidence-based guidelines, protocols, algorithms, and policies for practice (Brar, Boschma, & McCuaig, 2010). In addition, DNP-prepared nurses have the expertise to conduct and collaborate with clinical studies.

TABLE 1-1	Nurses' Participation in Research at Various Levels of Education
Educational Preparation	**Research Expectations and Competencies**
BSN	Read and critically appraise studies. Use best research evidence in practice with guidance. Assist with problem identification and data collection.
MSN	Critically appraise and synthesize studies to develop and revise protocols, algorithms, and policies for practice. Implement best research evidence in practice. Collaborate in research projects and provide clinical expertise for research.
DNP	Participate in evidence-based guideline development. Develop, implement, evaluate, and revise as needed protocols, policies, and evidence-based guidelines in practice. Conduct clinical studies, usually in collaboration with other nurse researchers.
PhD	Assume a major role, such as primary investigator, in conducting research and contributing to the empirical knowledge generated in a selected area of study. Obtain initial funding for research. Coordinate research teams of BSN, MSN, and DNP nurses.
Postdoctoral	Implement a funded program of research. Lead and/or participate in nursing and interdisciplinary research teams. Identified as experts in their areas of research. Mentor PhD-prepared researchers.

BSN, Bachelor of Science in Nursing; *DNP,* Doctor of Nursing Practice; *MSN,* Master of Science in Nursing; *PhD,* Doctor of Philosophy.

PhD-prepared nurses assume a major role in the conduct of research and the generation of nursing knowledge in a selected area of interest (Rehg & Smith-Battle, 2015; Smeltzer et al., 2015). These nurse scientists often coordinate research teams that include DNP-, MSN-, and BSN-prepared nurses to facilitate the conduct of rigorous studies in a variety of healthcare agencies and universities. Nurses with postdoctoral education have the expertise to develop highly funded programs of research. They lead interdisciplinary teams of researchers and sometimes conduct studies in multiple settings. These scientists often are identified as experts in selected areas of research and provide mentoring of new PhD-prepared researchers (see Table 1-1).

Abstract Thought Processes

As described earlier, **abstract thought processes** influence every aspect of the nursing world. In a sense, they link all aspects of nursing together. Without skills in abstract thought, we are trapped in a flat existence; we can experience the empirical world, but we cannot explain or understand it (Abbott, 1952). Through abstract thinking, however, we can test our theories (which explain the nursing world) and then include them in the body of scientific knowledge. Abstract thinking also allows scientific findings to be developed into theories (Charmaz, 2014; Smith & Liehr, 2013). Abstract thought enables both science and theories to be blended into a cohesive body of knowledge, guided by a philosophical framework, and applied in clinical practice (see Figure 1-1). Thus, abstract thought processes are essential for synthesizing research evidence and knowing when and how to use this knowledge in practice.

Three major abstract thought processes—introspection, intuition, and reasoning—are important in nursing (Silva, 1977; Thorne & Sawatzky, 2014). These thought processes are used in critically appraising and applying best research evidence in practice, planning and implementing research, and developing and evaluating theory.

Introspection

Introspection is the process of turning your attention inward toward your own thoughts. It occurs at two levels. At the more superficial level, you are aware of the thoughts you are experiencing. You have a greater awareness of the flow and interplay of feelings and ideas that occur in constantly changing patterns. These thoughts or ideas can rapidly fade from view and disappear if you do not quickly write them down. When you allow introspection to occur in more depth, you examine your thoughts more critically and in detail. Patterns or links between thoughts and ideas emerge, and you may recognize fallacies or weaknesses in your thinking. You may question what brought you to this point and find yourself really enjoying the experience.

Imagine the following clinical situation. You have just left Mark Smith's home. Mark has heart failure (HF) and has been receiving home health care for 2 weeks following his discharge from the hospital. Although Mark is managing his HF symptoms with medications, diet, and fluid restrictions, he is still reluctant to leave home for any length of time or to take trips. His wife is frustrated with this situation, and you are concerned that Mark is not feeling strong and in control of his life. You begin to review your nursing actions and to recall other patients who reacted in similar ways. What were the patterns of their behavior?

You have an idea: Perhaps the patient's behavior is linked to emotional distress, such as fear, anxiety, and depression related to his HF. You feel unsure about your ability to help the patient and family deal with this situation effectively. You recall other nurses describing similar reactions in their patients, and you wonder how many patients with HF have these emotional concerns. Your thoughts jump to reviewing the charts of other patients with HF and reading relevant ideas discussed in the literature. Research has been conducted on this topic recently, and you could critically appraise these findings to determine the level of evidence for possible use of the ideas in practice. If the findings are inadequate, perhaps other nurses would be interested in studying this situation with you.

Intuition

Intuition is an insight into or understanding of a situation or event as a whole that usually cannot be logically explained (Smith, 2009). Because intuition is a type of knowing that seems to come unbidden, it may also be described as a gut feeling, hunch, or sixth sense. Because intuition cannot be explained scientifically with ease, many people are uncomfortable with it. Some even say that it does not exist. Sometimes, therefore, the feeling or sense is suppressed, ignored, or dismissed as silly. However, intuition is not the lack of knowing; rather, it is a result of deep knowledge—tacit knowing or personal knowledge (Benner, 1984; Billay, Myrick, Luhanga, & Yonge, 2007). The knowledge is incorporated so deeply within that it is difficult to bring it consciously to the surface and express it in a logical manner (Thorne & Sawatzky, 2014). One of the most commonly cited example of nurses' intuition is their recognition of a patient's physically deteriorating condition. Odell, Victor, and Oliver (2009) conducted a review of the research literature and described nurses' use of intuition in clinical practice. They noted that nurses have an intuition or a knowing that something is not right with their patients by recognizing changes in behavior and physical signs. Through clinical experience and the use of intuition, nurses are able to recognize patterns of deviations from the normal clinical course and to know when to take action.

Intuition is generally considered unscientific and unacceptable for use in research. In some instances, that consideration is valid. For example, a hunch about significant differences between one set of scores and another set of scores is not particularly useful as an analysis technique (Grove & Cipher, 2017). However, even though intuition is often unexplainable, it has some important scientific uses. Researchers do not always need to be able to explain something in order to use it. A burst of intuition may identify a problem for study, indicate important concepts to be described, or link two ideas together in interpreting the findings. The trick is to recognize the feeling, value it, and hang on to the idea long enough to consider it. Some researchers keep a journal to capture elusive thoughts or hunches as they think about their phenomenon (singular) or phenomena (plural) of interest. Research **phenomena** are nurses' general ideas or thoughts of interest about behaviors, events, or experiences that often influence the conduct of their studies.

Imagine the following situation. You have been working in an oncology center for the past 3 years. You and two other nurses working in the center have been meeting with the acute care NP to plan a study to determine which factors are important for promoting positive patient outcomes in the center. The group has met several times with a nursing professor at the university, who is collaborating with the group to develop the study. At present, the group is concerned with identifying the outcomes that need to be measured and how to measure them.

You have had a busy morning. Mr. Williams, a patient, stops by to chat on his way out of the clinic. You listen, but not attentively at first. You then become more acutely aware of what he is saying and begin to have a feeling about one concept that should be studied. Although he didn't specifically mention fear of breaking the news about having cancer to his children, you sense that he is anxious about conveying bad news to his loved ones. You cannot really explain the origin of this feeling, and something in the flow of Mr. Williams' words has stimulated a burst of intuition. You suspect that other patients diagnosed with cancer face similar fear and hesitation about informing their family members of bad news, that they have cancer or that their cancer has spread. You believe the variable *fear of breaking bad news to loved ones* needs to be studied (phenomenon of interest). You feel both excited and uncertain. If the variable has not been studied, is it really significant? Somehow, you feel that it is important to consider.

Reasoning

Reasoning is the processing and organizing of ideas in order to reach conclusions. Through reasoning, people are able to make sense of their thoughts and experiences. This type of thinking is often evident in the verbal presentation of a logical argument in which all parts are linked together to reach a logical conclusion. Patterns of reasoning are used to develop theories and to plan and implement research. Barnum (1998) identified four patterns of reasoning as being essential to nursing: (1) problematic, (2) operational, (3) dialectic, and (4) logical. An individual uses all four types of reasoning, but one type of reasoning is often dominant over the others. Reasoning is also classified by the discipline of logic into inductive and deductive modes (Chinn & Kramer, 2015).

Problematic reasoning. **Problematic reasoning** involves (1) identifying a problem and the factors influencing it, (2) selecting solutions to the problem, and (3) resolving the problem. For example, nurses use problematic reasoning in the nursing process to identify diagnoses and to implement nursing interventions to resolve these problems. Problematic reasoning is also evident when one identifies a research problem and successfully develops a methodology to examine it (Creswell, 2014).

Operational reasoning. **Operational reasoning** involves identification of and discrimination among many alternatives and viewpoints. It focuses on the process (debating alternatives) rather than on the resolution. Nurses use operational reasoning to develop realistic, measurable health goals with patients and families. NPs and CNSs use operational reasoning to debate which pharmacological and nonpharmacological treatments to use in managing patient illnesses. In research, operationalizing a treatment for implementation and debating which measurement methods or data analysis techniques to use in a study require operational thought (Grove & Cipher, 2017; Waltz et al., 2010).

Dialectic reasoning. **Dialectic reasoning** involves looking at situations in a holistic way. A dialectic thinker believes that the whole is greater than the sum of the parts and that the whole organizes the parts. For example, a nurse using dialectic reasoning would view a patient as a person with strengths and weaknesses who is experiencing an illness, and not just as the *stroke in room 219*. Dialectic reasoning also involves examining factors that are opposites and making sense of them by merging them into a single unit or idea that is greater than either alone. For example, analyzing studies with conflicting findings and summarizing these findings to determine the current knowledge base for a research problem require dialectic reasoning. Analysis of data collected in qualitative research requires dialectic reasoning to gain an understanding of the phenomenon being investigated (Miles, Huberman, & Saldaña, 2014).

Logical reasoning. Logic is a science that involves valid ways of relating ideas to promote understanding. The aim of logic is to determine truth or to explain and predict phenomena. The science of logic deals with thought processes, such as concrete and abstract thinking, and methods of reasoning, such as logical, inductive, and deductive.

Logical reasoning is used to break the whole into parts that can be carefully examined, as can the relationships among the parts. In some ways, logical reasoning is the opposite of dialectic reasoning. A logical reasoner assumes that the whole is the sum of the parts and that the parts organize the whole. For example, a patient states that she is cold. You logically examine the following parts of the situation and their relationships: (1) room temperature, (2) patient's temperature, (3) patient's clothing, and (4) patient's activity. The room temperature is 65° F, the patient's temperature is 98.6° F, and the patient is wearing lightweight pajamas and drinking ice water. You conclude that the patient is cold because of external environmental factors (room temperature, lightweight pajamas, and drinking ice water). Logical reasoning is used frequently in quantitative and outcomes research to develop a study design, plan and implement data collection, and conduct statistical analyses. This type of reasoning is also used in qualitative and mixed methods research to analyze findings in the context of existing knowledge.

The science of logic also includes inductive and deductive reasoning. People use these modes of reasoning constantly, although the choice of types of reasoning may not always be conscious (Kaplan, 1964). **Inductive reasoning** moves from the specific to the general, whereby particular instances are observed and then combined into a larger whole or general statement (Chinn & Kramer, 2015). An example of inductive reasoning follows:

A headache is an altered level of health that is stressful.

A fractured bone is an altered level of health that is stressful.

A terminal illness is an altered level of health that is stressful.

Therefore, all altered levels of health are stressful.

In this example, inductive reasoning is used to move from the specific instances of altered levels of health that are stressful to the general belief that all altered levels of health are stressful. By testing many different altered levels of health through research to determine whether they are stressful, one can demonstrate support for the general statement that all types of altered health are stressful.

Deductive reasoning moves from the general to the specific or from a general premise to a particular situation or conclusion. A **premise** or **hypothesis** is a statement of the proposed relationship between two or more variables. An example of deductive reasoning follows:

PREMISES:

All human beings experience loss.

All adolescents are human beings.

CONCLUSION:

All adolescents experience loss.

In this example, deductive reasoning is used to move from the two general premises about human beings experiencing loss and adolescents being human beings to the specific conclusion, "All adolescents experience loss." However, the conclusions generated from deductive reasoning are valid only if they are based on valid premises. Consider the following example:

PREMISES:

All health professionals are caring.

All nurses are health professionals.

CONCLUSION:

All nurses are caring.

The premise that all health professionals are caring is not necessarily valid or an accurate reflection of reality. Research is a means to test and demonstrate support for or refute a premise so that valid premises can be used as a basis for reasoning in nursing practice.

Science

Science is a coherent body of knowledge composed of research findings and tested theories for a specific discipline (see Figure 1-1). Science is both a product (end point) and a process (mechanism to reach an end point) (Silva & Rothbart, 1984). An example from the discipline of physics is Newton's law of gravity, which was developed through extensive research. The knowledge of gravity (product) is a part of the science of physics that evolved through formulating and testing theoretical ideas (process). The ultimate goal of science is to explain the empirical world and thus to have greater control over it. To accomplish this goal, scientists must discover new knowledge, expand existing knowledge, and reaffirm previously held knowledge in a discipline. Health professionals integrate this evidence-based knowledge to control the delivery of care and thereby improve patient outcomes (EBP).

The science of a field determines the accepted process for obtaining knowledge within that field. Research is an important process for obtaining scientific knowledge in nursing. Some sciences rigidly limit the types of research that can be conducted to obtain knowledge. A valued method for developing a science is the traditional research process, or quantitative research. According to this process, the information gained from one study is not sufficient for its inclusion in the body of science. A study must be replicated several times and must yield similar results each time before that information can be considered to be sound empirical evidence (Brown, 2014; Chinn & Kramer, 2015).

Consider the research on the relationships among smoking, lung damage, and cancer. Numerous studies conducted on animals and humans over the past decades indicate causative relationships between smoking and lung damage and between smoking and lung cancer. Everyone who smokes experiences lung damage, and although not everyone who smokes develops lung cancer, smokers are at a much higher risk for cancer. Extensive, quality research has been conducted to generate empirical evidence about the health hazards of smoking, and this evidence guides the actions of nurses in practice. We provide smoking cessation programs, emotional support, and medications like nicotine patches, Zyban (bupropion hydrochloride), and Chantix (varenicline) to assist individuals to stop smoking. Because of this scientific evidence about the hazards of smoking, society has moved toward providing many smoke-free environments.

Findings from studies are systematically related to one another in a way that seems to best explain the empirical world. Abstract thought processes are used to make these linkages. The linkages are called *laws* or *principles*, depending on the certainty of the information and relationships within the linkage. Laws express the most certain relationships and provide the best research evidence for use in practice. The certainty depends on the amount of research conducted to test a relationship and, to some extent, on the skills of abstract thought processes in linking the research findings to form meaningful evidence. The truths or explanations of the empirical world reflected by these laws and principles are never absolutely certain and may be disproved by further research.

Nursing is in the process of developing a science for the profession, and additional original and replication studies are needed to develop the knowledge necessary for practice (Chinn & Kramer, 2015; Melnyk & Fineout-Overholt, 2015). As discussed earlier, nursing science is being developed using a variety of research methodologies, including quantitative, qualitative, mixed methods, and outcomes research (Creswell, 2014, 2015; Doran, 2011; Thorne & Sawatzky, 2014). The focus of this textbook is to increase your understanding of these different types of research used in the development and testing of nursing theory.

Theory

A **theory** is a creative and rigorous structuring of ideas that includes integrated concepts, existence statements, and relational statements that present a systematic view of a phenomenon (Chinn & Kramer, 2015; Smith & Liehr, 2013). A theory consists of a set of concepts that are defined and interrelated to present a view of a selected phenomenon. A classic example is the theory of stress developed by Selye (1976) to explain the physical and emotional effects of illness on people's lives. This theory of stress continues to be important in understanding the effects of health changes on patients and families. Extensive research has been conducted to detail the types, number, and severity of stressors experienced in life and the effective interventions for managing these stressful situations.

A theory is developed from a combination of personal experiences, research findings, and abstract thought processes. The theorist may use findings from research as a starting point and then organize the findings to best explain the empirical world. This is the process Selye used to develop his theory of stress. Alternatively, the theorist may use abstract thought processes, personal knowledge, and intuition to develop a theory of a phenomenon. This theory then requires testing through research to determine whether it is an accurate reflection of reality. Thus, research has a major role in theory development, testing, and refinement. Some forms of qualitative research focus on developing new theories or extending existing theories (Charmaz, 2014; Marshall & Rossman, 2016). Various types of quantitative research are often implemented to test the accuracy of theory. The study findings either support or fail to support the theory, providing a basis for refining the theory (Shadish et al., 2002).

Knowledge

Knowledge is a complex, multifaceted concept. For example, you may say that you *know* your friend John, *know* that the earth rotates around the sun, *know* how to give an injection, and *know* pharmacology. These are examples of knowing—being familiar with a person, comprehending facts, acquiring a psychomotor skill, and mastering a subject. There are differences in types of knowing, yet there are also similarities (Chinn & Kramer, 2015). Knowing presupposes order or imposes order on thoughts and ideas. People have a desire to know what to expect. There is a need for certainty in the world, and individuals seek it by trying to decrease uncertainty through knowledge. Think of the questions you ask a person who has presented some bit of knowledge: *Is it true? Are you sure? How do you know?* Thus, the **knowledge** that we acquire is expected to be an accurate reflection of reality.

Ways of Acquiring Nursing Knowledge

Nurses have historically acquired knowledge in a variety of ways, such as: (1) traditions, (2) authority, (3) borrowing, (4) trial and error, (5) personal experience, (6) role-modeling and mentorship, (7) intuition, (8) reasoning, and (9) research. Intuition, reasoning, and research were discussed earlier in this chapter; the other ways of acquiring knowledge are briefly described in this section.

Traditions. **Traditions** consist of "truths" or beliefs that are based on customs and past trends. Nursing traditions from the past have been transferred to the present by written and verbal communication and role-modeling and continue to influence the present practice of nursing. For example, some of the policies and procedures in hospitals and other healthcare facilities contain traditional ideas. In addition, some nursing interventions are transmitted verbally from one nurse to another over the years or by the observation of experienced nurses. For example, the idea of providing a patient with a clean, safe, well-ventilated environment originated with Florence Nightingale (1859).

However, traditions can also narrow and limit the knowledge sought for nursing practice. For example, tradition has established the time and pattern for providing baths, evaluating vital signs, and allowing patient visitation on many hospital units. The nurses on these units quickly inform new staff members about the accepted or traditional behaviors for the unit. Traditions are difficult to change because people with power and authority have accepted and supported them for a long time. Many traditions have not been tested for accuracy or efficiency and require research for continued use in practice.

Authority. An **authority** is a person with expertise and power who is able to influence opinion and behav-

ior. A person is thought of as an authority because she or he knows more in a given area than others do. Knowledge acquired from authority is illustrated when one person credits another person as the source of information. Frequently, nurses who publish articles and books or develop theories are considered authorities. Students usually view their instructors as authorities, and clinical nursing experts are considered authorities within their clinical settings. However, persons viewed as authorities in one field are not necessarily authorities in other fields. An expert is an authority only when addressing his or her area of expertise. Like tradition, the knowledge acquired from authorities sometimes has not been validated through research and is not considered the best evidence for practice.

Borrowing. As some nursing leaders have noted, knowledge in nursing practice is partly made up of information that has been borrowed from disciplines such as medicine, psychology, physiology, and education. **Borrowing** in nursing involves the appropriation and use of knowledge from other fields or disciplines to guide nursing practice (Marchuk, 2014; Walker & Avant, 2011).

Nursing practice has borrowed knowledge in two ways. For years, some nurses have taken information from other disciplines and applied it directly to nursing practice. This information was not integrated within the unique focus of nursing. For example, some nurses have used the medical model to guide their nursing practice, thus focusing on the diagnosis and treatment of physiological diseases with limited attention to the patient's holistic nature. This type of borrowing continues today as nurses use technological advances to focus on the detection and treatment of disease, to the exclusion of health promotion and illness prevention.

Another way of borrowing, which is more useful in nursing, is the integration of information from other disciplines within the focus of nursing. Because disciplines share knowledge, it is sometimes difficult to know where the boundaries exist between nursing's knowledge base and the knowledge bases of other disciplines. Boundaries blur as the knowledge bases of disciplines evolve (Thorne & Sawatzky, 2014). For example, information about self-esteem as a characteristic of the human personality is associated with psychology, but this knowledge also directs the nurse in assessing the psychological needs of patients and families. However, borrowed knowledge has not been adequate to answer many questions generated in nursing practice (Thorne, 2014).

Trial and error. **Trial and error** is an approach with unknown outcomes that is used in a situation of uncertainty when other sources of knowledge are unavailable. The nursing profession evolved through a great deal of trial and error before knowledge of effective practices was codified in textbooks and journals. The trial-and-error way of acquiring knowledge can be time-consuming, because multiple interventions might be implemented before one is found to be effective. There is also a risk of implementing nursing actions that are detrimental to a patient's health. Because each patient responds uniquely to a situation, however, uncertainty in nursing practice continues (Thorne & Sawatzky, 2014). Because of the uniqueness of patient response and the resulting uncertainty, nurses must use some trial and error in providing care. The trial-and-error approach to developing knowledge would be more efficient if nurses documented the patient and situational characteristics that provided the context for the patient's unique response.

Personal experience. **Personal experience** is the knowledge that comes from being personally involved in an event, situation, or circumstance. In nursing, personal experience enables one to gain skills and expertise by providing care to patients and families in clinical settings. The nurse not only learns but is able to cluster ideas into a meaningful whole. For example, APN students may be taught how to suture a wound in a classroom setting, but they do not *know* how to suture wounds until they observe other nurses suturing patients' wounds and actually suture several wounds themselves.

The amount of personal experience you have will affect the complexity of your knowledge base as a nurse. Benner (1984) described five levels of experience in the development of clinical knowledge and expertise that are important today. These levels of experience are (1) novice, (2) advanced beginner, (3) competent, (4) proficient, and (5) expert. *Novice* nurses have no personal experience in the work that they are to perform, but they have preconceived notions and expectations about clinical practice that are challenged, refined, confirmed, or contradicted by personal experience in a clinical setting. The *advanced beginner* has just enough experience to recognize and intervene in recurrent situations. For example, the advanced beginner nurse is able to recognize and intervene to meet patients' needs for pain management.

Competent nurses frequently have been on the job for 2 or 3 years, and their personal experiences enable them to generate and achieve long-range goals and plans (Benner, 1984). Through experience, the competent nurse is able to use personal knowledge to take conscious, deliberate actions that are efficient and orga-

nized. From a more complex knowledge base, the *proficient nurse* views the patient as a whole and as a member of a family and community. The proficient nurse recognizes that each patient and family have specific values and needs that lead them to respond differently to illness and health.

The *expert nurse* has had extensive experience and is able to identify accurately and intervene skillfully in a situation (Benner, 1984). Personal experience increases an expert nurse's ability to grasp a situation intuitively with accuracy and speed. Lyneham, Parkinson, and Denholm (2009) studied Benner's fifth stage of practice development and noted the links of intuition, science, knowledge, and theory to expert clinical practice. The clinical expertise of the nurse is a critical component of EBP. The expert RNs and APNs (CNSs, NAs, NMs, and NPs) have the greatest skill and ability to implement the best research evidence in practice to meet the unique values and needs of patients and families. The timelines for reaching these different stages of expertise vary with individual nurses, and some do not arrive at the highest level.

Role-modeling and mentorship. **Role-modeling** is learning by imitating the behaviors of an exemplar. An exemplar or role model knows the appropriate and rewarded roles for a profession, and these roles reflect the attitudes and include the standards and norms of behavior for that profession (ANA, 2010a). In nursing, role-modeling enables the novice nurse to learn from interacting with expert nurses or following their examples. Examples of role models are admired teachers, expert practitioners, researchers, and illustrious individuals who inspire students, practicing nurses, educators, and researchers through their examples.

An accentuated form of role-modeling is **mentorship**. In a mentorship, the expert nurse, or **mentor**, serves as a teacher, sponsor, guide, exemplar, counselor, and preceptor for the novice nurse (or **mentee**). Eller, Lev, and Feurer (2014, p. 815) conducted a qualitative study and described the following eight key components of an effective mentoring relationship: "(1) open communication and accessibility; (2) goals and challenges; (3) passion and inspiration; (4) caring personal relationship; (5) mutual respect; (6) exchange of knowledge; (7) independence and collaboration; and (8) role modeling." Both the mentor and the mentee or protégé invest time and effort, which often result in a close, personal mentor-mentee relationship. This relationship promotes a mutual exchange of ideas and aspirations relative to the mentee's career plans. The mentee assumes the values, attitudes, and behaviors of the mentor while gaining intuitive knowledge and personal experience.

Mentorship is important for building research competence in nursing.

To summarize, in nursing, a body of knowledge must be acquired (learned), incorporated, and assimilated by each member of the profession and collectively by the profession as a whole. This body of knowledge guides the thinking and behavior of the profession and of individual practitioners. It also directs further development and influences how science and theory are interpreted within the discipline (see Figure 1-1). This knowledge base is necessary in order for health professionals, consumers, and society to recognize nursing as a science.

Philosophy

Philosophy provides a broad, global explanation of the world. It is the most abstract and most all-encompassing concept in the model (see Figure 1-1). Philosophy gives unity and meaning to the world of nursing and provides a framework within which thinking, knowing, and doing occur (Chinn & Kramer, 2015; Rehg & Smith-Battle, 2015). Nursing's philosophical position influences its knowledge base. How nurses use science and theories to explain the empirical world depends on their philosophy. Ideas about truth and reality, as well as beliefs, values, and attitudes, are part of philosophy. Philosophy asks questions such as, "Is there an absolute truth, or is truth relative?" and "Is there one reality, or is reality different for each individual?"

Everyone's world is modified by her or his philosophy, as a pair of eyeglasses would modify vision. Perceptions are influenced first by philosophy and then by knowledge (Marchuk, 2014). For example, if what you see is not within your ideas of truth or reality, if it does not fit your belief system, you may not see it. Your mind may reject it altogether or may modify it to fit your philosophy. For example, you might believe that education is not effective in promoting smoking cessation, so you do not provide your patients this education. As you start to discover the world of nursing research, it is important to keep an open mind about the value of research and your future role in the development or use of research evidence in practice.

Philosophical positions commonly held within the nursing profession include the view that human beings are holistic, rational, and responsible. Nurses believe that people desire health, and health is considered to be better than illness. Quality of life is as important as quantity of life. Good nursing care facilitates improved patterns of health and quality of life (ANA, 2010a, 2010b). Although nurses' philosophies for practice and research vary, they are influenced by nursing's metaparadigm of the interactions among the constructs person,

health, environment, and nursing that are foundational to the profession (Fawcett, 1996; Smith & Liehr, 2013).

In nursing, truth is relative, and reality tends to vary with perception (Holt, 2014). For example, because nurses believe that reality varies with perception and that truth is relative, they would not try to impose their views of truth and reality on patients. Rather, they would accept patients' views of the world and help them seek health from within those worldviews, an approach that is a critical component of EBP.

SIGNIFICANCE OF RESEARCH IN BUILDING AN EVIDENCE-BASED PRACTICE FOR NURSING

The ultimate goal of nursing is to provide evidence-based care that promotes quality outcomes for patients, families, healthcare providers, and the healthcare system (Craig & Smyth, 2012; Doran, 2011; Melnyk & Fineout-Overholt, 2015). **Evidence-based practice** (EBP) evolves from the integration of the best research evidence with clinical expertise and patient needs and values (Sackett, Straus, Richardson, Rosenberg, & Haynes, 2000; Thorne & Sawatzky, 2014). The AACN (2012) developed the Quality and Safety Education for Nurses (QSEN) graduate level competencies to guide the preparation of future nurses and provide them with the advanced knowledge, skills, and attitudes needed to deliver, quality, safe health care. These graduate-level QSEN competencies include a focus on EBP with a similar definition, "the integration of best current evidence with clinical expertise and patient/family preferences and values for the delivery of optimal health care" (QSEN, 2014; Sherwood & Barnsteiner, 2012).

Figure 1-2 was developed to demonstrate the interrelationships between the three major concepts—best

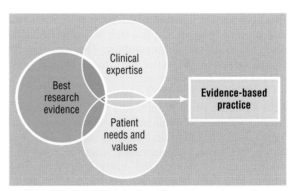

FIGURE 1-2 Model of evidence-based practice.

research evidence, clinical expertise, and patient needs—and values that are merged to produce EBP. **Best research evidence** is the empirical knowledge generated from the synthesis of quality study findings to address a practice problem. A team of expert researchers, healthcare professionals, policy makers, and consumers often synthesizes the best research evidence for developing standardized guidelines for clinical practice. For example, research related to the chronic health problem of high blood pressure (BP) or hypertension (HTN) has been conducted, critically appraised, and synthesized by experts to develop national practice guidelines. The "2014 Evidence-Based Guideline for the Management of High Blood Pressure in Adults" was reported by the members of the Eighth Joint National Committee (JNC 8; James et al., 2014). The Clinical Practice Guidelines for the Management of Hypertension in the Community were published by the American Society of Hypertension and the International Society of Hypertension in 2014 (Weber et al., 2014). HTN is diagnosed as a BP ≥ 140/90 mm Hg in adults who are less than 60 years of age. The guidelines vary for the diagnosis of HTN in individuals 60 years and older. The JNC 8 guideline indicated that HTN is diagnosed as a BP ≥ 150/90 mm Hg in persons 60 years of age or older (James et al., 2014). The American and International Societies of Hypertension indicated that HTN is diagnosed with a BP ≥ 140/90 mm Hg for persons less than 80 years of age and a BP ≥ 150/90 mm Hg for those 80 years and older (Weber et al., 2014). These guidelines are implemented by APNs, physicians, and other healthcare providers to ensure that individuals with HTN receive quality, cost-effective care. Many standardized guidelines are available through the Agency for Healthcare Research and Quality's National Guideline Clearinghouse at http://www.guidelines.gov (AHRQ, 2016) and professional organizations' websites (see Chapters 2 and 19).

Clinical expertise is the knowledge and skills of the healthcare professional providing care. A nurse's clinical expertise is determined by years of practice, current knowledge of the research and clinical literature, and educational preparation. The stronger the clinical expertise, the better the nurse's clinical judgment is in the delivery of quality care (Craig & Smyth, 2012; Eizenberg, 2010). The **patient's need(s)** might focus on health promotion, illness prevention, acute or chronic illness management, or rehabilitation (see Figure 1-2). In addition, patients bring values or unique preferences, expectations, concerns, and cultural beliefs to the clinical encounter. With EBP, patients and their families are encouraged to take an active role in managing their health care. In summary,

expert clinicians use the best research evidence available to deliver quality, cost-effective care to patients and families with specific health needs and values to achieve EBP (Brown, 2014; Craig & Smyth, 2012; Sackett et al., 2000).

Figure 1-3 provides an example of the delivery of evidence-based care to adult Hispanic women younger than 60 years of age with HTN (BP ≥ 140/90 mm Hg). In this example, the best research evidence for management of HTN is found in the clinical practice guidelines for the community developed by the American and International Societies of Hypertension (Weber et al., 2014) and the JNC 8 evidence-based guideline (James et al., 2014). Expert NPs and CNSs translate these guidelines to meet the needs (chronic illness management) and values of adult Hispanic women with HTN. The EBP outcomes for the Hispanic women are a BP < 140 mm Hg systolic and < 90 mm Hg diastolic who have knowledge of lifestyle modifications (LSM) and cardiovascular disease (CVD) risks and appropriate pharmacological management. The concepts in Figure 1-3 are discussed in more detail later in this chapter.

Focus of Research Evidence in Nursing

The empirical evidence in nursing focuses on description, explanation, prediction, and control of phenomena important to professional nursing. The following sections address the types of knowledge that need to be generated in these four areas as nursing moves toward EBP.

Description

Description involves identifying and understanding the nature of nursing phenomena and, sometimes, the relationships among them (Chinn & Kramer, 2015; Munhall, 2012). Through qualitative, quantitative, and mixed methods research, nurses are able to (1) explore and describe what exists in nursing practice, (2) discover new information and meaning, (3) promote understanding of situations, and (4) classify information for use in the discipline. Some examples of research evidence focused on description include the following:

- Identification of individuals' experiences related to a variety of health conditions and situations
- Description of the health promotion and illness prevention strategies used by various populations
- Determination of the incidence of a disease locally, nationally, and internationally
- Identification of the cluster of symptoms and responses for a particular disease

Andersen and Owen (2014) conducted a qualitative study to describe the process for helping people quit

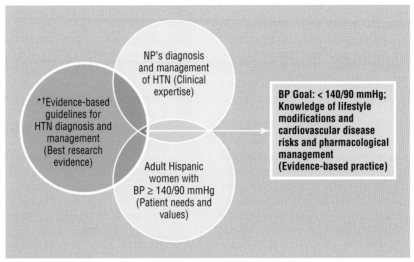

FIGURE 1-3 Evidence-based practice (EBP) for adult Hispanic women with hypertension (HTN). *NP*, nurse practitioner; *BP*, blood pressure.
*James, P. A., Oparil, S., Carter, B. L., Cushman, W. C., Dennison-Himmelfarb, C., Handler, J., et al. (2014). 2014 evidence-based guideline for the management of high blood pressure in adults: Report from the panel members appointed to the Eighth Joint National Committee (JNC 8). *Journal of American Medical Association, 311*(5), 507–520.
†Weber, M. A., Schiffrin, E. L., White, W. B., Mann, S., Lindholm, L. H., Kenerson, J. G., et al. (2014). Clinical practice guidelines for the management of hypertension in the community: A statement by the American Society of Hypertension and the International Society of Hypertension. *Journal of Clinical Hypertension, 16*(1), 14–26.

smoking. These researchers found that helping relationships for smoking cessation were very important for smokers to successfully quit. The findings from this study were organized into a model that focused on the concepts of qualities of the helper, building a helping relationship with the smoker, and constructing an environment supportive of nonsmoking. These concepts were important to smoking cessation and staying abstinent. This type of descriptive research is essential groundwork for future studies focused on explanation and prediction of nursing phenomena.

Explanation

Explanation clarifies the relationships among concepts and variables, which is accomplished through qualitative, quantitative, mixed methods, and outcomes research (Clark & Ivankova, 2016; Creswell, 2013, 2014; Marshall & Rossman, 2016). Research focused on explanation provides the following types of evidence essential for practice:
- Link of concepts to develop an explanation, model, or theory of a phenomenon in nursing

- Determination of the assessment data (both subjective data from the health history and objective data from physical examination) needed to address a patient's health need
- Link of assessment data to determine a diagnosis (both nursing and medical)
- Link of causative risk factors or etiologies to illness, morbidity, and mortality
- Determination of the relationships among health risks, health status, and healthcare costs

For example, Conley, Feder, and Redeker (2015) conducted a quantitative study to examine the relationships of pain, fatigue, and depression with functional performance in adults with stable heart failure (HF). The symptoms of pain, fatigue, and depression are common in individuals with HF and are present throughout all stages of the disease. Conley et al. (2015, p. 111) "found that while pain, fatigue, and depression were associated with decreased functional performance after controlling for demographic and clinical variables, these symptom variables were not associated with functional capacity. Thus, treatment of these symptoms through appropriate pharmacological or behavioral interventions and symptom management programs, may improve aspects of functional status in this population who are at high risk for poor function and excessive symptom burden." This study illustrates how explanatory research can identify relationships among nursing phenomena that are the basis for future research focused on prediction.

Prediction

Through **prediction**, one can estimate the probability of a specific outcome in a given situation (Chinn & Kramer, 2015; Shadish et al., 2002). However, predicting an outcome does not necessarily enable one to modify or control the outcome. It is through prediction that the risk of illness is identified and linked to possible screening methods that will identify the illness. Knowledge generated from research focused on prediction is critical for EBP and includes the following:

- Prediction of the risk for a disease in different populations
- Prediction of the accuracy and precision of a screening instrument, such as mammogram, to detect a disease
- Prediction of the prognosis once an illness is identified in a variety of populations
- Prediction of the impact of nursing actions on selected outcomes
- Prediction of behaviors that promote health, prevent illness, and increase longevity
- Prediction of the health care required based on a patient's need and values

Bortz, Ashkenazi, and Melnikov (2015) conducted a quantitative study to determine whether individuals' spirituality, purpose in life, and attitudes toward organ donation were predictive of their signing an organ donor card (SODC). These researchers found that a high purpose in life, positive attitudes toward organ donation, and low level of transcendental spirituality were predictive of SODC. Nurses are encouraged to take a leading role in educating and supporting people to facilitate organ donation. Predictive studies isolate independent variables that require additional research to ensure that their manipulation or control results in successful outcomes for patients, healthcare professionals, and healthcare agencies.

Control. If one can predict the outcome of a situation, the next step is to control or manipulate the situation to produce the desired outcome. Dickoff, James, and Wiedenbach (1968) described *control* as the ability to write a prescription to produce the desired results. Using the best research evidence, nurses could prescribe

specific interventions to meet the needs of patients. Nurses need this type of research evidence to provide EBP (see Figure 1-2). Research in the following areas is important for generating EBP in nursing:

- Testing interventions to improve the health status of individuals, families, and communities
- Testing management strategies to improve healthcare delivery
- Determination of the quality and cost-effectiveness of interventions
- Implementation of an evidence-based intervention to determine whether it is effective in managing a patient's health need (health promotion, illness prevention, acute and chronic illness management, and rehabilitation) and producing quality outcomes
- Synthesis of research evidence for use in practice.

As discussed earlier, the JNC 8 committee (James et al., 2014) and American and International Societies of Hypertension (Weber et al., 2014) provided national guidelines to control the incidence and severity of HTN in the adult population. These guidelines provide direction for the assessment, diagnosis, and management of HTN in adults. For adults 18 to 60 years of age, the goal is a BP of < 140/90 mm Hg. To achieve this goal, patients receive LSM education about balanced diet, exercise program, normal weight, and being a nonsmoker. They also need to be assessed for and educated about CVD risk factors of HTN, which are obesity, dyslipidemia, diabetes mellitus, cigarette smoking, physical inactivity, microalbuminuria, estimated glomerular filtration rate < 60 mL/min, and a family history of premature CVD. Pharmacological management is needed for adults with a BP ≥ 140/90 mm Hg (see Figure 1-3). In summary, healthcare providers work with adult clients to control their HTN using LSM education, CVD risk assessment, and appropriate pharmacological management. More details on the management of HTN with national guidelines are presented in Chapter 19.

Many more studies and research syntheses are needed to generate evidence for practice (Brown, 2014; Craig & Smyth, 2012; Melnyk & Fineout-Overholt, 2015). This need for additional nursing research provides you with many opportunities to be involved in the world of nursing research. This chapter introduced you to the world of nursing research and the significance of research in developing an EBP for nursing. The following chapters will expand your understanding of different research methodologies so you can critically appraise studies, synthesize research findings, and use the best research evidence available in clinical practice. This text also gives you a background for conducting research in collaboration with expert nurse researchers. We think you will find that nursing research is an exciting adventure that holds much promise for the future practice of nursing.

KEY POINTS

- This chapter introduces you to the world of nursing research.
- Nursing research is defined as a scientific process that validates and refines existing knowledge and generates new knowledge that directly and indirectly influences the delivery of EBP.
- This chapter presents a framework that links nursing research to the world of nursing and organizes the content presented in this textbook (see Figure 1-1). The concepts in this framework range from concrete to abstract and include concrete and abstract thinking, the empirical world (EBP), research, abstract thought processes, science, theory, knowledge, and philosophy.
- The empirical world is what we experience through our senses and is the concrete portion of our existence where nursing practice occurs.
- Research is a way to test reality, and nurses use a variety of research methodologies (quantitative, qualitative, mixed methods, and outcomes) to test their reality and generate knowledge.
- All nurses have a role in research—some are developers of research and conduct studies to generate and refine the knowledge needed for nursing practice, and others are consumers of research and use research evidence to improve their nursing practice.
- Three major abstract thought processes—introspection, intuition, and reasoning—are important in nursing.
- A theory is a creative and rigorous structuring of ideas that includes defined concepts, existence statements, and relational statements that are interrelated to present a systematic view of a phenomenon.
- Reliance on tradition, authority, trial and error, and personal experience is no longer an adequate basis for sound nursing practice.
- The goal of nurses and other healthcare professionals is to deliver evidence-based health care to patients and their families.
- EBP evolves from the integration of best research evidence with clinical expertise and patient needs and values (see Figure 1-2).
- The best research evidence is the empirical knowledge generated from the synthesis of quality studies to address a practice problem.

- The clinical expertise of a nurse is determined by years of clinical experience, current knowledge of the research and clinical literature, and educational preparation.
- The patient brings values—such as unique preferences, expectations, concerns, cultural beliefs, and health needs—to the clinical encounter, which are important to consider in providing evidence-based care.
- The knowledge generated through research is essential for describing, explaining, predicting, and controlling nursing phenomena.

REFERENCES

Abbott, E. A. (1952). *Flatland*. New York, NY: Dover.

Agency for Healthcare Research and Quality (AHRQ). (2016). *National guideline clearinghouse*. Retrieved February 9, 2016 from http://www.guideline.gov.

American Association of Colleges of Nursing (AACN). (2006). *AACN Position statement on nursing research*. Washington, DC: AACN. Retrieved April 13, 2015 from http://www.aacn.nche.edu/Publications/positions/NsgRes.htm.

American Association of Colleges of Nursing (AACN). (2016). *About AACN: Strategic plan*. Retrieved February 9, 2016 from http://www.aacn.nche.edu/about-aacn/strategic-plan.

American Association of Colleges of Nursing (AACN) QSEN Education Consortium. (2012). *Graduate-level QSEN competencies: Knowledge, skills, and attitudes*. Retrieved February 23, 2015 from http://www.aacn.nche.edu/faculty/qsen/competencies.pdf.

American Nurses Association. (2010a). *Nursing: Scope and standards of practice* (2nd ed.). Silver Spring, MD: Author.

American Nurses Association. (2010b). *Nursing's social policy statement: The essence of the profession*. Silver Spring, MD: Author.

American Nurses Association (ANA). (2016). *What is nursing?* Retrieved February 9, 2016 from http://www.nursingworld.org/EspeciallyForYou/What-is-Nursing.

Andersen, J. S., & Owen, D. C. (2014). Helping relationships for smoking cessation: Grounded theory development of the process of finding help to quit. *Nursing Research*, 63(4), 252–259.

Barnum, B. S. (1998). *Nursing theory: Analysis, application, evaluation* (5th ed.). Philadelphia, PA: Lippincott Williams & Wilkins.

Benner, P. (1984). *From novice to expert: Excellence and power in clinical nursing practice*. Menlo Park, CA: Addison-Wesley.

Billay, D., Myrick, F., Luhanga, F., & Yonge, O. (2007). A pragmatic view of intuitive knowledge in nursing practice. *Nursing Forum*, 42(3), 147–155.

Bortz, A. P., Ashkenazi, T., & Melnikov, S. (2015). Spirituality as a predictive factor for signing an organ donor card. *Journal of Nursing Scholarship*, 47(1), 25–33.

Brar, K., Boschma, G., & McCuaig, F. (2010). The development of nurse practitioner preparation beyond the master's level: What is the debate about? *International Journal of Nursing Education Scholarship, 7*(1), Article 9.

Brown, S. J. (2014). *Evidence-based nursing: The research-practice connection* (3rd ed.). Sudbury, MA: Jones and Bartlett.

Charmaz, K. (2014). *Constructing grounded theory* (2nd ed.). Los Angeles, CA: Sage.

Chinn, P. L., & Kramer, M. K. (2015). *Knowledge development in nursing: Theory and process* (9th ed.). St. Louis, MO: Mosby.

Clark, V. L. P., & Ivankova, N. V. (2016). *Mixed methods research: A guide to the field.* Los Angeles, CA: Sage.

Conley, S., Feder, S., & Redeker, N. S. (2015). The relationship between pain, fatigue, depression, and functional performance in stable heart failure. *Heart and Lung: The Journal of Critical Care, 44*(2), 107–112.

Craig, J. V., & Smyth, R. L. (2012). *The evidence-based practice manual for nurses* (3rd ed.). Edinburgh, Scotland: Churchill Livingstone.

Creswell, J. W. (2013). *Qualitative inquiry & research design: Choosing among five approaches* (3rd ed.). Thousand Oaks, CA: Sage.

Creswell, J. W. (2014). *Research design: Qualitative, quantitative, and mixed methods approaches* (4th ed.). Thousand Oaks, CA: Sage.

Creswell, J. W. (2015). *A concise introduction to mixed methods research.* Los Angeles, CA: Sage.

Dickoff, J., James, P., & Wiedenbach, E. (1968). Theory in a practice discipline: Practice oriented theory (Part I). *Nursing Research, 17*(5), 415–435.

Doran, D. M. (2011). *Nursing-sensitive outcomes: State of the science.* Sudbury, MA: Jones & Bartlett.

Eizenberg, M. M. (2010). Implementation of evidence-based nursing practice: Nurses' personal and professional factors? *Journal of Advanced Nursing, 67*(1), 33–42.

Eller, L. S., Lev, E. L., & Feurer, A. (2014). Key components of an effective mentoring relationship: A qualitative study. *Nurse Education Today, 34*(5), 815–820.

Fawcett, J. (1996). On the requirements for a metaparadigm: An invitation to dialogue. *Nursing Science Quarterly, 9*(3), 94–97.

Fawcett, J., & Garity, J. (2009). *Evaluating research for evidence-based nursing practice.* Philadelphia, PA: F. A. Davis.

Grove, S. K., & Cipher, D. (2017). *Statistics for nursing research: A workbook for evidence-based practice* (2nd ed.). St. Louis, MO: Saunders.

Holt, J. (2014). Nursing in the 21st century: Is there a place for nursing philosophy? *Nursing Philosophy, 15*(1), 1–3.

James, P. A., Oparil, S., Carter, B. L., Cushman, W. C., Dennison-Himmelfarb, C., Handler, J., et al. (2014). 2014 evidence-based guideline for the management of high blood pressure in adults: Report from the panel members appointed to the Eighth Joint National Committee (JNC 8). *Journal of American Medical Association, 311*(5), 507–520.

Kaplan, A. (1964). *The conduct of inquiry.* New York, NY: Harper & Row.

Kerlinger, F. N., & Lee, H. B. (2000). *Foundations of behavioral research* (4th ed.). Fort Worth, TX: Harcourt College Publishers.

Lyneham, J., Parkinson, C., & Denholm, C. (2009). Expert nursing practice: A mathematical explanation of Benner's 5th stage of practice development. *Journal of Advanced Nursing, 65*(11), 2477–2484.

Marchuk, A. (2014). A personal nursing philosophy in practice. *Journal of Neonatal Nursing, 20*(6), 266–273.

Marshall, C., & Rossman, G. B. (2016). *Designing qualitative research* (6th ed.). Los Angeles, CA: Sage.

Melnyk, B. M., & Fineout-Overholt, E. (2015). *Evidence-based practice in nursing & healthcare: A guide to best practice* (3rd ed.). Philadelphia, PA: Lippincott Williams & Wilkins.

Miles, M. B., Huberman, A. M., & Saldaña, J. (2014). *Qualitative data analysis: A methods sourcebook* (3rd ed.). Los Angeles, CA: Sage.

Morse, J. M. (2012). *Qualitative health research: Creating a new discipline.* Walnut Creek, CA: Left Coast Press.

Munhall, P. L. (2012). *Nursing research: A qualitative perspective* (5th ed.). Sudbury, MA: Jones & Bartlett Learning.

National League for Nursing (NLN). (2016). *About the NLN: Mission and goals.* Retrieved February 9, 2016 from http://www.nln.org/about/mission-goals.

Nightingale, F. (1859). *Notes on nursing: What it is, and what it is not.* Philadelphia, PA: Lippincott.

Odell, M., Victor, C., & Oliver, D. (2009). Nurses' role in detecting deterioration in ward patients: Systematic literature review. *Journal of Advanced Nursing, 65*(10), 1992–2006.

Quality and Safety Education for Nurses (QSEN) Institute. (2014). *Graduate-level competencies: Knowledge, skills, and attitudes (KSAs).* Retrieved February 23, 2015 from http://qsen.org/competencies/graduate-ksas/.

Rehg, E., & SmithBattle, L. (2015). On to the 'rough ground': Introducing doctoral students to philosophical perspectives on knowledge. *Nursing Philosophy, 16*(2), 98–109.

Riley, J. M., Beal, J., Levi, P., & McCausland, M. P. (2002). Revisioning nursing scholarship. *Journal of Nursing Scholarship, 34*(4), 383–389.

Sackett, D. L., Straus, S. E., Richardson, W. S., Rosenberg, W., & Haynes, R. B. (2000). *Evidence-based medicine: How to practice & teach EBM* (2nd ed.). London, England: Churchill Livingstone.

Selye, H. (1976). *The stress of life.* New York, NY: McGraw-Hill.

Shadish, W. R., Cook, T. D., & Campbell, D. T. (2002). *Experimental and quasi-experimental designs for generalized causal inference.* Chicago, IL: Rand McNally.

Sherwood, G., & Barnsteiner, J. (2012). *Quality and safety in nursing: A competency approach to improving outcomes.* Ames, IA: Wiley-Blackwell.

Silva, M. C. (1977). Philosophy, science, theory: Interrelationships and implications for nursing research. *Image-Journal of Nursing Scholarship, 9*(3), 59–63.

Silva, M. C., & Rothbart, D. (1984). An analysis of changing trends in philosophies of science on nursing theory development and testing. *Advances in Nursing Science, 6*(2), 1–13.

Smeltzer, S. C., Sharts-Hopko, N. C., Cantrell, M. A., Heverly, M. A., Nthenge, S., & Jenkinson, A. (2015). A profile of U.S. nursing faculty in research- and practice-focused doctoral education. *Journal of Nursing Scholarship, 47*(2), 178–185.

Smith, A. (2009). Exploring the legitimacy of intuition as a form of nursing knowledge. *Nursing Standard, 23*(40), 35–40.

Smith, M. J., & Liehr, P. R. (2013). *Middle range theory for nursing* (3rd ed.). New York, NY: Springer Publishing Company.

Thorne, S. (2014). Editorial: What constitutes core discipline knowledge? *Nursing Inquiry*, *21*(1), 1–2.

Thorne, S., & Sawatzky, R. (2014). Particularizing the general: Sustaining theoretical integrity in the context of an evidence-based practice agenda. *Advances in Nursing Science*, *37*(1), 5–18.

Walker, L. O., & Avant, K. C. (2011). *Strategies for theory construction in nursing* (5th ed.). Norwalk, CT: Appleton & Lange.

Waltz, C. F., Strickland, O. L., & Lenz, E. R. (2010). *Measurement in nursing and health research* (4th ed.). New York, NY: Springer Publishing Company.

Weber, M. A., Schiffrin, E. L., White, W. B., Mann, S., Lindholm, L. H., Kenerson, J. G., et al. (2014). Clinical practice guidelines for the management of hypertension in the community: A statement by the American Society of Hypertension and the International Society of Hypertension. *Journal of Clinical Hypertension*, *16*(1), 14–26.

Evolution of Research in Building Evidence-Based Nursing Practice

Susan K. Grove

http://evolve.elsevier.com/Gray/practice/

Initially, nursing research evolved slowly, from Florence Nightingale's investigations of patient morbidity and mortality in the nineteenth century to the studies of nursing education in the 1930s and 1940s. Nurses and nursing roles were the focus of research in the 1950s and 1960s. However, in the late 1970s and 1980s, many researchers designed studies aimed at improving nursing practice. This emphasis continued in the 1990s with research focused on describing nursing phenomena, testing the effectiveness of nursing interventions, and examining patient outcomes. The goal in this millennium is the development of evidence-based nursing practice.

Evidence-based practice (EBP) is the conscientious integration of best research evidence with clinical expertise and patient values and needs in the delivery of quality, cost-effective health care. Chapter 1 presents a model depicting the elements of EBP (see Figure 1-2) and a model of an example of EBP (see Figure 1-3). You probably have many questions about EBP because it is an evolving concept in nursing and health care. This chapter was developed to increase your understanding of how nursing research evolved over the past 160 years and of the current movement of the profession toward EBP. The chapter includes the historical events relevant to nursing research, identifies the methodologies used in nursing to develop research evidence, and concludes with a discussion of the best research evidence needed to build an EBP.

HISTORICAL DEVELOPMENT OF RESEARCH IN NURSING

Some people think that research is relatively new to nursing, but Florence Nightingale initiated nursing research more than 160 years ago (Nightingale, 1859). Following Nightingale's work (1840–1910), nursing research received minimal attention until the mid-1900s. In the 1960s, nurses gradually recognized the value of research, but few had the educational background to conduct studies until the 1970s. However, in the 1980s and 1990s, research became a major force in developing a scientific knowledge base for nursing practice. Today, nurses obtain federal, corporate, and foundational funding for their research; conduct complex studies in multiple settings; and generate sound research evidence for practice. Table 2-1 identifies key historical events that have influenced the development of nursing research and the movement toward EBP. These events are discussed in the following sections.

Florence Nightingale

Nightingale has been described as a researcher and reformer who influenced nursing specifically and health care in general. Nightingale, in her book *Notes on Nursing* (1859), described her initial research activities, which focused on the importance of a healthy environment in promoting the patient's physical and mental well-being. She identified the need to gather data on the environment, such as ventilation, cleanliness, temperature, purity of water, and diet, to determine their influence on the patient's health (Herbert, 1981).

Nightingale is also noted for her data collection and statistical analyses during the Crimean War. She gathered data on soldier morbidity and mortality rates and the factors influencing them and presented her results in tables and pie charts, a sophisticated type of data presentation for the period (Palmer, 1977). Nightingale was the first woman elected to the Royal Statistical Society (Oakley, 2010), and her research was highlighted

TABLE 2-1 Historical Events Influencing Research in Nursing

Year	Event
1850	Florence Nightingale recognized as first nurse researcher
1893	National League for Nursing (NLN) founded
1900	*American Journal of Nursing*
1923	First educational doctoral program for nurses, Teachers College, Columbia University
1929	First master's in nursing degree at Yale University
1932	Association of Collegiate Schools of Nursing formed to promote conduct of research
1950	American Nurses Association (ANA) study of nursing functions and activities
1952	First research journal in nursing, *Nursing Research*
1953	Institute of Research and Service in Nursing Education established
1955	American Nurses Foundation established to fund nursing research
1957	Southern Regional Educational Board (SREB), Western Interstate Commission on Higher Education (WICHE), Midwestern Nursing Research Society (MNRS), and New England Board of Higher Education (NEBHE) developed to support and disseminate nursing research
1963	*International Journal of Nursing Studies*
1965	ANA sponsors first nursing research conferences
1967	Sigma Theta Tau International Honor Society of Nursing publishes *Image*, now titled *Journal of Nursing Scholarship*
1970	ANA Commission on Nursing Research established
1972	Cochrane published *Effectiveness and Efficiency*, introducing concepts relevant to evidence-based practice (EBP)
	ANA Council of Nurse Researchers established
1973	First Nursing Diagnosis Conference held, becoming North American Nursing Diagnosis Association (NANDA)
1976	Stetler/Marram Model for Application of Research Findings to Practice published
1978	*Research in Nursing & Health* and *Advances in Nursing Science*
	WICHE Regional Nursing Research Development Project conducted
1979	*Western Journal of Nursing Research*
1980s–1990s	Methodologies developed to determine "best evidence" for practice by Sackett et al.
1982–1983	Conduct and Utilization of Research in Nursing (CURN) Project published
1983	*Annual Review of Nursing Research*
1985	National Center for Nursing Research (NCNR) established
1987	*Scholarly Inquiry for Nursing Practice*
1988	*Applied Nursing Research* and *Nursing Science Quarterly*
1989	Agency for Health Care Policy and Research (AHCPR) established
1990	*Nursing Diagnosis*, official journal of NANDA; now titled *International Journal of Nursing Terminologies and Classifications*
	American Nurses Credentialing Center (ANCC) implemented the Magnet Hospital Designation Program® for Excellence in Nursing Services
1992	*Healthy People 2000*
	Clinical Nursing Research
1993	NCNR renamed the National Institute of Nursing Research (NINR)
	Journal of Nursing Measurement
	Cochrane Collaboration initiated providing systematic reviews and EBP guidelines
1994	*Qualitative Health Research*
1999	AHCPR renamed Agency for Healthcare Research and Quality (AHRQ)
2000	*Healthy People 2010*
	Biological Research for Nursing

Continued

TABLE 2-1	Historical Events Influencing Research in Nursing—cont'd
Year	**Event**
2001	Stetler's published model "Steps of Research Utilization to Facilitate EBP"
	Institute of Medicine (IOM) report *Crossing the Quality Chasm: A New Health System for the 21st Century*
2002	Joint Commission revises accreditation policies for hospitals supporting EBP
	NANDA becomes international—NANDA-I
2004	*Worldviews on Evidence-Based Nursing*
2005	Quality and Safety Education for Nurses (QSEN) initiated
2006	American Association of Colleges of Nursing (AACN) statement on nursing research
2007	QSEN website (http://qsen.org/) launched featuring teaching strategies and resources
2011	ANA current research agenda
	NINR most current strategic plan
2012	Graduate QSEN Competencies online at http://qsen.org/competencies/graduate-ksas/.
2013	NINR mission statement refined
2014	*Healthy People 2020* available at U.S. DHHS website
2015–2016	AACN current mission and values
	AHRQ current mission and funding priorities
	NLN Missions and Goals

in the periodical *Scientific American* in 1984 (Cohen, 1984).

Through her research, Nightingale was able to instigate attitudinal, organizational, and social changes. She changed the attitudes of the military and society toward the care of the sick. The military began to view the sick as having the right to adequate food, suitable quarters, and appropriate medical treatment, a change that greatly reduced the mortality rate (Cook, 1913). Nightingale improved the organization of army administration, hospital management, and hospital construction. Because of Nightingale's research evidence and influence, society began to accept responsibility for testing public water, improving sanitation, preventing starvation, and decreasing morbidity and mortality rates (Palmer, 1977).

Early 1900s

From 1900 to 1950, research activities in nursing were limited, but a few national studies were conducted related to nursing education. These studies included the Nutting Report, 1912; Goldmark Report, 1923; and Burgess Report, 1926 (Abdellah, 1972; Johnson, 1977). On the basis of recommendations of the Goldmark Report, more schools of nursing were established in university settings. The baccalaureate degree in nursing provided a basis for graduate nursing education, with the first master's of nursing degree offered by Yale University in 1929. Teachers College at Columbia University offered the first Doctor in Education (EdD) for nurses

in 1923 to prepare teachers for the profession. The Association of Collegiate Schools of Nursing, organized in 1932 and later renamed the American Association of Colleges of Nursing (AACN), promoted the conduct of research to improve education and practice. This organization also sponsored the publication of the first research journal in nursing, *Nursing Research*, in 1952 (Fitzpatrick, 1978).

A research trend that started in the 1940s and continued in the 1950s focused on the organization and delivery of nursing services. Studies were conducted on the numbers and kinds of nursing personnel, staffing patterns, patient classification systems, patient and nurse satisfaction, and unit arrangement. Types of care such as comprehensive care, home care, and progressive patient care were evaluated for essential standards of care. These evaluations of care laid the foundation for the development of self-study manuals, which are similar to the quality assurance manuals of today (Gortner & Nahm, 1977).

Nursing Research in the 1950s and 1960s

In 1950, the American Nurses Association (ANA) initiated a 5-year study on nursing functions and activities. The findings were reported in *Twenty Thousand Nurses Tell Their Story*, and this study enabled the ANA to develop statements on functions, standards, and qualifications for professional nurses. Also during this time, clinical research began expanding as specialty groups, such as community health, psychiatric, medical-surgical, pediatric, and obstetrical nurses, developed standards of care. The research conducted by ANA and the specialty groups provided the basis for the nursing practice standards that currently guide professional nursing practice (Fitzpatrick, 1978).

Educational studies were conducted in the 1950s and 1960s to determine the most effective educational preparation for the registered nurse (RN). A nurse educator, Mildred Montag, developed and evaluated the 2-year nursing preparation (associate degree) in junior colleges. Student characteristics, such as admission and retention patterns and the elements that promoted success in nursing education and practice, were studied for both associate degree- and baccalaureate degree-prepared nurses (Downs & Fleming, 1979).

In 1953, an Institute for Research and Service in Nursing Education was established at Teachers College, Columbia University, which provided research-learning experiences for doctoral students (Werley, 1977). The American Nurses Foundation, chartered in 1955, was responsible for receiving and administering research funds, conducting research programs, consulting with nursing students, and engaging in research. In 1956, the Committee on Research and Studies was established to guide ANA research (See, 1977).

A Department of Nursing Research was established in the Walter Reed Army Institute of Research in 1957. This was the first nursing unit in a research institution that emphasized clinical nursing research (Werley, 1977). Also in 1957, the Southern Regional Educational Board (SREB), the Western Interstate Commission on Higher Education (WICHE), the Midwest Nursing Research Society (MNRS), and the New England Board of Higher Education (NEBHE) were created. These organizations remain actively involved today in promoting research and disseminating the findings. ANA sponsored the first of a series of research conferences in 1965, and the conference sponsors required that the studies presented be relevant to nursing and conducted by a nurse researcher (See, 1977). During the 1960s, a growing number of clinical studies focused on quality care and the development of criteria to measure patient outcomes. Intensive care units were being developed, promoting the investigation of nursing interventions, staffing patterns, and cost-effectiveness of care (Gortner & Nahm, 1977).

Nursing Research in the 1970s

In the 1970s, the nursing process became the focus of many studies, with investigations of assessment techniques, nursing diagnosis classification, goal-setting methods, and specific nursing interventions. The first

Nursing Diagnosis Conference, held in 1973, evolved into the North American Nursing Diagnosis Association (NANDA). In 2002, NANDA became international and is now known as NANDA-I. NANDA-I supports research activities focused on identifying appropriate diagnoses for nursing and generating an effective diagnostic process. NANDA's journal, *Nursing Diagnosis,* was published in 1990 and was later renamed *International Journal of Nursing Terminology and Classifications.* Details on NANDA-I can be found on their website at http://www.nanda.org/.

The educational studies of the 1970s evaluated teaching methods and student learning experiences. The National League for Nursing (NLN), founded in 1893, has had a major role in the conduct of research to shape nursing education. Over the last 20 years, a number of studies have been conducted to differentiate the practices of nurses with baccalaureate versus associate degrees. These studies, which primarily measured abilities to perform technical skills, were ineffective in clearly differentiating between the two levels of education. Currently, NLN provides programs, grants, and resources for the "advancement of the science of nursing education and to promote evidence-based nursing education and the scholarship of teaching" (NLN, 2016).

Primary nursing care, which involves the delivery of patient care predominantly by RNs, was the trend for the 1970s. Studies were conducted to examine the implementation and outcomes of primary nursing care delivery models. The number of nurse practitioners (NPs) and clinical nurse specialists (CNSs) with master's degrees increased rapidly during the 1970s. The NP, CNS, nurse midwifery, and nurse anesthetist roles have been researched extensively to determine their positive impact on productivity, quality, and cost of health care. In addition, those clinicians with master's degrees acquired the background to conduct research and to use research evidence in practice.

In the 1970s, nursing scholars began developing models, conceptual frameworks, and theories to guide nursing practice (Fawcett & DeSanto-Madeya, 2013). The works of these nursing theorists also provided frameworks for nursing studies. In 1978, a new journal, *Advances in Nursing Science,* began publishing the works of nursing theorists and the research related to their theories. The number of doctoral programs in nursing and the number of nurses prepared at the doctoral level greatly expanded in the 1970s (Jacox, 1980). Some of the nurses with doctoral degrees increased the conduct and complexity of nursing research; however, many doctorally-prepared nurses did not become actively involved in research. In 1970, the ANA Commission on Nursing Research was established; in turn, this commission established the Council of Nurse Researchers in 1972 to advance research activities, provide an exchange of ideas, and recognize excellence in research. The commission also prepared position papers on subjects' rights in research and on federal guidelines concerning research and human subjects (see Chapter 9), and it sponsored research programs nationally and internationally (See, 1977).

Federal funds for nursing research increased significantly, with a total of slightly more than $39 million awarded for research in nursing from 1955 to 1976. Even though federal funding for nursing studies increased, the funding was not comparable to the $493 million in federal research funds received by those conducting medical research in 1974 alone (de Tornyay, 1977).

Sigma Theta Tau, the International Honor Society for Nursing, sponsored national and international research conferences, and the chapters of this organization sponsored many local conferences to promote the dissemination of research findings. *Image* was a journal initially published in 1967 by Sigma Theta Tau. This journal, now titled *Journal of Nursing Scholarship*, includes many international nursing studies and global health-focused articles. A major goal of Sigma Theta Tau is to advance scholarship in nursing by promoting the conduct of research, communication of study findings, and use of research evidence in nursing. The addition of two new research journals in the 1970s, *Research in Nursing & Health* in 1978 and *Western Journal of Nursing Research* in 1979, also increased the communication of nursing research findings. However, the findings of many studies conducted and published in the 1970s were not being used in practice, so Stetler and Marram (1976) developed a model to promote the communication and use of research findings in practice.

Professor Archie Cochrane originated the concept of EBP with a book published in 1972 titled *Effectiveness and Efficiency: Random Reflections on Health Services*. Cochrane advocated the provision of health care based on research to improve quality of care and patient outcomes. To facilitate the use of research evidence in practice, the Cochrane Center was established in 1992, and the Cochrane Collaboration in 1993. The Cochrane Collaboration and Library house numerous EBP resources, such as systematic reviews of research and evidence-based guidelines for practice (discussed later in this chapter) (see the Cochrane Collaboration at http://www.cochrane.org/).

Nursing Research in the 1980s and 1990s

The conduct of clinical nursing research was the focus in the 1980s and 1990s. A variety of clinical journals (*Achieves of Psychiatric Nursing; Cancer Nursing; Dimensions of Critical Care Nursing; Heart & Lung; Journal of Obstetric, Gynecologic, and Neonatal Nursing; Journal of Pediatric Nursing;* and *Rehabilitation Nursing*) published a growing number of studies. One new research journal was started in 1987, *Scholarly Inquiry for Nursing Practice*, and two in 1988, *Applied Nursing Research* and *Nursing Science Quarterly*.

Even though the body of empirical knowledge generated through clinical research grew rapidly in the 1970s and 1980s, little of this knowledge was used in practice. Two major projects were launched to promote the use of research-based nursing interventions in practice: the Western Interstate Commission for Higher Education (WICHE) Regional Nursing Research Development Project and the Conduct and Utilization of Research in Nursing (CURN) Project. In these projects, nurse researchers, with the assistance of federal funding, designed and implemented strategies for using research findings in practice. The WICHE Project participants selected research-based interventions for use in practice and then functioned as change agents to implement the selected intervention in a clinical agency. Because of the limited amount of research that had been conducted, the project staff and participants had difficulty identifying adequate clinical studies with findings ready for use in practice (Krueger, Nelson, & Wolanin, 1978).

The CURN Project was a 5-year venture (1975–1980) directed by Horsley, Crane, Crabtree, and Wood (1983) to increase the utilization of research findings by (1) disseminating findings, (2) facilitating organizational modifications necessary for implementation, and (3) encouraging collaborative research that was directly transferable to clinical practice. Research utilization was seen as a process to be implemented by an organization rather than by an individual nurse. The project team identified the activities of research utilization to involve identification and synthesis of multiple studies in a common conceptual area (research base) as well as transformation of the knowledge derived from a research base into a solution or clinical protocol. The clinical protocol was then transformed into specific nursing actions (innovations) that were administered to patients. The implementation of the innovation was to be followed by clinical evaluation of the new practice to ascertain whether it produced the predicted result (Horsley et al., 1983). The clinical protocols developed during the project were published to encourage nurses in other healthcare agencies to use these research-based intervention protocols in their practice (CURN Project, 1981–1982).

To ensure that the studies were incorporated into nursing practice, the findings needed to be synthesized for different topics. In 1983, the first volume of the *Annual Review of Nursing Research* was published (Werley & Fitzpatrick, 1983). This annual publication contains experts' reviews of research in selected areas of nursing practice, nursing care delivery, nursing education, and the profession of nursing. The *Annual Review of Nursing Research* continues to be published to (1) expand the synthesis and dissemination of research findings, (2) promote the use of research findings in practice, and (3) identify directions for future research.

Many nurses obtained masters and doctoral degrees during the 1980s and 1990s, and postdoctoral education was encouraged for nurse researchers. The ANA (1989) stated that nurses at all levels of education have roles in research, which extend from reading research to conducting complex, funded programs of research (see Chapter 1). Another priority of the 1980s and 1990s was to obtain greater funding for nursing research. Most of the federal funds in the 1980s were designated for studies involving the diagnosis and cure of diseases. Therefore, nursing received a small percentage of the federal research and development funds (approximately 2% to 3%) as compared with medicine (approximately 90%), even though nursing personnel greatly outnumbered medical personnel (Larson, 1984). However, in 1985, the ANA achieved a major political victory when the National Center for Nursing Research (NCNR) was created within the National Institutes of Health (NIH). This center was created after years of work and two presidential vetoes (Bauknecht, 1986). The purpose of the NCNR was to support the conduct of basic and clinical nursing research and the dissemination of findings. With its creation, nursing research had visibility at the federal level for the first time. In 1993, during the tenure of its first director, Dr. Ada Sue Hinshaw, the NCNR became the National Institute of Nursing Research (NINR). This change in title reflected a change in status and enhanced the recognition of nursing as a research discipline with expanded funding.

Outcomes research emerged as an important methodology for documenting the effectiveness of healthcare services in the 1980s and 1990s. This type of research evolved from the quality assessment and quality assurance functions that originated with the professional standards review organizations (PSROs) in 1972. During the 1980s, William Roper, the director of the Health Care Finance Administration (HCFA), promoted outcomes research for determining the quality and cost effectiveness of patient care (Johnson, 1993).

In 1989, the Agency for Health Care Policy and Research (AHCPR) was established to facilitate the conduct of outcomes research (Rettig, 1991). The agency also had an active role in communicating research findings to healthcare practitioners and was responsible for publishing the first evidence-based national clinical practice guidelines in 1989. Several of these guidelines, including the latest research findings with directives for practice, were published in the 1990s. The Healthcare Research and Quality Act of 1999 reauthorized the AHCPR, changing its name to the Agency for Healthcare Research and Quality (AHRQ). This significant change positioned the AHRQ as a scientific partner with the public and private sectors to improve the quality and safety of patient care by promoting the use of the best research evidence available in practice (AHRQ, 2015). The AHRQ website (http://www.ahrq.gov/) is an excellent resource that includes healthcare information, research funding, research tools and data, and policies for professionals, patients, and consumers.

Building on the process of research utilization, physicians, nurses, and other healthcare professionals focused on the development of EBP during the 1990s. A research group led by Dr. David Sackett at McMaster University in Canada developed explicit research methodologies to determine the *best evidence* for practice. The term *evidence-based* was first used by David Eddy in 1990, with the focus on providing EBP for medicine (Craig & Smyth, 2012; Sackett, Straus, Richardson, Rosenberg, & Haynes, 2000).

In 1990, the ANA leaders established the American Nursing Credentialing Center (ANCC) and approved a recognition program for hospitals called the Magnet Hospital Designation Program® for Excellence in Nursing Services. This program has evolved over the last 20 years but has remained true to its commitment to promote research conducted by nurses in clinical settings and to support implementation of care based on the best current research evidence (ANCC, 2016).

Nursing Research in the 21st Century

The vision for nursing research in the 21st century includes conducting quality studies through the use of a variety of methodologies, synthesizing the study findings into the best research evidence, using this research evidence to guide practice, and examining the outcomes of EBP (Brown, 2014; Craig & Smyth, 2012; Doran, 2011; Melnyk & Fineout-Overholt, 2015). The focus on EBP has become stronger over the last decade. The

Council for the Advancement of Nursing Science was initiated in 2000 to expand the development of research evidence. In 2002, The Joint Commission on Accreditation of Healthcare Organizations (JCAHO, 2016) revised accreditation policies for hospitals to support the implementation of evidence-based health care. To facilitate the movement of nursing toward EBP in clinical agencies, Stetler (2001) developed her Research Utilization to Facilitate EBP Model (see Chapter 19 for a description of this model). The focus on EBP in nursing has resulted in the conduct of more biological studies and randomized controlled trials (RCTs) and the publication of *Biological Research for Nursing* in 2000 and *Worldviews on Evidence-Based Nursing* in 2004.

The AACN's (2006) most current position statement on nursing research is available online at http://www.aacn.nche.edu/publications/position/nursing-research. To ensure an effective research enterprise in nursing, the discipline must (1) create a research culture; (2) provide high-quality educational programs (baccalaureate, master's, practice-focused doctorate, research-focused doctorate, and postdoctorate) to prepare a workforce of nurse scientists; (3) develop a sound research infrastructure; and (4) obtain sufficient funding for essential research (AACN, 2006). In 2011, the ANA published a research agenda for the next 5 years that is compatible with the AACN (2006) research position statement. The current mission statement of AACN (2015) is focused on advancing nursing education, research, and practice.

Research Focused on Health Promotion and Illness Prevention

The focus of healthcare research and funding has expanded from the treatment of illness to include health promotion and illness prevention. *Healthy People 2000* and *Healthy People 2010,* documents published by the U.S. Department of Health and Human Services (U.S. DHHS 1992, 2000), have increased the visibility of health promotion goals and research. *Healthy People 2020* (U.S. DHHS, 2014) information is now available at the department's website, http://www.healthypeople.gov/2020/. Some of the new topics covered by *Healthy People 2020* include adolescent health; blood disorders and blood safety; dementias; early and middle childhood; genomics; global health; healthcare-associated infections; lesbian, gay, bisexual, and transgender health; older adults; preparedness; sleep health; and social determinants of health. In the next decade, nurse researchers will have a major role in the development of interventions to promote health and prevent illness in individuals, families, and communities.

Linking Quality and Safety Education for Nursing (QSEN) Competencies and Nursing Research

The Institute of Medicine (2001) published a report, *Crossing the Quality Chasm: A New Health System for the 21st Century,* that emphasized the importance of quality and safety in the delivery of health care. The Quality and Safety Education for Nurses (QSEN, 2012) initiative identified the following six essential competency areas for nursing education: patient-centered care, teamwork and collaboration, EBP, quality improvement, safety, and informatics. The QSEN (2012) program is focused on developing the requisite knowledge, skills, and attitude (KSA) statements for each of the competencies for pre-licensure and graduate education. The QSEN Institute website (http://qsen.org) was launched in 2007 featuring teaching strategies and resources to facilitate the accomplishments of the QSEN competencies in nursing educational programs.

The most current competencies for graduate nursing educational programs can be found online at http://qsen.org/competencies/graduate-ksas/ (QSEN, 2012; Sherwood & Barnsteiner, 2012). The QSEN (2012) EBP competency is defined as "integrating the best current evidence with clinical expertise and patient/family preferences and values for delivery of optimal health care." Graduate-level nursing students need to have KSAs to conduct critical appraisals of studies; summarize current research evidence; develop protocols, algorithms, and policies for use in practice based on research; and participate in the conduct of research activities. Your expanded knowledge of research is an important part of your developing an EBP and is necessary to accomplish the QSEN competencies.

Current Mission for the Agency for Healthcare Research and Quality

The AHRQ has been designated the lead agency supporting research designed to improve the quality of health care. "The Agency for Healthcare Research and Quality's (AHRQ) mission is to produce evidence to make health care safer, higher quality, more accessible, equitable, and affordable, and to work within the U.S. Department of Health and Human Services and with other partners to make sure that the evidence is understood and used" (AHRQ, 2015).

The AHRQ sponsors and conducts research that provides evidence-based information on healthcare outcomes, quality, cost, use, and access. This research information promotes effective healthcare decision making by patients, clinicians, health system executives, and policy makers. AHRQ identifies funding priorities and research findings on their website at http://

www.ahrq.gov/funding/index.html/. Currently, the AHRQ and NINR work collaboratively to promote funding for nursing studies. These agencies often issue joint calls for proposals for studies of high priority to both agencies.

National Institute of Nursing Research Mission and Strategic Plan

NINR is one of the most influential organizations committed to providing funding, support, and education for the purpose of advancing research in nursing. The current mission of NINR is as follows:

The mission of the National Institute of Nursing Research (NINR) is to promote and improve the health of individuals, families, communities, and populations. The Institute supports and conducts clinical and basic research and research training on health and illness across the lifespan to build the scientific foundation for clinical practice, prevent disease and disability, manage and eliminate symptoms caused by illness, and improve palliative and end-of-life care. (NINR, 2013)

The NINR Strategic Plan was published in 2011 and is available online at http://www.ninr.nih.gov/sites/ www.ninr.nih.gov/files/ninr-strategic-plan-2011.pdf. The plan was developed to provide a vision for nursing science for the next quarter century. This strategic plan includes an ambitious research agenda for nursing in order to meet current healthcare needs and future health challenges and priorities.

The NINR has also supported the development of nurse scientists in genetics and genomics and sponsored the Summer Genetics Institute to expand nurses' contributions to genetic research. The funding priorities, funding process, and current research findings are available on the NINR website at http://www.ninr.nih.gov/. With this professional support, nurses can conduct studies using a variety of research methodologies to generate the essential knowledge needed to promote EBP and quality health outcomes.

METHODOLOGIES FOR DEVELOPING RESEARCH EVIDENCE IN NURSING

Scientific method incorporates all procedures that scientists have used, currently use, or may use in the future to pursue knowledge (Kaplan, 1964). This broad definition dispels the belief that there is one way to conduct research and embraces the use of both quantitative and qualitative research methodologies in developing research evidence for practice.

Since the 1930s, many researchers have narrowly defined scientific method to include quantitative research. This research method is based in the philosophy of logical empiricism or positivism (Norbeck, 1987; Scheffler, 1967). Therefore, scientific knowledge is generated through an application of logical principles and reasoning whereby the researcher adopts a distant and noninteractive posture with the research subject to prevent bias (Borglin & Richards, 2010). Thus, **quantitative research** is best defined as a formal, objective, systematic study process implemented to obtain numerical data in order to answer a research question. This research method is used to describe variables, examine relationships among variables, and determine cause-and-effect interactions between variables (Kerlinger & Lee, 2000; Shadish, Cook, & Campbell, 2002).

Qualitative research is a systematic, interactive, subjective, naturalistic, scholarly approach used to describe life experiences, cultures, and social processes from the perspectives of the persons involved (Marshall & Rossman, 2016; Munhall, 2012). Qualitative research is not a new idea in the social and behavioral sciences (Baumrind, 1980; Glaser & Strauss, 1967). This type of research is conducted to explore, describe, and promote understanding of human experiences, situations, events, and cultures over time.

Comparison of Quantitative and Qualitative Research

The quantitative and qualitative types of research complement each other because they generate different kinds of knowledge that are useful in nursing practice. The problem and purpose to be studied determine the type of research to be conducted, and the researcher's knowledge of both types of research promotes accurate selection of the methodology for the problem identified (Creswell, 2013, 2014, 2016). Quantitative and qualitative research methodologies have some similarities because both require researcher expertise, involve rigor in implementation, and result in the generation of scientific knowledge for nursing practice. Some of the differences between the two methodologies are presented in Table 2-2. Some researchers include both quantitative and qualitative research methodologies in their studies, an approach referred to as **mixed methods research** (see Chapter 14; Creswell, 2014, 2015).

Philosophical Origins of Quantitative and Qualitative Research Methods

The quantitative approach to scientific inquiry emerged from a branch of philosophy called *logical positivism*, which operates on strict rules of logic, truth, laws,

TABLE 2-2   Characteristics of Quantitative and Qualitative Research Methods

Characteristic	Quantitative Research	Qualitative Research
Philosophical origin	Logical positivism, post-positivism	Naturalistic, interpretive, humanistic
Focus	Concise, objective, reductionistic	Broad, subjective, holistic
Reasoning	Logical, deductive	Dialectic, inductive
Basis of knowing	Cause-and-effect relationships	Meaning, discovery, understanding
Theoretical focus	Tests theory	Develops theory and frameworks
Researcher involvement	Control	Shared interpretation
Methods of measurement	Structured interviews, questionnaires, observations, scales, physiological measures	Unstructured interviews, observations, focus groups
Data	Numbers	Words
Analysis	Statistical analysis	Text-based analysis
Findings	Acceptance or rejection of theoretical propositions Generalization	Uniqueness, dynamic, understanding of phenomena, new theory, models, and/or frameworks

axioms, and predictions. Quantitative researchers hold the position that truth is absolute and that there is a single reality that one could define by careful measurement. To find truth as a quantitative researcher, you need to be completely objective, meaning that your values, feelings, and personal perceptions cannot enter into the measurement of reality. Quantitative researchers believe that all human behavior is objective, purposeful, and measurable. The researcher needs only to find or develop the *right* instrument or tool to measure the behavior.

Today, however, many nurse researchers base their quantitative studies on more of a post-positivist philosophy (Clark, 1998). This philosophy evolved from positivism but focuses on the discovery of reality that is characterized by patterns and trends that can be used to describe, explain, and predict phenomena. With post-positivism, "truth can be discovered only imperfectly and in a probabilistic sense, in contrast to the positivist ideal of establishing cause-and-effect explanations of immutable facts" (Ford-Gilboe, Campbell, & Berman, 1995, p. 16). For example, a preoperative educational intervention about deep breathing and ambulation decreases the *probability* of postoperative complications after abdominal surgery but does not prevent all complications in these patients. The post-positivist approach also rejects the idea that the researcher is completely objective about what is to be discovered but continues to emphasize the need to control environmental influences (Newman, 1992; Shadish et al., 2002).

Qualitative research is an interpretive methodological approach that values subjective science more than quantitative research does. Qualitative research evolved from the behavioral and social sciences as a method of understanding the unique, dynamic, holistic nature of human beings. The philosophical basis of qualitative research is interpretive, humanistic, and naturalistic and is concerned with helping those involved understand the meaning of their social interactions. Qualitative researchers believe that truth is both complex and dynamic and can be found only by studying persons as they interact with and within their sociohistorical settings (Marshall & Rossman, 2016; Miles, Huberman, & Saldaña, 2014; Munhall, 2012).

Focuses of Quantitative and Qualitative Research Methods

The focus or perspective for quantitative research is usually concise and reductionistic. **Reductionism** involves breaking the whole into parts so that the parts can be examined. Quantitative researchers remain detached from the study and try not to influence it with their values (objectivity). Researcher involvement in the study is thought to bias or sway the study toward the perceptions and values of the researcher, and biasing a study is considered poor scientific technique (Borglin & Richards, 2010; Shadish et al., 2002).

The focus of qualitative research is usually broad, and the intent is to reveal meaning about a phenomenon from the naturalistic perspective. The qualitative researcher has an active part in the study and acknowledges that personal values and perceptions may influence the findings. Thus, this research approach is subjective, because it assumes that subjectivity is essential for understanding human experiences (Morse, 2012; Munhall, 2012).

Uniqueness of Conducting Quantitative Research and Qualitative Research

Quantitative research is conducted to describe variables or concepts, examine relationships among variables, and determine the effect of an intervention on an outcome. Thus, this method is useful for testing a theory by testing the validity of the relationships that compose the theory (Chinn & Kramer, 2015; Creswell, 2014, 2016). Quantitative research incorporates logical, deductive reasoning as the researcher examines particulars to make generalizations about the universe.

Qualitative research generates knowledge about meaning through discovery. Inductive reasoning and dialectic reasoning are predominant in these studies. For example, the qualitative researcher studies the whole person's response to pain by examining premises about human pain and determining the meaning that pain has for a particular person. Because qualitative research is concerned with meaning and understanding, researchers using qualitative approaches may identify possible relationships among the study concepts, and these relational statements may be used to develop and extend theories.

Quantitative research requires control (see Table 2-2). The investigator uses control to identify and limit the problem to be researched and attempts to limit the effects of extraneous or other variables that are not the focus of the study. For example, as a quantitative researcher, you might study the effects of nutritional education on serum lipid levels (total serum cholesterol, low-density lipoprotein [LDL] cholesterol, high-density lipoprotein [HDL] cholesterol, and triglycerides). You would control the educational program by manipulating the type of education provided, the teaching methods, the length of the program, the setting for the program, and the instructor. The nutritional program might be consistently implemented with the use of a video shown to subjects in a structured setting. You could also control other extraneous variables, such as participant's age, history of cardiovascular disease, and exercise level, because these extraneous variables might affect the serum lipid levels. The intent of this control is to more precisely examine the effects of a nutritional education program (intervention) on the outcomes of serum lipid levels.

Quantitative research requires the use of (1) structured interviews, questionnaires, or observations; (2) scales; and (3) physiological measures that generate numerical data. Statistical analyses are conducted to reduce and organize data, describe variables, examine relationships, and determine differences among groups (Grove & Cipher, 2017). Control, precise measurement methods, and statistical analyses are used to ensure that the research findings accurately reflect reality so that the study findings can be generalized. **Generalization** involves the application of trends or general tendencies (which are identified by studying a sample) to the population from which the research sample was drawn. Researchers must be cautious in making generalizations, because a sound generalization requires the support of many studies with a variety of samples (Shadish et al., 2002).

Qualitative researchers use observations, interviews, and focus groups to gather data. Qualitative data take the form of words that are recorded on paper or electronically. For example, the researcher may ask study participants to share their experiences of powerlessness in the healthcare system and record their narrative responses. The interactions between the researcher and participants are guided by standards of rigor but are not controlled in the way that quantitative data collection is controlled. In some qualitative designs, researchers begin analyzing data during data collection (Miles et al., 2014).

Qualitative data are analyzed according to the qualitative approach that is being used. The intent of the analysis is to organize the data into a meaningful, individualized interpretation, framework, or theory that describes the phenomenon studied. Qualitative researchers recognize that their analysis and interpretations are influenced by their own perceptions and beliefs. The findings from a qualitative study are unique to that study, and it is not the researcher's intent to generalize the findings to a larger population (see Table 2-2). Qualitative researchers are encouraged to question generalizations and to interpret meaning based on individual study participants' perceptions and realities (Creswell 2014, 2016; Miles et al., 2014).

CLASSIFICATION OF RESEARCH METHODOLOGIES PRESENTED IN THIS TEXT

Research methods used frequently in nursing can be classified in different ways, so a classification system was developed for this textbook and is presented in Box 2-1. This textbook includes quantitative, qualitative, mixed methods, and outcomes research for generating nursing knowledge, which were supported in a study by Mantzoukas (2009). He researched the types of studies published from 2000 to 2006 in the top 10 nursing

BOX 2-1   **Classification of Research Methodologies for This Textbook**

Types of Quantitative Research
  Descriptive research
  Correlational research
  Quasi-experimental research
  Experimental research
Types of Qualitative Research
  Phenomenological research
  Grounded theory research
  Ethnographic research
  Exploratory-descriptive qualitative research
  Historical research
Mixed Methods Research
Outcomes Research

journals (*Advances in Nursing Science, International Journal of Nursing Studies, Journal of Advance Nursing, Journal of Clinical Nursing, Journal of Nursing Scholarship, Nursing Outlook, Nursing Research, Nursing Science Quarterly, Research in Nursing & Health,* and *Western Journal of Nursing Research*). Mantzoukas examined 2574 studies and found that 1323 (51.4%) were quantitative, 956 (37.2%) were qualitative, 57 (2.2%) were mixed methods studies, and 238 (9.2%) were studies based on secondary data analysis. Outcomes studies were probably included in the quantitative and secondary data analyses categories.

In this text, the quantitative research methods are classified into four categories: (1) descriptive, (2) correlational, (3) quasi-experimental, and (4) experimental (Kerlinger & Lee, 2000; Shadish et al., 2002). Types of quantitative research are used to test theories and generate and refine knowledge for nursing practice. Over the years, quantitative research has been the most frequently conducted methodology in nursing. Quantitative research methods are introduced in this section and described in more detail in Chapter 3.

The qualitative research methods included in this textbook are (1) phenomenological research, (2) grounded theory research, (3) ethnographic research, (4) exploratory-descriptive qualitative research, and (5) historical research (see Box 2-1; Charmaz, 2014; Creswell, 2013; Marshall & Rossman, 2016; Munhall, 2012). These approaches, all methodologies for discovering knowledge, are introduced in this section and described in depth in Chapters 4 and 12. Unit Two of this textbook focuses on understanding the research process and includes discussions of quantitative, qualitative, mixed methods, and outcomes research methodologies.

Quantitative Research Methods
Descriptive Research
Descriptive research provides an accurate portrayal or account of characteristics of a particular individual, situation, or group (Kerlinger & Lee, 2000). Descriptive studies offer researchers a way to (1) discover new meaning, (2) describe what exists, (3) determine the frequency with which something occurs, and (4) categorize information. Descriptive studies are usually conducted when little is known about a phenomenon and provide the basis for the conduct of correlational studies.

Correlational Research
Correlational research involves the systematic investigation of relationships between or among two or more variables that have been identified in theories, observed in practice, or both. If the relationships exist, the researcher determines the type (positive or negative) and the degree or strength of the relationships. In positive relationships, variables change in the same direction, either increasing or decreasing together. For example, the number of hours of sleep per day is positively related to a perception of being rested, which means as the hours of sleep increase, the perception of being rested increases. In a negative relationship, variables change inversely or in opposite directions. For example, hours of exercise per week is negatively related to a person's weight, which means as the hours of exercise per week increase, the lower the person's weight is. The primary intent of correlational studies is to *explain the nature of relationships, not to determine cause and effect.* However, correlational studies are the means for generating hypotheses to guide quasi-experimental and experimental studies that focus on examining cause-and-effect interactions (Shadish et al., 2002).

Quasi-Experimental Research
The purposes of **quasi-experimental studies** are (1) to identify causal relationships, (2) to examine the significance of causal relationships, (3) to clarify why certain events happened, or (4) a combination of these objectives (Shadish et al., 2002). These studies test the effectiveness of nursing interventions for possible implementation to improve patient and family outcomes in nursing practice.

Quasi-experimental studies are less powerful than experimental studies because they involve a lower level of control in at least one of three areas: (1) manipulation of the treatment or independent variable, (2) manipulation of the setting, and (3) assignment of subjects to groups. When studying human behavior, especially in clinical areas, researchers are commonly unable to manipulate or control certain variables. Subjects cannot be required to participate in research and are usually not selected randomly but on the basis of convenience. Thus, as a nurse researcher, you will probably conduct more quasi-experimental than experimental studies.

Experimental Research

Experimental research is an objective, systematic, controlled investigation conducted for the purpose of predicting and controlling phenomena. This type of research examines causality (Shadish et al., 2002). Experimental research is considered the most powerful quantitative method because of the rigorous control of variables. Experimental studies have three main characteristics: (1) a controlled manipulation of at least one treatment variable (independent variable), (2) administration of the treatment to some of the subjects in the study (experimental group) and not to others (control group), and (3) random selection of subjects or random assignment of subjects to groups, or both. Experimental studies usually are conducted in highly controlled settings, such as laboratories or research units in clinical agencies. An RCT is a type of experimental research that produces the strongest research evidence for practice from a single source or study (Melnyk & Fineout-Overholt, 2015).

Qualitative Research Methods
Phenomenological Research

Phenomenological research is a humanistic study of phenomena. The aim of phenomenology is to explore an experience as it is lived by the study participants and interpreted by the researcher. During the study, the researcher's experiences, reflections, and interpretations influence the data collected from the study participants (Creswell, 2013; Morse, 2012; Munhall, 2012). Thus, the participants' lived experiences are expressed through the researcher's interpretations that are obtained from immersion in the study data and the underlying philosophy of the phenomenological study. For example, phenomenological research might be conducted to describe the experience of living with heart failure or the lived experience of losing a family member in a flood.

Grounded Theory Research

Grounded theory research is an inductive research method initially described by Glaser and Strauss (1967). This research approach is useful for discovering what problems exist in a social setting and the processes people use to handle them. Grounded theory is particularly useful when little is known about the area to be

studied or when what is known does not provide a satisfactory explanation. Grounded theory methodology emphasizes interaction, observation, and development of relationships among concepts. Throughout the study, the researcher explores, proposes, formulates, and validates relationships among the concepts until a theory evolves. The basis of the social process within the theoretical explanation is described. The theory developed is *grounded in,* or has its roots in, the data from which it was derived (Charmaz, 2014).

Ethnographic Research

Ethnographic research was developed by anthropologists to investigate cultures through in-depth study of the members of the cultures. This type of research attempts to tell the story of people's daily lives while describing the culture in which they live. The ethnographic research process is the systematic collection, description, and analysis of data to develop a description of cultural behavior. The researcher (ethnographer) may live in or become a part of the cultural setting to gather the data. Ethnographic researchers describe, compare, and contrast different cultures to add to our understanding of the impact of culture on human behavior and health (Creswell, 2013; Wolf, 2012).

Exploratory-Descriptive Qualitative Research

Exploratory-descriptive qualitative research is conducted to address an issue or problem in need of a solution and/or understanding. Qualitative nurse researchers explore an issue or problem area using varied qualitative techniques with the intent of describing the topic of interest and promoting understanding. Although the studies result in descriptions and could be labeled as descriptive qualitative studies, most of the researchers are in the exploratory stage of studying the area of interest. This type of qualitative research usually lacks a clearly identified qualitative methodology, such as phenomenology, grounded theory, or ethnography. In this text, studies that the researchers identified as being qualitative without indicating a specific approach will be labeled as being exploratory-descriptive qualitative studies.

Historical Research

Historical research is a narrative description or analysis of events that occurred in the remote or recent past. Data are obtained from records, artifacts, or verbal reports. Initial historical research focused on nursing leaders, such as Nightingale and her contributions to nursing research and practice. Historical researchers enhance our understanding of nursing as a discipline and interpret its contributions to health care and society. In addition, the mistakes of the past can be examined to help nurses understand and respond to present situations affecting nurses and nursing practice. Thus, historical research has the potential to provide a foundation for and direct the future movements of the profession (Lundy, 2012).

Mixed Methods Research

Mixed methods research is conducted when the study problem and purpose are best addressed using both quantitative and qualitative research methodologies. Researchers might have a stronger focus on either a quantitative or a qualitative research method based on the purpose of their study. Sometimes quantitative and qualitative research methods are implemented concurrently or consecutively based on the knowledge to be generated. For example, researchers might examine the effectiveness of an intervention using quasi-experimental or experimental quantitative research and then conduct qualitative research to discover the participants' satisfaction with the intervention (Clark & Ivankova, 2016; Creswell, 2014, 2015). The different strategies for combining qualitative and quantitative research methods in mixed methods studies are described in Chapter 14.

Outcomes Research

The spiraling cost of health care has generated many questions about the quality and effectiveness of healthcare services and the patient outcomes. Consumers want to know what services they are buying and whether these services will improve their health. Healthcare policymakers want to know whether the care is cost-effective and of high quality. These concerns have promoted the proliferation during the past decade of **outcomes research**, which examines the results of care and measures the changes in health status of patients (AHRQ, 2015; Doran, 2011; Polit & Yang, 2016). Key ideas related to outcomes research are addressed throughout the text, and Chapter 13 contains a detailed discussion of this methodology. In summary, nurse researchers conduct a variety of research methodologies (quantitative, qualitative, mixed methods, and outcomes research) to develop the best research evidence for practice.

INTRODUCTION TO BEST RESEARCH EVIDENCE FOR PRACTICE

EBP involves the use of best research evidence to guide clinical decision making in practice. As a nurse, you make numerous clinical decisions each day that affect the health outcomes of your patients and their families.

By using the best research evidence available, you can make informed clinical decisions that will improve health outcomes for patients, families, and communities. This section introduces you to the concept of best research evidence for practice by providing (1) a definition of the term "best research evidence," (2) a model of the levels of research evidence available, and (3) a link of the best research evidence to evidence-based guidelines for practice.

Definition of Best Research Evidence

Best research evidence is a summary of the highest-quality, current empirical knowledge in a specific area of health care that is developed from a synthesis of quality studies in that area. The synthesis of study findings is a complex, highly structured process that is conducted most effectively by at least two researchers or even a team of expert researchers and healthcare providers. There are various types of research syntheses, and the type of synthesis conducted varies according to the quality and types of research evidence available. The quality of the research evidence available in an area depends on the number and strength of the studies. Replicating or repeating of studies with similar methodology adds to the quality of the research evidence. The strengths and weaknesses of the studies are determined by critically appraising the credibility or trustworthiness of the study findings (see Chapter 18).

The types of research commonly conducted in nursing were identified earlier in this chapter as quantitative, qualitative, mixed methods, and outcomes (see Box 2-1). The research synthesis process used to summarize knowledge varies for quantitative and qualitative research methods. In building the best research evidence for practice, the quantitative experimental study, such as an RCT, has been identified as producing the strongest research evidence for practice (Craig & Smyth, 2012; Spruce, Van Wicklin, Hicks, Conner, & Dunn, 2014).

The following processes are usually conducted to synthesize research in nursing and health care: (1) systematic review, (2) meta-analysis, (3) meta-synthesis, and (4) mixed methods systematic review. Depending on the quantity and strength of the research findings available, nurses and other healthcare professionals use one or more of these four synthesis processes to determine the current best research evidence in an area. Table 2-3 identifies the common processes used in research synthesis, the purpose of each synthesis process, the types of research included in the synthesis (sampling frame), and the analysis techniques used to achieve the synthesis of research evidence (Craig & Smyth, 2012;

TABLE 2-3 Processes Used to Synthesize Research Evidence

Synthesis Process	Purpose of Synthesis	Types of Research Included in the Synthesis (Sampling Frame)	Analysis for Achieving Synthesis
Systematic review	Systematically identify, select, critically appraise, and synthesize research evidence to address a particular problem in practice (Craig & Smyth, 2012; Higgins & Green, 2008; Whittemore, Chao, Jang, Minges, & Park, 2014).	Quantitative studies with similar methodology, such as randomized controlled trials (RCTs), and meta-analyses focused on a practice problem	Narrative and statistical
Meta-analysis	Pooling of the results from several previous studies using statistical analysis to determine the effect of an intervention or the strength of relationships (Higgins & Green, 2008; Whittemore et al., 2014).	Quantitative studies with similar methodology, such as quasi-experimental and experimental studies focused on the effect of an intervention, or correlational studies focused on selected relationships	Statistical
Meta-synthesis	Systematic compilation and integration of qualitative studies to expand understanding and develop a unique interpretation of the studies' findings in a selected area (Barnett-Page & Thomas, 2009; Finfgeld-Connett, 2010; Sandelowski & Barroso, 2007).	Original qualitative studies and summaries of qualitative studies	Narrative
Mixed methods systematic review	Synthesis of the findings from independent studies conducted with a variety of methods (quantitative, qualitative, and mixed methods) to determine the current knowledge in an area (Higgins & Green, 2008; Whittemore et al., 2014).	Variety of quantitative, qualitative, and mixed methods studies	Narrative and sometime statistical

Sandelowski & Barroso, 2007; Whittemore, Chao, Jang, Minges, & Parks, 2014).

A **systematic review** is a structured, comprehensive synthesis of the research literature conducted to determine the best research evidence available to address a healthcare question. A systematic review involves identifying, locating, appraising, and synthesizing quality research evidence for expert clinicians to use to promote an EBP (Craig & Smyth, 2012; Higgins & Green, 2008; Spruce et al., 2014). Teams of expert researchers, clinicians, and sometimes students conduct these reviews to determine the current best knowledge for use in practice. Systematic reviews are also used in the development of national and international standardized guidelines for managing health problems such as depression, hypertension, and type 2 diabetes. The processes for

critically appraising and conducting systematic reviews are detailed in Chapter 19.

A **meta-analysis** is conducted to statistically pool the results from previous studies into a single quantitative analysis that provides one of the highest levels of evidence about an intervention's effectiveness (Andrel, Keith, & Leiby, 2009; Craig & Smyth, 2012; Higgins & Green, 2008; Whittemore et al., 2014). The studies synthesized are usually quasi-experimental or experimental types of studies. In addition, a meta-analysis can be performed using correlational studies in order to determine the type (positive or negative) and strength of relationships among selected variables (see Table 2-3). Because meta-analyses involve statistical analysis to combine study results, the synthesis of research evidence is more objective. Some of the strongest evidence for using an intervention in practice is generated from a meta-analysis of multiple, controlled quasi-experimental and experimental studies. Thus, many systematic reviews conducted to generate evidence-based guidelines include meta-analyses. The process for conducting a meta-analysis is presented in Chapter 19.

Qualitative research synthesis is the process and product of systematically reviewing and formally integrating the findings from qualitative studies (Whittemore et al., 2014). No well-established process exists for synthesizing qualitative studies, but a variety of synthesis methods have appeared in the literature (Barnett-Page & Thomas, 2009; Finfgeld-Connett, 2010; Higgins & Green, 2008; Korhonen, Hakulinen-Viitanen, Jylhä, & Holopainen, 2013; Sandelowski & Barroso, 2007). In this text, the concept of meta-synthesis is used to describe the process for synthesizing qualitative research. **Meta-synthesis** is defined as the systematic compiling and integration of qualitative study results to expand understanding and develop a unique interpretation of study findings in a selected area. The focus is on interpretation rather than the combining of study results as with quantitative research synthesis (see Table 2-3). The process for conducting a meta-synthesis is presented in Chapter 19.

Over the past 10 to 15 years, nurse researchers have conducted mixed methods studies (previously referred to as triangulation studies) that include both quantitative and qualitative research methods (Creswell, 2014, 2015; Korhone et al., 2013). In addition, determining the current research evidence in an area might require synthesizing both quantitative and qualitative studies. Higgins and Green (2008) refer to this synthesis of quantitative, qualitative, and mixed methods studies as a **mixed methods systematic review** (see Table 2-3). Mixed methods systematic reviews might include a variety of study designs, such as quasi-experimental, correlational, and/or descriptive quantitative studies and different types of qualitative studies (Higgins & Green, 2008). Some researchers have conducted syntheses of quantitative and/or qualitative studies and called them integrative reviews of research, which usually lack specific content and reporting guidelines (Whittemore et al., 2014). In this text, the synthesis of a variety of quantitative and qualitative study findings is referred to as a mixed methods systematic review, which follows the guidelines presented by Higgins and Green (2008) and the Cochrane Collection. The value of these reviews depends on the application of rigorous standards during the synthesis process. The process for conducting a mixed methods systematic review is discussed in Chapter 19.

Levels of Research Evidence

The strength or validity of the best research evidence in an area depends on the quality and quantity of the studies conducted in the area. Quantitative studies, especially experimental studies like RCTs, are thought to provide the strongest research evidence from a single source. In addition, the conduct of studies with similar frameworks, research variables, designs, and measurement methods increases the strength of the research evidence generated in an area (Cohen, Thompson, Yates, Zimmerman, & Pullen, 2015). The levels of the research evidence can be visualized as a pyramid with the highest quality of research evidence at the top and the weakest research evidence at the base (Craig & Smyth, 2012; Higgins & Green, 2008; Melnyk & Fineout-Overholt, 2015). Many pyramids have been developed to illustrate the levels of research evidence in nursing, so Figure 2-1 was developed to identify the seven levels of evidence relevant to this text. Systematic reviews and meta-analyses of high-quality experimental studies (RCTs) provide the strongest or best research evidence for use by expert clinicians, administrators, and educators in nursing. Systematic reviews and meta-analyses of quasi-experimental and experimental studies also provide strong research evidence for managing practice problems (see Level I). Level II includes evidence from an RCT or experimental study, and Level III includes evidence from a quasi-experimental study. Nonexperimental correlational and cohort studies provide evidence for Level IV. Mixed methods systematic reviews of quantitative and qualitative studies and meta-syntheses of qualitative studies comprise the evidence for Level V (see Table 2-3 for a summary of these synthesis methods). Level VI includes a descriptive study or qualitative study, and these types of studies provide limited evidence for making changes in practice and are usually new areas of research (see Figure 2-1). The base of the pyramid includes the weakest evidence, which is generated from opinions of expert committees and authorities that are not based on research.

The levels of research evidence identified in Figure 2-1 help nurses determine the quality, trustworthiness, and validity of the evidence that is available for them to use in practice. Advanced practice nurses must seek out the best research knowledge available in an area to ensure that they promote health, prevent illness, and manage patients' acute and chronic illnesses with quality care (Butts & Rich, 2015; Craig & Smyth, 2012; Higgins & Green, 2008; Melnyk & Fineout-Overholt, 2015). The best research evidence generated from systematic reviews and meta-analyses is used most often to

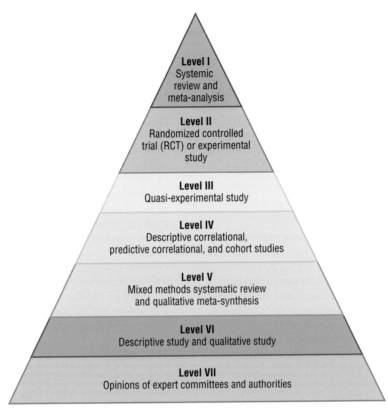

Level I
Systemic
review and
meta-analysis

Level II
Randomized controlled
trial (RCT) or experimental
study

Level III
Quasi-experimental study

Level IV
Descriptive correlational,
predictive correlational, and cohort studies

Level V
Mixed methods systematic review
and qualitative meta-synthesis

Level VI
Descriptive study and qualitative study

Level VII
Opinions of expert committees and authorities

FIGURE 2-1 Levels of evidence.

develop standardized or evidence-based guidelines for practice.

Introduction to Evidence-Based Practice Guidelines

Evidence-based practice guidelines are rigorous, explicit clinical guidelines that are based on the best research evidence available in an area. These guidelines are usually developed by a team or panel of expert researchers; expert clinicians (physicians, nurses, pharmacists, and other health professionals); and sometimes consumers, policymakers, and economists. The expert panel seeks consensus on the content of the guideline to provide clinicians with the best information for making clinical decisions in practice. However, expert clinicians must implement these generalized guidelines to meet the unique needs and values of the patient and family (Thorne & Sawatzky, 2014).

There has been a dramatic growth in the production of EBP guidelines to assist healthcare providers in building an EBP and in improving healthcare outcomes for patients, families, providers, and healthcare agencies.

Every year, new guidelines are developed, and some of the existing guidelines are revised when new research is published. These guidelines have become the **gold standard** (or standard of excellence) for patient care, and nurses and other healthcare providers are encouraged to incorporate these standardized guidelines into their practice. Expert national and international government agencies, professional organizations, and centers of excellence have made many of these evidence-based guidelines available online. When selecting a guideline for practice, be sure that a credible agency or organization developed the guideline and that the reference list reflects the synthesis of extensive research evidence.

An extremely important source for evidence-based guidelines in the United States is the National Guideline Clearinghouse (NGC), which was initiated in 1998 by the AHRQ. The Clearinghouse started with 200 guidelines and has expanded to contain more than 1500 EBP guidelines (see http://www.guideline.gov/). Another excellent source of systematic reviews and EBP guidelines is the Cochrane Collaboration and Library in the United Kingdom, which can be accessed at http://

www.cochrane.org/. The Joanna Briggs Institute has also been a leader in developing evidence-based guidelines for nursing practice (http://www.joannabriggs.edu.au/). In addition, professional nursing organizations, such as the Oncology Nursing Society (http://www.ons.org/) and the National Association of Neonatal Nurses (http://www.nann.org/), have developed EBP guidelines for their specialties. These websites will introduce you to some guidelines that exist nationally and internationally. Chapter 19 will help you critically appraise the quality of an EBP guideline and implement that guideline in your practice.

■ KEY POINTS

- Florence Nightingale initiated nursing research more than 160 years ago. Her work was followed by decades of limited research.
- During the 1950s and 1960s, research became a higher priority, with the development of graduate programs in nursing that increased the number of nurses with doctoral and master's degrees.
- Since the 1980s, the major focus of nursing research has been on the conduct of clinical research to improve nursing practice.
- Outcomes research emerged as an important methodology for documenting the effectiveness of healthcare service in the 1980s and 1990s.
- In 1989, the Agency for Health Care Policy and Research (later renamed the Agency for Healthcare Research and Quality [AHRQ]) was established to facilitate the conduct of outcomes research.
- The vision for nursing in the 21st century is the development of a scientific knowledge base that enables nurses to implement an EBP.
- Nursing research incorporates quantitative, qualitative, mixed methods, and outcomes research methodologies.
- Quantitative research is classified into four types for this textbook: descriptive, correlational, quasi-experimental, and experimental.
- Qualitative research is classified into five types for this textbook: phenomenological research, grounded theory research, ethnographic research, exploratory-descriptive qualitative research, and historical research.
- Mixed methods research is conducted when the study problem and purpose are best addressed using both quantitative and qualitative research methodologies.
- Outcomes research focuses on determining the results of care or a measure of the change in health status of the patient and family, as well as determining what variables are related to changes in selected outcomes.
- Best research evidence is a summary of the highest-quality, current empirical knowledge in a specific area of health care that is developed from a synthesis of high-quality studies (quantitative, qualitative, mixed methods, and outcomes) in that area.
- Research evidence in nursing and health care is synthesized using the following processes: (1) systematic review, (2) meta-analysis, (3) meta-synthesis, and (4) mixed methods systematic review (see Table 2-3).
- The levels of the research evidence can be visualized as a pyramid with the highest quality of research evidence at the top and the weakest research evidence at the base (see Figure 2-1).
- A team or panel of experts synthesizes the best research evidence to develop EBP guidelines.
- EBP guidelines have become the gold standard (or standard of excellence) for patient care, and nurses and other healthcare providers are encouraged to incorporate them into their practice.

REFERENCES

Abdellah, F. G. (1972). Evolution of nursing as a profession. *International Nursing Review*, 19(3), 219–235.

Agency for Healthcare Research and Quality (AHRQ). (2015). *About AHRQ: Mission & Budget*. Retrieved April 8, 2015 from http://www.ahrq.gov/cpi/about/index.html.

American Association of Colleges of Nursing (AACN). (2006). *AACN Position Statement: Nursing Research*. Retrieved April 8, 2015 from http://www.aacn.nche.edu/publications/position/nursing-research.

American Association of Colleges of Nursing (AACN). (2015). *Missions and values*. Retrieved April 8, 2015 from http://www.aacn.nche.edu/about-aacn/mission-values.

American Nurses Association (ANA). (1950). *Twenty thousand nurses tell their story*. Kansas City, MO: Author.

American Nurses Association (ANA). (1989). *Education for participation in nursing research*. Kansas City, MO: Author.

American Nurses Association (ANA). (2011). *American Nurses Association research agenda*. Retrieved April 8, 2015 from http://www.nursingworld.org/MainMenuCategories/ThePracticeofProfessionalNursing/Improving-Your-Practice/Research-Toolkit/ANA-Research-Agenda/Research-Agenda-.pdf.

American Nurses Credentialing Center (ANCC). (2016). *Magnet Recognition Program® overview*. Retrieved February 9, 2016 http://www.nursecredentialing.org/Magnet/ProgramOverview.aspx.

Andrel, J. A., Keith, S. W., & Leiby, B. E. (2009). Meta-analysis: A brief introduction. *Clinical & Translational Science*, 2(5), 374–378.

Barnett-Page, E., & Thomas, J. (2009). Methods for the synthesis of qualitative research: A critical review. *BMC*

Medical Research Methodology, 9, 1–11. doi:10.1186/147–2288–9–59. Available from http://www.biomedcentral.com/1471-2288/9/59.

Bauknecht, V. L. (1986). Congress overrides veto, nursing gets center for research. *American Nurse, 18*(1), 24.

Baumrind, D. (1980). New directions in socialization research. *American Psychologist, 35*(7), 639–652.

Borglin, G., & Richards, D. A. (2010). Bias in experimental nursing research: Strategies to improve the quality and explanatory power of nursing science. *International Journal of Nursing Studies, 47*(1), 123–128.

Brown, S. J. (2014). *Evidence-based nursing: The research-practice connection* (3rd ed.). Sudbury, MA: Jones and Bartlett Publishers.

Butts, J. B., & Rich, K. L. (2015). *Philosophies and theories for advanced nursing practice* (2nd ed.). Burlington, MA: Jones & Bartlett Learning.

Charmaz, K. (2014). *Constructing grounded theory* (2nd ed.). Los Angeles, CA: Sage.

Chinn, P. L., & Kramer, M. K. (2015). *Knowledge development in nursing: Theory and process* (9th ed.). St. Louis, MO: Mosby.

Clark, A. M. (1998). The qualitative-quantitative debate: Moving from positivism and confrontation to post-positivism and reconciliation. *Journal of Advanced Nursing, 271*(6), 1242–1249.

Clark, V. L. P., & Ivankova, N. V. (2016). *Mixed methods research: A guide to the field.* Los Angeles, CA: Sage.

Cohen, B. (1984). Florence Nightingale. *Scientific American, 250*(3), 128–137.

Cohen, M. Z., Thompson, C. B., Yates, B., Zimmerman, L., & Pullen, C. H. (2015). Implementing common data elements across studies to advance research. *Nursing Outlook, 63*(2), 181–188.

Conduct and Utilization of Research in Nursing (CURN) Project. (1981–1982). *Using research to improve nursing practice.* New York, NY: Grune & Stratton.

Cook, Sir E. (1913). *The life of Florence Nightingale* (Vol. 1). London, England: Macmillan.

Craig, J. V., & Smyth, R. L. (2012). *The evidence-based practice manual for nurses* (3rd ed.). Edinburgh, Scotland: Churchill Livingstone.

Creswell, J. W. (2013). *Qualitative inquiry & research design: Choosing among five approaches* (3rd ed.). Thousand Oaks, CA: Sage.

Creswell, J. W. (2014). *Research design: Qualitative, quantitative and mixed methods approaches* (4th ed.). Thousand Oaks, CA: Sage.

Creswell, J. W. (2015). *A concise introduction to mixed methods research.* Los Angeles, CA: Sage.

Creswell, J. W. (2016). *30 essential skills for the qualitative researcher.* Los Angeles, CA: Sage.

de Tornyay, R. (1977). Nursing research—the road ahead. *Nursing Research, 26*(6), 404–407.

Doran, D. M. (2011). *Nursing-sensitive outcomes: State of the science.* Sudbury, MA: Jones & Bartlett.

Downs, F. S., & Fleming, W. J. (1979). *Issues in nursing research.* New York, NY: Appleton-Century-Crofts.

Fawcett, J., & DeSanto-Madeya, S. (2013). *Contemporary nursing knowledge: Analysis and evaluation of nursing models and theories.* Philadelphia, PA: F. A. Davis Company.

Finfgeld-Connett, D. (2010). Generalizability and transferability of meta-synthesis research findings. *Journal of Advanced Nursing, 66*(2), 246–254.

Fitzpatrick, M. L. (1978). *Historical studies in nursing.* New York, NY: Teachers College Press.

Ford-Gilboe, M., Campbell, J., & Berman, H. (1995). Stories and numbers: Coexistence without compromise. *Advances in Nursing Science, 18*(1), 14–26.

Glaser, B. G., & Strauss, A. L. (1967). *The discovery of grounded theory: Strategies for qualitative research.* Chicago, IL: Aldine.

Gortner, S. R., & Nahm, H. (1977). An overview of nursing research in the United States. *Nursing Research, 26*(1), 10–33.

Grove, S. K., & Cipher, D. (2017). *Statistics for nursing research: A workbook for evidence-based practice* (2nd ed.). St. Louis, MO: Saunders.

Herbert, R. G. (1981). *Florence Nightingale: Saint, reformer or rebel?* Malabar, FL: Robert E. Krieger.

Higgins, J. P. T., & Green, S. (2008). *Cochrane handbook for systematic reviews of interventions.* West Sussex, England: Wiley-Blackwell and The Cochrane Collaboration.

Horsley, J. A., Crane, J., Crabtree, M. K., & Wood, D. J. (1983). *Using research to improve nursing practice: A guide; CURN Project.* New York, NY: Grune & Stratton.

Institute of Medicine. (2001). *Crossing the quality chasm: A new health system for the 21st century.* Washington, DC: National Academy Press.

Jacox, A. (1980). Strategies to promote nursing research. *Nursing Research, 29*(4), 213–218.

Johnson, J. E. (1993). Outcomes research and health care reform: Opportunities for nurses. *Nursing Connections, 6*(4), 1–3.

Johnson, W. L. (1977). Research programs of the National League for Nursing. *Nursing Research, 26*(3), 172–176.

Kaplan, A. (1964). *The conduct of inquiry: Methodology for behavioral science.* New York, NY: Chandler.

Kerlinger, F. N., & Lee, H. B. (2000). *Foundations of behavioral research* (4th ed.). Fort Worth, TX: Harcourt.

Korhonen, A., Hakulinen-Viitanen, T., Jylhä, V., & Holopainen, A. (2013). Meta-synthesis and evidence-based health care—a method for systematic review. *Scandinavian Journal of Caring Science, 27*(4), 1027–1034.

Krueger, J. C., Nelson, A. H., & Wolanin, M. A. (1978). *Nursing research: Development, collaboration, and utilization.* Germantown, MD: Aspen.

Larson, E. (1984). Health policy and NIH: Implications for nursing research. *Nursing Research, 33*(6), 352–356.

Lundy, K. S. (2012). Historical research. In P. L. Munhall (Ed.), *Nursing research: A qualitative perspective* (5th ed., p. 381397). Sudbury, MA: Jones & Bartlett Learning.

Mantzoukas, S. (2009). The research evidence published in high impact nursing journals between 2000 and 2006: A quantitative content analysis. *International Journal of Nursing Studies, 46*(4), 479–489.

Marshall, C., & Rossman, G. B. (2016). *Designing qualitative research* (6th ed.). Los Angeles, CA: Sage.

Melnyk, B. M., & Fineout-Overholt, E. (2015). *Evidence-based practice in nursing & healthcare: A guide to best practice* (3rd ed.). Philadelphia, PA: Lippincott Williams & Wilkins.

Miles, M. B., Huberman, A. M., & Saldaña, J. (2014). *Qualitative data analysis: A methods sourcebook* (3rd ed.). Los Angeles, CA: Sage.

Morse, J. M. (2012). *Qualitative health research: Creating a new discipline*. Walnut Creek, CA: Left Coast Press.

Munhall, P. L. (2012). *Nursing research: A qualitative perspective* (5th ed.). Sudbury, MA: Jones & Bartlett Learning.

National Institute of Nursing Research (NINR). (2011). *NINR Strategic Plan: Bringing science to life*. Retrieved April 8, 2015 from http://www.ninr.nih.gov/sites/www.ninr.nih.gov/files/ninr-strategic-plan-2011.pdf.

National Institute of Nursing Research (NINR). (2013). *NINR mission statement*. Retrieved April 8, 2015 from http://www.ninr.nih.gov/aboutninr/ninr-mission-and-strategic-plan#.VS1kWvnF-Ck.

National League for Nursing (NLN). (2016). *About the NLN: Missions and goals*. Retrieved February 9, 2016 from http://www.nln.org/about/mission-goals.

Newman, M. A. (1992). Prevailing paradigms in nursing. *Nursing Outlook, 40*(1), 10–13, 32.

Nightingale, F. (1859). *Notes on nursing: What it is, and what it is not*. Philadelphia, PA: Lippincott.

Norbeck, J. S. (1987). In defense of empiricism. *Image—Journal of Nursing Scholarship, 19*(1), 28–30.

Oakley, K. (2010). Nursing by the numbers. *Occupational Health, 62*(4), 28–29.

Palmer, I. S. (1977). Florence Nightingale: Reformer, reactionary, researcher. *Nursing Research, 26*(2), 84–89.

Polit, D. F., & Yang, F. M. (2016). *Measurement and the measurement of change*. Philadelphia, PA: Wolters Kluwer.

Quality and Safety Education for Nurses (QSEN) Institute. (2012). *Graduate-level competencies: Knowledge, skills, and attitudes (KSAs)*. Retrieved February 23, 2015 from http://qsen.org/competencies/graduate-ksas/.

Rettig, R. (1991). History, development, and importance to nursing of outcomes research. *Journal of Nursing Quality Assurance, 5*(2), 13–17.

Sackett, D. L., Straus, S. E., Richardson, W. S., Rosenberg, W., & Haynes, R. B. (2000). *Evidence-based medicine: How to practice & teach EBM* (2nd ed.). London, England: Churchill Livingstone.

Sandelowski, M., & Barroso, J. (2007). *Handbook for synthesizing qualitative research*. New York, NY: Springer.

Scheffler, I. (1967). *Science and subjectivity*. Indianapolis, IN: Bobbs-Merrill.

See, E. M. (1977). The ANA and research in nursing. *Nursing Research, 26*(3), 165–171.

Shadish, S. R., Cook, T. D., & Campbell, D. T. (2002). *Experimental and quasi-experimental designs for generalized causal inference*. Boston, MA: Houghton Mifflin Company.

Sherwood, G., & Barnsteiner, J. (2012). *Quality and safety in nursing: A competency approach to improving outcomes*. Ames, IA: Wiley-Blackwell.

Spruce, L., Van Wicklin, S. A., Hicks, R. W., Conner, R., & Dunn, D. (2014). Introducing AORN's new model for evidence rating. *AORN, 99*(2), 243–255.

Stetler, C. B. (2001). Updating the Stetler Model of research utilization to facilitate evidence-based practice. *Nursing Outlook, 49*(6), 272–279.

Stetler, C. B., & Marram, G. (1976). Evaluating research findings for applicability in practice. *Nursing Outlook, 24*(9), 559–563.

Thorne, S., & Sawatzky, R. (2014). Particularizing the general: Sustaining theoretical integrity in the context of an evidence-based practice agenda. *Advances in Nursing Science, 37*(1), 5–18.

The Joint Commission on Accreditation of Healthcare Organizations (JCAHO). (2016). *About The Joint Commission*. Retrieved February 9, 2016 from http://www.jointcommission.org/about_us/about_the_joint_commission_main.aspx.

U.S. Department of Health and Human Services (DHHS). (1992). *Healthy People 2000*. Washington, DC: Author.

U.S. Department of Health and Human Services (DHHS). (2000). *Healthy People 2010*. Washington, DC: Author.

U.S. Department of Health and Human Services (DHHS). (2014). *Healthy People 2020 topics and objectives*. Retrieved April 8, 2015 from http://www.healthypeople.gov/2020/topicsobjectives2020/default.

Werley, H. H. (1977). Nursing research in perspective. *International Nursing Review, 24*(3), 75–83.

Werley, H. H., & Fitzpatrick, J. J. (Eds.), (1983). *Annual review of nursing research* (Vol. 1). New York, NY: Springer.

Wolf, Z. (2012). Ethnography: The method. In P. L. Munhall (Ed.), *Nursing research: A qualitative perspective* (5th ed., pp. 285–338). Sudbury, MA: Jones & Bartlett Learning.

Whittemore, R., Chao, A., Jang, M., Minges, K. E., & Park, C. (2014). Methods for knowledge synthesis: An overview. *Heart and Lung: The Journal of Critical Care, 43*(5), 453–461.

Introduction to Quantitative Research

Suzanne Sutherland

ⓔ http://evolve.elsevier.com/Gray/practice/

Quantitative research counts or measures in order to answer a research question. Whether the original data the researcher obtains are numerical or language-based, a quantitative analysis always focuses on the data's counted or measured aspects: if the ultimate output of a study is the analysis of a count or a measurement, the research is quantitative. The results of quantitative research provide better understanding of one or more of the following three aspects of reality: incidence, connections between two ideas, and cause-and-effect relationships. The general public considers quantitative the only type of research, as it absorbs media reports such as, "Three dentists out of four recommend Brand A," "High school dropout rate is the result of poverty," and "Chocolate has been shown to prevent heart disease."

Quantitative research is empirical, meaning that it is able to be observed and measured or counted in some way. Logical positivism is a philosophy on which the scientific method is based. Logical positivists consider empirical discovery the only dependable source of knowledge. The natural sciences adhere to the logical positivist stance.

This chapter describes the scientific method and identifies several types of quantitative research and the distinctions among them. In addition, it elucidates the differences between basic and applied research, provides an explanation of the term "rigor" as it is used in quantitative research, explains what the term "control" means, and differentiates between control and comparison groups. Finally, it presents steps common to the quantitative research process.

THE SCIENTIFIC METHOD

The purpose of the scientific method is to develop knowledge by testing hypotheses. The method's roots can be traced to Ibn al-Haytham, a 10th-century Arabic scholar of mathematics, astronomy, and physics (Tokuhama-Espinosa, 2010). Early forms of the scientific method, using deduction and hypothetical reasoning, exist in the writings of 16th-century scientist Galileo and 17th-century mathematicians Keppler and Descartes (Hald, 1990). In the early 20th century, Karl Popper introduced the notion of falsifiability (Popper, 1968): if something is not able to be proven false, it is not in the realm of science. Popper argued that falsification cannot rely on one experiment but must be demonstrated in a different experiment, as well, because "non-reproducible single occurrences are of no significance to science" (Popper, 1968, p. 86).

The scientific method rests on the process of stating hypotheses, testing them, and then either disproving them or testing them more fully. The hypothesis-testing process involves several steps: identification of a research hypothesis, construction of the null hypothesis, sample size determination, choice of statistical test, setting of a decision point for the statistical test, data collection, statistical calculation, and decision making. This process is detailed in Box 3-1.

The principles of scientific research include the notion that measurement is never 100% accurate and that error intrudes in all measurement, to some extent. Because of this, one test of a hypothesis is never sufficient. What if the results were obtained in error, as a

BOX 3-1   The Hypothesis-Testing Process

After identification of a working research hypothesis, a null hypothesis is constructed. The researcher decides on sample size and statistical test to be used for testing the null hypothesis, and sets a decision point. Data are then collected. If the values calculated by the statistical test are greater than the preset decision point, it means that there is a difference between groups; if the values obtained are less than the decision point, it means that the groups are not all that different. If the statistical test reveals that the two groups are not very different, the null hypothesis is supported. The null hypothesis is not "proven true," merely supported, phrased as, "There is support for the null hypothesis." This would mean that the working research hypothesis is rejected.

If the statistical test reveals that the two groups are more different than the pre-set decision point, the researcher rejects the null hypothesis. There actually is a difference between groups, and the working research hypothesis is supported, phrased as, "There is support for the research hypothesis," never that it is proven or true.

When the null hypothesis is shown to be false through the data that the researcher collects, the null hypothesis is rejected, but the research hypothesis is not, however, "proven." The researcher can state only that there is evidence in support of the research hypothesis. In the scientific method, nothing is categorically proven. However, many accepted laws of science have never been disproven, and there is "ample evidence" in their support, which is as close as the scientific method comes to declaring that something is true.

fluke or accident? What if unusual numbers of extreme cases were included in the sample? Before research results are considered dependable, the same hypothesis should be retested in a subsequent study, called a **replication study**, in order to eliminate the very real possibility of error. Because so much nursing research consists of "stand-alone" efforts, generated either because of curiosity in one's own clinical area or due to the requirements of an advanced degree program, very little nursing research has been replicated. Replication of an existent study is a respected way to generate worthwhile, applicable research findings (Fitzpatrick & Kazer, 2012). Even if a study's findings are supported by a replication study, in order for the findings to be applied outside the location or setting in which the research was conducted, the population to which the findings are applied, or generalized, must be quite similar to the studies' samples.

Terminology: Methodology, Design, Method

In this text, **methodology** refers to the type of the research selected to answer the research question: quantitative research, qualitative research, outcomes research, or mixed-methods research. (These methodologies are also presented in Chapters 4, 13, and 14.) Clearly, if the research question is, "What are the three strongest predictors of immediate postoperative mortality after hip replacement?", the research methodology is quantitative. As a result of measurements performed by the researcher, the answer to this particular research question will be nested in its output of numerical data. The researcher's desired output determines a study's methodology.

Design in quantitative research refers to the researcher's way of answering a research question, with respect to several considerations, including number of subject groups, timing of data collection, and researcher intervention, if any. Various designs in quantitative research are described in Chapters 10 and 11. If the research question is, "What are the intergenerational economic effects of poverty?" many research designs would be appropriate for answering this question, including but not limited to predictive correlational design, cross-sectional descriptive design, and longitudinal correlational design.

Research **methods** are the specific ways in which the researcher chooses to conduct the study, within the chosen design. Most methods are conveniently listed in the Methods section of the research report and include details about the researcher's decision making related to important details like subject selection, choice of setting, attempts to limit factors that might introduce error, the manner in which a research intervention is strategized, ways in which data are collected, and choice of statistical tests. If a research question is, "What are the principal factors that determine a patient's decision to check out of a hospital against medical advice?", there are numerous methods with which the researcher might choose to conduct the study.

Decisions related to methodology, design, and methods represent the single most important step of the research process: designing the study.

TYPES OF QUANTITATIVE RESEARCH

Most disciplines divide quantitative research into two principal groups: interventional research and noninterventional research. The purpose of interventional research is to examine cause-and-effect relationships. In the classic experimental type of interventional research, the researcher does something to the interventional (experimental) group but not to the control group, in order to measure the amount of difference produced by the intervention. That something that the researcher does is called application of the independent variable. In this type of research, the independent variable is measurable, but usually it has only two potential values, corresponding to "Intervention" and "No Intervention." The dependent variable in interventional research *depends* upon the presence or absence of the independent variable. The **dependent variable** is the response, behavior, or outcome that is predicted and measured. In interventional research, changes in the dependent variable are presumed to be caused by the independent variable. The dependent variable, also, is measurable and has two or more potential values. Its values can be numerical, such as a number denoting heart rate, or non-numerical, such as "improved" and "not improved." The two types of interventional research discussed in this text are experimental and quasi-experimental. Interventional research always has a research hypothesis, either stated or implied.

In noninterventional research, the researcher does nothing to the research subjects except for what occurs in the process of measuring them, such as having them fill out a survey or submit to a blood draw. All noninterventional research is essentially descriptive (Cooper, 2012), in that it describes either variables or relationships between variables. However, in this text correlational research is presented as a distinct type of noninterventional research because of its applications for both prediction and model-testing. Correlational research often has a stated or implied research hypothesis; other descriptive research may or may not have a stated or implied hypothesis.

Descriptive Research

The general purpose of **descriptive research** is to explore and describe ideas, which in research are called phenomena, in real-life situations. Descriptive research is performed when collective knowledge about a phenomenon is incomplete: either no research has been conducted, or there is limited research knowledge. The underlying research questions in descriptive research are, "To what extent does this exist?" "What are the principal types of this?" and "What are the relative amounts of this?" There are many descriptive research designs, some of which are presented in Chapter 10. A few of these are the simple descriptive design, the comparative descriptive design, the longitudinal descriptive design, and the cross-sectional descriptive design. An example of descriptive research is Smeltzer et al.'s (2015) study examining the demographic characteristics and academic preparation of nursing faculty teaching in doctorate of philosophy (PhD) and doctorate of nursing practice (DNP) programs, as well as characteristics of role and work environment. The authors' intent was to describe United States (U.S.) nursing faculty, with regard to those attributes.

Correlational Research

In correlational research, the researcher measures the numerical strength of relationships between and among variables, in order to discover whether a change in the value of one is likely to occur when another increases or decreases. Bravais, Galton, Pearson, Yule, and Edgeworth were mathematicians and statisticians credited with substantial work in the development of the ideas of correlation and multiple correlation, and the formulas that measure the strength of relationships between and among variables (Hald, 1998; Johnson & Kotz, 1997). Correlational research in medicine dates from the early 20th century and has focused on relationships among interventions, diseases, symptoms, treatments, and outcomes. Nurses have conducted correlational research since the second part of the 20th century. In recent years, correlational research regarding outcomes and quality of care has burgeoned, due to the availability of computer-based data from both public and private databases.

In correlational research, one purpose of establishing a numerical relationship between variables is to allow prediction. For instance, correlational research in humans has documented the fact that excessive alcohol intake is related to liver and finally brain damage, and that the extent and severity of the damage are linked to nutritional deficits of thiamine and folate. In the emergency room, patients likely to be admitted who have a history of alcohol abuse are consequently administered their first of several "banana bags," yellow-colored intravenous fluids containing thiamine and folate, among other additives, to minimize chances of this predicted organ damage (Katz, 2012).

Correlational research establishes relationship strength by use of correlational formulas. Correlational formulas produce numbers varying from -1 through $+1$. A correlation between two variables of -1 is a perfect negative correlation (also called an inverse correlation): as one variable increases, the other decreases, and the amount of that increase is completely predictable. A correlation of $+1$ is a perfect positive correlation: as one variable increases in value, the value of the other variable also increases by a predictable amount. A correlation of 0 signifies no relationship at all. A correlational value near −1 signifies a strong negative relationship, and a value near +1 signifies a strong positive relationship. An example of this would be the relationship between number of times hospital staff cleaned their hands and bacterial counts of resistant organisms on hospital work surfaces. Another example would be the relationship between a community health department's number of accessible free immunization clinics and the immunization rate of children whose families have incomes below the poverty line. A value of 0 signifies no relationship at all. The correlational relationship between minutes of discharge teaching a nurse provides and significant long-term behavior change related to diet and exercise is close to 0, indicating almost no relationship at all.

The correlation statistic is usually referred to as r in published reports; for instance, a moderate negative correlation would be referred to as $r = -0.53$, and a strong positive one as $r = 0.82$. An example of correlational nursing research is Morrissy, Boman, and Mergler's (2013) study of predictors of affective well-being in nurses. Although optimism and anxiety were both contributory ($r = 0.38$, $r = -0.57$), the single strongest predictor of affective well-being was found to be depression ($r = -0.77$). The minus sign before 0.77 denotes a strong negative relationship: as depression decreases, affective well-being increases. There are three correlational research designs described in this text, all of which are clarified in Chapter 10. These are the simple correlational design, the predictive correlational design, and the model testing design.

Experimental Research

Ronald Fisher, an Englishman, was a noted mathematician, a pioneer statistician, and a theoretical geneticist, who contributed mightily to the development of modern experimental research. His practical insights about sampling and related to causation versus correlation, his invention of numerous statistical tests including the analysis of variance and Fisher's exact test, and his naming of the null hypothesis were unique. His writing was succinct and clear (Fisher, 1970).

Experimental research is one of the two principal design groups in interventional research. Its purpose is to test the null hypothesis by means of applying an intervention to experimental subjects but not to the control subjects, and then measuring the effect on a dependent variable. At least two separate groups must be present, one of which is a distinct control group that does not receive the intervention. In addition, in

experimental research, subjects must be randomly assigned to either the intervention group or the control group. Random assignment is the process of assigning subjects so that each has an equal opportunity of being in either group.

Basic research that tests the effect of an intervention is almost always experimental. Other experimental research is conducted outside labs, in healthcare settings not especially designed for basic research. Although these latter sites present a slightly higher potential for error, they maintain consistent specialized care for subjects, who are then treated in areas that address their particular health needs. Well-designed experimental research maintains as high a degree of precision, consistency, and sequestration of subjects from influences that might affect the research results as is possible in a real-world setting.

An example of experimental research is the study by Arvidsson, Bergman, Arvidsson, Fridlund, and Tingström (2013). The authors investigated the effectiveness of a self-care–promoting learning program for increasing quality of life, empowerment, and self-care ability for persons with rheumatic diseases. Although changes in health-related quality of life and self-care ability were found to be not statistically significant, empowerment was significantly increased in the experimental group. There are various experimental research designs described in this text, and these are clarified in Chapter 11. Four of these are the classic experimental design (pretest/posttest control group design), the experimental posttest-only control group design, the factorial design, and the Solomon four-group design.

Quasi-Experimental Research

Quasi-experimental research is the second principal design group in interventional research. *Quasi* experimental means similar, but not equivalent, to experimental. The purpose of **quasi-experimental research** is to test the hypothesis of a cause-and-effect relationship when an experimental design cannot or should not be used. As with experimental research, the structure of quasi-experimental research includes an independent variable and a dependent variable in a proposed cause-and-effect relationship. Unlike experimental research, however, quasi-experimental research is lacking in one or more of the other attributes of experimental research: (1) researcher-controlled manipulation of the independent variable, (2) the traditional type of control group, and (3) random assignment of subjects to group.

Sometimes, the use of quasi-experimental research is a fallback stance (Campbell & Stanley, 1963): something changes in a work setting, and the workers design a study to evaluate outcomes under the current condition, as opposed to the former condition. An example of this would be the case in which a new hospital-wide protocol for tracheostomy care is instituted, and nurses want to know whether the new protocol actually represents an improvement in terms of health, safety, or another measurable outcome. An experiment that randomly assigns some patients to the old protocol and some to the new protocol cannot be used, because it would be in violation of hospital standards: the new protocol is in place and must be used. In addition, presumably the new protocol was enacted based on the belief that it was preferable, so using the old protocol could be interpreted as less safe, more expensive, more time-consuming, or merely less preferred by healthcare workers. Consequently, a quasi-experimental design without random assignment and without a true control group might be employed because an experiment is not possible. A quasi-experimental study would provide research evidence about the quality of tracheostomy care under the new protocol, comparing it to data from existent medical records from the last few months under the old protocol. In other instances, the use of quasi-experimental research addresses problems of data interpretation that would occur with an experimental strategy. In all quasi-experimental research, the credibility of study conclusions is affected by the degree to which researchers can be clear, logical, creative, and intelligent in the comparisons they make.

In an actual quasi-experimental study, Smith and Holloman (2014) examined the effect of initiating an intervention using high school students to educate their peers about decreasing consumption of sugar-sweetened beverages and to initiate a 30-day beverage challenge. Measures made at the end of the intervention indicated a statistically significant decrease in the amount of sugar-sweetened beverages subjects consumed. There was no separate, distinct control group.

Many quasi-experimental research designs exist. Four of these are the one-group pretest-posttest design (Smith & Holloman, 2014), equivalence time-samples design (also called repeated reversal design), nonequivalent control group design, and crossover design (a counterbalanced design). Chapters 10 and 11 address the process of research design and the threats to design validity, as well as many types of descriptive, correlational, quasi-experimental, and experimental designs.

APPLIED VERSUS BASIC RESEARCH

A developing science, such as nursing, deserves a solid research foundation that includes both applied and basic inquiry (Wysocki, 1983). More important, if nurses do not participate in both basic and applied research in roles that transcend that of a research assistant, healthcare research will foster decisions that may overlook important facets of nursing practice. Instead of recognizing the contributions of nursing to patient outcomes, viewpoints will be promoted that are more consistent with the disciplines of those who do participate extensively in research, namely medicine, business, marketing, general science, and psychology. Nursing research is especially crucial in emerging areas of inquiry, such as those related to the evolving problems of healthcare delivery.

Basic research is scientific investigation directed toward better understanding, without any emphasis on application. Its purpose is to answer theoretical questions, not specific concrete ones. Within health-related fields, basic researchers seek to increase understanding of physiological or psychological processes by testing hypotheses that can answer general theoretical questions, not specific clinical-based ones.

Because basic research's findings are not applicable directly to a practice area, they must be tested with subsequent applied research in order to confirm that the findings are similar in specific practice settings in which the results are to be applied. Basic research's findings are, however, broadly generalizable because they are not limited to distinct clinical settings. In other words, the knowledge gained from these understandings can be used in many venues for informing clinical decisions and for generating research in those specific areas. Basic research may be qualitative or quantitative, but the most common type, by far, is quantitative. Basic research's quantitative questions are related to incidence, relationship, and cause.

Basic research is the opposite of applied research. It is conducted in a research lab or other artificial setting, often with paid human volunteers or with animals. Because it is often conducted in research labs on long tables or benches, it is sometimes referred to as bench research, or merely bench. In the physical sciences, some basic research uses the tissues of humans or animals. Basic research tests hypotheses and theories in progress, either confirming or refuting them. A refuted theory produces considerable discussion in a research lab, sometimes followed by revision of existent theory. After refutation of the working theory "A produces B," it could be revised as "A produces B, unless acted upon by C." This revised theory is then tested. Chapter 8 contains additional information about testing theories.

If it is limited to specific physiological processes, and to some psychological ones, basic research's findings are widely generalizable, after proper replication. "Severing the vas deferens of the rat results in sterility" would be widely generalizable to all rats and perhaps other species sharing the same general physiology. "Use of a nasogastric tube made with substance M instead of the usual silicone results in less discomfort on insertion" would be generalizable to persons of the same size and age as those in the basic research sample.

In interventional basic research, the research lab is designed to make certain that the conditions for experimental and control groups are identical. This makes it more likely that the research intervention is the only thing that affects the dependent variable's value. This type of research involves a high degree of precision, consistency of treatment, accuracy, calibration of instruments, and exactness in measurements.

An example of basic nursing research that served as a basis for the subsequent landmark study on children's procedural anxiety is Jean Johnson's work on information-giving and subsequent distress behaviors in response to pain. Johnson (1973) conducted basic research with human adults in lab settings, measuring volunteers' intensity of physical sensations and the degree of distress caused by these sensations when ischemic pain was applied by use of a blood pressure cuff inflated for up to 18 minutes. Volunteers were provided differing types of information prior to cuff application: sensory information about what they would feel (experimental group) or cognitive information about the physiology of the pain experience (control group). Johnson's (1973) basic research yielded information about the nature of distress in relation to information given about a painful procedure.

Applied Research

Applied research in nursing is a scientific investigation conducted to generate knowledge that is intended to have a direct influence upon practice. As opposed to basic research, the purpose of applied research is to answer specific questions, not general theoretical ones. Applied research may be qualitative or quantitative. Quantitative applied research questions are related to incidence, relationship, or cause.

The specific questions of applied research arise from practice situations. Consequently, applied research is conducted in practice settings quite similar to the settings in which the results will be applied. The majority of nursing research is applied, not basic. Applied research findings are directly applicable to a practice area. Because of this, its results are generalizable only to similar settings and circumstances, because the research that generated the findings was situated in a distinct clinical setting.

An example of applied research is Jean Johnson's landmark work with children in an orthopedics clinic, undergoing removal of plaster casts. After completing basic research, described previously, focusing on decreasing distress in adult human volunteers in a lab setting, by means of providing them information about the sensations they would experience, she conducted applied research in a clinic in which children's orthopedic casts were removed (Johnson, Kirchhoff, & Endress, 1975). Often, children are alarmed by the loud noises that occur during the procedure, as a circular plastic disc is applied to the cast surface and vibrated, causing the cast to crack open. The disc is not sharp and does not cause pain, but it looks like a small circular saw, engendering considerable apprehension. Johnson demonstrated that teaching about what children would see, feel, smell, and hear during cast removal decreased their distress behaviors of screaming, crying, and out-of-control behavior. The methods of Johnson et al.'s (1975) research are still applied today in pediatric areas for children undergoing procedures, and are known as sensory preparation.

Both basic and applied nursing studies have been funded at the national level by the National Institutes of Nursing Research (NINR). Although basic research is recognized by the NINR as one of its research priorities (NINR, 2012), many more requests for funding of applied research than for funding of basic research have been received by and funded by the NINR, over the years. In actuality, NINR program announcements for grant applications from March 2012 through March 2015, for instance, were overwhelmingly for applied, not basic, research (NINR, 2015), because most nursing research is applied research. The few nursing researchers conducting basic research tend to be those who work and teach in academic settings with major physiological research agendas and on-site laboratories.

RIGOR IN QUANTITATIVE RESEARCH

Rigor in quantitative research literally means hardness or difficulty, and it is associated with inflexible rules, strict logic, and unflagging effort. When applied to the quantitative research process, rigor implies a high degree of accuracy, consistency, and attention to all measurable aspects of the research. In rigorous quantitative research, deductions are flawlessly reasoned, and decisions are based on the scientific method. The first step to a rigorous study is a well-considered design with meticulously chosen methods. If a design is incorrect for a research question, the research will yield results that are not pertinent to the question. Even with a well-chosen design, there must be logical consistency among the various levels of the study, top to bottom: theoretical level, framework, hypothesis, variables, measurements, measurement levels including a range of potential values, and statistical tests chosen. Logic in research design is enhanced by using a process called substruction, a term coined by Hinshaw (1979) and later addressed by Dulock and Holzemer (1991) (Box 3-2).

After the design is decided upon, the study's specific methods must be carefully selected and enacted so as to produce precise, dependable results. Rigor implies the following:

- The sample is chosen in accordance with predetermined inclusion criteria.
- The site is chosen so as to eliminate intrusion of happenings that might affect results.
- Any research intervention is enacted the same way every time it is implemented.
- Measurements are made accurately with well-calibrated equipment.
- Data are recorded precisely.

BOX 3-2 Logic in Research Design

Gibbs (1972), a sociologist, observed that attention to connections between the theoretical and operational aspects of a study is essential for continuing the development of new knowledge. Within nursing, Hinshaw (1979) described, and later Dulock and Holzemer (1991) refined, the process of **theoretical substruction**, which is a way to ensure logic by comparing all levels of each variable, from very abstract through very concrete levels. This is accomplished by developing a diagram delineating constructs, concepts, variables, and measurement strategies, for easy review of logical consistency. Wolf and Heinzer (1999), instead of the terms "variable" and "measurement," used Gibbs' terms "referential" and "referent" (Figure 3-1). Each vertical set of terms must be logically consistent, from top to bottom.

Wolf and Heinzer (1999) recommended that substruction be used by all new researchers and by all students planning a research study. The exercise of constructing a diagram for each concept-variable set stimulates critical thinking and makes incongruence between the theoretical and operational aspects of the study more apparent. Despite its simplicity, the process produces "a condensed version of an investigation, a representation of the complexities of the infrastructure" (p. 37). It is an effective way to introduce rigor into a quantitative design.

- Statistical analyses are appropriately made with consideration of their assumptions.
- Interpretations are accurate and fair.
- Recommendations are made in accordance with guidelines for generalization.

CONTROL IN QUANTITATIVE RESEARCH

In a research context, the noun "control" is global and means little in itself. However, enacting control of, or controlling for, something refers to researcher actions intended to minimize the effects of extraneous variables. **Control** consists of design decisions made by the researcher to decrease the intrusion of the effects of extraneous variables that could alter research findings and consequently force an incorrect conclusion. The term "control" also is used to mean the researcher's enactment of an intervention, referred to as manipulative control (Kerlinger & Lee, 2000, p. 559).

An extraneous variable is something that is not the focus of a study; it has a potential effect on the study, though, making the independent variable appear more or less powerful than it really is in causing a change in the value of the dependent variable. While a study is in its early planning stages, the researcher makes adjustments in the research design and methods in order to attempt to control for the intrusion of extraneous variables that could alter the findings and consequently force an incorrect conclusion by the researcher. The end-goal of control of extraneous variables is one of the following: to eliminate or reduce an extraneous variable's effect upon perceived relationships between the study's principal variables, to eliminate the influence of an extraneous variable from calculations that measure relationships between the principal variables, or to permit the researcher to determine the magnitude and direction of an extraneous variable's effect. To reiterate, the purpose of enacting controls is to control for the effects of extraneous variables.

Random assignment, when a large sample is used, results in more or less equal distribution between subject groups of those characteristics that potentially might act as extraneous variables. Random assignment does not precisely control for extraneous variables: it merely makes their effects less powerful, provided that subjects with those variables are fairly evenly distributed between groups. The most common processes by which the researcher controls for extraneous variables before the study is conducted are selection of the study design, sampling strategy, selection of the intervention for experimental subjects, and choice of measurements for

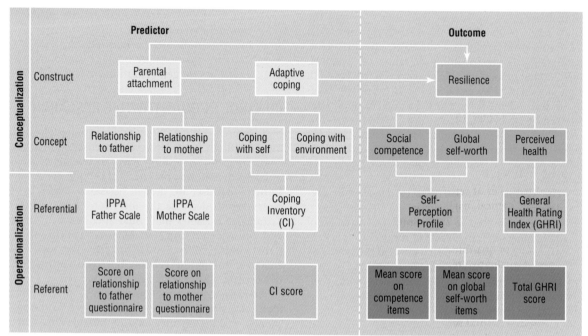

FIGURE 3-1 Substructure example of quantitative study, "Resilience of adolescents following parental death in childhood and its relationship to parental attachment and coping," *Inventory of Parent and Peer Attachment (IPPA)*. (Modified from Wolf, Z.R., & Heinzer, M.M. (1999). Substruction: Illustrating the connections from research question to analysis. *Journal of Professional Nursing, 15*(1), 33–37; adapted from Heinzer, M.M. (1993). Adolescent resilience following parental death in childhood and its relationship to parental attachment and coping. (Doctoral dissertation, Case Western Reserve University, 1993). *Dissertation Abstracts International, 55-01,* B6579.)

dependent variables. After study completion, the researcher tests for the effects of extraneous variables by means of a post hoc statistical analysis.

The extent to which the researcher controls for the effects of extraneous variables in the study's design is referred to as **internal validity**. Chapters 10 and 11 address the various types of design validity and the process for selecting an appropriate study design.

Sampling and Attrition

Whether humans, animals, plants, events, or venues, the individual participants in a study are called its **elements**. Collectively, all of the participants in a study constitute its sample. A study's sample is selected, in some way, from the population. **Sampling** is the process of selecting elements from the population. Sampling is addressed in detail in Chapter 15.

The manner in which a sample is chosen determines the degree to which a study's results are generalizable to the entire population. If a sample represents the population well, the answer to the research question pertains to the entire population. If the sample is not very representative of the population, then the answer to the research question pertains only to the sample or, at best, to only part of the population. Because random sampling methods represent the population well, random sampling allows generalization to a broader slice of the population than does non-random sampling.

It is desirable for a researcher to perform what is called a **power analysis** before finalizing plans for a study, in order to determine how large a sample is required for dependable statistical analysis. In an actual study, the wise researcher includes a few more subjects than the power analysis indicates, especially for research that has a lengthy data collection process or that impinges upon subjects' lives, because of the anticipated dropout rate, called **subject attrition**. When subjects decide to drop out of a study, the researcher, of course, must allow them to do so. If a study's attrition rate is high, its results can be affected. For instance, the subjects who decide to drop out of a 12-week study that pays volunteers to complete a lengthy questionnaire each week about stress might do so because of stress related to time commitments. The subjects with the highest stress levels may represent the bulk of the attrition list, leaving subjects with lower levels in the study, and making measurements of stress in the resultant sample artificially low. Chapter 15 contains more information about sampling, power analysis, and retaining subjects in a study.

Research Settings

There are three types of settings for conducting quantitative research: natural, partially controlled, and highly controlled. A **natural setting**, also called a naturalistic setting, is a real-life setting. Such settings are the common venues of quantitative descriptive research and of all types of qualitative research: control for extraneous variables is not an issue for these two types of research, because attribution of causation is not the goal of the research. Most frequently, correlational research is conducted in a natural setting.

A **highly controlled setting** is an artificially constructed environment, such as a research lab or a hospital unit especially constructed for research. The sole purpose for the setting's existence is the conduct of research. Strategies for preventing intrusion by the outside world potentially decrease the introduction of extraneous variables. For this reason, basic research's venue is most frequently a highly controlled artificial setting.

Virtually all quasi-experimental and experimental applied nursing research takes place in **partially controlled settings**. These are natural settings into which the researcher introduces various modifications, intended to control for the effects of selected extraneous variables.

CONTROL GROUPS VERSUS COMPARISON GROUPS

Control groups are constituted so as to control for the effects of potential extraneous variables. Random assignment establishes a control group that is very similar to the experimental group, with respect to factors that might affect the dependent variable. After a research intervention, if the value of the dependent variable is different in experimental and control groups, the implication is that the independent variable caused the change.

Nonrandom assignment establishes a control group that may or may not be very similar to the experimental group. If data collection is concurrent in the two groups, the researcher has at least controlled for the effects of external events, which would affect both groups similarly.

When a control group is lacking and the experimental group's data are compared with previous data at the same site under similar conditions, the study is said to use "historical controls," which means a historical control group. The term "historical comparison group" is sometimes used instead of "historical control group," because data collection is not concurrent and so external events can affect the groups differently. Other research uses a comparison group drawn from public sources, such as national morbidity and mortality data. Such a pool of data from multiple sources is merely a comparison: it doesn't control for anything.

Ultimately, the whole point of a control group is to control for the effect of extraneous variables. In the limitations section of a research report, the author of a study with a quasi-experimental design that uses nonrandomly selected groups should, in identifying the study's limitations, make a case for the degree to which the control group does control for extraneous variables. The reader should assess this limitation to generalizability, as well. If the researcher selects a nonintervention group in a way that does not control for the effect of any extraneous variables, that group, by default, is merely a comparison group.

STEPS OF THE QUANTITATIVE RESEARCH PROCESS

The quantitative research process consists of conceptualizing a research project, planning and implementing that project, and communicating the findings. Although Figure 3-2 sets forth the steps of the process as a list, the sequence of the activities is not arbitrary. This is especially true in earlier phases of a study, as the researcher re-examines the practicality of the design and adapts to changes both internal and external to the research. To illustrate the steps of the research process, several quotations from actual studies are included.

The Iterative Process

Iteration is a term used in mathematics and statistics and refers to repeating sequential operations, using early solutions in subsequent calculations, in order to produce a more accurate answer through successive approximation (Fry, 1941). In research, iteration refers to the ongoing process of revision of both design and methods while research is still in the planning stages, and to revision of interpretation during the latter phases of a study.

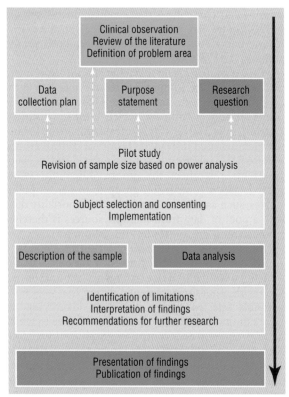

FIGURE 3-2 Steps of the quantitative research process.

More iterative activity seems to improve quality, as researchers re-examine various parts of the original proposed design and method (Sutcliffe & Maiden, 1992), increasing "the number of transitions between steps in the design process, the number of criteria considered, and the number of alternatives generated" (Adams & Atman, 1999, p. 11A6/13). Because of the interplay between student and advisor, the thesis and dissertation processes are highly iterative, by intention. As a graduate student, you can expect frequent revisions at many stages during design and analysis phases.

In most quantitative research, iteration laces lightly through the process as imagination and analysis are employed, involving both inductive and deductive reasoning. The initial research question "drives" the study methodology (Hoskins & Mariano, 2004): the research question, as asked, leads to a definite methodology and narrows the choice of potential designs. However, as fine-tuning proceeds, it may seem more productive to change the question a little, to add another question, to add a different measurement or strategy for data collection, to change to a different design, or perhaps to

change to a completely different methodology. This process of repeating the planning step, with reflection, coming back to it from time to time, is iteration.

The quantitative researcher explores thoughts about the phenomenon of interest creatively, considering new points of view and imaginative connections of ideas. Then these new thoughts are analyzed and assessed in light of what the researcher wants to learn, the researcher's professional and personal experience, and what is already known through research. Numerous other factors may affect the final design of the study, such as potentially extraneous variables, availability of subjects from the population of interest, overall practicality and feasibility of various research designs, potential research sites, anticipated time until study completion, and anticipated expenditures.

The interaction among these and other factors frequently requires balancing different priorities and competing goals. For example, as a beginning researcher, you may want to measure a physiological variable but lack the funds to purchase the needed equipment; as a result, you identify an alternative way to measure the variable. You may want to conduct a quasi-experimental study but lack the expertise or organizational support to implement the intervention and consequently decide to change to a correlational research design instead. There are no perfect studies: all researchers must choose the best design possible, given practical realities. Even after preliminary decisions have been made, each of these considerations influences decisions about subsequent aspects of the design. The challenge for you is to design and implement the best study, given the resources available.

Conducting a pilot study enables the researcher to re-enter the iterative process by conducting a smaller version of the study. From the pilot study, the researcher may decide, for example, to refine data collection instruments, revise strategies for access, add a tool or questionnaire, delete another one, include a larger sample, control for a potential extraneous variable, or add a second data collection period. If you choose to conduct a pilot study, you increase the potential scholarly value of your research.

Another iterative step occurs later in the process when addressing the "why" of the findings. Why did so many subjects prefer the control medication to the experimental medication? Can this be explained by reported side effects on a checklist, or is there something else out there that could better be captured by asking the subjects a couple more questions? Could collecting that additional data be accomplished with a mailed questionnaire, or could contact with subjects be made in another manner? Is there anything in the literature that explains why this happened? Exploring "why" is especially important for writing the Discussion section of the research report. Unanswered "why" questions can generate areas that the researcher recommends for further study. Failure to employ imagination with analysis while writing the Discussion section is eminently obvious to research advisors, thesis committee members, and peer reviewers when the manuscript of the findings is submitted for publication.

Formulating a Research Problem and Purpose

In nursing, a **research problem** is an area in which there is a gap in nursing's knowledge base. This gap may relate only to general understanding or it may have practice implications. Perhaps it represents an area in which theoretical knowledge is incomplete. It is, by implication, an area about which the researcher has some curiosity.

In a research proposal or research report, the problem statement addresses the current state of knowledge about a phenomenon for a given population, following the brief summary with a sentence that identifies the gap, such as, "However, little is known about . . ." Sometimes more information is added, such as, ". . . is a new concept and must be investigated," ". . . is not well described in the literature," ". . . is apparently related to Item L but this relationship has been neither defined nor quantified," ". . . may cause or be caused by Item O, but this causation has not yet been established." In clear language, the problem statement identifies the principal concepts upon which the study will focus.

Nursing practice is the most fertile source for identified nursing problems. The identified nursing problem at the outset of a research process can change through the iterative process. This is especially true for novice researchers. The problem so laboriously identified may not be a research problem, which is best described as the lack of related scientific knowledge, but rather a clinical problem, related to lack of incorporation of research findings into practice. For example, through reviewing the literature, you find sufficient prior research that could be used to develop evidence-based guidelines. Or in response to discussions with peers, you learn how a particular clinical problem is being addressed on other hospital units. The problem area may become amplified, truncated, or changed altogether. If you discover that potential funding or sponsorship of the planned study is available, you may choose to change or enlarge the problem area, so as to include items from a funding agency's statement of research opportunities, or a professional organization's priorities.

Frequently included in the problem statement is some rational argument for the reason the problem is significant to nursing. The significance can be social, psychological, physiological, cognitive, financial, humanistic, or philosophical. This rational argument is important for establishing the problem as being worthy of study, in a written application to a human subjects committee. It is equally important, though, to you as a researcher in that it establishes the need for the study: a first research study is time-consuming and very hard work, and you do not want to expend time and effort on a problem that will not contribute in a meaningful way to the body of nursing knowledge.

The research purpose is a short, usually one-sentence, statement. In a research proposal, it begins in the present tense, "The purpose of this research is to investigate . . . ," and, in a research report, in the past tense, "The purpose of this research was to demonstrate . . ." The purpose statement makes mention of the major variables, the population, and sometimes the setting, and it hints at the general type of study. For a research report on fungal infections in persons with a family history of diabetes who are not themselves diagnosed with the disease, the purpose statement might be, "The purpose of the enquiry was to determine whether, in the population of healthy elderly men, those with a positive family history of diabetes are afflicted more frequently with fungal infections than are those with a negative family history." The principal study variables are the incidence of fungal infections and a family history of diabetes; the population is healthy elderly men without diabetes; an outpatient setting is implied by the word "healthy." The general type of study is clearly noninterventional. The study purpose implies correlational research or descriptive research.

The research purpose states the reason the study was conducted, not the reason the research results were published. "The purpose of this report is to alert healthcare professionals to the overwhelming danger of over-the-counter medications containing opioids, for the elderly population" is not a research purpose. Chapter 5 presents in-depth information about research problems and purposes.

Fredericks and Yau (2013) identified the following problem and purpose for their study of a new postoperative teaching strategy for patients hospitalized for coronary artery bypass graft (CABG) or valvular replacement (VR):

Problem

"Across Canada, although resources to promote recovery are made available, more than a quarter of all CABG [coronary artery bypass graft] and/or VR [valvular replacement] patients are being readmitted to hospitals with postoperative complications experienced during the first three months of recovery (Guru, Fremes, Austin, Blackstone, & Tu, 2006). The most common causes of readmissions are postoperative infections (28%) and heart failure (22%; Hannan et al., 2003). The rate of hospital readmission following CABG and/or VR has significant implications for health care resource utilization, continuity of care across the system, and exacerbation of underlying cardiac condition (Guru et al., 2006). A possible reason for the high rate of readmission is patients may not be adequately prepared to engage in self-care during their home recovery period (Fredericks, 2009; Fredericks, Sidani, & Shugurensky, 2008; Harkness et al., 2005; Moore & Dolansky, 2001) resulting in the onset and/or exacerbation of complications, which can lead to hospital readmissions. Specifically, the quality of the patient education intervention received around the time of discharge may not be optimal in supporting patients up to 3 months following their hospital discharge. As a result, patients may not have the adequate knowledge to effectively engage in behaviors to prevent the development of complications leading to hospital readmissions." (Fredericks & Yau, 2013, p. 1253)

Purpose

"The purpose of this pilot study was to collect preliminary data to examine the impact of an individualized telephone education intervention delivered to patients following CABG and/or VR during their home recovery." (Fredericks & Yau, 2013, p. 1253)

The significance of this research problem is defensible, based on previous research. The problem statement indicated what was known and what was not known at the time the research was conducted, leading into the statement of the research purpose. The purpose also identified the population: patients who had experienced cardiac surgery. The focus of this study was clearly to examine the impact of the intervention of provision of individualized telephone education, the independent variable, in the setting of the home. The sentence immediately preceding the purpose identified the dependent variable, complications leading to hospital readmission.

Review of the Literature

A **review of the literature** is conducted to discover the most recent and most important information about a particular phenomenon, and to identify any knowledge gaps that exist. The problem statement is based on only a selected part of the researcher's fairly broad literature review. Although a review of the literature includes research reports, it may contain other non-research information, such as theories, clinical practice articles, and other professional sources. Often one or two theories are included in the research report, to help explain connections between and among study variables. Chapter 7 provides greater depth regarding the review of the literature.

Fredericks and Yau's (2013) literature review focused upon relevant literature regarding education for cardiovascular surgery patients. Orem's self-care model, one of nursing's grand theories, was included to some extent in the literature review, serving as the study's theoretical framework. The following is the literature review excerpted from the study:

"Within the current inpatient cardiovascular surgical (CVS) setting, education is provided for all patients who have had coronary artery bypass graft (CABG) and/or valvular replacement (VR) surgery (Jaarsma et al., 2000). The intended outcome of these education programs is the increased performance of self-care behaviors following hospital discharge (Johansson et al., 2004). Self-care is a process involving selection and performance of appropriate treatment strategies to enhance or maintain functioning (Orem, 2001). Thus, it is assumed, the more self-care behaviors an individual engages in, the more likely they will reduce the onset of complications and hospital readmissions following their hospital discharge.

"Typically, the content of patient education interventions are designed and delivered using either standardized or individualized techniques. Standardized patient education interventions involve delivering the same education material to all patients in its entirety regardless of whether it may be relevant or deemed to be useful by the individual . . . All patients receive the same information related to these topics, regardless of their personal learning needs.

"The effect of standardized patient education interventions in enhancing performance of self-care behaviors following heart surgery has been evaluated (Cebeci & Celik, 2008; Fredericks, 2009; Kummel et al., 2008; Marshall, Penckofer, & Llewellyn, 1986; Moore, 1995; Steele & Ruzicki, 1987). Results indicated minimal or nonsignificant effects of education on compliance with self-care instructions (Steele & Ruzicki, 1987), physical functioning (Moore, 1995), specifically, mobility, ambulation, and body care/movement, and symptom frequency (Marshall et al., 1986). These nonsignificant findings have been directly attributed to the standardized nature of the intervention.

"An alternative to standardized patient education interventions is individualized education, in which educational content is based on the perceived learning needs of the individual (Fox, 1998; Frantz & Walters, 2001) . . . However, inconsistent findings related to self-care behavior performance have been reported, in which studies did not attempt to control for biases, and used designs that were not tightly controlled (i.e., nonrandom allocation techniques; Beckie, 1989; Tranmer & Parry, 2004)." (Fredericks & Yau, 2013, pp. 1252–1253)

Frameworks

In research, ideas are called **concepts**. A **framework** is a combination of concepts and the connections between them, used to explain relationships. The explanation of the connection between concepts is a **relational statement**. In the statement, "Fatigue can impair performance," fatigue and performance are concepts. "Can impair" is the relational term that explains the connection between those concepts. A framework is an abstract version of the relationship between the study's variables. A framework's relational statements also are called propositions, and they are tested through research.

A theory is similar to a framework: both are abstract, both guide the development of research, and both are tested through quantitative research. A theory can exist by itself and be used to explain the concepts of various studies. A framework is linked to one given study, related to the major concepts being researched and the relationships among them. Because a framework provides an idea of how the concepts in a given study are related, it should both guide the research and help the reader of the research report understand the connections among study variables. Sometimes a framework is represented graphically as a diagram in a published research report. It may be called a map, a research framework, or a model of the framework. Chapter 8 provides an explanation of frameworks, theories, and related terms.

In published quantitative research reports, the framework often is absent or merely implied. This is especially true in physiological research published in clinical practice journals, such as *Heart and Lung: The Journal of Acute and Critical Care* and *American Journal of Critical Care*, as well as many United Kingdom-based journals. Merely because there is no framework in a published report does not mean that the study had no underlying framework. If a study has a stated or implied hypothesis, this means that at least a rudimentary framework must be present, as well, even if neither is explicated. On a practical level, if a researcher will use a hypothesis for a study, the research hypothesis should be formulated

before the theoretical framework is finalized, so that hypothesis and framework are congruent. This is imperative: the study framework must relate to the concepts and relational statements of the research. A framework that does not do this is gratuitous and consequently of no use for interpretation of the study findings.

If a framework is present in a quantitative research report, it may have been developed inductively by the authors from prior clinical observations. However, most stated frameworks in research reports are mid-range nursing theories or mid-range theories developed in related disciplines, such as psychology, physiology, or sociology (Smith & Liehr, 2013). Mid-range theories, also called middle-range theories, are those that are directly applicable to practice areas and, on the whole, are more easily explained, interpreted, and comprehended than are nursing's global grand theories addressing the identity and work of the nurse, because they are less abstract. Chapter 8 contains additional information about grand theories and middle-range theories.

The framework for a study by Berndt et al. (2012) determining predictors of short-term abstinence from smoking tobacco is identified and described in the following quote and model:

"To identify those factors that may cluster cardiac patients according to smoking characteristics on the one hand and that may predict smoking abstinence on the other hand, the Attitude-Social influence-Efficacy (ASE) model (de Vries & Mudde, 1998) was used (Figure 3-3). This model is grounded on several theories regarding health behavior, such as the Theory of Planned Behavior and Social Cognitive Theory (Ajzen, 1991; Bandura, 1986). The model postulates that behavior can be predicted by a behavioral intention, which is influenced by proximal factors, including attitudes, social influences, and self-efficacy expectancies. The impact of these 3 factors is assumed to be influenced by distal factors, such as demographic characteristics." (Berndt et al., 2012, p. 333)

The framework's model identifies the relationships that were examined in this study, and the description of the framework identifies the proposition that was tested.

Making Assumptions Explicit

An **assumption** is a belief that is accepted as true, without proof. The researcher maintains certain beliefs for the duration of the study; if false, these could compromise the believability of the results. Meaningful assumptions relate directly to the research process, the population, the sample, the intervention, the data

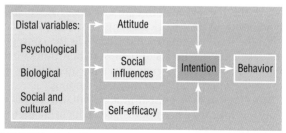

FIGURE 3-3 The Attitude-Social Influence-Efficacy Model (adapted from De Vries & Mudde, 1998). (Modified from Berndt, N., Bolman, C., Mudde, A., Verheugt, F., de Vries, H., & Lechner, L. (2012). Risk groups and predictors of short-term abstinence from smoking in patients with coronary heart disease. *Heart & Lung, 41*(4), 333; de Vries, H., & Mudde, A. N. (1998). Predicting stage transitions for smoking cessation applying the attitude-social influence-efficacy model. *Psychology and Health, 13*(2), 369–385.)

obtained in the course of conducting the research, or some other aspect of the study.

It is important that researchers make explicit their assumptions related to the conduct of the research. This involves a considerable amount of reflection on the researcher's part, in the nature of, "What is assumed in this research study? What is taken for granted as true? What are the beliefs that guide this study?" To reiterate, if the assumptions a researcher holds are not true, the findings will not be credible.

A hypothetical researcher designs a study to measure the relationship between a happy childhood and number of marriages in American adults who are now themselves parents. Study subjects are to be recruited online through a parent support chat room, and data collected anonymously using an online survey tool. In the study, each subject will self-rate childhood happiness on a 0- to 10-point scale and report number of marriages. The researcher's identified assumptions relate to how well the study variables will be measured. The assumptions are (1) subjects will honestly report number of marriages, and (2) subjects can remember their childhoods accurately enough to make an accurate assessment of childhood happiness. Each of these assumptions would affect the study's credibility, were it not true.

The researcher does not identify other assumptions. However, a theoretical assumption underlying the research is that divorce has some relationship to childhood happiness, and perhaps the relationship is causative. The findings of the research may contradict the

researcher's assumption. Another assumption, related to generalization of the results, is that the inhabitants of an online parent support chat room are fairly representative of the population of American adults who are parents. If this is not true, generalizability of the study results will be limited.

Research reports often do not identify assumptions. When assumptions are addressed, researchers tend to report only those that affect accurate measurement of variables.

Formulating Research Objectives, Questions, or Hypotheses

Quantitative research reports may or may not contain research objectives, research questions, and hypotheses. These three entities are less abstract and more concrete than the study purpose. In addition, they address smaller parts of the purpose, such as the relationship between only two variables, and identify the population of interest.

Research objectives often consist of a list of desired outcomes of the research. Some authors use the word "objective" instead of the word "purpose" in this case, the wording may be just as global as that of the study purpose. When the purpose is stated, a study's objectives (or aims) each address the outcome of a specific statistical test or comparison. For instance, a study's objectives might be "to establish the prevalence of methicillin-resistant *Staphylococcus aureus* (MRSA) in the general pediatric population in a major east-coast city," "to establish the prevalence of MRSA in the hospitalized pediatric trauma population in that city," and "to determine the association between number of prior hospital admissions and incidence of MRSA-positive status for the hospitalized pediatric population in that city." These particular objectives address variables, not concepts, and they specify the population to be studied. Objectives are objectives of the research study, not the ensuing application of the findings: an objective such as "to improve the health of patients and visitors through increasing awareness of the relationship between MRSA status and prior hospital admissions" is not an objective of the study.

Research questions are actual questions, such as "Is bar-code identification of the patient prior to administration of medications effective in decreasing the number of medication errors in a critical care setting in which each nurse cares for only one or two patients?" and "In ambulatory surgery areas, is requiring nurses to wear uniforms associated with increased patient satisfaction?" Each question addresses the relationship between variables in a defined population and setting.

Hypotheses are stated relationships between or among study variables. In a research report, the researcher may state them as either research hypotheses or null hypotheses, but the latter is far less common in nursing research. Hypotheses, either explicit or implied, are appropriate for all experimental and quasi-experimental research, and many correlational studies. If a study contains a hypothesis, there is also an implied framework.

Johnson's (1973) basic research contained a research hypothesis:

". . . preparatory information which reduces the incongruency between expected and experienced sensations is associated with less intense emotional response during painful stimulation." (Johnson, 1973, p. 271)

Chapter 6 examines the development of research objectives, questions, and hypotheses.

Defining Study Concepts and Variables

The researcher approaches a study using two levels of thinking. The first is the conceptual level, which deals with abstract ideas. The problem area description and the research framework contain concepts and their interrelationships. As long as these concepts and their interrelationships remain abstract, they cannot, at this early stage, be measured, because a conceptual definition makes a concept understandable but not measurable. It is much like a dictionary definition: it establishes the meaning of a concept, and that same conceptual definition can be used in multiple contexts. A study's purpose, objectives, and research question may be expressed at either the conceptual or the operational level.

The second level of thinking is the operational level, which deals with concrete ideas. Concepts are operationalized when they are made measurable. An **operational definition** establishes the means of measurement of a concept, converting it to a variable. A **variable** is a concept that has been made measurable for a particular study. If something cannot be measured, it is not a variable. Even an independent variable, which is applied to one group and not another, is measurable within the study's context: its two values are "applied" and "not applied."

The operational definition of a concept is chosen by the researcher for each individual study. The method of measurement that seems most practical, most accurate, or least invasive but still fulfills the researcher's need for

reliable and valid data is the one selected. For example, a novice researcher plans to measure the effect upon anxiety of a new method of teaching first-time outpatient colonoscopy patients about their upcoming procedures. The researcher wants to measure anxiety, which is a concept. In order to make it measurable, the researcher must operationally define it, so the researcher must choose a method of measurement. The researcher can think of four different ways to measure anxiety. The least invasive way to measure anxiety would be to ask patients to rate their anxiety on a 0- to 10-point scale, both before and after teaching occurs. (An aspect of concern might be quality of data. Does the researcher believe that this operationalization will produce reliable and valid data?) Another way might be to use an electronic device that measures how much patients' palms sweat, reflecting anxiety, both before and after teaching. (The principal point of concern is practicality. The researcher does not have much technical knowledge of how this machine works, and has no idea how to acquire it.) A third way might be to use vital sign measurements, taken every 10 minutes, to track patients' vital signs before, during, and after teaching, and while awaiting the procedure. (The concern with repeated vital sign measurements is that patients might become more anxious if they are constantly being measured.) A fourth way might be to administer the State-Trait Anxiety Inventory (STAI) (Spielberger, Gorsuch, & Lushene, 1970), a 40-item tool that measures both trait and state anxiety, both before and after the teaching occurs. (The main point of concern for the STAI is that it takes about 15 minutes to explain and administer, so patients would have to arrive early for their procedures.) The researcher must consider each strategy, along with the points of concern, and determine the best way to define operationally and, ultimately, to measure anxiety for this study.

A **hypothesis** is the expressed relationship between or among variables. Because it is essentially composed of variables and their interrelationships, the hypothesis exists at the operational level, as well. The research purpose and the objectives, questions, or hypotheses identify the concepts or variables that are examined in a study.

A variable can be defined both conceptually and operationally. In other words, the variable's meaning can be known and stated, and the variable's means of measurement in that particular study can be known and stated. Operational definitions establish each particular variable's means of measurement and must be articulated for each individual study; conceptual definitions are often used for several studies. For example, in one research study, the word "hope" may be conceptually defined as a feeling of positive expectation regarding future events. Hope might be operationally defined in the same study as the client's score on the Hope Index Scale (Obayuwana et al., 1982). In a different study, the conceptual definition that hope is a feeling of positive expectation regarding future events would still hold true, even if the operational measurement for that particular study were the Miller Hope Scale (Miller & Powers, 1988).

Brunetto et al. (2013) conducted research to determine correlational relationships among supervisor practices, employees' perceptions of well-being, and employee commitment, with a sample of nurses recruited from multiple hospitals in Australia and the U.S. The operational definitions of the study variables were noted in their aims statement: perceived organizational support, supervisor nurse relationships, teamwork, engagement, well-being, organizational commitment, and turnover intentions of nurses working in Australian and U.S. hospitals. Conceptual definitions were included within the literature review and discussed in light of the study framework. A study framework of social exchange theory (SET) was identified. Brunetto et al.'s (2013) definitions for perceived organizational support follow:

Perceived Organizational Support
Conceptual Definition

"Perceived organizational support (POS) is typical of a work-place relationship that can be explained using SET because it is assumed that, when the organization treats the employee well (access to resources, respect), the employee reciprocates, working hard to improve organizational effectiveness. Allen et al. (2003) argue that POS refers to employees' views about the extent to which the organization values their work and is concerned about them. POS is important because it has an impact on the quality of the supervisor–subordinate relationship (Wayne et al., 1997), predicts employee engagement (Saks, 2006), plus organizational commitment, citizenship behaviour and retention (Eisenberger et al., 2002)." (Brunetto et al., 2013, p. 2787)

Operational Definition

"Perceived Organizational Support was measured using the validated instrument by Eisenberger et al. (1997), including: 'My organisation cares about my opinion.' Well-being was measured using a four-item scale by Brunetto et al. (2011) including: 'Most days I feel a sense of accomplishment in what I do at work.'" (Brunetto et al., 2013, p. 2790)

Chapter 6 provides information about variables and both conceptual and operational definitions.

SELECTING A RESEARCH DESIGN

A **research design** is a general plan for implementation of a study, selected to answer a specific research question. Choice of a design commits the researcher to various details of the research process, which may include number of subject groups, methods of sample selection and assignment to group, sample size, type of research setting, whether the researcher performs an intervention, timing of the research intervention, duration of the research process, method of data collection, method of data analysis, statistical tests chosen, conclusions able to be drawn from the study results, and scope of recommendations made. Because alterations in design may be necessary between that first general plan and a study's actual implementation, there ensues a ripple effect for various elements of the study, which must be altered, as well, in order to maintain overall congruence with one another. For example, the research purpose and question must be edited to reflect changes in methodology and design.

Although one school of thought is that the research question "drives" the study methodology, the other school of thought is that it is undeniably true that the researcher phrases and asks that research question. In so doing, the researcher can phrase the question in a quantitative or a qualitative way. Then the researcher words the question, so as to indicate general design type. In quantitative studies, the words "cause" and "effect" hint at interventional research, indicating that an experimental or quasi-experimental design will be used; the words "associated," "related," and "correlated" herald correlational designs. The words "prevalence" and "incidence" hint at descriptive designs.

Choice of design for the new researcher is a fairly complex undertaking that involves iteration, as previously described. Choice of research design for an experienced researcher may be simpler because it depends, to some extent, upon the researcher's preferences and prior expertise. For instance, among nursing researchers, it is not likely that the noted qualitative phenomenology researcher Patricia Benner (1984, 2005, 2011, 2012) would pose a research question answerable only by a multisite experimental study, nor that the noted pain researcher Christine Miaskowski (1991, 2011, 2014a, 2014b, 2014c) would pose a research question answerable only by a qualitative phenomenological narrative. For each researcher, underlying philosophy, view of science, expertise, and experience support a specific type of research.

Defining the Population and Sample

The **population** is the set of all members of a defined group (Plichta & Kelvin, 2013). It contains the elements (humans, animals, plants, events, venues, substances) that share at least one characteristic. In a study, the population consists of an entire group of people or type of element that represents the focus of the research.

There are many ways a researcher might choose to define the population of a study. For example, a researcher wants to conduct a study to describe patients' responses to nurse practitioners as their primary care providers (PCPs). Some of the ways that the population might be defined are (1) all patients seen for their primary health care in healthcare clinics that employ nurse practitioners, (2) all patients who have already been under the care of nurse practitioners as their PCPs for at least a year, and (3) all adult patients covered by a health plan. The definition of the population would depend upon anticipated sampling criteria, type of research design, amount of time in which the study must be completed, method of data collection, costs, and researcher access. The part of the population to which the researcher has reasonable access is called the **accessible population**.

A **sample** is a subset of the accessible population that the researcher selects for participation in a study. Methods of selection are random sampling (probability sampling) or nonrandom sampling. In quantitative research, the size of the sample often is predetermined using a power analysis, so that there will be sufficient data for statistical testing.

Morrissy et al. (2013) conducted predictive correlational research in order to determine the effect of depression, optimism, and anxiety upon job-related affective well-being in graduate nurses. The following quote identifies the sample size, population, sampling criteria, and age and gender characteristics for their study. The research report does not name the sampling method used; if no mention of the sampling method is made by the study's authors, it is, by default, a convenience sample.

Participants

"Seventy participants (64 female, 6 male) took part in the current study. All participants were nurses in Brisbane, Australia who had transitioned from university to full-time work within the previous three years (2009–2011). Fifty-nine participants (84.3%) were aged 20–29 years, five participants (7.1%) were aged between 30–39 years, four participants (5.7%) were aged 40–49 years and 2 participants (2.9%) were aged 50 years or over." (Morrissy et al., 2013, p. 161)

Selecting Methods of Measurement

Measurement is the process of assigning "numbers to objects (or events or situations) in accord with some rule" (Kaplan, 1964, p. 177). An instrument is a device selected by the researcher to measure a specific variable. Examples of common measurement devices used in nursing research are behavioral observations such as whether or not a patient is capable of self-feeding, physiological devices such as the pulse oximeter, calculated laboratory tests such as sodium value, and patient self-rating scales such as the Beck Depression Inventory II (Beck, Steer, Ball, & Ranieri, 1996). Data collected with measurement devices range from the nominal level through the ratio level of measurement. At the nominal level of measurement, only named or category values are present, such as male/female or nurse specialties. The values are names, from the Latin term *nomina*. Before or during data entry, these category names are coded as numbers, for the process of descriptive statistical analysis. At the ratio level of measurement, using real numbers, there is an infinite array of possible values, such as - 4.821, 373, and 82$\frac{1}{2}$. Chapter 16 provides additional information on levels of measurement.

Proper use of an instrument in a study includes examination of its reliability and validity. **Reliability** assesses how consistently the measurement technique measures a concept. The **validity** of an instrument is the extent to which it actually reflects the abstract concept being examined (Waltz, Strickland, & Lenz, 2010). Chapter 16 introduces concepts of measurement and explains the different types of reliability and validity for instruments, and precision and accuracy for physiological measures (Ryan-Wenger, 2010). Chapter 17 provides a background for selecting measurement methods for a study.

Schulz et al. (2013) conducted a predictive correlational study of patients with implantable cardioverter defibrillators (ICDs), using various psychometric measures to determine correlations among patient anxiety over time, number of shocks delivered, and frequency of anti-tachyarrhythmia pacing. Their reported psychometric measures included the following, among other tools:

Psychometric Measures

"All psychometric measures were assessed at T0 and T1. The Spielberger STAI (Speilberger, Gorsuch & Lushene, 1970) consists of two self-report scales assessing state-anxiety (STAI-ST) and anxiety as a trait irrespective of the present situation (STAI-TR). For each item patients indicated on a 4-point scale (1 = not at all, 4 = very much) to what extent statements about aspects of anxiety applied to them. The STAI (Quek, Low, Razack, Loh, & Chua, 2004) offers high internal consistency (average Cronbach's alpha = .86).

"The Fear Questionnaire (FQ) (Marks & Mathews, 1979) has been designed to assess behavioral improvement of phobic patients during therapy. In the present study, it served to identify avoidance behavior caused by fear. Patients specified on an 8-point scale to what extent they avoided 15 agoraphobic situations. Internal consistency of the FQ is moderate (Cronbach's alpha = .35–.77) (Arrindell, Emmelkamp, & van der Ende, 1984) and retest reliability is considered high over a one-year period.

"Of note, it has been shown for the STAI and FQ that similar standards can be assumed when assessing individuals in the age range of ICD-patients (Stanley, Novy, Bourland, Beck, & Averill, 2001). For all psychometric measures, higher scores indicate higher symptom severity." (Schulz et al., 2013, p. 106–107)

The researchers listed and described psychometric instruments used for data collection. The reliability and validity of all listed instruments were provided. The researchers described a correlation between implantable cardioverter defibrillator (ICD) shocks within 1 year of implantation and subclinical anxiety 1 year after implantation. The research report would have been strengthened by inclusion of the calculation of reliability values for this specific study.

Developing a Plan for Data Collection and Analysis

A data collection plan in quantitative research is the researcher's plan for obtaining the output of various instruments, surveys, and measurements, including demographics. These data can be either numerical or language-based. If language-based, the data are converted to numbers for statistical analysis. When measurement is included in the study design, the plan for data collection addresses time, space, and materials needed for collection. For a study that examines data that were collected in the past, the plan for data

collection addresses access to preexistent charts, records, files, and raw data.

Planning data analysis in quantitative research occurs prior to implementation of the study. The plans for data analysis are based on (1) research hypotheses or questions (or research purpose, if hypotheses and questions are lacking) and (2) type and volume of data. Most researchers consult a statistician for assistance in developing analysis plans for complex research.

Implementing the Research Plan

Implementing the research plan involves preparation of data collection materials; sample selection; collection of demographic and baseline data; implementation of the intervention, if any; collection of data after intervention; data analysis; and interpretation of the findings.

Pilot Studies

Some studies are preceded by a pilot study; others are not. This is true of both quantitative and qualitative research. A **pilot study** is a smaller-sample study performed with the same research population, setting, intervention if any, and plans for data collection and analysis. The purpose of the usual pilot study is to determine whether the proposed methods are effective in locating and consenting subjects, and in collecting useful data. Most pilot studies are feasibility studies. Pilot research can determine whether subjects will actually consent to study participation, how many subjects really are available, how much time is required to gather data on one subject, how well instruments work, whether an intervention produces a measurable difference in the dependent variable, and how large that difference is. In addition, for quantitative studies, a statistical analysis of pilot results is often performed, so that the power analysis estimation of the number of subjects needed for statistical significance can be recalculated, assuring an adequate sample.

Some pilot studies reveal that no modifications to the methods are needed. In that case, the data obtained from the pilot study may be included in the actual study data set. At other times, through the iterative process, the researcher modifies the design based on information gained through the pilot study in order to (1) obtain a sample that is more representative; (2) obtain a sample that is able to provide more complete data; (3) select a larger sample than originally planned, because the magnitude of the difference in variable values is smaller than anticipated; (4) choose a different setting that will allow easier, more accurate, or more detailed data collection; (5) choose different instruments that are more accurate or less cumbersome to use, or that give unequivocal results; or (6) alter the data-recording method so that it captures data more precisely. Rarely, after a pilot study, the research project is abandoned because of unforeseen circumstances that pose undue risk or burden for subjects. Occasionally, a pilot study provides information resulting in the decision that conducting the full study would not be worth the expense and time involved to complete it.

A second kind of pilot study pretests some aspect of the study. Sometimes a pilot develops or refines an intervention or a measurement method. Other pilots test a data collection tool or even the entire data collection process. Sometimes a pilot study of a planned data collection instrument is conducted in order to obtain reliability and validity data. Again, information gained in this way allows the active process of iteration, for the purpose of creating a better and more effective research plan.

Conduction of pilot research is good insurance, especially for less-experienced researchers, expensive or lengthy studies, and studies with relatively unfamiliar designs. Although counterintuitive, taking time to conduct a pilot study may be practical in the long run, especially when a researcher's time is at a premium.

Some pilot studies are published because they contribute to general knowledge about a new phenomenon. A published pilot study showing merely observable differences between groups without statistical significance often includes a mention that replication with a larger-sample study might demonstrate statistically significant results.

When a pilot study is encountered in the literature, the reader of research must be skeptical about the term. Some reports focus on preliminary research and are followed by major studies with larger populations, representing true pilot research. Sometimes, however, the term "pilot" is merely a euphemism for an inadequate sample size. "The sample size was smaller than we desired," reported Horner, Piercy, Eure, and Woodard (2014, p. 200) in their research that tested the effect of mindfulness training for nursing staff upon their levels of mindfulness, compassion satisfaction, burnout, nurse stress, and patient satisfaction. In such instances, the researchers complete a study that ultimately shows no statistically significant differences because of an inadequate sample, but the authors often report, "the results were in the hypothesized direction" (Horner et al., 2014, p. 200), indicating that an intervention appeared promising. Especially if the research took advantage of a one-time opportunity to collect data, researchers may seek publication of the study as a pilot, even though subsequent research is not planned, provided that the reported interventions are benign and the topic is of general interest.

Data Collection

The process of data collection extends from before the first subject's data are obtained and ends as the last subject's data are obtained. In quantitative research, various instruments, surveys, and measurements yield numerical or language-based data. Prior to data collection, the researcher obtains permission for access to the research setting for the duration of the study. When this has been established, the researcher then obtains permission to collect data from human subjects, including approval of the consent form. That permission is obtained from the facility itself, if it has a committee for the protection of human subjects, usually called the **institutional review board** (IRB). The researcher may be required to complete training or certification related to data collection and ethical responsibilities to subjects. If the researcher is a student and is conducting research in a healthcare agency, the IRBs of both the university and agency must grant permission for the study to be conducted and approve all forms that will be given to subjects. The elapsed time for both processes may be weeks to months.

During data collection, study variables are measured through a variety of techniques, such as observation, interview, questionnaires, scales, and physiological measurement methods. The data are collected and then recorded systematically for each subject, often directly into a computer, facilitating retrieval and analysis (Ryan-Wenger, 2010). The procedure for data collection is usually identified in the Methods section of a study report.

Morrissy et al. (2013), for their study of the job-related affective well-being of nurses, provided this description of their data-collection process:

Procedure

"All participants read an outline of the nature of the study before completing demographic questions (age, gender, and time since transitioning to full-time work as a nurse to ensure that all participants had transitioned within the past three years) and the questionnaire. For online data collection, responses were saved in the researcher's Survey Monkey account and accessed via a password protected private computer. For collection of hard-copy questionnaires, participants were advised to return their surveys in a sealed envelope to their manager who then posted them back to the researcher. All steps of this procedure were reviewed and approved by appropriate ethical bodies." (Morrissy et al., 2013, p. 162)

Data Analysis

Data analysis in quantitative research is the reduction, organization, and statistical testing of information obtained in the data collection phase. In quantitative data analysis, study subjects are first analyzed in terms of preexistent demographics. Then statistical tests are applied to other data collected. Depending upon the research question, statistical tests employed may be descriptive, or they may examine correlation or causation. The tests are predetermined before any data collection takes place. Various computer software programs are available for conducting statistical analyses. Chapter 21 provides a table of software application programs.

Teman et al. (2015) conducted a retrospective cohort study to evaluate whether using inhaled nitric oxide (iNO) improved the outcomes of patients with hypoxemia who were being transported to a tertiary hospital. The researchers used frequencies and percentages to analyze subject demographics of interest, and diagnosis or cause for transfer, displayed in tables as characteristics, number and percentage (Table 3-1 and Table 3-2).

Responses to iNO for transfer are all displayed as numbers and percentages, with graphics and the results of statistical tests displayed in Figure 3-4. Analysis for differences was accomplished with the χ^2 test, in keeping with the research design's descriptive nature.

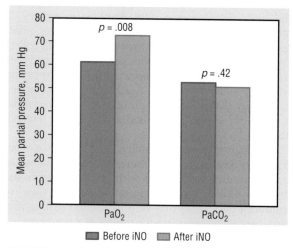

FIGURE 3-4 Change in arterial blood gas measurements after initiation of inhaled nitric oxide (iNO). (Modified from Teman, N. R., Thomas, J., Bryner, B. S., Haas, C. F., Haft, J. W., Park, P. K., et al. (2015). Inhaled nitric oxide to improve oxygenation for safe critical care transport of adults with severe hypoxemia. *American Journal of Critical Care, 24*(2), 115.)

TABLE 3-1   Baseline Demographics of 139 Patients Treated With Inhaled Nitric Oxide

Characteristic	Value*
Age ($n = 139$), mean (*SD*)	45.3 (15.7)
Men ($n = 139$)	84 (60)
White ($n = 93$)	74 (80)
Hypertension	50 (41)
Dyslipidemia	28 (23)
Diabetes mellitus	26 (21)
Previous known heart failure	14 (12)
Coronary artery disease	26 (21)
Pulmonary hypertension	6 (5)
Chronic obstructive pulmonary disease	15 (12)
History of smoking	48 (40)
Current smoker	34 (28)
Body mass index[†] ($n = 110$), mean (*SD*)	35.9 (11.7)

SD, standard deviation.

*Unless indicated otherwise, all values are number (%) of patients and $n = 121$.

[†]Calculated as weight in kilograms divided by height in meters squared.

From Teman, N. R., Thomas, J., Bryner, B. S., Haas, C. F., Haft, J. W., Park, P. K., et al. (2015). Inhaled nitric oxide to improve oxygenation for safe critical care transport of adults with severe hypoxemia. *American Journal of Critical Care, 24*(2), 110–117.

TABLE 3-2   Diagnosis or Cause for Transfer of 139 Patients Treated with Inhaled Nitric Oxide

Characteristic	No. (%)
Acute respiratory distress syndrome	110 (79)
Severe acute respiratory distress syndrome*	103 (74)
Cardiac failure	22 (16)
Other	7 (5)

*Ratio of Pao$_2$ to fraction of inspired oxygen ≤100 mm Hg.

From Teman, N. R., Thomas, J., Bryner, B. S., Haas, C. F., Haft, J. W., Park, P. K., et al. (2015). Inhaled nitric oxide to improve oxygenation for safe critical care transport of adults with severe hypoxemia. *American Journal of Critical Care, 24*(2), 110–117.

Statistical Analysis

"Categorical variables between survivors and nonsurvivors were compared by using χ^2 analysis. Two-sample t tests or Wilcoxon rank-sum tests were used to compare respiratory values before and after iNO therapy. Statistical significance was defined as a 2-sided p value less than 0.05." (Teman et al., 2015, p. 113)

Results

"Survival Flight treated 139 patients with iNO at referring hospitals, initiating iNO in 114 patients (82%) and continuing therapy that had previously been started in 25 patients (18%). Baseline characteristics of the patients treated with iNO are shown in Table 3-1. The underlying pathophysiological condition requiring iNO during transport was ARDS in 79% of patients, cardiac failure in 16%, and other causes in 5%. A total of 74% of patients had severe ARDS (P:F ratio ≤100) (Table 3-2).

Among the 102 patients, the mode of transport was helicopter in 66 (65%), ground in 33 (32%), and fixed-wing in 3 (3%). Mean iNO dose at transport was 33 (SD, 23) ppm. After arrival at the tertiary care center, 81 patients (79%) had treatment with iNO continued past the first day of admission. A total of 22 patients (22%) treated with iNO during transport required extracorporeal membrane oxygenation (ECMO) during admission at the tertiary care center; 9 of the 22 (41%) survived. Ultimately, 62 (60%) of the 102 patients treated with iNO during transport survived to discharge, including 67% of those who had cardiac failure and 60% of those who had ARDS . . .

Changes in arterial blood gas measurements from before iNO therapy to after iNO therapy are shown in Figure 3-3. Oxygenation improved significantly after iNO therapy was started, with an increase in mean PaO2 from 60.7 (SD, 20.2) mm Hg before to 72.3 (SD, 40.6) mm Hg after ($p = 0.008$) and a mean increase in the P:F ratio from 62.4 (SD, 26.1) before to 73.1 (SD. 42.6) after ($p = 0.03$). The P:F ratio continued to improve, with a mean of 109.7 (SD, 73.8) according to arterial blood gas analysis of blood obtained 6 to 8 hours after arrival at the tertiary care center ($p < 0.001$ relative to values before and after iNO therapy). No significant changes occurred in PaCO2 or pH . . ." (Teman et al., 2015, pp. 113–115)

Interpreting Research Outcomes

The results obtained from data analysis require interpretation to be meaningful. **Interpretation of research outcomes** involves (1) examining the results of data analysis, (2) explaining what the results mean, in light of current practice and previous research, (3) identifying study limitations, (4) forming conclusions in consideration of study limitations, (5) deciding on the appropriate recommendation for generalization of the findings, (6) considering the implications for nursing's body of knowledge, and (7) suggesting the direction of further research. All of these steps are related.

Limitations are aspects of the study that decrease the generalizability of the findings. These may or may not be results of problems or weaknesses of the study. There are four types of limitations, and they are related to the four types of validity discussed in Chapters 10 and 11. Construct limitations, sometimes called **theoretical limitations**, are failures of logic, related to the researcher's definitions or reasoning, which limit the ability to interpret study findings on the theoretical level, the application level, or both. Internal validity limitations amount to incomplete or poor control of important extraneous variables, and weaken the logical argument for the study's findings. External validity limitations refer to the actual population to which the study results can legitimately be generalized. Statistical limitations refer to inadequate or inappropriate statistical conclusions, often based on poor choices by the researcher.

Limitations can diminish the credibility of study findings and conclusions or restrict the population to which findings can be generalized. It is important to remember that quantitative research is generalized to populations similar with respect to the study variables and to other attributes or conditions that might have impacted the results.

Study conclusions provide a basis for identifying nursing implications and suggesting further studies (see Chapter 26). In the excerpt that follows, Fredericks and Yau (2013) presented their findings of the study described previously. They also discussed the applicability of the findings in terms of limitations, inability to formulate conclusions or suggest implications for practice without supportive research, and suggestions for further research:

Discussion

"The findings from this study provide preliminary evidence to indicate the delivery of an educational intervention to patients during their home recovery at multiple points in time may be beneficial in reducing the number of hospital readmissions and complications at 3 months following hospital discharge. Although a small sample size was used, the findings reinforce theoretical assumptions that suggest individualized patient education interventions, repeated over time, have more impact than standardized educational programs in enhancing patients' overall recovery experience (Guruge, 1999; Lauver et al., 2002) . . .

" . . . all of the study participants who were readmitted to hospitals were from the control group. This finding is similar to current trends (Guru et al., 2006) in that approximately a third of all individuals who are receiving only standardized, in-hospital patient education are being readmitted to hospitals for treatment and management of postoperative complications. This study serves as a foundation on which a larger clinical trial should be designed and implemented. In particular, a study designed in a similar manner, using a larger sample size, multiple sites, and strategies such as mailing out study reminder postcards or providing small . . . incentives to promote study retention should be incorporated into the design of a future trial.

"As the study findings were obtained from a small sample size, it may not be prudent to make significant revisions to existing patient education interventions at this time, until a more thorough examination of the impact of this intervention is carried out. However, this study does provide nurses with further evidence that underscores the need to continue to revise existing standardized, inpatient education . . . to continue to support patients following their hospital discharge . . . In conclusion, the findings with regard to the impact of the individualized telephone interaction are promising. Preliminary findings suggest the experimental intervention has an impact on reducing hospital readmission rates and complications during the initial home recovery period." (Fredericks & Yau, 2013, pp. 1262–1263)

Communicating Research Findings

Research is not considered complete until the findings have been communicated. **Communicating research findings** involves developing and disseminating a research report to appropriate audiences. The research report is disseminated through presentations and publication. (For further information, see Chapter 27.)

■ KEY POINTS

- Quantitative research, through counting or measuring, provides better understanding of one or more of the following three aspects of reality: incidence, connections between two ideas, and cause-and-effect relationships.
- The scientific method is the basis for decision making related to testing hypotheses.
- Basic research addresses general physiological or psychological responses, is broadly generalizable, and

cannot be applied to actual practice. Applied research is conducted in actual practice situations, is narrowly generalizable, and can be applied to practice.

- The two main design clusters of quantitative research are interventional and noninterventional. Interventional ones include experimental and quasi-experimental designs. Noninterventional ones include descriptive and correlational designs.
- Rigor in quantitative research refers to its degree of accuracy, consistency, and attention to all measurable aspects of the research.
- Control of extraneous variables is a design strategy whereby the researcher measures, eliminates, or decreases the effect of extraneous variables upon the dependent variable.
- The steps of the quantitative research process are fluid and punctuated by iterative reflection and redesign, as needed. Its steps need not occur in the order stated:
  - Choice of problem area and purpose
  - Review of the literature, identification of a research gap
  - Formulation of a research question, objective, or hypothesis.
  - Selection of a research design
  - Identification of a framework for the study if this is appropriate
  - Definition of study variables, both conceptually and operationally
  - Definition of population and sample
  - Choice of methods of measurement and data analysis
  - Formulation of a plan for data collection
  - Definition of how an intervention will be enacted
  - Implementation of a pilot study if one is to be employed
  - Revision based on the pilot study, if indicated
  - Implementation of the study itself
  - Analysis of data
  - Interpretation of outcomes
  - Communication of findings

REFERENCES

Adams, R. S., & Atman, C. J. (1999). Cognitive processes in iterative design behavior. *Frontiers in Education, 1*, 11A6/13–11A6/18.

Ajzen, I. (1991). The theory of planned behavior. *Organizational Behavior and Human Decision Processes, 50*(2), 179–211.

Allen, D., Shore, L., & Griffeth, R. (2003). The role of perceived organizational support and supportive human resource practices in the turnover process. *Journal of Management, 29*(1), 99–118.

Arrindell, W. A., Emmelkamp, P. M. G., & van der Ende, J. (1984). Phobic dimensions: I. Reliability and generalizability across samples, gender, and nations: The fear survey schedule (FSS-III) and the fear questionnaire (FQ). *Advances in Behaviour Research and Therapy, 6*(4), 207–253.

Arvidsson, S., Bergman, S., Arvidsson, B., Fridlund, B., & Tingström, P. (2013). Effects of a self-care promoting problem-based learning programme in people with rheumatic diseases: A randomized controlled study. *Journal of Advanced Nursing, 69*(7), 1500–1514.

Bandura, A. (1986). *Social foundations of thought and action: A social cognitive theory.* Englewood Cliffs, N.J.: Prentice-Hall.

Beck, A. T., Steer, R. A., Ball, R., & Ranieri, W. (1996). Comparison of Beck Depression Inventories—IA and -II in psychiatric outpatients. *Journal of Personality Assessment, 67*(3), 588–597.

Beckie, T. M. (1989). A supportive-educative telephone program: Impact on knowledge and anxiety after coronary artery bypass graft surgery. *Heart and Lung: The Journal of Critical Care, 18*(1), 44–55.

Benner, P. (1984). *From novice to expert: Excellence and power in clinical nursing practice.* Menlo Park, CA: Addison-Wesley.

Benner, P. (2005). Extending the dialogue about classification systems and the work of professional nurses. *American Journal of Critical Care, 14*(3), 242–243, 272.

Benner, P. (2011). Formation in professional education: An examination of the relationship between theories of meaning and theories of the self. *Journal of Medical Philosophy, 36*(4), 342–353.

Benner, P. (2012). Educating nurses: A call for radical transformation—how far have we come? *Journal of Nursing Education, 51*(4), 183–184.

Berndt, N., Bolman, C., Mudde, A., Verheugt, F., de Vries, H., & Lechner, L. (2012). Risk groups and predictors of short-term abstinence from smoking in patients with coronary heart disease. *Heart and Lung: The Journal of Critical Care, 41*(4), 332–343.

Brunetto, Y., Farr-Wharton, R., & Shacklock, K. (2011). Using the Harvard HRM model to conceptualise the impact of changes to supervision upon HRM outcomes for different types of public sector employees. *International Journal of Human Resource Management, 22*(3), 553–573.

Brunetto, Y., Xiong, M., Shriberg, A., Farr-Wharton, R., Shacklock, K., Newman, S., et al. (2013). The impact of workplace relationships on engagement, well-being, commitment and turnover for nurses in Australia and the USA. *Journal of Advanced Nursing, 69*(12), 2786–2799.

Campbell, D. T., & Stanley, J. C. (1963). Experimental and quasi-experimental designs for research on teaching. In N. L. Gage (Ed.), *Handbook of research on teaching* (pp. 171–246). Chicago, IL: Rand McNally.

Cebeci, F., & Celik, S. S. (2008). Discharge training and counselling increase selfcare ability and reduce post-discharge problems in CABG patients. *Journal of Clinical Nursing, 17*(3), 412–420.

Cooper, H. M. (2012). Introduction: Objectives of psychological research and their relations to research methods. In H. M. Cooper & P. M. Camic (Eds.), *APA handbook of research methods in psychology* (pp. xxiii–xliv). Washington, D.C.: American Psychological Association.

de Vries, H., & Mudde, A. N. (1998). Predicting stage transitions for smoking cessation applying the attitude-social influence-efficacy model. *Psychology and Health, 13*(2), 369–385.

Dulock, H. L., & Holzemer, W. L. (1991). Substruction: Improving the linkage from theory to method. *Nursing Science Quarterly, 4*(2), 83–87.

Eisenberger, R., Cummings, J., Armeli, S., & Lynch, P. (1997). Perceived organizational support, discretionary treatment and job satisfaction. *Journal of Applied Psychology, 82*(5), 812–820.

Eisenberger, R., Stinglhamber, F., Vandenberghe, C., Sucharask, I., & Rhoades, L. (2002). Perceived supervisor support: Contributions to perceived organizational support and employee retention. *Journal of Applied Psychology, 86*(3), 565–573.

Fisher, R. A. (1970). *Statistical methods for research workers* (14th ed.). New York, NY: Hafner Publishing Company.

Fitzpatrick, J. J., & Kazer, M. W. (2012). *Encyclopedia of nursing research* (3rd ed.). New York, NY: Springer Publishing Company, L.L.C.

Fox, V. J. (1998). Post-operative education that works. *Association of PeriOperative Registered Nurses Journal, 67*(5), 1010–1017.

Frantz, A., & Walters, J. (2001). Recovery from coronary artery bypass grafting at home: Is your nursing practice current? *Home Healthcare Nurse, 19*(7), 417–424.

Fredericks, S. (2009). Timing for delivering individualized patient education intervention to coronary artery bypass graft patients: An RCT. *European Journal of Cardiovascular Nursing, 8*(2), 144–150.

Fredericks, S., Sidani, S., & Shugurensky, D. (2008). The effect of anxiety on learning outcomes post-CABG. *Canadian Journal of Nursing Research, 40*(1), 127–140.

Fredericks, S., & Yau, T. (2013). Educational intervention reduces complications and rehospitalizations after heart surgery. *Western Journal of Nursing Research, 35*(10), 1251–1265.

Fry, T. C. (1941). Industrial mathematics. *The American Mathematical Monthly, 48*(6), 1–38.

Gibbs, J. (1972). *Sociological theory construction.* Hinsdale, IL: Dryden.

Guru, V., Fremes, S., Austin, P., Blackstone, E., & Tu, J. (2006). Gender differences in outcomes after hospital discharge from coronary artery bypass grafting. *Circulation, 113*(4), 507–516.

Guruge, S. (1999). *The effects of demographic outcomes on pre-operative teaching outcomes* (Unpublished master's thesis). Toronto, Ontario, Canada: University of Toronto.

Hald, A. (1990). *A history of probability and statistics before 1750.* New York, NY: John Wiley & Sons.

Hald, A. (1998). *A history of mathematical statistics from 1750 to 1930.* New York, NY: John Wiley & Sons, Inc.

Hannan, E. L., Racz, M. J., Walford, G., Ryan, T. J., Isom, O. W., Bennett, E., et al. (2003). Predictors of readmission for complications of coronary artery bypass graft surgery. *Journal of the American Medical Association, 290*(6), 773–780.

Harkness, K., Smith, K. M., Taraba, L., MacKenzie, C. L., Gunn, E., & Arthur, H. M. (2005). Effect of a postoperative telephone intervention on attendance at intake for cardiac rehabilitation after coronary artery bypass graft surgery. *Heart and Lung: The Journal of Critical Care, 34*(3), 179–186.

Heinzer, M. M. (1993). Adolescent resilience following parental death in childhood and its relationship to parental attachment and coping. (Doctoral dissertation, Case Western Reserve University, 1993). Dissertation Abstracts International, 55-01, B6579.

Hinshaw, A. S. (1979). Theroretical substruction: An assessment process. *Western Journal of Nursing Research, 1*(4), 319–324.

Horner, J. K., Piercy, B. S., Eure, L., & Woodard, E. K. (2014). A pilot study to evaluate mindfulness as a strategy to improve inpatient nurse and patient experiences. *Applied Nursing Research, 27*(3), 198–201.

Hoskins, C. N., & Mariano, C. (2004). *Research in nursing and health: Understanding and using quantitative and qualitative methods* (2nd ed.). New York, NY: Springer Publishing Company.

Jaarsma, T., Halfens, R., Abu-Saad, H., Dracup, K., Diederiks, J., & Tan, F. (2000). Self-care and quality of life with advanced heart failure: The effect of a supportive educational intervention. *Heart and Lung: The Journal of Critical Care, 29*(5), 319–330.

Johansson, K., Salantera, S., Heikkinen, K., Kuusisto, A., Virtanen, H., & Leino-Kilpi, H. (2004). Surgical patient education: Assessing the interventiona and exploring the outcomes from experimental and quasi-experimental studies from 1990 to 2003. *Clinical Effectiveness in Nursing, 8*(2), 81–92.

Johnson, J. E. (1973). Effects of accurate expectations about sensations on the sensory and distress components of pain. *Journal of Personality and Social Psychology, 27*(2), 261–275.

Johnson, J., Kirchhoff, K., & Endress, M. P. (1975). Altering chidlren's distress behavior during orthopedic cast removal. *Nursing Research, 24*(6), 404–410.

Johnson, N. L., & Kotz, S. (Eds.), (1997). *Leading personalities in statistical sciences.* New York, NY: John Wiley & Sons, Inc.

Kaplan, A. (1964). *The conduct of inquiry: Methodology for behavioral science.* New York, NY: Chandler.

Katz, K. D. (2012). Intravenous multivitamins ("banana bags") for emergency patients who may have nutritional deficits. *Annals of Emergency Medicine, 59*(5), 413–414.

Kerlinger, F. N., & Lee, H. B. (2000). *Foundations of behavioral research* (4th ed.). Fort Worth, TX: Harcourt College Publishers.

Kummel, M., Vahlberg, T., Ojanlatva, A., Karki, R., Mattila, T., & Kivela, S. L. (2008). Effects of an intervention on health behaviors of older coronary artery bypass (CAB) patients. *Archives of Gerontology and Geriatrics, 46*(2), 227–244.

Lauver, D. R., War, S. E., Heidrich, S. M., Keller, M. L., Bowers, B. J., Brennan, P. F., et al. (2002). Patient-centered interventions. *Research in Nursing & Health, 25*(4), 246–255.

Marks, I. M., & Mathews, A. M. (1979). Brief standard self-rating for phobic patients. *Behaviour Research and Therapy, 17*(3), 263–267.

Marshall, M., Penckofer, S., & Llewellyn, J. (1986). Structured post-operative teaching and knowledge and compliance of patients who had coronary artery bypass surgery. *Heart and Lung: The Journal of Critical Care, 15*(1), 76–82.

Miaskowski, C., Sutters, K. A., Taiwo, Y. O., & Levine, J. D. (1991). Comparison of the antinociceptive and motor effects of intrathecal opioid agonists in the rat. *Brain Research, 553*(1), 105–109.

Miaskowski, C., Penko, J. M., Guzman, D., Mattson, J. E., Bangsberg, D. R., & Kushel, M. B. (2011). Occurrence and characteristics of chronic pain in a community-based cohort of indigent adults living with HIV infection. *Journal of Pain, 12*(9), 1004–1016.

Miaskowski, C., Cataldo, J. K., Baggott, C. R., West, C., Dunn, L. B., Dhruva, A., et al. (2014a). Cytokine gene variations associated with trait and state anxiety in oncology patients and their family caregivers. *Supportive Care in Cancer, 17*(2), 175–184.

Miaskowski, C., Cooper, B. A., Melisko, M., Chen, L. M., Mastick, J., West, C., et al. (2014b). Disease and treatment characteristics do not predict symptom occurrence profiles in oncology outpatients receiving chemotherapy. *Cancer, 120*(15), 2371–2378.

Miaskowski, C., Paul, S. M., Cooper, B., West, C., Levine, J. D., Elboim, C., et al. (2014c). Identification of patient subgroups and risk factors for persistent arm/shoulder pain following breast cancer surgery. *European Journal of Oncology Nursing, 18*(3), 242–253.

Miller, J. F., & Powers, M. J. (1988). Development of an instrument to measure hope. *Nursing Research, 37*(1), 6–10.

Moore, S. (1995). A comparison of women's and men's symptoms during home recovery after coronary artery bypass surgery. *Heart and Lung: The Journal of Critical Care, 24*(6), 495–501.

Moore, S. M., & Dolansky, A. (2001). Randomized trial of a home recovery intervention following coronary artery bypass surgery. *Research in Nursing & Health, 24*(2), 93–104.

Morrissy, L., Boman, P., & Mergler, A. (2013). Nursing a case of the blues: An examination of the role of depression in predicting job-related affective well-being in nurses. *Issues in Mental Health Nursing, 34*(3), 158–168.

National Institute of Nursing Research (NINR) (2012). *Research and funding.* Retrieved April 7, 2016 from http://www.ninr.nih.gov/researchandfunding#.VwbwQzGaKuI.

National Institute of Nursing Research (NINR) (2015). *Research and funding: Program announcements.* Retrieved April 7, 2016 from http://www.ninr.nih.gov/researchandfunding/dea/oep/fundingopportunities/pas#.VRxGno6aKuI.

Obayuwana, A. O., Collins, J. L., Carter, A. L., Rao, M. S., Mathura, C. C., & Wilson, S. B. (1982). Hope Index Scale: An instrument for the objective assessment of hope. *Journal of the National Medical Association, 74*(8), 761–765.

Orem, D. E. (2001). *Nursing: Concepts of practice* (5th ed.). St. Louis, MO: C.V. Mosby.

Plichta, S. B., & Kelvin, E. (2013). *Munro's statistical methods for health care research.* Philadelphia: Wolters Kluwer/Lippincott Williams & Wilkins.

Popper, K. (1968). *The logic of scientific discovery.* New York, NY: Harper & Row, Publishers.

Quek, K. F., Low, W. Y., Razack, A. H., Loh, C. S., & Chua, C. B. (2004). Reliability and validity of the Spielberger State-Trait Anxiety Inventory (STAI) among urological patients: A Malaysian study. *Medical Journal of Malaysia, 59*(2), 258–267.

Ryan-Wenger, N. A. (2010). Evaluation of measurement precision, accuracy, and error in biophysical data for clinical research and practice. In C. F. Waltz, O. L. Strickland, & E. R. Lenz (Eds.),

Measurement in nursing and health research (4th ed., pp. 371–383). New York, NY: Springer Publishing Company.

Saks, A. M. (2006). Antecedents and consequences of employee engagement. *Journal of Managerial Psychology, 21*(7), 600–619.

Schulz, S. M., Massa, C., Grzbiela, A., Dengler, W., Wiedemann, G., & Pauli, P. (2013). Implantable cardioverter defibrillator shocks are prospective predictors of anxiety. *Heart and Lung: The Journal of Critical Care, 42*(2), 105–111.

Smeltzer, S. C., Sharts-Hopko, N. C., Cantrell, M. A., Heverly, M. A., Nthenge, S., & Jenkinson, A. (2015). A profile of U.S. nursing faculty in research- and practice-focused doctoral education. *Journal of Nursing Scholarship, 47*(2), 178–185.

Smith, L. H., & Holloman, C. (2014). Piloting "sodabriety": A school-based intervention to impact sugar-sweetened beverage consumption in rural Appalachian high schools. *Journal of School Health, 84*(3), 177–184.

Smith, M. J., & Liehr, P. R. (Eds.), (2013). *Middle range theory for nursing* (3rd ed.). New York, NY: Springer Publishing Company.

Spielberger, C. D., Gorsuch, R. L., & Lushene, R. E. (1970). *State-Trait Anxiety Inventory.* Palo Alto, CA: Consulting Psychologists Press.

Stanley, M. A., Novy, D. M., Bourland, S. L., Beck, J. G., & Averill, P. M. (2001). Assessing older adults with generalized anxiety: A replication and extension. *Behaviour Research and Therapy, 39*(2), 221–235.

Steele, J. M., & Ruzicki, D. (1987). An evaluation of the effectiveness of cardiac teaching during hospitalization. *Heart and Lung: The Journal of Critical Care, 16*(3), 306–311.

Sutcliffe, A. G., & Maiden, N. A. M. (1992). Analysing the novice analyst: Cognitive models in software engineering. *International Journal of Man-Machine Studies, 36*(5), 719–740.

Teman, N. R., Thomas, J., Bryner, B. S., Haas, C. F., Haft, J. W., Park, P. K., et al. (2015). Inhaled nitric oxide to improve oxygenation for safe critical care transport of adults with severe hypopxemia. *American Journal of Critical Care, 24*(2), 110–117.

Tokuhama-Espinosa, T. (2010). *Mind, brain, and education science: A comprehensive guide to the new brain-based teaching.* New York, NY: W. W. Norton & Company.

Tranmer, J. E., & Parry, M. J. E. (2004). Enhancing postoperative recovery of cardiac surgery patients: A randomized clinical trial of an advanced practice nursing intervention. *Western Journal of Nursing Research, 26*(5), 515–532.

Waltz, C. F., Strickland, O., & Lenz, E. R. (2010). *Measurement in nursing and health research.* New York, NY: Springer Publishing Company.

Wayne, S., Shore, L., & Liden, R. (1997). Perceived organizational support and leader-member exchange: A social exchange perspective. *Academy of Management Journal, 40*(1), 82–111.

Wolf, Z. R., & Heinzer, M. M. (1999). Substruction: Illustrating the connections from research question to analysis. *Journal of Professional Nursing, 15*(1), 33–37.

Wysocki, A. B. (1983). Basic versus applied research: Intrinsic and extrinsic considerations. *Western Journal of Nursing Research, 5*(3), 217–224.

4

Introduction to Qualitative Research

Jennifer R. Gray

http://evolve.elsevier.com/Gray/practice/

Qualitative research is a scholarly approach used to describe life experiences, cultures, and social processes from the perspectives of the persons involved. Qualitative researchers gain insights without measuring concepts or analyzing statistical relationships. Rather, they improve our comprehension of a phenomenon from the viewpoint of the people experiencing it. Qualitative researchers focus on "naturally occurring, ordinary events in natural settings" (Miles, Huberman, & Saldaña, 2014, p. 11). Qualitative research allows us to explore the depth, richness, and complexity inherent in the lives of human beings. Insights from this process build nursing knowledge by fostering understanding of patient needs and problems, guiding emerging theories, and describing cultural and social forces affecting health (Munhall, 2012).

Quantitative researchers determine the data collection and analysis procedures before the study begins. Deviating from those procedures, such as changing the sample or adding a question, is a threat to the rigor of the study. In contrast, qualitative research methods allow the researcher flexibility during data collection and analysis (Marshall & Rossman, 2016). For example, the researcher may adjust the interview or focus group questions during data collection in response to emergent patterns and themes. The ability to be responsive during a study does not mean that qualitative research lacks rigor. Qualitative researchers use systematic scholarly processes that require them to think abstractly and conceptually while analyzing data provided by participants (Miles et al., 2014).

Comprehending qualitative research methodologies will allow you to critically appraise published studies, use findings in practice, and develop skills needed to conduct qualitative research. Critical appraisal is necessary before you can incorporate qualitative research findings into the development of evidence-based practice guidelines (Hannes, 2011). Nurse researchers conducting qualitative studies contribute important information to our body of knowledge, information often unobtainable by quantitative means. For example, an instrument to measure the person's assessment of coping after a loss, a quantitative method, will provide valuable information but not have the individual richness of interviewing the person about coping after a loss, a qualitative method. Both the terminology and methods used in qualitative research are different from those of quantitative research and are reflections of the philosophical orientations or approaches supporting the various types of qualitative research. Each qualitative approach flows from beliefs and assumptions of a philosophical orientation that direct every aspect of the study from planning the study through reporting the findings.

This chapter presents a general overview of the following qualitative approaches: phenomenological research, grounded theory research, ethnographic research, exploratory-descriptive qualitative research, and historical research. These are the approaches and methods most frequently used by qualitative nurse researchers. Two other approaches, narrative analysis and case study methods, will be described briefly. Although each qualitative approach is unique, they share common ground. These commonalities constitute the perspective of the qualitative researcher.

PERSPECTIVE OF THE QUALITATIVE RESEARCHER

All scientists approach problems from a philosophical stance or perspective. The **philosophical perspective** of the researcher guides the questions asked and the methods selected for conducting a specific study (Birks & Mills, 2015). Both quantitative and qualitative researchers have philosophical perspectives (Roller & Lavrakas, 2015). In general, quantitative researchers ascribe to the philosophy of logical positivism that values logic, empirical data, and tightly controlled methods (see Chapter 3) (Kerlinger & Lee, 2000; Shadish, Cook, & Campbell, 2002). Researchers with logical positivist views think deductively, generate hypotheses, and seek to find truth as objectively as possible. Based on a philosophy of post-positivism, other quantitative researchers acknowledge that truth may exist, but can never be known fully (Hall, Griffiths, & McKenna, 2013). Post-positivism supports quantitative and qualitative research; however, qualitative research may also be based on constructivism, the belief that there are multiple realities. A person constructs reality within a context of time and place (Hall et al., 2013). Congruent with the values of post-positivism or constructivism, qualitative studies are based on a wide range of philosophies and traditions, such as phenomenology, symbolic interactionism, and hermeneutics, each of which espouses slightly different approaches to gaining new knowledge (Liamputtong, 2013).

Philosophy Describes a View of Science

Qualitative researchers ascribe to a view of science that values the uniqueness of the individual in context (Roller & Lavrakas, 2015). The philosophical perspective of the researcher is consistent with research questions that seek the participant's perspective of a phenomenon or experience. Figure 4-1 displays this idea, as the arrow on the left of the figure ("Philosophy") shapes and fits with the next arrow ("View of Science"). Qualitative researchers value rigorous but flexible methods of analysis to identify study findings. The findings contribute to our understanding of an experience using a discovery process that allows meaning to emerge (Patton, 2015).

The primary thinking process used in quantitative studies is deduction; in contrast, qualitative researchers use analytic strategies that are primarily inductively

driven (Streubert & Carpenter, 2011). In Chapter 1, you learned that **deductive thinking** begins with a theory or hypothesis that guides the selection of methods to gather data to support or refute the theory or hypothesis (Streubert & Carpenter, 2011). **Inductive thinking** involves putting insights and pieces of information together and identifying abstract themes or working from the bottom up. From this inductive process, meanings emerge. Because the perspective of each qualitative researcher is unique, the meanings drawn from the data vary from researcher to researcher, especially in the naming of the key ideas and describing these concepts and the relationships among them. The researcher keeps records of his or her thinking processes, analysis, findings, and conclusions so that others can audit or retrace the analysis and thinking processes that resulted in the researcher's conclusions. See Chapter 12 for additional information on qualitative data analysis.

Philosophy Guides Methods

The philosophies of science include an **epistemology,** a view of knowing and knowledge generation (Munhall, 2012). As a result, a researcher's philosophy directs how the research questions are asked and how data are collected and interpreted. Creswell (2013) emphasizes this point by stating that the assumptions of the specific philosophical approach cannot be separated from the methods. The different types of qualitative research are consistent with particular philosophical perspectives or traditions (Table 4-1). The philosophy shapes the view of science that in turn shapes the approaches and methods selected for the study (Streubert & Carpenter, 2011). A well-designed qualitative study is congruent at each stage with the underlying philosophical perspective

TABLE 4-1 **Philosophical Orientations Supporting Qualitative Approaches to Nursing Research**	
Philosophical and Theoretical Orientations	**Qualitative Approach**
Phenomenology	Phenomenological research
Symbolic interaction theory	Grounded theory research
Naturalism and ethical principles	Ethnographic research
Naturalistic and pragmatic perspectives	Exploratory-descriptive qualitative research
Historicism	Historical research

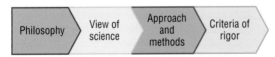

FIGURE 4-1 Valid science is based on congruence from philosophy to rigor.

or tradition as identified by the researcher (Corbin & Strauss, 2015).

Qualitative researchers in nursing and other health professions use open-ended and semi-structured methods to gather descriptions of health-related experiences from participants. These open-ended and semi-structured methods include interviews, focus groups, observation, and analysis of documents (Marshall & Rossman, 2016; Miles et al., 2014; Streubert & Carpenter, 2011). Usually, when oral methods are used, the researcher will capture the interaction by an audio or video recording so that a transcript of the communication can be prepared for analysis. The methods used in qualitative studies are discussed in detail in Chapter 12.

Philosophy Guides Criteria of Rigor

Scientific rigor is valued because it is associated with the worth or value of research findings. The **rigor** of qualitative studies is appraised differently from the rigor of quantitative studies because of differences in the underlying philosophical perspectives. Quantitative studies are considered rigorous when their procedures are prescribed before data collection, the sample is large enough to represent the population, and researchers maintain strict adherence to prescribed procedures during data collection and analysis. A quantitative researcher could replicate or repeat the work of another quantitative researcher with a similar study and expect to derive similar results. This is desirable because quantitative researchers define rigor to include objectivity and generalizability. Rigorous qualitative researchers are characterized by flexibility and openness while ensuring the methods used are congruent with the underlying philosophical perspective, data are collected with sensitivity and thoroughness, and analysis yields the perspective of the participants. The researcher's self-understanding is important because qualitative research is an interactive process shaped by the researcher's personal history, biography, gender, social class, race, and ethnicity, as well as by those of the study participants (Creswell, 2013; Marshall & Rossman, 2016; Patton, 2015). The researcher's self-awareness and understanding prevent the intrusion of personal biases about the phenomenon into the data analysis and interpretation processes. Critical appraisal of the rigor of qualitative studies is discussed in more detail in Chapter 18.

Gardner (2014) studied the phenomenon of mothering infants who were born with complex health conditions. Gardner's qualitative study provides an opportunity to apply the process shown in Figure 4-1.

The underlying philosophical tenets of grounded theory, symbolic interactionism, are evident in the study report. The researcher's description of the data collection and analysis is consistent with the criteria of rigor.

Gardner (2014) conducted the study of first-time mothers of fragile infants to "describe maternal and caregiving processes and practices in inexperienced mothers…" (p. 814). Using a grounded theory approach, Gardner interviewed eight mothers multiple times beginning two weeks after delivery and up to six months after the infant's discharge from the neonatal intensive care unit. Consistent with grounded theory principles, the researcher sought to describe the social processes used by the mothers to learn their new role while assuming responsibility for the care of a physiological unstable infant.

> "We conducted semistructured interviews about mothers' experiences and practices caring for their infants and about differences in these over time." (Gardner, 2014, p. 814-815)

Data analysis resulted in the grounded theory of 'getting the feel for it.' Gardner (2014) indicated that the theory "describes the shared problem, maternal process, context, strategy used, and consequences experienced by this group of new mothers" (p. 815). The participants "moved through a time-and-experience-mediated process" that shaped their "perceptions of mothering and caregiving" (Gardner, 2014, p. 815). Initially, the new mothers were overwhelmed with the tasks for which they were responsible because, in addition to learning to be mothers, they were also caring for the physical needs of their infants. On average, the mothers performed four complex medical procedures each day.

Gardner (2014) documented measures she implemented to protect the study's rigor. For example, the researcher increased the depth and richness of the data by interacting with the mothers over time, compared transcripts to the interview recordings to ensure accuracy, and relied on participant feedback to validate the emerging theory.

> "These strategies included prolonged involvement with participants, the use of multiple sites for participant recruitment, detailed audit trails of decision points in recruitment and data analysis, peer and expert audits, participant and expert feedback, and strategies for reflexivity. Reflexivity enhances the researcher's awareness of personal values and experiences that could influence the study and findings (Clancy, 2013)." (Gardner, 2014, p. 815)

This well-designed study was implemented with rigor. Specifying that reflexivity was used is a strength of the study. **Reflexivity** is the researcher's deep introspection and reflection on how his or her own biases and presence in the research situation may have affected how the data were collected, analyzed, and interpreted (Patton, 2015). Recruitment of participants continued until the core codes and the primary social process were established. Because of the richness of the quotations included in the article, gained through multiple interviews, nurses can gain insight into the mothers' experiences that may allow more empathetic and helpful interventions to support the parents in similar situations.

This example confirms that philosophy shapes one's view of science, which in turn shapes the methods used in a study and the criteria by which the rigor of the study will be evaluated (see Figure 4-1). Because qualitative studies emerge from several philosophies, an understanding of different approaches to qualitative research is needed as a foundation for appraising the rigor of research and making appropriate application of the findings.

APPROACHES TO QUALITATIVE RESEARCH

Five approaches to qualitative research commonly conducted and published in the nursing literature are phenomenological research, grounded theory research, ethnographic research, exploratory-descriptive qualitative research, and historical research (Figure 4-2). Although the five approaches share the commonalities already discussed, these approaches are different, in great part because researchers in different disciplines developed them. Psychologists and sociologists respectively developed the approaches known as phenomenological research (Giorgi, 2010) and grounded theory

research (Skeat, 2013). Anthropologists developed ethnography with its focus on culture (de Chesnay, 2014; Ladner, 2014). Exploratory-descriptive qualitative research has emerged from the disciplines of nursing and medicine and is focused on using the knowledge gained to benefit patients and families and improve health outcomes. Although no philosophy is formally linked to exploratory-descriptive qualitative research, its problem-solving approach is consistent with pragmatism (McDermid, n.d.). Historians developed methods to analyze source documents, artifacts, and interviews of witnesses to summarize the knowledge gained by studying the past (Lundy, 2012). Nurse researchers originally adopted historical methods to understand nursing's own history. Over time, they used historical methods to examine subsequent changes within nursing and health care. The common purpose among the methods, however, is to interpret the meaning of human experiences as constructed by the person (or persons) involved (Patton, 2015). The common experiences and patterns are described contextually within various philosophies and traditions.

To critically appraise the rigor of qualitative studies, you must understand that qualitative approaches are based on philosophical orientations or traditions that influence the study design from the wording of the research question through the interpretation of the data (see Table 4-1). Your appraisal of a study's rigor includes evaluating the extent to which the methods were consistent with the qualitative approach. To do this, you must be aware of guiding principles of the philosophical perspective of a study and use its criteria of rigor in your critical appraisal. The discussion of each approach will cover its philosophical perspective or orientation, methodology, and examples of how the method has been used to contribute to nursing knowledge.

Phenomenological Research

Phenomenology is both a philosophy and a research method. The purpose of **phenomenological research** is to describe experiences (or phenomena) from the participant perspective or, as frequently stated, capture the "lived experience" (Munhall, 2012; Patton, 2015). Phenomenology as a philosophical foundation undergirds the research methods of listening to individuals and analyzing verbal and nonverbal communication in order to gain a more comprehensive understanding of their experiences.

Philosophical Orientation

Phenomenologists perceive the person as being in constant interaction with the environment and making

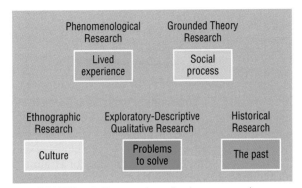

FIGURE 4-2 Focus of qualitative approaches.

meaning of experiences in that context. The world is shaped by the self and shapes the self. Beyond this, however, phenomenologists diverge in their beliefs about the person and the experience. The key philosophers who helped develop phenomenology are Husserl and Heidegger (Munhall, 2012).

A mathematician, Edmund Husserl (1859-1938), is considered the father of modern phenomenology (Phillips-Pula, Strunk, & Pickler, 2011). Departing from the positivist tradition of knowing, Husserl posited that **phenomena** make up the world of experience. These experiences cannot be explained by examining causal relations but need to be studied as the very things they are. Husserl wrote *Logical Investigations* (1901/1970), in which he developed his ideas about phenomena, contrasting human sciences (primarily psychology) and the basic or natural sciences (such as physics). Husserl articulated the importance of subjectivity (Staiti, 2014), the awareness of one's own being, feelings, and thoughts that can lead to self-understanding. The person experiencing his or her life must be the one to share the meaning of the experience. To describe the experience, the researcher must be open to the participant's worldview, set aside personal perspectives, and allow meanings to emerge. Setting aside one's beliefs during qualitative research is called **bracketing**.

Martin Heidegger (1889-1976) was a student of Husserl but expanded the goal of phenomenology from description of lived experience to the interpretation of lived experiences (Earle, 2010). The focus is on the meaning of the experience to the person experiencing it. Heidegger's seminal work was *Being and Time* (1927/1962). Heideggerian phenomenologists believe that the self exists within a body, or is **embodied** (Munhall, 2012). Experience cannot occur except through the body and its senses. Emotions and thoughts have physical sensations associated with them. **Embodiment** is "the unity of body and mind" that eliminates the "the idea of a subjective and objective world" (Munhall, 2012, p. 127). Building on the idea of embodiment, the person interprets experiences while they are occurring. Because of this, researchers who follow the philosophy proposed by Heidegger do not agree with Husserl's ideas on bracketing, taking the position that bracketing is not possible. One always remembers and is influenced by what one knows.

Heidegger also described situated freedom. To explain, you as a person are **situated** in specific context and time that shapes your experiences, paradoxically freeing and constraining your ability to establish meanings through language, culture, history, purposes, and values (Munhall, 2012). Part of your uniqueness is that you live in a historical, cultural, geographic, and temporal context. Consider the adolescent female athlete diagnosed with sarcoma who lives in 2017 in a U.S. urban area with availability of cancer treatment centers. Contrast the adolescent's perception with that of an 82-year-old man who lived on a farm in Europe in 1932 and was diagnosed with prostate cancer. Gender roles, availability of treatment, financial resources, geographical location, and historical era are only a few of the factors that would shape the cancer experience for these individuals. Each of them has only **situated freedom**, not total freedom. The adolescent has the freedom to choose physicians from among those who will accept her insurance. The older man may have the freedom only to choose whether he will use traditional herbs or not seek treatment at all. Until a disruption such as an unexpected diagnosis of cancer occurs, the person may not have considered the limits on meaning imposed by the context and the time.

Other philosophers have built on Husserl and Heidegger's perspectives and refined phenomenological methods. Merleau-Ponty (1945/2002) was among the French philosophers who further developed Heidegger's concepts. Colaizzi (1973), Giorgi (1985), and van Manen (1990) proposed procedural guidelines for phenomenological research (Streubert & Carpenter, 2011). The novice nurse researcher considering phenomenology should expand his or her knowledge in this area through immersion in the original writings of these philosophers (Munhall, 2012). Exploring the various philosophical stances within phenomenology will allow you to select a philosophy compatible with your perspective and a research question compatible with that particular point of view.

Despite the differences with the philosophical tradition, phenomenologists agree that there is no single reality. Each individual's experience is unique and ever-changing, according to the person's array of experiences. Reality is a subjective perception—a tenet that requires the researcher to listen, absorb, and elicit without judgment participants' subjective experiences in as much detail as possible. More information on the conduct of phenomenological research is provided in Chapter 12.

Phenomenology's Contribution to Nursing Science

Phenomenology has been the philosophical basis for many studies conducted by nurses. Bugel (2014) examined the lived experience of school-age siblings of children who were undergoing rehabilitation for a traumatic injury. Interviews with seven siblings revealed changes in their lives.

"The most significant change acknowledged by siblings was the change in the sibling relationship. At some point in the overall experience, siblings realized that they did, in fact, love their brother or sister." (Bugel, 2014, p.181)

Other changes occurred in the time spent with caring adults other than their parents and their daily routines. In addition, the children described the "constants" as being "sibling rivalry, school life, and having fun" (p. 182). Most poignant were the siblings' experiences of not being acknowledged by healthcare professionals, much less communicating with them about what had happened and the condition of the injured child. Their findings emphasize the importance of nurses focusing on the family as a unit when one member is injured.

Grounded Theory Research

Grounded theory research is an inductive research technique developed by Glaser and Strauss (1967) through their study of the experience of dying. The method's name means that the findings are grounded in the concrete world as experienced by participants, and grounded in the actual data. The data are interpreted, however, at a more abstract theoretical level. The desired outcome of grounded theory studies is a middle-range or substantive theory (Birks & Mills, 2015; Corbin & Strauss, 2015; Marshall & Rossman, 2016; Munhall, 2012).

Philosophical Orientation

Grounded theory is congruent with symbolic interaction theory, which holds many views in common with phenomenology. George Herbert Mead (1863-1931), a social psychologist, developed the principles of interaction theory that were posthumously published (Mead, 1934). His principles were shaped and refined by other social psychologists and became known as *symbolic interaction theory* (Crossley, 2010). Symbolic interaction theory explores how perceptions of interactions with others shape one's view of self and subsequent interactions. One's view of self is the context for subsequent interactions and thus shapes the meanings that are constructed. **Symbolic meanings** are different for each individual. We cannot completely know the symbolic meanings of another individual; however, individuals in the same group or society may hold common meanings, also called *shared meanings*. These shared meanings are embedded in catch phrases, beliefs, colloquialisms, and social behaviors, which present a core of belonging. Interactions among people may lead to redefinition of experiences, new meanings, and possibly a redefinition of self. Because of their theoretical importance, the interactions among the person and other individuals in social contexts are the focus of observation in grounded theory research.

Grounded Theory's Contribution to Nursing Science

Researchers using grounded theory contribute to nursing science by describing social processes at the heart of nursing care. Through careful analyses of the relationships among aspects of the social process, the researchers may describe an emerging theory through words, and often accompanied by a diagram. Grounded theory researchers examine experiences and processes with a breadth and depth not usually possible with quantitative research. The reader of the research report can intuitively verify these findings through her or his own experiences. The findings resonate with the reader.

Grounded theory researchers have contributed to our understanding of the patient experience across a wide range of settings. Davis et al. (2013) described women's thoughts and behaviors when having symptoms of acute coronary syndrome. Ramirez and Badger (2014) studied men suffering from depression and identified stages that men moved through from feeling different to confronting the illness and healing. Undergirding the stages was deep emotional pain. Ramirez and Badger developed a diagram of the stages of healing as a means of communicating their theory (Figure 4-3). Other grounded theory researchers have studied issues

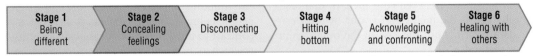

FIGURE 4-3 Men with depression navigating inward and outward: a grounded theory study. (Modified from Ramirez, J. L., & Badger, T. A. (2014). Men navigating inward and outward through depression. *Archives of Psychiatric Nursing, 28*(1), 21-28.)

facing nurses, such as caring for patients with substance abuse disorders (Morgan, 2014) and severe pain (Slayter, Williams, & Michael, 2015).

When theory is generated, that *grounded* and substantive theory can serve as a framework for understanding nursing interventions and generating quantitative studies. Grounded theory researchers interpret their results in terms of social processes; researchers using ethnography, the next qualitative approach, explore social interactions in the context of culture.

Ethnographic Research

Ethnographic research provides a framework for studying cultures. The term *culture* may mean a group that shares a common ancestral heritage, location, and social structure, or it can be applied to more loosely connected groups such as work cultures or organizational cultures. The word "ethnography" is derived by combining the Greek roots *ethno* (folk or people) and *graphy* (picture or portrait). **Ethnographies** are the written reports of a culture from the perspective of insiders. The insider's viewpoint is referred to as the **emic** perspective, as compared to the **etic** perspective, the views of someone from outside the culture (Marshall & Rossman, 2016). Initially, ethnographical research was limited to anthropology and the study of primitive, foreign, or remote cultures (Ladner, 2014; Liamputtong, 2013). Now, however, a number of other disciplines, including social psychology, sociology, political science, education, and nursing, promote cultural research using ethnography (Wolf, 2012).

Ethnography does not require travel to another country or region. Ethnography does require spending considerable time in the setting, studying, observing, and gathering data. **Participant observation** is the primary method of ethnographers (Patton, 2015) and is defined as being present and interacting with participants in routine activities. During these interactions, the researcher maintains the etic perspective, noting aspects of shared culture, including behaviors, rules, power structures, customs, and expectations.

A specific group or subculture is identified for study, such as women giving birth at home in Haiti or male nurses working in acute care settings. Ethnography can be used to describe and analyze aspects of the ways of life of a particular culture, even your own. In that case, ethnography allows the inclusion of your own experiences as data, which is not the case in the other major qualitative methods.

In a focused ethnography of healthy families who were members of a Northern Plains tribe of Native Americans, Martin and Yurkovich (2014) observed

family interactions, conducted focus groups, and interviewed community members.

"Almost all informants shared that a close-knit, healthy family is balanced in spiritual, emotional, physical, and social domains of their lives… Participants also identified that healthy families have the skills required to make adjustments during times of imbalance." (Martin & Yurkovich, 2014, p.60)

Their participants identified "close-knit" as the defining feature of healthy families. Martin and Yurkovich (2014) noted that participants described both healthy and unhealthy families in a "holistic manner, which reflected their Indigenous worldview" (p. 59).

Philosophical Orientation

Anthropologists seek to understand people: their ways of living, believing, acquiring information, transforming knowledge, and socializing the next generation. Studying a culture begins with the philosophical values of respecting, appreciating, and seeking to preserve the values and ways of life of the culture (Wolf, 2012). The philosophical bases of ethnography are naturalism and respect for others. The purpose of anthropological research is to describe a culture and explore "the meanings of social actions within cultures" (Wolf, 2012, p. 285).

Four schools of thought within ethnography, shown in Table 4-2, have emerged from different philosophical perspectives (Streubert & Carpenter, 2011). **Classic ethnography** seeks to provide a comprehensive description of a culture (Wolf, 2012), usually developed by researchers living for extended periods outside their own country in the environment being studied (de Chesnay, 2014). In contrast, **systematic ethnography** explores and describes the structures of the culture with an increased focus on specific groups, institutions, organizations, and patterns of social interaction. Because the study's scope is limited to a well-defined organizational culture, systematic ethnography is sometimes called **focused ethnography** (Streubert & Carpenter, 2011). **Interpretive ethnography** has as its goal understanding the values and thinking that result in behaviors and symbols of the people being studied (Streubert & Carpenter, 2011). In contrast to the descriptive goal of classical ethnography, researchers using interpretative ethnography are examining implications of behaviors and drawing inferences (de Chesnay, 2014). Wikberg, Eriksson, and Bondas (2012) conducted a study of new mothers from different

TABLE 4-2	**Four Types of Ethnography**	
Type	**Other Labels**	**Purpose**
Classic	Traditional	Describe a foreign culture through immersion in the culture for an extended period.
Systematic	Institutional	Describe the social organizational structure influencing a specific group of people.
Interpretative		Interpret the values and attitudes shaping the behaviors of members of a specific group, in order to promote understanding of the context of culture.
Critical	Disrupted	Examine the life of a group in the context of an alternative theory or philosophy, such as feminism or constructivism.

countries who were living in Finland. The researchers identified their study as an interpretive ethnography, based on their intent to compare the perspectives of mothers from different cultures.

The last type of ethnography, **critical ethnography**, has a political purpose of increasing the awareness of imbalances of power (de Chesnay, 2014), relieving oppression, and empowering a group of people to take action on their own behalf. Wolf (2012) calls this type of ethnography *disrupted* or *disruptive*, and identifies its philosophical foundation to be critical social theory (Fontana, 2004). O'Mahoney, Donnelly, Estes, and Bouchal (2012), Canadian researchers, conducted a critical ethnography of refugee and immigrant women who had postpartum depression. They interviewed 30 women who, by speaking out about their "individual experiences of social injustice and unequal social relations" (p. 736), hoped to improve the services available. Because ethnography can provide insight into societal issues affecting patients, the qualitative approach has resulted in significant contributions to nursing knowledge.

Ethnography's Contribution to Nursing Science

Madeline Leininger (1970), who earned her doctoral degree in anthropology, brought ethnography into nursing science by writing the first book linking nursing with anthropology and coining the term *ethnonursing*. She developed a framework for culture care that became the Sunrise Model (Clarke, McFarland, Andrews, & Leininger, 2009). The Sunrise Model identifies factors that affect health and illness, such as religion, income, kinship, education, values, and beliefs. Chapter 8 contains more information about the Theory of Culture Care developed by Leininger, so this section focuses on the method she developed to be consistent with ethnonursing.

Ethnonursing research values the unique perspective of groups of people within their cultural context that is influenced at the macro level by geographical location, political system, and social structures (see Table 4-1). Multiple levels of factors affect the culture and, consequently, the care expressions of the people. For example, a Vietnamese family who is the only Asian family in a small rural community in Georgia may have different care practices from those who live in New York City in a predominantly Vietnamese community. Leininger developed "enablers," sets of questions to guide the researcher's study of the culture (Leininger, 1997; 2002). The enablers provide a flexible framework for the researcher to use in order to collect and analyze the qualitative data. For example, one of the enablers is "Leininger's Observation-Participation-Reflection Enabler" (Leininger, 1997, p. 45), which reminds the researcher to use these three processes during a study. The method is naturalistic, meaning that the research is conducted in a natural setting without any attempt to control or alter the context. The researcher can be open to explore the insider perspective on health and well-being. As is true for other types of ethnography, the primary data collection method in ethnonursing research is participant observation (Douglas et al., 2010).

Exploratory-Descriptive Qualitative Research

Qualitative nurse researchers have conducted studies with the purpose of exploring and describing a topic of interest but, at times, have not identified or followed a specific qualitative methodology. Descriptive qualitative research is a legitimate method of research that may be the appropriate "label" for studies that have no clearly specified method or in which the method is specified but that ends with "a comprehensive summary of an event in the everyday terms of these events"

(Sandelowski, 2000, p. 336). Labeling a study as a specific type (grounded theory, phenomenology, or ethnographic) implies fixed categories of research with distinct boundaries, but the boundaries between methods are more appropriately viewed as permeable (Sandelowski, 2010). Although the studies result in descriptions and could be labeled as descriptive qualitative studies, most of the researchers are in the exploratory stage of studying the subject of interest. To decrease any confusion between quantitative descriptive studies and the discussion of this qualitative approach, we call this approach **exploratory-descriptive qualitative research**. In this book, studies without an identified qualitative method will be labeled as being exploratory-descriptive qualitative research.

Exploratory-descriptive qualitative studies are frequently conducted to address an issue or problem in need of a solution. For example, exercise had been clearly shown as being beneficial for patients with heart failure (HF), and providers were disappointed when HF patients did not comply with recommendations related to regular exercise (Albert, Forney, Slifcak, & Sorrell, 2015). Albert et al. (2015) designed their study to address a lack of understanding of "patients' perceptions of activity and exercise in relation to HF" (p. 3). Exploratory-descriptive qualitative researchers identify a specific lack of knowledge that can be addressed only through seeking the viewpoints of the people most affected.

Philosophical Orientation

The philosophical orientation that supports exploratory-descriptive qualitative studies undergirds most methods of qualitative inquiry. In contrast to the received view of reality that is the foundation for quantitative methods, all qualitative researchers ascribe to a perceived view of reality. The perceiver—the person living the experience—is the source and interpreter of information. A common assumption across qualitative approaches is that people express meaning in their language, decisions, and actions (Marshall & Rossman, 2016). When qualitative researchers explore and describe a phenomenon, they gather data from the perceptions and interpretations of the people and groups experiencing or affected by the phenomenon. Other qualitative experts call the general qualitative approach naturalistic inquiry. **Naturalistic inquiry** encompasses studies designed to study people and situations in their natural states (Sandelowski, 2000). Another philosophical orientation that may motivate some exploratory-descriptive qualitative researchers is pragmatism. William James and John Dewey took the rather obscure philosophical views of another philosopher, C. S. Peirce, and popularized them into an approach that focuses on the consequences of actions (McDermid, n.d.). Pragmatism, therefore, supports studies designed to gather data that become the information needed to solve a problem or offer a new strategy.

Exploratory-Descriptive Qualitative Research's Contribution to Nursing Science

Researchers who value the perspectives of participants may begin a program of research with qualitative methods to (1) begin development of interventions, (2) evaluate the appropriateness of an intervention following implementation, or (3) develop participants' definitions of concepts that researchers would like to measure. An example of a study conducted as a beginning point is the study conducted by Kitko, Hupcey, Gilchrist, and Boehmer (2013). They observed that left ventricular assistive devices (LVADs) were being implanted more frequently in persons with end-stage HF to increase cardiac output. Although the LVAD was a temporary treatment until a heart transplant for some patients, for others, the LVAD was destination therapy, or a permanent alternative to manage symptoms, improve quality of life, and extend life in persons who did not qualify for a heart transplant. Kitko et al. (2013) realized they lacked information about patient and caregiver needs during the transition from HF management to implantation of an LVAD as a destination therapy.

Kitko et al. (2013) interviewed 10 spousal caregivers to learn how to improve the "experiences and outcomes of both the patient and the spouse" (p. 196). The spouses described the role of caregiver that had involved, at first, providing care and support to a person with HF. As plans were made for placement of the LVAD, they were faced with learning additional skills required for post-implantation care. The spouses reported overwhelming fear and anxiety in the early months post LVAD implantation because they had to complete complex, daily care including dressing changes, charging batteries, monitoring vital signs, and activities of daily living. Kitko et al. (2013) noted that their study provided a description of how caregivers of patients with LVADS had adapted to their complex, demanding, and uncertain role.

> "...Caregivers also detailed how they had adapted to their new lives with an LVAD and how grateful they were that their spouses had a second chance." (Kitko et al., 2013, p.197)

Exploratory-descriptive qualitative studies have also been conducted to evaluate the cultural appropriateness of health messages, such as these three studies with African American samples. Beal (2015) conducted focus groups with African American women recruited from churches to identify their educational needs related to prevention and recognition of a stroke. Lem and Schwartz (2014) used interviews to elicit data from 13 African Americans with a diagnosis of HF. Lem and Schwartz learned that persons with HF knew little about the end stages of the illness. In another study with African American women, Jones (2015) conducted a qualitative study with mothers and daughters to learn more about their knowledge, beliefs, and attitudes related to breast cancer. Jones concluded that healthcare providers educating African American women appropriately will address fears about cancer, distrust of health care in general, and concerns that few treatments are available. Providers should also acknowledge the resources upon which the woman with breast cancer may rely, such as spirituality, social support, and family.

Historical Research

Historical research examines events of the past from the perspectives of the present day. Historians describe and analyze past events in the context of time, social structures, concurrent events, and key individuals. Their analyses can increase understanding and raise awareness of the societal forces shaping current events. Historical nursing research can provide continuity between the past and the present (Munhall, 2012) and facilitate learning from the past. Nurse researchers using historical methods have examined the events and people that shaped health in different settings and countries as well as nursing as a profession. For example, between 1930 and 1960, New Zealand nurse leaders wanted to improve the quality of care in hospitals. The nurse leaders developed and published standard instructions for nursing procedures (Wood & Nelson, 2013). With the current emphasis on evidence-based practice, Wood and Nelson wanted to learn how these nurse leaders had approached the pursuit of quality. They reviewed two primary sources of historical data: 20 years of records of the education committee of the New Zealand Nurses' Association and 30 years of issues of the national nursing journal. The leaders conducted national surveys of the ways in which different nursing procedures were performed, which resulted in a compilation of best practices based on expert opinion (Wood & Nelson, 2013). Similar to current principles of implementing evidence-based practice, the publica-

tions noted that standardization should not override the nurse's assessment of the patient's needs and well-being.

Philosophical Orientation

People and groups of people from the beginning of humankind have asked, "Where have we come from?" "Where are we going?" These questions often lead to an examination of past events to "prepare society for similar events in the future" (Streubert & Carpenter, 2011, p. 230). Historical researchers may use a biographical, intellectual, or social lens to examine the event or events they are studying. Using a biographical lens narrows the focus to key individuals living at a specific time, and whose actions influenced pivotal events. The intellectual lens is used to study ideas over time and the thinking of pivotal leaders. The social lens provides a description and analysis of everyday events and people living during a specific time (Streubert & Carpenter, 2011).

DeGuzman, Schminkey, and Koyen (2014) used a social lens to describe a volatile time in U.S. history. In 1967, racial relations were tense, and riots in Detroit, Michigan, destroyed property and neighborhoods. A few years prior, Nancy Milo had secured federal grants to build a community-based women's health clinic, Mom and Tots Center, in the neighborhood where she had grown up (DeGuzman et al., 2014). She worked closely with the community to understand and reduce infant and maternal mortality. As a result, during the riots when the neighborhood all around was heavily damaged, the Mom and Tots Center was untouched. DeGuzman et al. (2014) described the social context to Ms. Milo's work, including the Civil Rights Movement, the role of public health nurses, the introduction of the contraceptive pill, and a shift in funding the care for low-income women. Whichever lens or combination of lens the historical researcher uses, the goal is the same—to learn from the past.

A primary assumption of historical philosophy is that we can learn from the past and the knowledge gained can increase our understanding of the present and future. The philosophy of history is a search for wisdom. The historian examines what has been, what is, and what ought to be. Influenced by the values of the profession, historical nurse researchers may see themselves as stewards and teachers of the profession's rich heritage of commitment and leadership.

Historical Research's Contribution to Nursing Science

One example of nursing's rich heritage was the pioneering work done by Mary Breckinridge from 1925 to 1939

(Schminkey & Keeling, 2015). In the Appalachian region of Kentucky, Mary Breckinridge documented poor maternal and infant outcomes and started a "comprehensive assessment of births and deaths, conducted by registered nurses who had received midwifery training and certification in Great Britain" (Schminkey & Keeling, 2015, p. 48). The nurse midwives interviewed 1600 families living in Leslie County. Gradually, they became involved in the communities they were assessing, which laid a strong foundation for implementation of Ms. Breckinridge's next initiative, the Frontier Nursing Service. The Frontier Nursing Service opened eight nursing centers that included a clinic and a residence for the nurse midwives. The clinics were the location for primary health services, including inoculations for typhoid. Prenatal care was provided during home visits made by the nurse midwives. Prevention was the first goal; however, when that failed, the nurse midwives were trained to implement treatment in emergencies. Schminkey and Keeling (2015) documented the advanced procedures and outcomes of care by studying the Frontier Nursing Service records that comprise a Special Collection at the University of Kentucky's library. The researchers provide excerpts from a manual, *Medical Routines,* containing protocols for common situations that community healthcare providers might encounter. In emergencies, the nurse midwives could give ether to a mother so that they could turn an infant in breech or transverse position. They could administer medications to induce labor, stop seizures, and control hemorrhages. The nurse midwives of Leslie County prevented many deaths and improved the lives of their community. Schminkey and Keeling's study is a rigorous and interesting example of historical research.

Other Approaches to Qualitative Research

As you search the literature, you will see that qualitative researchers use other approaches in addition to those described in the chapter. Two additional approaches will be described briefly: narrative inquiry and case study method.

Narrative inquiry focuses on the story within the experiences of the participants (Patton, 2015). By analyzing the stories, the researcher learns how the participants construct their realities (Duffy, 2012; Marshall & Rossman, 2016). The philosophical foundation of narrative inquiry can be traced back to hermeneutics and phenomenology, but the method has been used by researchers from different philosophical and professional backgrounds (Howie, 2013). What these uses have in common are the desire to know how people create and reveal meaning in the stories they tell, how

the plot unfolds, and how metaphors are used in the story (Howie, 2013).

Sheilds et al. (2015) interviewed 32 people living with cancer, chronic kidney disease, or human immunodeficiency virus infection. Sheilds et al. (2015) interviewed each person up to four times over three years. Commonalities and differences were identified.

> "All the participants in the study described living with illness as a fine and delicate balance between a focus on living their lives and an awareness of death. Uncertainty was a continuous companion... These differences reflect trajectories of disease, personal stories and social constructions of illness." (Sheilds et al., 2015, p.210)

The stories of those living with these illnesses changed over time as the disease progressed or treatments changed. The findings remind nurses of the importance of listening to the stories of their patients facing life-threatening illnesses. Although Sheilds et al. (2015) interviewed their participants more than once every few months, conducting multiple interviews with each participant is not a requirement of the method.

Another frequently used method in nursing is the case study, and it has been widely used in medicine, as well. Case studies are frequently used for teaching and clinical purposes, but case studies as research are another method for qualitative researchers. Case studies have some similarities to historical research studies but are distinctive in that they focus on contemporary events (Yin, 2014). To use this method, the researcher identifies a distinct situation of interest in which decisions were made that shaped the situation (Yin, 2014). The researcher may decide to use the case study method to analyze "atypical cases that might lead to new understandings" (Abma & Stake, 2014, p. 1157). Various sources of evidence are analyzed with the goal of deriving a cohesive description incorporating multiple perspectives.

Mamier and Winslow (2014) used the case study approach to contrast the perspectives of a caregiver and a healthcare professional in a situation in which the caregiver was making a decision about her husband with Alzheimer's disease. The researchers interviewed the caregiver twice and the healthcare professional, a social worker, once about the placement decision. The caregiver described the continued physical decline of her husband and the lack of informal support she received from other family members. When her husband fell and had an extended hospital stay, she began to realize how difficult returning home with him would be.

"The tension between a perceived obligation and the experience of reaching one's personal limits created a dilemma for her leading to feelings of guilt and ambivalence." (Mamier & Winslow, 2014, p.15)

The social worker knew the caregiver through a support group. Through these interactions, the social worker identified additional triggers such as illnesses of other family members and the caregiver's own need for surgery that led to placement of the caregiver's husband. The professional maintained that there was no right or wrong time for placement and that the placement had to be the decision of the caregiver. One of the lessons in this case study was the professional's role in placement decisions.

"Of vital importance is that the professional have a clear understanding of where a caregiver is in his or her decision-making process. On the basis of understanding and interpreting the specific cues of the situation, the professional may play a vital role in guiding family caregivers in the preparatory work needed prior to a crisis." (Mamier & Winslow, 2014, p. 19)

As seen in this case study, in-depth descriptions can lead to increased understanding that provides nurses information to personalize care and improve outcomes. Qualitative researchers use approaches and methods that value the patient's and family's perspectives and contribute to evidence-based care.

▌ K E Y P O I N T S

- Qualitative research is a scholarly approach used to describe life experiences from the perspective of the persons involved.
- The philosophical foundation of qualitative research describes a view of science and guides both the selection of methods and the criteria of rigor.
- Qualitative researchers use open-ended methods to gather data, such as interviews, focus groups, observation, and examination of documents.
- The goal of phenomenological research is to describe experiences from the perspectives of the participants—to capture the lived experience. Phenomenology is the philosophy guiding these studies, a philosophy that began with the writings of Husserl.
- The goal of grounded theory research is to produce findings grounded in the data collected from and about the participants. The analysis results in a middle-range or substantive theory. Symbolic inter-

actionism is the underlying philosophical and theoretical perspective.
- Ethnographic research is the investigation of cultures through an in-depth study of the members of the culture. Nurse anthropologist Leininger developed the ethnonursing research method.
- Exploratory-descriptive qualitative research elicits the perceptions of participants to provide insights for understanding patients and groups, influencing practice, and developing appropriate programs for specific groups of people. In addition to the naturalistic orientation common to all qualitative research, exploratory-descriptive studies may be guided by the philosophy of pragmatism with a focus on problem solving.
- Historical research is designed to analyze the interaction of people, events, and social context that occurred in the remote or recent past. The goal of historical research in nursing is to tell a story from which the reader learns from the past for application in the present and future.
- Narrative inquiry and case study research are examples of other qualitative methods that may be used to answer research questions important to nurses.

REFERENCES

Abma, T., & Stake, R. (2014). Science of the particular: An advocacy of naturalistic case study in health research. *Qualitative Health Research, 24*(8), 1150–1161.

Albert, N., Forney, J., Slifcak, E., & Sorrell, J. (2015). Understanding physical activity and exercise behaviors in patients with heart failure. *Heart and Lung: The Journal of Critical Care, 44*(1), 2–8.

Beal, C. (2015). Stroke education needs of African American women. *Public Health Nursing, 32*(1), 24–33.

Birks, M., & Mills, J. (2015). *Grounded theory: A practice guide* (2nd ed.). Thousand Oaks, CA: Sage.

Bugel, M. (2014). Experiences of school-aged siblings of children with a traumatic injury: Changes, constants, and needs. *Pediatric Nursing, 4*(4), 179–186.

Clancy, M. (2013). Is reflexivity the key to minimizing problems of interpretation in phenomenological research? *Nurse Researcher, 20*(6), 12–16.

Clark, P. N., McFarland, M. R., Andrews, M. M., & Leininger, J. (2009). Caring: Some reflections on the impact of the culture care theory by McFarland & Andrews and a conversation with Leininger. *Nursing Science Quarterly, 22*(3), 233–239.

Colaizzi, P. F. (1973). *Reflection and research in psychology: A phenomenological study of learning.* Dubuque, IA: Kendall Hunt.

Corbin, J., & Strauss, A. (2015). *Basics of qualitative research: Techniques and procedures for developing grounded theory* (4th ed.). Thousand Oaks, CA: Sage.

Creswell, J. W. (2013). *Research design: Qualitative, quantitative, and mixed methods approaches* (4th ed.). Los Angeles, CA: Sage.

Crossley, N. (2010). Networks and complexity: Directions for interactionist research? *Symbolic Interaction, 33*(3), 341–363.

Davis, L., Mishel, M., Moser, D., Esposito, N., Lynn, M., & Schwartz, T. (2013). Thoughts and behaviors of women with symptoms of acute coronary syndrome. *Heart and Lung: The Journal of Critical Care, 42*(6), 428–435.

De Chesnay, M. (2014). Overview of ethnography. In M. de Chesnay, (Ed.) *Nursing research using ethnography* (pp. 1–14). New York, NY: Springer Publishing.

DeGuzman, P. B., Schminkey, D. L., & Koyen, E. A. (2014). "Civil unrest does not stop ovulation": Women's prenatal and family planning services in a 1960s Detroit neighborhood clinic. *Family & Community Health, 37*(3), 199–211.

Douglas, M. K., Kemppainen, J. K., McFarland, M. R., Papadopoulos, I., Ray, M. A., Roper, J. M., et al. (2010). Chapter 10: Research methodologies for investigating cultural phenomena and evaluating interventions. *Journal of Transcultural Nursing, 21*(Suppl. 1), 3737–4055.

Duffy, M. (2012). Narrative inquiry: The method. In P. L. Munhall (Ed.), *Nursing research: A qualitative perspective* (5th ed., pp. 421–440). Sudbury, MA: Jones & Bartlett.

Earle, V. (2010). Phenomenology as research method or substantive metaphysics? An overview of phenomenology's uses in nursing. *Nursing Philosophy, 11*(4), 286–296.

Fontana, J. S. (2004). A methodology for critical science in nursing. *Advances in Nursing Science, 27*(2), 93–101.

Gardner, M. (2014). Maternal caregiving and strategies used by inexperienced mothers of young infants with complex medical conditions. *Journal of Obstetric, Gynecologic, and Neonatal Nursing, 43*(6), 813–823.

Giorgi, A. (1985). *Phenomenology and psychological research.* Pittsburg, PA: Duquesne University Press.

Giorgi, A. (2010). Phenomenological psychology: A brief history and its challenges. *Journal of Phenomenological Psychology, 41*(2), 145–179.

Glaser, B. G., & Strauss, A. (1967). *The discovery of grounded theory: Strategies for qualitative research.* Chicago, IL: Aldine.

Hall, H., Griffiths, D., & McKenna, L. (2013). From Darwinism to constructivism: The evolution of grounded theory. *Nurse Researcher, 20*(3), 17–21.

Hannes, K. (2011). Critical appraisal of qualitative research. In J. Noyes, A. Booth, K. Hannes, J. Harris, S. Lewin, & C. Lockwood (Eds.), *Supplementary guidance for inclusion in qualitative research in Cochrane systematic reviews of interventions.* Available from http://cqrmg.cochrane.org/supplemental-handbook-guidance.

Heidegger, M. (1927/1962). *Being in time* (J. Macquarrie & E. Robinson, Trans.). New York, NY: Harper.

Howie, L. (2013). Narrative enquiry and health research. In P. Liamputtong (Ed.), *Research methods in health* (2nd ed., pp. 72–84). Melbourne, Australia: Oxford University Press.

Husserl, E. (1901/1970). *Logical investigations* (N. Findlay, Trans.). (Vol. 1). New York, NY: Routledge.

Jones, B. (2015). Knowledge, beliefs, and feelings about breast cancer: The perspectives of African American women. *The Association of Black Nursing Faculty Journal, 26*(1), 5–10.

Kerlinger, F. N., & Lee, H. P. (2000). *Foundations of behavioral research* (4th ed.). Fort Worth, TX: Harcourt College.

Kitko, L., Hupcey, J., Gilchrist, J., & Boehmer, J. (2013). Caring for a spouse with end-stage heart failure through implantation of a left-ventricular assist device as destination therapy. *Heart and Lung: The Journal of Critical Care, 42*(3), 195–201.

Ladner, S. (2014). *Practical ethnography: A guide to doing ethnography in the private sector.* Walnut Creek, CA: Left Coast Press.

Leininger, M. M. (1970). *Nursing and anthropology: Two worlds to blend.* New York, NY: Wiley.

Leininger, M. M. (1997). Overview of the Theory of Culture Care with the ethnonursing research method. *Journal of Transcultural Nursing, 8*(2), 32–54.

Leininger, M. M. (2002). Culture care theory: A major contribution to advance transcultural nursing knowledge and practices. *Journal of Transcultural Nursing, 13*(3), 189–192.

Lem, A., & Schwartz, M. (2014). African American heart failure patients' perspective on palliative care in the outpatient setting. *Journal of Hospice and Palliative Care Nursing, 16*(8), 536–542.

Liamputtong, P. (2013). *Qualitative research methods* (4th ed.). Oxford, UK: Oxford University Press.

Lundy, K. (2012). Historical research. In P. Munhall (Ed.), *Nursing research: A qualitative perspective* (5th ed.). Sudbury, MA: Jones & Bartlett.

Mamier, I., & Winslow, B. (2014). Divergent views of placement decision-making: A qualitative case study. *Issues in Mental Health Nursing, 35*(1), 13–20.

Marshall, C., & Rossman, G. B. (2016). *Designing qualitative research* (6th ed.). Thousand Oaks, CA: Sage.

Martin, D., & Yurkovich, E. (2014). "Close knit" defines a healthy Native American Indian family. *Journal of Family Nursing, 20*(1), 51–72.

McDermid, D. (n.d.) *Pragmatism.* Retrieved May 5, 2015 from *The Internet Encyclopedia of Philosophy.* http://www.iep.utm.edu/.

Mead, G. H. (1934). *Mind, self, and society.* Chicago, IL: University of Chicago Press.

Merleau-Ponty, M. (1945/2002). *Phenomenology of perception* (C. Smith, Trans.). London, England: Routledge Classics.

Miles, M., Huberman, A., & Saldaña, J. (2014). *Qualitative data analysis: A methods sourcebook* (3rd ed.). Los Angeles, CA: Sage.

Morgan, B. (2014). Nursing attitudes toward patients with substance use disorders in pain. *Pain Management Nursing, 15*(1), 165–175.

Munhall, P. L. (2012). *Nursing research: A qualitative perspective* (5th ed.). Sudbury, MA: Jones & Bartlett.

O'Mahoney, J., Donnelly, T., Estes, D., & Bouchal, S. (2012). Using critical ethnography to explore issues among immigrant and refugee women seeking help for postpartum depression. *Issues in Mental Health Nursing, 33*(11), 735–742.

Patton, M. (2015). *Qualitative research & evaluation methods* (4th ed.). Thousand Oaks, CA: Sage.

Phillips-Pula, L., Strunk, J., & Pickler, R. H. (2011). Understanding phenomenological approaches to data analysis. *Journal of Pediatric Health Care, 25*(1), 67–71.

Ramirez, J., & Badger, T. (2014). Men navigating inward and outward through depression. *Archives of Psychiatric Nursing, 28*(1), 21–28.

Roller, M., & Lavrakas, P. (2015). *Applied qualitative research design: A total quality framework approach.* New York, NY: Guilford Press.

Sandelowski, M. (2000). What happened to qualitative description? *Research in Nursing & Health, 23*(4), 334–340.

Sandelowski, M. (2010). What's in a name? Qualitative description revisited. *Research in Nursing & Health, 33*(1), 77–84.

Schminkey, D., & Keeling, A. (2015). Frontier nurse-midwives and antepartum emergencies, 1925-1939. *Journal of Midwifery & Women's Health, 60*(1), 48–55.

Shadish, W. R., Cook, T. D., & Campbell, D. T. (2002). *Experimental and quasi-experimental designs for generalization causal inference.* Chicago, IL: Rand McNally.

Sheilds, L., Molzahn, A., Bruce, A., Schick Makaroff, K., Stajduhar, K., Beuthin, R., et al. (2015). Contrasting stories of life-threatening illness: A narrative inquiry. *International Journal of Nursing Studies, 52*(1), 207–215.

Skeat, J. (2013). Using grounded theory in health research. In P. Liamputtong (Ed.), *Research methods in health* (2nd ed., pp. 101–131). Melbourne, Australia: Oxford University Press.

Slayter, S., Williams, A., & Michael, R. (2015). Seeking empowerment to comfort patients in severe pain: A grounded theory study of the nurse's perspective. *International Journal of Nursing Studies, 52*(1), 229–239.

Staiti, A. (2014). *Husserl's transcendental phenomenology: Nature, spirit, and life.* Cambridge, UK: Cambridge University Press.

Streubert, H., & Carpenter, D. (2011). *Qualitative research in nursing: Advancing the humanistic perspective* (5th ed.). Philadelphia, PA: Lippincott Williams & Wilkins.

van Manen, M. (1990). *Researching lived experience: Human science for an action sensitive pedagogy.* Ontario, Canada: Althouse Press.

Wikberg, A., Eriksson, K., & Bondas, T. (2012). Intercultural caring from the perspectives of immigrant new mothers. *Journal of Gynecological and Neonatal Nursing, 41*(5), 638–649.

Wolf, Z. E. (2012). Ethnography: The method. In P. L. Munhall (Ed.), *Nursing research: A qualitative perspective* (5th ed., pp. 285–338). Sudbury, MA: Jones & Bartlett.

Wood, P. J., & Nelson, K. (2013). Striving for best practice: Standardising New Zealand nursing procedures, 1930-1960. *Journal of Clinical Nursing, 22*(21–22), 3217–3224.

Yin, R. (2014). *Case study research: Design and methods.* Los Angeles, CA: Sage.

5

Research Problem and Purpose

Suzanne Sutherland

http://evolve.elsevier.com/Gray/practice/

Identifying a research problem is the first step toward conducting research. Frequently, the problem area a researcher chooses is the outgrowth of professional observation, for instance an awareness of an increase in the number of patients with pressure ulcers in a hospital unit over the past few months. External opportunities to conduct research also may stimulate thinking about a research problem, such as grant postings, agency calls for internal research, or requirements of graduate programs. The problem area is one about which the researcher has some curiosity, or else why would the inquiry take place at all?

The **research purpose** is the stated reason for conduct of a study. The purpose statement must be concise and specific if it is to direct the subsequent steps of the research process. **Research topics** are broad collections of ideas for potential research projects, related to one phenomenon of interest. Each identified research topic has many possible research purposes that might be identified.

This chapter defines and presents examples of research problems and purposes, identifies potential sources for research problems, and explains the process of formulating a research problem and purpose. In addition, it discusses criteria for determining the feasibility of a proposed study; discusses research topics, problems, and purposes for different methodologies; and provides examples of research problems and purposes from current published studies.

THE RESEARCH PROBLEM

Types of Research Problems and Gaps

A **research problem** is an area in which there is a gap in nursing's knowledge base. The gap can be one that relates to practice, such as the safest and most efficient way for a community emergency department to triage and establish prompt isolation in case of suspected exotic viruses such as severe acute respiratory syndrome (SARS) and Ebola, an area of inquiry currently in need of evidence on which to base best practices. Because of the scope of what is not known, many research studies are required to fill this particular gap.

Not all research addresses the "how-to" of practice, however. The research problem and identified gap may focus on understanding a process related to health, such as what the day-to-day experience is for families of children with hyperactivity (Moen, Hall-Lord, & Hedelin, 2014). Research that enhances understanding contributes to nursing's body of knowledge. It also allows the individual reader to accrue knowledge that might or might not have practical application to the art of practice.

A third type of gap relates to theory generation. Research that generates theory is qualitative, and only some types of qualitative research generate theory. (Research that tests theory is quantitative.) To some extent, new theory "informs" practice, such as research that addresses the theory gap surrounding challenges

BOX 5-1   **Essentials of the Research Problem Statement**

BOX 5-1   **Essentials of the Research Problem Statement**

- Summary of what is known about the phenomenon of interest, ending with the research gap
- Justification for the importance of addressing this knowledge gap (the significance statement)
- The population of interest (and sometimes the setting)

and needs of pregnant and parenting adolescents (Atkinson & Peden-McAlpine, 2014), ultimately giving the reader insight and understanding of process but not prescribing practice actions.

Elements That Comprise the Research Problem Statement

The research problem statement is usually several paragraphs in length, focuses on the principal concepts upon which the study will focus, and contains certain essentials (Box 5-1). The first of those essentials is a general summary of what is known about the phenomenon of interest, followed by a sentence that identifies a research gap. This general summary is often called a **background statement**. The beginning of a typical sentence identifying the research gap often begins with wording such as, "Nonetheless, there is inadequate knowledge about …"

The problem statement also includes a second essential component, a justification for the importance of addressing this knowledge gap, be it social, psychological, physiological, cognitive, financial, humanistic, or philosophical. This is sometimes called the **significance statement**. The stated justification implies that the study, or other studies that follow, will ameliorate the underlying issue described in the summary, partially enhancing humanity's wellness along health continua. There is often the implication that conduct of the study is the right thing to do: a modest amount of literary overemphasis accompanied by "must" or "should" is typical. The justification statement also serves as an important part of the researcher's application to a human subjects committee, also known as an **institutional review board** (IRB), for permission to conduct the study: research that consumes the time and energy of subjects should not be trivial or excessively redundant with what is already known. Finally, the research problem identifies a specific population, and sometimes a general setting.

A study by Happ et al. (2015) was conducted to describe mechanically ventilated intensive care unit (ICU) patients, in terms of their communication capa-

bility and communication needs. Its research problem discussion is presented as an example:

"Communication impairment presents a common, distressing problem for patients who receive mechanical ventilation (MV) during critical illness and for the clinicians who care for them (Carroll, 2004; Karlsson, Bergbom, & Forsberg, 2012; Khalaila et al., 2011; Menzel, 1998; Nelson et al., 2004; Rotondi et al. 2002). New hospital accreditation standards for patient communication include the communication disability acquired as a result of endotracheal or tracheal intubation during critical illness as a condition requiring provider assessment and accommodation (The Joint Commission, 2010). Augmentative and Alternative Communication (AAC) tools can be used successfully by clinicians and ICU patients to transmit or receive messages (Beukelman, Garrett, & Yorkston, 2007; Costello, 2000; Happ, Roesch, & Garrett, 2004; Radtke, Tate, & Happ, 2012; Radtke, Baumann, Garrett, & Happ, 2011; Stovsky, Rudy, & Dragonette, 1988). Our previous work showed significant improvements in nurse-patient communication with training and the use of AAC (Happ et al., 2014). Although measures of sedation, coma, and severity of illness are commonly reported in critical care research, few studies have documented the proportion of mechanically ventilated ICU patients who are awake, aware and responsive to verbal communication and who therefore could be served by these simple assistive communication tools. This information is necessary to (1) appropriately plan communication supplies and support programs, (2) prepare clinicians, and (3) provide benchmarking data from which to evaluate communication support initiatives in the ICU." (Happ et al, 2015, p. 45)

In this example, the research problem background discussion focused on an area of concern, communication needs, for a particular population, mechanically ventilated patients, in a selected setting, the ICU. Happ et al. (2015) clearly identified the significance of the problem, which is extensive as well as relevant to patients and to nursing. The conduct of the research is defensible, based on the identification of the research gap and the size of the population of patients who could quite probably benefit from research in this area. The problem background focused on key research related to communication in mechanically ventilated patients and tools available for patient use. The penultimate sentence in this example identified the gap in nursing's body of knowledge, which relates to practice. Prior to this study, there had been limited research describing how many mechanically ventilated ICU patients have the potential to communicate.

The research problem in this example gives rise to several concepts or research topics:

- Ability of ICU patients to communicate
- Quality of that communication
- Ability of ICU nurses to understand patients with and without communication assists
- Safety issues in ICUs related to impaired communication
- Nurses' knowledge regarding their hospitals' requirements for assessment and accommodation, relative to acquired impaired communication, when patients are intubated

Each of these topics includes an array of potential research purposes, for individual studies.

On a practical level, the original nursing problem area identified at the outset of a research process may require some alteration, augmentation, or refinement by the researcher, as a result of discoveries gleaned from various sources: discussions with peers, research findings uncovered during the literature review, logistic difficulties of site access, results of a pilot project, power analysis, and various unforeseen events. Potential external funding or sponsorship opportunities can cause a researcher to broaden the problem area first identified in order for the research to compete for funding or sponsorship.

THE RESEARCH PURPOSE

The **research purpose** is a clear, concise statement of the researcher's specific focus or aim: the reason the study was performed. The research purpose is a short statement, usually a single sentence. In a research proposal, the purpose statement is couched in the present tense, "The purpose of this research is to investigate …" and in a research report, in the past tense, "The purpose of this research study was to demonstrate …"

Often, the research purpose indicates the principal variables and setting, identifies the population, and hints at both methodology and design. A quantitative purpose statement addresses prevalence, measured connections between ideas, or a cause-and-effect relationship, ultimately to be analyzed by statistical analyses. A qualitative purpose statement addresses participants' reported experiences or the researcher's observations, within context, ultimately producing a narrative description. Variants of these, such as mixed-methods research and outcomes research, contain purpose statements that are similar to those found in ordinary quantitative and/ or qualitative reports.

Regardless of the type of research, a clear purpose statement is required in order to indicate what the study was designed to accomplish. Immediately after their research problem summary and identification of the research gap, Happ et al. (2015) stated their purpose, "to estimate the proportion of mechanically ventilated ICU patients who meet basic communication criteria and thus could potentially benefit from the use of assistive communication tools or referral for evaluation and intervention by a speech-language pathologist" (p. 45). This purpose statement suggests that Happ et al. conducted quantitative noninterventional research, in order to establish prevalence (the proportion of patients who met basic communication criteria) and to identify the characteristics of patients who did meet those criteria, as compared with those who did not. Happ et al. also found that some ICU patients were less likely to benefit by assistive communication devices: the authors reflected that this finding suggested "a need for unit-based programs and services targeted to the unique communication needs of specialty populations" (p. 49). This statement goes beyond the authors' stated purpose; however, it is good practice to present logical derivations of data analysis not foreseen in the original purpose statement.

SOURCES OF RESEARCH PROBLEMS

The nurse researcher who produces a series of related studies within a single problem area is at no loss for identification of a research purpose within that area. The novice researcher, however, especially a master's or doctoral student, may search not only for a purpose statement but also for an entire problem area. Rich sources for generating meaningful research are (1) clinical practice, (2) professional journals in one's area of expertise, (3) collaboration with faculty and nurse researchers, and (4) research priorities identified by funding agencies and specialty groups. Existent theory is a source of research problems for experienced researchers who are capable of generating studies that test all or part of that theory. Sources for refining research problem areas after they are initially generated are (1) discussions with peers and (2) literature review. Researchers often use multiple sources to identify and refine research problem areas and to define research purposes within an area.

Identifying a Problem Area
Clinical Practice
The practice of nursing, however expert, benefits by knowledge and evidence generated through research.

To be meaningful, however, knowledge and evidence obtained by research within a clinical area must emanate from the real concerns of clinical practice, not merely from external observations as to what those real concerns might be. Thus, nurses and nursing are the most fertile source for identifying problems that genuinely pertain to practice.

Potential problem areas can evolve from clinical observations. For example, a nurse working in an emergency department notes that in a 4-week period, three incidents have occurred in which patients' families have acted out and purposefully broken furniture and punched holes in the walls of the waiting room. These incidents have sparked clinical-based questions such as, "Is the emergency department waiting room a safe place for other clients? What can emergency department staff do to support families in crisis? What does the emergency department do now to help families manage stress? What is working and what isn't?"

The pediatric nurse's observation that adult siblings of autistic children seem to feel a responsibility for their affected brothers and sisters, over and above what is seen in other families, gives rise to questions such as, "What is the family dynamic when one of the children in a family is affected with autism? To what extent do unaffected siblings of autistic children co-parent? As adults, what are the limitations and enhancements related to having grown up with an autistic sibling?"

A nurse in a burn unit notes, "Most of the research findings for in-hospital management of burn injury have been derived from studies of patients in certain age ranges, and most of the subjects of those studies were men. Do the findings apply equally to elders and to women, or is the trajectory of healing somewhat different for these patients? Do findings apply, as well, to infants? What is the fate of skin grafts decades after the burn injury, in terms of skin integrity and normal function?"

A psychiatric mental health nurse practitioner (PMHNP) with a very busy practice, working long hours, wonders, "Are the other nurse practitioners in this same healthcare system exceptionally busy, like I am, and what kinds of hours do all of us work? Is there more mental illness in our system's population than there was 20 years ago? Is there a greater willingness to seek mental health treatment now than there was 20 years ago?"

All of these research questions are outgrowths of problem areas: stress and stress behaviors when a family member is ill, family dynamics when a child is affected with autism, treatment and healing of burns, and workload for PMHNPs. Each problem area was derived from on-the-job observations of patients, families, and the work of the nurse.

Professional Journals in One's Area of Expertise

On occasion, nurses who read professional journals are captivated by a certain article, either a research report or an essay discussing research reports about patient care or outcomes, in terms of best evidence. Sometimes the reaction of a nurse is, "I could have designed that study better," or "I wonder why they didn't get any information on *that* variable. I would have done so." At other times a case study of a patient, or an essay, inspires a nurse to design research on a certain topic. An essay about "proper" procedure may encourage a nurse to find out whether that "proper" procedure is indeed better in terms of patient safety, practicality, savings of time, cost-effectiveness, person-hours, or perhaps all or none of those variables.

Collaboration with Faculty and Nurse Researchers

For the graduate student searching for a problem area, conversations with nursing faculty members are invaluable, especially when the student cannot think of any problem area that would generate a research purpose with potentially meaningful results. Faculty advisors are adept at identifying areas that matter to students and suggesting those that are most fruitful to pursue. Some faculty members maintain their own programs of research and can suggest parallel research either using existent data or redesigning a proposed study to include an area of inquiry in which the student is interested.

A collaborative relationship is the norm between expert researchers and nurse clinicians. Because nursing research is critical for designation as a Magnet facility by the American Nurses Credentialing Center (ANCC, 2015), hospitals and healthcare systems employ nurse researchers for the purpose of guiding studies conducted by staff nurses. In many ways, this is the ideal supportive relationship: the clinician knows the problem area, and the researcher knows how to guide the clinician through the process of proposal writing, approval by nurse manager and medical team, IRB approval, selection of data collection strategies, and identification of appropriate methods of data analysis. Collaboration between nurse researchers and clinicians, and sometimes with researchers from other health-related disciplines, enhances the potential for generating evidence actually useful for practice. The opportunity to participate on an interdisciplinary research team is an informative experience and expands the nurse's knowledge of the research process, across disciplines.

Research Priorities Identified by Funding Agencies and Specialty Groups

Landmark research by Lindeman (1975) identified several research priorities related to clinical nursing interventions: stress, care of the aged, pain management, and patient education. Generating research evidence in these four areas continues to be a priority for nursing.

Since Lindeman's time, various funding agencies and professional organizations have identified nursing research priorities. Most professional organizations display their priorities on their websites. This allows new nurse researchers to use the guidance of their own individual professional organizations when selecting research problem areas.

For instance, the American Association of Critical-Care Nurses (AACN) has determined research priorities for the critical care specialty since the early 1980s (Lewandowski & Kositsky, 1983) and revised these priorities on the basis of patients' needs and changes in health care. Since 2012, the AACN research priorities have been (1) effective and appropriate use of technology to achieve optimal patient assessment, management and/or outcomes; (2) creation of a healing, humane environment; (3) processes and systems that foster the optimal contribution of critical care nurses; (4) effective approaches to symptom management; and (5) prevention and management of complications (AACN, 2015; Deutschman, Ahrens, Cairns, Sessler, & Parsons, 2012). In addition, the AACN (2015) has identified a particularly iconoclastic research agenda calling, among other things, for nurses to "move away from rituals in practice," establishment of a work culture that expects "nurses questioning their practice," and active broad sharing of research findings among "key stakeholders," including consumers, industry, and payers.

A significant funding agency for nursing research is the National Institute of Nursing Research (NINR). A major initiative of the NINR is the development of a national nursing research agenda that involves identifying nursing research priorities, outlining a plan for implementing priority studies, and obtaining resources to support priority projects. In 2015, the NINR's annual budget totaled more than $140,452,000, with approximately 68% of the budget allotted for extramural research grants, 3% for the centers programs in specialized areas, 3% for research career development and other research, 7% for predoctoral and postdoctoral training, 10% for research management and support, 3% for research and development contracts, and 6% for their intramural research program (NINR, 2015a). Intramural research is conducted at National Institutes of Health (NIH) research facilities, while extramural research is conducted by researchers who are not employees of NIH. Over the past few years, budgeted amounts available for extramural research project grants have decreased by 3%, reflecting increased costs and salaries. Competition for grants is brisk: NINR funded 11.6% of the proposals they received in 2014 (NIH, n.d.). The studies that are funded by the NINR are often those conducted by inter-professional teams at top-ranking research institutions.

Nonetheless, the NINR's research priorities are useful for guiding beginning researchers. The NINR (2015b) identified four priority research themes: (1) symptom science, including personalized health strategies; (2) wellness, including promotion of health and prevention of illness; (3) self-management to improve quality of life for persons with chronic illness; and (4) end-of-life care, including palliative care. These differed from previous research priorities in several respects, most notably in the prioritization of symptom science and elimination of health disparity from the listing.

Another federal agency that funds healthcare research is the Agency for Healthcare Research and Quality (AHRQ). Much of AHRQ's budget is earmarked for its internal programs; however, the budget for external grants is approximately half of NINR's total grant budget. Grants are more likely to be awarded to persons connected with academic programs. The research priorities heavily emphasize patient safety (AHRQ, 2015). In summary, funding organizations, professional organizations, and governmental healthcare organizations are fruitful sources for identifying priority research problems.

Refining the Research Problem Area

Once the initial identification of a research problem area occurs, in addition to conversations with one's thesis or dissertation advisors, there are two additional avenues useful for refinement of the problem area and narrowing of possible research purposes. These are discussions with peers and literature searches.

Discussions with Peers

Nobody knows everything. Even the cleverest researcher can benefit from discussions with peers throughout the research process. After a researcher decides upon a general problem area, discussions with peers can help refine that area. Peers almost invariably ask questions about problems that have not occurred to the researcher. When a researcher decides tentatively upon a research purpose, peers can critique the researcher's plan to produce a better, tighter purpose statement, or even suggest a more fruitful research design. The constructive criticism of a peer prepares you the researcher for the actual criticism you can expect when presenting the research results at a conference. Listen to those peers!

Literature Review

Hundreds of nursing journals are in print, and some of them publish research articles. Perusing articles in a research journal is helpful for refining problem areas and determining what is already known, versus what is needed for nursing's body of knowledge. Many journals contain a substantial amount of research; these are available online as well as in hard copy (Table 5-1).

You as a beginning researcher will almost always find published research in your planned problem area. Conclusion sections of published research contain authors' recommendations for subsequent research, indicating directions for verification of existent studies' findings, or exploration of the problem area in different ways. Designing a study based on these recommendations allows you to build on the work of others and expand what is known.

	Academic Journals	Clinical Practice Journals
20 to 40 Articles Annually	Journal of Research in Nursing Clinical Nursing Research	American Journal of Maternal Child Nursing
40 to 60 Articles Annually	Western Journal of Nursing Research Journal of Nursing Scholarship Nursing Research	Heart & Lung: The Journal of Acute and Critical Care Journal of Psychiatric and Mental Health Nursing Archives of Psychiatric Nursing
More than 60 Articles Annually	International Journal of Nursing Studies Applied Nursing Research	Journal of Pediatric Nursing

TABLE 5-1 Some of the Journals That Publish a Substantial Amount of Nursing Research

For example, a novice researcher working in an outpatient surgery center plans to study the incidence of patient anxiety prior to minor surgery performed in an outpatient setting, collecting data by postoperative mailed questionnaire. The assumption is that, based on the colloquial definition of minor surgery as a small, brief procedural intervention performed on someone else, the researcher expects to find that most surgical outpatients experience considerable anxiety. The researcher suspects that, for patients, the surgery is certainly not a minor event, especially in instances in which outcome is uncertain, such as biopsies.

The researcher performs a literature search and discovers that many studies have been conducted on the topic, for instance research performed in England, in which 82.4% of a sample of 674 surgical outpatients reported anxiety (Mitchell, 2012). The author also analyzed relationships between anxiety and gender, and between anxiety and type of anesthesia. The novice researcher can use these findings as evidence to support the significance of the topic, but also may decide to investigate similar variables such as gender and type of anesthesia. The researcher plans to add a few other variables, as well, based on literature review, such as number of miles from the surgery center to home, type of surgery, and whether the patient lives alone. After data collection, the researcher makes plans to review the subjects' medical records and adds biopsy results to the list of study variables, reflecting reports in the literature that indicate that the reason for outpatient surgery may affect anxiety. Because of information gained through literature review, the problem area will be slightly broadened.

Replication research. Karl Popper argued that one single experiment cannot provide definitive evidence because "non-reproducible single occurrences are of no significance to science" (Popper, 1968, p. 86). **Replication** involves repeating a research study to determine whether its findings are reproducible. Because one or two isolated small-sample studies do not constitute sufficient evidence on which to base practice, replication of previous research is a respected and essential way to advance the science of nursing.

The reason that replication is so important is that even well-conducted research can produce inaccurate findings. This is because statistical testing is based on probabilities, not certainties. In nursing research, the level of significance typically is set at $p < 0.05$ for the hypothesis testing process. This means that the researcher will allow for a 5% or lower probability of rejecting the null hypothesis when it is indeed true. When this happens, it is called a **Type I error**. The probability of accepting the null hypothesis when it is false is called a **Type II error** (Fisher, 1935). In nursing studies, the researcher usually allows a 20% or lower probability of the occurrence of a Type II error. (Chapter 21 provides further information regarding hypothesis testing, Type I error, and Type II error.)

A replication study serves several purposes besides confirmation of previous findings. It can extend generalizability if the replication study's population differs from that of the original research. If findings are similar in the replication study, they can then be applied to both populations. Replication research can improve upon the original study's methods using a more representative sample or an intervention that produces clearer results. Replication of qualitative research can lead to an expanded understanding of the phenomenon of interest, answering some of the "why" questions sparked by the original study.

Researchers who enact replications may do so because the original study's findings resonate with them and they hope to generate supportive evidence. Others are guarded in their enthusiasm, wondering whether replications with different settings or different subjects will affect the strength of the findings, and to what degree and in which direction. True skeptics may undertake a replication merely to challenge the findings or interpretations of original researchers. The occasional career researcher hones in very narrowly on a research problem area, conducting a series of sequential replication studies in order to strengthen evidence for practice.

Haller and Reynolds (1986) described several different types of replication. The first, **exact replication,** is an ideal, not a reality. In an exact replication, the replication study is identical to the original and is conducted solely to confirm the original study's results. Haller and Reynolds stated that "exact replication can be thought of as a goal that is essentially unobtainable" (p. 250) because it demands that everything be the same, including the sample, the site, and the time at which both studies are conducted. A second type, **concurrent** (or internal) **replication,** rare in nursing, is closely related because it uses a different site and, obviously, different subjects, but data collection occurs at the same time in both studies. When data collection takes place concurrently at two sites, it is far more common in nursing research for the results to be combined in one larger sample: the researchers analyze the different results in the two samples, including the combined results in one research report.

An **approximate** (or operational) **replication** is one of the two common replication strategies in nursing. Different researchers conduct the original research and the replication study adheres to the original design and methods as closely as possible. The purpose of an approximate replication is to determine whether findings are consistent "despite modest changes in research conditions" (Haller & Reynolds, 1986, p. 250), such as a different site and the subtle changes in distribution of subjects across ranges of age, culture, and gender. If replication results are consistent with the original findings, the evidence gleaned strengthens the likelihood that the results are generalizable.

If the findings generated in an approximate replication are not consistent with those of the original study, there are three possibilities: a Type I error (rejecting the null hypothesis in error) occurred in one or the other study, a Type II error (accepting the null hypothesis in error) occurred in one of the studies, or the changes in research methods such as setting and sample characteristics were responsible for the different findings. However, the reasons for the inconsistent results may not be immediately apparent. In the case of a Type I error, still another replication should be conducted. In the case of a possible Type II error, a post hoc power analysis should be conducted to determine whether the sample was too small, because that is the most common reason a Type II error occurs. If so, another replication with a larger sample should be conducted. In the third case, the methods that changed, such as constitution of the sample or nature of the setting, should be scrutinized to determine the reasons the results changed. Common sense dictates another replication in any of the three cases: more information is needed.

Systematic (or constructive) **replication,** the other common replication strategy in nursing, is conducted "under distinctly new conditions" (Haller & Reynolds, 1986, p. 250), and its goal is extension of the findings of the original study, most frequently to different settings or to clients with different disease processes. Different methods, such as means of subject selection, are common, and occasionally different research designs are employed. Successful systematic replication increases the generalizability of research findings, expanding the population to which results may be applied. An example would be an intervention to decrease anxiety, tested in various settings with diverse clients.

Even though most published nursing research does not consist of replication research, this is probably a reflection of the fact that most nursing research generated is not replication work. In 2003, Fahs, Morgan, and Kalman attributed the dearth of replication studies to various factors, among which was a decrease in the number of master's programs that required a thesis.

Over a decade later, this has been offset with a dramatic increase in doctorate of nursing practice (DNP) programs; in 2013 there were approximately three times as many DNP students as traditional doctorate of philosophy (PhD) nursing students (AACN, 2014). Although PhD dissertations usually consist of original research, in DNP programs the culminating projects, many of which include a research component, can be replication studies. This is expected to increase the number of replication studies submitted for publication.

TO SUMMARIZE: HOW TO DECIDE ON A PROBLEM AREA AND FORMULATE A PURPOSE STATEMENT

How to Decide on a Problem Area

For a new researcher, deciding on a problem area feels as final as sending out invitations to a wedding but, as it turns out, is far less stifling. As with many seemingly daunting tasks, it has identifiable steps, and there are four: (1) establish a focus by identifying one general area that is interesting, clinically or academically; (2) narrow the focus by imagining at least one general researchable topic within that area of interest; (3) find out what is known within a topic area by reviewing abstracts of research articles (and possibly skimming the discussion sections) of relevant literature; and (4) commit to discovery of what is not known by identifying a research problem area in which nursing's body of knowledge is not yet complete (Figure 5-1).

How to Formulate a Purpose Statement

Identifying a purpose statement begins with considering what is possible: (1) what is researchable, (2) which methodology is suitable, (3) whether plans are realistic, and (4) what is reasonable. The latter of these two considerations includes feasibility issues (Figure 5-2).

What Is Researchable

Some things cannot be known. "What is the meaning of life?" is not a researchable question, as stated. "To what degree does childhood loss of a parent to suicide cause adult depression?" is not, either, because familial depression may cloud the results. "How will early childhood sensory reintegration programs enable autistic persons to work and to live independently in 2035?" is still a matter of conjecture, and possibly science fiction (Moon, 2005). Although it is researchable, the question "In identical twins, what effect does showing systematic preference to one twin over the other have upon longitudinal growth in humans?" would not be approved, because of ethical considerations.

For a quantitative purpose and its related question to be researchable, the concepts or variables to be studied and their relational statement must be tangible, well-expressed, and ultimately measurable. For a qualitative purpose and its related question to be researchable, the ideas studied must be able to be expressed by the participants or observed by the researcher. Examples of researchable questions are: "Does an informational liaison between the surgical suite and the patient waiting

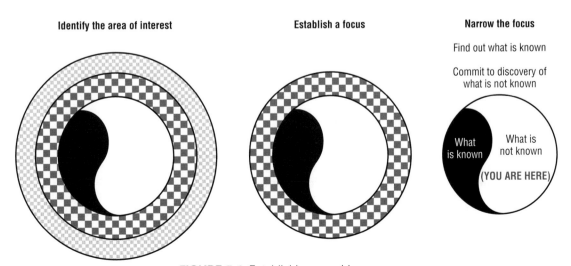

Identify the area of interest

Establish a focus

Narrow the focus

Find out what is known

Commit to discovery of what is not known

What is known

What is not known

(YOU ARE HERE)

FIGURE 5-1 Establishing a problem area.

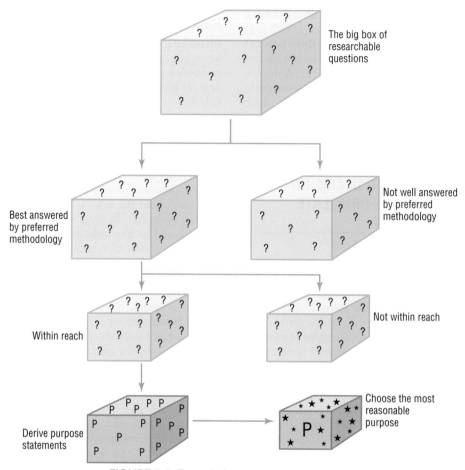

FIGURE 5-2 Formulating a purpose statement.

area increase families' satisfaction with the operative experience?" and "How do parents of toddlers hospitalized with pneumonia cope with the experience?"

Within your preferred problem area, now, formulate several research questions, ones to which you really would like answers and that are researchable.

Which Methodology Is Suitable

Both quantitative and qualitative methodologies have their limitations in terms of what research purposes they can address. Only concepts that can be measured can be studied quantitatively. If quantitative methodology is to be used, the elements of the concept being measured must be able to be measured, classified, or counted in some way. Quantitative methodologies do not lend themselves to philosophy or theology: whether or not dogs go to heaven is not a suitable area of inquiry for quantitative methodology. On a more concrete level,

to investigate quantitatively whether patients know whether their nurses like them or not, or are just faking sincerity while caring for them, and what nursing actions are perceived as evidence of caring and why, would be measurable by printed survey, but would be much more interesting and informative as a qualitative study.

Qualitatively speaking, anything is researchable, but some of these inquiries produce data decidedly less valuable than quantitative research could provide. For example, qualitative questions about the cost of one day's hospital stay in a community hospital, as opposed to a teaching hospital, would yield subjects' perceptions and opinions, whereas actual facts would be required to investigate this topic adequately. For patients after bariatric surgery, if the research purpose were to determine how many ounces of fluid the patients can drink without discomfort, this requires more than perceptions and opinions: quantitative measurement is the most meaningful way to address the research purpose.

Because the stated research purpose implies a methodology, the researcher must determine which methodology is to be used: quantitative, qualitative, or a combination. Then, the research purpose can be worded so that it is consistent with the desired methodology.

At this point, decide whether the few questions you have formulated in the problem area are best studied quantitatively or qualitatively (see Figure 5-2). If you have a preference for a quantitative versus a qualitative methodology, discard the ones that are not answerable by the preferred methodology.

Whether the Plans are Realistic

Although Browning (1895) observed that one's reach should exceed one's grasp, this is not necessarily the case when planning one's first research project. The researcher's grasp (see Figure 5-2) encompasses the realities of the research: actual access, individual aptitudes, mastery of the research process, and available support. For a thesis or dissertation, this is an essential question: what is realistically within my grasp?

When crafting a quantitative purpose, the researcher's ability to collect data is critical to consider. The research purpose should include only concepts that are measurable through access the researcher expects to have. Unless a researcher can arrange to have site access, for instance, an onsite project is impossible. Unless a researcher can obtain access to a preexistent data set, quantitative analysis of that set is not possible. If site access is granted only grudgingly, the researcher must assess the extent to which the agency will cooperate with the researcher. An unwilling manager, or unwilling staff, can make data collection difficult.

In a similar vein, access to adequate numbers of subjects is crucial. Suppose a clinic in a specialty area has only nine clients with the diagnosis that is the focus of proposed research. If quantitative analysis is planned with at least 30 subjects, additional sites for data collection must be pursued, or the design of the study altered. The research purpose must be reworded accordingly.

Mastery is an issue in settling on a research purpose. Conducting interviews in small villages in Nepal is not within the researcher's grasp, in terms of mastery, unless the researcher can speak Nepali or hire a full-time interpreter.

By the same token, if the researcher cannot speak the language of research, and has not mastered intricate research design, implementing a complex mixed methods study that uses new measurement tools devised specifically for the study, the researcher must have the support of a faculty member or nurse researcher familiar with the intricacies of these methodological tasks. The same applies for data analysis: the researcher must know how to perform statistical analyses if they are required by the research design, or be willing to employ a statistician. A faculty member or nurse researcher can provide a frank assessment as to whether the study proposal, as written, is a realistic goal.

At this point, take stock of your capabilities and review your options. Revise the list of potential research questions you have constructed, discarding those that are not realistically within your grasp.

What Is Reasonable

Somewhere between identification of a research problem and articulation of a purpose, the researcher must consider whether the envisioned study has even a remote chance of completion within the reasonable bounds of time and space. The principal questions that must be pondered relate to funding, time, subject recruitment, and ethical approval.

Funding is a consideration for most researchers. Unless money is no object, an extended six-month period living in London to conduct interviews with retired nurses about practice beliefs and trends in English hospitals, is not within the researcher's financial reach. If research requires specialized equipment for collection of physiological data, and the equipment cannot be used without charge, the amount a company will charge for rental will determine whether a study is feasible. However, other costs often are overlooked when a study is planned. All expenditures, including supplies, clinical lab charges, printed copies of copyrighted tools and scales, purchased data sets, equipment, mailing costs, researcher travel, parking, a statistician's fee, possibly the services of a typist, and subjects' fees or gifts (if any) for participation, must be tabulated ahead of time.

Approximate time for project completion should be decided upon in advance. The scope of a reasonable research project, especially for the novice researcher, must be consistent with completion of every step of the process within the allotted time. For theses and dissertations, the allotted time may be as short as a year. During that time, the student writes the research proposal for approval from academic review panels and IRBs, establishes agreements with a healthcare agency for access to subjects and data, recruits and consents subjects for participation, collects data, analyzes data, interprets the study findings, and writes the thesis or dissertation, according to the requirements of the university. The final step, revision of the manuscript into a publishable article or articles, may take quite a bit longer.

For a graduate student, it is important to limit the scope of the first research project so that it is manageable. A large, complex research purpose, with multiple variables and intricate methods of measurement and data analysis, cannot be completed reasonably in a small, set amount of time. A new researcher, quite properly, wants to know everything. It is difficult to limit that desire to knowing just a small portion of all the fascinating questions that pertain to the problem area. Trimming the purpose is important, however, because a large-scope research purpose commits a researcher to a lengthy period of data collection, data analysis, and interpretation. A good rule of thumb for a first study is to limit the anticipated time needed for collection, analysis, and interpretation of the data to a maximum of 6 months. Especially if the work is embedded in a graduate program, finishing is the goal.

Potential for difficulties recruiting subjects can lead to further amendments of the purpose statement. If the proposed research is such that potential subjects with an uncommon diagnosis will prove difficult to recruit, changes in the research methodology or design, or expansion of the problem to include patients with related diagnoses, may be necessary. Performing a pilot study is crucial in order to determine the approximate refusal rate by potential subjects. If very few subjects agree to participate, the purpose and even the problem area may have to be revisited and refined.

Gaining ethical approval by an IRB can require revision of the study purpose. In interventional quantitative research, some interventions may be questioned if they have the potential to cause disease, interfere with usual treatment, or use subjects that are currently involved in other approved research. For qualitative studies especially, the committee may determine that some topics encroach upon "overly sensitive areas" and should be excluded from the interview script. Usually, these changes do not require crafting a different study purpose, but they can lead to revisions in the purpose statement.

If you are still unable to decide on the study purpose, write out each potential research purpose statement. Each purpose should specify the study population and should imply a methodology and, for quantitative research, should hint at a design. Objectively investigate which of the listed study purposes are actually feasible, considering access to subjects and data, subject availability, funding required to complete the research, and time required to complete the research versus time available. Make certain of study feasibility. Usually one

of the study purposes will appeal to you more than the others, because of its clinical applicability, or its importance to wellness. If none is preferred, choose the one that is achievable in the most reasonable amount of time (see Figure 5-2).

In truth, feasibility issues can plunge a novice researcher back into the iterative process for refinement of purpose and sometimes even problem area. Although this process may consume more time than desired, rethinking and refining are vastly preferable to discovering mid-study that the research cannot be completed.

EXAMPLES OF RESEARCH TOPICS, PROBLEMS, AND PURPOSES FOR DIFFERENT TYPES OF RESEARCH

Quantitative Research

Quantitative research reports contain problems and purposes that reflect the different foci of each type of quantitative research. Examples from published research of topics, problems, and purposes for the four principal types of quantitative research are presented in Table 5-2. The research purpose often hints at the type of quantitative design that will be chosen, by use of words like effect, association, and identification.

Descriptive research measures prevalence: of a single variable, of the characteristics within populations, of two different variables that may or may not be related, of groups within a population, and so forth. For example, Curtis and Glacken (2014) conducted descriptive research of Irish public health nurses' job satisfaction. They used a national survey to collect data about job satisfaction and contributing factors. The authors found that low levels of satisfaction characterized their subjects. The subjects attributed their low levels of satisfaction to pay and to task-related activities. Professional status, interaction, and autonomy were found to be contributory to high levels of satisfaction.

Correlational research measures connections between ideas, and the direction (positive or negative) and strength of those connections. In their correlational study, Burk, Grap, Munro, Schubert, and Sessler (2014b) examined the relationships between ICU patients' development of agitation and various demographic and clinical characteristics. Agitation was identified as an issue because of its potential for fostering clinically adverse happenings. The authors measured relationships between agitation and many other preexistent factors, attempting to identify variables that would predict agitation in ICUs. The strongest clinical predictor of agitation present on admission was the use of restraints; the strongest demographic predictor of agitation 24 hours before the event was psychiatric diagnosis.

Both quasi-experimental research and experimental research are conducted to establish evidence for a cause-and-effect relationship: whether the independent variable appears to be effective in causing a change in the dependent variable. An example of a quasi-experimental study is Ramadi, Stickland, Rodgers, and Haennel's (2015) research, conducted to address a knowledge gap of whether an exercise intervention would improve physical activity of a specific group of patients. The rehabilitation program proved to be effective in some respects.

An example of experimental research is Shelton, Freeman, Fish, Bachman, and Richardson's (2015) study designed to address the research problem of whether computer-based education might improve surrogates' knowledge about the informed consent process for genomics research. The results indicated that the authors' experimental method of instruction by computer module was superior to the usual method in terms of surrogate decision makers' understanding of 8 of the 13 elements of informed consent.

Qualitative Research

Qualitative research reports contain problems and purposes. Examples from published research of topics, problems, and purposes for the five principal types of qualitative research discussed in this text are presented in Table 5-3. As with quantitative studies, the qualitative research purpose sometimes hints at the study design. It is not uncommon for the title of a qualitative study to mention the name of the methodology or design that the study employs.

Phenomenological research investigates participants' experiences, and often the meaning those experiences hold for them. Problem statements and purpose statements reflect this emphasis on participants' experiences. Trauma nurses are exposed to tragedy and the effects of violence on a daily basis. Freeman, Fothergill-Bourbonnais, and Rashotte (2014) conducted a phenomenological study to explore their experiences in this professional role. Within the essential theme of seeing through cloudy situations, the authors identified four sub-theme clusters that characterized the work of being a trauma nurse: (1) being on guard all the time, (2) being caught up short, (3) facing the challenge, and (4) sharing the journey. The recurrent issues of fear and workplace violence lace through the sub themes.

Grounded theory research investigates a human process within a sociological focus, and some grounded theory research produces theory. Problem statements and purpose statements identify the shared human process and sometimes the intention to generate theory. In their study, entitled "Advancing adolescent maternal development: A grounded theory," Atkinson and Peden-McAlpine (2014) presented substantive theory, grounded in data obtained from 30 public health nurses. Data collection was accomplished through email communication or telephone communication, in which the public health nurses related their accounts of how public health nursing interventions assist in promoting maternal development in at-risk adolescents. Examples of behaviors of incomplete, intermediate, and advanced maternal development were provided and integrated into a theoretical model. Case management was used extensively, to promote client self-efficacy.

Ethnographic research examines individuals within cultures, identifying the membership requirements, expected behaviors, enacted behaviors, and rules of the shared culture. The problem statement and purpose statement identify the culture of interest. These cultures can be actual societal groups, loose associations of persons sharing common experiences, or unconnected individuals who share a common experience. The latter is the case in Higham and Davies' (2013) study, conducted to explore fathers' experiences when their children were hospitalized. The results described fathers' roles in times of sudden acute child illness. Results included: "Fathers were observed undertaking a range of protective behaviours and discussed the importance of protecting their children and partners" (p. 1393); "Providing has long been regarded as central to the father role. In this study providing behaviours included: ensuring that others' needs were met, providing care, and working" (p. 1394); and "Most of the fathers discussed how they and the child's mother had participated in the overall care of the ill child and wider family. Fathers participated by: sharing the caring, assisting with clinical care, and in decision-making" (p. 1395).

Exploratory-descriptive qualitative research is the broad term that includes qualitative descriptive work in which a specific methodology is not mentioned as serving as a foundation for the study. Problem statements and purpose statements often address the desire to increase knowledge of a process or situation. An example is Pettersson, Hedström, and Höglund's (2014) study of nurses' experiences with, and perceptions of, do-not-resuscitate orders. The inquiry was accomplished through "a qualitative descriptive methodology" (p. 902). The authors listed their findings as, "the nurses strived for good nursing care through balancing harms and goods and observing integrity and quality of life as

TABLE 5-2   Quantitative Research: Topics, Problems, and Purposes

Type of Research	Research Topic	Research Problem and Purpose
Descriptive research	Irish public health nurses' job satisfaction; demographics and job factors that are contributory	*Title of study:* "Job satisfaction among public health nurses: A national survey" (Curtis & Glacken, 2014, p. 653) *Problem:* "Research on job satisfaction continues to increase. A computer search undertaken on PsycINFO using the keywords *job satisfaction* in 2004 produced 18,600 papers and dissertations while a similar search in 2010 yielded 27,458 documents. Evidence also suggests several correlates of job satisfaction. Notable among these are absenteeism and turnover (Cohen & Golan 2007; Jones 2008), productivity (Lin et al., 2009; Westover et al., 2009; Whitman et al., 2010), commitment to care (Baernholdt & Mark, 2009) and emotional stress (Ruggiero, 2005). Despite this growing interest, however, relatively few studies have explored job satisfaction among public health nurses (PHNs). Those that have indicate that the main stressors predictive of high levels of job dissatisfaction include demands of the job, lack of communication, changing working environment, and career development (Doncevic et al., 1998; Kolkman et al., 1998; Rout Rani, 2000). Job dissatisfaction suggests a problem in either the job or the person and it is important that managers assess their organisations to identify the root of the problem." (Curtis & Glacken, 2014, pp. 653–654) *Purpose:* The purpose of this study was "'to establish current level of job satisfaction among public health nurses and identify the main contributing variables/factors to job satisfaction among this population …'" (Curtis & Glacken, 2014, p. 653)
Correlational research	Agitation, critical care, predictors on admission, predictors 24 hours before onset of agitation	*Title of study:* "Predictors of agitation in critically ill adults" (Burk, Grap, Munro, Schubert, & Sessler, 2014b) *Problem:* "One of the more frequent complications in the intensive care unit (ICU) is agitation. Agitation is associated with poorer outcomes, including longer ICU stay, longer duration of mechanical ventilation, higher rate of self-extubation, increased use of resources, and increased ICU costs (Burk et al., 2014a; Fraser, Prato, Riker, Berthiaume, & Wilkins, 2000; Gardner, Sessler, & Grap, 2006; Jaber et al., 2005; Woods et al., 2004). Studies (Fraser, Prato, Riker, Berthiaume, & Wilkins, 2000; Gardner, Sessler, & Grap, 2006; Jaber et al., 2005; Sessler, Rutherford, Best, Hart, & Levenson, 1992; Woods et al., 2004) indicate that 42% to 71% of critically ill patients experience agitation. Recognizing the impact of agitation, the Society of Critical Care Medicine recently updated its sedation and analgesia guidelines (Barr et al., 2013) to include agitation, emphasizing the need for prompt identification of this complication. Potential causes of agitation in critically ill patients are numerous; however, data on factors predictive of agitation are limited. Because agitation is often identified after overtly agitated behavior is observed, a critical barrier to progress has been the lack of identification of the precursors of agitation. Empirically based information would help care providers identify patients at risk for agitation and also predict agitation, providing an opportunity to implement preventive strategies." (Burk et al., 2014b, p. 415) *Purpose:* "The purpose of this study was to examine the relationship between demographic and clinical characteristics of critically ill patients in the development of agitation." (Burk et al., 2014b, p. 415)

TABLE 5-2   Quantitative Research: Topics, Problems, and Purposes—cont'd

Type of Research	Research Topic	Research Problem and Purpose
Quasi-experimental research	Supervised exercise rehabilitation program, cardiopulmonary patients, possible improvement in amount of daily exercise	*Title of study:* "Impact of supervised exercise rehabilitation on daily physical activity of cardiopulmonary patients" (Ramadi, Stickland, Rodgers, & Haennel, 2015, p. 9) *Problem:* "It is well known that there is an inverse linear relationship between amount of aerobic physical activity (PA) and mortality in patients with cardiopulmonary disorders. In fact, regular aerobic PA of moderate to vigorous intensity has been associated with a lower risk of all-cause mortality, respiratory-related hospitalizations and mortality, as well as the incidence of and mortality from cardiovascular disease (Garber et al., 2011; Garcia-Aymerich, Lange, Benet, Schnohr & Antó, 2006; Haapanen, Miilunpalo, Vuori, Oja, & Pasanen, 1996; Haennel & Lemire, 2002; Leon, Connett, Jacobs, & Rauramaa, 1987). Consequently, aerobic PA is considered a core component of cardiopulmonary rehabilitation programs (American Association of Cardiopulmonary Resuscitation, 1999; Nici et al., 2006). While an improved exercise capacity is considered one of the benchmark outcomes associated with completion of an exercise rehabilitation (ER) program (Lacasse, Martin, Lasserson, & Goldstein, 2007; Maines et al., 1997), research suggests that this increased exercise capacity may not be indicative of a more active lifestyle following completion of the ER program (van den Berg-Emons, Balk, Bussmann & Stam, 2004). Indeed the impact of ER programs on the objectively measured quantity and quality of daily PA in cardiopulmonary patients is not completely understood." (Ramadi et al., 2015, p. 9) *Purpose:* "Therefore, the purpose of this study was to use a multisensor device to objectively assess the impact of a supervised ER program on the quantity and quality of daily PA of patients with cardiopulmonary disorders." (Ramadi et al., 2015, p. 9)
Experimental research	Computer-based education module for family members, relative to informed consent for genomics research, family understanding of the process for, and elements of, informed consent	*Title of study:* "A computer-based education intervention to enhance surrogates' informed consent for genomics research" (Shelton, Freeman, Fish, Bachman, & Richardson, 2015, p. 149) *Problem:* "Patients in the intensive care unit (ICU) often are unable to give informed consent because of cognitive or physical impairments due to illness, trauma, or sedation (Arnold & Kellum, 2003, Luce et al., 2004). In such circumstances, a patient's family member or proxy is asked to serve as a surrogate and provide informed consent on behalf of the patient (Bein, 1991; Coppolino & Ackerson, 2001). With increasing frequency, surrogates of ICU patients are being asked to provide consent for crucial genomics research (Cobb & O'Keefe, 2004; Luce, 2003). This type of research has an immediate aspect (Freeman et al., 2012; Freeman et al., 2010); any delay in consent for enrollment in the study may result in a missed opportunity to collect transient and perhaps vital clinical data (Harvey, Elbourne, Ashcroft, Jones, & Rowan (2006); Luce, 2009). Furthermore, genomics research is complex and has inherent ethical, legal, and social implications (Collins, Green, Guttmacher, & Guyer, 2003; Collins, 2007). Without a basic understanding of the process of informed consent related to genomics research, surrogates may be poorly prepared to consent for their loved ones to participate in the studies (Azoulay et al., 2005). … The computer-based educational interventions used in [various] studies included video, CD-ROM, and slide presentations, yet no single approach has been more effective than another (Campbell, Goldman, Boccia, & Skinner, 2004)." (Shelton et al., 2015, p. 149) *Purpose:* "The purpose of this pilot study was to examine the effectiveness of a new, computer-based education module on the understanding of patients' surrogates about the process of informed consent for genomics research in the ICU." (Shelton et al., 2015, p. 149)

TABLE 5-3 Qualitative Research: Topics, Problems, and Purposes

Type of Research	Research Topic	Research Problem and Purpose
Phenomenological research	The work of being a trauma nurse, the meaning of being a trauma nurse, what trauma nurses find rewarding in their practice, what difficulties they encounter, the factors that facilitate or hinder being a trauma nurse	*Title of study:* "The experience of being a trauma nurse: A phenomenological study" (Freeman, Fothergill-Bourbonnais, & Rashotte, 2014) *Problem:* "In 2008–2009, over 14,000 patients were hospitalised with a major injury across eight provinces that contributed data to the Canadian National Trauma Registry Comprehensive Data Set (Canadian Institute of Health Information, 2011). Of these cases, 11% died, either in the emergency department or after admission to hospital. Patients with these injuries spent over 212,000 hospital days in the participating facilities, with an average length of stay of 15 days. Trauma nurses are faced with the challenge of meeting the cognitive, physical and emotional demands of patients with major traumatic injuries (Von Rueden, 1991). They need to be knowledgeable about mechanisms of injury and potential complications; they are challenged to frequently and suddenly alter their nursing care priorities because patients' needs and physiological status often change quickly. They also require skill in helping families work through the stress and emotional devastation that accompanies a sudden severe injury. Despite daily exposure to patient and family crisis situations with the emotional toll this may take (Von Rueden et al., 2010), patients and families perceive that trauma nurses demonstrate caring behaviours (Clukey et al., 2009; Hayes & Tyler-Ball, 2007). Only a few studies have attempted to examine trauma nursing and these were conducted within an emergency department context (Clukey et al., 2009; Curtis, 2001; Morse and Proctor, 1998). No studies were found that examined trauma nursing within a trauma unit context or that explored the meaning of being a trauma nurse." (Freeman et al., 2014, p. 7) *Purpose:* "The purpose of this study was to explore the lived experience of being a trauma nurse in a designated trauma unit." (Freeman et al., 2014, p. 7)
Grounded theory research	Adolescent maternal development, theory generation based on data, foundational theory to support nursing care of pregnant and parenting adolescents	*Title of study:* "Advancing adolescent maternal development: A grounded theory" (Atkinson & Peden-McAlpine, 2014) *Problem:* "More than 80 percent of teen pregnancies are unplanned (Finer & Henshaw, 2006). Compared to older mothers, adolescent mothers and their children have higher rates of adverse health and social outcomes including infant morbidity and mortality, preterm birth, low birth weight, unintentional injuries, failure to complete high school, and poverty (Chen et al., 2005; Folkes-Skinner & Meredith, 1997; Flynn, 1999; Flynn, Budd, & Modelski, 2008; Koniak-Griffin & Turner-Pluta, 2001; Koniak-Griffin, Anderson, Verzemnieks, & Brecht, 2000; Koniak-Griffin et al., 2003; Nguyen, Carson, Parris, & Place, 2003). The birth rate for adolescent females age 15–19 years began to rise in 2005, reaching 42.5 births per 1000 in the U.S. in 2007 (Centers for Disease Control & Prevention [CDC], 2010). Beginning in 2007, the birth rate for adolescent females age 15–19 years began to decline, reaching 33.3 births per 1000 women in 2011 (CDC, 2012). Research supporting a theoretical basis for the nursing care of pregnant and parenting adolescents is lacking in the literature. The weak theoretical base for the public health nursing care of pregnant and parenting adolescents, the high rate of unintended adolescent pregnancies, and the poor health and social outcomes associated with adolescent pregnancy provide firm incentives for researchers to develop a stronger evidence-base for public health nursing practice intended to improve adolescent pregnancy outcomes." (Atkinson & Peden-McAlpine, 2014, p. 168) *Purpose:* "The purpose of this study was to identify the problems, challenges, and needs specific to pregnant and parenting adolescents in a state public health nurse (PHN) home visiting program, and to determine the process by which these problems, challenges, and needs are resolved within the context of the program." (Atkinson & Peden-McAlpine, 2014, p. 168)

TABLE 5-3   Qualitative Research: Topics, Problems, and Purposes—cont'd

Type of Research	Research Topic	Research Problem and Purpose
Ethnography research	Fathers' roles during their child's unplanned acute care hospitalization, expected cultural roles of fathers during children's hospitalization	*Title of study:* "Protecting, providing, and participating: Fathers' roles during their child's unplanned hospital stay, an ethnographic study" (Higham & Davies, 2013, pp. 1390–1391). *Problem:* "There has been a global trend in recent decades for fathers to become more involved in all aspects of their children's lives (Lamb 2000, Flouri 2005), including health care. In recent years, fathers' experiences in relation to childhood long-term illness have been investigated, including diabetes (Sullivan-Bolyai et al., 2006), cancer (McGrath & Chesler, 2004), and kidney disease (Swallow et al., 2011), in addition to neonatal and paediatric intensive care (Board 2004). Whilst research concerning fathers has increased, Isacco and Garfield (2010) claim that healthcare research with fathers has focused on severe and atypical situations. Mothers' and fathers' experiences have been compared in relation to long-term illness (for example Hobson & Noyes, 2011) and planned surgery (Tourigny et al., 2004), but little research has addressed fathers in short stay acute inpatient care. Yet in England, 7% of children experience an inpatient stay annually, the majority unplanned (Shribman 2007), with increasing rates of emergency admissions and decreasing lengths of stay (Department of Health, 2009)." (Higham & Davies, 2013, pp. 1390–1391) *Purpose:* "The purpose of this study was therefore to explore fathers' experiences following their child's unplanned admission to hospital." (Higham & Davies, 2013, p. 1391)
Exploratory-descriptive qualitative research	Nurses' experiences of Do Not Resuscitate orders, oncology and hematology patients at end-of-life, nurses' involvement in decision-making, nurses' involvement in ongoing discussion	*Title of study:* "Striving for good nursing care: Nurses' experiences of do not resuscitate orders within oncology and hematology care" (Pettersson, Hedström, & Höglund, 2014, p. 902) *Problem:* "DNR orders are important to study within oncology and hematology care, as they are frequently made, yet often a difficult decision to make. Although studies of DNR decisions within oncology and hematology units have been performed in some countries (Jezewski & Finnell, 1998; Kim et al., 2007; Levin et al., 2008; Olver & Eliott, 2008), Swedish studies on the subject are scarce. In particular, research focusing on the specific role of the nurse in relation to these decisions is lacking." (Pettersson et al., 2014, p. 904) *Purpose:* "The aim of this study was to investigate hematology and oncology nurses' experiences and perceptions of DNR orders, in order to achieve a deeper understanding of the nurses' specific role in these decisions." (Pettersson et al., 2014, p. 904)
Historical research	Early twentieth-century New Zealand, the sick poor, the "deserving" poor, home-care nursing of the chronically ill poor	*Title of study:* "Sunless lives': District nurses' and journalists' co-construction of the 'sick poor' as a vulnerable population in early twentieth-century New Zealand" (Wood & Arcus, 2012) *Problem:* "A generic definition of vulnerable populations, such as those offered by Flaskerud and Winslow (1998) and Mechanic and Tanner (2007), focus on factors that differentiate one group from another in terms of life expectancy, mortality and morbidity, noting in particular the impact of few resources and increased risk. Precisely how these factors are configured to identify vulnerable populations, however, varies in different locations and time periods (Flaskerud et al., 2002). We become so used to current situations and our own contexts that it is difficult to recognise the process at work in constructing a population group as vulnerable. Considering how social groups in past times were characterised as vulnerable offers this fresh perspective." (Wood & Arcus, 2012, p. 145) *Purpose:* "… the intention of this research was therefore to identify the meaning of vulnerability as a term associated with the sick poor …" (Wood & Arcus, 2012, p. 145)

important values." (p. 902). Hindrances the nurses experienced in their goal for providing good care were "unclear and poorly documented decisions, uninformed patients and relatives, and disagreements among the caregivers and family" (p. 902). The nurses in the study expressed a need for an ongoing discussion on do-not-resuscitate decisions, "including all concerned parties" (p. 902).

Historical research tells a story of the past, from the point of view of persons living in the time during which the research was conducted. In keeping with that particular orientation, purposes in historical research usually focus on a definite time but, beyond that, can scrutinize everything from a person or an event, to a public building, or even a discussion of the new meaning of a word or expression. Exemplifying the last, Wood and Arcus (2012) conducted historical research to clarify the concept "sick poor" and its implication of vulnerability, in early twentieth-century New Zealand. The research revealed that the term was intended to identify a subgroup of the poor with chronic conditions, the so-called "deserving" poor, who needed help on an ongoing basis from the newly created district nursing services. In addition, charitable groups provided assistance and, eventually, hired nurses for the work. Nurses wrote essays for a newspaper, *Kai Tiaki*, describing their work with clients who were clearly in need of assistance. All of this was important in establishing the new face of

worthiness on the part of the poor, as opposed to the more traditional Anglo-Saxon position that the poor were unmotivated and unwilling to help themselves.

Mixed Methods Research

Mixed methods research reports contain problems and purposes that reflect the combined approach of two methods. In Table 5-4, an example is presented of the topic, problem, and purpose for Beischel's (2013) mixed methods study of student characteristics and anxiety in a high-fidelity simulation (HFS) learning environment. Please note that, as is the case in some mixed methods reports, after a single purpose statement, Beischel (2013) provided two purpose statements, one quantitative and the other qualitative. Each represented a different arm of the study. The quantitative design for the research was quasi-experimental, and the qualitative design was exploratory-descriptive. The exploratory-descriptive design is used frequently in mixed methods studies. Beischel's (2013) research resulted in modification of the theoretical model tested in the quantitative portion of the study. Student anxiety was found not to be statistically significant in affecting cognitive learning outcomes in the HFS environment. However, the qualitative phase of the study revealed that despite the lack of statistically significant quantitative findings, students perceived that anxiety did indeed "negatively affect their learning and ability to perform" (Beischel, 2013, p. 240).

TABLE 5-4   Mixed Methods Research: Topics, Problems, and Purposes

Type of Research	Research Topic	Research Problem and Purpose
Mixed methods research (explanatory sequential design: model-testing with structural equation modeling, followed by exploratory-descriptive qualitative)	The relationships among students' learning and lifestyle characteristics, learning styles, cognitive learning outcomes, and anxiety state, during a high-fidelity simulation (HFS) experience; students' explanations of these factors	*Title of study:* "Variables affecting learning in a simulation experience: A mixed methods study" (Beischel, 2013, p. 226) *Problem:* "… health education scholars are calling for research to determine the effectiveness of using high-fidelity simulation (HFS) as a teaching method. Yet, before empirically determining the efficacy of simulation, it is important to explore variables with potential to affect the educational outcome of simulation experiences. The literature suggests that there are many variables that affect learning such as environment, nutrition, emotions, gender, sleep, culture, learning styles, and previous learning experiences … However, there are no studies to date examining variables affecting learning in a simulated environment." (Beischel, 2013) *Purpose:* "The primary purpose of this study was to test a hypothesized model describing the direct effects of learning variables on anxiety and cognitive learning outcomes in a high-fidelity simulation (HFS) experience. The secondary purpose was to explain and explore student perceptions concerning the qualities and context of HFS affecting anxiety and learning. (Beischel, 2013)

TABLE 5-5	Outcomes Research: Topics, Problems, and Purposes	
Type of Research	**Research Topic**	**Research Problem and Purpose**
Outcomes research (quasi-experimental in design)	Non-ventilator hospital-acquired pneumonia rates before and after the intervention of enhanced basic oral nursing care	*Title of study:* "Basic nursing care to prevent nonventilator hospital-acquired pneumonia" (Quinn et al., 2014, p. 11) *Problem:* "Nonventilator hospital-aquired pneumonia (NV-HAP) is an underreported and understudied disease, with potential for measurable outcomes, fiscal savings, and improvement in quality of life ... U.S. hospitals are required to monitor ventilator-associated pneumonia; however, there are currently no requirements to monitor NV-HAP. The limited studies available indicate that NV-HAP is an emerging factor in prolonged hospital stays and significant patient morbidity and mortality ..." (Quinn et al., 2014, p. 11) *Purpose:* "The purpose of our study was to (a) identify the incidence of NV-HAP in a convenience sample of U.S. hospitals and (b) determine the effectiveness of reliably delivered basic oral nursing care in reducing NV-HAP." (Quinn et al., 2014, p. 11)

Outcomes Research

Reports of outcomes studies contain problems and purposes that are almost identical to those found in quantitative research. The exception is that sometimes the word "outcomes" is included in the purpose statement. In Table 5-5, an example is presented of the topic, problem, and purpose for Quinn et al.'s (2014) outcomes research study of the effectiveness of enhanced oral care in the prevention of non-ventilator-associated pneumonia (NVAP) in hospitalized patients. The study design was quasi-experimental. The overall incidence of NVAP at four inpatient hospital facilities decreased by 37% after the intervention of enhanced oral care was initiated.

▌ KEY POINTS

- A research problem is an area in which there is a gap in nursing's knowledge base. The typical research problem includes background, a problem statement, and a justification for the significance of research in the area.
- The major source for nursing research problems is clinical nursing practice. Other good sources are discussions with peers, review of professional journals, and research priorities identified by specialty groups and professional organizations. Theories are fruitful sources for research problems for experienced researchers.
- Replication is essential for the development of evidence-based knowledge for practice and consists of four types: exact, approximate, concurrent, and systematic.

- The research purpose is the stated reason for conduct of a study. The purpose usually hints at whether the study will be interventional or noninterventional, and sometimes at the study design. Typically it mentions the population and the study's variables or factors of interest.
- Once the research purpose is decided upon, the research question can be formulated. If appropriate, a research hypothesis can then be developed to further direct the study.
- The feasibility of research problem and purpose is determined by access to research subjects and data, availability of sufficient numbers of willing potential subjects, researcher expertise or ability to collaborate with knowledgeable others, financial resources that will cover the costs of the study, sufficient time for study completion, a manageable-sized purpose, and ethical approval from human subjects committees.
- If a purpose and problem present major feasibility concerns, the wise researcher revisits the iterative process and redesigns the study.

REFERENCES

AACN. (2015). *AACN's research vision and mission.* Retrieved February 16, 2016 from http://www.aacn.org/wd/practice/content/research/research-mission-and-vision.content?menu=practice.

AACN. (2014). *Annual Report 2014.* American Association of Colleges of Nursing. Retrieved February 16, 2016 from http://www.aacn.nche.edu/aacn-publications/annual-reports/AnnualReport14.pdf.

Agency for Healthcare Research and Quality. (2015). *AHRQ research funding priorities and special emphasis notices.* Retrieved February

16, 2016 from http://www.ahrq.gov/funding/priorities-contacts/special-emphasis-notices/index.html.

American Association of Cardiopulmonary Resuscitation (1999). *Guidelines for cardiac rehabilitation and secondary prevention programs* (Vol. 3). Champaign, IL: Human Kinetics.

American Nurses Credentialing Center (ANCC). (2015). *Magnet© Program: Overview.* Retrieved May 16, 2015 from http://www.nursecredentialing.org/Magnet/ProgramOverview.

Arnold, R. M., & Kellum, J. (2003). Moral justifications for surrogate decision making in the intensive care unit: Implications and limitations. *Critical Care Medicine, 31*(5), S347–S353.

Atkinson, L. D., & Peden-McAlpine, C. J. (2014). Advancing adolescent maternal development: A grounded theory. *Journal of Pediatric Nursing, 29*(2), 168–176.

Azoulay, E., Pochard, F., Kentish-Barnes, N., Chevray, S., Aboab, J., Adrie, C., et al., FAMIREA Study Group (2005). Risk of post-traumatic stress symptoms in family members of intensive care unit patients. *American Journal of Respiratory and Critical Care Medicine, 171*(9), 987–994.

Baernholdt, M., & Mark, B. A. (2009). The nurse work environment, job satisfaction and turnover rates in rural and urban nursing units. *Journal of Nursing Management, 17*(8), 994–1001.

Barr, J., Fraser, G. L., Puntillo, K., Ely, E. W., Gélinas, C., Dasta, J. F., et al. (2013). Clinical practice guidelines for the management of pain, agitation, and delirium in adult patients in the intensive care unit. *Critical Care Medicine, 41*(1), 263–306.

Bein, P. M. (1991). Surrogate consent and the incompetent experimental subject. *Food, Drug, Cosmetic Law Journal, 46*(5), 739–771.

Beischel, K. P. (2013). Variables affecting learning in a simulation experience: A mixed methods study. *Western Journal of Nursing Research, 35*(2), 226–247.

Beukelman, D., Garrett, K., & Yorkston, K. (2007). *Augmentative communication strategies for adults with acute or chronic medical conditions.* Baltimore, MD: Paul H. Brookes Publishing Co.

Board, R. (2004). Father stress during a child's critical care hospitalization. *Journal of Pediatric Health Care, 18*(5), 244–249.

Browning, R. (1895). *The complete poetic and dramatic works of Robert Browning. "Andrea del Sarto."* Boston: Houghton Mifflin and Company.

Burk, R. S., Grap, M. J., Munro, C. L., Schubert, C. M., & Sessler, C. N. (2014a). Agitation onset, frequency, and associated temporal factors in the adult critically ill. *American Journal of Critical Care, 23*(4), 296–304.

Burk, R. S., Grap, M. J., Munro, C. L., Schubert, C. M., & Sessler, C. N. (2014b). Predictors of agitation in critically ill adults. *American Journal of Critical Care, 23*(5), 414–422.

Campbell, F. A., Goldman, B. D., Boccia, M. L., & Skinner, M. (2004). The effect of format modifications and reading comprehension on recall of informed consent information by low-income parents: A comparison of print, video, and computer-based presentations. *Patient Education Counseling, 53*(2), 205–216.

Canadian Institute of Health Information (CIHI) (2011). *National Trauma Registry 2011 report: Hospitalization for major injury in Canada. March 2011.* Retrieved January 9, 2011 from http://secure.cihi.ca/cihiweb/products/NTRCDS20082009AnnualReport.pdf.

Carroll, S. M. (2004). Nonvocal ventilated patients' perceptions of being understood. *Western Journal of Nursing Research, 26*(1), 85–103.

Centers for Disease Control and Prevention [CDC] (2010). *National Center for Health Statistics, Fast Stats: Teen Births.* Retrieved November 6, 2010 from http://www.cdc.gov/nchs/fastats/teenbrth.htm.

Centers for Disease Control and Prevention [CDC] (2012). *National Vital Statistics Reports.* Retrieved February 16, 2016 from www.cdc.gov/nchs/data/nvsr/nvsr62/nvsr62_01.pdf.

Chen, M., James, K., Hsu, L., Chang, S., Huang, L., & Wang, E. K. (2005). Health-related behavior and adolescent mothers. *Public Health Nursing, 22*(4), 280–288.

Clukey, L., Hayes, J., Merrill, A., & Curtise, D. (2009). Helping them understand: Nurses' caring behaviors as perceived by family members of trauma patients. *Journal of Trauma Nursing, 16*(2), 73–80.

Cobb, J. P., & O'Keefe, G. E. (2004). Injury research in the genomic era. *Lancet, 363*(9426), 2076–2083.

Cohen, A., & Golan, R. (2007). Predicting absenteeism and turnover intentions by past absenteeism and work attitudes: An empirical examination of female employees in long-term nursing care facilities. *Career Development International, 12*(5), 416–432.

Collins, F. (2007). *The threat of genetic discrimination to the promise of personalized medicine. Testimony before the Subcommittee on Health, Committee on Energy and Commerce, US House of Representatives hearing on HR 493, the Genetic Information Nondiscrimination Act of 2007.* Retrieved April 9, 2016 from https://www.genome.gov/Pages/Newsroom/SpeechesAndTestimony/CollinsGINATestimony030807.pdf.

Collins, F. S., Green, E. D., Guttmacher, A. E., & Guyer, M. S. (2003). A vision for the future of genomics research. *Nature, 422*(6934), 835–847.

Coppolino, M., & Ackerson, L. (2001). Do surrogate decision makers provide accurate consent for intensive care research? *Chest, 119*(2), 603–612.

Costello, J. (2000). AAC intervention in the intensive care unit: The Children's Hospital Boston model. *AAC Augmentative and Alternative Communication, 16*(3), 137–153.

Curtis, E. A., & Glacken, M. (2014). Job satisfaction among public health nurses: A national survey. *Journal of Nursing Management, 22*(5), 653–663.

Curtis, K. (2001). Nurses' experiences of working with trauma patients. *Nursing Standard, 16*(9), 33–38.

Department of Health (2009). *Trends in children and young people's emergency care: Statistics.* London: Department of Health.

Deutschman, C. S., Ahrens, T., Cairns, C. B., Sessler, C. N., & Parsons, P. E. (2012). Multisociety task force for critical care research: Key issues and recommendations. *American Journal of Critical Care, 21*(1), 15–23.

Doncevic, S. T., Romelsjo, A., & Theorell, T. (1998). Comparison of stress, job satisfaction, perception of control and health among district nurses in Stockholm and pre-war Zagreb. *Scandinavian Journal of Social Medicine, 26*(2), 106–114.

Fahs, P. S., Morgan, L. L., & Kalman, M. (2003). A call for replication. *Journal of Nursing Scholarship, 35*(1), 67–71.

Finer, L., & Henshaw, S. K. (2006). Disparities in rates of unintended pregnancy in the United States, 1994 and 2001. *Perspectives on Sexual and Reproductive Health, 38*(2), 90–96.

Fisher, R. A. (1935). *The design of experiments.* Edinburgh, Scotland: Oliver & Boyd.

Flaskerud, J., Lesseer, J., Dixon, E., Anderson, N., Conde, F., Kim, S., et al. (2002). Health disparities among vulnerable populations: Evolution of knowledge over five decades in *Nursing Research* publications. *Nursing Research, 51*(2), 74–85.

Flaskerud, J., & Winslow, B. (1998). Conceptualising vulnerable populations health-related research. *Nursing Research, 47*(2), 69–78.

Flouri, E. (2005). *Fathering and child outcomes.* Oxford: Wiley Blackwell.

Flynn, L. (1999). The adolescent parenting program: Improving outcomes through mentorship. *Public Health Nursing, 16*(3), 182–189.

Flynn, L., Budd, M., & Modelski, J. (2008). Enhancing resource utilization among pregnant adolescents. *Public Health Nursing, 25*(2), 140–148.

Folkes-Skinner, J., & Meredith, E. (1997). Young mothers: Teenage mothers and their experiences of services. *Health Visitor, 70*(4), 139–140.

Fraser, G. L., Prato, B. S., Riker, R. R., Berthiaume, D., & Wilkins, M. L. (2000). Frequency, severity, and treatment of agitation in young versus elderly patients in the ICU. *Pharmacotherapy, 20*(1), 75–82.

Freeman, B. D., Kennedy, C. R., Bolcic-Jankovic, D., Eastman, A., Iverson, E., Shehane, E., et al. (2012). Considerations in the construction of an instrument to assess attitudes regarding critical illness gene variation research. *Journal of Empirical Research on Human Research Ethics, 7*(1), 58–70.

Freeman, B. D., Kennedy, C. R., Frankel, H. L., Clarridge, B., Bolcic-Jankovic, D., Iverson, E., et al. (2010). Ethical considerations in the collection of genetic data from critically ill patients: What do published studies reveal about potential directions for empirical ethics research? *Pharmacogenomics Journal, 10*(2), 77–85.

Freeman, L., Fothergill-Bourbonnais, F., & Rashotte, J. (2014). The experience of being a trauma nurse: A phenomenological study. *Intensive and Critical Care Nursing, 30*(1), 6–12.

Garber, C. E., Blissmer, B., Deschenes, M. R., Franklin, B. A., Lamonte, M. J., Lee, I. M., et al., American College of Sports Medicine (2011). American College of Sports Medicine position stand. Quantity and quality of exercise for developing and maintaining cardiorespiratory, musculoskeletal, and neuromotor fitness in apparently healthy adults: Guidance for prescribing exercise. *Medicine and Science in Sports and Exercise, 43*(7), 1334–1359.

Garcia-Aymerich, J., Lange, P., Benet, M., Schnohr, P., & Antó, J. M. (2006). Regular physical activity reduces hospital admission and mortality in chronic obstructive pulmonary disease: A population based cohort study. *Thorax, 61*(9), 772–778.

Gardner, K., Sessler, C. N., & Grap, M. J. (2006). Clinical factors associated with agitation [abstract]. *American Journal of Critical Care, 15*(3), 330–331.

Haapanen, N., Miilunpalo, S., Vuori, I., Oja, P., & Pasanen, M. (1996). Characteristics of leisure time physical activity associated with decreased risk of premature all-cause and cardiovascular disease mortality in middle-aged men. *American Journal of Epidemiology, 143*(9), 870–880.

Haennel, R. G., & Lemire, F. (2002). Physical activity to prevent cardiovascular diseases. How much is enough? *Canadian Family Physician, 48*(1), 65–71.

Haller, K. B., & Reynolds, M. A. (1986). Using research in practice: A case for replication in nursing: Part II. *Western Journal of Nursing Research, 8*(2), 249–252.

Happ, M. B., Garret, K. L., Tate, J. A., DiVirgilio, D., Houze, M. P., Demirci, J. R., et al. (2014). Effect of a multi-level intervention of nurse-patient communication in the intensive care unit: Results of the SPEACS trial. *Heart and Lung: The Journal of Critical Care, 43*(2), 89–98.

Happ, M., Roesch, T., & Garrett, K. (2004). Electronic voice-output communication aids for temporarily nonspeaking patients in a medical intensive care unit: A feasibility study. *Heart and Lung: The Journal of Critical Care, 33*(2), 92–101.

Happ, M. B., Seaman, J. B., Nilsen, M. L., Sciulli, A., Tate, J. A., Saul, M., et al. (2015). The number of mechanically ventilated ICU patients meeting communication criteria. *Heart and Lung: The Journal of Critical Care, 44*(1), 45–49.

Harvey, S. E., Elbourne, D., Ashcroft, J., Jones, C. M., & Rowan, K. (2006). Informed consent in clinical trials in critical care: Experience from the PAC-Man study. *Intensive Care Medicine, 32*(12), 2020–2025.

Hayes, J., & Tyler-Ball, S. (2007). Perceptions of nurses' caring behaviors by trauma patients. *Journal of Trauma Nursing, 14*(4), 187–190.

Higham, S., & Davies, R. (2013). Protecting, providing, and participating: Fathers' roles during their child's unplanned hospital stay: An ethnographic study. *Journal of Advanced Nursing, 69*(6), 1390–1399.

Hobson, I., & Noyes, J. (2011). Fatherhood and children with complex needs: Qualitative study of fathering, caring and parenting. *BMC Nursing, 10*(1), 5.

Isacco, A., & Garfield, C. (2010). Child healthcare decision-making: Examining "conjointness" in paternal identities among resident and non-resident fathers. *Fathering, 8*(1), 109–130.

Jaber, S., Chanques, G., Altairac, C., Sebbane, M., Vergne, C., Perrigault, P. F., et al. (2005). A prospective study of agitation in a medical-surgical ICU: Incidence, risk factors, and outcomes. *Chest, 128*(4), 2749–2757.

Jezewski, M., & Finnell, D. (1998). The meaning of DNR status: Oncology nurses' experiences with patients and families. *Cancer Nursing, 21*(3), 212–221.

Joint Commission (2010). *New and revised standards and EPs for patient-centered communication-Hospital accreditation program.* Retrieved from http://www.jointcommission.org/NR/rdonlyres/26D4ABD6-3489-4101-B397-56C9ER7CC7FB/0/Post_PatientCenteredCareStandardsEPs_20100609.pdf.

Jones, C. (2008). Revisiting nurse turnover costs. *Journal of Nursing Administration, 38*(1), 11–18.

Karlsson, V., Bergbom, I., & Forsberg, A. (2012). The lived experiences of adult intensive care patients who were conscious during mechanical ventilation: A phenomenological-hermeneutic study. *Intensive and Critical Care Nursing, 28*(1), 6–15.

Khalaila, R., Zbidat, W., Anwar, K., Bayya, A., Linton, D. M., & Syiri, S. (2011). Communication difficulties and psychoemotional distress in patients receiving mechanical ventilation. *American Journal of Critical Care, 20*(6), 470–479.

Kim, D. Y., Lee, K. E., Nam, E. M., Lee, H. R., Lee, K.-W., Kim, J. H., et al. (2007). Do-not-resuscitate orders for terminal patients with cancer in teaching hospitals of Korea. *Journal of Palliative Medicine, 10*(5), 1153–1158.

Kolkman, P. M. E., Luteijn, A. J., Masiiro, R. S., Bruney, V., Smith, R. J. A., & Meyboom-de Jong, B. (1998). District nursing in Dominica. *International Journal of Nursing Studies, 35*(5), 259–264.

Koniak-Griffin, D., Anderson, N. L. R., Verzemnieks, I., & Brecht, M. L. (2000). A public health nursing early intervention program for adolescent mothers: Outcomes from pregnancy through 6 weeks postpartum. *Nursing Research, 49*(3), 130–138.

Koniak-Griffin, D., Merzemnieks, I. L., Anderson, N. L. R., Brecht, M., Lesser, J., Kim, S., et al. (2003). Nurse visitation for adolescent mothers: Two-year infant health and maternal outcomes. *Nursing Research, 52*(2), 127–136.

Koniak-Griffin, D., & Turner-Pluta, C. (2001). Health risks and psychosocial outcomes of early childbearing: A review of the literature. *The Journal of Perinatal & Neonatal Nursing, 15*(2), 1–17.

Lacasse, Y., Martin, S., Lasserson, T. J., & Goldstein, R. S. (2007). Meta-analysis of respiratory rehabilitation in chronic obstructive pulmonary disease. A Cochrane systematic review. *Europa Medicophysica, 43*(4), 475–485.

Lamb, M. (2000). The history of research on father involvement: An overiew. *Marriage and Family Review, 29*(2), 23–42.

Leon, A. S., Connett, J., Jacobs, D. R., Jr., & Rauramaa, R. (1987). Leisure-time physical activity levels and risk of coronary heart disease and death. The Multiple Risk Factor Intervention Trial. *Journal of the American Medical Association, 258*(17), 2388–2395.

Levin, T. T., Li, Y., Weiner, J. S., Lewis, F., Bartell, A., Piercy, J., et al. (2008). How do-not-resuscitate orders are utilized in cancer patients: Timing relative to death and communication training implications. *Palliative Support Care, 6*(4), 341–348.

Lewandowski, A., & Kositsky, A. M. (1983). Research priorities for critical care nursing: A study by the American Association of Critical Care Nurses. *Heart and Lung: The Journal of Critical Care, 12*(1), 35–44.

Lin, C. P., Chiu, C. K., & Joe, S.-W. (2009). Modelling perceived job productivity and its antecedents considering gender as a moderator. *Social Science Journal, 46*(1), 192–200.

Lindeman, C. A. (1975). Delphi survey of priorities in clinical nursing research. *Nursing Research, 24*(6), 434–441.

Luce, J. M. (2003). Research ethics and consent in the intensive care unit. *Current Opinion in Critical Care, 9*(6), 540–544.

Luce, J. M. (2009). Informed consent for clinical research involving patients with chest disease in the United States. *Chest, 135*(4), 1061–1068.

Luce, J. M., Cook, D. J., Martin, T. R., Angus, D. C., Boushey, H. A., Curtis, J. R., American Thoracic Society, et al. (2004). The ethical conduct of clinical research involving critically ill patients in the United States and Canada: Principles and recommendations. *American Journal of Respiratory and Critical Care Medicine, 170*(12), 1375–1384.

Maines, T. Y., Lavie, C. J., Milani, R. V., Cassidy, M. M., Gilliland, Y. E., & Murgo, J. P. (1997). Effects of cardiac rehabilitation and exercise programs on exercise capacity, coronary risk factors, behavior, and quality of life in patients with coronary artery disease. *Southern Medical Journal, 90*(1), 43–49.

McGrath, P., & Chesler, M. (2004). Fathers' perspectives on the treatment for pediatric hematology: Extending the findings. *Issues in Comprehensive Pediatric Nursing, 27*(1), 39–61.

Mechanic, D., & Tanner, J. (2007). Vulnerable people, groups, and populations: Societal view. *Health Affairs, 26*(5), 1220–1230.

Menzel, L. K. (1998). Factors related to the emotional responses of intubated patients to being unable to speak. *Heart and Lung: The Journal of Critical Care, 27*(4), 245–252.

Mitchell, M. (2012). Influence of gender and anaesthesia type on day surgery anxiety. *Journal of Advanced Nursing, 68*(5), 1014–1025.

Moen, O. L., Hall-Lord, M. L., & Hedelin, B. (2014). Living in a family with a child with attention deficit hyperactivity disorder: A phenomenographic study. *Journal of Clinical Nursing, 23*(21–22), 3166–3175.

Moon, E. (2005). *The speed of dark.* New York, NY: Balantine Books.

Morse, J., & Proctor, A. (1998). Maintaining patient endurance: The comfort work of trauma nurses. *Clinical Nursing Research, 7*(3), 250–274.

National Institutes of Health. (n.d.). *Research project success rates by NIH institute for 2014.* Retrieved February 16, 2016 from https://report.nih.gov/sucess_rates/.

National Institute of Nursing Research (NINR). (2015a). *Fiscal Year 2015 Budget.* Retrieved February 16, 2016 from https://www.ninr.nih.gov/sites/www.ninr.nih.gov/files/cj2015_0.pdf.

National Institute of Nursing Research (NINR). (2015b). *NIH National Institute of Nursing Research.* Almanac. Retrieved April 9, 2016 from http://www.nih.gov/about/almanac/organization/NINR.htm.

Nelson, J. E., Meier, D. E., Litke, A., Natale, D. A., Siegel, R. E., & Morrison, R. S. (2004). The symptom burden of chronic critical illness. *Critical Care Medicine, 32*(7), 1527–1534.

Nguyen, J. D., Carson, M. L., Parris, K. M., & Place, P. (2003). A comparison pilot study of public health field nursing home visitation program interventions for pregnant Hispanic adolescents. *Public Health Nursing, 20*(5), 412–418.

Nici, L., Donner, C., Wouters, E., Zuwallack, R., Ambrosino, N., Bourbeau, J., et al. (2006). American Thoracic Society/European Respiratory Society statement on pulmonary rehabilitation. *American Journal of Respiratory and Critical Care Medicine, 173*(12), 1390–1413.

Olver, I., & Eliott, J. A. (2008). The perceptions of do-not-resuscitate policies of dying patients with cancer. *Psycho-Oncology*, *17*(4), 347–353.

Pettersson, M., Hedström, M., & Höglund, A. T. (2014). Striving for good nursing care: Nurses' experiences of do not resuscitate orders within oncology and hematology care. *Nursing Ethics*, *21*(8), 902–915.

Popper, K. (1968). *The logic of scientific discovery*. New York, NY: Harper & Row, Publishers.

Quinn, B., Baker, D. L., Cohen, S., Stewart, J. L., Lima, C. A., & Parise, C. (2014). Basic nursing care to prevent nonventilator hospital-acquired pneumonia. *Journal of Nursing Scholarship*, *46*(1), 11–19.

Radtke, J. V., Baumann, B. M., Garrett, K. L., & Happ, M. B. (2011). Listening to the voiceless patient: Case reports in assisted communication in the intensive care unit. *Journal of Palliative Medicine*, *14*(6), 791–795.

Radtke, J. V., Tate, J. A., & Happ, M. B. (2012). Nurses' perceptions of communication training in the ICU. *Intensive and Critical Care Nursing*, *28*(1), 16–25.

Ramadi, A., Stickland, M. K., Rodgers, W. M., & Haennel, R. G. (2015). Impact of supervised exercise rehabilitation on daily physical activity of cardiopulmonary patients. *Heart and Lung: The Journal of Critical Care*, *44*(1), 9–14.

Rotondi, A. J., Chelluri, L., Sirio, C., Mendlesohn, A., Schulz, R., Belle, S., et al. (2002). Patients' recollections of stressful experiences while receiving prolonged mechanical ventilation in an intensive care unit. *Critical Care Medicine*, *30*(4), 746–752.

Rout Rani, U. (2000). Stress amongst district nurses: A preliminary investigation. *Journal of Clinical Nursing*, *9*(2), 303–309.

Ruggiero, J. S. (2005). Health, work variables, and job satisfaction among nurses. *Journal of Nursing Administration*, *35*(5), 254–263.

Sessler, C. N., Rutherford, L., Best, A., Hart, R., & Levenson, J. (1992). Agitation in a medical intensive care unit: Prospective analysis and risk factors [abstract]. *Chest*, *102*(2_S), 191S.

Shelton, A. K., Freeman, B. D., Fish, A. F., Bachman, J. A., & Richardson, L. I. (2015). A computer-based education intervention to enhance surrogates' informed consent for genomics research. *American Journal of Critical Care*, *24*(2), 148–155.

Shribman, S. (2007). *Making better: For children and young people*. London: Department of Health.

Stovsky, B., Rudy, E. B., & Dragonette, P. (1988). Comparison of two types of communication methods used after cardiac surgery with patients with endotracheal tubes. *Heart and Lung: The Journal of Critical Care*, *17*(3), 281–289.

Sullivan-Bolyai, S., Rosenburg, R., & Bayard, M. (2006). Fathers' reflections on parenting young children with type 1 diabetes. *Maternal-Child Nursing*, *31*(1), 24–31.

Swallow, V., Lambert, H., Santacroce, S., & Macfadyn, A. (2011). Fathers and mothers developing skills in managing children's long-term conditions: How do their accounts compare? *Child: Care, Health and Development*, *37*(4), 512–523.

Tourigny, J., Ward, V., & Lepage, T. (2004). Fathers' behavior during their child's ambulatory surgery. *Issues in Comprehensive Pediatric Nursing*, *27*(2), 69–81.

van den Berg-Emons, R., Balk, A., Bussmann, H., & Stam, H. (2004). Does aerobic training lead to a more active lifestyle and improved quality of life in patients with chronic heart failure? *European Journal of Heart Failure*, *6*(1), 95–100.

Von Rueden, K. R. (1991). The physical, personal and cognitive demands of trauma nursing. *Critical Care Nurse*, *11*(6), 9.

Von Rueden, K., Hinderer, K., McQuillan, K., Marray, M., Logan, T., Kramer, B., et al. (2010). Secondary traumatic stress in trauma nurses: Prevalence and exposure, coping and personal/ environmental characteristics. *Journal of Trauma Nursing*, *17*(4), 191–200.

Westover, J. H., Westover, A. R., & Westover, L. A. (2009). Enhancing long-term worker productivity and performance: The connection of key work domains to job satisfaction and organisational commitment. *International Journal of Productivity and Performance Management*, *59*(4), 372–387.

Whitman, D. S., Van Rooy, D. L., & Viswesvaran, C. (2010). Satisfaction, citizenship behaviours, and performance in work units: A meta-analysis of collective construct relations. *Personnel Psychology*, *63*(1), 41–81.

Wood, P. J., & Arcus, K. (2012). 'Sunless lives': District nurses' and journalists' co-construction of the 'sick poor' as a vulnerable population in early twentieth-century New Zealand. *Contemporary Nurse*, *42*(2), 145–155.

Woods, J. C., Mion, L. C., Connor, J. T., Viray, F., Jahan, L., Huberr, C., et al. (2004). Severe agitation among ventilated medical intensive care unit patients: frequency, characteristics and outcomes. *Intensive Care Medicine*, *30*(6), 1066–1072.

6

Objectives, Questions, Variables, and Hypotheses

Suzanne Sutherland

http://evolve.elsevier.com/Gray/practice/

Beyond defining the study purpose, some researchers choose also to set specific objectives, aims, or both for a study. These are merely smaller segments of the overall purpose.

After problem and purpose have been established, the research question is decided upon. If that question is not stated in the research report, it is implied, and the reader can derive it from the purpose statement and the researcher's stated methodology and design. Next, the principal ideas in the research question are defined conceptually, so that the meaning of each is clear. Conceptually defining an idea establishes its abstract significance, much as a dictionary definition does.

In quantitative research, principal research concepts are defined operationally, as well as conceptually. Operationally defining a concept translates it into a variable and provides a definition of how the researcher will quantify that variable during the course of a study. In order for meaningful quantitative research to be conducted, its variables must be able to be counted or measured.

A researcher may generate a hypothesis from the research question, to be used as part of the process of statistical testing. If research is interventional, there is always a hypothesis, either explicit or implied. Correlational research may contain a stated hypothesis, as well; simple descriptive research seldom does so. Hypotheses are classified in four different ways: causal versus noncausal, simple versus complex, directional versus nondirectional, and null versus research.

This chapter focuses upon objectives, questions, definitions of variables, and hypotheses. Objectives and aims, and their relationship to the research purpose, are described. Research questions, their phrasing, and their constituent parts are presented. Differences between conceptual and operational definitions of variables are reviewed, as well as the means of constructing both. Types of variables are explained. The differences among the principal types of research hypotheses, and their uses in hypothesis testing, are elucidated.

LEVELS OF ABSTRACTION

The levels of abstraction encountered in a research report are the conceptual level, also called the abstract or theoretical level, and the operational level, also called the concrete level (Dulock & Holzemer, 1991). The research purpose is expressed at the conceptual level: it does not reveal details of how concepts of a study will be measured but merely states them and sometimes identifies their relationship to one another. (See Figure 3-1 in Chapter 3.)

The research question is slightly more tangible. It identifies the study population and the concepts that are to be the study's principal variables, as well as posited relationships among those variables. However, the research question does not define the manner in which variables will be measured so, in a technical sense, the research question exists at the conceptual level, as well. It does represent a bridge, of sorts, between abstract and concrete levels.

In quantitative research, measurement occurs at the operational level. At this level are variables, relationships among variables including the study hypothesis, the specifics of measurement, such as tools and scales, and statistical analyses. Quantitative data that the researcher classifies, counts, and measures are

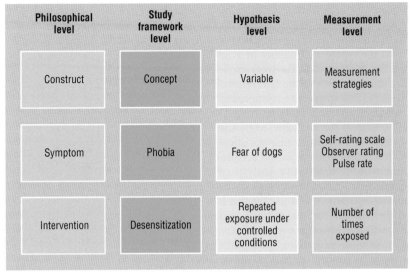

FIGURE 6-1 Substruction of treatment for fear of dogs. (Steps of analysis, as described by Dulock, H. L., & Holzemer, W. L. [1991]. Substruction: Improving the linkage from theory to method. *Nursing Science Quarterly, 4*[2], 83-87.)

concrete, as well. Figure 6-1 displays the construct, concept, variable, and measurement levels of quantitative research.

PURPOSES, OBJECTIVES, AND AIMS

When the author of a research study states a purpose, an objective, or an aim, this is merely an explication of intention. All three terms, *purpose*, *objective*, and *aim*, refer to what the researcher intends to accomplish through this study—the reason the study is to be performed. In this respect, the three terms are at least seriously overlapping and perhaps synonymous. In fact, thesaurus entries (Roget & Dutch, 1962) list the three as synonyms for one another. This is why purposes, objectives, and aims are so confusing for beginning students. "What's the difference?" you ask. Great question: in reality, minimal, if any.

In its classic form, the abstract of a nursing research report contains a statement of the study's overall purpose, and this is reiterated at the end of the literature review, following the identification of the research gap. In a study of the experience of feeling disappointed, Bunkers (2012) stated the purpose in the abstract of the report: "The purpose of the study was to enhance understanding of the lived experience of feeling disappointed" (p. 53), reiterating it with similar wording at the end of the literature review, "The purpose of the

study was to understand the lived experience of feeling disappointed" (p. 54).

Within the methods section, or immediately after the purpose statement, a research report sometimes contains a listing of two or more objectives of the research. In their report of a feasibility study to examine team clinical supervision (TCS) in acute care, O'Connell, Ockerby, Johnson, Smenda, and Bucknall (2013) stated their purpose: "The purpose of this study was to explore the implementation and evaluation of TCS for nurses and midwives working in acute settings" (p. 332). The objectives the authors listed were to "(1) validate recruitment and consent procedures, (2) test the appropriateness of instruments used during the study, (3) determine sample size for the main study, and (4) explore the acceptability of the intervention to participants" (p. 332). When authors articulate both purpose and objectives, all of the objectives considered together should be equivalent to the purpose statement, or at least a logical outgrowth of it, as is true in this example. Often each objective refers to a different part of the study, or to a statistical consideration of certain variables and their interrelationships.

Aims in a research study pertain to the desired output of a study, from the researcher's point of view. The aims might be sequential steps in the research process. In a study by Yun, Kang, Lee, and Yi (2014), the stated purpose was: "... to examine the relationship between perceived work environment and workplace bullying among Korean intensive care units (ICU) nurses" (p. 219). The aims of the study were "to (a) investigate the work environment and the extent of bullying in ICU nurses, (b) investigate the differences in the work environment and bullying in accordance to the characteristics of ICU nurses, and (c) investigate the relationship between the work environment and bullying in ICU nurses" (p. 220). It is common for each aim to be the outgrowth of one method of analysis or one statistical test. In this example, descriptive analysis would accomplish the first aim, comparative descriptive analysis of bullying and nurse characteristics would accomplish the second, and correlational tests would address the third.

You may be confused about the distinctions and overlaps among these with good reason: over the years, distinctions among purposes, objectives, and aims have tended to blur. Authors choose whichever one or more of these terms they desire in order to inform the reader of the intent of conducting a study, producing the state of a distinction without a difference. To further muddy the waters, in the *International Journal of Nursing Studies* and some other research journals, the prescribed heading within each abstract requires "objectives," not purpose. Some authors do indeed state an objective or objectives in the designated space, as directed (Mallidou, Cummings, Schalm, & Estabrooks, 2013). Undeterred by the header, after the word "objectives" in the abstract, other authors state their purpose (Alexis, 2015; Huang, Chen, Liang, & Miaskowski, 2015; Osafo, Knizek, Akotia, & Hjelmeland, 2012; Yun et al., 2014), their aim or aims (Baum & Kagan, 2015; Poutiainen, Levälahti, Hakulainan-Viitanen, & Laatikainen, 2015), or both their purpose and their aims (Solodiuk, 2013). In the same manner, the cue word "aim" in an abstract template is sometimes used by the author to state a purpose (Arvidsson, Bergman, Arvidsson, Fridlund, & Tingstrom, 2013). Nonetheless, if a study does state a research purpose, the objectives/aims that subsequently appear all emanate from that purpose statement.

Formulating Objectives or Aims in Quantitative Studies

Objectives or aims in quantitative studies are developed on the basis of the research problem and purpose, in order to clarify a study's goals. The objectives or aims use the same major variables identified in the purpose statement, possibly adding a few extra, and examine these within the same population.

Vermeesch et al. (2013) conducted predictive correlational research to evaluate the contribution of self-esteem to the relationship between stress and depressive symptoms in Hispanic women. The following excerpts from that study demonstrate the fluency and cohesiveness among problem, purpose, and objectives:

Research Problem
"Self-esteem has been defined as a continuum of self-worth (Rosenberg, 1965). Self-esteem is inversely related to depressive symptoms among Hispanic women (González-Guarda, Peragallo, Vasquez, Urrutia, & Mitrani, 2009; Rosenberg, 1965). Various researchers have concluded that self-esteem is inversely related to depressive symptoms in Hispanics (De Santis et al., 2012; González-Guarda et al., 2009). ... Several studies described herein before have linked stressors unique to Hispanics and self-esteem to depression, but only one study was found that attempted to link these constructs using a stress process model in which self-esteem mediated the link between stress and depressive symptoms (Land & Hudson, 2004)." (Vermeesch et al., 2013, pp. 1327–1328)

Research Purpose
"The current study was designed to expand the understanding of Hispanic stress, self-esteem, and depressive symptoms and the Stress Process Model for Hispanic women." (Vermeesch et al., 2013, p. 1328)

Research Objectives
"The objectives of the current study were to (a) evaluate the relationship of Hispanic stress and self-esteem to depressive symptoms among Hispanic women and (b) examine whether self-esteem mediated the relationship between Hispanic stress and depression." (Vermeesch et al., 2013, p. 1328)

In this example, the identified problem provided a basis for the purpose statement. The objectives were derived from the purpose, indicating specific statistical analyses to measure (1) relationships between stress and depressive symptoms, and between self-esteem and depressive symptoms; and (2) the relationship between stress and depression, at varying levels of self-esteem. The first objective focused on correlations between pairs of variables, and the statistical tests were selected so as to measure linear regression (the amount and direction of the relationship between two variables). The second objective focused on correlations among three variables, and the statistical test was selected so as to evaluate multiple regression (the relationships among all three stated variables as they influenced the values of the others).

Formulating Objectives or Aims in Qualitative Studies

In qualitative research, objectives or aims also are developed on the basis of the research problem and purpose, in order to clarify a study's goals. The objectives or aims use the same major concepts identified in the purpose statement and examined within the same population.

The following excerpts are from an ethnographic study investigating interruptions in hospital nurses' work (Sørensen & Brahe, 2013):

Research Problem

"We now know that the nurse's work is driven by interruptions. ... A study among 1870 nurses in Denmark showed that rising workloads increased the risk of error and that one out of two nurses were concerned about making mistakes, a risk which they attributed primarily to interruptions (Søndergaard, 2010). ... It has been shown that nurses are interrupted more frequently than other staff groups (Paxton et al., 1996; Brixey et al., 2007; Biron et al., 2009) and that the interruptions are often instigated by nurse colleagues (Kreckler et al., 2008). Brixey et al. (2007) have warned of the consequences of our poor understanding of the nature of interruptions and their causes and effects." (Sørensen & Brahe, 2013, pp. 1274–1275)

Research Purpose

"The purpose of the study was to investigate interruptions as they occur in clinical nursing practice in a typical hospital surgery ward in Denmark." (Sørensen & Brahe, 2013, p. 1275)

Research Aims

"... to investigate interruptions as they occur in clinical nursing practice in a typical hospital surgery ward in Denmark. A further aim was to improve our understanding of the impact of interruptions in nurses' work." (Sørensen & Brahe, 2013, p. 1275)

In this study, the problem statement indicated that there was poor understanding of the nature of interruptions and their causes and effects. The stated purpose was to investigate such interruptions. The aims reiterated the purpose as the first aim, and added a second aim directed toward understanding the impact of interruptions. Both aims identified the principal phenomenon of interest, interruptions in the hospital nurse's work. The researchers identified the nature of hospital workplace interruptions for the nurse, most of which were not patient-initiated and were centered around administration of medications. The researchers also identified the nurse's quandary as being accessible versus being focused on the job (Sørensen & Brahe, 2013).

HOW TO CONSTRUCT RESEARCH QUESTIONS

Even if a researcher does not state all of them, each purpose, objective, and aim has a corresponding question associated with it. The wording of those particular questions indicates the methodology and design of each specific line of inquiry.

What exactly is a research question? A **research question** is a concise, interrogative statement that is worded in the present tense and includes one or more of a study's principal concepts. Research questions are actual queries that address variables, and sometimes the relationships among them, within a population.

A research question has three parts: a questioning part such as "what is," "what are," "is there," or "are there"; a word that indicates what the researcher wants to know about the study variables or population; and the naming of the population, and the variables if appropriate. The principal research question is often merely a rewording of the research purpose. In quantitative designs, the research question hints heavily at the type of design that is to be used, implying incidence, connections between ideas, and cause-and-effect relationships, and perhaps even containing the exact words "incidence," "prevalence," "correlation," "relationship," "predict," "cause," or "effect." In Table 6-1, a quantitative research question's components are listed. In Table 6-2, the same quantitative research questions, their associated purposes, and their probable designs are listed.

In qualitative designs, the research question implies understanding the cultural context that acts as a platform for human behavior and experience, understanding human behavior and experience within a social context, generating theory, describing the lived experience and possibly the meaning of that experience to the study participants, telling the story of the past, or relating basic narrative descriptive information. It may even contain the exact words *lived experience, culture, society, history,* or *narrative.* In Table 6-3, a qualitative research question's components are listed. Sometimes the research question hints at a specific design; at other times, the question implies only that the qualitative methodology will be employed. Sometimes the population is not named in qualitative research purposes and questions, especially if the researcher is attempting to define a concept that transcends one particular population. In Table 6-4, qualitative research questions, their

TABLE 6-1   A Quantitative Research Question's Components

The Questioning Part	What the Researcher Wants to Know	Population	Research Question
What are	Characteristics	Population X	What are the characteristics of population X?
What is	Incidence of B	Population X	What is the incidence of B in population X?
Is there	Incidence of C	Populations X_1 and X_2	Is there a different incidence of C in population X_1 than there is in population X_2?
What is	Correlation between D and E	Population Y	What is the correlation between D and E in population Y?
Which...predict	Correlation between J and the predictor variables F, G, H, and I	Population Z	Which variables (F, G, H, I, etc.) predict the presence of variable J, in population Z?
Does......cause	Causal relationship between K and L	Population Z	In population Z, does K cause L?

TABLE 6-2   Quantitative Research Questions, Purposes, and Probable Designs

Research Question	Research Purpose	Probable Design
What are the characteristics of population X?	The purpose of this study is to identify the characteristics of population X.	Descriptive
What is the incidence of B in population X?	The purpose of this study is to discover the incidence or amount of B in population X.	Descriptive
Is there a different incidence of C present in population X_1 than there is in population X_2?	The purpose of this study is to compare the incidence of C in population X_1 with the incidence in population X_2.	Descriptive
What is the correlation between D and E in population Y?	The purpose of this study is to measure the correlation between D and E in population Y.	Correlational
Which variables (F, G, H, I, etc.) predict the presence of variable J, in population Z?	The purpose of this study is to establish which of the variables F, G, H, and I predict variable J, in population Z.	Correlational
In population Z, does K cause L?	The purpose of this study is to determine whether K causes L, in population Z.	Causational (experimental or quasi-experimental)

TABLE 6-3   A Qualitative Research Question's Components

The Questioning Part	What the Researcher Wants to Know	Population	Research Question
What are	Characteristics of the culture and the nature of its members, experiencing E	Population W	What are the characteristics of the culture of population W and the nature of its members experiencing E?
What are	Experiences and perspectives of individuals in the situation F (and the related concepts and processes)	Population V	What are the (concepts and processes that characterize the) experiences and perspectives of individuals of population V, in the situation F?
What is	Lived experience of persons with the characteristics G	Population U	What is the lived experience of persons with G (in the population U)?
What is	Story of occurrences related to the concept L, during the ____ time period	Population S	What is the story of occurrences related to the concept L, during the ____ time period, within the population S?
What are	Collective perceptions about J	Population Q	What are the collective perceptions about J, in the population Q?

TABLE 6-4 **Qualitative Research Questions, Purposes, and Probable Designs**		
Research Question	**Research Purpose**	**Probable Design**
What are the characteristics of the culture of population W and the nature of its members experiencing E?	The purpose of this study is to identify the characteristics of the culture of population X, and the nature of its members experiencing E.	Ethnography
What are the (concepts and processes that characterize the) experiences and perspectives of individuals of population V, in the situation F?	The purpose of this study is to identify the (concepts and processes that characterize the) experiences and perspectives of individuals of population V, experiencing F.	Grounded theory research
What is the lived experience of persons with G (in the population U)?	The purpose of this study is to discover the lived experience of persons with G (in population U).	Phenomenology
What is the story of occurrences related to the concept L, during the ____ time period, within the population S?	The purpose of this study is to tell the story of occurrences related to L that occurred during the ____ time period, in population S.	Historical research
What are the collective perceptions about J, in the population Q?	The purpose of this research is to present qualitative data related to J in population Q.	Exploratory-descriptive qualitative research

associated purposes, and their probable designs are listed.

Formulating Questions in Quantitative Studies

If a research question is present in a quantitative research report, it is likely to be a restatement of the research purpose. If more than one research question is present, the questions often relate to the study's individual objectives or aims.

Fredericks and Yau (2013) conducted an experimental comparative pilot study to test a new method of postoperative teaching for cardiac surgery patients. The following excerpts from this study demonstrate how their research purpose was generated from the stated problem, and then phrased as a research question.

Problem

"Across Canada, although resources to promote recovery are made available, more than a quarter of all CABG [coronary artery bypass graft] and/or VR [valve replacement] patients are being readmitted to hospitals with postoperative complications experienced during the first three months of recovery (Guru, Fremes, Austin, Blackstone, & Tu, 2006). The most common causes of readmissions are postoperative infections (28%) and heart failure (22%; Hannan et al., 2003). The rate of hospital readmission following CABG and/or VR has significant implications for health care resource utilization, continuity of care across

the system, and exacerbation of underlying cardiac condition (Guru et al., 2006). A possible reason for the high rate of readmission is patients may not be adequately prepared to engage in self-care during their home recovery period (Fredericks, 2009; Fredericks, Sidani, & Shugurensky, 2008; Harkness et al., 2005; Moore & Dolansky, 2001) resulting in the onset and/or exacerbation of complications, which can lead to hospital readmissions. Specifically, the quality of the patient education intervention received around the time of discharge may not be optimal in supporting patients up to 3 months following their hospital discharge. As a result, patients may not have the adequate knowledge to effectively engage in behaviors to prevent the development of complications leading to hospital readmissions." (Fredericks & Yau, 2013, p. 1253)

Purpose

"The purpose of this pilot study was to collect preliminary data to examine the impact of an individualized telephone education intervention delivered to patients following CABG and/or VR during their home recovery." (Fredericks & Yau, 2013, p. 1253)

Research Question

"Does individualized telephone patient education have more impact in reducing the rate of complications and hospital readmissions during the first 3 months following hospital discharge for CABG and/or VR than standardized patient education?" (Fredericks & Yau, 2013, p. 1253)

Fredericks and Yau's (2013) research question was essentially the purpose statement, rearranged as a query, adding a mention of standardized patient education as the usual treatment. Both purpose and question identified the population of coronary artery bypass grafting (CABG) and valve replacement (VR) patients, and the researchers' intent to discover whether an independent variable, individualized telephone patient education, caused a decreased incidence of two dependent variables, complications and hospital readmissions in the first three months after hospital discharge, as contrasted with the control condition, standardized patient education. Fredericks and Yau's (2013) intervention group and control group demonstrated a statistically significant difference in complications and hospital readmissions at 12 weeks.

Formulating Questions in Qualitative Studies

Among published reports for studies using the major qualitative nursing research methodologies, few include stated research questions. We undertook a focused literature search of nursing publications for the 42-month period January 2012 through June 2015; our inquiry revealed that only about 3% (6 of 183) of study reports using a phenomenological, ethnographic, or grounded theory design presented a research question.

If questions are included in qualitative research reports, they tend to have a broader and more global phrasing than questions in quantitative reports, underscoring an experience, a feeling, a perception, or a process, and only sometimes mentioning the population of interest. This may be due to the intuitive basis of the art of discovery during qualitative inquiry, which emphasizes collective themes, codes, essences, and truths, rather than counted values.

Bunkers (2012) conducted a phenomenological study in which the focus was to better understand the lived experience of feeling disappointed. Typical of qualitative inquiries that investigate the global meaning of a concept, no population was specified in the research purpose or question. The following excerpts from this study demonstrate how the research purpose was generated from the stated problem and then phrased as a research question.

Research Problem

"Feeling disappointed can be intimately involved in experiencing challenges to health and quality of life. Plutchik (1991) suggested that feeling disappointed is composed of the primary emotions of sorrow and surprise. A frightening diagnosis of disease can surface feelings of both sorrow and surprise and can shatter a person's sense of well-being. …

Although the emotion of disappointment has been studied in multiple disciplines in the natural sciences, there are no known published studies on the lived experience of feeling disappointed in the nursing literature from a human science perspective. The importance of feeling disappointed in matters of health and quality of life underscores the necessity to understand the meaning of feeling disappointed and for this study to be conducted." (Bunkers, 2012, pp. 53–54)

Research Purpose

"The purpose of this article was to investigate the lived experience of feeling disappointed." (Bunkers, 2012, p. 54)

Research Question

"What is the structure of the lived experience of feeling disappointed?" (Bunkers, 2012, p. 54)

Bunkers' (2012) research question was essentially the purpose statement, reworded according to the language of phenomenology. Although the nine participants in the study were 46 to 80 years of age, and all recruited from a foot care clinic, neither purpose nor question identified the population specifically. The author's recommendations for further study did not include similar studies with other populations: it seems that the feeling of disappointment was perceived by the researcher as being universal rather than situated within a given smaller population and because of this, the researcher did not adjudge the findings as being specific only to one similar-aged or medically similar population.

VARIABLES IN QUANTITATIVE VERSUS QUALITATIVE RESEARCH

Although variables have been defined, traditionally, as qualities that vary within a research study, it is more helpful to think of them as concepts that can be measured, yielding at least two different "values," either numeric or non-numeric. Abstract concepts can be defined so that they can be measured, some well, some not so well. For instance, "dog happiness" can be defined as how many times a companion dog wags its tail in one minute, calling to mind the paraphrased truism that just because something can be measured does not mean that it should be measured.

Because the researcher's task is to choose the best measurement for a specific study, a researcher might choose to measure an abstract concept in more than one way, when that concept is measured infrequently in research. For instance, fear might be measured in two different ways during a study about initiation of chemotherapy: the subject's statement of being afraid or unafraid, and percentage elevation of heart rate. During data analysis, it might be determined that the percentage elevation of heart rate is a more sensitive measure than the subject's statement, and that lower levels of fear are not captured as well by the subject's statement.

Sometimes quantitative measurements of several different aspects of a concept are summed, particularly when the researcher is not confident that a single measure will capture the concept but is reasonably sure that, taken together, several measures will be successful. For instance, hospital patient acuity ratings, made for purposes of refining in-unit staff assignments or assisting supervisors in allotting staff to various areas, are based on summed multiple measures.

At the outset of a qualitative research study, on the other hand, abstract concepts are described and sometimes defined but they are not operationalized, since they will not be measured, and they will not necessarily assume more than one value. Because of this, qualitative research does not refer to concepts as variables, except in the special case of grounded theory research, in which the sole central concept revealed at the end of the study through data analysis is sometimes called the core variable.

Concepts in Qualitative Research

There are two types of concepts found in qualitative research. The first is the concept on which the research is focused: the topic the researcher explores. The topic of the research is, of course, known to the researcher at the outset, and is named in the study purpose and research question. This foundational topic is known in both quantitative and qualitative research as the phenomenon, the phenomenon of interest, the study focus, the concept of interest, and the central issue, among other terms. In this chapter it is referred to as the **phenomenon of interest**. An example of a phenomenon of interest is found in Westphal, Lancaster, and Park's (2014) descriptive qualitative study of workarounds, which the authors described as "changes in work patterns to accomplish patient care goals" (p. 1002), and the reason nurses were observed to use them. Work-arounds, in this study, were the phenomenon of interest.

The second type of concept found in qualitative research is specific to qualitative inquiry. It is the

emergent concept, which is what the researcher discovers during the process of studying the phenomenon of interest. Emergent concepts in Westphal et al.'s (2014) study were reported as the research results. The emergent concepts were infection prevention and control, medication management, and workload, all of which emerged from categories identified during data analysis. The word **theme** was used by Westphal et al. (2014) for these concepts. Theme is the term most commonly used in qualitative research reports for concepts that emerge during the conduct of a study. Those themes represent the study results, especially in phenomenology and exploratory descriptive research, although the words *essences* and *truths* are sometimes seen in phenomenology, as are other terms specific to that type of inquiry. Names for emergent concepts used in grounded theory research are factors, factors of interest, categories, codes, and core variable, among others. Ethnography tends to use the word *themes*, and occasionally *factors*. These terms all refer to the emergent concepts—the discoveries—of the research.

Types of Variables in Quantitative Research
Demographic Variables

One type of variable is found in all quantitative and most qualitative nursing research reports, and that is the demographic variable. **Demographic variables** are subject characteristics measured during a study and used to describe a sample. In nursing research, common demographic variables are age, gender, and ethnicity, which define the population represented by the sample. Thorough description of the sample guides the researcher in making appropriate generalizations, conclusions, and recommendations at the study's end. For hospital-based studies, additional demographic variables typically include medical diagnosis, acuity, and length of stay. In non-hospital settings, educational level, income, and occupation may be included as demographics, especially when provision of services is a study focus.

To obtain data about demographic variables, researchers either access existent records or ask subjects to complete an information sheet. After study completion, demographic information is analyzed to provide what are called the **sample characteristics**, or occasionally the sample demographics. In a quantitative research report, sample characteristics almost invariably are presented at the beginning of the Results section, in a table, sometimes accompanied by a narrative. For their study of the effect of exercise rehabilitation on the daily physical activity of cardiopulmonary patients, Ramadi, Stickland, Rodgers, and Haennel (2015) presented demographics in a table (p. 11), reproduced as Table 6-5:

TABLE 6-5 Baseline Sample Demographics and Clinical Characteristics

Demographics	
Age (years)	74.6 (6.2)
Male	22 (59.5%)
BMI (kg/m^2)	28.3 (5.6)
Primary Diagnosis	
Anterior MI	2 (5.4%)
NSTEMI	8 (21.6%)
STEMI	6 (16.2%)
Asthma	3 (8.1%)
Bronchiectasis	1 (2.7%)
Lung cancer	1 (2.7%)
COPD	12 (32.4%)
Pulmonary fibrosis	4 (10.8%)

BMI, body mass index; *COPD*, chronic obstructive pulmonary disease; *MI*, myocardial infarction; *NSTEMI*, non-ST segment elevation myocardial infarction; *STEMI*, ST segment elevation myocardial infarction.
Data are presented as mean (standard deviation) or as the absolute number (percentage).
From Ramadi, A., Stickland, M. K., Rodgers, W. M., & Haennel, R. G. (2015). Impact of supervised exercise rehabilitation on daily physical activity of cardiopulmonary patients. *Heart and Lung: The Journal of Critical Care, 44*(1), 9–14.

Qualitative sample characteristics seldom are presented as tables. Calvin, Engebretson and Sardual (2014) investigated understanding of end-of-life decision-making processes in family members of hemodialysis patients, presenting the sample characteristics narratively:

"The sample of 18 was self-identified as Black (10), Hispanic (6), and White (2) and 14 were female. Ages of participants ranged from 21 to 67 years, with a mean age of 42. Hemodialysis patients' ages ranged from 29 to 76, with a mean age of 55. The age of 1 female patient was unknown. Seven participants were spouses of the patient, 7 were adult children of the patient, 1 was a parent, 1 was a sibling, 1 was a niece, and 1 was a daughter-in-law. Sixteen participants were recruited from outpatient dialysis centers and 2 from an inpatient dialysis unit." (Calvin et al., 2014, p. 1362)

Independent and Dependent Variables

The terms "independent variable" and "dependent variable" are used in two different ways in nursing research. In experimental and quasi-experimental research, they are used to denote the cause and effect of a researcher intervention. In predictive correlational research, they are used to mean potential predictors and their outcome. So an independent variable is either a cause or a predictor, depending on the research design. A dependent variable is the entity that it is the researcher's intent to produce, modify, or predict.

Interventional research designs: independent and dependent variables. Quantitative research is either interventional or noninterventional. Interventional research includes experimental and quasi-experimental designs. Interventional experimental research, in which the researcher enacts an intervention upon the experimental group and not the control group, has two principal types of variables, the independent variable and the dependent variable. The **independent variable** is the intervention or treatment that the researcher applies to the experimental group but not to the control group. The tricky thing about independent variables in true experimental research is that they must have been intentionally enacted by the researcher, not by nature, not by chance, for the research to be considered experimental. For example, the civilian mortality rate in Europe due to influenza in the two-year period 1918-1920 that characterized the Great Flu Pandemic was much higher than it was in 2012-2014, partially because of modern flu immunizations and modern treatment of critically ill patients. Immunizations and sophisticated treatment were not available in the early part of the 20th century, and the mortality rate in Europe is estimated to have been between 10% and 20% of those affected (Taubenberger & Morens, 2006). Research comparing these two periods cannot be termed interventional because the researcher did not cause modern-day Europeans to be vaccinated or cause modern critical care units to be constructed. The **dependent variable** is so called because it depends on the action of the independent variable. The dependent variable is defined as the result or outcome that is the study's focus.

As described earlier, Fredericks and Yau (2013) tested the effect upon complications and hospital readmissions of an individualized education intervention given to cardiac surgery patients above and beyond the usual care, delivered at two points in time following hospital discharge. In this experimental study, the individualized education intervention was enacted by the researchers upon the experimental group, not the control group, making the educational intervention the independent variable. Complication rate and hospital readmission rate depended on whether patients received the individualized education intervention. Consequently, complication rate and hospital readmission rate were the study's dependent variables.

Frequently, a study's purpose statement identifies both independent and dependent variables, such as "The purpose of this study was to examine the effect of an asthma education program on schoolteachers' knowledge" (Kawafha & Tawalbeh, 2015, p. 425). In this case, the independent variable (enacted by the research team, for members of the experimental group) was an asthma education program. The dependent variable was schoolteachers' knowledge. If Kawafha and Tawalbeh's (2015) purpose statement had been worded, "the purpose of this study was to determine the effect on school teachers' knowledge of an asthma education program," the independent variable would still be the researchers' intervention of an asthma education program. (The order in which the variables are stated does not determine which is independent and which is dependent: the action of the researcher remains the independent variable.)

Predictive correlational design: independent and dependent variables. Predictive correlational research also uses the terms "independent" and "dependent" variables, not to denote causation but in a different way. The variable whose value the researcher is attempting to predict is the dependent variable, sometimes called the outcome variable; the researcher tests one or more other variables to discover whether they predict the value of the dependent variable, and to what extent they do so. Those predictors are called independent variables. Vermeesch et al. (2013) conducted predictive correlational research on the contribution of self-esteem to the relationship between stress and depressive symptoms in Hispanic women. In their study, the dependent or outcome variable was depression, and an independent or predictor variable was stress.

Extraneous variables in interventional and correlational studies. **Extraneous variables** are variables that are not central to a study's research purpose: they are not identified as either independent or dependent variables. An extraneous variable has a potential effect on the results, however, making the independent variable appear more or less powerful than it really is in its effect on the value of the dependent variable.

An example of an extraneous variable in health research is an unrelated medical condition that makes a study's dependent variables greater or smaller in value. Lester, Bernhard, and Ryan-Wenger (2012) developed a tool to measure urogenital atrophy in breast cancer survivors. One of the steps in the process was to obtain self-reported symptoms in 168 women with and 166 women without breast cancer. Exclusion criteria were women with a "history of pelvic, perineal, or intravaginal radiation therapy, and/or previous history of other cancer(s)" (p. 78), because this type of history could produce some of the same symptoms being measured, which then would be falsely attributed to side effects of treatment for breast cancer.

When conducting your own study, with an active imagination, you as the researcher will be able to identify a number of potentially extraneous variables that might have an effect on your study's findings. Because of limitations of time and space, however, you will need to make adjustments in the research design and methods in order to attempt to control for the intrusion of only the extraneous variables that are most likely to alter the research findings and consequently force an incorrect conclusion. See Table 6-6 for further information about the goals of controlling for extraneous variables. (For additional information on the effects of extraneous variables and researcher-enacted controls, see Chapters 10 and 11.)

Confounding variables in interventional studies. A **confounding variable** is a special subtype of extraneous variable, but it is unique in that it is embedded in the study design because it is intertwined with the independent variable. Substruction (Dulock & Holzemer, 1991) reveals that, in the case of a confounding variable, the concept underlying the independent variable was not operationalized narrowly enough to exclude a second "piggybacked" variable. An example of this would be an experiment with knee-replacement patients, in which the control group receives physical therapy three times a day, and the experimental group receives a new, different style of physical therapy, also three times a day. A specially trained physical therapist from a renowned clinic is brought to the experimental site for four weeks and performs all physical therapy for the experimental subjects. The control subjects receive physical therapy from whichever therapist is on duty that day. Aside from the difference in type of therapy, are the two groups treated equally? You may already have discerned an important difference: the control group's therapist varies from day to day, according to scheduling, whereas the experimental group subjects see the same therapist every day. If patients feel more comfortable and try to achieve more while working with a familiar therapist, this may skew the study results in favor of the new therapy, making it appear more powerful than it actually is. A second and more serious problem is present as well, though: the therapist from the renowned clinic, although very knowledgeable, has a very jarring personality and a sarcastic sense of humor, which she uses frequently to criticize the efforts of patients and nursing staff members. The hospital's physical therapists are appalled, observing, "If we treated patients and nurses that way, we'd be out of a job." This second confounding variable may skew the study results in favor of the control therapy, making the new therapy seem less powerful than it actually is.

Confounding variables cannot be controlled for, once the study is underway. However, an astute researcher may be able to foresee that one may be present and design the study differently, to avoid the problem. In order to control for unequal treatment for the control group, one strategy would be to train the hospital's physical therapy staff and have them apply the old therapy to the control group and the new therapy to the experimental group. Can you think of any other strategies that would be effective in controlling for this particular confounding variable?

Other Variables Encountered in Quantitative Research

Many other types of variables are named in quantitative research reports. Four of them discussed here pertain to design and several to measurement (Table 6-7).

Research variable is a default term used to refer to a variable that is the focus of a quantitative study but that is not identified as an independent or a dependent variable. Research variables include those stated in the research purpose and question. The design of a study containing research variables is either descriptive or correlational. Happ et al. (2015), in their study concerning the proportion of mechanically ventilated patients who could potentially be served by assistive communication tools and speech-language consultation, used a quantitative descriptive design. The variables in their study were neither predictive nor causative and, consequently, are most appropriately termed research variables.

Modifying variables, when present, are those that change the strength and sometimes the direction of a relationship between other variables. In van der Kooi, Stronks, Thompson, DerSarkissian, and Onyebuchi's (2013) correlational study of the relationship between persons' educational attainment and their self-rated

---

TABLE 6-6   Controlling for Extraneous Variables: The Goals

BEFORE AND DURING THE STUDY	
Goal	**Strategy**
Reduce or eliminate extraneous variables' effects on relationships among the study's principal variables.	• Modify the study's inclusion criteria to eliminate potential subjects possessing a specific extraneous variable. • Use a large sample with random assignment to groups, so that subjects with extraneous variables will be equally distributed between groups.*
Reduce or eliminate the influence of extraneous variables on calculations that measure relationships.	• Measure the effects of extraneous variables and mathematically remove those effects from statistical calculations.
Establish the magnitude and direction of extraneous variables' effects.	• Treat extraneous variables as predictor variables in statistical calculations.
AFTER COMPLETION OF DATA COLLECTION	
Confirm that the effects of potentially extraneous variables were the same in all groups.	• Compare groups to determine whether they demonstrate the same proportion of potentially extraneous variables (post-hoc data analysis).*

*If the groups have approximately the same proportion of subjects with a certain extraneous variable, the researcher can conclude that that particular variable's effects were "controlled for" by the research design and methods.

TABLE 6-7   Other Design Variables

Type of Variable	**Description**
Research variable	Neither an independent nor a dependent variable; the focus of a quantitative research study that is neither causative nor predictive
Modifying variable	A variable that changes the strength, and possibly the direction, of a relationship between other variables
Mediating variable	A variable that is an intermediate link in the relationship between other variables
Environmental variable	A characteristic of the study setting

health, the level of development of the country was found to be a modifying variable: as the level of development of the country increased, the relationship between educational attainment and self-rated health became even stronger.

Mediating variables are intermediate variables that occur as links in the chain between independent and dependent variables. Often they provide insight as to the relationship between the independent and dependent variables, especially in physiological research. For example, in their research of self-efficacy, social support, and other psychosocial variables in patients with diabetes and depression, Tovar, Rayens, Gokun and Clark (2015) found that self-efficacy was an important link between other variables' relationships, reporting that their findings "suggest complete mediation via self-efficacy and some types of social support" (p. 1405).

Environmental variables are those that emanate from the research setting. In a healthcare milieu, they include but are not limited to temperature, ambient noise, lighting, rules regulating the length of nurses' breaks, floor surface covering, actions of other clients, and furniture. Unless they interfere with interventional research, no attempt is made to control for their effects. However, if the researcher assesses an environmental variable as potentially interfering with data collection, such as the presence of a delusional client who intrudes into an interview room and interrupts the flow of conversation during qualitative interviewing of acute care patients, the researcher can control for the variable by relocating interviews to a room further away from acute care areas.

Variables Pertaining to Measurement

There are many variable names that pertain to measurement. These are infrequently encountered in the purposes, objectives, aims, questions, and hypotheses segment of the research report, and are usually encountered in the Methods and Results sections. Some of these are listed in Table 6-8.

A dichotomous or binary variable, sometimes called a Bernoulli variable, is one with only two possible values, such as dead-alive, yes-no, truth-dare, present-absent, pregnant-not pregnant, or left-right. Dichotomous variables are a subtype of nominal variables. A **nominal** or **categorical variable** is one with values that are names or categories, not numbers with real mathematical values, such as married-partnered-divorced-widowed-single, Type 1-Type 2-Type 3, or dog-cat-parrot-piranha. A **continuous** or **ratio variable**, such as age, can have an infinite number of values because it allows for fractions and decimal values, whereas a discrete variable,

TABLE 6-8 Variables Pertaining to Measurement

Type of Variable	Other Name	Description
Dichotomous	Binary, Bernoulli	The variable has only two possible values.
Nominal*	Categorical	Values are names or categories, not real numbers.
Continuous	Ratio	Values use the real number scale, including the values between numerals.
Discrete		Numeric values used are not continuous.

*From the Latin *nomina*, which means name.

such as number of times hospitalized, does not have potential values in the "gaps" between numbers. Because of this, when reporting the average or mean of a set of values of a continuous variable, a decimal or fractional value may be used, whereas the mean of several values of a discrete variable should be rounded to a whole number. Of the following demographic variables, half are continuous and half discrete: current age, number of children in one's family of origin, income in the previous 12 months, length of time employed at current job, number of motor vehicle accidents in the past five years, and stage of tumor.

DEFINING CONCEPTS AND OPERATIONALIZING VARIABLES IN QUANTITATIVE STUDIES

A variable can be defined both conceptually and operationally, revealing both its meaning and its means of measurement in a particular study. A conceptual definition might be used for several studies (see Chapter 3 for further clarification and example).

Conceptual Definitions

A **conceptual definition** identifies the meaning of an idea. Regardless of methodology, a study's principal concepts require some amount of conceptual definition, first so that the researcher is crystal-clear as to what is being studied, and second so that the eventual audience for the research results will understand what was investigated. A conceptual definition can be derived from a theorist's definition of a variable or developed through concept analysis. However, a definition also may be drawn from the theoretical piece of the literature review (see Chapter 8, for potential sources of conceptual definitions). Alternatively, the conceptual definition may be drawn from previous publications on the same topic, a medical dictionary, and even a standard dictionary, and then synthesized by the researcher so as to encompass the study's intended focus.

In quantitative research, conceptual definitions of the principal variables seldom appear in the published report, unless the study focuses on concepts and their interactions, which occurs in a predictive correlational design. If conceptual definitions do appear, they can be found in the Literature Review/Background or Methods section of the report.

Defining Concepts in Qualitative Research

In qualitative research, it is typical for the phenomenon of interest to be conceptually defined quite thoroughly. This definition appears in the Introduction, in the Review of the Literature section or, less frequently, in the Results or Conclusions section when definition of the phenomenon of interest was the solitary goal of the research. If a definition is interlaced in discussions of its meaning as revealed in other publications, it is derived from the literature or other sources. If it appears later in the report, the definition emanates from the research data and represents at least part of the study results.

As described earlier in the chapter, Bunkers (2012) used phenomenological inquiry "to enhance understanding of the lived experience of feeling disappointed" (p. 53). After considerable discussion of works from sociology, psychotherapy, philosophy, education, communications, and social science describing disappointment, the author synthesized a conceptual definition of this phenomenon of interest as, "From a human becoming perspective, a synthetic definition of feeling disappointed is the following: feeling disappointed expresses the loss of an expected good fortune surfacing discontent and regret while engaging with others in forging on" (Bunkers, 2012, p. 55), which appears near the end of the section reviewing the literature.

Operational Definitions in Quantitative Research

The conceptual level of thinking is the first and higher level; the second level is the operational level (Dulock & Holzemer, 1991). Operationally defining a concept converts it to a variable and establishes how it will be

measured in that particular study. The researcher selects the **operational definition** that results in a measurement that is best for that study.

Because concepts in qualitative research are not measured during the research process, it makes little sense to define them operationally. Quantitative research, though, does involve measurement, so each variable that will be measured must be operationally defined, revealing the way in which it will be measured.

In the research report of their correlational study of supervisor practices, employees' perceptions of well-being, and employee commitment, Brunetto et al. (2013) presented these ways of measuring perceived organizational support, employee engagement, and organizational commitment, actually using the word "operationalized," which is unusual in a report:

"Perceived Organizational Support was measured using the validated instrument by Eisenberger et al. (1997), including: 'My organisation cares about my opinion.' Well-being was measured using a four-item scale by Brunetto et al. (2011a) including: 'Most days I feel a sense of accomplishment in what I do at work.'

Employee Engagement was operationalized as employees' positive work-related state of fulfillment and was measured using a nine-item scale from Schaufeli and Bakker (2003) (reflective measure), including: 'Time flies when I'm working.'

Organizational Commitment: using the eight-item scale from Allen and Meyer (1990), we measured nurses' commitment to their organizations (reflective measure), including: 'I feel a strong sense of belonging to this hospital.'" (Brunetto et al., 2013, p. 2790)

Although they did not use the word *operationalization*, Vermeesch et al. (2013) presented the ways they measured variables:

"Hispanic stress was measured using the Hispanic Stress Inventory (HSI; Cervantes et al., 1991). ... Self-esteem was measured using the RSE (Rosenberg, 1965). ... Depressive symptoms were assessed with the CES-D (Radloff, 1977)." (Vermeesch et al., 2013, pp. 1329–1330)

A succinct format in which to present operational definitions is the general statement, "The variable _____ was operationally defined as _____ measured with the _____ ..." and then stating other particulars such as "by the research assistant at 10 a.m., in the outpatient orthopedics clinic, immediately after completion of the patient demographic instrument." More specifics about who will measure, when the measurement will be performed, and where the measurement will be obtained are especially important in physiological studies. When stating how variables will be measured for all master's theses and dissertations, students should provide as much detail as possible regarding who, when, and where, articulating these within the operational definition.

HYPOTHESES

A **hypothesis** is a stated relationship between or among variables, within a specified population. It uses the same variables originally identified as concepts in the research purpose and subsequently given operational definitions. It uses the same population identified in the purpose and research question. It uses the same relationships identified in the purpose and question, if a relationship is stated, focusing on the association between variables if the research is correlational, or on causation if one variable is proposed to cause another. The wording of the hypothesis can almost dictate specific designs, through use of phrases like "over time" or "demonstrating incrementally larger effects with repeated applications." Along with measurement strategies, the hypothesis determines appropriate statistical tests for the study. Because the hypothesis is the stated relationship among variables, like the variables, it exists at the concrete level.

The scientific method rests on the process of stating a hypothesis, testing it, and rejecting or accepting the hypothesis. The hypothesis-testing process involves several steps, the first two of which are identification of a research hypothesis and construction of the corresponding null hypothesis. Even if a hypothesis is not identified in a research report, when a study is experimental or quasi-experimental, a hypothesis is present. Most correlational research and some quantitative descriptive research studies use hypotheses as well.

The purpose of the hypothesis statement is to begin the logical process of hypothesis testing (see Chapter 3). Consequently, phrasing and accuracy make a difference. Through careful substruction (Dulock & Holzemer, 1991), the researcher makes certain that there is coherency between the hypothesis's posited relationships among variables and the study's identified theoretical framework. If the theoretical framework is not coherent with the hypothesis, a new framework should be chosen, or a framework newly developed, using the hypothesis as a jumping-off point (Box 6-1).

BOX 6-1 Creating a Framework From the Study Hypothesis

To demonstrate the process of creating a framework, imagine that infection with a newly identified widespread global virus World ABCD produces initial disinhibition (the brain does not inhibit behaviors in its usual way), followed by difficulties with executive function (diminished wisdom and poorly considered decision making), then loss of some gross motor skills, loss of cognitive acquisitions like arithmetic and ability to read, and finally confusion, impaired manual dexterity, and speech impairment. Onset of symptoms is gradual and progressive, peaking in severity at about eight weeks after infection. Recovery from the virus takes several months, during which the symptoms abate, in reverse order to the way in which they appeared, with speech impairment resolving first and disinhibition last.

A therapist working with patients notes that their recoveries parallel normal human development and devises a therapy program that uses developmentally appropriate teaching for anticipatory guidance after patients emerge from confusion, to guide them in re-acquisition of cognitive and gross motor skills, and subsequently incorporates dialectical behavior therapy in assisting patients with their executive functioning and inhibition of impulses, until they are fully recovered. The therapist decides to study the patients' outcomes, in terms of adaptation, safety, and social disasters, comparing them with patients in a nearby sister facility that uses the traditional therapy model. The therapist-researcher uses the hypothesis that anticipatory guidance assists patients to be safer and more socially appropriate while they return to "adult" status, and helps their families support them through the final stages of becoming successfully self-governing and progressively less in need of supervision and guidance.

The therapist-researcher had originally chosen a theoretical framework of neuro-rehabilitation used in post-stroke recovery, but notes that the patients with World ABCD do not rehabilitate in the same way, nor with the same outcomes. After an initial period of panic, the researcher decides to construct a framework from the study hypothesis, based loosely on physiological neuro-development and on psychological studies of decision making between ages 10 and 25 years, also constructing a map showing loss of function and recovery as mirror-images of one another, and calling the idea the World ABCD De-Development and Re-Development Framework.

Types of Hypotheses

There are four categories used to describe hypotheses, reflecting types of relationships, number of variables, direction of the posited relationship, and use in the process of hypothesis testing. They are (1) causative versus associative, (2) simple versus complex, (3) directional versus nondirectional, and (4) null versus research.

Causal versus Associative Hypotheses

Relationships in hypotheses may be identified as associative or causal (Figure 6-2). A **causal hypothesis** proposes a cause-and-effect relationship between variables, in which one causes the other. The cause is the independent variable; the result is the dependent variable.

McCain, Del Moral, Duncan, Fontaine, and Piño (2012) presented their causal hypothesis for the effect of the semidemand feeding method on amount of time it took infants to learn to nipple-feed, "... the hypothesis that preterm infants with bronchopulmonary dysplasia who transitioned from gavage to nipple feeding with the semidemand method would achieve nipple feeding sooner and be discharged from hospital sooner than control infants who received standard care" (p. 380). Norris, Hughes, Hecht, Peragallo, and Nickerson (2013) also used a causal hypothesis in their research as, "... the hypothesis that playing an avatar-based virtual reality technology game can strengthen peer resistance skills, and early adolescent Hispanic girls will have a positive response to this game" (p. 25). In general, a causal hypothesis mentions the independent variable first and then the dependent variable or variables.

An **associative hypothesis** presents a non-causative relationship between or among variables. None of the variables are posited to cause any of the other variables: two or more of them merely may vary in unison.

Toscano (2012) tested a new tool intended to identify violence in dating relationships in college women, offering an associative hypothesis for its relationship with various existent measurement instruments, "... results from the Danger Assessment (DA) tool and the Abuse Assessment Screen (AAS) will be highly correlated with concepts from the Theory of Female Adolescents' Safety as Determined by the Dynamics of the Circle (TFASDC)" (p. 81). Lin, MacLennan, Hunt, and Cox (2015) investigated the quality of Taiwanese nurses' working lives in relation to transformational leadership styles, identifying seven hypotheses in their work. The first two hypotheses listed in the article, and both associative, are (1) "Transformational leadership styles are related to nursing mental health outcomes" and (2) "The higher the level of transformational leadership, the higher the level of perceived supervisor support" (p. 2).

Simple versus Complex Hypotheses

Hypotheses may be simple or complex (Figures 6-3 and 6-4). A **simple hypothesis** predicts the relationship between only two variables. It may be either causal or associative. In Dobson's (2015) study, assessing the effect of using guided imagery (GI) upon self-efficacy, in children with sickle cell disease (SCD), the author stated her simple hypothesis: "Children with SCD who use guided imagery will have greater disease-specific self-efficacy following training with GI, than they had prior to training" (p. 385). The two variables were guided imagery and disease-specific self-efficacy. The intervention of GI was successful in improving children's disease-specific self-efficacy.

Edmunds, Sekhobo, Dennison, Chiasson, and Stratton (2014) "... tested their simple hypothesis that early enrollment in the Special Supplemental Nutrition Program for Women, Infants and Children (WIC) is associated with a reduced risk of rapid infant weight

FIGURE 6-2 Causal hypothesis versus associative hypothesis. Note that the "arrow of causation" points from the independent variable toward the dependent variable.

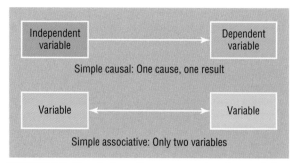

FIGURE 6-3 Simple hypotheses: causal and associative.

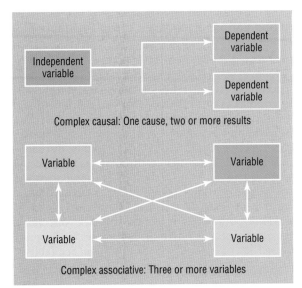

FIGURE 6-4 Complex hypotheses: causal and associative.

gain (RIWG)" (p. S35). The two variables were early enrollment in WIC and RIWG. The results revealed that the variables were associated.

A **complex hypothesis** predicts the relationship among three or more variables. It may be either causal or associative. In interventional research, this means one independent variable and two or more dependent variables; in correlational research, this merely indicates that three variables or more will be examined. McCain et al. (2012), in their experimental study of the effect of the semidemand feeding method on earlier ability to nipple-feed and resultant earlier discharge from the hospital stated their complex hypothesis as, "… the hypothesis that preterm infants with bronchopulmonary dysplasia who transitioned from gavage to nipple-feeding with the semidemand method would achieve nipple feeding sooner and be discharged home from hospital sooner than control infants who received standard care" (p. 380). The independent variable was the semidemand method of feeding, and the dependent variables were time until achievement of nipple-feeding and discharge home. Rodwell, Brunetto, Demir, Shacklock, and Farr-Wharton's (2014) study presented the complex hypothesis: "Isolating behaviors will be linked directly and indirectly to the health and work outcomes of decreased job satisfaction, increased psychological strain, and increased intention to quit," in their correlational study of abusive supervision and nurses' intention to quit their jobs (p. 359). The variables examined in this complex hypothesis were

isolating behaviors, job satisfaction, psychological strain, and intention to quit.

Nondirectional Versus Directional Hypotheses

A **directional hypothesis** states the nature or direction of a proposed relationship between variables. If a researcher anticipates the direction of the proposed relationship, increase versus decrease, more versus less, the hypothesis includes directional wording. In their correlational study of abusive supervision, Rodwell et al.'s (2014) hypothesis, "Isolating behaviors will be linked directly and indirectly to the health and work outcomes of decreased job satisfaction, increased psychological strain, and increased intention to quit" (p. 359), is a directional one, predicting a decrease in job satisfaction, an increase in psychological strain, and an increase in the intention to quit.

Apostolo, Cardoso, Rosa, and Paul (2014) stated the hypothesis, in their experimental study of the effect of cognitive stimulation therapy (CST) on cognition and depressive symptoms of elder adults in nursing homes (NH) as, "… we hypothesize that elderly residents in NHs who received 14 sessions of CST will achieve improved cognition and depressive symptoms" (p. 158). Their hypothesis was directional, specifying improvement in the dependent variables of cognition and depressive symptoms.

A **nondirectional hypothesis**, as the definition implies, does not specify the direction of the relationship between and among variables. If the researcher does not anticipate any particular direction of the proposed relationship, increase versus decrease, more versus less, the hypothesis will be worded nondirectionally. Del-Pino-Casado, Frías-Osuna, Palomino-Moral, and Martínez-Riera (2012) in their study of differences between male and female informal caregivers of elders, presented the hypothesis, "There are gender differences in subjective burden among informal caregivers of older people" (p. 349), not specifying whether the subjective burden would be higher in female or in male caregivers. Wang, Zhan, Zhang, and Xia (2015) in their research of blame attribution in cancer diagnosis presented the hypothesis, "Participants' blame attributions to cancer patients are associated with participants' educational level, personal/family history of cancer, and personal unhealthy behaviours," (p. 1601) in which the associations were not identified as positive or negative in direction.

Null Versus Research Hypotheses

The **null hypothesis** (H_0), also referred to as a **statistical hypothesis**, is used for statistical testing and interpretation of results. Even if the null hypothesis is not stated, it may be derived by stating the opposite of the research hypothesis. A null hypothesis can be simple or complex, associative or causal. Although seen infrequently, occasionally a null hypothesis is phrased so that it mentions direction, and can thus be argued to be directional, such as the null hypothesis that the independent variable does not increase the magnitude of the dependent variable.

Killion et al. (2014) studied the relationship in health science educators between use of smart devices and burnout. Their null hypothesis was "… that there would be no statistically significant effects of increased connectivity … on burnout scores" (p. 150). Results of the study allowed rejection of the null hypothesis in favor of the unstated alternative hypothesis, also called the research hypothesis: "there will be statistically significant effects of increased connectivity on burnout scores." More accurately phrased as the unstated relationship between the study variables, the research hypothesis or alternative hypothesis would be "In health science educators, increased connectivity through smart device use is positively related to job burnout."

Secomb, McKenna, and Smith (2012) used a pretest-posttest experimental design to study the effect on cognitive scores of nursing students, randomly assigned to either self-instructed activities, or to instructor-facilitated activities, in simulation laboratory learning environments. Their null hypothesis was: "There is no significant difference in nursing students' cognitive gain scores between self-instructed simulation activities in computer-based learning environments and facilitated simulation activities in instructor-led skills laboratory learning environments" (p. 3479).

A **research hypothesis** is the alternative hypothesis (H_1 or H_a) to the null, and it represents the research's posited results. The research hypothesis states that "there is a relationship" between two or more variables, and that relationship can be simple or complex, nondirectional or directional, and associative or causal. As such, it is opposite to the null hypothesis. All of the hypotheses presented previously are research hypotheses, except for those of Killion et al. (2014) and Secomb et al. (2012).

Researchers have different beliefs about when to state a research hypothesis versus a null hypothesis in a research report. A few list both of them. Although some researchers state the null hypothesis because it is more consistent with the reporting of statistical analyses, the vast majority of articles present the research hypothesis only. This is a matter of style: the reader of a report can easily construct one hypothesis, given the other.

Putting Various Hypothesis Types Together

A single study can be described in terms of all four of these paired descriptions of hypotheses. For instance, McCain et al.'s (2012) hypothesis for their study on preterm infants and transition to nipple feeding was "… the hypothesis for this study that preterm infants with bronchopulmonary dysplasia who transitioned from gavage to nipple feeding with the semidemand method would achieve nipple feeding sooner and be discharged from hospital sooner than control infants who received standard care" (p. 380). Of the choices, causal or associative, simple or complex, directional or nondirectional, and null or research, one can identify McCain et al.'s (2012) hypothesis as a causal, complex, directional, research hypothesis. Given the hypotheses for the previous articles, how would you identify them? See Table 6-9 for the classifications.

Testing Hypotheses

Hypotheses exist for the purpose of testing them. After testing, using proper statistical procedures, they are the researcher's basis for reporting results, identifying findings, and forming both conclusions and generalizations. Hypotheses are evaluated in the hypothesis-testing process, described in Chapter 3. To learn more about selecting appropriate statistical tests and a level of significance for testing hypotheses, see Chapters 21 through 25.

As described in Chapter 3, the results of hypothesis testing are described with unique wording. Research findings do not "prove" hypotheses true or false: instead, "there is evidence" for their support. After a series of studies of the same hypothesis with identical positive findings, the word "proven" is still not used; instead, "there is considerable evidence" in support of the hypothesis. If a null hypothesis is "accepted," that acceptance is always provisional. The same is true for the "rejection" of a null hypothesis: falsification of a hypothesis by a single test, according to Popper (1968), cannot stand unsupported, because "non-reproducible single occurrences are of no significance to science" (p. 86). Replication is essential, whether rejection or acceptance is the outcome for a single study.

Mixed Methods Research and Outcomes Research

As observed in Chapter 5, because of its incorporation of two different designs, mixed methods research may contain more than one stated purpose (Beischel, 2013). When only a single purpose is stated, however, two objectives or aims may be identified, clarifying the two distinct

TABLE 6-9	**Hypothesis Types in Research**				
Authors, Year	**Hypothesis**	**Causal or Associative**	**Simple or Complex**	**Directional or Nondirectional**	**Null or Research**
Apostolo, Cardoso, Rosa, and Paul (2014)	"… we hypothesize that elderly residents in NHs who received 14 sessions of CST will achieve improved cognition and depressive symptoms" (p. 158)	Causal	Complex	Directional	Research
Dobson (2015)	"Children with SCD who use guided imagery will have greater disease-specific self-efficacy following training with GI, than they had prior to training" (p. 385).	Causal	Simple	Directional	Research
Edmunds, Sekhobo, Dennison, Chiasson, & Stratton (2014)	"… tested the hypothesis that early enrollment in the Special Supplemental Nutrition Program for Women, Infants and Children (WIC) is associated with a reduced risk of rapid infant weight gain (RIWG)" (p. S35)	Associative	Simple	Directional	Research
Killion et al. (2014)	"… that there would be no statistically significant effects of increased connectivity … on burnout scores" (p. 150)	Associative	Simple	Nondirectional (but direction is implied in the article)	Null
McCain, Del Moral, Duncan, Fontaine, & Piño (2012)	"… the hypothesis for this study that preterm infants with bronchopulmonary dysplasia who transitioned from gavage to nipple feeding with the semidemand method would achieve nipple feeding sooner and be discharged from hospital sooner than control infants who received standard care" (p. 380)	Causal	Complex	Directional	Research

Continued

TABLE 6-9 **Hypothesis Types in Research—cont'd**

Authors, Year	Hypothesis	Causal or Associative	Simple or Complex	Directional or Nondirectional	Null or Research
Norris, Hughes, Hecht, Peragallo, & Nickerson (2013)	"… the hypothesis that playing an avatar-based virtual reality technology game can strengthen peer resistance skills, and early adolescent Hispanic girls will have a positive response to this game" (p. 25)	Causal	Complex	Directional	Research
Rodwell, Brunetto, Demir, Shacklock, & Farr-Wharton (2014)	"Isolating behaviors will be linked directly and indirectly to the health and work outcomes of decreased job satisfaction, increased psychological strain, and increased intention to quit" (p. 359)	Associative	Complex	Directional	Research
Secomb, McKenna, and Smith (2012)	"There is no significant difference in nursing students' cognitive gain scores between self-instructed simulation activities in computer-based learning environments and facilitated simulation activities in instructor-led skills laboratory learning environments" (p. 3479)	Causal	Simple	Nondirectional (but direction is implied in the article)	Null
Toscano (2012)	"… results from the Danger Assessment (DA) tool and the Abuse Assessment Screen (AAS) will be highly correlated with concepts from the Theory of Female Adolescents' Safety as Determined by the Dynamics of the Circle (TFASDC)" (p. 81)	Associative	Complex	Nondirectional as stated (but implied in text that this is a positive correlation, since this research tested a new tool, against two others)	Research

parts of the inquiry. Mixed methods research with one quantitative and one qualitative design can contain either one or more than one research question, although inclusion of two questions is preferred, for clarity (Creswell, 2014). Variables that will be used for the quantitative part of the study require both conceptual and operational definition. Hypotheses are included if the quantitative portion of the study involves hypothesis testing.

Outcomes research, because it uses quantitative designs, follows the guidelines presented in this chapter for quantitative research in respect to objectives, aims, research questions, definition of variables, and hypothesis testing. The exception is that objectives, aims, and questions often contain the word outcomes.

▮ KEY POINTS

- The research problem and purpose are stated abstractly. The research question is the bridge between abstract and conceptual levels. Variables, the relationships among them, the study hypothesis, the specifics of measurement, and quantitative data are concrete because they are consistent with classification, counting, or measurement.
- A research question is a concise, interrogative statement that is worded in the present tense and includes one or more of the study's principal concepts. The principal research question is usually a rewording of the study's purpose.
- In research, a concept is one focus of a study. The principal focus of a study, quantitative or qualitative, is the phenomenon of interest. A variable is a concept that has been made measurable for a particular quantitative study.
- Demographic variables are subject characteristics measured during a study and used to describe a sample.
- The independent variable is the intervention or treatment that the researcher applies to the experimental group but not to the control group. In predictive correlational research, an independent variable is a predictor of the value of the dependent variable.
- The dependent variable is the result or outcome that is the study's focus.
- An extraneous variable is not central to the study's research purpose but has a potential effect on the results, making the independent variable appear more or less powerful than it really is in its effect on the value of the dependent variable.
- A confounding variable is a special subtype of extraneous variable that is intertwined with the independent variable.

- Research variable is a default term used to refer to variables that are the focus of a quantitative study but that are not independent or dependent variables.
- Modifying variables, when present, are variables that change the strength and sometimes the direction of a relationship between other variables.
- Mediating variables are intermediate variables that occur as links in the chain between independent and dependent variables.
- Environmental variables are those that emanate from the research setting.
- A conceptual definition makes a concept understandable, revealing its meaning. An operational definition makes a concept measurable, indicating the way it will be measured in a particular study.
- A hypothesis is a stated relationship between or among variables, within a specified population.
- Hypotheses can be described in terms of four categories: (1) associative versus causal, (2) simple versus complex, (3) nondirectional versus directional, and (4) null versus research.

REFERENCES

Alexis, O. (2015). Internationally recruited nurses' experiences in England: A survey approach. *Nursing Outlook, 63*(3), 238–244.

Allen, N. J., & Meyer, J. P. (1990). The measurement and antecedents of affective, continuance, and normative commitment to the organization. *Journal of Occupation Psychology, 63*(1), 1–18.

Apostolo, J. L. A., Cardoso, D. F. B., Rosa, A. I., & Paul, C. (2014). The effect of cognitive stimulation on nursing home elders: A randomized controlled trial. *Journal of Nursing Scholarship, 46*(3), 157–166.

Arvidsson, S., Bergman, S., Arvidsson, B., Fridlund, B., & Tingstrom, P. (2013). Effects of a self-care promoting problem-based learning programme in people with rheumatic diseases: A randomized controlled study. *Journal of Advanced Nursing, 69*(7), 1500–1514.

Baum, A., & Kagan, I. (2015). Job satisfaction and intent to leave among psychiatric nurses: Closed versus open wards. *Archives of Psychiatric Nursing, 29*(4), 213–216.

Beischel, K. P. (2013). Variables affecting learning in a simulation experience: A mixed methods study. *Western Journal of Nursing Research, 35*(2), 226–247.

Biron, A. D., Loiselle, C., & Lavoie-Tremblay, M. (2009). Work interruptions and their contributions to medication administration errors: An evidence review. *Worldviews on Evidence-based Nursing, 6*(2), 70–86.

Brixey, J., Robinson, D., Turley, J., & Zhang, J. (2007). Initiators of interruption in workflow: The role of MDs and RNs. *Information Technology in Health Care, 130*, 103–109.

Brunetto, Y., Farr-Wharton, R., & Shacklock, K. (2011a). Using the Harvard HRM model to conceptualise the impact of changes to supervision upon HRM outcomes for different types of public sector employees. *International Journal of Human Resource Management, 22*(3), 553–573.

Brunetto, Y., Xiong, M., Shriberg, A., Farr-Wharton, R., Shacklock, K., Newman, S., et al. (2013). The impact of workplace relationships on engagement, well-being, commitment and turnover for nurses in Australia and the USA. *Journal of Advanced Nursing, 69*(12), 2786–2799.

Bunkers, S. S. (2012). The lived experience of feeling disappointed: A Parse research method study. *Nursing Science Quarterly, 25*(1), 53–61.

Calvin, A. O., Engebretson, J. C., & Sardual, S. A. (2014). Understanding of advance care planning by family members of persons undergoing hemodialysis. *Western Journal of Nursing Research, 36*(10), 1357–1373.

Cervantes, R. C., Padilla, A. M., & Salgado de Snyder, N. (1991). The Hispanic Stress Inventory: A culturally relevant approach to psychosocial assessment. *Psychological Assessment, 3*(3), 438–447.

Creswell, J. W. (2014). *Research design: Qualitative, quantitative and mixed methods approaches* (4th ed.). Thousand Oaks, CA: Sage.

del-Pino-Casado, R., Frias-Osuna, A., Palomino-Moral, P. A., & Martinez-Riera, J. R. (2012). Gender differences regarding informal caregivers of older people. *Journal of Nursing Scholarship, 44*(4), 349–357.

De Santis, J. P., Gonzalez-Guarda, R., & Vasquez, E. P. (2012). Psychosocial and cultural correlates of depression among Hispanic men with HIV infection: A pilot study. *Journal of Psychiatric and Mental Health Nursing, 19*(10), 860–869.

Dobson, C. (2015). Outcome results of self-efficacy in children with sickle disease pain who were taught to use guided imagery. *Applied Nursing Research, 28*(4), 384–390.

Dulock, H. L., & Holzemer, W. L. (1991). Substruction: Improving the linkage from theory to method. *Nursing Science Quarterly, 4*(2), 83–87.

Edmunds, L. S., Sekhobo, J. P., Dennison, B. A., Chiasson, M. A., & Stratton, H. H. (2014). Association of prenatal participation in a public health nutrition program with healthy infant weight gain. *American Journal of Public Health, 104*(S1), S35–S42.

Eisenberger, R., Cummings, J., Armeli, S., & Lynch, P. (1997). Perceived organizational support, discretionary treatment and job satisfaction. *Journal of Applied Psychology, 82*(5), 812–820.

Fredericks, S. (2009). Timing for delivering individualized patient education intervention to coronary artery bypass graft patients: An RCT. *European Journal of Cardiovascular Nursing, 8*(2), 144–150.

Fredericks, S., Sidani, S., & Shugurensky, D. (2008). The effect of anxiety on learning outcomes post-CABG. *Canadian Journal of Nursing Research, 40*(1), 127–140.

Fredericks, S., & Yau, T. (2013). Educational intervention reduces complications and rehospitalizations after heart surgery. *Western Journal of Nursing Research, 35*(10), 1251–1265.

González-Guarda, R. M., Peragallo, N., Vasquez, E. P., Urrutia, M. T., & Mitrani, V. B. (2009). Intimate partner violence, depression, and resource availability among a community sample of Hispanic women. *Issues in Mental Health Nursing, 30*(4), 227–236.

Guru, V., Fremes, S., Austin, P., Blackstone, E., & Tu, J. (2006). Gender differences in outcomes after hospital discharge from coronary artery bypass grafting. *Circulation, 113*(4), 507–516.

Hannan, E. L., Racz, M. J., Walford, G., Ryan, T. J., Isom, O. W., Bennett, E., et al. (2003). Predictors of readmission for complications of coronary artery bypass graft surgery. *Journal of the American Medical Association, 290*(6), 773–780.

Happ, M. B., Seaman, J. B., Nilsen, M. L., Sciulli, A., Tate, J. A., Saul, M., et al. (2015). The number of mechanically ventilated ICU patients meeting communication criteria. *Heart and Lung: The Journal of Critical Care, 44*(1), 45–49.

Harkness, K., Smith, K. M., Taraba, L., MacKenzie, C. L., Gunn, E., & Arthur, H. M. (2005). Effect of a postoperative telephone intervention on attendance at intake for cardiac rehabilitation after coronary artery bypass graft surgery. *Heart and Lung: The Journal of Critical Care, 34*(3), 179–186.

Huang, H. P., Chen, M.-L., Liang, J., & Miaskowski, C. (2015). Changes in and predictors of severity of fatigue in women with breast cancer: A longitudinal study. *International Journal of Nursing Studies, 51*(4), 582–592.

Kawafha, M. M., & Tawalbeh, L. I. (2015). The effect of asthma education program on knowledge of school teachers: A randomized controlled trial. *Western Journal of Nursing Research, 37*(4), 425–440.

Killion, J. B., Johnston, J. N., Gresham, J., Gipson, M., Vealé, B. L., Behrens, P. I., et al. (2014). Smart device use and burnout among health science educators. *Radiologic Technology, 86*(2), 144–154.

Kreckler, S., Catchpole, K., Bottomley, M., Handa, A., & McCulloch, P. (2008). Interruptions during drug rounds: An observational study. *British Journal of Nursing, 17*(21), 1326–1330.

Land, H., & Hudson, S. (2004). Stress, coping, and depressive symptomatology in Latina and Anglo Aids caregivers. *Psychology & Health, 19*(5), 643–666.

Lester, J., Bernhard, L., & Ryan-Wenger, N. (2012). A self-report instrument that describes urogenital atrophy in breast cancer survivors. *Western Journal of Nursing Research, 34*(1), 72–96.

Lin, P.-Y., MacLennan, S., Hunt, N., & Cox, T. (2015). The influences of nursing transformational leadership style on the quality of nurses' working lives in Taiwan: A cross-sectional quantitative study. *BMC Nursing, 14*(1), 33. Retrieved February 18, 2016 from http://bmcnurs.biomedcentral.com/articles/10.1186/s12912-015-0082-x.

Mallidou, A. A., Cummings, G. G., Schalm, C., & Estabrooks, C. A. (2013). Health care aides use of time in a residential long-term care unit: A time and motion study. *International Journal of Nursing Studies, 50*(9), 1229–1239.

McCain, G. C., Del Moral, T., Duncan, R. C., Fontaine, J. L., & Piño, L. D. (2012). Transition from gavage to nipple feeding for preterm infants with bronchopulmonary dysplasia. *Nursing Research, 61*(6), 380–387.

Moore, S. M., & Dolansky, A. (2001). Randomized trial of a home recovery intervention following coronary artery bypass surgery. *Research in Nursing & Health, 24*(2), 93–104.

Norris, A. E., Hughes, C., Hecht, M., Peragallo, N., & Nickerson, D. (2013). Randomized trial of a peer resistance skill-building game for Hispanic early adolescent girls. *Nursing Research, 62*(1), 25–35.

O'Connell, B., Ockerby, C. M., Johnson, S., Smenda, H., & Bucknall, T. K. (2013). Team clinical supervision in acute hospital wards: A feasibility study. *Western Journal of Nursing Research, 35*(3), 330–347.

Osafo, J., Knizek, B. L., Akotia, C. S., & Hjelmeland, H. (2012). Attitudes and psychologists and nurses toward suicide and suicide prevention in Ghana: A qualitative study. *International Journal of Nursing Studies, 49*(6), 691–700.

Paxton, F., Heaney, D. J., Howie, J. G., & Porter, A. M. (1996). A study of interruption rates for practice nurses and GPs. *Nursing Standard, 10*(43), 33–36.

Plutchik, R. (1991). *The emotions: Facts, theories, and a new model* (rev. ed). New York: University Press of America.

Popper, K. R. (1968). *The logic of scientific discovery*. New York: Harper & Row, Publishers.

Poutiainen, H., Levälahti, E., Hakulainan-Viitanen, T., & Laatikainen, T. (2015). Family characteristics and health behaviour as antecedants of school nurses' concerns about adolescents' health development: A path model approach. *International Journal of Nursing Studies, 52*(5), 920–929.

Radloff, L. S. (1977). The CES-D Scale: A self-report depression scale for research in the general population. *Applied Psychological Measurement, 1*(3), 385–401.

Ramadi, A., Stickland, M. K., Rodgers, W. M., & Haennel, R. G. (2015). Impact of supervised exercise rehabilitation on daily physical activity of cardiopulmonary patients. *Heart and Lung: The Journal of Critical Care, 44*(1), 9–14.

Rodwell, J., Brunetto, Y., Demir, D., Shacklock, K., & Farr-Wharton, R. (2014). Abusive supervision and links to nurse intentions to quit. *Journal of Nursing Scholarship, 46*(5), 357–365.

Roget, P. M., & Dutch, R. A. (Eds.), (1962). *The Original Roget's Thesaurus of English Words and Phrases* (Americanized ed.). New York: Longmans, Green & Co./Dell Publishing Co., Inc.

Rosenberg, M. (1965). *Society and the adolescent self-image*. Princeton, NJ: Princeton University Press.

Schaufeli, W., & Bakker, A. (2003). *UWES Utrecht Work Engagement Scale: Preliminary manual*. Utrecht: Utrecht University, Occupational Health Psychology Unit.

Secomb, J., McKenna, L., & Smith, C. (2012). The effectiveness of simulation activities on the cognitive abilities of undergraduate third-year nursing students: A randomised controlled trial. *Journal of Clinical Nursing, 21*(23–24), 3475–3484.

Solodiuk, J. C. (2013). Parent described pain responses in nonverbal children with intellectual disability. *International Journal of Nursing Studies, 50*(8), 1033–1044.

Søndergaard, B. (2010). Sygeplejersker frygter at begå fejl [Nurses are afraid of making mistakes]. *Sygeplejersken, 17*, 23–25, (in Danish).

Sørensen, E. E., & Brahe, L. (2013). Interruptions in clinical nursing practice. *Journal of Clinical Nursing, 23*(9–10), 1274–1282.

Taubenberger, J. K., & Morens, D. M. (2006). 1918 influenza: Mother of all pandemics. *Emerging Infectious Diseases, 12*(1), 15–22.

Toscano, S. E. (2012). Exploration of a methodology aimed at exploring the characteristics of teenage dating violence and preliminary findings. *Applied Nursing Research, 25*(2), 81–88.

Tovar, E., Rayens, M. K., Gokun, Y., & Clark, M. (2015). Mediators of adherence among adults with comorbid diabetes and depression: The role of self-efficacy and social support. *Journal of Health Psychology, 20*(11), 1405–1415.

van der Kooi, A. L. F., Stronks, K., Thompson, C. A., DerSarkissian, M., & Onyebuchi, A. A. (2013). The modifying influence of country development on the effect of individual educational attainment on self-rated health. *Research and Practice, 103*(11), e49–e54.

Vermeesch, A. L., Gonzales-Guarda, R. M., Hall, R., McCabe, B. E., Cianelli, R., & Peragallo, N. P. (2013). Predictors of depressive symptoms among Hispanic women in south Florida. *Western Journal of Nursing Research, 35*(10), 1325–1338.

Wang, L. D.-L., Zhan, L., Zhang, J., & Xia, Z. (2015). Nurses' blame attributions towards different types of cancer: A cross-sectional study. *International Journal of Nursing Studies, 52*(10), 1600–1606.

Westphal, J., Lancaster, R., & Park, D. (2014). Work-arounds observed by fourth-year nursing students. *Western Journal of Nursing Research, 36*(8), 1002–1028.

Yun, S., Kang, J., Lee, Y.-O., & Yi, Y. (2014). Work environment and workplace bullying among Korean intensive care unit nurses. *Asian Nursing Research, 8*(3), 219–225.

7

Review of Relevant Literature

Jennifer R. Gray

ⓔ http://evolve.elsevier.com/Gray/practice/

New knowledge is being generated constantly. Experts in the 1960s estimated that scientific knowledge doubled every 13 to 15 years (Larsen & von Ins, 2010). Currently, it is estimated that knowledge is doubling every two years (Frické, 2014). Fortunately, electronic bibliographical databases have been developed that can be searched to identify and retrieve publications on a specific topic (Aveyard, 2014). Relevant literature is easily found, but then the challenge lies in selecting the most relevant sources from a very large number of articles. The tasks of reading, critically appraising, analyzing, and synthesizing can become formidable. Tools to manage the complexity of writing a literature review can make the endeavor feasible. The goal of this chapter is to provide basic knowledge and skills about how to write a literature review, beginning with answers to some preliminary questions that the student may have, related to that task. The chapter is designed primarily for the nurse with little experience in writing a review of the literature.

GETTING STARTED: FREQUENTLY ASKED QUESTIONS

What Is a Literature Review?

The **literature review** of a research report is an interpretative, organized, and written presentation of what the study's author has read (Aveyard, 2014). The purpose of conducting a review of the literature is to discover the most recent, and the most relevant, information about a particular phenomenon. The literature review provides an answer to the question "What is known on this topic?" The literature review may be a synthesis of research findings, an overview of relevant

theories, or a description of knowledge on a topic (Paré, Trudel, Jaana, & Kitsiou, 2015). Developing the ability to write coherently about what you have found in the literature requires time and planning. You will organize the information you find into sections by themes, trends, or variables. The purpose is not to list all of the material published, but rather to evaluate, interpret, and synthesize the sources you have read. There are four principal reasons a nurse may conduct a literature review. First, for a nursing student, writing a review of the literature is a course requirement, as in "generate a literature review." Second, as an end-program goal, especially at the master's level, some programs assign a capstone project that includes a substantial literature summary. The third reason is that a literature review is part of the formal research proposal and subsequent report that represents the summative requirement at the end of a master's or doctoral program. Fourth, nurses in practice may be seeking answers to clinical problems and include their review of the literature as part of a proposal to administrators to implement changes.

What Is the "Literature"?

The **literature** consists of all written sources relevant to the selected topic. It consists of printed and electronic newspapers, encyclopedias, conference papers, scientific journals, textbooks, other books, theses, dissertations, and clinical journals. Websites and reports developed by government agencies and professional organizations are included as well. For example, if you were writing a paper on diabetes mellitus, statistics about the prevalence and cost of the disease could be obtained from publications by the Centers for Disease Control and Prevention (CDC) and the World Health Organization

(WHO). Not every source that you find, however, will prove valid and legitimate for scholarly use. The website of a company that sells insulin may not be an appropriate source for diabetes statistics. Users contribute to and edit some online encyclopedias and blogs, such as Wikipedia (Curnalia & Ferris, 2014). There is debate as to whether Wikipedia is an appropriate source for course assignments and scholarly papers (Haigh, 2011). Wikipedia is helpful for gathering preliminary information on a topic. The preliminary information can be used to identify keywords and authors in a subsequent search for professional sources. Wikipedia is not peer-reviewed and most teachers do not accept Wikipedia references as support for information for a formal paper. Scholarly papers and graduate course assignments may require that you use exclusively peer-reviewed professional literature as source material.

Peer review is the process whereby a scholarly abstract, paper, or book is read and evaluated by one or more experts, who make recommendations as to its worth to the professional discipline. Peer review is used for many journal submissions, and also for abstracts submitted for podium or poster presentation at professional conferences: these are accepted or rejected by the journal editor or conference presentation coordinator, on the basis of peer review.

What Types of Literature Can I Expect to Find?

You will be able to find a wide variety of literature because of bibliographical databases. A **bibliographical database** is an "an electronic version of a bibliographic index" (Tensen, 2013, p. 57) or compilation of citations. The database consists of computer data, collected and arranged to be searchable and automatically retrievable. The database may be a broad collection of citations from a variety of disciplines or may consist of citations relevant to a specific discipline or field. Sometimes the latter are called subject-specific electronic databases (Aveyard, 2014). The Cumulative Index to Nursing and Allied Health Literature (CINAHL) is a subject-specific database widely used in nursing.

When searching, you will find two broad types of literature that are cited in the review of literature for a research study: theoretical and empirical. **Theoretical literature** consists of concept analyses, models, theories, and conceptual frameworks that support a selected research problem and purpose. **Empirical literature** is comprised of knowledge derived from research. The quantity of empirical literature depends on the study problem and the number of research reports available. Extensive empirical literature can be found related to common illnesses and health

processes: caring for a person with Alzheimer disease, making health promotion and prevention decisions, or coping with cancer treatment. For newer topics or rare diseases, less literature may be available. When searching for empirical literature, you may find seminal and landmark studies. **Seminal studies** are the studies that prompted the initiation of a field of research. For example, Sacks (2013) published a systematic literature review of suffering and included the findings of a seminal paper published by Cassel (1982). Chickering and Gamson (1987) wrote seminal papers in the area of effective teaching and were included in the review conducted by Parker, McNeill, and Howard (2015). **Landmark studies** are published research that led to an important development or a turning point in a certain field of study. For example, Grabbe's (2015) paper on attachment theory included a review of the literature, in which the author applied attachment theory to primary care. Grabbe cited Bowlby's (1980) landmark theory of attachment as an important development in understanding human development. By citing seminal or landmark papers on their topics, Sacks (2013), Parker et al. (2015), and Grabbe (2015) indicated their awareness of how knowledge has developed as a result of research that has changed their respective fields of study.

Literature is disseminated in several different formats. **Serials** are published over time or may be published in multiple volumes at one time but do not necessarily have recurrent and predictable publication dates. **Periodicals** are subsets of serials with predictable publication dates, such as journals. Periodicals are published over time and are numbered sequentially. This sequential numbering is seen in the year, volume, issue, and page numbering of a journal. The reference for the article by Parker et al. (2015) is as follows:

Parker, R., McNeill, J., & Howard, J. (2015). Comparing pediatric simulation and traditional clinical experience: Student perceptions, learning outcomes, and lessons for faculty. *Clinical Simulation in Nursing, 11*(3), 188-193.

The reference indicates that the article was published in the 11th volume, the 3rd issue, on pages 188-193 in the periodical, *Clinical Simulation in Nursing*. Next year, the periodical will be identified as volume 12 and the first issue will begin again with page number 1. Some journals are published in electronic form only. Because of the high costs of publishing and distributing a printed journal, a publishing company risks losing money unless there is a large market for that journal. Faculty members at some universities have established online journals in particular specialty areas for smaller potential audiences. Online journals may have more current information on your topic than you will find in traditional journals, because the time to review the manuscript is shorter and accepted manuscripts can be published quickly. Articles submitted to printed journals are usually under review for 8 to 12 weeks and, if accepted, may not be seen in print for up to a year. Because of competition from online journals, some print journals are releasing their accepted articles online before publication.

Some online journals are considered open-source. This means that their articles are available online to anyone searching the Internet, instead of access being limited to those persons with a subscription to the journal. When you use a journal published online only, be sure to check the journal description to discover whether the journal is peer-reviewed.

Monographs, such as books, hardcopy conference proceedings, and pamphlets, are written and published for a specific purpose and may be updated with a new edition, as needed. Researchers may present their findings at a national or international conference prior to publishing them, so searching conference proceedings can increase awareness of cutting-edge knowledge in a research area. **Textbooks** are monographs written as resource materials for educational programs. Many books and textbooks are now available in a digital format known as **eBooks** (Tensen, 2013). You may be familiar with digital books in the mass publication literature that are available for download onto special reading devices, such as Kindle or Nook. In the same way, scholarly books and articles can be downloaded to a reading device, cell phone, tablet, laptop, or other computer. Books that in the past would have been difficult to obtain through interlibrary loan are now available 24 hours a day, 7 days a week as eBooks.

To develop the significance and background section of a proposal, you might choose search for **government reports** for the United States (U.S.) and other countries, if appropriate to the topic of the review. A researcher developing a study on nursing interventions related to non-communicable disease in low-resource countries would search Ministry of Health websites for those countries. For example, researchers proposing an intervention study related to malaria in Uganda, East Africa, must be aware of the Uganda government's standards and treatment guidelines for malaria. Researchers developing smoking cessation programs for adolescents living in rural communities would do well to consult the Healthy People 2020 website for the national goals related to smoking cessation among adolescents (http://www.healthypeople.gov/2020/default.aspx/). They may also find it productive to explore health-related rural agencies such as the Federal Office of Rural Health Policy to find reports and position papers relevant to adolescents in rural areas (Health Resources and Services Administration, 2016).

Position papers are disseminated by professional organizations and government agencies to promote a particular viewpoint on a debatable issue. Position papers, along with descriptions of clinical situations, may be included in a discussion of the background and significance of a research problem. For example, a researcher developing a proposal on the health status of recently arrived migrants needs to review the website of the International Organization for Migration (IOM), which has a position paper available online, *Health of Migrants: The Way Forward* (IOM, 2012).

Master's theses and doctoral dissertations are valuable literature as well and are available electronically through ProQuest, a collection of dissertations and theses (http://www.dc4.proquest.com/en-US/default.shtml). A **thesis** is a research project completed as part of the requirements for a master's degree. A **dissertation** is the written report of an extensive research project completed as the final requirement for a doctoral degree. Theses and dissertations can be found by searching ProQuest and other library databases, such as CINAHL. Most PhD dissertations represent original research, not replication studies.

The published literature contains primary and secondary sources. A **primary source** is written by the person who originated, or is responsible for generating, the ideas published (Aveyard, 2014). A research publication authored by the person or people who conducted the research is a primary source. A theoretical book or paper written by the theorist who developed that theory or conceptual content is a primary source. A **secondary source** summarizes or quotes content from primary sources. (In historical research, primary and secondary source materials have slightly different definitions. See Chapter 12). Thus, authors of secondary sources interpret the works of researchers and theorists, paraphrase the information, and cite the primary articles in their papers. You must read secondary sources with caution, knowing that the secondary authors' interpretations may have been influenced by their own perceptions and biases. Sometimes authors have spread errors and misinterpretations by using secondary sources rather than primary sources (Aveyard, 2014). You should use primary sources as much as possible when writing literature reviews. However, secondary sources are properly used in several instances. Box 7-1 lists situations in which it is appropriate to cite a

BOX 7-1 Situations in Which Using Secondary Sources Is Appropriate

1. The primary source has been destroyed or cannot be accessed.
2. The primary source is located at such a distance that the cost of travel to review it would be prohibitive.
3. The primary source is written in a language not currently spoken, or in one that the researcher has not mastered.
4. The primary publication is written in unfamiliar jargon that is very difficult to decipher, but a secondary source analyzes and simplifies the material.
5. The secondary source contains creative ideas or a unique organization of information not found in the primary source.

secondary source. **Citation** is the act of quoting or paraphrasing a source within the body of a paper, using it as an example, or presenting it as support for a position taken.

Why Write a Review of the Literature?

Literature reviews require time and energy. Before making that investment, be sure you understand the purpose of the review. You may be reviewing the literature as part of writing a formal paper in a course, or you may be examining published research to discover evidence for use in practice, either to make a change or to oppose a proposed change. At other points in your career, you may be reviewing the literature to write a research proposal. Understanding the purpose for reviewing the literature can guide your efforts and yield a high-quality product. In the next sections, each of these purposes is described.

Writing a Course Paper

While reading the syllabus for a course, you learn one of the course assignments involves a literature review. The professor indicates that you will review published sources on a selected topic, analyze what you read, and write a formal paper that includes those sources. Reviews of the literature for a course assignment vary depending on the level of educational program, the purpose of the assignment, and the expectations of the instructor. The depth, scope, and breadth of a literature review increase as you move from undergraduate courses to master's level courses to doctoral courses.

The role for which you are preparing also will shape the review. For a paper in a nurse practitioner course, you might review pharmacology and pathology reference texts in addition to journal articles. In a nursing education course, you may review neurological development, cognitive science, and general education publications to write a paper on a teaching strategy. For a course about clinical information systems in a Doctorate of Nursing Practice (DNP) program, the review might extend into computer science and hospital management literature. For a theory course in a Doctorate of Philosophy of Nursing (PhD) program, your review may need to include all of the publications of a specific theorist, or you might be expected to write a review of 5 to 10 theories that pertain to one area of nursing inquiry.

For each of these papers, clarify with your professor the publication years and the type of literature to be included. The professor also may indicate the acceptable length of the written review of the literature. Reviews of the literature for course assignments tend to focus on what is known, the strength of the evidence, and the implications of the knowledge. Discussion board postings in a course may also require citations of peer-review literature.

Evaluating Clinical Practice

Another reason to review the literature is to determine whether clinical practice is consistent with the latest research evidence. In this context, it is necessary to identify all studies that provide evidence of a particular nursing intervention, critically appraise the strength of each individual study's research processes, synthesize the findings of all the studies, and provide an analytic summary. In addition to primary source research reports, any existing systematic literature reviews of the collective evidence for or against a particular intervention should also be included. In addition, the search should include existing evidence-based practice guidelines. Evidence-based practice guidelines are based on prior syntheses of the literature about the nursing intervention in question. Literature syntheses related to promoting evidence-based nursing practice are described in detail in Chapter 19.

DEVELOPING A QUALITATIVE RESEARCH PROPOSAL

From perusal of the literature, you have identified a research problem and have chosen to address that problem by conducting a qualitative study. The literature also provides information that you may use to establish the significance of the research problem (Marshall & Rossman, 2016). At this point, you need to select the type of qualitative study you plan to conduct, because the purpose and timing of the literature review varies by the type of study (see Chapter 12). In general, phenomenologists believe that no further literature review should be undertaken until after the data have been collected and analyzed, so that the knowledge of the results of prior studies in the area does not intrude upon the researcher's interpretation of the text of interviews and other data.

Classical grounded theory researchers begin with "tabula rasa," a blank slate, an attempt to know as little as possible about the area of study before they begin the research. The purpose of a brief literature review prior to beginning the study is to discover whether this particular study has been performed before. As the process progresses, the researchers collect and analyze all data before they return to the literature, so that the entirety of the analysis is grounded in their data, not in the literature (Charmaz, 2014). When the core concept or process has been identified and data analysis is complete, the researcher theoretically samples the literature for extant theories that may assist in explaining and extending the emerging theory (Munhall, 2012). In historical research, the initial review of the literature helps the researcher define the study questions and make decisions about relevant sources. The ensuing data collection for a historical study is an intense review of published and unpublished documents that the researcher has found to be relevant to the event and time being studied. Because the work of historical research includes painstaking review of literature, documents, artifacts, the arts, and other resources, review of the literature is ongoing throughout the research process.

The role of the literature review for ethnographic research is similar to the role of the literature review for quantitative research. The process of ethnographic research includes extensive preparation before data collection in order to familiarize oneself with the culture, and this includes a detailed review of the literature. The literature review provides a background for both conducting the study and interpreting the findings.

Researchers who plan to conduct exploratory descriptive qualitative study frequently have conducted an extensive review of the literature and found a dearth of research on the topic of interest. The lack of knowledge on the topic supports the need for an exploratory descriptive qualitative study. Following data collection, the researcher will compare the findings to the literature. Consequently, review of the literature in exploratory-descriptive research usually occurs before and after data collection. Chapter 12 describes in more

detail the role of the literature review in qualitative research.

DEVELOPING A QUANTITATIVE RESEARCH PROPOSAL

Quantitative research studies are shaped by the review of literature, whether descriptive, correlational, quasi-experimental, or experimental in design. Outcomes research and the quantitative portion of mixed methods research are also shaped by the review of the literature in the same way that quantitative research is. Based on review of the literature, you decide a quantitative (or outcomes or mixed methods) study is the best way to address a particular research problem. You plan a study to add knowledge in the area of the identified gap. For example, earlier researchers found that an intervention reduced hospital-acquired infections among postoperative patients who had no history of diabetes mellitus. After thorough review of the literature, you identify a specific gap in knowledge: the intervention's efficacy has not yet been tested with diabetic, postoperative patients. You decide to replicate the earlier study with a sample of postoperative diabetic patients. After data collection is complete, you analyze the data and then you again use the literature to compare your findings to those of earlier studies, as well as to other related studies. Your goal is to integrate knowledge from the literature with new information obtained from the study in progress.

Table 7-1 describes the role of the literature throughout the development and implementation of a quantitative study. The types of sources needed and the way you search the literature vary throughout the study. The introduction section uses relevant sources to summarize the background and significance of the research problem. The Review of the Literature section includes both theoretical and empirical sources that document current knowledge of the problem. The researcher develops the framework section from theoretical literature. If little theoretical literature is found, the researcher may choose to develop a tentative theory to guide the study based on findings of previous research studies (see Chapter 8 for more information), and on the posited relationships in the current study's research hypothesis. In the Methods section, the design, sample, measurement methods, treatment, and data collection processes of the planned study are described. Research texts, describing standards of methodological rigor, and previous studies are cited in this section. In the Results section, the researcher cites sources for the different types of statistical analyses conducted and the computer software used to conduct these analyses.

TABLE 7-1 Literature in the Quantitative Research Proposal and Report

Phase of the Research Process	How Literature Is Used and Its Role
Research topic	• Narrow topic by reading widely about what is known and what is not known; identify relevant concepts.
Statement of the research problem, including background and significance of the problem	• Search books and articles to provide an overview of the topic. • Search government reports and other documents to find facts about the size, cost, and consequences of the research problem. • Synthesize literature to identify the specific gap in knowledge that this study will address.
Research framework	• Find and read relevant frameworks. • Develop conceptual definitions of concepts.
Purpose; research questions or hypotheses	• Based on review of literature and research problem, state the purpose of the study. • Decide whether there is adequate evidence to state a hypothesis.
Review of the literature	• Find evidence to support why the selected methods are appropriate. • Summarize current empirical knowledge that is related to the topic.
Methodology	• Compare research designs of reviewed studies to select the most appropriate design for the proposed study. • Identify possible instruments or measures of variables. • Describe performance of measures in previous studies. • Provide operational definitions of concepts. • Develop sampling strategies based on what has been learned from studies in the literature.
Findings	• Refer to statistical textbooks to explain the results of the data analysis.
Discussion	• Compare the findings with those of previously reviewed studies. • Return to the literature to find new references to interpret unexpected findings. • Refer to theory sources to relate the findings to the research framework.
Conclusions	• On the basis of previous literature and the current study's findings, draw conclusions. • Discuss implications for nursing clinical practice, administration, and education.

The discussion section of the research report begins with what the results mean, in light of the results of previous studies. Conclusions are drawn that are a synthesis of the findings from previous studies and from the current study.

PRACTICAL CONSIDERATIONS FOR PERFORMING A LITERATURE REVIEW

How Long Will the Review of the Literature Take?

The time required to review the literature is influenced by the problem studied, the available sources, and the reviewer's goals. The literature review for a topic that is focused and somewhat narrow may require less time than one for a broader topic. The difficulty experienced

identifying and locating sources and the number of sources to be located also influence the time involved, as does the intensity of effort.

You, as a novice reviewer, will require more time to find the relevant literature than an experienced searcher would require. Consequently, you may underestimate the time needed for the review. Finding 20 relevant sources may take 10 to 15 hours. Usually reading and synthesizing the articles or reports take twice as long as finding the sources (20 to 30 hours). Graduate students new to the process may need three times as long for reading and developing a detailed synthesis. As searching skills are refined, and the synthesis process becomes more familiar, the required time decreases. Often, performing a literature review is limited by the time that the reviewer can commit to the task. The best strategy is to begin as early as possible and stay focused on the purpose of the review, so as to use time efficiently and prepare the best review possible given the circumstances.

How Many Sources Do I Need to Review?

Many students ask, "How many articles should I have? How many years back should I look to find relevant information?" The answer to both those questions is an emphatic, "It depends." Faculty for master's courses commonly require use of full-text articles published in the previous 5 to 10 years, describing studies relevant to the concepts or variables in the proposed study. Seminal and landmark studies should be included, even though they may have been published prior to the time frame the instructor designates. Doctoral students must conduct thorough reviews for course papers, with expectations for increasing analytic sophistication throughout their programs (Wisker, 2015). If you are writing a research proposal for a thesis or dissertation, the literature review will be required to be comprehensive, which means that it will include most or all of the literature that is pertinent to the topic. A comprehensive review includes all of the key papers in a given field of interest. After some initial searches, it is important to discuss what exists in that particular sphere of the literature with the course instructor, thesis chairperson, or dissertation chairperson, who will help you determine a reasonable time period and scope for the review.

Am I Expected to Read Every Word of the Available Sources?

No. If researchers attempted to read every word of every source that is somewhat related to a selected problem, they would be well-read but would not complete the course assignment or develop their study proposals. With the availability of full-text online articles, the researcher can easily become "lost in the literature" and forget the focus of the review. Becoming a skilled reviewer of the literature involves finding a balance and learning to identify the most pertinent and relevant sources. On the other hand, you cannot critically appraise and synthesize what you have not read. Avoid being distracted by information in the article that is not relevant to your topic. Learn to read with a purpose.

STAGES OF A LITERATURE REVIEW

The stages of a literature review reflect a systems model. Systems have input, throughput, and output. The *input* consists of the sources that you find through searching the literature. The *throughput* consists of the processes you use to read, critically appraise, analyze, and synthesize that literature. The written literature review is the

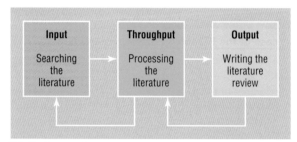

FIGURE 7-1 Systems model of the review of the literature.

output of these processes (Figure 7-1). The quality of the input and throughput will determine the quality of the output. As a result, attention to detail at each stage is critical to producing a high-quality literature review. Although these stages are presented here as sequential, you will move back and forth between stages. Through an iterative process you expand, refine, and clarify the written review (Wisker, 2015). For example, during the analysis and synthesis of sources, you identify that the studies you cite were conducted only in Europe. You might go back, search the literature again, and specifically search for studies conducted on the topic in other countries. When reading your literature review in progress, you may identify a problem with the logic of the presentation. To resolve it, you will return to the processing stage to rethink and edit the review.

Searching the Literature

Before writing a literature review, you must first perform an organized literature search to identify sources relevant to the topic of interest, keeping in mind the purpose of the review. Whether you are a student, a nurse in clinical practice, or a nurse researcher, the goal is to develop a search strategy to retrieve as much of the relevant literature as possible, given the time and financial constraints of the project (Aveyard, 2014).

Because of the magnitude of available literature, start by setting inclusion criteria. For example, your teacher may have specified that only peer-reviewed or scholarly sources are acceptable. You can set the search engine to retrieve only articles that meet that criterion. As mentioned earlier, other inclusion criteria may be the year of publication or a keyword. A **keyword** is a term or short phrase that is characteristic of a specific type or topic of research. For example, keywords for a study of women's adaptation to a diagnosis of multiple sclerosis might include *women, coping,* and *multiple sclerosis.* Consider consulting with an information professional, such as a subject specialist librarian, to develop a literature search strategy (Booth, Colomb, & Williams, 2008; Tensen, 2013). Often these consultations can be performed via email or a Web-based meeting, eliminating the need for travel.

Develop a Search Plan

Before beginning a search, you must consider exactly what information you seek. A written plan helps avoid duplication of effort. Your initial search should be based on the widest possible interpretation of the topic. This strategy enables you to envision the extent of the relevant literature. As you see the results of the initial efforts and begin reading the material, you will refine the topic and then narrow the focus for subsequent searches.

As you work through the literature, add selected search terms to the written plan, such as keywords and other words and phrases that you discover while reviewing pertinent references (Aveyard, 2014). For each search, record (1) the name of the database, (2) the date, (3) search terms and searching strategy, (4) the number and types of articles found, and (5) an estimate of the proportion of retrieved citations that were relevant. Table 7-2 is an example of a chart that you can use to record what sources you accessed and how you conducted the search. Some databases allow you to create an account and save a search history online (i.e., the record of what and how you searched). You also may want to export the results of each search to a Word document on a computer or external device, such as a flash drive.

Select Databases to Search

There are different types of bibliographical databases. Library electronic databases contain titles, authors, publication dates, and locations for hardcopy books and documents, government reports, and reference books. A library database also includes a searchable list of the journals to which the library maintains a subscription: electronic, paper, or both. Databases typically comprise citations that include authors, title, journal, keywords, and usually an abstract of each article. For example, nursing's subject-specific electronic database, CINAHL, contains an extensive listing of nursing publications and uses more nursing terminology as subject headings than would a non-nursing journal. With the greater focus on interdisciplinary research, nurse researchers must be consumers of the literature available from the National Library of Medicine (MEDLINE), government agencies, and professional organizations. Table 7-3 provides descriptions of commonly used bibliographical databases relevant to nursing.

When two bibliographical databases are provided by the same company, such as EBSCO Publishing, a simultaneous search of more than one database can be performed to save time. Usually the search engine will combine the results into a single list and automatically delete duplications. You also can change the order in which the results of the search are shown. For example, with EBSCO Publishing databases, you can sort the citations by relevance, date descending (most current first), or date ascending (oldest to more recent).

Search Strategies

Keywords

When a keyword is typed into the search box of an online search engine, such as MEDLINE or CINAHL, each reference on the resultant list contains that keyword. **Subject terms** are standardized phrases and are more formal than keywords. Most databases have a thesaurus for the database in which you can find subject terms. You can also combine subject terms and keywords to expand or focus the literature review. For instance, a search for *heart attack* may yield a few articles. Adding the terms *myocardial infarction, MI,* or *cardiovascular event* may result in a longer list of articles. In contrast, adding the term *women* to the previous search would result in fewer articles, because the search would eliminate studies with samples that were all men.

TABLE 7-2 **Plan and Record for Searching the Literature**				
Database Searched	**Date of Search**	**Search Strategy and Limiters**	**Number and Type of Articles Found**	**Estimate of Relevant Articles**
Cumulative Index to Nursing and Allied Health Literature (CINAHL)				
MEDLINE				
Academic Search Premier				
Cochrane Library				

TABLE 7-3   Bibliographical Databases

Name of Database	Description of the Database by the Publisher*
Cumulative Index of Nursing and Allied Health Literature (CINAHL)	"Comprehensive source of full text for nursing & allied health journals, providing full text for more than 770 journals"
MEDLINE	"Information on medicine, nursing, dentistry, veterinary medicine, the health care system, pre-clinical sciences, and much more" Created and provided by the National Library of Medicine Uses Medical Subject Headings (MeSH terms) for indexing and searching of "citations from over 4,800 current biomedical journals"
PubMed	Free access to Medline that provides links to full-text articles when available
PsychARTICLES	15,000 "full-text, peer-reviewed scholarly and scientific articles in psychology" Limited to journals published by the American Psychological Association (APA) and affiliated organizations
PsychINFO	"Scholarly journal articles, book chapters, books, and dissertations, is the largest resource devoted to peer-reviewed literature in behavioral science and mental health" Supported by APA Covers over 3 million records
Academic Search Complete	"Comprehensive scholarly, multi-disciplinary full-text database, with more than 8,500 full-text periodicals, including more than 7,300 peer-reviewed journals"
Health Source Nursing/ Academic Edition	"Provides nearly 550 scholarly full text journals focusing on many medical disciplines" Also includes 1,300 patient education sheets for generic drugs
Psychological and Behavioral Sciences Collection	"Comprehensive database covering information concerning topics in emotional and behavioral characteristics, psychiatry & psychology, mental processes, anthropology, and observational & experimental methods" 400 journals indexed

*Direct quotations from EBSCO Publishing descriptions of the databases, available at http://www.ebscohost.com/academic/.

A simple way to begin identifying a database's standardized subject terms is to search using one of your keywords and display full records of a few relevant citations. The records, in addition to the citations and abstracts of the articles, will include subject terms. The subject terms for the article are listed near the end of the abstract. Examine the terminology used to describe the major concepts in these articles, and use the same terms to refine additional searches and reveal related articles. Frequently, word-processing programs, dictionaries, and encyclopedias are helpful in identifying synonymous terms and subheadings. Using a combination of keywords and formal subject terms may result in targeted search results.

The format and spelling of search terms can yield different results. Truncating words can allow you to locate more citations related to that term. For example, authors might have used terms such as *intervene, intervenes, intervened, intervening, intervention,* or *intervener.*

To capture all of these terms, you can use a truncated term in your search, such as *interven, interven*,* or *interven$.* The form or symbol used to truncate a search term depends on the rule of the search engine you are using. On the other hand, avoid shortening a search word to fewer than four or five letters. If you shorten intervene to *inte**(four letters), the search will contain all articles using the words *internal, interstellar, intestine, integral, integrity, intellect, intemperance, intensity, internecine, intervertebral, intern,* and *intermittent,* to name a few, taking the searcher far afield from *intervene.* Also, pay attention to variant spellings. You may need to search, for example, by *orthopedic* or *orthopaedic* (British spelling). For irregular plurals, such as *woman* and *women,* enter both woman and women into the search.

Authors

If you identify an author who has published on your topic, you can find additional articles written by the same person by including the name as an author term, not a keyword term, during your search. Recognize that some databases list authors only under first and middle initials, whereas others use full first names. Using a general search engine such as Google or Yahoo, search by the author's name, and you may find a personal or university website with a list of their publications.

You may also want to find other researchers who cited the author, and this is especially true for authors who published seminal or landmark studies. Some bibliographical databases allow you to search the citations and find recent publications in which the author is cited. Web of Science is one such database that combines the *Science Citation Index, Social Science Citation Index, Arts & Humanities Index*, as well as indexes of conference proceedings (Thomson Reuters, 2016). Indexes such as Web of Science may require that your library subscribe to their services, however. To learn more about the index, you may want to check out their Facebook page (https://www.facebook.com/WebofScience.ThomsonReuters) or their website, http://wokinfo.com/. Several other databases, depending on the company, may also have a function for searching the references of articles.

Complex Searches

A complex search of the literature combines two or more concepts or synonyms in one search. There are several ways to arrange terms in a database search phrase or phrases. The three most common ways are by using (1) Boolean operators, (2) locational operators (field labels), and (3) positional operators. **Operators** are words with specific functions that permit you to group ideas, select places to search in a database record, and show relationships within a database record, sentence, or paragraph. Examine the Help screen of a database carefully to determine whether the operators you want to use are available and how they are used.

The **Boolean operators** are the three words AND, OR, and NOT. In most search engines, the words must be capitalized for them to function in this way. Use AND when you want to search for the presence of two or more terms in the same citation. For example, to find studies in which medication adherence of hypertensive patients has been studied, you might search by "medication adherence AND hypertension." The Boolean operator OR is most useful with synonymous terms or concepts, such as *compliance* and *adherence*. Use OR when you want to search for the presence of either of two terms in the same search. Use NOT when you want to search for one idea but not another in the same citation. NOT is used less frequently because doing so may result in missing relevant publications.

Locational operators (field labels) identify terms in specific areas or fields of a record. These fields may be parts of the simple citation, such as the article title, author, and journal name, or they may be from additional fields provided by the database, such as subject headings, abstracts, cited references, publication type notes, instruments used, and even the entire article. In some databases, these specific fields can be selected by means of a drop-down menu in the database input area. In other databases, specific coding can be used to do the same thing. Do not assume that the entire article is being searched when you are using the default search; the default is usually looking for your terms in the title, abstract, and/or subject fields. You may choose to search for a concept only within the abstract of articles.

Positional operators are used to look for requested terms within certain distances of one another. Availability and phrasing of positional operators are highly dependent on the database search software. Common positional operators are NEAR, WITH, and ADJ; they also are often required to be capitalized and may have numbers associated with them. A positional operator is most useful in records with a large amount of information, such as those with full-text articles attached. Positional operators may be used simultaneously with locational operators, either in an implied way or explicitly. For example, ADJ is an abbreviation for adjacent; it specifies that one term must be next to another, and must appear in the order entered. "ADJ2" commands that there must be no more than two intervening words between the two search terms, and that they appear in the order entered. NEAR does not define the specific order of the terms; the command "term1 NEAR1 term2" requires that the first term occur first and within two words of the second term. WITH often indicates that the terms must be within the same sentence, paragraph, or region (such as subject headings) of the record.

Limit Your Search

There are several strategies that will limit a search if, after performing Boolean searches, the list of references is unmanageably long. The limits you can impose vary with the database. In CINAHL, for example, the search may be limited to a single language such as English. You can also limit the years of your search, to coincide with an instructor's requirement that publications older than five years cannot be cited in a course paper. Searches can be limited to find only papers that are research reports, review papers, or patient education materials. Adding a certain population or intervention to the search strategy is another option that both shortens

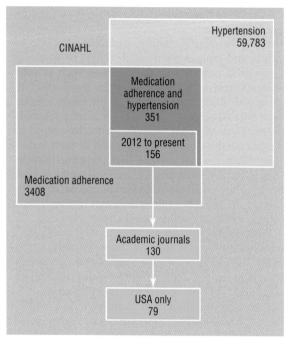

FIGURE 7-2 Example of search using operators.

the list of references and increases their applicability. Figure 7-2 is a display of the results of a literature search in which the Boolean operator AND was used to combine searches for medication adherence and hypertension. When the search resulted in more references than could be reviewed in the time the reviewer had available, the search was further limited by additional characteristics: years of publication, type of journals, and geographical location.

Search the Internet

In some cases, you may have to subscribe to an online journal to gain access to its articles. Some electronic journals are listed in available bibliographical databases, and you can access full-text articles from an electronic journal through the database. However, many electronic journals are not yet included in bibliographical databases or may not be in the particular database you are using. Ingenta Connect (http://www.ingenta.com) is a commercial website that allows you to search more than 11,000 publications from many disciplines. Publications available through Ingenta include both those that are free to download and those that require the reader to buy the article.

Metasearch engines, such as Google, also allow you to search the Internet. Online documents retrieved

within Google are listed based not on relevance to your topic, but on the number of times an individual document has been viewed (Hyman & Schulman, 2015). Google Scholar is a specialized tool that allows you to focus your search on research and theoretical publications. With the exception of articles in online-only journals, scholarly sources are published first in print and may be available online a few years later. Thus, online reference may be older, but may point you to seminal and landmark studies or help you identify subject terms for new searches. Government reports and publications by professional organizations also may be found by searching the Internet.

Prior to using a reference from the Internet that has not been subjected to peer review, you must evaluate the accuracy of its information and the potential for bias on the part of its author. There is no screening process for information placed on the World Wide Web, and it is almost devoid of primary sources. Thus, you find a considerable amount of misinformation, as well as accurate information that you might not be able to access in any other way. It is important to check the source of any information you obtain from the Web so that you can determine whether it is appropriate for inclusion in a scholarly article.

Locate Relevant Literature

Within each database that you choose to use, conduct your search of **relevant literature** by implementing the strategies described in this chapter. Most databases provide short records that include abstracts of the articles, allowing you to get some sense of their content so you may judge whether the information is useful in relation to your selected topic. If you find the information to be an important reference, save it to a file on your computer or in an online folder maintained by your employer or university, and/or move it to a reference management program (next section). It is often practical at the end of a search session to use a flash drive for storage of promising articles, and for the list of references searched and databases accessed, to avoid duplicating these steps in a subsequent search. At this point in the process, do not try to examine all of the citations listed; merely save them.

It is rare for a scholar to be able to identify every relevant literature source. The most extensive retrievals of literature are funded projects focused on defining evidence-based practice or developing clinical practice guidelines (see Chapter 19). For the most comprehensive of these projects, a literature review coordinator manages the literature review process and has funds to employ several full-time, experienced, professional librarians as literature searchers. When extensive literature reviews are completed, the results are published so that you may have access to synthesis and the citations from the reviewed journal articles.

Systematically Record References

Bibliographical information on a source should be recorded in a systematic manner, according to the format that you will use in the reference list. The purpose for carefully citing sources is that readers can retrieve references for themselves, confirming your interpretation of the findings, or gathering additional information on the topic, if they so desire. Many journals and academic institutions use the format developed by the American Psychological Association (APA) (2010). Computerized lists of sources usually contain complete citations for references, which must be saved electronically so you have the information needed in case you decide to cite a particular article, including its publication details in your reference list. The 6th edition of the APA's *Publication Manual* (2010) provides revised guidelines for citing electronic sources and direct quotations from electronic sources. The APA standard for direct quotations of five or more words is to cite the page of the publication in which the quotation appears. Citing direct quotations from electronic sources has posed unique challenges and may require a paragraph number or a Web address. We present references in this text in APA format, expect for modifying how multiple authors are cited and not including digital object identifiers (DOIs).

DOIs have become the standard for the International Standards Organization (http://www.doi.org/) but have not yet received universal support. The use of DOIs seems to be gaining in credibility because the DOI "provides a means of persistent identification for managing information on digital networks" (APA, 2010, p. 188). CrossRef is an example of a registration agency for DOIs that enables citations to be linked to the DOI across databases and disciplines (http://www.crossref.org/).

Each citation on the reference list is formatted as a paragraph with a *hanging indent,* meaning that the first line is on the left margin and subsequent lines are indented. If you do not know how to format a paragraph this way, search the Help tool in your word-processing program to find the correct command to use. When you retrieve an electronic source in portable document format (pdf), you cite the source as if you had made a copy of the print version of the article. Electronic sources available only in html format (Web format) do not have page numbers for the citation. The APA standard is to provide the URL (uniform resource locator)

for the home page of the journal from which the reader could navigate and find the source (APA, 2010). Providing the URL that you used to retrieve the article is not helpful because it is unique to the path you used to find the article and reflects your access to search engines and bibliographical databases.

Use Reference Management Software

Reference management software can make tracking the references you have obtained through your searches considerably easier. You can use such software to conduct searches and to store the information on all search fields for each reference obtained in a search, including the abstract. Within the software, you can store articles in folders with other similar articles. For example, you may have a folder for theory sources, another for methodological sources, and a third for relevant research topics. When you export search results from the bibliographical database to your reference management software, all of the needed citation information and the abstract are readily available to you electronically when you write the literature review. As you read the articles, you also can insert comments about each one into the reference file.

Reference management software has been developed to interface directly with the most commonly used word-processing software. It organizes the reference information using the specific citation style you stipulate. For instance, you may be familiar with APA format but want to submit a manuscript to a journal that uses another bibliographical style. Within a reference management program, a reference list or bibliography can be generated in a different format—in this case, the format required by the journal. A mere keystroke or two will insert citations into your paper. The four most commonly used software packages, along with websites that contain information about them, are as follows:

- EndNote (http://www.endnote.com/) is compatible with Windows and Macintosh computers and allows you to access your saved materials from multiple electronic devices.
- RefWorks (www.refworks.com/) operates from the Web and can be accessed free by students and faculty if their respective universities maintain licenses for usage.
- Reference Manager (http://www.refman.com/) operates on your personal computer or you can use it to make your databases accessible to others in a Web environment.
- Bookends (http://www.sonnysoftware.com/) is a reference manager for Macintosh users that

allows users to search bibliographical databases and download citations and full-text articles. Searches can also be downloaded to other Apple products, such as iPhone and iPad.

Saved Searches and Alerts

When working on a research project in which the literature review may take months, or engaged in a field of study that will interest you for years, repeating the same search periodically, using the same strategy, is both necessary and time-consuming. Many databases, however, permit you to create an account in which you can save the original search strategy so that the same search will be initiated with just a few clicks, without having to enter the entire strategy again. You can also arrange for email notification of any new articles that fit your saved search strategy. Another option available from many journals is to register to have the table of contents of new issues sent automatically by email. Examine the help function of the database or journal home page to determine the available options.

PROCESSING THE LITERATURE

The processes of reading and critically appraising sources promote understanding of a research problem. They involve skimming, comprehending, analyzing, and synthesizing content from sources. Skills in reading and critically appraising sources are essential to the development of a high-quality literature review.

Reading

Skimming a source is quickly reviewing a source to gain a broad overview of its content. When you retrieve an article, you quickly read the title, the author's name, and an abstract or introduction. Then you read the major headings and sometimes one or two sentences under each heading. Next, you glance at any tables and figures. Finally, you review the conclusion or summary section. Skimming enables you to make a preliminary judgment about the value of a source, relative to your area of review, and to determine whether the source is primary or secondary. You may choose to review the citations listed in secondary sources to identify primary sources the authors cited, but secondary sources are seldom cited in a research proposal, review of the literature, or research report.

Comprehending a source requires that you read all of it carefully. This is necessary for key references that you have retrieved. Focus on understanding major concepts and the logical flow of ideas within the source. Highlight the content you consider important or make notes in the margins. Notes might be recorded on photocopies or electronic files of articles, indicating where the information will be used in developing a research proposal, review of the literature, or research report.

The kind of information you highlight or note in the margins of a source depends on the type of study or source. Information that you might note or highlight from the theoretical sources are relevant concepts, definitions of those concepts, and relationships among them. Notes recorded in the margins of empirical literature might include relevant information about the researcher, such as whether the author is a major researcher of a selected problem, as well as comparisons with other studies by the same author. For a research article, the research problem, purpose, framework, data collection methods, study design, sample size, data collection, analysis techniques, and findings are usually noted or highlighted. You may wish to record quotations with quotation marks (including page numbers) for possible use in the written review. This is essential for avoiding accidental plagiarism. The final decision whether to use a direct quote or paraphrase the information can be made later. You might also record your own thoughts about the content while you are reading a source.

At this point, you will identify relevant categories for sorting and organizing sources. These categories will ultimately guide you in writing the review of literature section, and some may even be major headings in the review.

Appraising and Analyzing Sources for Possible Inclusion in a Review

Through analysis, you can determine the value of a source for a particular review. Analysis must take place in two stages. The first stage involves the critical appraisal of individual studies. The steps of appraising individual studies is detailed in Chapter 18. During the critical appraisal process, you will identify relevant content in the articles and evaluate the rigor of the studies.

Conducting an **analysis of sources** to be used in a research proposal, review of the literature, or research report requires some knowledge of the subject to be critiqued, some knowledge of the research process, and the ability to exercise judgment in evaluation (Pinch, 1995, 2001). However, the critical appraisal of individual studies is only the first step in developing an adequate review of the literature. A literature review that is a series of paragraphs, in which each paragraph is a description of a single study with no link to other studies being reviewed, does not provide evidence of adequate analysis and synthesis of the literature.

Analysis requires not taking the "text at face value" and being able to tolerate the uncertainty (Hyman & Schulman, 2015, p. 64) until you can identify the common elements and contradictions in the text. Analysis involves rewording and re-analyzing the information that you find, literally making it your own (Garrard, 2011). Pinch (1995), a nurse, published a strategy to synthesize research findings using a literature summary table. Pinch (2001) developed a modified table for translating research findings into clinical innovations. We modified this table by adding two columns that are useful in sorting information from studies into categories for analysis (Table 7-4). When using reference management software, tables can be generated from information you entered into the software about each individual study. Curnalia and Ferris (2014) provide examples of other table formats for annotations and for different approaches to analyzing and comparing references during the review.

The second stage of analysis involves making comparisons among studies. This analysis allows you to critically appraise the existing body of knowledge in relation to the research problem. From your appraisal, you will be able to summarize important points that will shape your research proposal (Box 7-2). Different researchers may have approached the examination of the problem from different perspectives. They may have organized the study from different theoretical perspectives, asked different questions related to the problem, selected different variables, or used different designs. Pay special attention to conflicting findings, as they may

provide clues for gaps in knowledge that represent researchable problems.

Sorting Your Sources

Relevant sources are organized for inclusion in the different sections of a research proposal or research report. See Table 7-1 to review contributions of the literature to each part of the research process. The sources for a course assignment or review related to a clinical problem can be sorted for different sections of the paper. For example, in the introduction of the assignment, include information from sources that provide background and significance for the study. Research reports can be grouped by concepts that were studied, populations included, or similar findings.

Synthesizing Sources

In a literature review, **synthesis of sources** involves clarifying the meaning obtained from the sources as a whole. Integration refers to "making connections between ideas, theories, and experience" (Hart, 2009, p. 8). Through synthesis and integration, one can cluster and connect ideas from several sources to develop a personal overall view of the topic. Garrard (2011) describes this personal level of knowledge as ownership, as "being so familiar with what has been written by previous researchers that you know clearly how this area of research has progressed over time and across ideas" (p. 7).

Synthesis is the key to the next step of the review process, which is developing the logical argument that supports the research problem you intend to address. Booth et al. (2008) describe the process of constructing an argument as beginning with stating a claim and identifying supporting reasons. The reviewer must also include adequate information so that the reader agrees that the reasons are relevant to the claim. The reviewer provides evidence to support each of the reasons. Thinking at this level and depth prepares you for outlining the written review. Figure 7-3 provides a visual representation of an argument that can be developed through a written review. The writer/reviewer supports each claim with evidence so that the reader can accept the reviewer's conclusion. For example, the reviewer has synthesized several sources related to medication adherence and is presenting the argument for developing patient-

---

BOX 7-2   Critical Questions to Answer From a Synthesis of the Literature

- What theoretical formulations have been used to identify concepts and the relationships among them?
- What methodologies have researchers used to study the problem?
- What methodological flaws were found in previous studies?
- What is known about the problem?
- What are the most critical gaps in the knowledge base?

TABLE 7-4   Literature Summary Table

Author and Year	Purpose	Framework	Sample	Measurement	Treatment	Results	Findings

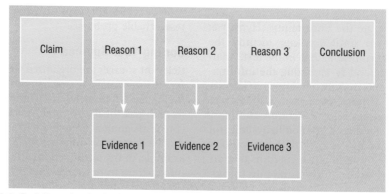

FIGURE 7-3 Building the logical argument. (Adapted from Booth, W. C., Colomb, G. G., & Williams, J. M. (2008). *The craft of research* (3rd ed.). Chicago, IL: University of Chicago Press.)

focused medication adherence intervention. The following outline could be developed for this argument.

Claim 1: Interventions to promote medication adherence must incorporate the hypertensive patient's perspective.

Reason 1: Provider-focused interventions have not resulted in long-term improvement in medication adherence.

> *Evidence 1:* Description of studies of provider-focused interventions and their outcomes

Reason 2: Patients who do not adhere to an externally imposed medication regimen (the target population) may be less likely to use an intervention that is externally imposed.

> *Evidence 2:* Description of studies in which patients failed to return for appointments during a trial of an electronic device to promote adherence

Reason 3: Medication adherence requires behavior change that must be incorporated into the patient's life.

> *Evidence 3:* Theoretical principles of behavior change that recommend individualization of interventions to meet unique patient needs

Conclusion 1: Using a participatory approach to develop individual strategies for promoting medication adherence is an important first step to improving patient outcomes.

WRITING THE REVIEW OF LITERATURE

Writing Suggestions

Clear, correct, and concise are the 3 Cs of good writing (Curnalia & Ferris, 2014). If you have followed the steps for reviewing the literature in this chapter, you are ready to demonstrate your synthesis and ownership of the literature by clearly presenting your argument. Rather than using direct quotes from an author, you should paraphrase his or her ideas. Paraphrasing involves expressing ideas clearly and in your own words; the ability to paraphrase is an indication of understanding what you have read (Hyman & Schulman, 2015). In paraphrasing, the author of the review connects the meanings of these sources to the proposed study, being careful to present the information correctly. Last, the reviewer combines, or clusters, the meanings obtained from all sources to establish the current state of knowledge for the research problem (Pinch, 1995, 2001).

Each paragraph has three components: a theme sentence, sentences with evidence, and a summary sentence. Start each paragraph with a theme sentence that describes the main idea of the paragraph or makes a claim. Concisely present the relevant studies as evidence of the main idea or claim, and end the paragraph with a concluding sentence that connects to the next claim and next paragraph.

Organization of Written Reviews

The purpose of the written literature review is to establish a context for a research proposal, review of the literature, or research report. The literature review for a research proposal or research report may have four major sections: (1) the introduction, (2) a discussion of theoretical literature, (3) a discussion of empirical literature, and (4) a summary. The introduction and summary are standard sections, but you will want to organize the discussion of sources in a way that makes sense for the topic.

Introduction

By reading the introduction of a literature review, the reader should learn the purpose of the study and the organizational structure of the review. The reader also should gain an appreciation of why the topic is important and significant. You should make clear in this section what you will and will not discuss in the review: the scope of the review. If you are taking a particular position or developing a logical argument for a particular perspective, make this position clear in the introduction.

Discussion of Theoretical Literature

The theoretical literature section contains concept analyses, models, theories, and conceptual frameworks that support the study. In this section, you will present the concepts, definitions of concepts, relationships among concepts, and assumptions. You will analyze these elements to build the theoretical basis for the study. This section of the literature review may be used to present the framework for the study and may include a conceptual map that synthesizes the theoretical literature (see Chapter 8 for more details on developing frameworks).

Discussion of Empirical Literature

The presentation of empirical literature should be organized by concepts or organizing topics, instead of by studies. The findings from the studies should logically build on one another so that the reader can understand how the body of knowledge in the research area evolved. Instead of presenting details about purpose, sample size, design, and specific findings for each study, the researcher presents a synthesis of findings across studies. Conflicting findings and areas of uncertainty are explored. Similarities and differences in the studies should be identified. Gaps and areas needing more research are discussed. A summary of findings in the topic area is presented, along with inferences, generalizations, and conclusions drawn from review of the literature. A conclusion is a statement about the state of knowledge in relation to the topic area. This should include a discussion of the strength of evidence available for each conclusion.

The reviewer who becomes committed to a particular viewpoint on the research topic must maintain the ethical standard of intellectual honesty. The content from reviewed sources should be presented honestly, not distorted to support a selected problem. Reviewers may read a study and wish that the researchers had studied a slightly different problem or designed the study differently. However, the reviewers must recognize their own opinions and must be objective in presenting

information. The defects of a study must be addressed, but it is not necessary to be highly critical of another researcher's work. The criticisms must focus on the content that is in some way relevant to the proposed study and should be stated as possible or plausible explanations, so that the criticisms are more neutral and scholarly than negative and blaming.

Summary

Through the literature review, you will present the evidence and reveal the research problem—what is not known about the particular concept or topic. The summary of the review consists of a concise presentation of the current knowledge base for the research problem. The gaps in the knowledge base are identified. The summary concludes with a statement of how the findings from the current study contribute to the body of knowledge in this field of research.

Refining the Written Review

You complete the first draft of your review of the literature and breathe a sigh of relief before moving onto the next portion of the assignment or research proposal. Before moving on, you need to read, evaluate, and refine your review. Set the review aside for 24 hours and then read it aloud. In this way, you may identify missing words and awkward sentences that you might overlook when reading silently. Ask a fellow student or a trusted colleague to read your work and provide constructive feedback. Use the criteria and guiding questions in Table 7-5 to evaluate the quality of the literature review.

Checking References

Sources that will be cited in a paper or recorded in a reference list should be cross-checked two or three times to prevent errors. Questions that will identify common errors are displayed in Box 7-3. To prevent these errors, check all of the citations within the text of the literature review and each citation in the reference list. Typing or keyboarding errors may result in inaccurate information. You may have omitted some information, planning to complete the reference later, and then forgotten to do so. Downloading citations from a database directly into a reference management system and using the system's manuscript formatting functions reduce some errors but do not eliminate all of them. Use your knowledge and skills to enhance your technology use; relying on technology will not ensure a quality manuscript.

TABLE 7-5   Characteristics of High-Quality Literature Reviews

Criteria	Guiding Questions
Coverage	Did the writer provide evidence of having reviewed sufficient literature on the topic? Does the review indicate that the writer is sufficiently well informed about the topic and has identified relevant studies?
Understanding	Does the written review indicate that the writer has understood and synthesized what is known about the topic? Have similarities and differences within the synthesized literature been described?
Coherence	Does the writer make a logical argument related to the significance of the topic and the gap to be addressed by the proposed study?
Accuracy	Does the writer's attention to detail give the reader confidence in the conclusions of the review?

BOX 7-3   Checking to Avoid Common Reference Citation Errors

- Does every source cited in the text have a corresponding citation on the reference list?
- Is every reference on the reference list cited in the text?
- Are names of the authors spelled the same way in the text and in the reference list?
- Are the years of publication cited in the text the same as the years of publication that appear on the reference list?
- Does every direct quotation have a citation that includes the author's name, year, and page number?
- Are the citations on the reference list complete so that the reference can be retrieved?

▌ KEY POINTS

- A literature review consists of all written sources relevant to the selected topic. It is an interpretative, organized, and logically written presentation of what the study's author has read.

- Reviewing the existing literature related to a research topic is a critical step in the research process.
- One of the goals of reviewing the literature is identifying a gap in the literature. Information from the literature review guides the development of the statement of the research problem.
- Two types of literature predominate in the review of literature for research: theoretical and empirical.
- Theoretical literature consists of concept analyses, models, theories, and conceptual frameworks that support a selected research problem and purpose.
- Empirical literature is comprised of relevant studies in journals and books as well as unpublished studies, such as master's theses and doctoral dissertations.
- With use of a systems approach, the three major stages of a literature review are searching the literature (input), processing the literature (throughput), and writing the literature review (output).
- Searching the literature begins with a written plan for the review that is maintained as a search history during the first stage of the literature review.
- Searching the literature requires use of bibliographical databases. Using a reference management system may be helpful for organizing retrieved sources and creating reference lists.
- Processing the literature requires the researcher to read, critically appraise, analyze, and synthesize the information that has been retrieved.
- The well-written literature review presents a logical argument for why the research question should be studied and for the specific way of studying it that is being proposed.

REFERENCES

American Psychological Association. (2010). *Publication manual of the American Psychological Association* (6th ed.). Washington, DC: Author.

Aveyard, H. (2014). *Doing a literature review in health and social care: A practical guide* (3rd ed.). Berkshire, EN: Open University Press.

Booth, W. C., Colomb, G. G., & Williams, J. M. (2008). *The craft of research* (3rd ed.). Chicago, IL: University of Chicago Press.

Bowlby, J. (1980). *Attachment and loss. Vol. 3: Loss: Sadness and depression.* New York: Basic Books.

Cassel, E. (1982). The nature of suffering and the goals of medicine. *New England Journal of Medicine, 306*(11), 639–645.

Charmaz, K. (2014). *Constructing grounded theory* (2nd ed.). Thousand Oaks, CA: Sage.

Chickering, A., & Gamson, Z. (1987). Seven principles for good practice in undergraduate education. *AAHE Bulletin, 39*(7), 3–7.

Curnalia, R., & Ferris, A. (2014). *CSI: Concepts, sources, integration: A step-by-step guide to writing your literature review in communication studies.* Dubuque, IA: Kendall Hunt Publishing.

Frické, M. (2014). Big data and its epistemology. *Journal of the Association for Information Science and Technology*, 66(4), 651–661.

Garrard, J. (2011). *Health sciences literature review made easy: The matrix method* (3rd ed.). Sudbury, MA: Jones & Bartlett.

Grabbe, L. (2015). Attachment-informed care in a primary care setting. *Journal for Nurse Practitioners*, 11(3), 321–327.

Haigh, C. (2011). Wikipedia as an evidence source for nursing and healthcare students. *Nurse Education Today*, 31(2), 135–139.

Hart, C. (2009). *Doing a literature review: Releasing the social science imagination*. Los Angeles, CA: Sage.

Hyman, G., & Schulman, M. (2015). *Thinking on the page: A college student's guide to effective writing*. Cincinnati, OH: Writer's Digest Books.

International Organization of Migration. (2012). Health of migrants*: The way forward*. Retrieved on April 9, 2016 from <https://www.iom.int/files/live/sites/iom/files/What-We-Do/docs/Health-of-Migrants-Info-Sheet_2012.pdf>.

Larsen, P. O., & von Ins, M. (2010). The rate of growth in scientific publication and the decline in coverage provided by Scientific Citation Index. *Scientometrics*, 84(3), 575–603.

Marshall, C., & Rossman, G. (2016). *Designing qualitative research* (6th ed.). Thousand Oaks, CA: Sage.

Munhall, P. L. (2012). *Nursing research: A qualitative perspective* (5th ed.). Sudbury, MA: Jones & Bartlett.

Paré, G., Trudel, M.-C., Jaana, M., & Kitsiou, S. (2015). Synthesizing information systems knowledge: A typology of literature reviews. *Information & Management*, 52(2), 183–199.

Parker, R., McNeill, J., & Howard, J. (2015). Comparing pediatric simulation and traditional clinical experience: Student perceptions, learning outcomes, and lessons for faculty. *Clinical Simulation in Nursing*, 11(3), 188–193.

Pinch, W. J. (1995). Synthesis: Implementing a complex process. *Nurse Educator*, 20(1), 34–40.

Pinch, W. J. (2001). Improving patient care through use of research. *Orthopaedic Nursing*, 20(4), 75–81.

Sacks, J. (2013). Suffering at the end of life: A systematic review of the literature. *Journal of Hospice and Palliative Nursing*, 15(5), 286–297.

Tensen, B. L. (2013). *Research strategies for the digital age* (4th ed.). Boston, MA: Wadsworth.

Thomson Reuters. (2016). *Web of Science*. Retrieved April 9, 2016 from <http://ipscience.thomsonreuters.com/product/web-of-science/>.

U. S. Department of Health & Human Services. (2016). *Rural health policy*. Retrieved April 8, 2016 from <http://www.hrsa.gov/ruralhealth/policy/index.html>.

Wisker, G. (2015). Developing doctoral authors: Engaging with theoretical perspectives through the literature review. *Innovations in Education and Teaching International*, 52(1), 64–74.

8

Frameworks

Jennifer R. Gray

http://evolve.elsevier.com/Gray/practice/

"Scientists formulate theories, test theories, accept theories, reject theories, modify theories, and use theories as guides to understanding and predicting events in the world around them" (Jaccard & Jacoby, 2010, p. 3). Nurse researchers are among those scientists who use theory. A theoretical **framework** is an abstract, logical structure of meaning that guides the development of a study and enables the researcher to link the findings to the body of knowledge in nursing (Meleis, 2012). Theoretical frameworks are used in quantitative and outcomes research, sometimes in qualitative research, and rarely in mixed methods studies. In quantitative studies, the framework may be a testable theory or may be a tentative theory developed inductively from published research or clinical observation. Most outcomes studies are based on Donabedian's theory of quality of care (Donabedian, 1987). In most qualitative studies, the researcher will identify a philosophical perspective, but may not identify a formal theoretical framework (see Chapters 4 and 12). In grounded theory research, concepts and the relationships among them play central roles because the researcher often develops a theory as an outcome of the study.

Almost every quantitative study has a theoretical framework, although some researchers do not identify or describe the framework in the report of the study. Often, the theoretical framework can be inferred from research questions or hypotheses. For example, researchers may use their knowledge of anatomy and physiology to guide a study without identifying a framework, although both the language and the reasoning the researcher uses are consistent with known facts of anatomy and physiology. Others may study self care and not link the concept to Orem's Theory of Self Care (2001), despite using terms from that theory. Ideally, the framework of a quantitative study is carefully structured, clearly presented, and well integrated with the methodology. One aspect of critically appraising studies is identifying the theoretical framework and evaluating the extent to which the framework is congruent with the study's methodology. Your ability to understand the study findings will depend on your ability to understand the logic within the framework and determine how the findings might be used. In addition, when developing a quantitative study, the theoretical framework should be described.

After introducing relevant terms, this chapter describes processes used to examine and appraise the components of theories and presents approaches to identifying or developing a framework to guide a study.

INTRODUCTION OF TERMS

The first step in understanding theories and frameworks is to become familiar with theoretical terms and their application. These terms are concept, relational statement, conceptual model, theory, middle-range theory, and study framework.

Concept

A **concept** is a term that abstractly describes and names an object, a phenomenon, or an idea, thus providing it with a distinct identity or meaning. As a label for a phenomenon or a composite of behavior or thoughts, a concept is a concise way to represent an experience or state (Meleis, 2012). Concepts are the basic building blocks of theory (Figure 8-1). An example of a concept is the term "anxiety." The concept brings to mind a feeling of uneasiness in the stomach, a rapid pulse rate, and troubling thoughts about future negative outcomes.

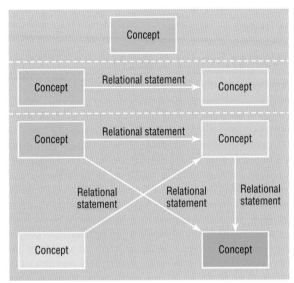

FIGURE 8-1 Concepts, relational statements, and theories.

Another example of a concept is patient, which denotes a person receiving healthcare services. Think about all the different ways that people receive health care. In many of these settings, the recipients are called patients. The concept of patient encompasses millions of people from widely divergent nationalities, health conditions, and living situations, all of whom share the common characteristic of receiving care.

Concepts can vary in their levels of abstraction. At high levels of abstraction, concepts that naturally cluster together are called constructs. For example, a construct associated with the concept of anxiety might be "emotional responses." Within the same construct, hope, anger, fear, and optimism could be identified. Another construct is health care, which includes the concepts of treatment, prevention, health promotion, palliative care, and rehabilitation, to name a few.

Relational Statements

A **relational statement** is the explanation of the connection between or among concepts (Fawcett & DeSanto-Madeya, 2013; Walker & Avant, 2011). Relational statements provide the structure of a framework (see the middle section of Figure 8-1). Clear relational statements are essential for constructing an integrated framework that guides the development of a study's objectives, questions, and hypotheses. The types of relationships described determine the study design and indicate the types of statistical analyses that may be used

to answer the research question. Mature theories, such as physiological theories, have measurable concepts and clear relational statements that can be tested through research.

Conceptual Models

A **conceptual model**, one type of which is known as a grand theory, is a set of highly abstract, related constructs. A conceptual model broadly explains phenomena of interest, expresses assumptions, and reflects a philosophical stance. Nurse scholars have expended time and effort to debate the distinctions among definitions of theory, conceptual model, conceptual framework, and theoretical framework (Chinn & Kramer, 2015; Fawcett & DeSanto-Madeya, 2013; Higgins & Moore, 2000; Meleis, 2012). For example, Watson's theory of caring (1979) has been identified as a metatheory (Higgins & Moore, 2000), a theory (Meleis, 2012), a philosophy (Alligood, 2010), and a conceptual model (Fitzpatrick & Whall, 2005). Most of nursing's grand theories, such as Watson's, are global and offer theoretical, almost philosophical, explanations of what nursing should be, and what the vital parts of nursing should entail. They are explanations of nursing as a whole. In this textbook, we use the terms "conceptual model" l and "conceptual framework" interchangeably. We have deliberately chosen not to contribute to the scholarly debate, but to provide the information needed to use concepts, relational statements, and theories.

Theory

A **theory** consists of a set of defined concepts and relational statements that provide a structured way to think about a phenomenon (see the portion of Figure 8-1 below the lowest dashed line). Theories are developed to describe, explain, or predict a phenomenon or outcome (Goodson, 2015). As discussed earlier, relational statements clarify the relationship that exists between or among concepts. It is the individual statement within a theory that is tested through research, not the entire theory. Thus, identifying and categorizing the statements (relationships among the concepts) within the theory are critical to the research endeavor: one or more of these relationships forms the basis of the study's framework.

Scientific theories are those for which repeated studies have validated relationships among the concepts (Goodson, 2015). These theories are sometimes called laws for this reason. Although few nursing and psychosocial theories have been validated to this extent, physiological theories have this level of validation through research and can provide a strong basis for nursing studies.

Middle-Range Theories

Middle-range theories present a partial view of nursing reality. Proposed by Merton (1968), a sociologist, middle-range theories are less abstract and address more specific phenomena than do the grand theories (Peterson, 2009). They apply directly to practice, with a focus on explanation of the specifics of condition, symptom, diagnosis, or process, and on implementation. They differ from grand theories because they are concerned with aspects of nursing, not its totality. Because of the narrower focus, middle-range theories can provide a framework to guide a research study.

Middle-range theories may be developed from grand theories in nursing through substruction. For example, Pickett, Peters, and Jarosz (2014) identified Orem's Theory of Self Care (2001) as a grand theory that was applicable to weight management. Pickett et al. (2014, p. 243) "deduced from the assumptions and concepts of the theory" to construct their middle-range theory of weight management. Middle-range theory may also be developed inductively from research findings, such as grounded theory studies. Others emanate from practice, or from existent theory in related fields. Whatever their source, middle-range theories are sometimes called **substantive theories** because they are more concrete than grand theories.

Research Frameworks

A research framework is the theoretical structure guiding a specific study. One way to describe the research framework is to present a map or diagram of its concepts and relational statements. Diagrams of research frameworks are **conceptual maps** (Fawcett, 1999; Newman, 1979, 1986). A conceptual map summarizes and integrates visually the theoretical structure of a study. A narrative explanation allows us to grasp the essence of a phenomenon in context. A research framework should be supported by references from the literature. The framework may have been derived from research findings or be an adaptation of a theory, so the literature is available to support the explanation. If the framework has emerged from clinical experiences, a search of the literature may reveal supporting studies or theories. Frameworks vary in complexity and accuracy, depending on the available body of knowledge related to the phenomena being described.

Building on your initial knowledge of these theoretical terms, the next sections will revisit each one and

provide additional description of analyzing concepts, statements, and theories.

UNDERSTANDING CONCEPTS

Concepts are often described as the building blocks of theory: useful, in an amorphous sort of way, but difficult to tack down because of their abstractness. To make a concept concrete, the researcher must identify how it can be measured. The concept's operational definition is a statement of how it will be measured (see Chapters 3 and 6). A concept made measurable is referred to as a **variable**. The word *variable* implies that the values associated with the term can vary from one instance to another. A variable related to anxiety might be "palmar sweating," which the researcher can measure by assigning a numerical value to the amount of sweat on the subject's palm. In Chapter 3, substruction was described in relation to linking concepts and variables when designing a study. To review this principle and provide examples, Figure 8-2 shows examples of the links among constructs, concepts, and variables. On the left of the figure is the template of the construct-to-variable continuum. The other two sets of shapes are examples of a construct, concept, and variable. Notice that a concept may have multiple ways of being measured. For example, to measure anxiety, a researcher may assess palmar sweating, ask subjects to complete the State-Trait Anxiety Scale, or observe subjects and complete a checklist of behaviors such as pacing, wringing of hands, and verbalizing concerns.

Defining concepts allows us to be consistent in the way we use a term in practice, apply it to theory, and measure it in a study. A conceptual definition differs from the **denotative** (or dictionary) **definition** of a word. A **conceptual definition** (connotative meaning)

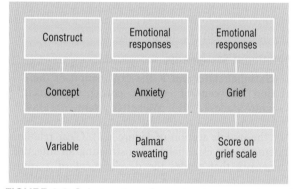

FIGURE 8-2 Substruction of constructs, concepts, and variables.

is more comprehensive than a denotative definition because it includes associated meanings the word may have. For example, a connotative definition may associate the term *fireplace* with images of comfort and warmth, whereas the denotative definition would be a rock or brick structure in a house designed for burning wood. Conceptual definitions may be found in theories, but can also be established through concept synthesis, concept derivation, or concept analysis (Walker & Avant, 2011).

Concept Synthesis

In nursing, many phenomena have not yet been identified as discrete entities. Recognizing, naming, and describing these phenomena are critical steps to understanding the process and outcomes of nursing practice. In your clinical practice, you may notice a pattern of behavior or find a pattern or theme in empirical data and select a name to represent the pattern. The process of describing and naming a previously unrecognized concept is **concept synthesis**. Nursing studies often involve previously unrecognized and unnamed phenomena that must be named and carefully defined, so that study readers can understand their meanings and functions. Smith, Swallow, and Coyne (2015) conducted a concept synthesis of family-centered care and partnership-in-care. They reviewed 30 studies that used one or both of the concepts to find common elements. They integrated the shared elements into a framework of pediatric nurses' involvement with families of children with long-term health conditions.

Concept Derivation

Concept derivation may occur when the researcher or theorist finds no concept in nursing to explain a phenomenon (Walker & Avant, 2011). Concepts identified or defined in theories of other disciplines can provide insight. In **concept derivation**, a concept is transposed from one of field of knowledge to another. If a conceptual definition is found in another discipline, it must be examined to evaluate its fit with the new field in which it will be used. The conceptual definition may need to be modified so that it is meaningful within nursing and consistent with nursing thought (Walker & Avant, 2011). For example, Manojlovich and Sidani (2008) identified four attributes of dose through concept analysis: purity, amount, frequency, and duration. Using these attributes, they examined the literature of medicine and behavioral therapy to derive a dose concept relevant to nurse staffing. Purity as a component of nurse dose was defined as concentration of nursing knowledge on a hospital unit. Amount was defined as the "total number

of nurses available to provide care" (p. 315). The authors also provided definitions of frequency and duration in terms of nurse staffing and linked each aspect of nurse dose to patient outcomes. These attributes of nurse staffing could be helpful in developing an outcomes study. Concept derivation is a creative process that can be fostered by thinking deeply and having a willingness to learn about processes and theories in other disciplines.

Concept Analysis

Concept analysis is a strategy that identifies a set of characteristics essential to defining the connotative meaning of a concept. Several approaches to concept analysis have been described in the nursing and health care literature. Because the approaches have varying philosophical foundations and products, nurse theorists and researchers must select the concept analysis approach that best suits their purposes in a specific situation (Table 8-1). A frequently used approach to concept analysis is the process proposed by Walker and Avant (2011). The procedure guides the scholar to explore the various ways the term is used and to identify a set of characteristics that clarify the range of objects or ideas to which that concept may be applied (Walker & Avant, 2011). These essential characteristics, called defining attributes or criteria, provide a means to distinguish the concept from similar concepts and provide a foundation for determining whether an instrument has construct validity (see Chapters 10 and 16). Clinicians analyze concepts as a means to improve practice, such as Robson and Troutman-Jordan (2014) who analyzed the concept of cognitive reframing as a nursing intervention. Nurses can use cognitive reframing to help patients and their families change their perception of a diagnosis or situation to a more positive view. A more positive view may promote behavior change and well-being (Robson & Troutman-Jordan, 2014).

Educators may conduct concept analysis to expand their knowledge of a concept and its implications for their teaching strategies. Page-Cutrara (2015) published a concept analysis of prebriefing in clinical simulation. Her purpose was to increase nurse educators' understanding of this element, used to improve student learning. When researchers are new to a topic or phenomenon, they may analyze both central and related concepts to develop a clear conceptual definition, which is the basis for selecting an appropriate operational definition (see Chapters 3 and 6). Petersen (2014, p. 1243), as a doctoral student, conducted a concept analysis of "spiritual care of the child with cancer at the end of life." The resulting antecedents, attributes, and consequences are listed in Box 8-1.

TABLE 8-1	Methods of Concept Analysis
Type of Concept Analysis (Author[s], Date)	**Unique Characteristics**
Principle-based method (Hupcey & Penrod, 2005)	Analysis guided by linguistic, epistemological, pragmatic, and logical principles
Ordinary use approach (Wilson, 1963)	Foci of analysis are exemplars (cases) used to identify criteria, antecedents, and consequences
Evolutionary method (Rodgers, 2000)	Contextual analysis of how the concept has developed over time in different settings
Hybrid method (Schwartz-Barcott & Kim, 2000)	Contextual analysis and data collection in the field leading to conclusions about how concept has developed over time in different settings
Linguistic, pragmatic approach (Walker & Avant, 2011)	Analysis of explicit and implicit concept definitions in the literature to identify criteria, antecedents, and consequences for use in practice and research
Simultaneous analysis method (Haase, Britt, Coward, Leidy, & Penn, 1992)	Examines closely related concepts to distinguish their unique meanings as well as areas of overlap

EXAMINING STATEMENTS

Understanding the statements in a theory is essential for ensuring consistency among research framework, study design, and statistical analyses. In addition to relational statements that involve two or more concepts,

statements can also be non-relational and involve a single concept. A non-relational statement indicates a concept exists or defines the concept. See Box 8-2. The first two statements are nonrelational statements about concepts in a study of self care related to dysmenorrhea of adolescent girls (Wong, Ip, Choi, & Lam, 2015). The authors also included several relational statements supported by research findings of published studies.

BOX 8-1   Spiritual Care of the Child With Cancer at End of Life: Antecedents, Attributes, and Consequences

Antecedents
- Spiritual distress
- Existential questions at end of life

Attributes
- Assessing the child's spiritual needs
- Assisting the child to express feelings and concerns
- Guiding the child in strengthening relationships
- Helping the child to be remembered
- Assisting the child to find meaning and purpose
- Aiding the child find hope

Consequences
- Peaceful death
- Spiritual growth
- Relationship of trust
- Enhanced end-of-life care

Data from Petersen, C. (2014). Spiritual care of the child with cancer at end of life: A concept analysis. *Journal of Advanced Nursing, 70*(6), 1243–1253.

BOX 8-2   Examples of Nonrelational and Relational Statements

Nonrelational Statements
"Patterns of living encompass all the actions people perform daily (Orem, 2001)."

"Family system factors are commonly defined as mother's and father's occupation and education, living situation, marital status, birth order, and social and emotional support (Moore & Pichler, 2000)."

Relational Statements
"Availability of resources influences the means to meet self-care measures (Orem, 2001)."

"… BCF [basic conditioning factors] may influence an individual's ability to participate in self-care activities or modify the kind or amount of self-care required."

Statements from Wong, C., Ip, W., Choi, K., & Lam, L. (2015). Examining self-care behaviors and their associated factors among adolescent girls with dysmenorrhea: An application of Orem's self-care deficit nursing theory. *Journal of Nursing Scholarship, 47*(3), 219–227.

Characteristics of Relational Statements

As stated earlier, a relational statement is the explanation of the connection between concepts. Relational statements in a research framework can be described by their characteristics. **Relational statements** describe the direction, shape, strength, sequencing, probability of occurrence, necessity, and sufficiency of a relationship (Walker & Avant, 2011). One statement may have several of these characteristics; each characteristic is not exclusive of the others. Statements may be expressed as words in a sentence (language form), as shapes and arrows (diagram form), or as equations (mathematical form). In nursing, the language and diagrammatic forms of statements are used most frequently and are shown in Figures 8-3 and 8-4. Figure 8-3 displays simple statements of relationships among spiritual perspective, social support, and coping, including a dotted arrow to indicate a relationship about which less is known. Figure 8-4 provides language and diagrammatic forms of a more complex statement among the previous concepts with the addition of perceived stress. Diagrams can be constructed to show how relationships are moderated by another concept, such as the change in the arrow between perceived stress and coping: the arrow is darker and heavier until spiritual perspective and social support modify the relationship. You can infer that the relationship between perceived stress and coping changes due to the influence of spiritual perspective and social support.

Direction

The **direction of a relationship** may be positive, negative, or unknown (Fawcett, 1999). The letters A and B in parentheses in the following paragraphs indicate concepts. A **positive linear relationship** implies that as one concept changes (the value or amount of the concept increases or decreases), the second concept will also change in the same direction (Figure 8-5). For example, in the Wong et al. (2015) study of adolescent girls, presented earlier in the chapter, the researchers proposed the statement, "As maternal education level increases (A), self care related to dysmenorrhea (B) increases," which expresses a positive relationship. Another positive relationship tested in the study was "As self care agency (A) decreases, self care behaviors decrease (B).

A **negative linear relationship** implies that as a concept changes, the other concept in the statement changes in the opposite direction. For example, instead of the positive relationship that was proposed between

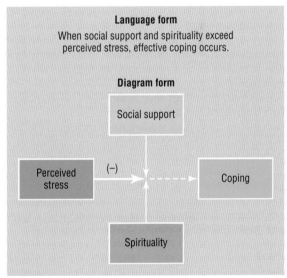

FIGURE 8-4 Language and diagram forms of a complex statement.

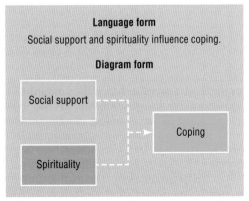

FIGURE 8-3 Language and diagram forms of a simple statement.

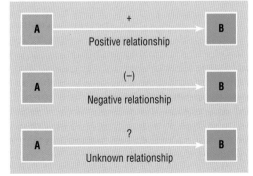

FIGURE 8-5 Directions of relational statements.

maternal education and self care, Wong et al. (2015) found a negative relationship that can be stated, "As maternal education (A) increased, self care behaviors (B) decreased." Another negative relationship from the study findings was that, "As pain intensity decreased, self care behaviors increased."

The nature of the relationship between two concepts may be unknown because it has not been studied or because there have been conflicting findings from two or more studies. For example, consider two studies of coping and social support. Tkatch et al. (2011) found that the number of people in the social networks of African American patients in cardiac rehabilitation (*N* = 115) and their health-related social support were both weakly, but statistically significantly, related to coping efficacy. In contrast, Jackson et al. (2009) found nonsignificant relationships between social support and coping in a longitudinal study of 88 parents of children with brain tumors. From the findings, we can conclude that, although there is some evidence that a relationship may exist between these two concepts, the findings from the two studies do not agree.

Conflicting findings may result from differences in the researchers' definitions and measurements of the two concepts in various studies. Another reason for conflicting findings might have been an unidentified variable changed the relationship between coping and social support. A third possibility is that the findings of one of the studies reflect Type I or Type II error. Whatever the reason, conflicting findings about a relationship between concepts can be indicated diagrammatically by a question mark, the third example shown in Figure 8-5.

Shape

Most relationships are assumed to be linear, and so initial statistical tests are conducted to identify linear relationships. In a **linear relationship**, the relationship between two concepts remains consistent regardless of the values of each of the concepts. For example, if the value of B increases by 1 point each time the value of A increases by 2 points, then the values continue to increase proportionally whether the values are 2 and 4 or 200 and 400. We can diagram relationships between concepts using a vertical axis and a horizontal axis, with each axis representing the score on one of the concepts. Each subject's paired scores on the two concepts are plotted as a dot on the diagram. If the relationship between the concepts is linear, most of the dots will be clustered around a straight line, as shown in Figure 8-6.

Relationships also can be curvilinear or form some other shape. In a **curvilinear relationship**, the relationship between two concepts varies according to the

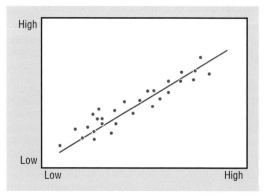

FIGURE 8-6 Linear relationship.

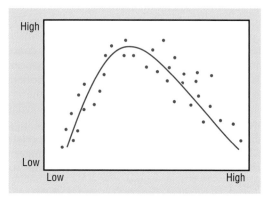

FIGURE 8-7 Curvilinear relationship.

relative values of the concepts. Kubicek, Korunka, and Tement (2014) found that the irritation of eldercare workers (nurses, nursing assistants, and orderlies) was lower when medium levels of job control were found. Workers with low and high job control were found to have more irritation and less work engagement, indicating a curvilinear relationship as shown in Figure 8-7.

Strength

The **strength of a relationship** is the amount of variation explained by the relationship. If two concepts are related, some of the variation in one concept may be found to be associated with variation in another concept (Fawcett, 1999). Usually, researchers determine the strength of a linear relationship between concepts through correlational analysis. The mathematical result of the analysis is a correlation coefficient such as the following: $r = 0.35$. The statistic r is the result obtained by performing the statistical procedure known as

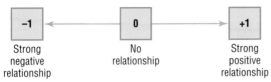

FIGURE 8-8 Strength of relationships.

Pearson's product-moment correlation (see Chapter 23). A value of 0 indicates no relationship, whereas a value of +1 or −1 indicates a perfect relationship (Figure 8-8). The closer that the correlation is to +1 or −1, the stronger the relationship between the variables.

When the correlation is large, a greater portion of the variation can be explained by the relationship; in others, only a moderate or a small portion of the variation can be explained by the relationship. For example, Kamitani, Fukuoka, and Dawson-Rose (2015) found a relationship of $r = -0.36$ ($p < 0.01$) between self-rated health and HIV stigma among Asians living with HIV infection who had little or no insurance ($n = 67$). The strength of the relationship meant that a small portion of the variance in health was explained by variations in perceived HIV stigma. Details on statistically determining linear relationships in studies are presented in Chapter 23

Whether the relationship is positive or negative does not have an impact on the strength of the relationship. For example, $r = -0.36$ is as strong as $r = +0.36$. The closer the r-value is to 1 or −1, the stronger the relationship. Stronger relationships are more easily detected, even in a small sample. Weaker relationships may require larger samples to be detected. This idea will be explored further in the chapters on sampling, measurement, and data analysis.

Sequential Relationships

The amount of time that elapses between one concept and another is stated as the sequential nature of a relationship. If the two concepts occur simultaneously or are measured at the same time, the relationship is **concurrent** (Fawcett, 1999). When there is a change in one concept, there is change in the other at the same time (Table 8-2). If a change in one concept now influences changes in second concept at a later time, the relationship is **sequential**. In a study with 162 Iranian women with breast cancer, Rohani, Abedi, Omranipour, and Languis-Eklof (2015) found that sense of coherence at diagnosis was related positively to health-related quality of life six months later, a sequential relationship. These relationships are diagrammed in Figure 8-9.

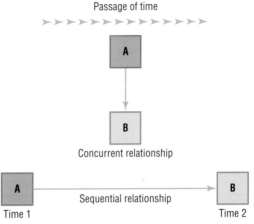

FIGURE 8-9 Sequencing of relationships.

TABLE 8-2 Characteristics of Relationships

Type of Relationship	Descriptive Statement
Positive linear	As A increases, B increases. As A decreases, B decreases.
Negative linear	As A increases, B decreases. As A decreases, B increases.
Unknown linear	As A changes, B may or may not change.
Curvilinear	At a specific level, as A changes, B changes to a similar degree. At another specific level, as A changes, B changes to a greater or lesser extent.
Concurrent	When A changes, B changes at the same time.
Sequential	After A changes, B changes.
Causal	If A occurs, B always occurs.
Probabilistic	If A occurs, then probably B occurs.
Necessary	If A occurs, and only if A occurs, B occurs. If A does not occur, B does not occur.
Sufficient	If A occurs, and if A alone occurs, B occurs.
Substitutable	If A_1 or A_2 occurs, B occurs.
Contingent	If A occurs, then B occurs, but only if C occurs.

Probability of Occurrence

A relationship can be deterministic or probabilistic depending on the degree of certainty that it will occur. **Deterministic** (or **causal**) **relationships** are statements of what always occurs in a particular situation. Scientific laws are an example of deterministic relationships (Fawcett, 1999). A causal relationship is expressed as follows:

If A, then always B.

A **probability statement** expresses the probability that something will happen in a given situation (Fawcett, 1999). For example, patients identified at admission to be a high fall risk had a 17% higher probability of falling during the hospitalization than patients identified as low or medium fall risk (Cox et al., 2015). This relationship is expressed as follows:

If A, then probably B.

This probability could be expressed mathematically as follows:

$$p > 0.17.$$

The p is a symbol for probability. The $>$ is a symbol for "greater than." This mathematical statement asserts that there is more than a 17% probability that the second event will occur.

Necessity

In a **necessary relationship**, one concept must occur for the second concept to occur (Fawcett, 1999). For example, one could propose that if sufficient fluids are administered (A), and only if sufficient fluids are administered, the unconscious patient will remain hydrated (B). This relationship is expressed as follows:

If A, and only if A, then B.

In a **substitutable relationship**, a similar concept can be substituted for the first concept and the second concept will still occur (see Table 8-2). For example, a substitutable relationship might propose that if tube feedings are administered (A_1), or if hyperalimentation is administered (A_2), the unconscious patient can remain hydrated (B). This relationship is expressed as follows:

If A_1, or if A_2, then B.

Sufficiency

A **sufficient relationship** states that when the first concept occurs, the second concept will occur, regardless of the presence or absence of other factors (Fawcett, 1999). A statement could propose that if a patient is immobilized in bed longer than a week, he or she will lose bone calcium, regardless of anything else. This relationship is expressed as follows:

If A, then B, regardless of anything else.

A **contingent relationship** will occur only if a third concept is present. For example, a statement might

claim that if a person experiences a stressor (A), the person will manage the stress (B), but only if she or he uses effective coping strategies (C). The third concept, in this case effective coping strategies, is referred to as an **intervening** (or **mediating**) **variable**. Intervening variables can affect the occurrence, strength, or direction of a relationship. A contingent relationship can be expressed as follows:

If A, then B, but only if C.

Being able to describe relationships among the concepts is an important first step in identifying, evaluating, and developing research frameworks. Table 8-2 provides a summary of the characteristics of relational statements. Remember that each statement may have multiple descriptive characteristics.

Levels of Abstraction of Statements

Statements about the same two conceptual ideas can be made at various levels of abstractness. The relational statements found in conceptual models and grand theories (**general propositions**) are at a high level of abstraction. Relational statements found in middle-range theories (**specific propositions**) are at a moderate level of abstraction. **Hypotheses**, which are a form of statement, consisting of an expressed relationship between variables, are at the concrete level, representing a low level of abstraction. As statements become less abstract, they become narrower in scope (Fawcett, 1999).

Statements at varying levels of abstraction that express relationships between or among the same conceptual ideas can be arranged in hierarchical form, from general to specific. This arrangement allows you to see (or evaluate) the logical links among the various levels of abstraction. In Chapter 3, abstract concepts were linked to more concrete concepts through substruction. Linking general propositions to more specific propositions is the same process of substruction and links the relationships expressed in the framework with the hypotheses, research questions, or objectives that guide the methodology of the study (McQuiston & Campbell, 1997; Trego, 2009). The following excerpts provide an example of the more abstract theoretical proposition that provided the basis for four hypotheses that were tested in a study by de Guzman et al. (2013). These researchers studied the risk of falls with older Filipinos living at home ($n = 125$) and based their study hypotheses on Pender's Health Promotion Model (1996) and McGill's Model of Nursing (Gottlieb & Rowat, 1987). From the theories, they proposed a model that increased autonomy, increased environmental safety, increased social support, and decreased depression are associated with increased risk for falls. The researchers stated the hypotheses but the propositions were embedded in the related theoretical discussion. The following proposition and hypothesis are provided as an example.

Proposition

Having a support system, such as being married or having significant others providing care, is related to having assistance with activities of daily living. Having assistance with activities of daily living is protective.

Hypothesis

"H2: The better the support system, the lesser the risk for fall incidence." (de Guzman et al., 2013, p. 672)

Based on the study results, de Guzman et al. (2013) revised the model, finding that only increased environmental safety and decreased depression were significantly related to a lower risk for falls.

GRAND THEORIES

Most disciplines have several conceptual models, each with a distinctive vocabulary. Table 8-3 lists a few of the conceptual models or grand theories in nursing. Each theory provides an overall picture, or gestalt, of the phenomena they explain. In addition to concepts specific to the theory, nurse theorists include the metaparadigm or domain concepts of nursing: person, health, environment, and nursing (Chinn & Kramer, 2015; Fawcett, 1985). Each theorist may define the domain concepts differently to be consistent with the other concepts and propositions of the theory. For example, Roy (1988) defined health as restoring or maintaining adaptation by activating cognator and regulator systems and using

one of four adaptive modes (Roy & Andrews, 2008). Consistent with her theory of self care, Orem (2001) defined health as the extent to which persons can meet their own universal, developmental, and health-related self-care requisites. Most grand theories are not directly testable through research and thus cannot be used alone as the framework for a study (Fawcett, 1999; Walker & Avant, 2011). Application of grand nursing theories to research is discussed later in the chapter. For detailed information about grand nursing theories, refer to the primary sources written by the theorist and reference books about nursing theory (Fawcett & DeSanto-Madeya, 2013; McEwen & Wills, 2014).

MIDDLE-RANGE THEORIES

Middle-range theories are useful in both research and practice. Middle-range theories are less abstract than grand theories and closer to the day-to-day substance of clinical practice, a characteristic that explains why they can be called substantive theories. As a result, middle-range theories guide the practitioner in understanding the client's behavior, enabling interventions that are more effective. Because of their usefulness in practice, some writers refer to middle-range theories as **practice theories**.

Middle-range theories have been developed from grand nursing theories, clinical insights, and research findings. Mefford and Alligood (2011) combined health promotion principles with Levin's Conservation Theory (1967), an older grand nursing theory, to develop a theory of health promotion for preterm infants. Middle-range theories may be developed by combining a nursing and a non-nursing theory. Some middle-range theories have been developed from clinical practice guidelines,

TABLE 8-3 Selected Grand Nursing Theories	
Author (Year)	**Descriptive Label of the Theory**
King, Imogene (1981)	Interacting Systems Theory of Nursing (includes middle-range theory of Goal Attainment)
Leininger, Madeline (1997)	Transcultural Nursing Care, Sunrise Model of Care
Orem, Dorothea (2001)	Self-Care Deficit Theory of Nursing
Neuman, Betty (Neuman & Fawcett, 2002)	Systems Model of Nursing
Newman, Margaret (1986)	Health as Expanding Consciousness
Parse, Rosemarie (1992)	Human Becoming Theory
Rogers, Martha E (1970)	Unitary Human Beings
Roy, Calista (1988)	Adaptation Model
Watson, Jean (1979)	Philosophy and Science of Caring

such as Good and Moore's (1996) theory of acute pain following surgery. Kolcaba's Theory of Comfort (1994) is an example of a middle-range theory developed over time. Kolcaba's clinical experiences motivated her to analyze the concept of comfort (Kolcaba & Kolcaba, 1991) and continue to refine the theory. Several research instruments have been developed to measure different types of comfort (http://www.thecomfortline.com/). Often grounded theory studies result in a middle-range theory, such as Baumhover's (2015) middle-range theory of family members' awareness of a critical care patient's imminent death. Through her grounded theory study, Baumhover identified six key categories and a core category labeled "death imminence awareness" (p. 153). Another example of a middle-range theory emanating from a grounded theory study is the Noiseux and Ricard's (2008) middle-range theory of recovery in schizophrenia. Carr's (2014) theory of family vigilance was developed from the findings of three ethnographic studies the author conducted in hospitals.

Middle-range theories are used more commonly than grand theories as frameworks for research. For example, Mefford and Alligood (2011) tested their middle-range theory of health promotion for preterm infants in their study using clinical data from neonatal units. Another study built upon a middle-range theory was Chism and Magnan' (2009) study of nursing students' perspectives on spiritual care and their expressions of spiritual empathy. Chism (2007) had previously developed the theory upon which the study was based, the Middle-Range Theory of Spiritual Empathy, as part of her doctoral study. Covell and Sidani (2013a, b) identified empirical indicators for the concepts in Covell's (2008) nursing intellectual capitol theory, evaluated the propositions among the concepts, and found mixed support for the relationships.

A specific type of middle-range theory is intervention theory. Intervention theories seek to explain the dynamics of a patient problem and exactly how a specific nursing intervention is expected to change patient outcomes (Wolf, 2015). Using two theories, Peek and Melnyk (2014) developed an intervention theory for a coping intervention to help mothers with the cancer diagnosis of a child. The self-regulation theory of Johnson (1999) was the basis for providing the mothers anticipatory guidance about the expected behaviors and emotions of a child with cancer. At the same time, the control theory of Carver and Scheier (1982) was used as the basis for equipping the mothers with "education, information, and behavior skills development of parent behaviors specific to this novel situation" (Peek & Melnyk, 2014, p. 204).

APPRAISING THEORIES AND RESEARCH FRAMEWORKS

Nurses examine and evaluate theories to determine their applicability for practice and usefulness for research. The evaluation of theories is complicated by the availability of several sets of evaluative criteria (Meleis, 2012). From these, we have selected the following for inclusion in the critical appraisal of research frameworks in published studies (Box 8-3).

Critical Appraisal of a Research Framework

During the process of critically appraising a study, the first task related to the research framework is to describe it. This task is easier when the researchers have explicitly identified the framework. For example, Rodwell, Brunetto, Demir, Shacklock, and Farr-Wharton (2014) based their study on the concepts and relationships of a theory of stress, appraisal, and coping (Lazarus & Folkman, 1984). They applied the theory to abusive supervision and nurses' intention to quit their jobs in Australian hospitals. The hypothesized model drawn from the theory was consistent with their study aim: "Examine forms of abusive supervision … and their links to health and work outcomes of nurses, including job satisfaction, psychological strain, and intentions to quit" (Rodwell et al., 2014, p. 359).

Other researchers, such as Moon, Phelan, Lauver, and Bratzke (2015), did not identify frameworks in their study of heart failure (HF) and sleep quality. However, Moon et al. began their research report by presenting findings from other studies of patients with HF related to sleep quality and cognitive function. Cognitive function is an issue for HF patients because poor cognition may decrease their ability to manage their medications and impair self-care, both of which have been shown to contribute to mortality and morbidity. The researchers also noted that magnetic resonance imaging (MRI) tests have shown changes in cerebral structures of patients with HF, presumably due to poor cerebral blood flow.

BOX 8-3   Critical Appraisal of Research Frameworks

- Identify and describe the theory.
- Examine the logical structure of the framework.
- Evaluate extent to which the framework guided the methodology of the study.
- Decide the extent to which the researcher connected the findings to the framework.

These relational statements were not tested but provided the rationale for studying cognitive function in this sample. The following statements describe possible relationships among the concepts.

> "Cross sectional studies have documented a relationship between poor sleep quality, excessive daytime sleepiness (EDS), and cognitive function." (Moon et al., 2015, p. 212)
>
> "... self reported poor sleep quality is associated with reduced prefrontal cortex function." (p. 213)
>
> "Daytime symptoms ... of disturbed sleep and sleep disorders may be related to cognitive function as well." (p. 213)

Describing the research framework may be easier if you draw a diagram of the concepts and relationships among them. For the Moon et al. (2015) study, Figure 8-10 presents our diagram of the concepts and relationships among the concepts. In the figure, the constructs of sleep quality, daytime alertness, and cognitive function and the relationships among them are shown. Another aspect of describing the theory is to find or infer the conceptual and operational definitions of the variables related to the concepts in the framework. Table 8-4 includes the conceptual and operational definitions of the three concepts in the research framework.

Following your description of the framework, you are ready to examine the logical structure of the framework. Meleis's (2012) criteria for critically appraising theories include assessing the clarity and consistency of the logical structure. When the following questions about clarity and consistency can be answered *yes*, the framework has a strong logical structure:

1. Are the definitions of concepts consistent with the theorist's definitions? This question is asked only if the researchers link their framework to a parent theory. (The **parent theory** is the theory from which the researchers have selected the constructs for their study.)
2. Do the concepts reflect constructs identified in the framework? Some frameworks may not identify constructs and may be comprised of only concepts.

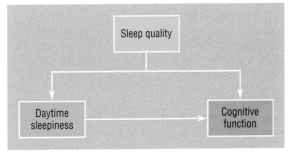

FIGURE 8-10 Research framework inferred from Moon et al. (2015).

TABLE 8-4	Conceptual and Operational Definitions for Study of Sleep Quality, Daytime Sleepiness, and Cognitive Function of Patients With Heart Failure	
Concept	**Conceptual Definition**	**Operational Definition**
Sleep quality	Multidimensional concept that includes "general quality of one's sleep, duration of sleep, the time required to fall asleep (sleep latency), the percent of time spent in bed asleep (sleep efficiency), disrupted sleep, and use of sleep medication" (Buysse, Reynolds, Monk, Berman, & Kupfer, 1989, as cited in Moon et al., 2014, p. 212).	Scale and subscale scores on the Pittsburgh Sleep Quality Index (Buysse et al., 1989) that measures use of sleep medication, daytime dysfunction, and the quality, latency, duration, efficiency, disturbance of sleep (Moon et al., 2015, p. 213)
Daytime sleepiness	Decreased alertness, desire to rest, and decreased attention related to sleep deprivation (inferred from Moon et al., 2014)	Self-reported likelihood of falling asleep in daily situations on the Epworth Sleepiness Scale (Johns, 1991, 1993)
Cognitive function	Mental ability as indicated by "immediate memory, visual/spatial construction, language, attention, and delayed memory" ... "complex visual scanning, attention, processing speed, and executive function" (Moon et al., 2014, p.213-214)	Scores on the separate components of the "Repeatable Battery for the Assessment of Neuropsychological Status (RBANS)" (Randolph, Tierney, Mohr, & Chase, 1998, as cited in Moon et al., 2015, p. 213)

Data from Moon, C., Phelan, C., Lauver, D., & Bratzke, L. (2015). Is sleep quality related to cognition in individuals with heart failure? *Heart & Lung, 44*(3), 212–218.

3. Do the variables reflect the concepts identified in the framework?
4. Are the conceptual definitions validated by references to the literature?
5. Are the propositions (relational statements) logical and defensible?

The next step in critically appraising a study framework is to evaluate the extent to which the framework guided the methodology by asking the following questions:

1. Do the operational definitions reflect the conceptual definitions?
2. Do the hypotheses, questions, or objectives reflect the constructs and/or concepts in the propositions of the framework?
3. Is the design appropriate for testing the propositions of the framework?

When a framework guides the methodology of a study, the answer to these questions will be *yes.* Some researchers may describe a theory or theories to provide context for their study but fail to use the framework to guide the methodology. Bond et al. (2011) conducted a study of how nurse researchers use theory by reviewing research reports in seven leading journals over 5 years. In 837 of the 2184 research reports (38%), the researchers included a theoretical framework, either a nursing theory or a theory from another discipline. Of these 837 reports, 93% contained evidence that the theory had been integrated into the study methodology. Bond et al. documented that, when identified, the study framework most likely will be used to guide the methodology.

The final step in critically appraising a study framework is to decide the extent to which the researcher connected the findings to the framework by asking the following questions:

1. Did the researcher interpret the findings in terms of the framework?
2. Are the findings for each hypothesis, question, or objective consistent with the relationships proposed by the framework?

Even in studies clearly guided by a research framework, the findings may not be discussed in terms of the framework. Findings that are consistent with the framework are evidence of the framework's validity, and this point should be noted in the discussion. When the findings are not consistent with the research framework, researchers should discuss the possible reasons for this disconnect. One reason may be a lack of construct

validity (see Chapters 10, 11, and 16). The instruments used may not have measured the constructs/concepts of the study framework adequately and accurately. Other possible reasons are that the framework was based on assumptions that were not true for the population being studied and that the framework did not represent the reality of the phenomena being studied in this specific sample.

DEVELOPING A RESEARCH FRAMEWORK FOR STUDY

Developing a framework is one of the most important steps in the research process but, perhaps, also one of the most difficult. A research report in a journal often contains only a brief presentation of the study framework because of page limitations, hardly equivalent to the prolonged work the researchers expended to develop a framework for the study.

As a new researcher, assume you have identified a research problem and are thinking about the proposed study's methodology. You need a research framework but where do you start? This section presents three basic approaches to beginning the process of constructing a study framework: (1) identify an existing theory from nursing or another discipline, (2) synthesize a framework from research findings, and (3) propose a framework from clinical practice. The final steps of constructing a research framework are discussed after the presentation of the approaches.

Identifying and Adapting an Existing Theory

Take another look at the research reports you have read related to your topic. Which theories have others used when studying this area? In your exploration, include studies on your topic of interest that have been conducted with populations other than your own. For example, researchers have used several health behavior and psychological theories to guide studies related to medication adherence. Gulley and Boggs (2014) described predictors of physical activity, based on the theory of planned behavior (Fishbein & Ajzen, 2010). As described earlier, Gulley and Boggs found positive relationships among concepts of the theory and physical exercise among adolescents. Kamitani et al. (2015) used the Information-Motivation-Behavioral Skills model (Fisher, Fisher, Amico, & Harman, 2006) in their study of the relationships among HIV stigma, knowledge of acute coronary syndrome, perceived risk for coronary disease, and perceived ability to access health care among Asians living with HIV infection. Wong et al. (2015), as mentioned earlier in the chapter, researched adolescent girls' self-care related to dysmenorrhea, using Orem's self-care theory (2001) as their framework. Existing theories can provide insights into how the topic has been studied and the range of perspectives available on a given research topic.

When trying to find a theory that pertains to your variables and relational statements, you may choose to review theory textbooks and middle-range theory publications to examine the applicability of other nursing theories that might provide insight into your research problem (McEwen & Wills, 2014). Before making a final decision about a theory, you should read primary sources written by the theorists to ensure that your topic is a good fit with the theory's concepts, definitions of concepts, assumptions, and propositions.

Synthesis From Research Findings

Developing a theory or a framework from research findings is the most accepted strategy of theory development (Meleis, 2012). The research-to-theory strategy, an inductive approach, begins by identifying relevant studies. Charette et al. (2015) were concerned about the high levels of pain and anxiety that adolescents reported after surgery to correct scoliosis. The levels and prolonged nature of pain and anxiety following the surgery hindered physical activity and recovery. The researchers reviewed the research literature, identified relevant studies, and found support for the following relationships:

- Spinal fusion, the corrective surgery for scoliosis, is associated with prolonged, severe postoperative pain and anxiety.
- Guided imagery is associated with decreased anxiety and postoperative pain.
- Provision of information and assisting coping through guided imagery and relaxation are more effective in reducing pain and anxiety than either intervention alone (Charette et al., 2015).

Based on these research findings, Charette et al. (2015) developed an intervention that combined "guided imagery, relaxation, and education to decrease postoperative pain and anxiety related to spinal fusion" (p. 212). Figure 8-11 is a visual model of these relationships. The research team tested the intervention in a randomized clinical trial pilot study of its effects on pain, anxiety, coping, and daily activities compared to usual postoperative care. As predicted, the intervention group reported less overall pain at discharge, two weeks post-discharge, and at the one-month follow-up visit, when compared to the usual care group. The team's next planned steps are to repeat the study with a larger sample over a longer follow-up period.

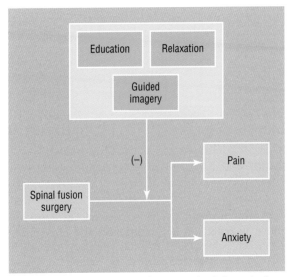

FIGURE 8-11 Research framework inferred from Charette et al. (2015).

Proposing a Framework From Practice Experiences

As members of a practice discipline, nurses may develop research frameworks from their clinical experiences. Nurses in practice can make generalizations about patients' responses as they provide care to different types of patients. Nurses who reflect on practice may, over time, realize underlying principles of human behavior that guide their choices of interventions. Meleis (2012) noted that a nurse may have nagging questions about why certain situations persist, or wonder how to improve patient or organizational outcomes, which can lead to development of tentative theories. For example, a novice researcher who worked in a newborn intensive care unit might become convinced from her clinical experiences that a mother's frequent visits to the hospital might be related to her infant's weight gain. The nurse's ideas could be diagrammed as the lower set of relationships shown in Figure 8-12.

The relationship the nurse identified consisted of two concrete ideas: number of mother visits and weight gain. From the perspective of research, these ideas are variables. Instead of starting with a framework and linking the concepts of the framework to possible study variables, she was starting with variables and needed to identify the concepts that the variables represented. The nurse reviewed the literature and looked for explanations for why visits by the mother were important and what happened when a mother visited the baby. As she reflected on what she read, she realized that maybe the

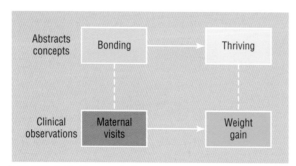

FIGURE 8-12 Research framework from clinical practice.

visits promoted bonding or attachment. The nurse continued to reflect on her experiences and remembered that when babies failed to gain weight or lost weight, they were sometimes labeled as "failing to thrive." Wording that more positively, she decided the concept related to weight gain was thriving. On the basis of her clinical experiences and her thinking processes, the nurse began to learn more about theories of bonding and used what she learned to develop a framework for a study related to bonding and thriving of newborns in neonatal intensive care units (see Figure 8-12).

Research frameworks rarely develop from only one source of knowledge. Nurse researchers often combine existing theories, research findings, and insights from their clinical experiences into a framework for a study. For example, to study adherence to blood pressure medications among older Chinese immigrants, Li, Wallhagen, and Froelicher (2010) derived their model from four sources: Becker's Health Belief Model (1974), findings from preliminary studies, hypertension literature, and clinical experience. Rishel (2014) described combining her clinical experience as a pediatric bone marrow transplant nurse with her review of the literature when she began to explore parents' end-of-life decisions. Later in her career as a researcher, she proposed a middle-range theory of the process of parental decision making.

Study frameworks begun in these ways are considered tentative theory until research findings provide evidence to support the relationships as diagrammed. **Tentative theories** are those that are developed from other theories, research findings, and clinical practice and that, as yet, do not have evidence to support their relational statements. Whatever your approach to beginning the process, once you can identify possible concepts and relationships, you are ready to move through the remainder of the process to develop the framework that is explicated in the final research report.

Defining Relevant Concepts

Concepts are selected for a framework on the basis of their relevance to the phenomenon of interest. The concepts included in the research framework should reflect the problem statement and the literature review of the proposal. Each concept included in a framework must be defined conceptually. Conceptual definitions may be found in existing theoretical works and quoted in the proposal with sources cited. Conceptual definitions also may be found in published concept analyses, previous studies using the concept, or the literature associated with an instrument developed to measure the concept. Although the instrument itself is an operational definition of the concept, often the writer provides a conceptual definition on which the instrument development was based. (See Chapter 6 for more extensive discussion of conceptual and operational definitions for study variables.) When acceptable conceptual definitions are not available, you should perform concept synthesis or concept analysis to develop them.

Developing Relational Statements

The next step in framework development is to link all of the study concepts through relational statements. If you began with an existing theory, the author may have identified theoretical propositions already. If you synthesized research findings, you have evidence that supports relationships between or among some or all of the concepts. This evidence supports the validity of each relational statement. This support must include a discussion of previous quantitative, qualitative and mixed methods research that have examined the proposed relationship, or published observations from the perspective of clinical practice.

Extracting relational statements from the written description of an existing theory, published research, or clinical literature can be a daunting task. The following procedure describes how to do so: Select the portion of the theory, research report, or clinical literature that discusses the relationships among concepts relevant to your study. Write single sentences that link concepts. Change each sentence to a diagram of the relationship, similar to those presented earlier in the chapter (see Figures 8-3 and 8-4). Continue this process until all of the relationships in the text have been expressed as simple diagrams or small maps.

If statements relating the concepts of interest are not available in the literature, statement synthesis is necessary. Develop statements that propose specific relationships among the concepts you are studying. You may gain the knowledge for your statement synthesis through clinical observation and integrative literature review (Walker & Avant, 2011).

Developing Hierarchical Statement Sets

A **hierarchical statement set** is composed of a specific proposition (relational statement) at the conceptual level and a hypothesis or research question, representing concrete relationships among variables. The specific proposition may be preceded by a more general proposition when an existing theory was the source of the framework (see example earlier in the chapter). The proposition is listed first, with the hypothesis or research question immediately following. In some cases, more than one hypothesis or research question may be developed for a single proposition. The statement set indicates the link between the framework and the methodology. The following is an example:

- Anxiety is intensified by a lack of information about the future (construct level).
- Patients' anxiety is reduced when information about a procedure is provided (concept level).
- Preoperative teaching provided several days prior to a procedure and repeated in the preoperative phase produces lower self-rated anxiety than the usual method of preoperative teaching (hypothesis/variable level).

Constructing a Conceptual Map

A conceptual map is the visual representation of a research framework. With the concepts defined and the relational statements diagrammed, you are ready to represent the framework for your study in a visual manner. The resultant map may be limited to only the concepts that you are studying or may be inclusive of other related concepts that are not going to be studied or measured at this time. When the map includes concepts that are not included in the specific study being proposed, you must clearly identify the concepts in the map that will be measured in the study.

From a practical standpoint, first arrange the relational statements you have diagrammed from left to right with outcomes located at the far right. Concepts that are elements of a more abstract construct can be placed in a frame or box. To show a group of closely interrelated concepts, enclose the concepts in a frame or circle (see Figure 8-12 as an example). Second, using lines and arrows, link the concepts in a way that is consistent with the statement diagrams you previously developed. Every concept should be linked to at least one other concept. Third, examine the framework diagram for completeness by asking yourself the following questions:

1. Are all of the concepts in the study also included on the map?
2. Are all of the concepts on the map defined?
3. Does the map clearly portray the framework and its phenomenon of interest?
4. Does the map accurately reflect all of the statements?
5. Is there a statement for each of the links portrayed by the map?
6. Is the sequence of links in the map accurate?
7. Do arrows point from cause to effect, reflecting direction of relationship?

Developing a well-constructed conceptual map requires repeated tries, but persistence pays off. You may need to reexamine the statements identified. Are there some missing links? Are some of the links inaccurately expressed?

As the map takes shape and begins to seem right, show it to trusted colleagues. Can that person follow your logic? Does that person agree with your links? Can missing elements be identified? Can you explain the map aloud? Seek out individuals who have experienced the phenomenon you are mapping. Does the process depicted seem valid to those individuals? Find someone more experienced than you in conceptual mapping to examine your map closely and critically.

The product of the creative and critical thinking that you have expended in the development of your research framework may provide a structure for one study or become the basis for a program of research. Continue to consider the framework as you collect and analyze data and interpret the findings. While you wait to hear whether your proposal has been funded or while your data are being collected, use the time to expand the written description of the framework and the evidence supporting its relationships into a manuscript for publication (see Chapter 27). When disseminated, your research framework has the potential to make a valuable contribution to nursing knowledge.

■ KEY POINTS

- A concept is a term that abstractly describes and names an object or a phenomenon, thus providing it with a distinct identity or meaning.
- A relational statement is the explanation of the connection between concepts.
- A conceptual model or grand theory broadly explains phenomena of interest, expresses assumptions, and reflects a philosophical stance.
- A theory is a set of concepts and relational statements explaining the relationships among them.
- Scientific theories have significant evidence and their relationships may be considered laws.

- Substantive theories are less abstract, can easily be applied in practice, and may be called middle-range theories.
- Middle-range theories may be developed from qualitative data, clinical experiences, clinical practice guidelines, or more abstract theories.
- Tentative theories are developed from research findings and clinical experiences, and they have not yet been validated.
- A framework is the abstract, logical structure of meaning that guides the development of the study and enables the researcher to link the findings to the body of knowledge used in nursing.
- Relational statements are the core of the framework; it is these statements that are examined through research.
- Relational statements can be described by their linearity, timing, and type of relationships.
- Almost every study has a theoretical framework, either implicit or explicit.
- The steps of critically appraising a research framework are (1) describing its concepts and relational statements, (2) examining its logical structure, (3) evaluating the extent to which the framework guided the methodology, and (4) determining the extent to which the researcher linked the findings back to the framework.
- The logical adequacy of a research framework is the extent to which the relational statements are clear and used consistently.
- The framework should be well integrated with the methodology, carefully structured, and clearly presented, whether the study is physiological or psychosocial.
- Research frameworks may start with existing theories, research findings, and/or clinical experiences.
- The remaining steps of the process are (1) selecting and defining concepts, (2) developing statements relating the concepts, (3) expressing the statements in hierarchical fashion, and (4) developing a conceptual map.
- Concepts and relational statements can be diagrammed as a conceptual map, in order to visually represent the research framework.
- Developing a framework for a study is one of the most important steps in the research process.

REFERENCES

Alligood, M. R. (2010). *Nursing theory: Utilization & application* (4th ed.). Maryland Heights, MO: Mosby Elsevier.

Baumhover, N. (2015). The process of death imminence awareness by family members of patients in adult critical care. *Dimensions of Critical Care, 34*(3), 149–160.

Becker, M. (1974). The Health Belief Model and sick role behavior. *Health Education Monographs, 2*(4), 409–462.

Bond, A., Eshah, N., Bani-Khaled, M., Hamad, A., Habashneh, S., Kataua, H., et al. (2011). Who uses nursing theory? A univariate descriptive analysis of five years' research articles. *Scandinavian Journal of Caring Sciences, 25*(2), 404–409.

Buysse, D., Reynolds, C., Monk, T., Berman, S., & Kupfer, D. (1989). The Pittsburgh Sleep Quality Index (PSQI): A new instrument for psychiatric research and practice. *Psychiatry Research, 28*(2), 193–213.

Carr, J. (2014). A middle range theory of family vigilance. *Medsurg Nursing, 23*(4), 251–255.

Carver, C., & Scheier, M. (1982). Control theory: A useful conceptual framework for personality-social, clinical, and health psychology. *Psychological Bulletin, 92*(1), 111–135.

Charette, S., Lacbance, J., Charest, M., Villeneuve, D., Theroux, J., Joncas, J., et al. (2015). Guided imagery for adolescent post-spinal fusion pain management: A pilot study. *Pain Management Nursing, 16*(3), 211–220.

Chinn, P. L., & Kramer, M. K. (2015). *Integrated theory and knowledge development in nursing* (9th ed.). St. Louis, MO: Elsevier.

Chism, L. (2007). *Spiritual empathy: A model for spiritual well-being.* Unpublished dissertation, Oakland University, Rochester, MI.

Chism, L., & Magnan, M. (2009). The relationship of nursing students' spiritual care perspectives to their expressions of spiritual empathy. *Journal of Nursing Education, 48*(11), 597–605.

Covell, C. (2008). The middle range theory of nursing intellectual capital. *Journal of Advanced Nursing, 63*(1), 94–103.

Covell, C., & Sidani, S. (2013a). Nursing intellectual capital theory: Operationalization and empirical validation of concepts. *Journal of Advanced Nursing, 69*(8), 1785–1796.

Covell, C., & Sidani, S. (2013b). Nursing intellectual capital theory: Testing selected propositions. *Journal of Advanced Nursing, 69*(11), 2432–2445.

Cox, J., Thomas-Watkins, C., Pajarillo, E., DeGennaro, S., Cadmus, E., & Martinez, M. (2015). Factors associated with falls in hospitalized adult patients. *Applied Nursing Research, 28*(2), 78–82.

De Guzman, A., Garcia, J., Garcia, M., German, M., & Grajo, A. (2013). A multinomial regression model for risk for falls (RFF) factors among Filipino elderly in a community setting. *Educational Gerontology, 39*(9), 669–683.

Donabedian, A. (1987). Some basic issues in evaluating the quality of health care. In L. T. Rinke (Ed.), *Outcome measures in home care* (Vol. I, p. 338). New York, NY: National League for Nursing. (Original work published 1976).

Fawcett, J. (1985). Theory: Basis for the study and practice of nursing education. *Journal of Nursing Education, 24*(6), 226–229.

Fawcett, J. (1999). *The relationship of theory and research* (3rd ed.). Philadelphia, PA: F. A. Davis.

Fawcett, J., & DeSanto-Madeya, S. (2013). *Contemporary nursing knowledge: Analysis and evaluation of nursing models and theories* (3rd ed.). Philadelphia: F.A. Davis.

Fishbein, M., & Ajzen, I. (2010). *Predicting and changing behavior: The reasoned action approach.* New York, NY: Psychology Press.

Fisher, J., Fisher, W., Amico, K., & Harman, J. (2006). An information-motivation-behavioral skills of model of adherence to antiretroviral theory. *Health Psychology, 25*(4), 462–473.

Fitzpatrick, J. J., & Whall, A. J. (2005). *Conceptual models of nursing: Analysis and application* (4th ed.). Upper Saddle River, NJ: Pearson Prentice Hall.

Good, M., & Moore, S. (1996). Clinical practice guidelines as a new source of middle-range theory: Focus on pain. *Nursing Outlook, 44*(2), 74–79.

Goodson, P. (2015). Theory as practice. In J. Butts & K. Rich (Eds.), *Philosophies and theories for advanced nursing practice* (2nd ed., pp. 71–108). Burlington, MA: Jones & Bartlett.

Gottlieb, L., & Rowat, K. (1987). The McGill model of nursing: A practice-derived model. *Advances in Nursing Science, 9*(4), 51–61.

Gulley, T., & Boggs, D. (2014). Time perspective and the Theory of Planned Behavior: Moderate predictors of physical activity among central Appalachian adolescents. *Journal of Pediatric Health Care, 28*(5), e41–e47.

Haase, J., Britt, T., Coward, D., Leidy, N., & Penn, P. (1992). Simultaneous concept analysis of spiritual perspective, hope, acceptance, and self-transcendence. *Image: Journal of Nursing Scholarship, 24*(2), 141–147.

Higgins, P., & Moore, S. (2000). Levels of theoretical thinking in nursing. *Nursing Outlook, 48*(4), 179–183.

Hupcey, J., & Penrod, J. (2005). Concept analysis: Examining the state of the science. *Research for Theory and Nursing Practice, 19*(2), 197–208.

Jaccard, J., & Jacoby, J. (2010). *Theory construction and model-building skills: A practical guide for social scientists.* New York, NY: Guilford Press.

Jackson, A., Enderby, K., O'Toole, M., Thomas, S., Ashley, D., & Gedye, R. (2009). The role of social support in families coping with childhood brain tumor. *Journal of Psychosocial Oncology, 27*(1), 1–24.

Johns, M. (1991). New method for measuring daytime sleepiness: The Epworth Sleepiness Scale. *Sleep, 14*(6), 540–545.

Johns, M. (1993). Daytime sleepiness, snoring, and obstructive sleep apnea: The Epworth Sleepiness Scale. *Chest, 103*(1), 30–36.

Johnson, J. (1999). Self-regulation theory and coping with physical illness. *Research in Nursing & Health, 22*(6), 436–448.

Kamitani, E., Fukuoka, Y., & Dawson-Rose, C. (2015). Knowledge, self-efficacy, and self-perceived risk for cardiovascular disease among Asians living with HIV: The influence of HIV stigma and acculturation. *Journal of Nurses in AIDS Care, 26*(4), 443–453.

King, I. (1981). *A theory for nursing: Systems, concept, and process.* New York, NY: Delmar.

Kolcaba, K. (1994). A theory of holistic comfort for nursing. *Journal of Advanced Nursing, 19*(6), 1176–1184.

Kolcaba, K., & Kolcaba, R. (1991). An analysis of the concept of comfort. *Journal of Advanced Nursing, 16*(11), 1301–1310.

Kubicek, B., Korunka, C., & Tement, S. (2014). Too much job control? Two studies of curvilinear relations between job control

and eldercare workers' well-being. *International Journal of Nursing Studies, 51*(12), 1644–1653.

Lazarus, R., & Folkman, S. (1984). *Stress, appraisal, and coping.* New York, NY: Springer.

Leininger, M. M. (1997). Overview of the Theory of Culture Care with the ethnonursing research method. *Journal of Transcultural Nursing, 8*(2), 32–54.

Levin, M. (1967). Four conservation principles of nursing. *Nursing Forum, 6*(1), 45–59, 7.

Li, W.-W., Wallhagen, M., & Froelicher, E. (2010). Factors predicting blood pressure control in older Chinese immigrants to the United States of America. *Journal of Advanced Nursing, 66*(10), 2202–2212.

Manojlovich, M., & Sidani, S. (2008). Nurse dose: What's in a concept? *Research in Nursing & Health, 31*(4), 310–319.

McEwen, M., & Wills, E. M. (2014). *Theoretical basis for nursing* (4th ed.). Philadelphia, PA: Lippincott Williams & Wilkins.

McQuiston, C., & Campbell, J. (1997). Theoretical substruction: A guide for theory testing research. *Nursing Science Quarterly, 10*(3), 117–123.

Mefford, L., & Alligood, M. (2011). Testing a theory of health promotion for preterm infants based on Levine's conservation model of nursing. *Journal of Theory Construction and Testing, 15*(2), 41–47.

Meleis, A. I. (2012). *Theoretical nursing: Development and progress* (5th ed.). Philadelphia, PA: Wolters Kluwer/Lippincott Williams & Wilkins.

Merton, R. K. (1968). *Social theory and social structure.* New York, NY: Free Press.

Moon, C., Phelan, C., Lauver, D., & Bratzke, L. (2015). Is sleep quality related to cognition in individuals with heart failure? *Heart and Lung: The Journal of Critical Care, 44*(3), 212–218.

Moore, J., & Pichler, V. (2000). Measurement of Orem's basic conditioning factors: A review of published research. *Nursing Science Quarterly, 13*(2), 137–142.

Neuman, B., & Fawcett, J. (2002). *The Neuman Systems Model* (4th ed.). Upper Saddle River, NJ: Prentice-Hall.

Newman, M. (1979). *Theory development in nursing.* Philadelphia, PA: F.A. Davis.

Newman, M. (1986). *Health as expanding consciousness.* St. Louis, MO: Mosby.

Noiseux, S., & Ricard, N. (2008). Recovery as perceived by people with schizophrenia, family members and health professionals: A grounded theory. *International Journal of Nursing Studies, 45*(8), 1148–1162.

Orem, D. E. (2001). *Nursing: Concepts for practice* (6th ed.). St. Louis, MO: Mosby Year-Book Inc.

Page-Cutrara, K. (2015). Prebriefing in nursing simulation: A concept analysis. *Clinical Simulation in Nursing, 11*(7), 335–340.

Parse, R. (1992). Human becoming: Parse's theory of nursing. *Nursing Science Quarterly, 5*(1), 35–42.

Peek, G., & Melnyk, B. (2014). A coping intervention for mothers of children diagnosed with cancer: Connecting theory and research. *Applied Nursing Research, 27*(3), 202–204.

Pender, N. (1996). *Health promotion in nursing practice* (3rd ed.). Stamford, CT: Appleton & Lange.

Petersen, C. (2014). Spiritual care of the child with cancer at end of life: A concept analysis. *Journal of Advanced Nursing, 70*(6), 1243–1253.

Peterson, S. (2009). Introduction to the nature of nursing knowledge. In S. J. Peterson & T. S. Bredow (Eds.), *Middle-range theories: Application to nursing research* (2nd ed., pp. 3–45). Philadelphia, PA: Wolters Kluwer/Lippincott Williams & Wilkins.

Pickett, S., Peters, R., & Jarosz, P. (2014). Toward a middle range theory of weight management. *Nursing Science Quarterly, 27*(3), 242–247.

Randolph, C., Tierney, M., Mohr, E., & Chase, T. (1998). Repeatable Battery for the Assessment of Neuropsychological Status (RBANS): Preliminary clinical validity. *Journal of Clinical and Experimental Neuropsychology, 20*(3), 310–319.

Rishel, C. (2014). An emerging theory on parental end-of-life decision making as a stepping stone to new research. *Applied Nursing Research, 27*(4), 261–264.

Robson, J., & Troutman-Jordan, M. (2014). A concept analysis of cognitive reframing. *Journal of Theory Construction & Testing, 18*(2), 55–59.

Rodwell, J., Brunetto, Y., Demir, D., Shacklock, K., & Farr-Wharton, R. (2014). Abusive supervision and links to nurse intentions to quit. *Journal of Nursing Scholarship, 46*(5), 357–365.

Rodgers, B. L. (2000). Concept analysis: An evolutionary view. In B. L. Rodgers (Ed.), *Concept development in nursing: Foundations, techniques, and applications* (2nd ed., pp. 77–102). Philadelphia, PA: W. B. Saunders.

Rogers, M. E. (1970). *An introduction to the theoretical basis of nursing.* Philadelphia, PA: Davis.

Rohani, C., Abedi, H., Omranipour, R., & Languis-Eklof, A. (2015). Health-related quality of life and the predictive role of sense of coherence, spirituality, and religious coping in a sample of Iranian women with breast cancer: A prospective study with comparative design. *Health and Quality of Life Outcomes, 13,* Article 40.

Roy, C. (1988). An explication of the philosophical assumptions of the Roy Adaptation Model. *Nursing Science Quarterly, 1*(1), 26–34.

Roy, C., & Andrews, H. A. (2008). *Roy's Adaptation Model for Nursing* (3rd ed.). Stamford, CT: Appleton & Lange.

Schwartz-Barcott, D., & Kim, H. S. (2000). An expansion and elaboration of the hybrid model of concept development. In B. L. Rogers & K. Knafl (Eds.), *Concept development in nursing: Foundations, techniques, and applications* (pp. 129–159). Philadelphia: W. B. Saunders.

Smith, J., Swallow, V., & Coyne, I. (2015). Involving parents in managing their child's long-term condition—A concept synthesis of family-centered care and partnership in care. *Journal of Pediatric Nursing, 30*(1), 141–159.

Tkatch, R., Artinian, N., Abrams, J., Mahn, J., Franks, M., Keteyian, S., et al. (2011). Social networks and health outcomes among African American cardiac rehabilitation patients. *Heart and Lung: The Journal of Critical Care, 40*(3), 193–200.

Trego, L. (2009). Theoretical substruction: Establishing links between theory and measurement of military women's attitudes toward menstrual suppression during military operations. *Journal of Advanced Nursing, 65*(7), 1548–1559.

Walker, L. O., & Avant, K. C. (2011). *Strategies for theory construction in nursing* (5th ed.). Boston, MA: Prentice Hall.

Watson, J. (1979). *Nursing: The philosophy and science of caring.* Boston, MA: Little Brown and Company.

Wilson, J. (1963). *Thinking with concepts.* Cambridge, England: Cambridge University Press.

Wolf, L. (2015). Research as problem solving: Theoretical frameworks as tools. *Journal of Emergency Nursing, 41*(1), 83–85.

Wong, C., Ip, W., Choi, K., & Lam, L. (2015). Examining self-care behaviors and their associated factors among adolescent girls with dysmenorrhea: An application of Orem's self-care deficit nursing theory. *Journal of Nursing Scholarship, 47*(3), 219–227.

9

Ethics in Research

Jennifer R. Gray

ⓔ http://evolve.elsevier.com/Gray/practice/

Many factors affected your decision to be a nurse but, for most of you, a key motivation was the desire to help others. Nursing as a profession is firmly based on the ethical principles of respect for persons, beneficence, and justice. These ethical principles that guide clinical practice must also be the standards for the conduct of nursing research (Manton et al., 2014). In research endeavors, the application of ethics begins with identifying a study topic and continues through publication of the study findings.

Ethical research is essential for generating evidence for nursing practice, but what does the ethical conduct of research involve? This question has been debated for many years by researchers, politicians, philosophers, lawyers, and even research subjects. The debate continues, probably because of the complexity of human rights issues; the focus of research in new, challenging arenas of technology and genetics; the complex ethical codes and regulations governing research; and the various interpretations of these codes and regulations. Unfortunately, specific standards of ethical research were developed only in response to historical events in which the rights of subjects were egregiously violated, or the behavior of research scientists was blatantly dishonest.

To provide an understanding of the rationale for today's human subject protection requirements, this chapter begins by reviewing some of these historical events, and the mandates and regulations for ethical research that were generated as a result of them. One of these regulations, the Health Insurance Portability and Accountability Act (HIPAA), was enacted in 2003 to protect the privacy of an individual's health information. HIPAA has had an important impact on researchers and institutional review boards (IRBs) in universities and healthcare agencies. The chapter also discusses the

actions essential for conducting research in an ethical manner through protection of the rights of human subjects. This includes making an unbiased assessment of the potential benefits and risks inherent in a study, and assuring that informed consent is obtained properly. The submission of a research proposal for institutional review is also presented.

An ethical problem that has received increasing attention since the 1980s is researcher misconduct, also called **scientific misconduct.** Scientific misconduct is the violation of human rights during a study. Scientific misconduct also includes falsifying results or behaving dishonestly when disseminating the findings. Misconduct has occurred during all study phases, including reporting and publication of studies. The Office of Scientific Enquiry Review and the Office of Scientific Enquiry were founded in 1989 and 2009, respectively, to manage this problem. In 1992 the two offices were combined as the Office of Research Integrity under the auspices of the U.S. Department of Health and Human Services (DHHS) (ORI, 2012). Many disciplines, including nursing, have experienced episodes of research misconduct that have affected the quality of research evidence generated and disseminated. A discussion of current ethical issues related to research misconduct and to the use of animals in research concludes the chapter.

HISTORICAL EVENTS AFFECTING THE DEVELOPMENT OF ETHICAL CODES AND REGULATIONS

The ethical conduct of research has been a focus since the 1940s because of mistreatment of human subjects in selected studies. Although these are not the only examples of unethical research, five historical experimental projects have been publicized for their unethical treatment of subjects and will be described in the order in which the projects began: (1) the syphilis studies in Tuskegee, Alabama (1932–1972); (2) Nazi medical experiments (1941–1946) and resulting trials at Nuremberg; (3) the sexually transmitted infection study in Guatemala (1946–1948); (4) the Willowbrook State School study (1955–1970); and (5) the Jewish Chronic Disease Hospital study (1963–1965). More recent examples are included in the chapter, in relation to specific aspects of research. Although these five projects were biomedical and the primary investigators were physicians, there is evidence that nurses were aware of the research, identified potential subjects, delivered treatments to subjects, and served as data collectors in all of them. The five projects demonstrate the importance of ethical conduct for anyone reviewing, participating in, and conducting nursing or biomedical research. As indicated earlier, these and other incidences of unethical treatment of subjects and research misconduct in the development, implementation, and reporting of research were important catalysts in the formulation of the ethical codes and regulations that direct research today. In addition, the concern for privacy of patient information related to the electronic storage and exchange of health information, has resulted in Health Information Portability and Accountability Act (HIPAA) privacy regulations (Olsen, 2003). HIPAA did not require anything that was not required in the course of routine nursing practice before its instigation; however, it addressed both electronic data security and consequences of failure to protect such data.

Tuskegee Syphilis Study

In 1932, the U.S. Public Health Service (U.S. PHS) initiated a study of syphilis in black men in the small, rural town of Tuskegee, Alabama (Brandt, 1978; Reverby, 2012; Rothman, 1982). The study, which continued for 40 years, was conducted to determine the natural course of syphilis in black men. The research subjects were organized into two groups: one group consisted of 400 men who had untreated syphilis, and the other was a control group of approximately 200 men without syphilis. Many of the subjects who consented to participate in the study were not informed about the purpose and procedures of the research. Some individuals were unaware that they were subjects in a study. Some of the study participants were subjected to spinal taps and told the procedure was

treatment for their "bad blood" (Reverby, 2012), which is a term that was used colloquially to refer to syphilis and other diseases of the blood. Untreated syphilis is the most damaging of the bacterial venereal diseases, with degeneration occurring over the course of many years from cardiac lesions, brain deterioration, or involvement of other organ systems, as well as severe effects in affected fetuses.

By 1936, study results indicated that the group of men with syphilis experienced more health complications than did the control group. Ten years later, the death rate of the group with syphilis was twice as high as that of the control group. The subjects with syphilis were examined periodically but were never administered penicillin, even after it became accepted as standard treatment for the disease in the 1940s (Brandt, 1978). Published reports of the Tuskegee syphilis study first started appearing in 1936, and additional papers were published every 4 to 6 years. In 1953, Nurse Eunice Rivers was the first author on a publication about the study procedures to retain subjects over time (Rivers, Schuman, Simpson, & Olansky, 1953). At least 13 articles were published in medical journals reporting the results of the study. In 1969, the U.S. Centers for Disease Control (CDC) reviewed the study and decided that it should continue. In 1972, a story describing the study published in the *Washington Star* sparked public outrage. Only then did the U.S. Department of Health, Education, and Welfare (DHEW) stop the study. An investigation of the Tuskegee syphilis study found it to be ethically unjustified. In 1997, President Clinton publicly apologized for the government's role in this event (Baker, Brawley, & Marks, 2005; Reverby, 2012).

Nazi Medical Experiments

From 1933 to 1945, the Third Reich in Europe implemented atrocious, unethical activities (Steinfels & Levine, 1976). The programs of the Nazi regime were intended to produce a population of racially pure Germans. In addition to encouraging population growth among the Aryans (originally persons of Indo-European descent but interpreted by Hitler as those of European origin, especially those of Nordic descent, which he considered the purest race), Nazi military personnel sterilized people they regarded as racial enemies, such as the Jews. In addition, Nazis killed various groups of people whom they considered racially impure, such as insane, deformed, senile, and homosexual individuals. Most notably, the Nazis targeted all Jews for imprisonment and systematic genocide, resulting in millions of deaths. In addition, it is estimated that almost a quarter million Germans who were physically or mentally handicapped (Jacobs, 2008) and 300,000 psychiatric patients (Foth, 2013) were killed. Research subjects were members of these same "valueless" groups.

The medical experiments involved exposing subjects to high altitudes, freezing temperatures, malaria, poisons, spotted fever (typhus), and untested drugs and operations, usually without anesthesia (Steinfels & Levine, 1976). For example, subjects were exposed to freezing temperatures or immersed in freezing water to determine how long German pilots could survive if shot down over the North Sea. Identical twins were forced to be subjects of experiments in which one would be infected with a disease and both killed for postmortem examination of their organs to determine differences due to the disease. These medical experiments purportedly were conducted to generate knowledge to benefit Aryans at the cost of suffering and death for prisoners in no position to give consent. In addition to the atrocities and coercion, however, studies were poorly designed and conducted. As a result, little if any useful scientific knowledge was generated.

The Nazi experiments violated ethical principles and rights of the research participants. Researchers selected subjects on the basis of race, affliction, or sexual orientation, demonstrating an unfair selection process. The subjects also had no opportunity to refuse participation; they were prisoners who were coerced or forced to participate. Frequently, study participants were killed during the experiments or sustained permanent physical, mental, and social damage (Levine, 1986; Steinfels & Levine, 1976). The doctors who propagated the mistreatment of human subjects were brought to trial, along with other Nazi soldiers and officers, in Nuremberg, Germany, beginning in 1945.

Nuremberg Code

At the conclusion of the trials of Nazi doctors involved in research, the defense presented 10 guidelines for appropriate research with human subjects, which collectively became known as the **Nuremberg Code** (1949). Among the principles were the following: (1) subjects' voluntary consent to participate in research; (2) the right of subjects to withdraw from studies; (3) protection of subjects from physical and mental suffering, injury, disability, and death during studies; and (4) an assessment of the benefits and risks in a study. The Nuremberg Code (1949), formulated mainly to direct the conduct of biomedical research worldwide, forms the basis for protection for all human subjects, regardless of a researcher's disciplinary affiliation.

Declaration of Helsinki

The members of the World Medical Association (WMA) were understandably alarmed by the actions of Nazi researchers during World War II. The General Assembly of the WMA drafted a document called the **Declaration of Helsinki** in 1964. The Declaration of Helsinki (WMA, 1964) has subsequently been reviewed and amended, with the last amendment being approved in 2013 (WMA, 2008; 2013). The Declaration forms the foundation for current research protection practices, such as research ethics committees.

A research ethics committee must review proposed human subject research for possible approval; if the study is approved, the committee is responsible for continuing to monitor its methods and outcomes as well as reviewing and approving any alterations in the research plan before such changes are implemented. The declaration also differentiates therapeutic research from nontherapeutic research. **Therapeutic research** gives the patient an opportunity to receive an experimental treatment that might have beneficial results. **Nontherapeutic research** is conducted to generate knowledge for a discipline: the results from the study might benefit future patients with similar conditions but will probably not benefit those acting as research subjects. Box 9-1 contains several ethical principles from the declaration. The complete document can be found on the WMA's website (http://www.wma.net/en/).

BOX 9-1   Key Ideas of the Declaration of Helsinki

1. Well-being of the individual research subject must take precedence over all other interests.
2. Investigators must protect the life, health, privacy, and dignity of research subjects.
3. A strong, independent justification must be documented prior to exposing healthy volunteers to risk of harm, merely to gain new scientific information.
4. Extreme care must be taken in making use of placebo-controlled trials, which should be used only in the absence of existing proven therapy.
5. Clinical trials must focus on improving diagnostic, therapeutic, and prophylactic procedures for patients with selected diseases without exposing subjects to any additional risk of serious or irreversible harm.

From Declaration of Helsinki. (1964, 2013). *WMA Declaration of Helsinki-Ethical Principles for Medical Research Involving Human Subjects.* Retrieved July 13, 21015 from http://www.wma.net/en/30publications/10policies/b3/.

Worldwide, most institutions in which clinical research is conducted have adopted the Declaration of Helsinki. It has been revised, with the most recent revision increasing protection for vulnerable populations and requiring compensation for subjects harmed by research (WMA, 2013). However, neither this document nor the Nuremberg Code has prevented some investigators from conducting unethical research (Beecher, 1966; ORI, 2012). Remember that the Tuskegee study continued after the declaration was first released.

Guatemala Sexually Transmitted Disease Study

Beginning in 1946, a U.S. Public Health employee, Dr. John C. Cutler, conducted a study in Guatemala in which subjects were intentionally exposed to syphilis and other sexually transmitted diseases. The subjects were "sex workers, prisoners, mental patients, and soldiers" (Reverby, 2012, p. 8). Initially, subjects were to be given penicillin or an arsenic compound (the treatment prior to penicillin) between exposure and infection to determine the prophylactic efficacy of each medication. The records for the study are incomplete, and it is not known how many persons actually developed an infection, died from the infection, or were harmed by the administered treatment (Reverby, 2012). The researchers suppressed information about their interventions and findings because they anticipated negative publicity due to the unethical nature of the study. After Dr. Cutler left in 1948, the U.S. PHS continued to fund researchers to monitor the research subjects and conduct serological testing through 1955 (Presidential Commission, 2011).

In 2010, Reverby (2012) was reviewing the records of researchers who participated in the Tuskegee study and found the papers of Dr. Cutler in which the Guatemala study was described. She shared her discovery with the CDC, and, subsequently, President Obama was informed. A public apology ensued. The Presidential Commission for the Study of Bioethical Issues was charged to conduct an investigation that resulted in a report confirming the facts of the Guatemala study (Presidential Commission, 2011).

Willowbrook Study

From the mid-1950s to the early 1970s, Dr. Saul Krugman at Willowbrook State School, a large institution for cognitively impaired persons in Brooklyn, New York, conducted research on hepatitis A (Rothman, 1982). The subjects, all children, were deliberately infected with the hepatitis A virus. During the 20-year study, Willowbrook closed its doors to new inmates because of overcrowded conditions. However, the research ward continued to admit new inmates. To gain a child's admission to the institution, parents were required to give permission for the child to be a study subject. Hepatitis A affects the liver, producing vomiting, nausea, and tiredness, accompanied by jaundice.

From the late 1950s to early 1970s, Krugman's research team published several articles describing the study protocol and findings. Beecher (1966) cited the Willowbrook study as an example of unethical research. The investigators defended exposing the children to the virus by citing their own belief that most of the children would have acquired the infection after admission to the institution. They based their belief on the high hepatitis infection rates of children during their first year of living at Willowbrook. The investigators also stressed the benefits that the subjects received on the research ward, which were a cleaner environment, better supervision, and a higher nurse-patient ratio (Rothman, 1982). Despite the controversy, this unethical study continued until the early 1970s.

Jewish Chronic Disease Hospital Study

Another highly publicized example of unethical research was a study conducted at the Jewish Chronic Disease Hospital in the 1960s. The U.S. PHS, the American Cancer Society, and Sloan-Kettering Cancer Center funded the study (Nelson-Marten & Rich, 1999). Its purpose was to determine the patients' rejection responses to live cancer cells. Twenty-two patients were injected with a suspension containing live cancer cells that had been generated from human cancer tissue (Levine, 1986).

Most of the patients and their physicians were unaware of the study. An extensive investigation revealed that the patients were not informed they were research subjects. They were informed that they were receiving an injection of cells, but the word cancer was omitted (Beecher, 1966). In addition, the Jewish Chronic Disease Hospital's IRB never reviewed the study. The physician directing the research was an employee of the Sloan-Kettering Institute for Cancer Research, and there was no indication that this institution had reviewed the research project (Hershey & Miller, 1976). The study was considered unethical and was terminated, with the lead researcher found to be in violation of the Nuremberg Code (1949) and the Declaration of Helsinki (WMA General Assembly, 1964). This research had the potential to cause study participants serious or irreversible harm and possibly death, reinforcing the importance of conscientious institutional review and ethical researcher conduct.

EARLY U.S. GOVERNMENT RESEARCH REGULATIONS

U.S. Department of Health, Education, and Welfare

Dr. Henry Beecher (1966) published a paper with 22 examples of experimental treatments implemented without patient consent, raising concerns that the interests of science could override the interests of the patient. Federal funding by the National Institutes for Health for research grew rapidly from less than a million dollars in 1945 to over $435,000,000 in 1965 (Beecher, 1966). This influx of funds along with newly discovered advances in medical treatment raised the potential for increased numbers of research violations. As unethical harmful research continued, it became clear that additional controls were necessary. In 1973, the DHEW published its first set of regulations intended to protect human subjects. Clinical researchers were required to be compliant with the new stricter regulations for human research, with additional regulations to protect persons with limited capacity to consent, such as ill, cognitively impaired, or dying individuals (Levine, 1986). All research proposals involving human subjects were required to undergo full institutional review, a task that became overwhelming and greatly prolonged the time required for study approval. Even studies conducted by nurses and other health professionals that involved minimal or no risks to study participants were subjected to full board review. Despite the advancement of the protection of subjects' rights, the government recognized the need for additional strategies to manage the extended time now required for study approval.

National Commission for the Protection of Human Subjects of Biomedical and Behavioral Research

Because of the problems related to the DHEW regulations, the National Commission for the Protection of Human Subjects of Biomedical and Behavioral Research (1978) was formed. The commission's charge was to identify basic ethical principles and develop guidelines based on these principles that would underlie the conduct of biomedical and behavioral research involving human subjects. The commission developed what is now called the Belmont Report (available at http://www.hhs.gov/ohrp/archive/belmontArchive.html). This report identified three **ethical principles** as relevant to research involving human subjects: respect for persons, beneficence, and justice (Havens, 2004). The **principle of respect for persons** holds that persons have the right to self-determination and the freedom to participate or not participate in research. The **principle of beneficence** requires the researcher to do good and avoid causing harm. The **principle of justice** holds that human subjects should be treated fairly. The commission developed ethical research guidelines based on these three principles, made recommendations to the U.S. DHHS, and was dissolved in 1978. However, the three ethical principles are still followed for all federally supported research, whether implemented in the U.S. or internationally.

Subsequent to the work of the commission, the U.S. DHHS developed federal regulations in 1981 to protect human research subjects, which have been revised as needed over the past 35 years (U.S. DHHS, 1981). The first of these was the *Code of Federal Regulations* (CFR), Title 45, Part 46, Protection of Human Subjects (2009), with the most recent edition being available online. An arm of the DHHS is the Federal Drug Administration (FDA) and its research activities are governed by CFR Title 21, Food and Drugs, Part 50, Protection of Human Subjects (U.S. FDA, 2010a), and Part 56, Institutional Review Boards (IRBs; U.S. FDA, 2010b). The DHHS regulations are known as the **Common Rule**. The Common Rule is the name given to the regulations because they were applicable across multiple DHHS agencies.

The two codified regulations have similar requirements for human subjects research that are applied in different types of studies. Biomedical and behavioral studies conducted in the United States are still governed by the U.S. DHHS (2009) Protection of Human Subjects Regulations. Physicians and nurses conducting clinical trials to generate new drugs and refine existent drug treatments must comply with FDA regulations. Boxes 9-2 and 9-3 provide the specific types of research for which each administrative entity is responsible.

These regulations are interpreted and enforced by the Office for Human Research Protection (OHRP), an agency within the U.S. DHHS (2012). In addition to providing guidance and regulatory enforcement, the OHRP develops educational programs and materials, and provides advice on ethical and regulatory issues related to biomedical and social-behavior research.

STANDARDS FOR PRIVACY FOR RESEARCH DATA

The privacy and confidentiality of health information became a greater concern for patients and the public

BOX 9-2   Research Regulated by DHHS: CFR Title 45, Part 46, Protection of Human Subjects

1. Studies conducted by, supported by, or otherwise subject to regulations by any federal department or agency
2. Research conducted in educational and healthcare settings
3. Research involving the use of biophysical measures, educational tests, survey procedures, scales, interview procedures, or observation
4. Research involving the collection or study of existing data, documents, records, pathological specimens, or diagnostic specimens.

Summarized from U.S. DHHS (2009). *Code of Federal Regulations, Title 45 Public Welfare, Department of Health and Human Services, Part 46, Protection of Human Subjects.* Retrieved March 24, 2016 from http://www.hhs.gov/ohrp/humansubjects/guidance/45cfr46.html.

BOX 9-3   Research Regulated by the FDA: CFR Title 21, Parts 50 and 56

- Studies that test
  1. Drugs for humans
  2. Medical devices for human use
  3. Biological products for human use
  4. Human dietary supplements
  5. Electronic healthcare products used with humans
- Responsibility for the management of new drugs and medical devices

Data from U.S. Food and Drug Administration (2015). *Code of Federal Regulations, Title 21 Food and Drugs, Department of Health and Human Services, Part 50 Protection of Human Subjects* and *Part 56 Protection of Human Subjects.* Retrieved March 24, 2016 from https://www.accessdata.fda.gov/scripts/cdrh/cfdocs/cfcfr/CFRSearch.cfm.

with the advent of electronic transfer of data. In 2003, the U.S. DHHS developed regulations titled the Privacy Rule (U.S. DHHS, 2003), also known as Standards for Privacy of Individually Identifiable Health Information. The HIPAA Privacy Rule established the category of protected health information (PHI), which allows covered entities, such as health plans, healthcare clearinghouses, and healthcare providers that transmit health information, to use or disclose PHI to others only in certain situations. You are probably familiar with the application of the HIPAA Privacy Rule in clinical practice. It also applies to research conducted in a healthcare facility that accesses PHI and research that involves the collection of PHI (U.S. DHHS, 2010). An individual must provide his or her signed permission, or authorization, before his or her PHI can be used or disclosed for research purposes.

Any study you propose with human subjects must comply with federal regulations pertaining to PHI, whether it is a funded or unfunded study. Thus, this chapter covers these regulations in the sections on protecting human rights, obtaining informed consent, and institutional review of research.

PROTECTION OF HUMAN RIGHTS

Human rights are claims and demands that have been justified in the eyes of an individual or by the consensus of a group of individuals. These rights are necessary for the self-respect, dignity, and health of an individual (Fry, Veatch, & Taylor, 2011). The American Nurses Association Code of Ethics for Nurses (ANA, 2015) provides guidelines for protecting the rights of human subjects in biological and behavioral research, founded on the ethical principles of beneficence, nonmaleficence, autonomy, and justice. The human rights that require protection in research are (1) the right to self-determination; (2) the right to privacy; (3) the right to anonymity and confidentiality; (4) the right to fair treatment or justice; and (5) the right to protection from discomfort and harm (ANA, 2010; Fry et al., 2011).

Right to Self-Determination

The **right to self-determination** is based on the ethical principle of respect for persons. This principle holds that because humans are capable of self-determination, or making their own decisions, they should be treated as autonomous agents who have the freedom to conduct their lives as they choose without external controls. As a researcher, you treat prospective subjects as **autonomous agents** when you inform them about a proposed study and allow them to choose voluntarily whether or not to participate. In addition, subjects have the right to withdraw from a study at any time without penalty (Fry et al., 2011). Conducting research ethically requires that research subjects' right to self-determination not be violated and that persons with diminished autonomy have additional protection during the conduct of research (U.S. DHHS, 2009).

Preventing Violation of Research Subjects' Right to Self-Determination

A subject's right to self-determination can be violated through the use of (1) coercion; (2) covert data collection; or (3) deception. **Coercion** occurs when one person intentionally presents another with an overt threat of harm or the lure of excessive reward to obtain his or her compliance. Some subjects feel coerced to participate in research because they fear that they will suffer harm or discomfort if they do not participate. For example, some patients believe that their medical or nursing care will be negatively affected if they do not agree to be research subjects, a belief that may be reinforced if a healthcare provider is the one who attempts to recruit them for a study. Sometimes students feel forced to participate in research to protect their grades or prevent negative relationships with the faculty conducting the research. Other subjects feel coerced to participate in studies because they believe that they cannot refuse the excessive rewards offered, such as large sums of money, specialized health care, special privileges, and jobs. In the case of parents of children at Willowbrook State School, the promise of specialized education in a setting to which they otherwise would not have had access represented coercion. Most nursing studies do not offer excessive rewards to subjects for participating. A researcher may offer reasonable payment for time and transportation costs, such as $10 to $30, or a gift certificate for this amount. An IRB will evaluate whether a proposed payment is coercive based on the effort and time required to participate in a study (Fawcett & Garity, 2009; Fry et al., 2011).

An individual's right to self-determination can also be violated if he or she becomes a research subject without realizing it. Some researchers have exposed persons to experimental treatments without their knowledge, a prime example being the Jewish Chronic Disease Hospital study. With **covert data collection**, subjects are unaware that research data are being collected because the investigator's study collects data involving normal activity or routine health care (Reynolds, 1979). Studies in which observation is used to collect data, such as ethnographic research, are especially challenging because the researcher does not want to interfere with what would normally happen by identifying that observational data are being collected. Covert data collection can occur if subjects' behaviors are public. For example, a researcher could observe and record the number of people walking down a street who are smoking. However, covert data collection is considered unethical when research deals with sensitive aspects of an individual's behavior, such as illegal conduct, sexual behavior, and drug use (U.S. DHHS, 2009). In keeping with the HIPAA Privacy Rule (U.S. DHHS, 2003), the use of any type of covertly collected data would be questionable, and it would be illegal if PHI data were being used or disclosed.

The use of **deception** in research also can violate a subject's right to self-determination. Deception is misinforming subjects of the study's purpose (Kelman, 1967). A classic example of deception is the Milgram (1963) study, in which subjects thought they were administering electric shocks to another person. The subjects were unaware that the person being shocked was really a professional actor who pretended to feel pain. Some subjects experienced severe mental tension, almost to the point of collapse, because of their participation in this study (Shamoo & Resnik, 2015).

Covert data collection can be approved by an IRB in situations in which the research is essential, provided that the data cannot be obtained any other way (Athanassoulis & Wilson, 2009) and the subjects will not be harmed. On a clinical unit, what would happen if the researcher indicated the study was related to whether nurses were complying with hand washing guidelines? Instead the researcher might inform the nurses that the study's purpose is to observe the number and types of interruptions they experience during their shift. In the rare situations in which covert data collection is allowable, subjects must be informed of the deception once the study is completed, provided full disclosure of the study activities that were conducted (APA, 2010; Fry et al., 2011; U.S. DHHS, 2009), and given the opportunity to withdraw their data from the study.

Protecting Persons With Diminished Autonomy

Some persons have **diminished autonomy** or are vulnerable and less advantaged because of legal or mental incompetence, terminal illness, or confinement to an institution (Fry et al., 2011). These persons require additional protection of their right to self-determination, because they have a decreased ability, or an inability, to give informed consent. In addition, these persons may be vulnerable to coercion and deception because of limited or impaired reasoning. The U.S. DHHS (2009) has identified certain groups of individuals who require additional protection in the conduct of research, including pregnant women, human fetuses, neonates, children, mentally incompetent persons, and prisoners. Researchers must justify including subjects with diminished autonomy in a study, and the need for justification increases as the subjects' risk and vulnerability increase. However, in many situations, the knowledge needed to provide evidence-based care to these vulnerable populations can be gained only by studying them. "Vulnerable populations or groups have an equal right to have their condition represented and addressed in research" (Sweet et al., 2014, p. 261), despite the challenges this may pose for the researcher.

In addition to the federal laws regulating research with subjects with diminished autonomy, an international body, the Council for International Organizations of Medical Sciences (CIOMS), has developed international ethical guidelines for biomedical research, first published in 1982 (CIOMS, 2013). In 2000, a formal consultation was completed to provide information on emerging issues related to genomics research and clinical trials in low-resource countries (Gallagher, Gorovitz, & Levine, 2000). CIOMS has implemented working groups to revise their ethical guidelines. Researchers must evaluate each prospective subject's capacity for self-determination and must protect subjects with diminished autonomy during the research process (ANA, 2010, APA, 2010; U.S. DHHS, 2009).

Legally or mentally incompetent subjects. Neonates and children (minors), the cognitively impaired, and unconscious patients are legally or mentally incompetent to give informed consent. These individuals lack the ability to comprehend information about a study or to make decisions regarding participation in or withdrawal from the study. Their vulnerability ranges from minimal to absolute. The use of persons with diminished autonomy as research subjects is more acceptable if several conditions exist. When the research is therapeutic, there is less concern because the subjects have the potential to benefit directly from the experimental process (U.S. DHHS, 2009). Research with persons with diminished autonomy is more acceptable when the researcher is willing to use both vulnerable and nonvulnerable individuals as subjects. Another positive factor is the situation in which preclinical and clinical studies have been conducted and the researchers now have more data upon which to base the assessment of potential risks to subjects. Research with vulnerable groups is also more acceptable when risk is minimal and the consent process is strictly followed to protect the rights of the prospective subjects (U.S. DHHS, 2009).

Neonates. A neonate is defined as a newborn and is further identified as either viable or nonviable on delivery. Viable neonates are able to survive after delivery, if given the benefit of available medical therapy, and can independently maintain a heartbeat and respiration. A nonviable neonate is a newborn who after delivery, although living, is not able to survive (U.S. DHHS, 2009). Neonates are extremely vulnerable and require extra protection to determine their involvement in

---

BOX 9-4 **Conditions to Be Met for Approval of Research With Neonates**

- Scientifically appropriate study
- Data available from preclinical and clinical study to assess potential risk to neonates
- Potential to provide important biomedical knowledge that cannot be obtained by other means
- No additional risk to the neonate
- Potential to enhance the probability of the neonate's survival
- Both parents fully informed about the research and give consent
- Research team has no part in determining the viability of the neonate

Summarized from U.S. DHHS (2009). *Code of Federal Regulations, Title 45 Public Welfare, Department of Health and Human Services, Part 46, Protection of Human Subjects.* Retrieved March 24, 2016 from http://www.hhs.gov/ohrp/humansubjects/guidance/45cfr46.html.

---

research. However, research may involve viable neonates, neonates of uncertain viability, and nonviable neonates when the conditions identified in Box 9-4 are met. In addition, for the nonviable neonate, the vital functions of the neonate should not be artificially maintained because of the research, and the research should not terminate the heartbeat or respiration of the neonate (U.S. DHHS, 2009).

Children. The unique vulnerability of children means that their safety must be balanced with the need for research to improve their care (Hunfeld & Passchier, 2012). Because of maturity levels, consent involving children must focus not only on assuring that they understand their rights but also on comprehension of the study, as well (Hunfeld & Passchier, 2012). To that end, special ethical and regulatory considerations exist for research involving children (U.S. DHHS, 2009). Federal regulations contain two stipulations for obtaining informed consent: the research must be of minimal risk, and both the assent of the child (when capable) and the consent of the parent or guardian must be obtained (U.S. DHHS, 2009). For therapeutic research, IRBs can approve studies with children when more than minimal risk is present, provided that potential benefit exists for the child, or when the experimental treatment is similar to usual care and the findings have potential benefit for others. Studies that do not meet these stipulations but have the potential for significant contribution to knowledge that may benefit other children with the same condition can be submitted to DHHS for special review and possible approval (U.S. DDHS, 2005). In all cases, procedures to obtain assent and parental permission must be implemented.

Assent means a child's affirmative agreement to participate in research. A sample assent form is provided in Box 9-5. **Permission to participate in a study** means

---

BOX 9-5 Sample Assent Form for Children Ages 6 to 12 Years: Pain Interventions for Children With Cancer

Oral Explanation

I am a nurse who would like to know whether relaxation, special ways of breathing, and using your mind to think pleasant things help children like you to feel less afraid and feel less hurt when the doctor has to do a bone marrow aspiration or spinal tap. Today, and the next five times you and your mom and/or dad come to the clinic, I would like for you to answer some questions about the things in the clinic that scare you. I would also like you to tell me about how much pain you felt during the bone marrow or spinal tap. In addition, I would like to videotape (take pictures of) you and your mom and/or dad during the tests. The second time you visit the clinic I would like to meet with you and teach you special ways to relax, breathe, and use your mind to imagine pleasant things. You can use the special imagining and breathing during your visits to the clinic. I would ask you and your mom and/or dad to practice the things I teach you at home between your visits to the clinic. At any time you could change your mind and not be in the study anymore.

To Child

1. I want to learn special ways to relax, breathe, and imagine.
2. I want to answer questions about things children may be afraid of when they come to the clinic.
3. I want to tell you how much pain I feel during the tests I have.
4. I will let you videotape me while the doctor does the tests (bone marrow and spinal taps).

   If the child says YES, have him/her put an "X" here:

   _____

   If the child says NO, have him/her put an "X" here:

   _____

   Date: _____
   Child's signature: _____

From Broome, M. E. (1999). Consent (assent) for research with pediatric patients. *Seminars in Oncology Nursing, 15*(2), 101.

---

that the parent or guardian agrees to the participation of the child or ward in research (U.S. DHHS, 2009). If a child does not assent to participate in a study, he or she should not be included as a subject even if the parent or guardian gives permission.

At what age is a child or adolescent able to give consent? Unfortunately, the legal definitions of the minor status of a child are statutory and vary from state to state and country to country (Leibson & Koren, 2015). A child who is no longer a minor can give consent. A child's competency to assent is usually governed by age, and research evidence supports the standard of a child over 9 years of age being capable of sufficient understanding to give assent (Leibson & Koren, 2015; Ondrusek, Abramovitch, Pencharz, & Koren, 1998). Children who are developmentally delayed, have a cognitive impairment, suffer an emotional disorder, or are physically ill must be considered on an individual basis (Broome, 1999; Broome & Stieglitz, 1992). The social context of the study, the child's relationship with parents and with care providers, and the presence of a learning disability can also affect the child's ability to give assent. When designing a study in which children will be subjects, it is helpful to seek consultation with the primary IRB to which you will submit the study for approval. Some IRBs have developed assent guidelines specific for their facilities.

Adolescents should have a stronger role than do children in the consent process. Even among adolescent subjects in research, however, understanding their rights and grasping the meaning of the study itself has been found to be less than desired (Grootens-Wiegers, de Vries, & van den Broek, 2015). Grady et al. (2014) studied the perceptions of assent/consent among adolescents enrolled in clinical research and their parents. Approximately 40% of the sample believed that the decision for an adolescent to participate should be jointly made by parents and adolescent.

Assent and consent require that both child and parents be informed about the study. The information shared with the child about the study should be appropriate for the child's age and culture. In the assenting process, the child must be given developmentally appropriate information on the study purpose, expectations, and benefit-risk ratio (discussed later). Media-enhanced presentations and play activities have been used as a means of providing information about the study. A group of researchers in the Netherlands conducted a participatory study to develop and test comic strips for the purpose of providing information about research participation (Grootens-Wiegers, de Vries, van Beusekom, van Dijck, & van den Broek, 2015). With the input of children at each stage of development, the comic strips evolved and, in their final version, were found to have the potential for increasing children's knowledge about research. Linder et al. (2013) described using an iPad in pediatric research for providing study information, documenting assent and parental permission, and collecting data. Another research team conducted a field-test of story-boarding and word searches as two approaches to providing, and evaluating the acquisition of, information about a research study (Kumpunen, Shipway, Taylor, Aldiss, & Gibson, 2012). Continued research is needed for development and testing of innovative strategies for providing informed consent information to children and adults.

A child who assents to participate in a study should sign the requisite form and be given a copy. Consistent with adult research procedures, the researcher must give the child the opportunity to ask questions and to withdraw from the study if he or she so desires (Broome, 1999; Schwenzer, 2008). Legally, a non-assenting child can be a research subject if the parents give permission, even if some potential for harm exists. Chwang (2015) argues, however, that including children in a study who have not given consent is every bit as unethical as including non-consenting adults in a study.

Assent becomes more complex if the child is bilingual, because the researchers must determine the most appropriate language to use for the consent process for the child and the parents. Rew, Horner, and Fouladi (2010) conducted a study of school-aged children's health behaviors to determine whether they were precursors of adolescents' health-risk behaviors. Because the sample included Hispanic and non-Hispanic children and their parents, cover letters to parents, assent and consent forms, and all other research documents were available in English and Spanish versions that had been developed through an extensive process of forward and backward translation by independent researchers. The researchers also sought input from community members who reviewed the documents for readability and clarity. Additional information was provided in parent and researcher meetings at the schools involved in the study (Rew et al., 2010). Assent of the children and permission of the parents were documented. All of these activities promoted the ethical conduct of this study according to the U.S. DHHS (2009) regulations. The researchers found that girls have more health-focused behaviors than boys, health behaviors decreased from grades 4 to 6, and the school environment was important for promoting health behaviors.

Adults with diminished capacity. Certain adults have a diminished capacity for, or are incapable of,

giving informed consent because of mental illness (Beebe & Smith, 2010), cognitive impairment, or a comatose state (Simpson, 2010). Persons are said to be incompetent if a qualified healthcare provider judges them to have attributes that designate them as incompetent (U.S. DHHS, 2009). Incompetence can be temporary (e.g., intoxication), permanent (e.g., advanced senile dementia), or transitory (e.g., behavior or symptoms of psychosis). Because of diminished capacity to absorb, retain, and use information provided about a study, the potential research subject has a diminished ability to protect himself or herself from possible harm (Eriksson, 2012).

If an individual is judged incompetent and incapable of consent, you must seek approval from the prospective subject and his or her legally authorized representative. A **legally authorized representative** means an individual or other body authorized under law to consent on behalf of a prospective subject to his or her participation in research. This is often a spouse or close relative, if the potential subject has made no legal designation. If no spouse or close relative can be accessed, a legal representative can be appointed by the state. A legally authorized representative may also be called a proxy. However, individuals can be judged incompetent and can still assent to participate in certain minimal-risk research if they have the ability to understand what they are being asked to do, to make reasonably free choices, and to communicate their choices clearly and unambiguously (Sweet et al., 2014; U.S. DHHS, 2009).

A number of people in intensive care units and nursing homes experience some level of cognitive impairment. These individuals must be assessed for their capacity to give consent to participate in research (Sweet et al., 2014). The assessment needs to include the following elements: the potential subject understands the study information, can develop a belief about the information, displays reasoning ability, and understands what choices are available. Simpson (2010) reviewed the literature and found that the MacArthur Competency Assessment Tool for Clinical Research (MacCAT-CR) is one of the strongest instruments available for assessing an individual's capacity to give informed consent. Using this instrument or similar tools, researchers can make a sound decision about a subject's ability to consent to research versus contacting the legal representative for permission.

Some individuals are permanently incompetent due to the advanced stages of dementia and Alzheimer's disease, and their legal guardians must give permission for their participation in research. Often families or guardians of these patients are reluctant to give consent for their participation in research. However, nursing research is needed to establish evidence-based interventions for comforting and caring for these individuals. Families and guardians may be assisted in decision making by following either the **best interest standard** which involves doing what is best for the individual on the basis of balancing risks and benefits, or the **substituted judgment standard** which involves determining the course of action that incompetent individuals would take if they were capable of making a choice (Beattie, 2009).

Jones, Munro, Grap, Kitten, and Edmond (2010) conducted a quasi-experimental study to determine the effect of toothbrushing on bacteremia risk in mechanically ventilated adults. These researchers described their process for obtaining consent from their study participants in the following study excerpt:

> "The subjects who met inclusion criteria were assessed for ability to provide informed consent through gesturing or writing. If subjects had medications that impaired cognition or were unable to provide informed consent due to their illness, the legally authorized representative provided informed consent" (Jones et al., 2010, p. S58).

Jones et al. (2010) developed a process for determining the cognitive competence of their potential research participants and obtained appropriate consent on the basis of their assessments. Competent subjects were given the right to self-determination regarding study participation. For the other subjects, legal representatives consented. The researchers found that the toothbrushing intervention did not cause transient bacteremia in their sample of ventilated patients.

Other vulnerable populations. Although mentally competent to consent, pregnant women, terminally ill persons, and hospitalized or imprisoned persons are considered vulnerable populations for the purposes of research. The researcher must take additional precautions to protect their rights.

Pregnant women. Pregnant women require additional protection in research because of the potential risks to their fetuses (Schwenzer, 2008). Federal regulations define pregnancy as encompassing the period of time from implantation until delivery. "A woman is assumed to be pregnant if she exhibits any of the pertinent presumptive signs of pregnancy, such as missed menses, until the results of a pregnancy test are negative or until delivery" (U.S. DHHS, 2009, 45 CFR Section 46.202). Research conducted with pregnant women can occur only after studies have been done with animals to assess the potential risk to the mother and the fetus

(Schwenzer, 2008). Studies are needed with nonpregnant women to determine if the intervention poses risks to the mother, which could also affect the fetus. The research should have the potential for direct benefit to the woman or the fetus. If an investigation is thought to provide a direct benefit only to the fetus, the consent of the pregnant woman and father must be obtained. In addition, studies with pregnant women should include no inducements to terminate the pregnancy (U.S. DHHS, 2009).

Terminally ill subjects. When conducting research focusing on terminally ill subjects, two factors to consider are who will benefit from the research and whether it is ethical to conduct research on individuals who are unlikely to benefit from the study (U.S. DHHS, 2009). Participating in research could have greater risks and minimal or no benefits for these subjects. In addition, the dying subject's condition could affect the study results and lead the researcher to misinterpret the results. Another consideration is that terminally ill patients have very little time remaining to them, and it may not be fair to ask them to spend time on a study instead of spending it with family and engaged in activities with which they would prefer to fill their remaining days. Nonetheless, it is important to conduct end-of-life studies in palliative care to generate evidence that will improve care for terminally ill persons (Abernathy et al., 2014; Sweet et al., 2014).

Some terminally ill individuals are willing subjects because they believe that participating in research is a way to contribute to society before they die. Others want to take part in research because they believe that the experimental process will benefit them. For example, individuals with AIDS might want to participate in AIDS research to gain access to experimental drugs and hospitalized care. Researchers studying populations with serious or terminal illnesses are faced with ethical dilemmas as they consider the rights of the subjects and their responsibilities in conducting quality research (Fry et al., 2011; U.S. DHHS, 2009).

Subjects who are hospitalized or imprisoned. Hospitalized patients have diminished autonomy because they are ill and are confined in settings that are controlled by healthcare personnel (Levine, 1986). Some hospitalized patients feel obliged to be research subjects because they want to assist a particular practitioner (nurse or physician) with his or her research. Others feel coerced to participate because they fear that their care will be adversely affected if they refuse. Some of these hospitalized patients are survivors of trauma (such as auto accidents, gunshot wounds, or physical and sexual abuse) who are very vulnerable and often have decreased decision-making capacities (Irani & Richmond, 2015; Yamal et al., 2014). When conducting research with these patients, you must pay careful attention to the informed consent process and make every effort to protect these subjects from feelings of coercion and harm (U.S. DHHS, 2009).

Prisoners have diminished autonomy to consent for research because of their confinement. They may feel coerced to participate in research because they fear harm if they refuse or because they desire the benefits of special treatment, monetary gain, or relief from boredom. In the past, prisoners were used for drug studies in which the medications had no health-related benefits and, instead, potential harmful side effects. Current regulations regarding research involving prisoners require that "the risks involved in the research are commensurate with risks that would be accepted by nonprisoner volunteers and procedures for the selection of subjects within the prison are fair to all prisoners and immune from arbitrary intervention by prison authorities or prisoners" (U.S. DHHS, 2009, Section 46.305). Some IRBs prohibit the use of hospitalized prisoners as subjects.

Right to Privacy

Privacy is an individual's right to determine the time, extent, and general circumstances under which personal information is shared with or withheld from others. This information consists of one's attitudes, beliefs, behaviors, opinions, and records. The federal government enacted the Privacy Act of 1974 to control potential infringement of privacy, related to information collected by the government, or held in federal agencies' records. The Act has four important provisions for the researcher: (1) data collection methods must be strategized so as to protect subjects' privacy; (2) data cannot be gathered from subjects without their knowledge; (3) individuals have the right to access their records; and (4) individuals may prevent access by others to existent federal data (U.S. DHHS, 2009). The intent of this act was to prevent the **invasion of privacy** that occurs when private information is shared without an individual's knowledge, or against his or her will. Invading an individual's privacy might cause loss of dignity, friendships, or employment or create feelings of anxiety, guilt, embarrassment, or shame (Pritts, 2008).

The **HIPAA Privacy Rule** expanded the protection of an individual's privacy, specifically his or her protected individually identifiable health information, extending the protection to data held by private entities. It described the ways in which those entities covered by the rule can use or disclose this informa-tion. "**Individually identifiable health information** (IIHI) is information that is a subset of health information, including demographic information collected from an individual, and: (1) is created or received by healthcare provider, health plan, or healthcare clearinghouse; and (2) [is] related to past, present, or future physical or mental health or condition of an individual, the provision of health care to an individual, or the past, present, or future payment for the provision of health care to an individual, and that identifies the individual; or with respect to which there is a reasonable basis to believe that the information can be used to identify the individual" (U.S. DHHS, 2003, 45 CFR, Section 160.103).

According to the HIPAA Privacy Rule, IIHI is PHI that is transmitted by electronic media, maintained in electronic media, or transmitted or maintained in any other form or medium. Thus, the HIPAA privacy regulations must be followed when a nurse researcher wants to access data from a covered entity, such as reviewing a patient's medical record in clinics or hospitals. HIPAA also applies when an instrument developer requests that researchers who use the instrument share their data with the developer. Researchers can comply with this request by accessing a limited data set that has been de-identified (Sarpatwari, Kesselheim, Malin, Gagne, & Schneeweiss, 2014). De-identification consists of removing 18 items from patient records before they are released to other agencies or to researchers. These 18 items include name, contact information, identification numbers, photographs, biometrics, and other elements by which a subject could potentially be identified (Box 9-6).

The U.S. DHHS developed the following guidelines to help researchers, healthcare organizations, and healthcare providers determine the conditions under which they can use and disclose IIHI:

- The PHI has been "de-identified" under the HIPAA Privacy Rule. (De-identifying PHI is defined in the following section.)
- The data are part of a limited data set, and a data use agreement with the researcher(s) is in place.
- The individual who is a potential subject for a study authorizes the researcher to use and disclose his or her PHI.
- A waiver or alteration of the authorization requirement is obtained from an IRB or a privacy board (U.S. DHHS, 2007a).

The first two items are discussed in this section of the chapter. The authorization process is discussed in the section on obtaining informed consent, and the waiver or alteration of authorization requirement is covered in the section on institutional review of research.

BOX 9-6 18 Elements That Could Be Used to Identify an Individual to Relatives, Employer, or Household Members

1. Names
2. All geographical subdivisions smaller than a state
3. All elements of dates (except year) for dates directly related to an individual
4. Telephone numbers
5. Facsimile numbers
6. Electronic mail (e-mail) addresses
7. Social security numbers
8. Medical record numbers
9. Health plan beneficiary numbers
10. Account numbers
11. Certificate/license numbers
12. Vehicle identifiers and serial numbers, including license plate numbers
13. Device identifiers and serial numbers
14. Web universal resource locators (URLs)
15. Internet protocol (IP) address numbers
16. Biometric identifiers, including fingerprints and voiceprints
17. Full-face photographic images and any comparable images
18. Any other unique identifying number, characteristic, or code, unless otherwise permitted by the Privacy Rule for De-identification (U.S. DHHS, 2007b). For additional detail, see http://privacyruleandresearch .nih.gov/pr_08.asp.

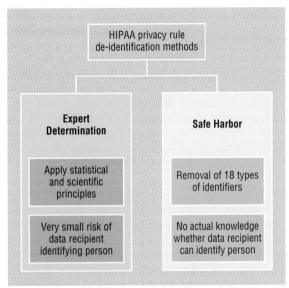

FIGURE 9-1 Use of PHI: Two methods of de-identifying data. (Data from the HIPAA Privacy Rule.)

De-Identifying Protected Health Information Under the Privacy Rule

Covered entities, such as healthcare providers and agencies, can allow researchers access to health information if the information has been de-identified, either by applying statistical methods (expert determination) or removing information (safe harbor) (Figure 9-1). The covered entity can apply statistical methods that experts agree render the information unidentifiable. The statistical method used for de-identification of the health data must be documented. Safe harbor is certifying that the 18 elements for identification have been removed or revised to ensure the individual is not identified. The covered entity has done what it could to make the information de-identified, but has no information whether in fact, the individuals could still be identified. No matter the method used, you must retain this certification information for six years. It is important to note that the element concerning biometrics may be interpreted to include DNA results and other particularized physiological variants, such as unusual laboratory and histological markers.

Limited Data Set and Data Use Agreement

With the use of electronic health records, data about patients are being generated at each health encounter. In addition, large studies may produce data that could be reused to answer other research questions. **Secondary data analysis** is data analysis that reuses data collected for a previous study or for other purposes, such as data in clinical or administrative databases (Johantgen, 2010). Under certain conditions, researchers and covered entities (healthcare provider, health plan, and healthcare clearinghouse) may use and disclose a limited data set to a researcher for a study, without an individual subject's authorization or an IRB waiver. These data sets are considered PHI, and the parties involved must have a data use agreement. The **data use agreement** limits how the data set may be used and how it will be protected, including identification of the researcher who is permitted to use the data set. The researcher receiving the data is not allowed to use or disclose the information in any way that is not permitted by the agreement, is required to protect against the unintended use or disclosure of the information, and must agree not to contact any of the individuals in the limited data set. Other members of the research team such as statisticians and research assistants are held to the same standards (U.S. DHHS, 2003).

Using secondary analysis of data from the Heart Failure (HF) Quality of Life Registry database, Riegel et al. (2011) conducted a study to establish whether confidence and activity status determined HF patients' self-care performance. The researchers found three levels of self-care performance: (1) novice in self-care with limited confidence and few activity restrictions; (2) inconsistent in self-care abilities; and (3) expert with confidence in self-care abilities. The researchers ensured the PHI of the individuals in the database was ethically managed, as described in the following excerpt:

"By prior consensus of investigators in the HF Quality of Life Registry, study samples are enrolled using comparable inclusion and exclusion criteria, as well as the same variables and measures whenever possible. All data are stored at one site, where one of the investigators has volunteered to integrate newly acquired data. The only identifiers in the data set are site (e.g., Cleveland Clinic) and the specific study name, as more than one study is common at each site. No protected health information [PHI] is included in the database. All requests to use the full database are viewed and approved by the lead investigators. For this analysis, five samples enrolled at three different sites in the United States between 2003 and 2008 were used" (Riegel et al., 2011, p. 133).

Right to Anonymity and Confidentiality

On the basis of the right to privacy, the research subject has the right to anonymity and the right to assume that all data collected will be kept confidential. **Anonymity** means that even the researcher cannot link a subject's identity to that subject's individual responses (APA, 2010; Fry et al., 2011). For studies that use de-identified health information or data from a limited data set, subjects are anonymous to the researchers, as described by Riegel et al. (2011).

In most studies, researchers desire to know the identity of their subjects and promise that their identity will be kept confidential. **Confidentiality** is the researcher's management of private information shared by a subject that must not be shared with others without the authorization of the subject. Confidentiality is grounded in the premises that patients own their own information, and that only they can decide with whom to share all or part of it (Pritts, 2008). When information is shared in confidence, the recipient (researcher) has the obligation to maintain confidentiality. Researchers, as professionals, have a duty to maintain confidentiality consistent with their profession's code of ethics (Shamoo & Resnick, 2015).

Breach of Confidentiality

A **breach of confidentiality** can occur when a researcher, by accident or direct action, allows an unauthorized person to gain access to a study's raw data. Confidentiality can be breached in the reporting or publishing phases of a study, especially in qualitative studies, in which a subject's identity is accidentally revealed, violating the subject's right to anonymity (Morse & Coulehan, 2015; Munhall, 2012a). Breaches can harm subjects psychologically and socially as well as destroy the trust they had in the researcher who promised confidentiality. Breaches can be especially harmful to a research participant when they involve religious preferences, sexual practices, employment, personal attributes, or opinions that may be considered positive or negative, such as racial prejudices. For example, a university researcher conducted a study of nurses' stressful life events and work-related burnout in an acute care hospital. One of the two male participants in the study was a nurse who is being treated for an anxiety disorder. Reporting that one of the male nurses in the study was being treated for an anxiety disorder would violate his confidentiality and potentially cause harm. Nurse administrators might be less likely to promote a nurse who has an anxiety disorder. There are limits to confidentiality that occur when a subject reveals current drug use, child abuse, or specific intent to harm oneself or others. The informed consent document must describe the specific limitations on confidentiality.

Maintaining confidentiality includes not allowing health professionals to access data the researcher has gathered about patients in the hospital. Sometimes, family members or close friends will ask to see data collected about a specific research subject. Sharing research data in these circumstances is a breach of confidentiality. When requesting consent for study participation, you should assure the potential subject that you will not share the raw information with healthcare professionals, family members, and others in the setting. However, you may elect to share the research report, including a summary of the data and findings from the study, with healthcare providers, family members, and other interested parties.

Maintaining Confidentiality

Researchers have a responsibility to protect the anonymity of subjects and to maintain the confidentiality of data collected during a study. You can protect confidentiality giving each subject a code number. Keep a master list of the subjects' names and their code numbers in a locked place; for example, subject Maria Brown might be assigned the code number "001." All of the instruments and forms that Maria completes and the data you collect about her during the study will be identified with the "001" code number, not her name. The master list of subjects' names and code numbers should be kept separate from the data collected, to protect subjects' anonymity. You should not staple signed consent forms and authorization documents to instruments or other data collection tools, as this would make it easy for unauthorized persons to readily identify the subjects and their responses. Consent forms are appropriately stored with the master list of subjects' names and code numbers. When entering the collected data into a computer, code numbers instead of names should be used for identification. Data should be stored in a secure place on a flash drive, in the researcher's computer, or on a website. In the study by Rew et al. (2010) that was introduced earlier in this chapter, the school-aged children participating in the study of their health behaviors completed a questionnaire on the computer, and their data were saved by research assistants to a secure website. These actions ensured that all data were kept confidential during and after completion of the study but were readily retrievable by researchers for purposes of data analysis.

Another way to protect your subjects' anonymity is to have subjects or study participants generate their own identification codes (Yurek, Vasey, & Havens, 2008). With this approach, each subject generates an individual code from personal information, such as the first letter of a mother's name, the first letter of a father's name, the number of brothers, the number of sisters, and middle initial. Thus, the code would be composed of three letters and two numbers, such as "BD21M." This code would be used on each form that the subject completes. Subject-generated identification codes are often used when data will be collected repeatedly over time. The premise is that the elements of the code do not change and the subject can generate the same code each time. However, using subject-generated codes has been found to have mixed results. Although the specific components of the ID number were selected for their stability, the subject may not remember, for example, whether they included half-sisters in the number of sisters or whether they used a parent's legal name or nickname.

Maintaining confidentiality of participants' data in qualitative studies often requires more effort than in quantitative research. "The very nature of data collection in qualitative investigation makes anonymity impossible" (Streubert & Carpenter, 2011, p. 64). The small number of participants used in a qualitative study and the depth of detail gathered on each participant requires planning to ensure confidentiality (Morse & Coulehan, 2015). Informed consent documents should contain details about how the data will be identified,

who will have access to the data, and how the findings will be reported (Sanjari, Bahramnezhad, Fomani, Shoghi, & Cheraghi, 2014). In addition, it is important to communicate that direct quotes from the interview will be included in both professional publications and presentations. Sometimes qualitative participants inappropriately equate confidentiality with secrecy.

Researchers should take precautions during data collection and analysis to maintain confidentiality in qualitative studies. The interviews conducted with participants frequently are recorded and later transcribed, so participants' names should not be mentioned during the recording. Some researchers ask participants to identify pseudonyms by which they will be identified during the interview and on transcripts. Depending on the methods of the study, the researcher may return descriptions of interviews or observations to participants to allow them to correct inaccurate information or remove any information that they do not want included. Researchers must respect participants' privacy as they decide how much detail and editing of private information are necessary to publish a study while maintaining the richness and depth of the participants' perspectives (Munhall, 2012a).

Participants have the right to know whether anyone other than you will be transcribing interview information. In addition, participants should be informed on an ongoing basis that they have the right to withhold information. By allowing other researchers to critically appraise the rigor and credibility of a qualitative study, an audit trail is produced. Allowing others to examine the data to confirm the study findings may create a dilemma regarding the confidentiality of participants' data, however, so you must inform subjects if other researchers will be examining their data to ensure the credibility of the study findings (Munhall, 2012a). When reporting findings, the researcher must ensure that quotations provided to support the trustworthiness of the findings do not contain identifying information (Streubert & Carpenter, 2011).

In quantitative research, the confidentiality of subjects' information must be ensured during the data analysis process. The data collected should undergo group analysis so that an individual cannot be identified by his or her responses. If subjects are divided into groups and a group has less than five members, the results for that group should not be reported. For example, a researcher conducts a study with nurses and collects demographic data. In reporting the results by demographic groups, if only a few men participated, the results by gender should not be reported. In writing the research report, you should describe the findings in such a way that an individual or a group of individuals cannot be identified from their responses.

Right to Fair Treatment

The right to **fair treatment** is based on the ethical principle of justice. This principle holds that each person should be treated fairly and should receive what he or she is due or owed. In research, the selection of subjects and their assignment to experimental or control group should be made impartially. In addition, their treatment during the course of a study should be fair.

Fair Selection of Subjects

In the past, injustices in subject selection have resulted from social, gender, cultural, racial, and sexual biases in society. For many years, research was conducted on categories of individuals who were thought to be especially suitable as research subjects, such as the poor, uninsured patients, prisoners, slaves, peasants, dying persons, and others who were considered undesirable (Reynolds, 1979). Researchers often treated these subjects carelessly and had little regard for the harm and discomfort they experienced. The Nazi medical experiments, the Tuskegee syphilis study, and the Willowbrook study all exemplify unfair subject selection and treatment.

More recently, concerns were raised about the exclusion of women from biomedical studies, especially women of childbearing age. The greatest fear was not that female hormones would obscure the effects of a medication or treatment, but a potential fetus would be harmed (Stevens & Pletsch, 2002). The exclusion of women to avoid harming a fetus or interfering with childbearing also excluded women from the potential benefits of new medications and treatments, for herself and her fetus. In 1986, the National Institutes of Health (NIH) implemented a policy requiring the inclusion of women and minorities in federally funded studies. This policy became law in 1993 as part of the NIH Revitalization Act (NIH Office of Research on Women's Health, 2015).

The selection of a population and the specific subjects to study should be fair so that the risks and benefits of the study are distributed fairly (Shamoo & Resnick, 2015). Subjects should be selected for reasons directly related to the problem being studied. Too often subjects are selected because the researcher has easy access to them. The Common Rule requires equitable selection of subjects (U.S. DHHS, 2009). Children, women, minorities, and persons who speak other languages cannot be excluded based solely on their demographic characteristics. Researchers seeking federal funding must describe in their proposals plans to recruit subjects from different groups who have been traditionally underrepresented in research. The researchers must remember, if a study poses risk, no demographic group should bear an unfair burden of that risk.

Another concern with subject selection is that some researchers select certain people as subjects because they like them and want them to receive the specific benefits of a study. Other researchers have been swayed by power or money to make certain individuals subjects so that they can receive potentially beneficial treatments. Random selection of subjects can eliminate some of the researcher bias that might influence subject selection. For a study that poses potential benefit, no demographic group should be deprived of participation solely because of that demographic classification. The researcher should make every effort to include fair representation, across demographic characteristics.

A current concern in the conduct of research is finding an adequate number of appropriate subjects to take part in certain studies, especially an adequate number of minority and female subjects. As a solution to this problem in the past, some biomedical researchers have offered finder's fees to healthcare providers for identifying research subjects. For example, investigators studying patients with lung cancer would give a physician a fee for every patient with lung cancer the physician referred to them. However, the HIPAA Privacy Rule requires that individuals give their authorization before PHI can be shared with others. Thus, healthcare providers cannot recommend individuals for studies without first seeking the permission of the patients. Researchers can obtain a partial waiver from the IRB or privacy board so that they can obtain PHI necessary to recruit potential subjects (U.S. DHHS, 2003). This makes it more difficult for researchers to find subjects for their studies; however, researchers are encouraged to work closely with their IRBs and healthcare agencies to ensure fair selection and recruitment of adequate-sized samples.

Fair Treatment of Subjects

Researchers and subjects should have a specific agreement about what a subject's participation involves and what the role of the researcher will be (APA, 2010). While conducting a study, you should treat the subjects fairly and respect that agreement. If the data collection requires appointments with the subjects, be on time for each appointment and terminate the data collection process at the agreed-upon time. You should not change the activities or procedures that a subject is to perform unless you obtain the subject's consent.

The benefits promised the subjects should be provided. For example, if you promise a subject a copy of the study findings, you should deliver on your promise when the study is completed. In addition, subjects who participate in studies should receive equal benefits, regardless of age, race, and socioeconomic status. When possible, the sample should be representative of the study population and should include subjects of various ages, ethnic backgrounds, and socioeconomic levels. Treating subjects fairly and respectfully facilitates the data collection process and decreases the likelihood that subjects will withdrawal from a study (Fry et al., 2011; McCullagh, Sanon, & Cohen, 2014). Thanking subjects for their participation is always appropriate: they have given you their time and their honesty.

Right to Protection from Discomfort and Harm

The right to **protection from discomfort and harm** is based on the ethical principle of beneficence, which holds that one should do good and, above all, do no harm. Therefore, researchers should conduct their studies to protect subjects from discomfort and harm and try to bring about the greatest possible balance of benefits in comparison with harm. Discomfort and harm can be physiological, emotional, social, or economic in nature. In his classic text, Reynolds (1979) identified the following five categories of studies, which are based on levels of discomfort and harm: (1) no anticipated effects; (2) temporary discomfort; (3) unusual levels of temporary discomfort; (4) risk of permanent damage; and (5) certainty of permanent damage. Each level is defined in the following discussion.

No Anticipated Effects

In some studies, neither positive or negative effects are expected. For example, studies that involve reviewing patients' records, students' files, pathology reports, or other documents have no anticipated effect on the subjects. In these types of studies, the researcher does not interact directly with research subjects. Even in these situations, however, there is a potential risk of invading a subject's privacy. The HIPAA Privacy Rule requires that the agency providing the health information de-identify the 18 essential elements (see Box 9-6 and Figure 9-1), which could be used to identify an individual, to promote subjects' privacy during a study.

Temporary Discomfort

Studies that cause temporary discomfort are described as minimal-risk studies, in which the discomfort encountered is similar to what the subject would experience in his or her daily life, and which ceases with the termination of the study. Many nursing studies require subjects to complete questionnaires or participate in interviews, which usually involve minimal risk. Physical discomforts of such research might be fatigue, headache, or muscle tension. Emotional and social risks might entail the anxiety or embarrassment associated with responding to certain questions. Economic risks might consist of the time spent participating in the study or travel costs to the study site. Participation in many nursing studies is considered a mere inconvenience for the subject, with no foreseeable risks of harm.

Most clinical nursing studies examining the impact of a treatment involve minimal risk. For example, your study might involve examining the effects of exercise on the blood glucose levels of patients with non-insulin dependent diabetes. During the study, you ask the subjects to test their blood glucose level one extra time per day. There is discomfort when the blood is drawn and a risk of physical changes that might occur with exercise. The subjects might also experience anxiety and fear in association with the additional blood testing, and the testing is an added expense. Diabetic subjects in this study would experience similar discomforts in their daily lives, and the discomforts would cease with the termination of the study.

Unusual Levels of Temporary Discomfort

In studies that involve unusual levels of temporary discomfort, the subjects commonly experience discomfort both during the study and after its termination. For example, subjects might experience a deep vein thrombosis (DVT), prolonged muscle weakness, joint pain, and dizziness after participating in a study that required them to be confined to bed for seven days to determine the effects of immobility. Studies that require subjects to experience failure, extreme fear, or threats to their identity or to act in unnatural ways involve unusual levels of temporary discomfort. In some qualitative studies, participants are asked questions that reopen old emotional wounds or involve reliving traumatic events (Munhall, 2012a; Streubert & Carpenter, 2011). For example, asking participants to describe a sexual assault experience could precipitate feelings of extreme fear, anger, and sadness. In these types of studies, you should make arrangements prior to the study to have appropriate professionals available for referrals should the participants become upset. During the interview, you would need to be vigilant about assessing the participants' discomfort and refer them for appropriate professional intervention as necessary. If a participant appears upset during a qualitative interview, the researcher should ask questions such as "Do you want to pause for a moment?" or "Do you want to talk about something else for awhile?" or "Do you want to stop this interview?" Most participants will decline, and some may say they want to continue because it is important for them to tell their story.

Risk of Permanent Damage

In some studies, subjects have the potential to suffer permanent damage: this potential is more common in biomedical research than in nursing research. For example, medical studies of new drugs and surgical procedures have the potential to cause subjects permanent physical damage. However, nurses have investigated topics that have the potential to damage subjects permanently, both emotionally and socially. Studies examining sensitive information, such as HIV diagnosis, sexual behavior, child abuse, or drug use, can be risky for subjects. These types of studies have the potential to cause permanent damage to a subject's personality or reputation. There are also potential economic risks, such as reduced job performance or loss of employment.

Certainty of Permanent Damage

In some research, such as the Nazi medical experiments and the Tuskegee syphilis study, subjects experienced permanent damage. Conducting research that will permanently damage subjects is highly questionable and must be scrutinized carefully, regardless of the benefits gained. One exception might be a study that investigates a medical procedure that potentially cures a life-threatening condition but causes permanent damage to hearing, to peripheral sensation, or to vision. Frequently, in studies that cause permanent damage, other people, not the subjects, will receive the benefits of the study. Studies causing permanent damage to subjects, without a concomitant gain, violate the Nuremberg Code (1949).

BALANCING BENEFITS AND RISKS FOR A STUDY

Researchers and reviewers of research must examine the balance of benefits and risks in a study. To determine this balance or **benefit-risk ratio**, you must first predict the most likely outcomes of your study. The outcomes of a study are predicted on the basis of previous research, clinical experience, and theory. What are the benefits and risks, both actual and potential, of these outcomes? As the researcher, your goal is to maximize the benefits and minimize the risks (Figure 9-2).

Assessment of Benefits

The probability and magnitude of a study's potential benefits must be assessed. A **research benefit** is defined as something of health-related, psychosocial, or other value to a subject, or something that will contribute to

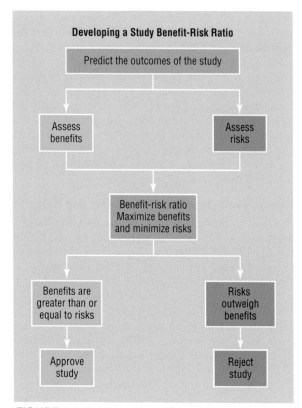

FIGURE 9-2 Balancing benefits and risks of a study.

the acquisition of knowledge for evidence-based practice. Money and other compensations for participation in research are not benefits but, rather, are remuneration for research-related inconveniences (U.S. DHHS, 2009). In study proposals and informed consent documents, the research benefits are described for the individual subjects, subjects' families, and society.

The type of research conducted, whether therapeutic or nontherapeutic, affects the potential benefits for the subjects. In therapeutic nursing research, the individual subject has the potential to benefit from the procedures, such as skin care, range of motion, touch, and other nursing interventions, that are implemented in the study. The benefits might include improvement in the subject's physical condition, which could facilitate emotional and social benefits. The subject also may benefit from the additional attention of and interaction with a healthcare professional. In addition, knowledge generated from the research might expand the subjects' and their families' understanding of health. The conduct of nontherapeutic nursing research does not benefit the subject directly but is important to generate and refine nursing knowledge for practice. Subjects who understand the lack of therapeutic benefit for them frequently will participate because of altruism and the desire to help others with their condition (Irani & Richmond, 2015). By participating in research, subjects have an opportunity to know the findings from a particular study (Fry et al., 2011).

Assessment of Risks

You must assess the type, severity, and number of risks that subjects might experience by participating in your study. The risks involved depend on the purpose of the study and the procedures used to conduct it. Research risks can be physical, emotional, social, or economic in nature and can range from no risk or mere inconvenience to the risk of permanent damage (Reynolds, 1979). Studies can have actual (known) risks and potential risks for subjects. As mentioned earlier, subjects in a study of the effects of prolonged bed rest have the actual risk of transient muscle weakness and the potential risk of DVT. Some studies contain actual or potential risks for the subjects' families and society. You must determine the likelihood of the risks and take precautions to protect the rights of subjects when implementing your study.

Benefit-Risk Ratio

The benefit-risk ratio is determined on the basis of the maximized benefits and the minimized risks. The researcher attempts to maximize the benefits and minimize the risks by making changes in the study purpose or procedures or both (Rubin, 2014). If the risks entailed by your study cannot be eliminated or further minimized, you must justify their existence. If the risks outweigh the benefits, the IRB is unlikely to approve the study and you probably need to revise the study or develop a new one. If the benefits equal or outweigh the risks, you can usually justify conducting the study, and an IRB will probably approve it (see Figure 9-2).

HUMAN SUBJECT PROTECTION IN GENOMICS RESEARCH

Special challenges to protecting subjects' right of self determination and informed consent are studies in the field of genomics research. The Human Genome Project funded by NIH recognized from the onset the ethical and legal dilemmas of genomic research. As a result, program funding has included funding specifically for the study of these issues (McEwen, Boyer, & Sun, 2013). "No other area of biomedical research has sustained such a high commitment, backed by dollars, to the examination of ethical issues" (McEwen et al., 2013, p. 375). Despite this investment, many issues remain unresolved.

Several highly publicized cases have increased awareness as well as fear among the public. In 1951, Henrietta Lacks, an African American woman, only 31 years of age, was diagnosed with cervical cancer. She was admitted to the hospital for the standard treatment (Jones, 1997). The specimens collected were taken to the laboratory of a scientist named Dr. Gey. Dr. Gey was trying to identify and reproduce a cell line for research purposes (Jones, 1997), and generously provided the cell line to other researchers free of charge. These researchers, building on Dr. Gey's research, developed a cell line from those especially hardy tumor cells that was successfully used in research (Bledsoe & Grizzle, 2013; Skloot, 2010). The highly effective treatments, such as the polio vaccine and in vitro fertilization, that were developed using the cell line were extremely profitable for the researchers and the institutions with which they were associated, and resulted in literally billions of dollars being made by selling the cell line to other researchers (McEwen et al., 2013). Mrs. Lacks died never knowing her tumor cells were used for research, and her family only learned of her contribution to science in 2010.

In 1990, researchers began collecting blood specimens of members of an isolated Native American Indian tribe, the Havasupai, who lived in the Grand Canyon (Caplan & Moreno, 2011). Diabetes mellitus was a devastating disease among their tribe, and the researchers proposed a study to identify genetic clues of disease susceptibility. However, the researchers used the blood specimens to study other topics, such as schizophrenia and tribal origin (McEwen et al., 2013). The tribe sued Arizona State University, the employer of the original researcher, and was awarded a settlement in 2010. Part of the settlement was the release of the remaining blood samples to the tribe to be disposed of in a culturally appropriate way. A related case occurred with the people of the First Nations in Canada. Researchers collected genetic materials to study arthritis in 2006, and the subjects asked later for the specimens to be returned, based on cultural beliefs (Brief & Illes, 2010).

Among the unresolved issues in genomics research are de-identification of data, subjects withdrawing from a study, additional studies being conducted with specimens already collected, return of information to the research subject if beneficial to the subject, and ownership of specimens. There is concern that, by its very nature, genomic data cannot be completely de-identified (Terry, 2015). Genetic data de-identified (18 elements removed) has the potential of being combined with data from genetic genealogy databases and other publicly available demographic data to re-identify a subject (McEwen et al., 2013). Pending rule changes in the Common Rule will require informed consent in genomic studies to include the possibility of re-identification (Bledsoe & Grizzle, 2013; U.S. DHHS, 2015b).

De-identification may go beyond the individual in some cultures. Brief and Illes (2010) describe their preparation to conduct a study on early-onset Alzheimer's disease with people of the First Nations. Using a community participatory research approach involving tribal elders and other members of the community, Brief and Illes (2010) addressed potential issues prior to beginning the study. One of these was whether publications and presentations could identify the community in which the study was conducted. The research team has decided not to reveal the name of the specific community. Discussions are ongoing, however, because some tribe members would like their contributions to be acknowledged (Brief & Illes, 2010).

As noted earlier, use of genomic data in secondary studies has caused legal and ethical problems. With de-identified data, although technically possible, it would be extremely expensive and time-consuming to re-consent all subjects for a future study. The recommendation at this time is for researchers gathering genetic data to obtain consent for further use of the data and to specify whether the specimen will be added to a tissue bank (Terry & Terry, 2001).

The costs of re-identification also affect the issue of whether to contact subjects when their genetic data reveal potential health problems (McEwen et al., 2013). De-identification is usually viewed as desirable; however, it makes contacting subjects more difficult. Contacting subjects could potentially harm the subjects, for example, if the information involves an unpreventable disease (Wendler & Rid, 2015). Women have had their ovaries removed based on genetic test results indicating a higher risk for ovarian cancer when, in fact, the tests were inaccurate (Kushner, 2014). Harm may ensue when information provided is incorrect.

OBTAINING INFORMED CONSENT

Obtaining informed consent from human subjects is essential for the conduct of ethical research in the United States (U.S. FDA, 2010a; U.S. DHHS, 2009) and internationally (CIOMS-WHO, 2009). Informing is the transmission of essential ideas and content from the investigator to the prospective subject. Consent is the prospective subject's agreement, after assimilating essential information, to participate in a study as a subject. The phenomenon of **informed consent** was formally defined in the first

principle of the Nuremberg Code as follows: "the person involved should have legal capacity to give consent; should be so situated as to be able to exercise free power of choice, without the intervention of any element of force, fraud, deceit, duress, over-reaching, or other ulterior form of constraint or coercion; and should have sufficient knowledge and comprehension of the elements of the subject matter involved, as to enable him to make an understanding and enlightened decision" (Nuremberg Code, 1949, p. 181). Prospective subjects, to the degree they are capable, should have the opportunity to choose whether or not to participate in research. With careful accommodations, a study's subjects may include persons with cognitive impairment (Simpson, 2010), a diagnosis of psychosis (Beebe & Smith, 2010), or dementia (Beattie, 2009).

The definition of informed consent from the Nuremberg Code provides a basis for the discussion of consent in all subsequent research codes and has general acceptance in the research community. Informed consent involves the researcher disclosing essential information and the potential subject being mentally competent and able to comprehend that information. The subject must also freely volunteer to participate. This section describes the elements of informed consent and the methods of documenting consent.

Information Essential for Consent

Informed consent requires the researcher to disclose specific information to each prospective subject. In addition to the elements that are required by federal regulations (Box 9-7), the IRB or agency may have additional elements that they require (U.S. FDA, 2010a; U.S. DHHS, 2009).

Introduction of Research Activities

Each prospective subject is provided a statement that he or she is being asked to participate in research and a description of the purpose and the expected duration of participation in the study. In clinical nursing research, the patient, serving as a subject, must know which nursing activities are research activities and which are routine nursing interventions. If at any point the prospective subject disagrees with the researcher's goals or the intent of the study, he or she can decline participation or withdraw from the study.

Prospective subjects also must receive a complete description of the procedures to be followed and identification of any procedures in the study that are experimental (U.S. FDA, 2010a; U.S. DHHS, 2009). Thus, researchers need to describe the research variables and the procedures or mechanisms that will be used to observe, examine, manipulate, or measure these variables. In addition, they must inform prospective subjects about when the study procedures will be implemented, how many times, and in what setting.

Research participants also need to know the funding source(s) of a study, such as specific individuals, organizations, or companies. For example, researchers studying the effects of a specific drug must identify any sponsorship by a pharmaceutical company. If the study is being conducted as part of an academic requirement, researchers should share that information also (Fry et al., 2011).

Description of Risks and Discomforts

Prospective subjects must be informed about any foreseeable risks or discomforts (physical, emotional, social, or economic) that might result from the study (U.S. DHHS, 2009; U.S. FDA, 2010b). They also must know how the risks of a study were minimized and the benefits maximized. If a study involves greater than minimal risk, it is a good idea to encourage prospective subjects to consult another person regarding their participation, such as a friend, family member, or another nurse. In addition, researchers may require a delay between discussing the study and signing the informed consent document so that subjects can thoughtfully consider their decision before agreeing.

Description of Benefits

You should describe any benefits to the subject or to others that may be expected from the research. The study might benefit the current subjects or might generate knowledge that will provide evidence-based care to patients and families in the future (U.S. DHHS, 2009; U.S. FDA, 2010a).

Disclosure of Alternatives

Study participants must receive a disclosure of alternatives related to their participation in a study. They must be informed about appropriate, alternative procedures or courses of treatment, if any, that might be advantageous to them (U.S. DHHS, 2009). For example, nurse researchers examining the effect of a distraction intervention on the chronic pain of patients with osteoarthritis would need to make potential subjects aware of other alternatives for pain management available to them.

Assurance of Anonymity and Confidentiality

Prospective subjects must be assured that the confidentiality of their records and PHI will be maintained during and following their study participation (U.S. FDA, 2010a; U.S. DHHS, 2003, 2009). Thus, subjects need to know that their responses and the information obtained from their records during a study will be kept confidential and that their identities will remain anonymous in presentations, reports, and publications of the study findings. Any limits to confidentiality, such as the researcher's need to reveal anything the subject reports about ongoing child abuse, must also be disclosed to the prospective subject before participation begins if relevant to the study. Depending on the study design, participants' identities may be made anonymous to the researchers, to decrease the potential for bias.

Compensation for Participation in Research

For research involving more than minimal risk, prospective subjects must be given an explanation as to whether any compensation or medical treatment, or both, would be available if injury should occur. If medical treatments are available, the person obtaining consent must describe the type and extent of the treatments. Female prospective subjects need to know whether the study treatment or procedure may involve potential risks to them or their fetuses if they are or may become pregnant during the study (U.S. DHHS, 2009; U.S. FDA, 2010a). Potential subjects also need to know whether they will receive a small financial payment ($10 to $30), or other equivalent incentive, to compensate them for time and effort related to study participation.

Offer to Answer Questions

As a conscientious researcher, you need to offer to answer any questions that the prospective subjects may have during the consent process. Study participants also need an explanation of whom to contact for answers to questions about the research during the conduct of the study and of whom to contact in the event of a research-related problem or injury, as well as how to do so (U.S. DHHS, 2009; U.S. FDA, 2010a). The healthcare facility or university IRB to which you are submitting your materials will have specific contact information to include.

Noncoercive Disclaimer

A **noncoercive disclaimer** is a statement that participation is voluntary and refusal to participate will involve no penalty or loss of benefits to which the subject is entitled (U.S. DHHS, 2009; U.S. FDA, 2010a). This statement can facilitate a more positive relationship between you and your prospective subjects, especially if the relationship has a potential for coercion.

Option to Withdraw

Subjects may discontinue participation in, or may withdraw from, a study at any time without penalty or loss of benefits (Rubin, 2014). However, at the time of consent, researchers do have the right to ask subjects whether they think that they will be able to complete the study, to decrease the number of subjects withdrawing early. There may be circumstances under which the subject's participation may be terminated by the researcher without regard to the subject's consent (U.S. DHHS, 2009). For example, if a particular treatment becomes potentially dangerous to a subject, you as a researcher have an obligation to discontinue the subject's participation in the study. Thus, it is necessary to describe for prospective subjects the circumstances under which they might be withdrawn from the study, and to make a general statement about the circumstances that could lead to termination of the entire project. This is especially important in therapeutic research.

Consent to Incomplete Disclosure

In some studies, subjects experience **incomplete disclosure** of study information, or are not completely informed of the study purpose, because that knowledge would alter their actions. However, prospective subjects must know that certain information is being withheld deliberately. You, the researcher, must ensure that there are no undisclosed risks to the subjects that are more than minimal and that their questions are truthfully answered regarding the study. Subjects who are exposed to nondisclosure of information must know when and how they will be debriefed about the study. Subjects are **debriefed** by informing them of the actual purpose of

the study and the results that were obtained. At this point, subjects have the option to have their data withdrawn from the study. If the subjects experience adverse effects related to the study, you must make every attempt to compensate or alleviate the effects (APA, 2010; U.S. DHHS, 2009).

Comprehension of Consent Information

Informed consent implies not only the imparting of information by the researcher but also the comprehension of that information by the subject. Studies examining subjects' levels of comprehension of consent information have found their comprehension to be limited (Erlen, 2010). Potential subjects' comprehension of the consent depends on time pressure, literacy, language, the complexity of the study, and the clarity of its explanation. Federal regulations require that information given to subjects or their representatives be expressed in a language they can understand (U.S. DHHS, 2009; U.S. FDA, 2010a). Consequently, healthcare facilities may require that the researcher make the consent form available in the most common languages spoken by their patients. Depending on the geographic area, the consent form may need to be translated into Vietnamese, French, Spanish, or another language. Thus, the consent information must be written and verbalized in lay terminology, not professional jargon, and must be presented without the use of biased terms that might coerce a subject into participating in a study. The reading level of the consent form should be at or below fifth-grade level (National Quality Forum, 2005). When likely that some subjects may have limited reading ability, the researcher may read the consent aloud to all subjects to avoid embarrassment. Kim and Kim (2015) compared a simplified version of informed consent to the standard version with the outcome variable being comprehension of the study's purposes and processes. The authors found that comprehension was higher in the group that received the simplified version of the consent.

Researchers can take steps to determine the prospective subjects' level of comprehension by having them complete a survey or questionnaire examining their understanding of consent information (Cahana & Hurst, 2008). Montalvo and Larson (2014) conducted a systematic review of studies that assessed subjects' comprehension of the study in which they were asked to participate. Based on the review, the authors recommended that researchers routinely assess the health literacy and comprehension of potential subjects

In qualitative research, participants might comprehend their participation in a study at the beginning, but unexpected events or consequences might occur during the study to obscure that understanding (Sanjari et al. 2014). These events might precipitate a change in the focus of the research and the type of participation by the participants. For example, the topics of an interview might change with an increased need for participants to address these emerging topics. Thus, informed consent is an ongoing, evolving process in qualitative research, even though it does not involve actual signature of new consent forms to accompany each change in focus. The researcher must verbally renegotiate the participants' consent and determine their comprehension of that consent as changes occur in the study, discussing evolving information, and requesting their participation in verifying and exploring new information. By continually clarifying and determining the comprehension of participants, you will establish trust with them and promote the conduct of an ethical study (Munhall, 2012a).

Competence to Give Consent

Autonomous individuals, who are capable of understanding and weighing the benefits and risks of a proposed study, are competent to give consent. The researcher may assess the competence of the subject by using a formal assessment of decisional capacity (Beattie, 2009).

As described earlier, diminished capacity to comprehend may be related to a subject's health, age, or educational status, and in hospitalized patients may be transient and related to treatments and medications. However, when this is the case, the researcher makes every effort to present information at a level prospective subjects can understand, so that they can consent or assent to the research, whichever is appropriate to their status. In addition, researchers need to present essential information clearly for consent to the legally authorized representative, if one is required, such as the conservator, parent, or guardian of the prospective subject (U.S. DHHS, 2009). (See previous discussion related to vulnerable populations.)

Voluntary Consent

Voluntary consent means that the prospective subject has decided to take part in a study of his or her own volition without coercion or any undue influence. Voluntary consent is obtained after the prospective subject has been given essential information about the study and has shown comprehension of this information (U.S. DHHS, 2009; U.S. FDA, 2010a). Some researchers, because of their authority, expertise, or power, have the potential to coerce subjects into participating in research.

Researchers need to ensure that their persuasion and compensation of prospective subjects are not coercive.

Documentation of Informed Consent

The standard is that informed consent is presented formally and requires the signature of the subject and a witness. There are lower-risk studies, however, in which signatures and/or written consent can be waived, with the approval of the IRB.

Written Consent Waived

Requirements for written consent or the participants' signatures on their consent forms may be waived in research that "presents no more than minimal risk of harm to subjects and involves no procedures for which written consent is normally required outside of the research context" (U.S. DHHS, 2009, 45 CFR Section 46.117c). For example, if you were using questionnaires to collect low risk data, obtaining a signed consent form from subjects might not be necessary. The subject's completion of the questionnaire may serve as consent. The top of the questionnaire might contain a statement such as "Your completion of this questionnaire indicates your consent to participate in this study." In other low risk studies, data may be collected by mail or online and, after the text of the consent is presented, the subject then signifies consent by completing the questionnaire.

Written consent also is waived when the only record linking the subject and the research would be the consent document and the principal risk is the harm that could result from a breach of confidentiality. The subjects must be given the option of signing or not signing a consent form, and the subject's wishes govern whether the consent form is signed (U.S. DHHS, 2009). However, the four elements of consent—disclosure, comprehension, competence, and voluntarism—are essential in all studies, whether written consent is waived or required.

Written Consent Documents

Short-form written consent document. The short-form consent document includes the following statement: "The elements of informed consent required by Section 46.116 [see the section on information essential for consent] have been presented orally to the subject or the subject's legally authorized representative" (U.S. DHHS, 2009, 45 CFR Section 46.117b). The researcher must develop a written summary of what is to be said to the subject in the oral presentation, and the summary must be approved by an IRB. When the oral presentation is made to the subject or to the subject's representative, a witness is required. The subject or representative must sign the short-form consent document. The

Study title: The Needs of Family Members of Critically Ill Adults
Investigator: Linda L. Norris, R.N.

   Ms. Norris is a registered nurse studying the emotional and social needs of family members of patients in the Intensive Care Units **(research purpose)**. Although the study will not benefit you directly, it will provide information that might enable nurses to identify family members' needs and to assist family members with those needs **(potential benefits)**.
   The study and its procedures have been approved by the appropriate people and review boards at The University of Texas at Arlington and X hospital **(IRB approval)**. The study procedures might cause fatigue for you or your family **(potential risks)**. The procedures include: (1) responding to a questionnaire about the needs of family members of critically ill patients and (2) completing a demographic data sheet **(explanation of procedures)**. Participation in this study will take approximately 20 minutes **(time commitment)**. You are free to ask any questions about the study or about being a subject and you may call Ms. Norris at (999) 999-9999 (work) or (999) 999-9999 (home) if you have further questions **(offer to answer questions)**.
   Your participation in this study is voluntary; you are under no obligation to participate **(alternative option and voluntary consent)**. You have the right to withdraw at any time and the care of your family member and your relationship with the healthcare team will not be affected **(option to withdraw)**.
   The study data will be coded so they will not be linked to your name. Your identity will not be revealed while the study is being conducted or when the study is reported or published. All study data will be collected by Ms. Norris, stored in a secure place, and not shared with any other person without your permission **(assurance of anonymity and confidentiality)**.

I have read this consent form and voluntarily consent to participate in this study.

(If Appropriate)

_____   _____
Subject's Signature   Date   Legal Representative   Date

I have explained this study to the above subject and have sought his/her understanding for informed consent

_____
Investigator's Signature   Date

FIGURE 9-3 Sample consent form. Words in parentheses and **boldface** identify common essential consent information and would not appear in an actual form.

witness must sign both the short-form and a copy of the summary, and the person actually obtaining consent must sign a copy of the summary. Copies of the summary and short form are given to the subject and the witness; the researcher retains the original documents and must keep these documents for 3 years after the end of the study. Short-form written consent documents may be used in studies that present minimal or moderate risk to subjects.

   Formal written consent document. The written consent document or **consent form** includes the elements of informed consent required by the U.S. DHHS (2009) and U.S. FDA (2010a) regulations (see the previous section on information essential for consent). The IRBs of most healthcare facilities and universities maintain their own templates for the informed consent document with specific requirements, such as detailed headings, suggested wording, and contact information. A sample consent form is presented in Figure 9-3 with the essential consent information. The subject can read the consent form, or the researcher can read it to the subject; however, it is wise also to explain the study to the subject, using different words, in a conversational manner, which encourages questions. The subject signs the form, and the investigator or research assistant collecting the data witnesses it. This type of consent can be used for minimal- to moderate-risk studies. All persons signing the consent form must receive a copy. The researcher keeps the original for 3 years in a secure location, such as a locked file cabinet in a locked room.

   Studies that involve subjects with diminished autonomy require a written consent form. If these prospective subjects have some comprehension of the study and agree to participate as subjects, they must sign the consent form. However, each subject's legally authorized representative also must sign the form. The representative indicates his or her relationship to the subject under the signature (see Figure 9-3).

The written consent form used in a high-risk study often contains the signatures of two witnesses, the researcher, and an additional person. The additional person signing as a witness is present to observe the informed consent process, to assure that it adheres to specifications, and must not be otherwise connected with the study. The best witnesses are research advocates or patient ombudspersons employed by the institution. Sometimes nurses are asked to sign a consent form as a witness for a biomedical study. They must know the study purpose and procedures and the subject's comprehension of the study before signing the form as a witness (Fry et al., 2011). The role of the witness is more important in the consent process if the prospective subject is in awe of the investigator and does not feel free to question the procedures of the study.

Jones (2015) conducted a qualitative study of African American women's perspectives on breast cancer. She recruited women who had survived at least a year since diagnosis and their mothers ($n = 14$) to explore their experiences. The themes that emerged were "issues of mistrust of the medical community," "limited treatment options," "knowledge deficit for screening," and "it's a death sentence" (Jones, 2015, pp. 6, 7). Jones (2015) reported a typical approach to the protection of human subjects, but narrowed the inclusion criteria to include only women with cancer who had completed their treatment. Jones (2015, p. 5) indicated her rationale for the criterion to be completion of treatment so "the individuals would be stabilized medically and free from any discomfort that might occur as a result of cancer care." To obtain approval from the IRB of her institution, she ensured that the consent form stated the study was voluntary and responses were confidential. Each woman signed the informed consent form and received a copy.

Recording of the Consent Process

A researcher might elect to document the consent process through audio- or video-recordings. These methods document what was said to the prospective subject, and record the subject's questions and the investigator's answers. Recordings can be time-consuming and costly, and thus not appropriate for studies of minimal or moderate risk. If your study is considered high risk, it is advisable to document the consent process completely, because doing so might protect you and

---

BOX 9-8   Requirements for Authorization to Release PHI for Research

- Types of PHI to be used, such as medical diagnosis or assessment data, identified in an understandable way
- Name of researcher who will use the PHI
- How the PHI will be used in this specific study
- Authorization expiration date, which may be the end of the study or "none" if data will become part of a research database or repository
- Signature of the subject, legal representative if appropriate, and date (see Privacy Rule, 45 CFR Section 164.508[c][1], U.S. DHHS, 2004)

---

your subjects. Both of you would retain a copy of the recording.

Authorization for Research Uses and Disclosure

The HIPAA Privacy Rule provides individuals the right, as research subjects, to authorize covered entities (healthcare provider, health plan, and healthcare clearinghouse) to use or disclose their PHI for research purposes. This authorization is regulated by HIPAA and is separate from the informed consent that is regulated by the U.S. DHHS (2009) and the U.S. FDA (2010a). The authorization information can be included as part of the consent form, but it is probably best to have two separate forms. The authorization focuses on privacy risks and states how, why, and with whom PHI will be shared. The key ideas required on the authorization form when used for research are included in Box 9-8.

INSTITUTIONAL REVIEW

An **institutional review board (IRB)** is a committee that reviews research to ensure that all investigators are conducting research ethically. All hospital-based research must be submitted to the hospital's IRB, which will then determine whether it is high risk, moderate risk, minimal risk, or exempt from review. This is true, as well, of research that does not involve patients. Even though some research clearly falls under the category of "exempt from review" it must, nonetheless, be submitted to the IRB, which then will declare it exempt. Requiring review of all studies is necessary because, in the past, studies that should have been reviewed escaped notice. Universities, hospital corporations, and many managed care centers maintain IRBs to promote the conduct of ethical research and protect the rights of prospective subjects at these institutions, as required since 1974.

Federal regulations require that the members of an IRB evaluate the study for protection of human subjects, including processes for obtaining informed consent. Federal regulations stipulate the membership, functions, and operations of an IRB (U.S. DHHS, 2009, 45 CFR Sections 46.107–46.115; U.S. FDA, 2010b, 21 CFR Sections 56.101–56.124).

Each IRB has at least five members of various backgrounds (cultural, economic, educational, professional, gender, racial) to promote a complete, scholarly, and fair review of research that is commonly conducted in an institution. If an institution regularly reviews studies with vulnerable subjects, such as children, neonates, pregnant women, prisoners, and mentally disabled persons, the IRB should include one or more members with knowledge about and experience in working with these individuals. The members must have sufficient experience and expertise to review a variety of studies, including quantitative, qualitative, and mixed methods research. IRB members may be less familiar with qualitative methodologies and the qualitative component of mixed method studies, requiring the researcher to provide additional explanation (Munhall, 2012b). Any IRB member who has a conflict of interest with a research project being reviewed must excuse himself or herself from the review process, except to provide information requested by the IRB. The IRB also must include members who are not affiliated with the institution and whose primary concern is nonscientific, such as an ethicist, a lawyer, or a minister (U.S. DHHS, 2009; U.S. FDA, 2010b). IRBs in hospitals are often composed of physicians, nurses, lawyers, scientists, clergy, and community laypersons.

In 2009, U.S. FDA and U.S. DHHS regulations were revised to require all IRBs to register through a system maintained by the DHHS. The registration information includes contact information for the IRB's institution and the official who oversees its activities, the number of active protocols involving federally regulated products reviewed during the preceding 12 months, and a description of the types of products involved in the protocols reviewed (U.S. DHHS, 2009; U.S. FDA, 2010b). The IRB registration requirement was implemented to make it easier for the DHHS to supervise and communicate information to IRBs. This rule was made effective in July of 2009 and requires each IRB to renew its registration every three years.

Levels of Reviews Conducted by Institutional Review Boards

Federal guidelines apply to universities and healthcare agencies, so that their IRBs function in a similar way in the review of research (U.S. DHHS, 2009; U.S. FDA, 2010b). Faculty members and students must receive IRB approval from their universities and the agencies or hospitals in which the study is to be conducted. The functions and operations of an IRB involve the review of research at three different levels of scrutiny: (1) exempt from review, (2) expedited review, and (3) full board review. *The IRB chairperson and/or committee, not the researcher, decide the level of the review.*

Studies are usually **exempt from review** if they pose no apparent risks for research subjects. Studies usually considered exempt from IRB review, according to federal regulations are identified in Box 9-9. For example, studies by nurses and other health professionals that have no foreseeable risks or are a mere inconvenience for subjects may be identified as exempt from review by the chairperson of the IRB committee. In other states or regions, these same studies may be evaluated to be expedited studies. Studies incorporating previously collected data from which PHI has been de-identified are usually exempt as well (U.S. DHHS, 2004).

Studies that have some risks, which are viewed as minimal, are expedited in the review process. **Minimal risk** means "that the risks of harm anticipated in the proposed research are not greater, considering probability and magnitude, than those ordinarily encountered in daily life or during the performance of routine physical or psychological examinations or tests" (U.S. DHHS, 2009, 45 CFR Section 46.102). Expedited review procedures can also be used to review minor changes in previously approved research. Under **expedited IRB review** procedures, the review may be carried out by the IRB chairperson or by one or more experienced reviewers designated by the chairperson from among members of the IRB. In reviewing the research, the reviewers may exercise all of the authorities of the IRB except disapproval of the research. If the reviewer does not believe the research should be approved, the full committee must review the study. Only the full committee can disapprove a study (U.S. DHHS, 2009; U.S. FDA, 2010b). Box 9-10 identifies research that usually qualifies for expedited review.

A study involving greater than minimal risk to research subjects requires a **complete IRB review** also called a full board review. To obtain IRB approval, researchers must ensure that ethical principles are upheld. Risks must be minimized, and those risks must be reasonable when compared to benefits of participation. Consistent with justice, the selection of subjects must be fair and equitable. Informed consent must be obtained from each subject or legal representative and documented appropriately. In addition, the researcher

---

BOX 9-9   Research Qualifying for Exemption From Review

1. Conducted in established or commonly accepted educational settings, involving normal educational practices
2. Involving the use of educational tests, survey procedures, interview procedures or observation of public behavior, unless:
   - Recorded in such a manner that human subjects can be identified, directly or through identifiers
   - Disclosure of the human subjects' responses could reasonably place the subjects at risk of criminal or civil liability
   - Disclosure of the human subjects' responses could reasonably be damaging to the subjects' financial standing, employability, or reputation
3. Research involving the use of educational tests, survey procedures, interview procedures, or observation of public behavior that is not exempt
   - Exempt if human subjects are elected or appointed public officials or candidates for public office
   - Federal statute(s) require(s) without exception that the confidentiality of the personally identifiable information will be maintained throughout the research and thereafter.
4. Involving the collection or study of existing data, documents, records, pathological specimens, or diagnostic specimens if publicly available or recorded by the investigator in such a manner that subjects cannot be identified, directly or through identifiers
5. Conducted by or subject to the approval of department or agency heads, and which are designed to study, evaluate, or examine
   - Public benefit or service programs
   - Procedures for obtaining benefits or services under those programs
   - Possible changes in or alternatives to those programs or procedures
   - Possible changes in methods or levels of payment for benefits or services under those programs
6. Taste and food quality evaluation and consumer acceptance studies when:
   - Wholesome foods without additives are consumed
   - Food is consumed that contains a food ingredient at or below the level and for a use found to be safe
   - Food consumed contains an agricultural chemical or environmental contaminant at or below the level found to be safe by the FDA or other federal agency

Adapted from U.S. Department of Health and Human Services (U.S. DHHS, 2009). *Protection of human subjects. Code of Federal Regulations, Title 45, Part 46*. Retrieved March 24, 2016 from http://www.hhs.gov/ohrp/policy/ohrpregulations.pdf/.

BOX 9-10   Research Qualifying for Expedited Institutional Review Board Review

Expedited review for studies with no more than minimal risk involving:

1. Collection of hair, collection of nail clippings, extraction of deciduous teeth, and extraction of permanent teeth if extraction needed
2. Collection of excreta and external secretions (sweat, saliva, placenta removed at delivery, and amniotic fluid at rupture of the membrane)
3. Recording of data from subjects 18 years of age or older using noninvasive procedures routinely employed in clinical practice with exception of X-rays
4. Collection of blood samples by venipuncture from healthy, non-pregnant subjects 18 years of age or older (amount not >450 mL in an 8-week period, no more than two times per week)
5. Collection of dental plaque and calculus using accepted prophylactic techniques
6. Voice recordings made for research purposes such as investigations of speech defects
7. Moderate exercise by healthy volunteers
8. The study of existing data, documents, records, pathological specimens, or diagnostic specimens
9. Behavior or characteristics of individuals or groups, with no researcher manipulation. Research will not increase stress of subjects.
10. Drugs or devices for which an investigational new drug exemption or an investigational device exemption is not required

Summarized from U.S. Department of Health and Human Services (U.S. DHHS, 2009). *Protection of human subjects. Code of Federal Regulations, Title 45, Part 46*. Retrieved March 24, 2016 from http://www.hhs.gov/ohrp/policy/ohrpregulations.pdf/.

must have a plan to monitor data collection, protect privacy, and maintain confidentiality (U.S. DHHS, 2009, 45 CFR 46.111; U.S. FDA, 2010b, 21 CFR 56.111).

Every research report must indicate that the study had IRB approval and whether the approval was from a university and/or clinical agency. All of the reports used as examples in this chapter indicated the studies had appropriate IRB approval. For example, Riegel et al. (2011) provided the following description of their IRB approval. This study involved a secondary data analysis using a national database of HF patients to determine their levels of self-care performance. These researchers ensured the studies in the database had IRB approval and that they obtained IRB approval from their university.

"All studies had been approved by local institutional review boards. In each, eligibility was confirmed by a trained nurse research assistant who then explained study requirements and obtained written informed consent. This secondary analysis was approved by the institutional review board of the University of Pennsylvania" (Riegel et al., 2011, p. 134).

Influence of HIPAA Privacy Rule on Institutional Review Boards

Under the HIPAA Privacy Rule, an IRB or an institutionally established privacy board can act on requests for a waiver or an alteration of the requirement to have signed HIPAA authorization from each subject in a study (U.S. DHHS, 2013). If an IRB and a privacy board both exist in an agency, the approval of only one board is required, and is customarily the IRB for research projects. Researchers can choose to obtain a signed form from potential subjects authorizing the release of PHI to the researcher, can ask for a partial or complete waiver, or propose an alteration of the authorization requirement. Some studies are not possible without some degree of waiver or alteration in the requirement to authorize release of PHI. A partial waiver, discussed earlier, may be needed so that the researcher can obtain PHI to identify and recruit potential subjects. As noted earlier, informed consent may be waived by an IRB for a low risk study or when the signed informed consent document would be the link of the subject to his or her data. When an IRB has granted a waiver of documented informed consent, it can also give a researcher a complete waiver of the need for PHI authorization. An altered authorization requirement occurs when an IRB approves a request that some but not all of the required 18 elements be removed from health information that

is to be used in research. A waiver or alteration of the authorization requirement may occur when certain conditions are met, including that the researcher's plan provides steps to protect the PHI from misuse. In addition, the PHI must be destroyed as soon as possible, and the researcher assures the IRB that the PHI will not be reused or disclosed to any other person (U.S. DHHS, 2013).

The healthcare provider, health plan, or healthcare clearinghouse cannot release the PHI to the researcher until the following documentation has been received: (1) the identity of the approving IRB, (2) the date the waiver or alteration was approved, (3) IRB documentation that the criteria for waiver or alteration have been met, (4) a brief description of the PHI to which the researcher has been granted access or use, (5) a statement as to whether the waiver was approved under normal or expedited review procedures, and (6) the signature of the IRB chair or the chair's designee.

RESEARCH MISCONDUCT

The goal of research is to generate sound scientific knowledge, which is possible only through the honest conduct, reporting, and publication of studies. As described in this chapter, extensive federal regulations have been developed and enforced in research. Since the 1980s, a number of fraudulent studies have been conducted and published in prestigious scientific journals and researchers have submitted reports of fabricated data. In response to the increasing incidences of scientific misconduct, the federal government developed the Office of Research Integrity (ORI) in 1989 within the U.S. DHHS. The ORI was instituted to supervise the implementation of the rules and regulations related to research misconduct and to manage any investigations of misconduct.

The ORI's website contains a growing list of persons found to have falsified or fabricated research reports. For example, in May 2015 (ORI, 2015a), Ryan Asherin, "former Surveillance Officer and Principal Investigator, Oregon Health Authority, Public Health Division," was found by the Office of Research Integrity to have "falsified and/or fabricated fifty-six (56) case report forms (CRFs) while acquiring data on the incidence of *Clostridium difficile* infections in Klamath County, Oregon. Specifically, the Respondent (1) fabricated responses to multiple questions on the CRFs for patient demographic data, patient health information, and *Clostridium difficile* infection data, including the diagnoses of toxic megacolon and ileus and the performance of a colectomy, with no evidence in patient medical records to support the responses; and (2) falsified the CRFs by omitting data on the CRFs that clearly were included in patient medical records" (ORI, 2015a).

Research misconduct has also been documented in nursing (Fierz et al., 2014). For example, Habermann, Broome, Pryor, and Ziner (2010) asked 266 research coordinators, predominately registered nurses, whether they had firsthand knowledge of scientific misconduct in the past year. The types and frequencies of research misconduct the coordinators reported included: 50% protocol violations, 26.6% consent violations, 13.9% fabrication, 5.2% financial conflict of interest, and 5% falsification. Fierz et al. (2014) recommended promoting scientific integrity through mentoring, training, and role modeling.

Role of the ORI in Promoting the Conduct of Ethical Research

The most current regulations implemented by the ORI (2005) are CFR 42, Parts 50 and 93, Policies of General Applicability. The ORI was responsible for defining important terms used in the identification and management of research misconduct. **Research misconduct** was defined as "the fabrication, falsification, or plagiarism in processing, performing, or reviewing research, or in reporting research results. It does not include honest error or differences in opinion" (ORI, 2005, 42 CFR Section 93.103). **Fabrication in research** is the making up of results and the recording or reporting of them. **Falsification of research** is manipulating research materials, equipment, or processes or changing or omitting data or results such that the research is not accurately represented in the research record. Fabrication and falsification of research data are two of the most common acts of research misconduct managed by the ORI (2015b) over the past 5 years. **Plagiarism** is the appropriation of another person's ideas, processes, results, or words without giving appropriate credit, including those obtained through confidential review of others' research proposals and manuscripts.

Currently, the ORI promotes the integrity of biomedical and behavioral research in approximately 4000 institutions worldwide (ORI, 2012). The office applies federal policies and regulations to protect the integrity of the U.S. PHS's extramural and intramural research programs. The extramural program provides funding to research institutions, and the intramural program provides funding for research conducted within the federal government. Box 9-11 contains a summary of the functions of the ORI.

To be classified as research misconduct, an action must be intentional and involve a significant departure

---

BOX 9-11   Functions of the Office of Research Integrity

- Developing policies, procedures, and regulations related to responsible conduct of research and to the detection, investigation, and prevention of research misconduct
- Monitoring research misconduct investigations
- Making recommendations related to findings and consequences of investigations of research misconduct
- Assisting the Office of the General Counsel (OGC) to present cases before the U.S. DHHS appeals board
- Providing technical assistance to institutions responding to allegations of research misconduct
- Implementing activities and programs to teach responsible conduct of research, promote research integrity, prevent research misconduct, and improve the handling of allegations of research misconduct
- Conducting policy analyses, evaluations, and research to build the knowledge base in research misconduct, research integrity, and prevention and to improve the DHHS research integrity policies and procedures
- Administering programs for
  - Maintaining institutional assurances
  - Responding to allegations of retaliation against whistle blowers
  - Approving intramural and extramural policies and procedures
  - Responding to Freedom of Information Act and Privacy Act requests

Summarized from Office of Research Integrity (ORI, 2005). *Public Health Services Policies on Research Misconduct. Code of Federal Regulations, Title 42, Parts 50 and 93. Policies of General Applicability.* Retrieved March 24, 2016 from https://ori.hhs.gov/sites/default/files/42_cfr_parts_50_and_93_2005.pdf.

---

from acceptable scientific practices for maintaining the integrity of the research record. When an allegation is made, it must be proven by a preponderance of evidence. The ORI has a section on its website titled, "Handling Misconduct," which includes a summary of the allegations and investigations managed by its office from 1994 to 2012 (ORI, 2015b). When research misconduct was documented, the actions taken against the researchers or agencies have included disqualification to receive federal funding for periods ranging from 18 months to 8 years. Other actions taken may be that the researcher can conduct only supervised research and all data and sources must be certified.

The researcher's publications may be corrected or retracted (ORI, 2015b).

Role of Journal Editors and Researchers in Preventing Scientific Misconduct

Editors of journals also have a major role in monitoring and preventing research misconduct in the published literature (World Association of Medical Editors [WAME], n.d.). WAME has identified data falsification, plagiarism, and violations of legal and regulatory requirements as some types of scientific misconduct. (See Chapter 27 for more information on ethical practices for authorship.)

Preventing the publication of fraudulent research requires the efforts of authors, coauthors, research coordinators, reviewers of research reports for publication, and editors of professional journals (Hansen & Hansen, 1995; Hawley & Jeffers, 1992; WAME, n.d.). Authors who are primary investigators for research projects must be responsible in their conduct and the conduct of their team members, from data collection through publication of research. Coauthors and coworkers should question and, if necessary, challenge the integrity of a researcher's claims. Sometimes, well-known scientists' names have been added to a research publication as coauthors to give it credibility. Individuals should not be listed as coauthors unless they were actively involved in the conduct and publication of the research (International Council of Medical Journal Editors [ICMJE], 2014). Similarly, supervisors and directors of hospital units should not be included as last author as a "courtesy" for a publication unless they were actively involved in at least one phase of the research.

Research coordinators in large, funded studies have a role to promote integrity in research and to identify research misconduct activities. These individuals are often the ones closest to the actual conduct of the study, during which misconduct often occurs. In the Habermann et al. (2010) study introduced earlier, research coordinators had firsthand experiences with both scientific misconduct and research integrity. Research coordinators often learned of the misconduct firsthand, and the principal investigator was usually identified as the responsible party. The actions noted were protocol violations, consent violations, fabrication, falsification, and financial conflict of interest. Thus, Habermann et al. (2010) recommended that the definition of research misconduct might need to be expanded beyond fabrication, falsification, and plagiarism.

Peer reviewers have a key role in determining the quality and publishability of a manuscript. They are considered experts in the field, and their role is to examine research for inconsistencies and inaccuracies. Editors must monitor the peer review process and must be cautious about publishing manuscripts that are at all questionable (ICMJE, 2014; WAME, n.d.). Editors also must have procedures for responding to allegations of research misconduct. They must decide what actions to take if their journal contains an article that has proven to be fraudulent. Usually, fraudulent publications require retraction notations and are not to be cited by authors in future publications (ORI, 2005).

The publication of fraudulent research is a growing concern in medicine and nursing (Habermann et al., 2010; ICMJE, 2014). The shrinking pool of funds available for research and the greater emphasis on research publications for retention in academic settings could lead to a higher incidence of fraudulent publications. However, the ORI (2012; 2015b) has made major advances in addressing research misconduct and the management of fraudulent publications by: (1) identifying appropriate ORI responses to acts of research misconduct, (2) developing a process for notifying funding agencies and journals of acts of research misconduct, and (3) providing for public disclosure of incidents of research misconduct.

Each researcher is responsible for monitoring the integrity of his or her research protocols, results, and publications. In addition, nursing professionals and journal editors must foster a spirit of intellectual inquiry, mentor prospective scientists regarding the norms for good science, and stress quality, not quantity, in publications (Fierz et al., 2014).

ANIMALS AS RESEARCH SUBJECTS

The use of animals as research subjects is a controversial issue of growing interest to nurse researchers. A small but increasing number of nurse scientists are conducting physiological studies that require the use of animals. Many scientists have expressed concerns that the animal rights' movement could threaten the future of health research. The goal of animal rights' groups is to raise the consciousness of researchers and society to ensure that animals are treated humanely in the conduct of research. Some animal rights' organizations have the expressed purpose of eliminating animal research (Bennett, 2014) and have tried to frighten the public with distorted stories about inhumane treatment of animals in research. Some of the activist leaders have made broad comparisons between human life and animal life and have disseminated misinformation about the care that research animals receive. Some of these activists have progressed to serious vandalism of laboratories and intimidation of researchers (Animal rights and wrongs, 2011). Even more damage is being done to research through lawsuits that have blocked the conduct of research and the development of new research centers.

The use of animals in research is a complicated issue that requires careful ethical consideration by investigators, in view of the knowledge that is needed to manage healthcare problems (Carbone, 2012). Two important questions must be addressed when the use of animals for research is considered: should animals be used as subjects to answer this specific research question, and, if animals are used in the study, what mechanisms ensure that they are treated humanely? Some studies require the use of animals to answer the research question. Animals are more commonly used in laboratory studies that involve investigation of high-risk physiological variables. Approximately 26 million animals were used in research in 2010 with about 25 million of these being mice, rats, fish, and birds (Hastings Center, 2012). However, there is some evidence that other models may be preferable to animal research (Gilbert, 2012). The Institute of Medicine (2011) (now called the Health and Medicine Division) released a report containing the conclusion that the research on chimpanzees was no longer necessary. As a result, the NIH has indicated that they intend to decrease funding of studies that use chimpanzees as subjects (HMD, 2013).

The second question, concerning humane treatment, also must be answered. At least five separate sets of regulations exist to protect research animals from mistreatment. Federal government, state governments, independent accreditation organizations, professional societies, and individual institutions work to ensure that research animals are used only when necessary and only under humane conditions. At the federal level, animal research is conducted according to the guidelines of U.S. PHS Policy on Humane Care and Use of Laboratory Animals, which was adopted in 1986, and was recently updated (U.S. DHHS, 2015a).

Any institution proposing research involving animals must have a written Animal Welfare Assurance statement acceptable to the U.S. PHS that documents compliance with the U.S. PHS policy. Every assurance statement is evaluated by the National Institutes of Health's Office for Protection from Research Risks (OPRR) to determine the adequacy of the institution's proposed program for the care and use of animals in activities conducted or supported by the U.S. PHS (Office of Laboratory Animal Welfare, 2015). The Institute for Laboratory Animal Welfare (2011) publishes a guidebook with specific instructions on what elements must be included in an animal-use protocol.

Much like an institutional assurance for human subjects' research, an institution can seek an assurance for the care and use of research animals. Assurance statements are in compliance with U.S. PHS policy. In addition, more than 950 institutions in 40 countries have obtained accreditation by the Association for the Assessment and Accreditation of Laboratory Animal Care (AAALAC, 2015), which demonstrates the commitment of these institutions to ensure the humane treatment of animals in research. Nurse researchers interested in using animals for research must be trained in their care and appropriate use.

■ KEY POINTS

- The ethical conduct of research starts with the identification of the study topic and continues through the publication of the study to assure that valid research evidence is developed for practice.
- Discussions of ethics and research must continue because of (1) the complexity of human rights issues; (2) the focus of research in new, challenging arenas of technology and genetics; (3) the complex ethical codes and regulations governing research; and (4) the variety of interpretations of these codes and regulations.
- Two historical documents that have had a strong impact on the conduct of research are the Nuremberg Code and the Declaration of Helsinki.
- U.S. federal regulations direct the ethical conduct of research. These regulations include (1) general requirements for informed consent, (2) documentation of informed consent, (3) IRB review of research, (4) exempt and expedited review procedures for certain kinds of research, and (5) criteria for IRB approval of research.
- The Council for International Organizations of Medical Sciences revises and updates ethical guidelines for biomedical research conducted internationally.
- Public Law 104–191, the HIPAA, was implemented in 2003 to protect individuals' health information.
- Conducting research ethically requires protection of the human rights of subjects. Human rights are claims and demands that have been justified in the eyes of an individual or by the consensus of a group of individuals. The human rights that require protection in research are (1) self-determination, (2) privacy, (3) anonymity or confidentiality, (4) fair treatment, and (5) protection from discomfort and harm.
- The rights of research subjects can be protected by balancing benefits and risks of a study, securing informed consent, and submitting the research for

institutional review. The onus of responsibility for protection of research subjects is borne by the lead researcher.

- To balance the benefits and risks of a study, its type, level, and number of risks are examined, and its potential benefits are identified. If possible, risks must be minimized and benefits maximized to achieve the best possible benefit-risk ratio.
- Informed consent involves the transmission of essential information, comprehension of that information, competence to give consent, and voluntary consent of the prospective subject.
- In institutional review, a committee of peers (IRB) examines each study for ethical concerns. The IRB conducts three levels of review: exempt, expedited, and full board.
- The process for accessing PHI must be completed according to the HIPAA Privacy Rule.
- Research misconduct includes fabrication, falsification, and plagiarism during the conduct, reporting, or publication of research. The ORI was developed to investigate and manage incidents of research misconduct to protect the integrity of research in all disciplines.
- Another current ethical concern in research is the use of animals as subjects. The U.S. PHS Policy on Humane Care and Use of Laboratory Animals provides direction for the conduct of research with animals as subjects.

REFERENCES

Abernathy, A., Capell, W., Aziz, N., Ritchie, C., Prince-Paul, M., Bennett, R., et al. (2014). Ethical conduct of palliative care research: Enhancing communication between investigators and institutional review boards. *Journal of Pain and Symptom Management*, 48(1), 1211–1221.

American Nurses Association (ANA) (2010). *The nurse's role in ethics and human rights: Protecting and promoting individual worth, dignity, and human rights in practice settings (Revised Position Statement)*. Retrieved March 24, 2016 from http://www.nursingworld.org/MainMenuCategories/EthicsStandards/Ethics-Position-Statements/-Nursess-Role-in-Ethics-and-Human-Rights.pdf.

American Nurses Association (ANA) (2015). *Code of ethics for nurses with interpretive statements*. Washington, DC: American Nurses Association.

American Psychological Association (APA) (2010). *Ethical principles of psychologists and code of conduct*. Washington, DC: American Psychological Association. Retrieved June 20, 2011 from http://www.apa.org/ethics/code/index.aspx/.

Animal rights and wrongs. (2011). *Nature*, 470(7335). Retrieved March 24, 2016 from http://www.nature.com/nature/journal/v470/n7335/full/470435a.html.

Association for the Assessment and Accreditation of Laboratory Animal Care International (AAALAC) (2015). *About AAALAC*. Retrieved July 20, 2015 from http://www.aaalac.org/about/index.cfm.

Athanassoulis, N., & Wilson, J. (2009). When is deception in research ethical? *Clinical Ethics*, 4(1), 44–49.

Baker, S., Brawley, O., & Marks, L. (2005). Effects of untreated syphilis in the Negro male, 1932–1972: Closure comes to the Tuskegee study, 2004. *Urology*, 65(6), 1259–1262.

Beattie, E. (2009). Research participation of individuals with dementia: Decisional capacity, informed consent, and considerations for nurse investigators. *Research in Gerontological Nursing*, 2(2), 94–102.

Beebe, L. H., & Smith, K. (2010). Informed consent to research in persons with schizophrenia spectrum disorders. *Nursing Ethics*, 17(4), 425–434.

Beecher, H. K. (1966). Ethics and clinical research. *New England Journal of Medicine*, 274(24), 1354–1360.

Bennett, A. (2014). *Animal research: The bigger picture and why we need psychologists to speak out*. American Psychological Association. Retrieved July 18, 2015 from http://www.apa.org/science/about/psa/2012/04/animal-research.aspx.

Bledsoe, M., & Grizzle, W. (2013). Use of human specimens in research: The evolving United States regulatory, policy, and scientific landscape. *Diagnostic Histopathology*, 15(9), 322–330.

Brandt, A. M. (1978). Racism and research: The case of the Tuskegee Syphilis Study. *Hastings Center Report*, 8(6), 21–29.

Brief, E., & Illes, J. (2010). Tangles of neurogenetics, neuroethics, and culture. *Neuron*, 68(2), 174–177.

Broome, M. E. (1999). Consent (assent) for research with pediatric patients. *Seminars in Oncology Nursing*, 15(2), 96–103.

Broome, M. E., & Stieglitz, K. A. (1992). The consent process and children. *Research in Nursing & Health*, 15(2), 147–152.

Cahana, A., & Hurst, S. A. (2008). Voluntary informed consent in research and clinical care: An update. *Pain Practice*, 8(6), 446–451.

Caplan, A., & Moreno, J. (2011). The Havasu 'Baaja tribe and informed consent. *The Lancet*, 377(9766), 621–622.

Carbone, L. (2012). The utility of basic animal research. Special report. *Hastings Center Report*, 42(6), S12–S15.

Chwang, E. (2015). Against harmful research on non-agreeing children. *Bioethics*, 29(6), 431–439.

Council for International Organizations of Medical Sciences (CIOMS) (2013). *CIOMS: About us*. Retrieved July 10, 2015 from http://www.cioms.ch/about/frame_about.htm/.

Council for International Organizations of Medical Sciences in Collaboration with the World Health Organization (CIOMS-WHO). (2009). *International ethical guidelines for epidemiological studies*. Author: Geneva.

Eriksson, S. (2012). On the need for improved protections for incapacitated and non-benefitting research subjects. *Bioethics*, 26(1), 15–21.

Erlen, J. A. (2010). Informed consent: Revisiting the issues. *Orthopaedic Nursing*, 29(4), 276–280.

Fawcett, J., & Garity, J. (2009). *Evaluation research for evidence-based practice*. Philadelphia, PA: F. A. Davis.

Fierz, K., Gennaro, S., Dierickx, K., Van Achterbert, T., Morin, K., De Geest, S., et al. (2014). Scientific misconduct: Also an issue in nursing science? *Journal of Nursing Scholarship, 46*(4), 271–280.

Foth, T. (2013). Understanding 'caring' through biopolitics: The case of nurses under the Nazi regime. *Nursing Philosophy, 14*(4), 284–294.

Fry, S. T., Veatch, R. M., & Taylor, C. (2011). *Case studies in nursing ethics* (4th ed.). Sudbury, MA: Jones & Bartlett Learning.

Gallagher, J., Gorovitz, S., & Levine, R. (2000). *Biomedical research ethics: Updating international guidelines: A consultation.* Geneva, Switzerland: Council of International Organizations of Medical Sciences.

Gilbert, S. (2012). Progress in the animal research war. *Hastings Center Report, 42*(6), S2–S3.

Grady, C., Wiener, L., Abdoler, E., Trauernicht, E., Zadeh, S., Diekema, D., et al. (2014). Assent in research: The voices of adolescents. *Journal of Adolescent Health, 54*(5), 515–520.

Grootens-Wiegers, P., de Vries, M., van Beusekom, M., van Dijck, L., & van den Broek, J. (2015). Comic strips help children understand medical research: Targeting the informed consent procedure to children's needs. *Patient Education and Counseling, 98*(4), 518–524.

Grootens-Wiegers, P., de Vries, M., & van den Broek, J. (2015). Research information for minors: Suitable formats and readability. A systematic review. *Journal of Paediatrics and Child Health, 51*(5), 505–511.

Habermann, B., Broome, M., Pryor, E. R., & Ziner, K. W. (2010). Research coordinators' experiences with scientific misconduct and research integrity. *Nursing Research, 59*(1), 51–57.

Hansen, B. C., & Hansen, K. D. (1995). Academic and scientific misconduct: Issues for nursing educators. *Journal of Professional Nursing, 11*(1), 31–39.

Hawley, D. J., & Jeffers, J. M. (1992). Scientific misconduct as a dilemma for nursing. *Image—Journal of Nursing Scholarship, 24*(1), 51–55.

Hastings Center (2012). *Animals used in research in US.* Retrieved July 9, 2015 from http://animalresearch.thehastingscenter.org/facts-sheets/animals-used-in-research-in-the-united-states/.

Havens, G. (2004). Ethical implications for the professional nurse of research involving human subjects. *Journal of Vascular Nursing, 22*(1), 19–23.

Health and Medicine Division (2013). *NIH announces plans to reduce its use of chimpanzees in NIH-funded biomedical research: Action taken.* Retrieved July 28, 2016 from http://nationalacademies.org/hmd/reports/2011/chimpanzees-in-biomedical-and-behavioral-research-assessing-the-necessity/action-taken.aspx.

Hershey, N., & Miller, R. D. (1976). *Human experimentation and the law.* Germantown, MD: Aspen.

Hunfeld, J., & Passchier, J. (2012). Participation in medical research: A systematic review of the understanding and experience of children and adolescents. *Patient Education and Counseling, 87*(3), 268–275.

Institute of Medicine (2011). *Report brief: Chimpanzees in biomedical and behavioral research: Assessing the necessity.* Retrieved July 28, 2016 from http://www.nationalacademies.org/hmd/~/media/Files/%20Report%20Files/2011/Chimpanzees/chimpanzeereportbrief.pdf.

International Council of Medical Journal Editors (2014). *Recommendations for the conduct, reporting, editing, and publication of scholarly work in medical journals.* Retrieved July 18, 2015 from http://www.icmje.org/icmje-recommendations.pdf.

Irani, E., & Richmond, T. (2015). Reasons for and reservations about research participation in acutely injured adults. *Journal of Nursing Scholarship, 47*(2), 161–169.

Jacobs, S. (2008). Revisiting hateful science: The Nazi "contribution" to the journey of antisemitism. *Journal of Hate Studies, 7*(1), 47–75.

Johantgen, M. (2010). Using existing administrative and national database. In C. Waltz, O. Strickland, & W. Lenz (Eds.), *Measurement in nursing and health research* (4th ed., pp. 241–250). New York: Springer.

Jones, B. (2015). Knowledge, beliefs, and feelings about breast cancer: The perspective of African American women. *Association of Black Nursing Faculty (ABNF) Journal, 26*(1), 5–10.

Jones, D. J., Munro, C. L., Grap, M. J., Kitten, T., & Edmond, M. (2010). Oral care and bacteremia risk in mechanically ventilated adults. *Heart and Lung: The Journal of Critical Care, 39*(6S), S57–S65.

Jones, H. W. (1997). Record of the first physician to see Henrietta Lacks at the Johns Hopkins Hospital: History of the HeLa cell line. *American Journal of Obstetrics and Gynecology, 176*(6), s227–s228.

Kelman, H. C. (1967). Human use of human subjects: The problem of deception in social psychological experiments. *Psychological Bulletin, 67*(1), 1–11.

Kim, E., & Kim, S. (2015). Simplification improves understanding of informed consent information in clinical trials regardless of health literacy level. *Clinical Trials, 12*(3), 232–236.

Kumpunen, S., Shipway, L., Taylor, R., Aldiss, S., & Gibson, F. (2012). Practical approaches to seeking assent from children. *Nurse Researcher, 19*(2), 23–27.

Kushner, J. (2014). The ethics of personalized medicine. *Personalized Medicine Universe, 3*, 42–45.

Leibson, T., & Koren, G. (2015). Informed consent in pediatric research. *Pediatric Drugs, 17*(1), 5–11.

Levine, R. (1986). *Ethics and regulations of clinical research* (2nd ed.). Baltimore, MD: Urban & Schwarzenberg.

Linder, L., Ameringer, S., Erickson, J., Macpherson, C., Stegenga, K., & Linder, W. (2013). Using an iPad in research with children and adolescents. *Journal of Specialists in Pediatric Nursing, 18*(2), 158–164.

Manton, A., Wolf, L., Baker, K., Carman, M., Clark, P., Henderson, D., et al. (2014). Ethical considerations in human subjects research. *Journal of Emergency Nursing, 40*(1), 92–94.

McCullagh, M., Sanon, M., & Cohen, M. (2014). Strategies to enhance participant recruitment and retention in research involving a community-based population. *Applied Nursing Research, 27*(4), 249–253.

McEwen, J., Boyer, J., & Sun, K. (2013). Evolving approaches to the ethical management of genomic data. *Trends in Genetics, 29*(6), 375–382.

Milgram, S. (1963). Behavioral study of obedience. *Journal of Abnormal and Social Psychology, 67*(4), 371–378.

Montalvo, W., & Larson, E. (2014). Participant comprehension of research for which they volunteer: A systematic review. *Journal of Nursing Scholarship, 46*(6), 423–431.

Morse, J., & Coulehan, J. (2015). Maintaining confidentiality in qualitative publications. *Qualitative Health Research, 25*(2), 151–152.

Munhall, P. L. (2012a). Ethical considerations in qualitative research. In P. L. Munhall (Ed.), *Nursing research: A qualitative perspective* (5th ed., pp. 491–502). Sudbury, MA: Jones & Bartlett Learning.

Munhall, P. L. (2012b). Institutional review of qualitative research proposals: A task of no small consequence. In P. L. Munhall (Ed.), *Nursing research: A qualitative perspective* (5th ed., pp. 503–515). Sudbury, MA: Jones & Bartlett Learning.

National Commission for the Protection of Human Subjects of Biomedical and Behavioral Research (1978). *Belmont report: Ethical principles and guidelines for research involving human subjects (DHEW Publication No. [05] 78–0012).* Washington, DC: U.S. Government Printing Office.

National Institutes of Health Office of Research on Women's Health (2015). *Background: Inclusion of women and minorities in research.* Retrieved July 7, 2015 from http://orwh.od.nih.gov/research/inclusion/background.asp.

National Quality Forum (2005). *Implementing a national volunteer consensus standard for informed consent.* Washington, DC: Author.

Nelson-Marten, P., & Rich, B. (1999). A historical perspective on informed consent in clinical practice and research. *Seminars in Oncology Nursing, 15*(2), 81–88.

Nuremberg Code (1949). *Trials of War Criminals before the Nuremberg Military Tribunals under Control Council Law No. 10* (Vol. 2, pp. 181–182). Washington, D.C.: U.S. Government Printing Office. Retrieved July 7, 2015 from http://www.hhs.gov/ohrp/archive/nurcode.html.

Office for Laboratory Animal Research (2011). *Guide for the care and use of laboratory animals* (8th ed.). Washington, DC: National Academies Press.

Office of Laboratory Animal Welfare (OLAW) (2011). *For researchers and institutions: Good animal care and good science go hand-in-hand.* Retrieved July 15, 2015 from http://grants.nih.gov/grants/policy/air/researchers_institutions.htm/.

Office of Laboratory Animal Welfare (OLAW) (2015). *Obtaining an assurance.* Retrieved July 15, 2015 from http://grants.nih.gov/grants/olaw/obtain_assurance.htm.

Office of Research Integrity (ORI) (2005). *Public Health Service Policies on Research Misconduct.* Code of Federal Regulations, Title 42, Parts 50 and 93, Policies of General Applicability. Retrieved July 7, 2015 from http://ori.dhhs.gov/documents/FR_Doc_05–9643.shtml.

Office of Research Integrity (ORI) (2012). *About ORI—History.* Retrieved March 23, 2016 from http://ori.dhhs.gov/about/history.shtml/.

Office of Research Integrity (ORI) (2015a). *Case summaries - Case summary Ryan Asherin.* Retrieved March 23, 2016 from http://ori.hhs.gov/content/case-summary-asherin-ryan.

Office of Research Integrity (ORI) (2015b). *Handling misconduct—Case summaries.* Retrieved March 23, 2016 from http://ori.dhhs.gov/misconduct/cases/.

Olsen, D. (2003). Methods: HIPAA privacy regulations and nursing research. *Nursing Research, 52*(5), 344–348.

Ondrusek, N., Abramovitch, R., Pencharz, P., & Koren, G. (1998). Empirical examination of the ability of children to consent to clinical research. *Journal of Medical Ethics, 24*(3), 158–164.

Presidential Commission for the Study of Bioethical Issues (2011). *"Ethically impossible:" STD research in Guatemala 1946-1948.* Retrieved July 10, 2015 from http://www.bioethics.gov.

Pritts, J. (2008). *The importance and value of protecting the privacy of health information: The roles of the HIPAA Privacy Rule and the Common Rule in health research.* National Academy of Science Paper. Retrieved March 24, 2016 from http://iom.nationalacademies.org/~/media/Files/Activity%20Files/Research/HIPAAandResearch/PrittsPrivacyFinalDraftweb.ashx.

Reverby, S. (2012). Ethical failures and history lessons: The U.S. Public Health Service research studies in Tuskegee and Guatemala. *Public Health Reviews, 43*(1), 1–18.

Rew, L., Horner, S. D., & Fouladi, R. T. (2010). Factors associated with health behaviors in middle childhood. *Journal of Pediatric Nursing, 25*(3), 157–166.

Reynolds, P. D. (1979). *Ethical dilemmas and social science research.* San Francisco, CA: Jossey-Bass.

Riegel, B., Lee, C. S., Albert, N., Lennie, T., Chung, M., Song, E. K., et al. (2011). From novice to expert: Confidence and activity status determine heart failure self-care performance. *Nursing Research, 60*(2), 132–138.

Rivers, E., Schuman, S., Simpon, L., & Olansky, S. (1953). Twenty years of followup experience in a long-range medical study. *Public Health Reports, 68*(4), 391–395.

Rothman, D. J. (1982). Were Tuskegee and Willowbrook "studies in nature"? *Hastings Center Report, 12*(2), 5–7.

Rubin, S. (2014). The clinical trials nurse as subject advocate for minority and culturally diverse research subjects. *Journal of Transcultural Nursing, 25*(4), 383–387.

Sanjari, M., Bahramnezhad, F., Fomani, F., Shoghi, M., & Cheraghi, A. (2014). Ethical challenges of researchers in qualitative studies: The necessity to develop a specific guideline. *Journal of Medical Ethics and History of Medicine, 7*(14), 1–6.

Sarpatwari, A., Kesselheim, A., Malin, B., Gagne, J., & Schneeweiss, S. (2014). Ensuring patient privacy in data sharing for postapproval research. *The New England Journal of Medicine, 137*(17), 1644–1649.

Schwenzer, K. (2008). Protecting vulnerable subjects in clinical research: Children, pregnant women, prisoners, and employees. *Respiratory Care, 53*(10), 1342–1349.

Shamoo, A., & Resnik, R. (2015). *Responsible conduct of research* (3rd ed.). New York, NY: Oxford University Press.

Simpson, C. (2010). Decision-making capacity and informed consent to participate in research by cognitively impaired individuals. *Applied Nursing Research, 23*(4), 221–226.

Skloot, R. (2010). *The immortal life of Henrietta Lacks.* New York, NY: Crown Publishing.

Steinfels, P., & Levine, C. (1976). Biomedical ethics and the shadow of Naziism. *Hastings Center Report, 6*(4), 1–20.

Stevens, P., & Pletsch, P. (2002). Informed consent and the history of inclusion of women in clinical research. *Health Care for Women International, 23*(8), 809–819.

Streubert, H., & Carpenter, D. (2011). *Qualitative research in nursing: Advancing the humanistic imperative.* Philadelphia, PA: Lippincott Williams & Wilkins.

Sweet, L., Adamis, D., Meagher, D. J., Davis, D., Currow, D. C., Bush, S. H., et al. (2014). Ethical challenges and solutions regarding delirium studies in palliative care. *Journal of Pain and Symptom Management, 48*(2), 259–271.

Terry, N. (2015). Developments in genetic and epigenetic data protection in behavioral and mental health spaces. *Behavioral Sciences & Law, 33*(5), 653–661.

Terry, S., & Terry, P. (2001). A consumer perspective on informed consent and third-party issues. *Journal of Continuing Education in the Health Professions, 21*(4), 256–264.

U.S. Department of Health and Human Services (DHHS). (1998). *Informed consent checklist: Basic and additional elements.* Retrieved March 26, 2016 from Office for Human Subjects Protection website http://www.hhs.gov/ohrp/regulations-and-policy/guidance/checklists/index.html.

U.S. Department of Health and Human Services (U.S. DHHS) (1981, January 26). *Final regulations amending basic HHS policy for the protection of human research subjects.* Code of Federal Regulations, Title 45, Part 46.

U.S. Department of Health and Human Services (U.S. DHHS) (2003). *Health information privacy: Summary of the HIPAA Privacy Rule.* Retrieved July 12, 2015 from http://www.hhs.gov/ocr/privacy/hipaa/understanding/summary/index.html/.

U.S. Department of Health and Human Services (U.S. DHHS) (2004). *Institutional review boards and the HIPAA Privacy Rule.* Retrieved July 11, 2015 from http://privacyruleandresearch.nih.gov/irbandprivacyrule.asp/.

U.S. Department of Health and Human Services (U.S. DHHS) (2005). *Children involved as subjects in research: Guidance on the HHS 45 CFR 46.407 ("407") review process.* Retrieved July 13, 2015 from http://www.hhs.gov/ohrp/policy/populations/guidance_407process.html.

U.S. Department of Health and Human Services (U.S. DHHS) (2007a). *How do other privacy protections interact with the privacy rule?* Retrieved July 12, 2015 from http://privacyruleandresearch.nih.gov/pr_05.asp/.

U.S. Department of Health and Human Services (U.S. DHHS) (2007b). *How can covered entities use and disclose protected health information for research and comply with the Privacy Rule?* Retrieved July 12, 2015 from http://privacyruleandresearch.nih.gov/pr_08.asp/.

U.S. Department of Health and Human Services (U.S. DHHS) (2009). *Protection of human subjects.* Code of Federal Regulations, Title 45, Part 46. Retrieved July 12, 2015 from http://www.hhs.gov/ohrp/policy/ohrpregulations.pdf.

U.S. Department of Health and Human Services (U.S. DHHS) (2010). *HIPAA Privacy Rule Information for researchers: Overview.* Retrieved July 12, 2015 from http://privacyruleandresearch.nih.gov/.

U.S. Department of Health and Human Services (U.S. DHHS) (2012). *Office for Human Research Protections (OHRP).* Retrieved March 24, 2016 from http://www.hhs.gov/ohrp/.

U.S. Department of Health and Human Services (U.S. DHHS) (2013). *HIPAA Administrative Simplification.* Retrieved March 24, 2015 from http://www.hhs.gov/sites/default/files/ocr/privacy/hipaa/administrative/combined/hipaa-simplification-201303.pdf.

U.S. Department of Health and Human Services (U.S. DHHS) (2015a). *Public Health Service policy on humane care and treatment of laboratory animals.* Retrieved from July 15, 2015 http://grants.nih.gov/grants/olaw/references/PHSPolicyLabAnimals.pdf.

U.S. Department of Health and Human Services (U.S. DHHS) (2015b). *Regulatory changes in the ANPRM [Advanced Notice of Proposed Rulemaking].* Retrieved March 24, 2015 from http://www.hhs.gov/ohrp/humansubjects/anprmchangetable.html.

U.S. Food and Drug Administration. (2015). *Code of Federal Regulations, Title 21 Food and Drugs,* Department of Health and Human Services, Part 50 Protection of Human Subjects. Retrieved March 24, 2016 from https://www.accessdata.fda.gov/scripts/cdrh/cfdocs/cfcfr/CFRSearch.cfm?CFRPart=50.

U.S. Food and Drug Administration (FDA) (2010a). *Protection of human subjects (informed consent).* Code of Federal Regulations, Title 21, Part 50. Retrieved July 15, 2015 from http://www.accessdata.fda.gov/scripts/cdrh/cfdocs/cfcfr/CFRsearch.cfm?CFRPart=50/.

U.S. Food and Drug Administration (FDA) (2010b). *Institutional review boards.* Code of Federal Regulations, Title 21, Part 56. Retrieved July 12, 2015 from http://www.accessdata.fda.gov/scripts/cdrh/cfdocs/cfcfr/CFRsearch.cfm?CFRPart=56/.

Wendler, D., & Rid, A. (2015). Genetic research on biospecimens poses minimum risk. *Trends in Genetics, 31*(1), 11–15.

World Association of Medical Editors [WAME] (n.d.). *About WAME.* Retrieved July 19, 2015 from http://www.wame.org/.

World Medical Association (WMA) General Assembly (1964). *Declaration of Helsinki (1964).* Helsinki, Finland: Author. Retrieved June 20, 2011 from http://www.cirp.org/library/ethics/helsinki/.

World Medical Association (WMA) General Assembly (2008). *World Medical Association Declaration of Helsinki: Ethical principles for medical research involving human subjects.* Seoul, Korea: Author. Retrieved July 11, 2015 from http://www.wma.net/en/30publications/10policies/b3/.

World Medical Association (2013). *Press release: WMA publishes its revised Declaration of Helsinki.* Retrieved March 24, 2016 from http://www.wma.net/en/40news/20archives/2013/2013_28/.

Yamal, J., Robertson, C., Rubin, M., Benoit, J., Hannay, H., & Tilley, B. (2014). Enrollment of racially/ethnically diverse participants in traumatic brain injury trials: Effect of availability of exception from informed consent. *Clinical Trials, 11*(2), 187–194.

Yurek, L., Vasey, J., & Havens, D. (2008). The use of self-generated identification codes in longitudinal research. *Evaluation Review, 32*(5), 435–452.

10

Quantitative Methodology: Noninterventional Designs and Methods

Suzanne Sutherland

ⓔ http://evolve.elsevier.com/Gray/practice/

The researcher's process of planning and creating proposed research is referred to as designing the study: this process includes selecting the general type of research to be conducted, choosing its specific subtype, and, finally, deciding on the particulars of the actual conduct of the research. Designing is a multistep endeavor that is the single most important component in producing a study that is appropriate to the discipline, well grounded, credible, precise, and useful. For this reason, it is time-consuming because it involves considerable reflection.

Designing a study includes three decisions: what the research methodology will be, what research design will be employed, and what research methods will be selected. Collectively, these represent the researcher's plan for conducting the study. In the literature, the three terms, "methodology," "design," and "methods," are used in an overlapping manner and often are substituted for one another, to the chagrin of the well-prepared reader who really understands what each term means.

The **research methodology** represents the major type of research used for a study. For the purpose of designing research, methodology types are quantitative and qualitative. All existent designs used for nursing research can be classified as quantitative, qualitative, or mixed. Quantitative and qualitative methodologies emanate from research traditions of other disciplines and are reflective of philosophies, logic, structures, strategies, and general rules embedded in those traditions. Outcomes research is founded on the same philosophies as quantitative research but has the unique characteristic that its focus is on quality of care. Mixed methods research refers to research with more than one

methodological type or more than one research design. The vast majority of mixed methods studies use one quantitative design and one qualitative, as described in Chapter 14.

Research design is the researcher's choice of the best way in which to answer a research question, with respect to several considerations, including number of subject groups, timing of data collection, and researcher intervention, if any. Quantitative research may be interventional or noninterventional, as displayed in the algorithm, Figure 10-1. Interventional designs test the effect of an intentional action, called an intervention, on a measured result. Interventional research includes both experimental and quasi-experimental designs. Noninterventional designs count and measure characteristics about the phenomenon of interest and the study variables as they exist naturally, without intentional intervention. Noninterventional research in this text is divided into descriptive designs and correlational designs. Although correlational research is noninterventional, it is distinct from descriptive research because its focus is to describe relationships between and among variables, whereas the intent of descriptive research is to describe the variables themselves (see Figure 10-1).

Within the four subdivisions of experimental, quasi-experimental, correlational, and descriptive research lie the specific designs of quantitative research, like the predictive correlational design, the Solomon four-group design, and the one-group pretest-posttest design. In most research reports, it is assumed that the reader knows, for instance, that a cross-sectional design is descriptive in nature, that the one-group pretest-posttest design is quasi-experimental research, and that the

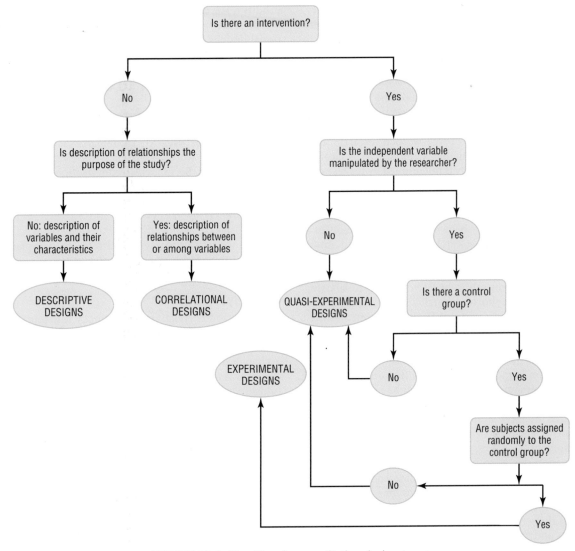

FIGURE 10-1 Algorithm for quantitative design types.

Solomon four-group design is experimental. Authors of published research reports identify the name of the specific design used but may or may not identify the major subdivision of quantitative research methodology to which a design belongs. The reader unfamiliar with a certain design usually can determine its major subdivision within the report's context; however, it is sometimes necessary to refer to a textbook or an online resource for clarification, especially for complex or rare designs.

The researcher chooses the methodology and design that seem best able to provide a meaningful answer to the proposed study's research question. In quantitative research, the answer is provided through statistical analysis of quantitative research's output, numerical data. For reasons of clear communication, the researcher should state the research methodology and design clearly near the beginning of the research report, be it a publication or a presentation, so that the consumer of research knows what to expect.

After methodology and design are decided upon, the researcher defines the study methods. The **methods** are the specific ways in which the researcher chooses to conduct the study, within the chosen design. These are the details of the endeavor, the bare bones of inquiry, and include how the research site or sites will be selected, which subjects should be included, how those subjects will be recruited and consented, what data collection tools will be used, how data will be collected, how any interventions will be enacted, how data will be organized, and how data will be analyzed. The methods of a study are reported in the Methods section of the proposal or research report.

For the vast majority of well-worded research questions, the choice of a suitable methodology is clear. If the choice of methodology is not implied by the research question, the researcher should reword the question until it indicates the methodology more clearly.

For well-worded research questions the design is implied, but there may be several suitable designs for a given question. The research question should imply whether the researcher will enact an intervention in order to answer that question. For example, the question, "Will administration of IV vitamin C to laboring mothers result in shorter labors?" suggests that laboring mothers will be administered IV vitamin C in an interventional study, using one of the experimental or quasi-experimental research designs. In a similar manner, the question, "Is there a relationship between vegan diet and postpartum hemorrhage?" implies that one of the correlational designs very probably will be used.

As for methods, there are numerous potential research method strategies, some better, some worse, for answering a particular question. Review of existent research publications, identification of available subjects, inquiries as to possible research settings, refinement of research objectives, timeline constraints, and need for precision are considerations for selection of the specific methods for a study. The best researcher considers all elements that might diminish the accuracy of the results and the believability of the conclusions, and then designs the study within the realities of available time and practicality.

Intrinsically, no one quantitative research design is superior to any other. The best design for a given question is the one that best answers that pressing question, providing results marked by accuracy, timeliness, and practical utility. In a problem area in which very little is known, descriptive research may be the perfect design choice. In an area in which there is already considerable knowledge, including several correlational or interventional studies, an interventional design may be the best choice, building logically upon previous information.

This chapter introduces concepts important in the design of noninterventional quantitative research, and explains how the various types of quantitative design validity relate to noninterventional research. The chapter concludes with a presentation of various noninterventional designs, both descriptive and correlational, their uses, their salient features, and examples of each.

CONCEPTS RELEVANT TO QUANTITATIVE RESEARCH DESIGNS

Research design uses many terms with specific meanings within a science context. In research literature, the meaning of the words is distinctly different than their meaning would be in casual conversation. Several of these terms—*causality, multiple causality, probability, bias, measurement, manipulation, control, partitioning, prospective versus retrospective,* and *validity*—present varied aspects within different design types. Their importance to noninterventional research is explained here, and their implications for interventional research are presented in Chapter 11.

Causality

Causality and correlation are distinctly different. **Causality** refers to a cause-and-effect relationship (Shadish, Cook, & Campbell, 2002), in which one variable causes a change in another. Interventional research tests the stated or implied hypothesis of a cause-and-effect relationship between variables, in which a researcher enacts an intervention that causes a change in the dependent variable. Noninterventional research describes variables as they exist, sometimes examining the relationship or association between variables but never establishing causality. In noninterventional research, a researcher does not enact an intervention in order to measure its effect: in noninterventional research, all that a researcher does is classify, count, measure, and retrieve data.

According to the 18th-century philosopher Hume (1999), many conditions must be present for a causational relationship to exist. One of these, a strong relationship between the proposed cause and effect, may be present in non-causational relationships, as well: in and of itself, that strong relationship cannot be the sole criterion of causation. An example of this is the relationship between work stress and home stress: one type of stress cannot be said to cause the other, just because they are related.

Another condition that must be present is that the proposed cause must occur earlier in time than the proposed result (Hume, 1999). In the same way, the timing of variables so that a proposed cause always precedes an effect may be present in non-causational relationships, as well: in and of itself, preceding something else in time is not enough to conclude that a causational relationship exists. An example of this is the correlation between scores on the Scholastic Aptitude Test (SAT) and academic success in college: scoring well on the SAT does not cause subsequent academic success.

Both the reader and the designer of research must be clear on these points. Causality is discussed at some length in Chapter 11: Quantitative Methodology: Interventional Designs and Methods.

Multiple Causality

Multiple causality, *multifactorial causation, multicausation,* and *multicausality* are terms derived from epidemiology and medicine. They refer to the case in which two or more variables combine in causing an effect (Acheson, 1970; Stein & Susser, 1970). Again, cause relates to interventional research. However, noninterventional research sometimes explores relationships among many variables, so that a theory of possibilities can be constructed through use of a model-testing design, a correlational strategy discussed later in this chapter. After a new model is constructed and affirmed through demonstration of strong relationships among variables, the model can provide the theoretical basis for a subsequent interventional study.

Probability and Prediction

Prediction is the offering of an opinion or guess about an unknown or future event, amount, outcome, or result. Prediction is sometimes 100%: if the head is separated from the body, clinical death will result. More often, prediction is based on probabilities. Probabilities are likelihoods, expressed as percentages. For instance, it is predicted that a first-time offender convicted of a crime against property will be arrested again for a similar crime within 5 years, and that probability is greater than 82% (National Institute of Justice, 2014). This means that after an individual convicted of a crime against property is released from incarceration, it is probable that the person will be rearrested, but it is not a certainty. For every six persons, on average, the dire prediction of re-conviction will fail for one of them. Prediction of outcomes is important in healthcare research because of the multifactorial nature of human health and illness. For nurses in all areas ranging from critical care through ambulatory settings, it is clinically desirable to be able to predict adverse patient events before they occur.

Bias

The word **bias** is derived from a French word that means slant or oblique. In common parlance, it refers to a point of view that differs from truth; it slants away from the square, the objective, the balanced, leaning to one side. In designing research, it is important to be aware of bias emanating from decisions made during this phase of the study, because many aspects of the design process are subject to bias. The researcher can hold a biased view. Measurements made can lean in a certain direction. For example, systematic error occurs when a scale is not calibrated correctly and all measurements are skewed by the same amount. Subjects selected may not represent a population well, introducing bias into the analysis. The research assistant assigning a number to subjects' behaviors may rate some individuals higher than others for reasons of personal bias such as preconception, perceptual problems, poor technique, and fatigue. Measurements always contain a certain amount of error, as well. This is why replication of results is so essential in increasing believability.

Potentially, all quantitative research designs are affected by bias. An important concern in designing a study is to identify possible sources of bias early in the process and eliminate those that are susceptible to modification by using better-trained observers, more precisely calibrated instruments, stronger statistical analyses, more intelligently selected samples, and operational definitions that are worded more specifically.

Measurement

Measurement refers to the process whereby some sort of value is assigned to a variable (see Chapters 3 and 16 for further detail). The tools of measurement, such as questionnaires, calipers, blood pressure cuffs, and printed inventories, must do their job well. When you as a researcher decide upon a certain measurement for a variable in your study, you want it to be appropriate for that variable's conceptual definition, and you want it to prove both accurate and consistent over time. These attributes of accuracy and consistency refer to that measurement's validity and reliability. In addition, precision is essential, so that you can be sure that the value obtained is measured with a specificity that is adequate for meaningful statistical analysis. If you decide to measure systolic blood pressure as one of three values, low (0 to 80), medium (81 to 160), or high (161 to 240), your statistical analysis will be nonsensical: a more precise measurement is indicated. Choice of measurement method and that method's validity, reliability, and precision all determine the quality of the raw data you so laboriously obtain during the data collection process.

Manipulation

Manipulation is another word for intervention. It refers to the quantitative researcher's action of changing the value of the independent variable in order to measure its effect on the dependent variable. Researcher manipulation is present in interventional research, but never present in noninterventional research.

In some types of basic descriptive research, however, measures may be made of subjects under different artificially produced conditions in order to describe characteristics. This does not constitute manipulation. New readers of research may mistake this type of research as interventional when it is indeed descriptive. Even though the researcher introduces something that changes subjects' responses, if description is the only goal, the research is noninterventional. For instance, a basic cognitive researcher describing differences in test scores in a threatening environment as opposed to a safe one might introduce frightening sounds and sights into the testing environment, in order to produce the condition of "threat." The basic researcher's intent is not to quantify the effect of lab milieu on scores: the intent is to describe subjects' test performance under two different conditions, both of which the researcher has simulated in the lab setting.

Control

Control in research design means control for the effects of potentially extraneous variables (Campbell & Stanley, 1963; Shadish et al., 2002). This is a serious issue for interventional research. However, researchers using noninterventional designs also can choose to control for possibly extraneous variables that might interfere with results by broadening a study's exclusion criteria, so as to eliminate subjects with a characteristic that might introduce bias by means of an extraneous variable. An example of this would be a study that measures pre-procedural anxiety before routine colonoscopy. A researcher might decide to exclude potential subjects who have experienced accidental colon perforation during a previous colonoscopy, anticipating that their anxiety scores might be atypically elevated.

Prospective Versus Retrospective

Prospective is a term that means looking forward, whereas **retrospective** means looking backward, usually in relationship to time. Within research studies, these terms are used most frequently to refer to the timing of data collection. Are the data obtained in "real time," with measurements being obtained by the research team, or are the study data retrieved from data collected at a prior time for a different purpose?

Much of noninterventional research in health care uses retrospective data, drawn from health records archived in electronic databases. This is especially true

of outcomes research (Chapter 13), which examines various aspects of quality of care using predominantly correlational and descriptive designs to analyze preexistent data. Data collection in noninterventional research can be either prospective or retrospective because, by definition, it lacks researcher intervention. In nursing research, prospective data collection has a somewhat better chance of being accurate than does retrospective. This is partially because you as a researcher, by your presence, example, and passionate curiosity about the phenomenon of interest, encourage staff through role-modeling to be rigorous in measurement and data collection. You observe staff as they collect data, or perhaps collect the data yourself.

Many nurse researchers choose prospective data collection so that they can obtain data with fewer errors. The accuracy of retrospective data depends on the meticulousness of those who entered those data originally. Researchers using retrospective data must examine the raw data and "clean" it, if necessary, before it is analyzed. An example would be a database containing demographic information, in which the value for Number of Live Children Born for one subject is 444. It is likely that the person entering data "stuttered" when tapping in the number. The error in that piece of data means that it must be discarded, or corrected if the actual value can be confirmed, because the number 444 is not a reasonable value for the variable.

Epidemiologists use noninterventional strategies extensively to track disease outbreaks and patterns. Within their field, prospective research is considered a stronger design choice than retrospective, because the preexistence of a disease before data collection begins can be ruled out, making a stronger case for the hypothesis that exposure (whether that exposure is to a virus, a bacterium, a protozoan, radiation, or another potentially harmful entity) eventually causes the disease or condition in question.

Data collection in experimental research, however, must be prospective because the researcher enacts an intervention in real time. This is not to say that the research team does not access current data from the medical record for real-time studies. A researcher collecting arterial blood pressure data in critically ill infants using a new protocol for administration of vasopressors such as dobutamine might collect data over a 24-hour period for several days. Nurses on the various shifts would record arterial blood pressure at least hourly, as is common practice, and the research team would retrieve that information during daily data collection. Although information retrieval of the infants' electronic chart data does look back in time over the preceding

24-hour period, this study would be considered prospective because it is generated and recorded at the same time that infants are hospitalized.

Partitioning

Partitioning, also called **event-partitioning** or **treatment-partitioning**, is a strategy in which the researcher analyzes subjects according to a variable that could be regarded as dichotomous but actually has several different values. This method of analysis is useful when subjects are different from one another in respect to a certain characteristic, such as an exposure, a medication, or a repeated occurrence, and the researcher wants to examine the results in relation to increments of this difference. The strategy can be used in noninterventional research to create subdivisions of the amount of any event that occurs naturally in subjects during the period over which data are collected, as well as in the past. Examples of partitioning in noninterventional research might be found in descriptive or correlational designs in which the researcher examines the incidence of chronic obstructive pulmonary disease (COPD) in relationship to cigarette smoking status. For example, in a simple cross-sectional study, each subject's status as a smoker or nonsmoker might be compared with the presence of COPD and how long it has existed. However, if the researcher has historical information about duration and magnitude of cigarette smoking over the years, the researcher could classify subjects not only as smokers/nonsmokers but also as 5 to 9 pack-year smokers, 10 to 14 pack-year smokers, 15 to 19 pack-year smokers, and so forth. Having this additional detail would allow the researcher to make a more accurate evaluation of disease rates for people with varying amounts of exposure to cigarette smoking's negative effects. A longitudinal study like this one that evaluates the incidence of a disease over time in relation to duration of exposure would be strengthened by partitioning of this sort that roughly establishes cohorts that are equivalent in terms of amount of exposure, corresponding to "dose received."

DESIGN VALIDITY FOR NONINTERVENTIONAL RESEARCH

Design validity, in research, is the degree to which an entity that the researcher believes is being performed, evaluated, measured, or represented is actually what is being performed, evaluated, measured, or represented. Validity of a study is roughly analogous to truthfulness. Validity is an important concern during study design and has several facets (Cook & Campbell, 1986; Shadish et al., 2002): construct validity, internal validity, external validity, and statistical conclusion validity. A factor or condition that decreases the validity of research results is called a **threat to validity**.

Threats to design validity are discussed at length in Chapter 11, because they are of special concern for interventional research. However, design validity does affect noninterventional research, as well. Because validity problems decrease believability of research results, the validity of a study is an important consideration for the usefulness of those results. Each of the four facets of validity can be linked to the limitations of the study that a researcher identifies and lists in a research report's final Discussion section. Limitations to a study are limitations to generalization—essentially limitations to the research's usefulness, due to limited validity.

Construct Validity

The first aspect of design validity is construct validity (Table 10-1). **Construct validity** in quantitative research relates to whether a study measures all aspects of the concepts it purports to measure (Waltz, Strickland, & Lenz, 2010). This is a direct result of how well the researcher has conceptually defined and then operationalized a study's variables. For example, if the topic of the research is satisfaction with the hospital experience, the way the researcher may choose to measure this is with a single question, "Would you please provide a number on a 0- to 10-point scale that represents how satisfied you were with your hospitalization?" The researcher asks patients this question as they are discharged, when they are in the wheelchair on their way out of the hospital. This may not be an optimal operationalization of satisfaction with the hospital experience, partially because it is asked at a time at which the patient is focused in the moment and not given a chance to reflect and analyze previous hospital days and reflect on different aspects of the hospitalization. In addition, a nurse or other hospital employee is present steering the wheelchair, and responses may reflect a desire not to insult the employee. The data collected would measure only the patient's immediate perception and would not provide hospital administration with specific information that would guide changes if satisfaction ratings proved low, nor with information about positive actions of healthcare workers that should be encouraged if ratings were high. Most measurements of satisfaction with the hospital experience are made days or weeks after patients have been discharged. They consist of several focused questions that measure individual aspects of the hospital stay. For instance, the questions in the Hospital Consumer Assessment of Healthcare Providers and Systems

TABLE 10-1	**Design Validity for Noninterventional Research**			
Type of Design Validity	**Meaning**	**Target Point in Noninterventional Designs**	**Related Aspects**
Construct validity	How well the researcher defines the study concepts	Conceptual and operational definitions Substruction	Timing of measurement, persons present during measurement, number of measurements
Internal validity	Whether relationships among variables are truly present or whether they have been acted upon by extraneous variables	Identification of subject inclusion and exclusion criteria Operational definitions Timing and number of measurements	Biased samples Sample heterogeneity versus homogeneity Data collection that reflects seasonal or diurnal variation
External validity	Whether results can be generalized back to the population from which the sample was obtained	Means of sample selection Recruitment Single-site vs. multisite	Subject attrition, especially for extended data-collection
Statistical conclusion validity	Whether the sample is of sufficient size Whether correct statistical tests are used	Sample size determination Data analysis	Power analysis Consultation with statistician

(HCAHPS) survey focus on, among other things, physician communication, nurse communication, information provided about medications, information provided about hospital discharge, responsiveness to patient needs, pain control, noise of surroundings, and cleanliness, as well as an overall impression of care (CMMS, 2012).

The way a variable is operationally defined affects generalization (Shadish et al., 2002), because after the findings are analyzed, generalization is made to situations supporting similar operational definitions of that same variable. If the variable is operationalized too broadly, it may include parts of other related concepts that undermine the study's logic.

Internal Validity

Internal validity reflects design-embedded decisions about how dependent variables and research variables are measured and how those values might be influenced by extraneous variables. **Internal validity** is an assessment of the degree to which the measured relationships among variables are truly due to their interaction, and the degree to which other intrusive variables might have accounted for the measured value (Campbell, 1957). Internal validity is primarily concerned with study operations (Shadish et al., 2002), for instance the way data

measurements are strategized. An example of this in correlational research would be a 2-day study undertaken by dietary services in a hospital, measuring which main courses patients request most often and relationships among their choices, ages, and genders. If a busload of seniors who are also vegetarians should be involved in an accident and hospitalized at the research site during the same 2-day period, research conducted may attribute preference for non-meat entrées to age rather than to pre-illness dietary pattern.

In a similar vein, internal validity in descriptive and correlational research may be affected when research results are subject to seasonal or diurnal variation. If a study in the emergency department of a hospital with a large trauma population is conducted in summer, there would be a disproportionately large number of patients with head injuries and burn injuries. These traumatic classifications peak, respectively, in the early summer and midsummer (Hultman et al., 2012; Sethi et al., 2014). In a similar way, a study of the safety of hospital parking areas might show quite different results at 9:00 in the morning as opposed to midnight.

Similarly, natural fluctuations that can be anticipated in any phenomenon should be compensated for in the research design by collecting data that averages results over a longer period of time. Another example of this would be the types of surgery performed on children and adolescents at a large teaching hospital. Let us assume that there is orthopedic-spinal specialist at this particular hospital who performs many complex scoliosis repairs. This type of surgery is typically postponed until linear growth has ceased. Consequently, patients are usually in high school, during which time prolonged absences from school are to be avoided. Recovery from spinal surgery is lengthy and painful (Charette et al., 2015). Because of this, many surgeries for scoliosis correction occur during summer vacation. If you were conducting research to describe the frequencies of various types of pediatric surgery performed at the hospital annually and accessed inpatient surgery records for a 3-month period, June through August, your research results would reflect a disproportionately elevated number of scoliosis repair cases in the sample.

Sometimes a researcher identifies a potentially extraneous variable that exists in an identifiable portion of the population and, for that reason, decides to narrow the study's inclusion criteria in order to exclude that subpopulation. Physiological studies of women's endocrine values might be conducted using only women who were not pregnant and not receiving any hormone supplements. For that reason, the researcher might be inclined to set inclusion criteria that subjects must be between 30 and 40 years of age, must have had had tubal ligations, and must still be menstruating. The sample in this case would be homogeneous for age and absence of pregnancy. In research, a sample with a high degree of **homogeneity** includes participants who are similar with respect to one or more characteristics. A sample with a high degree of **heterogeneity** is a varied sample, with respect to at least one characteristic. Homogeneous samples allow generalization to a similar homogeneous population; heterogeneous samples allow broader generalization.

External Validity

External validity is the extent to which study findings can be generalized beyond the sample included in the study. It reflects design-resultant decisions that determine the population to which research results can be generalized (Campbell, 1957). External validity is due, in large part, to sampling strategy, because the population to which results can be generalized is the population represented by the sample. Large numbers of subjects who decline participation in a study, or a large proportion of subjects who drop out of a study, also can limit generalization of the findings (for further detail, see Chapters 15 and 26). Selecting a large random sample allows generalization of study findings to the population. Nonrandom sampling may or may not allow this generalization.

An example of random sampling that allows generalization might be research in which half of the nurses in British Columbia, Canada, are sent a brief mailed survey instrument to be returned with their annual applications for relicensure. The half that receives the mailed survey is randomly selected. The mailed survey instrument consists of only three questions that ask the subject's age, number of years in practice, and anticipated year of retirement. Ninety-nine percent of the nurses return the surveys with their applications. Because the targeted sample was not only drawn from the population but was half of the entire population, and the response consisted of almost the entire targeted sample, results can be generalized to all nurses in British Columbia. This study, consequently, is said to have excellent external validity.

Problems with recruitment and sample attrition also affect external validity. Regarding recruitment, if the return rate in the imagined study above had been only 1% or 2% of the population, generalization to all nurses in British Columbia would not have been possible. A very small return of the original randomly selected sample cannot be said to be random any longer. In that case, the external validity of the research would be said to be limited. Similarly, if a study design includes random sampling from a large population in which repeated data collection extends over a long period of time, the greater the subject attrition, the less likely it is that the final sample will be representative of the entire population of interest (for further information about attrition, see Chapter 15).

Statistical Conclusion Validity

Statistical conclusion validity is the degree to which the researcher makes proper decisions about the use of statistics, so that conclusions about relationships and differences drawn from analyses are accurate reflections of reality (Cook & Campbell, 1979; Shadish et al., 2002). Incorrect decisions produce inaccurate conclusions. The two most important considerations for noninterventional research methods, in relation to statistical conclusion validity, are (1) selection of an adequately large sample so that true relationships among variables are revealed, avoiding the threat of inadequate statistical power; and (2) use of the correct statistical tests, given the nature of the study variables.

To avoid the threat of inadequate statistical power in noninterventional research, termed inaccurate effect size estimation (Shadish et al., 2002), a power analysis should be performed, providing an estimate of the number of subjects needed, so that a difference, if it really exists, will be revealed through statistical testing. Then if a statistical test fails to reject the null hypothesis, the researcher can be fairly certain that there was little difference between groups studied. If the sample is too small, and there is failure to reject the null hypothesis, the researcher cannot discern whether this was due to no real relationship between variables or to Type II error (inability to detect a difference due to small sample size). There are online applications that estimate how large a sample is needed for a research project, given the amount of difference anticipated for a given relationship (Lenth, 2006–2009), as well as texts that provide information on power analysis and demonstrate how to perform power calculations, for use with different types of statistical techniques (Grove & Cipher, 2017). If interactions among variables are subtle and small in magnitude, a larger sample is necessary. Statistical power is discussed in Chapter 15. Use of correct statistical tests, with the assumptions of each, is discussed in Chapters 21 through 25.

DESCRIPTIVE RESEARCH AND ITS DESIGNS

Descriptive research is conducted in a natural setting to answer a research question related to incidence, prevalence, or frequency of occurrence of a phenomenon of interest and its characteristics. It is customarily the first quantitative research strategy used to count and classify newly emergent phenomena and their attributes. Without the answers to questions of "What?" or "How much?" that descriptive research provides, it is difficult to construct more complex designs that predict outcomes or establish evidence of causation.

Descriptive designs are of varying levels of complexity, the more involved of them containing more than two variables, with data collection that takes place at more than one time. However, for all types of descriptive and correlational research, simple or complex, there is no researcher intervention, and there is no attempt to demonstrate causality. Figure 10-2 is an algorithm of various descriptive study designs, which are explained in the following sections. Fourteen research reports, some of which have been introduced in previous chapters, are included in Table 10-2, to exemplify various commonly used descriptive and descriptive correlational designs. Descriptive correlational research uses statistical tests to establish both incidence and association. For the purposes of this chapter, descriptive correlational studies are considered descriptive in nature if their primary purpose is to describe variables, and correlational in nature if their primary purpose is to describe relationships between variables.

There are four commonly occurring descriptive research designs: descriptive, comparative descriptive, descriptive longitudinal, and descriptive cross-sectional. The terms "prospective," "retrospective," and "partitioning" are treated here as modifiers of those four basic designs.

Descriptive Design

A research question of "What is?" or "To what degree?" often can be answered quite adequately using a descriptive design, sometimes called a simple descriptive design. Other descriptive designs can best be understood as variations of the simple descriptive design (Table 10-3). The purpose of simple descriptive research is to describe the phenomenon of interest and its component variables within one single subject group, sometimes called a **cohort**. This is accomplished through the use of descriptive statistics (see Chapter 22). In this design, data collection for all subjects occurs within the same time frame, over a span of minutes, hours, days, weeks, or months.

An example of descriptive research is Smeltzer et al.'s (2015) study of nursing faculty in the United States (U.S.), teaching in nursing programs that offered the Doctor of Philosophy (PhD) degree, the Doctor of Nursing Practice (DNP) degree, or both. The authors' purpose was "to profile" (p. 178) nursing faculty, a purpose entirely consistent with a descriptive design. Smeltzer et al. (2015) collected data through an electronic survey. "Samples of schools were drawn until 1,197 faculty members had been invited to participate, and 642 (54%) responses were received, of which 554 (46.3%) surveys were complete" (p. 180). The researchers' survey questions related to their phenomenon of interest, the characteristics of faculty members teaching in doctoral programs, and focused on the "demographics, commitments of time to facets of the faculty role, and components of the doctoral faculty role" (p. 181). Data were analyzed descriptively, using a data analysis computer program.

Smeltzer et al.'s (2015) findings were that (1) younger faculty were more likely to teach in DNP programs, (2) PhD programs employed predominantly PhD-prepared faculty, (3) DNP-prepared faculty more often maintained some external employment in clinical settings, (4) PhD-prepared faculty were more heavily involved in research and grant-writing, and (5) PhD-prepared faculty received more research support both from their institutions and from external sources. Based on the results, and the continuing trend among PhD-prepared faculty that "senior faculty members with research experience are aging out of the system faster

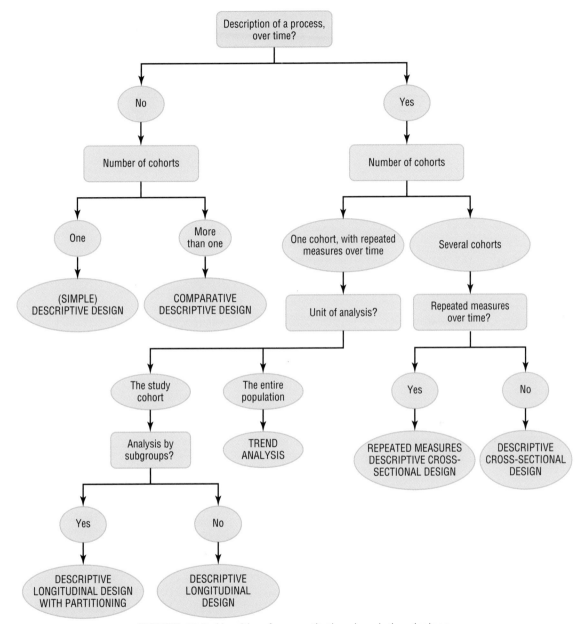

FIGURE 10-2 Algorithm for quantitative descriptive designs.

than the next generation can be developed" (p. 184), Smeltzer et al. expressed concern for the continuing development of the scientific discipline of nursing, also recommending that strategic planning be used to best develop existent faculty for roles in research. The researchers' conclusions are in keeping with the data and do not overreach the boundaries of the design. Because of the huge sample used and the high response rate to

their survey, the authors' generalization to all U.S. universities with PhD and DNS programs was appropriate.

Comparative Descriptive Design

Exactly as in simple descriptive research, the purpose of the comparative descriptive design is to describe, to answer the question of "What is?" or "To what degree?" The difference between the two designs, however, is that

TABLE 10-2   Studies Identified by Their Authors as Descriptive or Descriptive Correlational Designs

Authors (Year)	Design Identified by Researcher/Actual Design	Phenomenon of Interest	Other Variables	Data Collection
Alexis (2015)	"Descriptive survey"/ Descriptive	Internationally registered nurses' perceptions of discrimination while working in England	Support, adjustment to the new environment	Survey (questionnaire)
Alkubat, Al-Zaru, Khater, & Ammouri, 2013	"Descriptive correlational"/ Descriptive	Perceived learning needs of Yemeni patients after coronary artery bypass graft surgery	Demographics	In-person interview
Curtis & Glacken (2014)	"Quantitative descriptive"/ Descriptive	Job satisfaction among public health nurses	Professional status, interaction, autonomy, age, tenure	Survey
del-Pino-Casado, Frias-Osuna, Palomino-Moral, & Martinez-Riera (2012)	"Cross-sectional survey"/Descriptive cross-sectional	Gender differences regarding informal caregivers of older people	Intensity of care, duration of caregiving, subjective burden, satisfaction with caregiving	Secondary analysis of national survey
Ducharme et al. (2015)	"Comparative descriptive"/ Comparative descriptive	Characteristics of early- versus late-onset dementia family caregivers	Relationship, employment, education, preparedness, awareness of services	Prospective interview at cognition clinics; no specific statistical program cited
Happ et al. (2015)	"Retrospective longitudinal observational study"/Descriptive (not longitudinal)	The proportion of mechanically ventilated intensive care patients who meet basic communication criteria	Diagnosis, age, prognosis	Retrospective records review
Killion et al. (2014)	"Survey research design"/Descriptive	Burnout, smart device use	Stress	Survey via Survey Monkey
Layte, Sexton & Savva (2013)	"Cross-sectional study"/Descriptive cross-sectional	Quality of life in older age	—	Face interviews and self-completed questionnaires
Moon, Phelan, Lauver, & Bratzke (2015)	"Descriptive correlational, cross-sectional"/ Correlational	Sleep quality and its relationship to cognition, in persons with HF	Excessive daytime sleepiness	Secondary analysis of results of 8 standardized tests and chart data

TABLE 10-2   Studies Identified by Their Authors as Descriptive or Descriptive Correlational Designs—cont'd

Authors (Year)	Design Identified by Researcher/Actual Design	Phenomenon of Interest	Other Variables	Data Collection
Smeltzer et al. (2015)	"Descriptive"/ Descriptive	Nursing faculty in the U.S. teaching in PhD and DNP programs	Faculty roles in research (development of nursing science)	Survey, electronic, through Survey Monkey
Son, Thomas, & Friedmann (2013)	"Secondary data analysis"/ Descriptive longitudinal	Changes in coping for spouses of MI patients	Age of spouse, time since MI	Secondary analysis
Teman et al. (2015)	"Retrospective cohort study"/Descriptive	Effectiveness and safety of iNO before and during transport	Hypoxemia	Retrospective records review from institutional database
Wang, Zhan, Zhang, & Xia (2015)	"Cross-sectional survey"/Descriptive	Oncology nurses' blame attributions, different types of cancer	Nurse subspecialty work area	Survey by anonymous questionnaire
Yun, Kang, Lee, & Yi (2014)	"Cross-sectional descriptive study"/ Descriptive cross-sectional	Perceived work environment, workplace bullying	—	Survey with written questionnaire

DNP, Doctorate of Nursing Practice; *HF*, heart failure; *iNO*, inhaled nitric oxide; *MI*, myocardial infarction; *PhD*, Doctorate of Philosophy.

TABLE 10-3   Basic Descriptive Designs

Type of Design	Purpose	Number of Groups	Data-Collection Periods, During Which Each Subject Is Measured	Predominant Statistics
Descriptive (simple descriptive)	To describe the phenomenon of interest and related variables	One	One	Descriptive
Comparative descriptive	To describe the phenomenon of interest and related variables	Two, and sometimes more	One	Inferential
Longitudinal descriptive	To describe the phenomenon of interest and related variables over time	One	Two or more	Inferential
Cross-sectional descriptive (classical)	To describe the phenomenon of interest and related variables as a function of time	One with at least two subgroups in differing stages of a process	One	Inferential

in comparative descriptive research two distinct groups are described and compared in terms of their respective variables. An example of this type of research is Ducharme et al.'s (2015) comparative descriptive study, conducted for the purpose of describing and comparing characteristics of family caregivers of persons with early- versus late-onset dementia. The convenience sample consisted of 96 family caregivers. Data, collected through individual interviews at cognition clinics in Canada, were analyzed descriptively. Results indicated that caregivers of persons under age 60 with dementia were more likely to be spouses, continued to maintain employment, were better educated, "perceived themselves as better prepared to deal with future needs," and were "better informed about services" (Ducharme et al., 2015, p. 1) than were the caregivers of persons over 70 years of age. The researchers' conclusions were drawn from the data and from other studies of the same population. The authors made an appropriate, conservatively worded recommendation: "Our study provides data that highlight certain intergroup differences that should be taken into consideration in order to offer services tailored to the needs of each group" (p. 7). The study's conclusions and recommendations are data-based, in keeping with the design, and worded as advisories rather than generalizations, again consistent with the study's sample size and sampling type.

Researchers also use the comparative descriptive design to compare "before" and "after" states related to changes in clinical products, utilization, or protocols, and to other externally driven passive events. For instance, a comparative descriptive design would be suitable for evaluating the effect of a new protocol for maintaining patency of arterial lines, by comparing arterial line patency before and after the change. Many researchers report this type of investigation as quasi-experimental research; however, strictly speaking, if the change in protocol was not enacted by the researchers, the study is noninterventional—namely, comparative descriptive research.

Designs That Capture Change Across Time

Time-dimensional designs are used extensively within the discipline of epidemiology, to examine change over time, in relation to disease occurrence. In nursing research, the change over time that is studied is likely to be the result of a positive change such as normal development, learning, or self-enacted change in lifestyle, or the result of a negative change such as disease progression, exposure, aging, or other deteriorative process. Although samples in this type of research are called **cohorts** by epidemiologists, healthcare research

also uses the term "cohort" to apply to a sample that is studied at a single point in time (Teman et al., 2015).

Time-dimensional designs are useful in establishing patterns and trends in relation to potential precipitating factors and, consequently, can be precursors to interventional research. Interventional research is not appropriate for investigation of certain health problems, however. For instance, it would not be ethical to conduct a study to determine the effects of applying potentially harmful substances or treatments. In this case, the information gained from time-dimensional research, if repeatedly replicated, is convincing in implying causation. Examples of this type of cumulative evidence are studies in humans that examine the development of skin cancer in relation to sun exposure, of lung cancer in relation to cigarette smoking, of heart disease in relation to methamphetamine use, and of deterioration of both cognitive and physical capabilities in relation to chronic stress. Even though time-dimensional studies establish descriptive and correlational evidence, they only imply causation (Campbell & Stanley, 1963; Shadish et al., 2002). However, findings of time-dimensional research can generate evidence for designing subsequent interventional research.

Within noninterventional research, there are two principal types of time-dimensional studies: (1) longitudinal research and (2) cross-sectional research. Either of these can be descriptive or correlational in type. Both types of time-dimensional research can be conducted either retrospectively or prospectively.

Longitudinal Designs

Longitudinal designs examine changes in the same subjects over time. In other disciplines, these are called panel designs or cohort analyses (Figure 10-3). The purpose of longitudinal designs is to examine changes in a variable over time, within a defined group. Because of this focus on tracking changes, many descriptive longitudinal studies employ some correlational statistical methods, such as linear regression or multiple regression analysis (see Chapter 24), as well as descriptive statistics, to describe changes over time. Multiple regression analysis is a statistical procedure that examines many variables from a data set in conjunction with one another, so that their combined effects as well as their individual effects on the principal variable of interest can be understood fully.

Longitudinal research that is retrospective merely involves accessing data and transcribing values that reflect measured increments of time in the past. An example of this is research that uses data from the U.S.

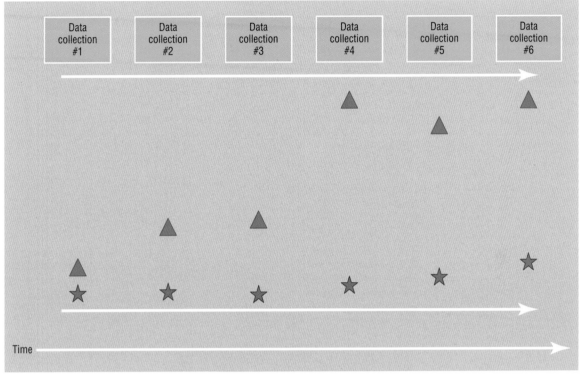

▲ Variable A mean value   ★ Variable B mean value

FIGURE 10-3 Descriptive longitudinal design.

Census. Longitudinal research could be conducted to determine life span in various socioeconomic groups. A researcher with access to census data could conduct data collection for such a study in a relatively short period of time. Not so, however, for prospective longitudinal research. In prospective longitudinal research, samples must be relatively large, because attrition over time is expected. For this reason, if a power analysis is used to calculate optimal sample size, more subjects should be recruited than needed (Grove & Cipher, 2017). A "captive" sample—for instance four consecutive semester-cohorts in an undergraduate nursing program, committed to finishing the program—is less apt to have high attrition rates than would a sample of persons working for a fast-food chain. Chapter 15 discusses sampling and retention of subjects.

Consultation with a statistician is recommended for longitudinal research, because data analysis is more complex than it would be in simple descriptive research. Analyses commonly used are repeated measures of analysis of variance, multiple regression analysis, and other

complicated methods (see Chapters 24 and 25 for additional detail about statistical tests). Although some aspects of a descriptive longitudinal study may include tests of association, if its statistical treatment is predominantly descriptive, the research is considered descriptive longitudinal in design, because its stated purpose is to describe change in variables of interest over time.

Son, Thomas, and Friedmann (2013) conducted longitudinal research "to examine changes in coping for spouses of post-MI [myocardial infarction] patients over time" (p. 1011). The researchers described spouses' 2-year trajectory of coping, using data collected in a previous clinical trial of automated external defibrillators in the home setting. Principal study findings were that coping was better for older spouses and worse in the presence of anxiety or depression. Coping worsened over time, with the most rapid declines in spouses of patients who had experienced an MI more recently.

Longitudinal designs may be broadened by partitioning (Figure 10-4). A university nurse surveys nursing

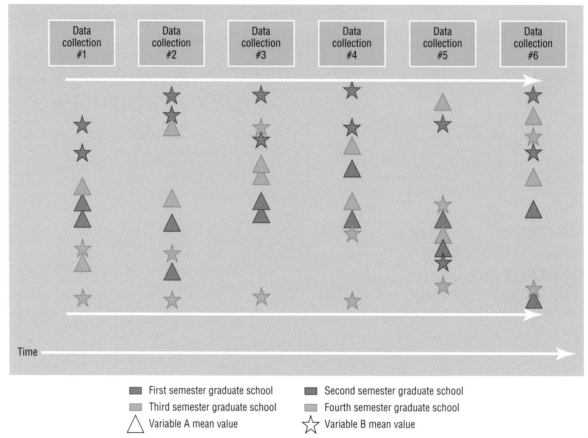

FIGURE 10-4 Descriptive longitudinal design with partitioning.

students in a four-semester master's program to determine how they self-rate their stress. The nurse decides also to survey the nursing students during the semester before they begin the program and the semester after they finish. If the nurse also partitions the students, so as to examine each student cohort over time, it can be determined how stress levels fluctuate for nursing graduate students semester to semester. In this way, the researcher could identify one semester as being especially stressful, or one class as being composed of particularly high-stress or low-stress people, as well as controlling for situational stressors that could affect students, both as class groups, and as peers in the same department. This adjustment makes a longitudinal study into a kind of hybrid longitudinal/cross-sectional study, certainly more work for the researcher but yielding more meaningful data.

A **trend design**, also called a trend analysis, is a variation of the longitudinal design. It is used extensively in

epidemiology to examine changes across time in incidence, usually incidence of disease. Measurements in trend designs occur at similarly spaced intervals—monthly, yearly, or every 5 years, for instance. In this respect, they are similar to longitudinal designs, but in trend designs a somewhat different sample from the population is selected each time that data are collected. Samples usually are large, sometimes entire populations, and the sole aim is to measure incidence of one or more related variables within that population. Research on health in an entire nation, such as research emanating from the Healthy People initiatives, uses trend designs. Currency for immunization against polio is an example of a variable that might be studied using a trend design.

Campbell and Stanley (1963) described a "pre-experimental" design, named the "one-shot case study." Case study research (Box 10-1) shares features of both qualitative descriptive and quantitative descriptive research.

BOX 10-1 Case Study Research: Quantitative or Qualitative?

Case study research provides a report of data collected over an extended period. It is structurally a mini-version of longitudinal research, the difference being that a single individual, or occasionally one family or tiny cohort, is measured and sometimes remeasured in order to demonstrate change. Campbell and Stanley (1963) described the "one-shot case study" as a pre-experimental design, stating, "Such studies have such a total absence of control [of extraneous variables] as to be of almost no scientific value" (p. 6), and that can be perceived as meaning no significant quantitative value. Most texts regard case study research, even if it includes numeric data, as qualitative because its results pertain only to its own participants. In addition, it has a narrative tone because it invariably presents data using an account that describes the case and its importance in a story-like format. In an evidence-based practice sense, because of the inability to generalize its results, case study research serves only to enlighten the reader, as does qualitative research or expert opinion, thereby informing practice and perhaps providing inspiration for subsequent quantitative inquiry. This text considers case study research qualitative.

Cross-Sectional Designs

Cross-sectional designs, in their classical form, examine change over time but, in order to do so, they employ data from different groups of subjects in various stages of a process, with all data collected at about the same time. The purpose of cross-sectional designs is to examine changes in a variable over time by comparing its value in several groups that are in different phases of a process (Figure 10-5). The assumption of the design is that the process for change in that variable is similar across groups.

Prospective cross-sectional research has the advantage of a fairly rapid time of data collection, as compared with prospective longitudinal research. Its primary disadvantage is that it demands a fairly large sample, so that measurements truly reflect changes in the characteristics of the phenomenon of interest, and not merely differences inherent in individual small groups. As with longitudinal research, because of the study aim of tracking changes, many descriptive cross-sectional studies are actually a combination of descriptive and correlational research, using regression analyses to describe changes across different values of the variables of interest. As long as the

purpose is to describe the variables, and the statistics are predominantly descriptive, the research is considered descriptive cross-sectional.

An example of descriptive cross-sectional research is Layte, Sexton, and Savva's (2013) study on quality of life in adults 50 years and older. Using prospectively collected data within the larger Irish Longitudinal Study of Ageing, the authors examined changes in the four dimensions of quality of life at older ages—control, autonomy, self-realization, and pleasure—and compared them with demographics, physical health, mental health, social participation, and socioeconomics. Quality of life increased until the late sixties, and then declined in persons over the remainder of their life span, with social participation making a somewhat larger contribution but with all four dimensions contributing to quality of life (Layte et al., 2013).

Cross-sectional research can be designed so that all subjects are measured at least twice. This variation is referred to as a repeated-measures cross-sectional design.

Much research identified as cross-sectional in healthcare literature, and some within nursing literature, focuses less on change across time and more on change across other entities, such as diagnostic categories (Wang, Zhan, Zhang, & Xia, 2015) and illness severity (Moon, Phelan, Lauver, & Bratzke, 2015). The term "cross-sectional" is used sometimes when authors refer to a mixed or heterogeneous sample, with few exclusion criteria. It may be that, given its current evolution, a better contemporary definition for this subtype of research, when changes across time are not a focus of study, would be mixed-sample descriptive/correlational research.

Confusion About the Term Descriptive Correlational Design

The **descriptive correlational design** has been considered a subtype of correlational research, with its primary purpose being to examine relationships between and among variables. The label of the design, unfortunately, has led students and researchers alike to draw the false conclusion that even one test of correlation in a descriptive research report reclassifies a study as a descriptive correlational design. To clarify, in this edition the term for research design that examines relationships between and among variables will now be **correlational design**, and it is referred to occasionally as **simple correlational design**. To reiterate, in descriptive designs, the overall purpose of the study is to describe its variables, and the predominant type of statistical analysis for the study results is descriptive.

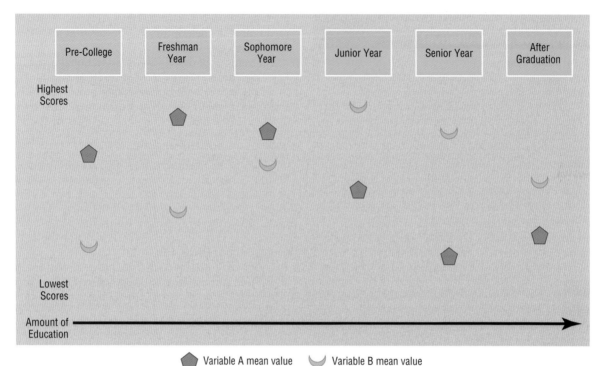

Pre-College **Freshman Year** **Sophomore Year** **Junior Year** **Senior Year** **After Graduation**

Highest Scores

Lowest Scores

Amount of Education

⬠ Variable A mean value   ⌣ Variable B mean value

FIGURE 10-5 Descriptive cross-sectional design.

An example of research termed by its authors descriptive correlational research but that is primarily descriptive is Alkubat, Al-Zaru, Khater, and Ammouri's (2013) study of perceived learning needs of Yemeni patients after coronary artery bypass surgery. While still hospitalized, 120 patients completed a 44-item questionnaire about their learning needs. The researchers found that patients' learning needs were highest between 24 and 48 hours after surgery; that the learning needs of men were more extensive than those of women; that older patients needed less information than middle-aged and young patients; and that educated and employed patients had higher learning needs. Statistics employed in data analysis were predominantly descriptive.

Research that has the stated purpose of establishing the strength and direction of relationships, but which is identified by its authors as descriptive correlational in design, is more properly termed correlational research and is discussed in the following section. In correlational research designs, the primary purpose of the study is to describe the relationships between and among variables, and the predominant statistical analysis for the study results is correlational.

CORRELATIONAL DESIGNS

Correlational research is conducted in order to establish the direction and the strength of relationships between or among variables, as they exist in a natural setting. The outcome of correlational research may be (1) the description of relationships between or among variables, (2) the ability to predict values of one variable based on the values of the other, or (3) the confirmation of the individual relationships within a proposed theoretical model. All three types of correlational research can be valuable precursors to interventional research, because strength of relationship is one requisite for establishment of causation. However, correlational studies also can provide important evidence for practice and confirmation of theory, in and of themselves.

Correlational designs, like descriptive designs, are of varying levels of complexity, the more involved of them containing many variables and testing several relationships. Data collection can take place at one time or extend over weeks or months, and it can take place at one site or many sites. Studies can be retrospective or prospective, longitudinal or cross-sectional, in their strategies of data-collection. Figure 10-6 displays the principal types

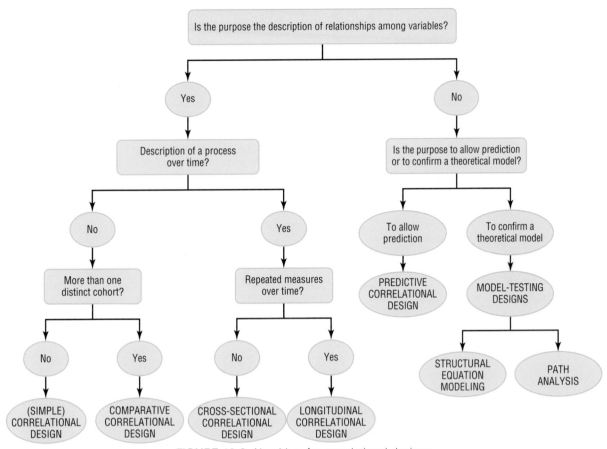

FIGURE 10-6 Algorithm for correlational designs.

of correlational designs. Research reports already introduced in previous chapters are included in Table 10-4, with a few additions, to exemplify commonly used correlational designs.

There are three principal types of correlational research described in this text: the simple correlational design, the predictive correlational design, and the model-testing designs. They differ in their respective purposes: to describe relationships, to enable prediction, and to confirm theoretical models. The simple correlational design and the predictive correlational design both use the statistical process of linear regression, which measures the strength of a relationship between pairs of variables. In addition, the predictive correlational design and model-testing designs use multiple regression analyses, which measure the strength of relationships among three or more variables as they interact with one another.

Simple Correlational Designs

Studies identified by their researchers as descriptive correlational in design but that have a stated purpose to describe relationships between variables are now termed **correlational design** or simple correlational design. The statistics used to establish the results are predominantly correlational, although descriptive statistics are used to describe sample characteristics and the distribution of individual variables. Data are collected either prospectively or retrospectively. There is no researcher intervention. Like descriptive designs, the correlational design group has several design types that are a variation on the basic design (Table 10-5).

An example of (simple) correlational research is Dahn, Alexander, Malloch, and Morgan's (2014) study of the relationship between recidivism and the type of violation for which the Arizona Board of Registered Nursing (BON) initially had disciplined nurses. Data

TABLE 10-4 **Studies Identified by Their Authors as Correlational Designs**

Authors (Year)	Design Identified by Researcher/Actual Design	Phenomenon of Interest	Other Variables	Data Collection
Baum & Kagan (2015)	"Cross-sectional quantitative design"/ (Simple) correlational, cross-sectional	Psychiatric nurses' job satisfaction and intention to leave	Closed versus open wards	Questionnaire, hand-delivered
Brunetto et al. (2013)	"Multigroup structural equation modeling analysis"/Structural equation modeling	Workplace relationships and turnover	Engagement, well-being, organizational commitment	Self-report survey
Burk, Grap, Munro, Schubert, & Sessler (2014)	(Not named)/ Predictive correlational	Agitation in critically ill adults, potential predictors	Psychiatric diagnosis, illicit substance use, physical status, lab values, height	Prospective with records review
Côté, Gagnon, Houme, Abdeljelil, & Gagnon's (2012)	"Predictive correlational"/ Predictive correlational	Nurses' intention to integrate research evidence into clinical decision-making	Moral norm, normative beliefs, perceived behavioral control, past behavior	Hand-distributed questionnaire
Dahn, Alexander, Malloch, & Morgan (2014)	"Retrospective quantitative descriptive correlational"/ (Simple) correlational	Type of violation for nurse disciplinary action (BRN) and recidivism	—	Retrospective from database
Hjelm, Broström, Riegel, Årestedt, & Strömberg (2015)	"Descriptive cross-sectional"/Predictive correlational, cross-sectional	Cognitive function and self-care in patients with chronic heart failure	Symptoms of depression, psychomotor speed	Interview and examination, prospective
Huang, Chen, Liang, & Miaskowski (2014)	"Observational prospective... longitudinal" Correlational, longitudinal	Fatigue severity in breast cancer	Depressive symptoms, symptom distress, receipt of chemotherapy	Self-assessment questionnaire, repeated over one year
Li, Inouye, Davis, & Arikaki (2013)	"Structural equation modeling"/Structural equation modeling	Diabetes health indicators in Asian and Pacific Islander adults with DM2, psychological and physiological factors	Diet, exercise, foot care, and depression most important	Secondary analysis of data from RCT
Lin, MacLennan, Hunt, & Cox (2015)	"Cross-sectional quantitative"/ Model-testing	Nursing transformational leadership style, quality of nurses' working lives	Workplace support from supervisor, organizational commitment, job satisfaction	Self-report paper questionnaire

TABLE 10-4 Studies Identified by Their Authors as Correlational Designs—cont'd

Authors (Year)	Design Identified by Researcher/Actual Design	Phenomenon of Interest	Other Variables	Data Collection
Moon, Phelan, Lauver, & Bratzke (2015)	"Descriptive correlational, cross-sectional"/ Correlational	Sleep quality and its relationship to cognition, in persons with HF	Excessive daytime sleepiness	Secondary analysis of results of 8 standardized tests and chart data
Poutiainen, Levälahti, Hakulinen-Viitanen, & Laatikainen (2015)	"Path modeling, cross-sectional"/ Path modeling path analysis	Family characteristics, health behaviors, school nurses' concerns about adolescents' health and development	Smoking among parents and adolescents (boys), paternal education, single mother (girls)	Secondary analysis of data from Children's Health Monitoring (LATE) Study
Rodwell, Brunetto, Demir, Shacklock, & Farr-Wharton (2014)	"Cross-sectional survey"/Model-testing	Abusive supervision and nurse intentions to quit	Job satisfaction, psychological strain	Paper survey
van der Kooi, Stronks, Thompson, DerSarkissian, & Arah (2013)	(Not named) / Model-testing	Human Development Index (HDI), education, self-reported health	—	Secondary analysis of World Health Survey Data
Vermeesch et al. (2013)	(Not named— "predictive") / Model-testing	Hispanic stress, self-esteem, depression	—	Secondary analysis of a randomized trial

BRN, Board of Registered Nursing; *DM2*, diabetes mellitus 2; *HF*, heart failure; *RCT*, randomized controlled trial.

TABLE 10-5 Basic Correlational Designs

Type of Design	Purpose	Number of Groups	Data-Collection Periods, During Which Each Subject Is Measured	Predominant Statistics
Correlational (simple correlational)	To describe the relationships between and among variables	One	One	Correlational: such as Pearson r, linear regression
Comparative correlational (rare)	To describe the relationships between and among variables	Two, and sometimes more (distinct and different)	One	Correlational: such as Pearson r, linear regression
Longitudinal correlational	To describe the relationships between and among variables, over time	One	Two or more	Correlational: such as Pearson r, linear regression
Cross-sectional correlational (classical)	To describe the relationships between and among variables, as a function of time	One with at least two subgroups in differing stages of a process	One	Correlational: such as Pearson r, linear regression

were obtained from the Arizona BON data bank. The researchers found no associations between type of violation and recidivism. Statistics used to analyze the variables that were the focus of the research were correlational.

Another example of correlational research is Moon et al.'s (2015) study of the relationship between sleep quality and cognition in patients with heart failure. The study's stated objective was "to examine how self-reported sleep quality and daytime symptoms are associated with selected domains of cognitive function among individuals with heart failure (HF)" (p. 212). The researchers found that, although sleep quality and daytime symptoms were not associated with cognitive functioning overall, increased daytime dysfunction was associated with both reduced attention and poorer executive function. Moon et al. (2015) speculated that this association might be due to speed of information processing. Statistics employed in data analysis were almost exclusively correlational.

Predictive Designs

The **predictive correlational design** is used to establish strength and direction of relationships between or among variables, with the intention of predicting the value of one of the variables based on the value of the other variable(s). A researcher uses a predictive correlational design when a relationship has been described previously, and when the ability to predict the presence and value of one of the study variables is of interest, either for potential application to clinical practice or for use in subsequent research. When predictive correlational research examines multiple variables and their potential interactions with one another, both linear and multivariate statistical tests are used to determine which predictors are most powerful. When more than one predictor is tested, a final equation is presented that best explains the change in the value of the dependent variable. The total amount of change in the value of the dependent variable explained by the predictor variables is called the **variance**, and it is represented as R^2. (See Chapter 24 for clarification of the concept of explained variance, R^2.)

The ability to predict confers clinical benefits. For clients with recurrent severe depression being treated through a mental health clinic, consider how helpful it would be for the healthcare team to be cognizant of identified symptoms that were indicative of exacerbation of the disease. Knowledge of the symptoms and findings most likely to lead to self-destructive acts would help psychiatric mental health nurse practitioners and other healthcare professionals to predict impending crises in a timely manner, allowing the healthcare team to intervene to decrease harm.

Predictive correlational research is often the prelude to construction of a theoretical model (see Chapter 8). After construction, the resultant model would then be evaluated for the statistical strength of the relationships within it, using a model-testing design (see the following section).

Prediction also is useful as a precursor to interventional research. For example, in a hospital practice setting, a "bundled" intervention consisting of seven different time-consuming nursing actions is discovered to be effective in treatment or prevention. Predictive correlational research could reveal which of the seven strategies were likely to be most powerful for preventing complications or for contributing to cure. With this information, nurse administrators could design a "modified bundle," consisting of the three or four most powerful interventions. This modified bundle would be the focus of research, in which patient outcomes were measured and compared with outcomes of the full "bundled" intervention. If the two outcomes were not statistically different, policy could be changed. Nurses could then spend their time and effort performing nursing actions that contributed most strongly to restoration or maintenance of health. A secondary advantage might be decrease in the cost of care delivery.

Predictive correlational research uses the terms "independent" and "dependent" to refer to its principal variables. The **independent variable** or variables are also called predictors. The **dependent variable** or outcome variable is the one whose value or occurrence the researcher wants to be able to predict.

An example of predictive correlational research is Côté, Gagnon, Houme, Abdeljelil, and Gagnon's (2012) study of nurses working in a university hospital in Quebec, Canada. The purpose of the research was to identify statistical predictors of nurses' intention to integrate research evidence into their practice. Data were collected by means of a printed questionnaire made available to 600 nurses at the work site. Initial return rate was 353 and, after removing questionnaires that were incomplete, 336 were finally analyzed, representing a 56% return, which is a moderate to high figure for questionnaire research (see Chapter 17). The researchers found that the "moral norm, normative beliefs, perceived behavioural control, and past behaviour" (p. 2289) were the strongest predictors of the dependent variable, intention to integrate research evidence into practice. Statistics used to analyze interactions among variables were correlational.

Model-Testing Designs

Model-testing designs use correlational research for measurement of proposed relationships within a theoretical model (see Chapter 8). The primary model-testing designs used within nursing research are path analyses and structural equation modeling (SEM). An early antecedent of SEM was development of the path diagram, a drawing of the linear associations among variables, developed in the early 1920s by mathematicians (Wright, 1934). At that time, the correlation represented by each "path" or connection between variables was calculated by hand; a computer now performs these calculations. In **path analysis**, the relationship between each pair of variables in a model is tested for its strength and direction (Pearl, 2010), yielding a correlational value (Norris, 2013).

SEM also tests theoretical relationships within a model. Its complex calculations, however, also allow the researcher to identify the best model that explains interactions among variables, yielding the greatest explained variance. SEM is capable of analyzing models with two-way paths between variables, as well as determining how three or more variables interact, using multiple regression analysis (Norris, 2013).

In model-testing designs, the researcher sets the level of statistical significance. Relationships that are within that level, the stronger relationships, are retained in the model. Relationships that are weaker than the set point (greater than the p-level set by the researcher) are removed from the model. The model may involve correlation, proposed causation, or both. If a model with causative elements is supported by model-testing research, the model can provide the framework for subsequent interventional study.

Because a number of variables may be examined in such research, samples must be large enough to provide statistical power. Previously, the rule of thumb was that 10 subjects were required for each variable tested. With model testing, however, the sample must be even larger because statistical relationships are complex, multilevel, and interacting. Researchers conducting studies for model testing use large samples. In the seven articles listed in Table 10-4 that used model-testing designs, sample sizes were 207 (Li, Inouye, Davis, & Arikaki, 2013), 250 (Rodwell, Brunetto, Demir, Shacklock, & Farr-Wharton, 2014), 548 (Vermeesch et al., 2013), 651 (Lin, MacLennan, Hunt, & Cox, 2015), 1006 (Poutiainen, Levälahti, Hakulinen-Viitanen, & Laatikainen, 2015), 1228 (Brunetto et al., 2013), and, by far the largest, 217,642 (van der Kooi, Stronks, Thompson, DerSarkissian, & Arah, 2013) for a sample that accessed World Survey Data (p. e49). Because of the large sample sizes required, model-testing and predictive correlational research frequently use data collected in previous studies or for public purposes (census data, for example). If a study uses data collected in this manner, it is called a secondary analysis (see Chapter 17). **Secondary analysis** is a strategy in which a researcher performs an analysis of data collected and originally analyzed by another researcher or agency.

Publications that report model-testing research usually provide a preliminary conceptual map of potential relationships and interactions among them to be tested. Figure 10-7 from Poutiainen et al.'s (2015) article is an example of a preliminary conceptual map of such a model. Near the end of the article, the final map (Figure 10-8), with correlations and levels of significance, is displayed for the variables maternal smoking, child smoking, family type, and school nurses' concerns (Poutiainen et al., 2015). Some maps are more complex than others. The lines drawn between concepts are sometimes called paths, yielding one name for such studies, a path analysis.

Variables examined in model-testing research are referred to as exogenous (literally "grown from outside") and endogenous ("grown within"). Exogenous variables

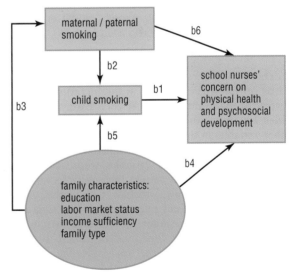

FIGURE 10-7 Map of conceptual model for path analysis. (Adapted from Poutiainen, H., Levälahti, E., Hakulainan-Viitanen, T., & Laatikainen, T. (2015). Family characteristics and health behaviour as antecedents of school nurses' concerns about adolescents' health development: A path model approach. *International Journal of Nursing Studies, 52*(5), 922.)

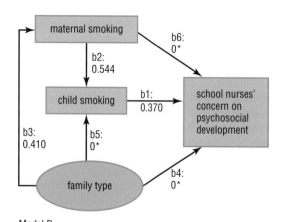

Model D
Indirect effects:
b3*b2*b1 = 0.083
b2*b1 = 0.201
b3*b2 = 0.223

Model fit:
$\chi^2 = 2.977$, df = 3, p = 0.395

FIGURE 10-8 Map of path analysis of one aspect of the conceptual model. (Adapted from Poutiainen, H., Levälahti, E., Hakulainan-Viitanen, T., & Laatikainen, T. (2015). Family characteristics and health behaviour as antecedents of school nurses' concerns about adolescents' health development: A path model approach. *International Journal of Nursing Studies*, *52*(5), 926.)

are chosen by the researcher to be included in the model, based on information found in the literature, existent theory, or the researcher's experience. **Exogenous variables** are those whose values influence the values of other variables in the model (Norris, 2013). The causes of the exogenous factors are not explained by the model.

Endogenous refers to variables whose values are influenced, and possibly caused, by exogenous variables and other endogenous variables within the model (Norris, 2013). **Residual** refers to effects of unknown variables, some unmeasurable or even unknown, which are not included in the final model (Pearl, 2010). The residual is equivalent to the total "unexplained variance," the amount of change in endogenous variables not "explained" or "accounted for" by the terms in the model. The amount of change "explained" by the model is represented by R^2. The residual is what remains, and it is represented as $(1 - R^2)$.

An example of model-testing research is Rodwell et al.'s (2014) study of abusive supervision and the intention to quit, in a sample of 250 Australian nurses.

The authors examined relationships among their phenomenon of interest and five other variables: isolation, task attacks, personal attacks, psychological strain, and job satisfaction. The results included the findings that "personal abuse had personal and health impacts," whereas "work-focused abuse had work-oriented effects" (p. 357). The researchers' recommendation for application was that "the results can be used to devise programs aimed at educating and supporting supervisors and their subordinates to adhere to zero tolerance policies of antisocial workplace behaviors and encourage reporting incidents" (p. 363).

■ KEY POINTS

- Designing a research study involves deciding upon three components: the research methodology, the research design, and the research methods. The best methodology, design, and methods are the ones that provide a meaningful answer to the proposed study's research question.
- For the vast majority of well-worded research questions, the choice of a suitable methodology is clear.
- Choice of a quantitative design first involves deciding between interventional and noninterventional. Noninterventional designs are descriptive or correlational. They describe and may establish correlation; they never establish causation.
- Methods of a study define the way subjects will be recruited, sites will be chosen, and data will be collected, recorded, and analyzed.
- Causality, multiple causality, probability, bias, measurement, prospective versus retrospective, partitioning, and validity are concepts relevant to both interventional and noninterventional quantitative research.
- Design validity is based upon how well the researcher has (1) defined study concepts (construct validity), (2) eliminated potentially extraneous variables (internal validity), (3) chosen a sample so that results can be generalized back to the population (external validity), and (4) made appropriate statistical choices (statistical conclusion validity).
- Extraneous variables are variables other than the study variables that potentially affect the value of the dependent variable(s), making the independent variable appear more powerful or less powerful than it actually is.
- Descriptive research describes the phenomenon of interest and its related variables. Correlational research describes the relationships between and among variables.

- Secondary data analysis uses a data set collected and originally analyzed in a previous study.
- Algorithms are helpful both for identification of a study's design and for decision making relative to planned research.

REFERENCES

Acheson, R. M. (1970). Epidemiology of serum uric acid and gout: An example of the complexities of multifactorial causation. *Proceedings of the Royal Society of Medicine, 63*(2), 193–197.

Alexis, O. (2015). Internationally recruited nurses' experiences in England: A survey approach. *Nursing Outlook, 63*(3), 238–244.

Alkubat, S. A., Al-Zaru, I. M., Khater, W., & Ammouri, A. A. (2013). Perceived learning needs of Yemeni patients after coronary artery bypass graft surgery. *Journal of Clinical Nursing, 22*(7–8), 930–938.

Baum, A., & Kagan, I. (2015). Job satisfaction and intent to leave among psychiatric nurses: Closed versus open wards. *Archives of Psychiatric Nursing, 29*(4), 213–216.

Brunetto, Y., Xiong, M., Shriberg, A., Farr-Wharton, R., Shacklock, K., Newman, S., et al. (2013). The impact of workplace relationships on engagement, well-being, commitment and turnover for nurses in Australia and the USA. *Journal of Advanced Nursing, 69*(12), 2786–2799.

Burk, R. S., Grap, M. J., Munro, C. L., Schubert, C. M., & Sessler, C. N. (2014). Agitation onset, frequency, and associated temporal factors in the adult critically ill. *American Journal of Critical Care, 23*(4), 296–304.

Campbell, D. T. (1957). Factors relevant to the validity of experiments. *Psychological Bulletin, 54*(4), 297–312.

Campbell, D. T., & Stanley, J. C. (1963). Experimental and quasi-experimental designs for research on teaching. In N. L. Gage (Ed.), *Handbook of research on teaching* (pp. 171–246). Chicago, IL: Rand McNally.

Centers for Medicare and Medicaid Services (CMMS). (2012). *Hospital Consumer Assessment of Healthcare Providers and Systems CAHPS® Hospital Survey.* Accessed 05.03.16 at http://www.hcahps.org/home.aspx.

Charette, S., Lacbance, J., Charest, M., Villeneuve, D., Theroux, J., Joncas, J., et al. (2015). Guided imagery for adolescent post-spinal fusion pain management: A pilot study. *Pain Management Nursing, 16*(3), 211–220.

Cook, T. D., & Campbell, D. T. (1979). *Quasi-experimentation: Design and analysis issues for field settings.* Boston: Houghton Mifflin Company.

Cook, T., & Campbell, D. (1986). The causal assumptions of quasi-experimental practice. *Synthese, 68*(1), 141–180.

Côté, F., Gagnon, J., Houme, P. K., Abdeljelil, A. B., & Gagnon, M. P. (2012). Using the theory of planned behaviour to predict nurses' intention to integrate research evidence into clinical decision-making. *Journal of Advanced Nursing, 68*(10), 2289–2298.

Curtis, E. A., & Glacken, M. (2014). Job satisfaction among public health nurses: A national survey. *Journal of Nursing Management, 22*(5), 653–663.

Dahn, J. M., Alexander, R., Malloch, K., & Morgan, S. A. (2014). Does a relationship exist between the type of initial violation and recidivism? *Journal of Nursing Regulation, 5*(3), 4–8.

del-Pino-Casado, R., Frias-Osuna, A., Palomino-Moral, P. A., & Martinez-Riera, J. R. (2012). Gender differences regarding informal caregivers of older people. *Journal of Nursing Scholarship, 44*(4), 349–357.

Ducharme, F., Lachance, L., Kergoat, M. J., Coulombe, R., Antoine, P., & Pasquier, F. (2015). A comparative descriptive study of characteristics of early- and late-onset dementia family caregivers. *American Journal of Alzheimer's Disease and Other Dementias, 31*(1), 1–9.

Grove, S. K., & Cipher, D. J. (2017). *Statistics for nursing research: A workbook for evidence-based practice* (2nd ed.). St. Louis, MO: Elsevier.

Happ, M. B., Seaman, J. B., Nilsen, M. L., Sciulli, A., Tate, J. A., Saul, M., et al. (2015). The number of mechanically ventilated ICU patients meeting communication criteria. *Heart and Lung: The Journal of Critical Care, 44*(1), 45–49.

Hjelm, C. M., Broström, A., Riegel, B., Årestedt, K., & Strömberg, A. (2015). The association between cognitive function and self-care in patients with chronic heart failure. *Heart and Lung: The Journal of Critical Care, 44*(2), 113–119.

Huang, H. P., Chen, M. L., Liang, J., & Miaskowski, C. (2014). Changes in and predictors of severity of fatigue in women with breast cancer: A longitudinal study. *International Journal of Nursing Studies, 51*(4), 582–592.

Hultman, C. S., Tong, W. T., Surrusco, M., Roden, K. S., Kiser, M., & Cairns, B. A. (2012). To everything there is a season: Impact of seasonal change on admissions, acuity of injury, length of stay, throughput, and charges at an accredited, regional burn center. *Annals of Plastic Surgery, 69*(1), 30–34.

Hume, D. (1999). *A treatise of human nature: Being an attempt to introduce the experimental method of reasoning into moral subjects.* Kitchener, Ontario, CAN: Batoche Books.

Killion, J. B., Johnston, J. N., Gresham, J., Gipson, M., Vealé, B. L., Behrens, P. I., et al. (2014). Smart device use and burnout among health science educators. *Radiologic Technology, 86*(2), 144–154.

Layte, R., Sexton, E., & Savva, G. (2013). Quality of life in older age: Evidence from an Irish cohort study. *Journal of the American Geriatric Society, 61*(S2), S299–S305.

Lenth, R. V. (2006–2009). *Java applets for power and sample size [computer software].* Retrieved March 5, 2016 from http://www.stat.uiowa.edu/~rlenth/Power.

Li, D., Inouye, J., Davis, J., & Arakaki, R. F. (2013). Associations between psychosocial and physiological factors and diabetes health indicators in Asian and Pacific Islander adults with type 2 diabetes. *Nursing Research and Practice, 2013.* Retrieved March 5, 2016 from http://www.hindawi.com/journals/nrp/2013/703520/.

Lin, P. Y., MacLennan, S., Hunt, N., & Cox, T. (2015). The influences of nursing transformational leadership style on the quality of nurses' working lives in Taiwan: A cross-sectional quantitative study. *BMC Nursing, 14*, 33. Retrieved March 5, 2016 from http://www.ncbi.nlm.nih.gov/pubmed/25991910.

Moon, C., Phelan, C. H., Lauver, D. R., & Bratzke, L. C. (2015). Is sleep quality related to cognition in individuals with heart failure? *Heart and Lung: The Journal of Critical Care, 44*(3), 212–218.

National Institute of Justice. (2014). *Recidivism.* Retrieved July 20, 2015 from http://www.nij.gov/topics/corrections/recidivism/pages/welcome.aspx#statistics.

Norris, A. E. (2013). Path analysis. Structural equation modeling. In S. B. Plichta & E. Kelvin (Eds.), *Statistical methods for health care research* (6th ed., pp. 399–443). Philadelphia, PA: Lippincott Williams & Wilkins.

Pearl, J. (2010). The foundations of causal inference. *Sociological Methodology, 40*(1), 75–XII.

Poutiainen, H., Levälahti, E., Hakulainan-Viitanen, T., & Laatikainen, T. (2015). Family characteristics and health behaviour as antecedents of school nurses' concerns about adolescents' health development: A path model approach. *International Journal of Nursing Studies, 52*(5), 920–929.

Rodwell, J., Brunetto, Y., Demir, D., Shacklock, K., & Farr-Wharton, R. (2014). Abusive supervision and links to nurse intentions to quit. *Journal of Nursing Scholarship, 46*(5), 357–365.

Sethi, R. K. V., Kozin, E. D., Fagenholz, P. J., Lee, D. J., Shrime, M. G., & Gray, S. T. (2014). Epidemiological survey of head and neck injuries and trauma in the United States. *Otolaryngology-Head and Neck Surgery, 151*(5), 776–784.

Shadish, S. R., Cook, T. D., & Campbell, D. T. (2002). *Experimental and quasi-experimental design for generalized causal inference.* Boston, MA: Houghton Mifflin Company.

Smeltzer, S. C., Sharts-Hopko, N. C., Cantrell, M. A., Heverly, M. A., Nthenge, S., & Jenkinson, A. (2015). A profile of U.S. nursing faculty in research- and practice-focused doctoral education. *Journal of Nursing Scholarship, 47*(2), 178–185.

Son, H., Thomas, S. A., & Friedmann, E. (2013). Longitudinal changes in coping for spouses of post-myocardial infarction patients. *Western Journal of Nursing Research, 35*(8), 1011–1025.

Stein, Z., & Susser, M. (1970). Mutability of intelligence and epidemiology of mild mental retardation. *Review of Educational Research, 40*(1), 29–67.

Teman, N. R., Thomas, J., Bryner, B. S., Haas, C. F., Haft, J. W., Park, P. K., et al. (2015). Inhaled nitric oxide to improve oxygenation for safe critical care transport of adults with severe hypopxemia. *American Journal of Critical Care, 24*(2), 110–117.

van der Kooi, A. L. F., Stronks, K., Thompson, C. A., DerSarkissian, M., & Arah, O. A. (2013). The modifying influence of country development on the effect of individual educational attainment on self-rated health. *Research and Practice, 103*(11), e49–e54.

Vermeesch, A. L., Gonzales-Guarda, R. M., Hall, R., McCabe, B. E., Cianelli, R., & Peragallo, N. P. (2013). Predictors of depressive symptoms among Hispanic women in south Florida. *Western Journal of Nursing Research, 35*(10), 1325–1338.

Waltz, C. F., Strickland, O. L., & Lenz, E. R. (2010). *Measurement in nursing and health research.* New York, NY: Springer Publishing Company.

Wang, L. D. L., Zhan, L., Zhang, J., & Xia, Z. (2015). Nurses' blame attributions towards different types of cancer: A cross-sectional study. *International Journal of Nursing Studies, 52*(10), 1600–1606.

Wright, S. (1934). The method of path coefficients. *The Annals of Mathematical Statistics, 5*(3), 161–215.

Yun, S., Kang, J., Lee, Y. O., & Yi, Y. (2014). Work environment and workplace bullying among Korean intensive care unit nurses. *Asian Nursing Research, 8*(1), 219–225.

11

Quantitative Methodology: Interventional Designs and Methods

Suzanne Sutherland

The researcher commits to the quantitative methodology and decides to conduct interventional research, and the process of design begins. Interventional research is somewhat more complicated to design than is noninterventional, principally because delivery of the intervention and collection of data require more steps.

Next, the researcher defines the intervention and the expected results conceptually and operationally. At this point, the researcher scrutinizes the design in progress and decides whether experimental research is feasible for both setting and circumstances. The researcher also must make a judgment as to whether experimental research will produce the clearest answer to the research question. The goal is a study that will be credible, precise, timely, and appropriate to nursing. If experimental research is chosen, both design and methods are finalized, including site, subjects, recruitment, the consenting process, data collection tools, data collection strategies, enactment of interventions, organization of data, and data analysis. Details about the chosen methods are specified in the Methods section of the proposal and research report.

If conducting an experiment is not feasible, or impractical, or likely to produce questionable results, the researcher selects instead a quasi-experimental design. In quasi-experimental research, many extraneous variables can intrude, producing error. Because of this, choosing a specific quasi-experimental design involves identification of extraneous variables likely to present themselves, for each potential design, and selection of the design that offers the best chance of accurate study results.

This chapter begins with concepts relevant to interventional research design, including threats to validity and strategies for controlling those threats. Various experimental designs are presented, with examples of each. Several quasi-experimental designs used frequently for nursing research are described, focusing on their inherent issues for validity, and examples are included. Several algorithms specifying distinguishing features of various designs are displayed. These are useful for differentiating among designs of published research and for identifying the most suitable designs for a planned study.

CONCEPTS RELEVANT TO INTERVENTIONAL RESEARCH DESIGN

Several concepts introduced in Chapter 10 are of special concern when designing interventional research. They are random selection versus random assignment, causality and its emergence in modern research, multiple causality, manipulation, control, control versus comparison groups, and validity. A few concepts that relate to maintenance of consistency in the interventional research process are discussed at the end of the chapter.

Random Selection Versus Random Assignment
Random Selection
When the intent is to generalize findings to an entire target population, the researcher uses random selection to select the study sample. This means that the researcher selects the elements from the accessible population according to a random number table, a computer

program, a coin toss, a hat draw, or some other method in which the researcher has no control over whether any given element is chosen. In random selection, every element of the accessible population has an equal chance of being selected. The resultant random sample, if large enough, will have the characteristics of the accessible population and almost the same proportions of those characteristics. (See Chapter 15 for a thorough explanation of populations and samples, and ways in which random sampling may be performed.)

Random sampling is a tactic that increases external validity—the extent to which results are generalizable to the population. Although a study that uses a random sample has better external validity than one that does not, experimental design does not require random sampling.

Random Assignment

Random assignment occurs after study subjects have been selected and have agreed to participate in a study. Whether a study's method of selection is random or nonrandom does not affect the process of random assignment. The two are different strategies. Random assignment is the process of assigning each member of the sample (the research subject) to one of the groups, so that each subject has the chance of being in a certain group. The researcher makes the assignment blindly, according to a random number table, a coin toss, or some other predetermined method. For a simple experimental study, the groups to which the subjects are assigned are called the intervention (or treatment, or experimental, or interventional) group and the control group.

Random assignment is a tactic that increases internal validity, not external. If the subjects who receive the experimental intervention and the subjects who do not have been randomly assigned to group, they are very similar to one another. This allows the researcher to be relatively certain that the difference in their behaviors, lab values, or clinical course is due to the effects of the experimental intervention. Random assignment is a requisite of experimental design. In the medical literature, random assignment is called randomization, and the subjects are referred to as "randomized" or "fully randomized."

Causality and Its Emergence in Modern Research

Causality is another word for causation. It refers to a cause-and-effect relationship. Association is not the same as causality. The purpose of an interventional design is to examine whether causation exists between variables. The independent variable in a study is the proposed cause, and the dependent variable is measured in order to quantify the independent variable's hypothesized effect.

Although the philosopher Hume predated the logical positivist philosophical movement by almost 200 years, his ideas are fundamental to stances taken by the movement (Hume, 1999). Logical positivists believe that logic is based on facts and reasoning. Hume made a significant contribution to interventional research by asserting that causation depends upon eight separate conditions. The three conditions most frequently attributed to him are contiguity, succession, and conjunction. Cause and effect are required to be near one another in space and time (contiguous), effect must succeed cause (succession), and cause and effect must be joined (conjunction) (Hume, 1999). However, Hume also specified in a fourth condition that an effect always had to be produced by the same cause, and that the occurrence of the cause always produced the effect, describing an exclusive relationship between cause and effect. Hume also observed that our understanding that a certain cause produces an effect is inferred, not innately known; after this inference, the relationship must be tested. These ideas are somewhat analogous to theorizing or hypothesizing, followed by quantitative testing.

A philosophical group known as essentialists dates from the time of Plato and Aristotle. The essentialists proposed two adjectives for causality: necessary and sufficient (Cartwright, 1968). The proposed cause must be **necessary** for the effect to occur. (The effect cannot occur unless the cause first occurs.) The proposed cause must also be **sufficient** (requiring no other factors) for the effect to occur. This means that causation is not present if a cause seems to result in an effect only some of the time. An example of necessary is the cause-and-effect relationship between the gene for cystic fibrosis and the disease of cystic fibrosis: it is necessary that a person receives the gene for cystic fibrosis from each parent (cause) in order for the disease to be present (effect). This particular cause is also sufficient for the person to have the disease, cystic fibrosis: as far as it is known, no second gene or condition is required for development of the disease.

John Stuart Mill, more than two millennia after Plato and Aristotle, suggested a third idea related to causation: there must be no alternative explanations for why a change in one variable seems to lead to a change in a second variable. In the research report, the researcher should address the possibility of alternative explanations for the study results, expressed as **rival hypotheses** (Campbell & Stanley, 1963; Shadish et al., 2002). For example, a researcher conducts a study of linear growth in 14-year-old boys, in which each subject is administered a multivitamin daily for 12 months. At the study's conclusion, the researcher notes that the subjects have grown an average of three inches during the year, attributing the growth to multivitamin administration. An example of a rival hypothesis, in the case of this study, would be that the subjects grew an average of three inches during the year because 14 years of age is a typical period of rapid growth for adolescent boys. A perceptive reader could argue that the boys would have grown that much without the intervention. Rival hypotheses are an important focus of the Discussion section of the research report.

Multiple Causality

Multiple causality refers to the case in which two or more causes acting together produce an effect. This idea was raised by Hume but not as fully developed as was his writing on single causes. Modern epidemiology, pathophysiology, and medicine have engaged in extensive research examining multiple causality over the past century.

If two or more causative factors are examined at the same time, the research uses a design that tests for multiple causality. Because of the complexity of humans and their interaction with the environment, many factors may be involved in causing an effect. Multiple regression analysis is the statistical strategy used to examine several factors in relation to one another. However, some experimental designs allow a researcher to examine the effects of two different variables, analyzing the contribution of each independently and the combined effect of both of them, in comparison with a control group. This allows the researcher to evaluate the ways they are additive in effect. One of these is the Fisher factorial design (Campbell & Stanley, 1963; Shadish et al., 2002).

Although a number of interrelating variables often combine to cause an effect, a single research study need not examine them all. An example is research in the mid-twentieth century focusing on neural tube defects (NTDs), which are believed to be caused by a number of interacting factors. In studies examining causation, not multiple causation, daily oral supplementation with folic acid was demonstrated to decrease the incidence of NTDs in populations with a high birthrate of this group of related disorders. Later, in a series of animal studies, one of the proposed genes causing neural tube malformation was identified, again in a single cause, single effect model. Later research in humans suggested up to 200 genes that may be causative for NTD, the most promising of which is the MTHFR gene, which regulates folic acid absorption (Greene, Stanier, & Copp, 2009). The presence of the MTHFR gene makes neural tube malformations more likely to occur; daily dosing with folic acid makes them less likely to occur.

Manipulation

Manipulation is one of the hallmarks of experimental research, and it is absent from noninterventional research. Manipulation in interventional research means that the researcher enacts an intervention that alters the value of the independent variable, then measures the resultant effect on one or more dependent variables. The most common values for the independent variable are "present" and "absent": present for the experimental group and absent for the control group. Manipulation in an experiment must be due to the researcher's action, the intervention. Research that measures a naturally occurring change is not, strictly speaking, interventional, because the researcher did not intervene—did not change the value of the independent variable.

Control

Control in research design means control for the effects of potentially extraneous variables, a serious issue for interventional research. Exerting controls does not mean "being in control of" the subjects' experience. Exerting control merely means either eliminating the effect of an extraneous variable or measuring its effect on the dependent variable. The term **highly controlled setting** almost always implies a research lab or a hospital unit especially designed for the conduct of research. In these environments, intrusion is minimized, and extraneous variables such as sound, light, and temperature are regulated. Basic research usually takes place in a highly controlled environment.

Control for the Effects of Extraneous Variables

Control for the effects of extraneous variables through the research design is the most straightforward way of making sure they do not affect the researcher's conclusions related to the effect of the independent variable on the dependent variable. Use of random assignment is the most generically efficient way to control for the effects of extraneous variables. When it is not feasible to control for the effects of known extraneous variables through design, though, it is possible to measure them in the course of the study. After data collection is complete, the researcher analyzes the effects of one or more extraneous variables by measuring their relationships with the dependent variable. This is a fallback position when it is not possible to control for extraneous variables through design.

The ability of random assignment with a large sample to control for the effects of extraneous variables is a powerful tool in research. The truth of the strategy is that if the sample is large, random assignment of subjects to treatment and control groups controls for the effects of most extraneous variables quite well, but not necessarily all extraneous variables. Even though the groups are assumed to be quite similar, researchers often compare the experimental group characteristics and control group characteristics and provide a table of these in the research report, with the percentage distribution in each per group, for confirmation of their sameness. An example would be an examination of the proportion of men versus women in both groups. This is called a **post hoc test** or post hoc analysis, from the Latin *after this one*. When "Table 1, Characteristics of the Sample" appears in a research report, with a note at the foot of the table stating, "Differences among groups were found not to be statistically significant," this represents a post hoc analysis for the distribution of potentially extraneous demographic variables. The researcher may measure other possibly extraneous variables as well, such as medical diagnoses or number of people in the household, on the suspicion that they too might intrude significantly upon the results. These are displayed either with the demographics or in a different table.

Control Groups and Comparison Groups

Control groups in experimental research control for the effects of potential extraneous variables. The traditional control group is randomly assigned in this type of research. If a change occurs in the dependent variable in the treatment (experimental) group and not in the randomly assigned control group, the researcher can be fairly confident that the independent variable caused the change in the dependent variable, and that the change was not merely the result of an uncontrolled-for extraneous variable. The presence of a randomly assigned control group is a requirement of experimental designs.

Quasi-experimental research can be said to use a control group when the researcher is able to obtain a group that is very similar to the experimental group. That control group might be obtained by random assignment, by matching, or by using subjects as their own controls. The reason these are considered control groups is that they control, at least to some extent, for the effects of extraneous variables. They do the job a control group should do. The point of differentiation, however, is whether the "control group" actually controls for anything.

Comparison groups are groups created for the purpose of comparison, and they are not products of random assignment. When a researcher identifies one of the groups in a study as a control group, but it does not control for any extraneous variables, the group is by default a comparison group. This is the case in which research data are compared with national norms or averages, or with standard universal values, such as serum sodium levels. These norms or averages are included for purposes of comparison, not control.

In some healthcare disciplines, "comparison group" has become synonymous with "nonrandomly assigned group," regardless of the group's effectiveness at controlling for extraneous variables. We do not support that position universally. As with almost everything, truth lies in the mid-ground. Control groups in experimental studies, by virtue of poor conceptual definitions or methodological difficulties, may not control very well for extraneous variables. On the other hand, some quasi-experimental designs control for the effects of more extraneous variables than does the most frequently used experimental design. In that case, these quasi-experimental designs' groups are quite properly termed control groups.

Because the purpose of a control group is to control for the effect of extraneous variables, a researcher using a nonrandomly selected "control" group should discuss the group in the study's limitations. The researcher must make a case for the degree to which the control group in the study actually controlled for extraneous variables. The reader of research should assess this limitation to validity, as well, especially if the authors of a research report did not do so.

An example is a study design in which data collection occurs simultaneously in both groups, and groups are not randomly assigned. The treatment group consists of all patients who are seen in an outpatient clinic on Tuesdays and Fridays; the control group consists of all patients seen at the same clinic on Mondays and Thursdays. Statistical analysis reveals that all demographics are statistically very similar between the groups. In addition, data collection is to proceed simultaneously, so external factors affecting patients would affect both groups equally. Is this a control group or a comparison group?

Prospective Versus Retrospective

Prospective is a term that means looking forward, whereas **retrospective** means looking backward, usually in relationship to time. Data collection in experimental research is prospective because the researcher enacts the research intervention in real time and then measures its effect. Prospective refers to measurements of the dependent variable that occur after the beginning of the experiment. In a prospective experimental design, a researcher may retrospectively collect demographic data from the medical record but is still said to be conducting prospective experimental research if the intervention and measurements of the dependent variable occur in real time.

Quasi-experimental research legitimately may rely on retrospectively collected measurements of the dependent variable. This strategy is most common for designs with passively enacted interventions, and for designs that involve non-concurrent data collection in experimental and control/comparison groups. (See the following descriptions of quasi-experiment designs.)

Partitioning

Partitioning, an analysis strategy, is used for interventional research, as well as noninterventional. In interventional studies, partitioning refers to subdividing a variable into subsets for the purpose of analysis. If this is related to the independent variable, as is sometimes the case, the researcher's intervention is applied in the usual way to the experimental group and not the control group. If little or no difference between groups is noted in the analysis phase, the research may note that after the independent variable was applied, subjects chose to perform an action one or more times. Those performing it more frequently exhibited a greater change in the dependent variable than did other subjects.

An example of this might be the intervention of a nurse attending half of the marathon races in a large area and presenting a mass onsite teaching intervention related to the benefits of consistent and frequent hydration with an appropriate rehydration solution during the race. In the analysis phase, no statistically significant differences are noted in the number of runners requiring medical treatment for dehydration at the end of the races, when the nurse-teaching marathons are compared with no-teaching marathons. However, the researcher notes a difference between runners who consistently and frequently stop to self-hydrate at the one-per-mile hydration stations and those who do not. In this example, when the researcher examines various levels of the desired behavior, partitioning the racers into occasional, medium, and frequent rehydration groups, a difference is evident, and this is the case across all races. The independent variable did not account for the difference in the dependent variable, but subjects' utilization of the touted resource certainly did.

Partitioning also can be applied to a variable with several values that is neither an independent nor a dependent variable but that seems to have a gradated effect on the dependent variable. In this case, the "treatment" or "event" can be a condition, exposure, or medication not enacted by the researcher, such as smoking history or number of apneic episodes per day. In this case, the partitioned event occurs naturally, as it does in noninterventional research, with the researcher applying an intervention, as well. The dependent variable is analyzed according to both the intervention and the naturally "partitioned" dose. An example would be patient response to a new medication designed to improve breathlessness related to chronic obstructive lung disease. The researcher might choose to partition the variable of years since initial symptoms, analyzing data in terms of how many years the subjects had complained of breathlessness. The treatment may well be determined to be most effective in subjects in whom the symptom has been present for the shortest amount of time.

VALIDITY FOR INTERVENTIONAL RESEARCH

Validity is the truthfulness of a research study. The validity of an interventional study represents the extent to which the study tests its underlying hypothesis, allowing support for the conceptual level of the study, its theoretical framework. **Design validity** is an important concern that the researcher addresses by choices made during interventional study design. It has four major facets (Cook & Campbell, 1986): construct validity, internal validity, external validity, and statistical conclusion validity (Table 11-1). A factor or condition that decreases the validity of research results is termed a **threat to validity** (Campbell & Stanley, 1963). These four facets of validity are the basis for the "limitations" to generalization of the study, which appear in the Discussion section of the research report.

As a caveat, one must not assume that because a certain design usually controls for a certain threat to validity, it always does so. Individual studies must be scrutinized for particularized threats, arising not only from their designs but also from their methods.

Construct Validity

The first aspect of design validity is construct validity (Table 11-1). Construct validity represents the extent to which a study's operational definitions reflect its conceptual definitions and constructs, and how well the research process adheres to the operational definitions, consistently and predictably for the duration of the study (Campbell, 1957). It is especially important in interventional research to have a complete and detailed

TABLE 11-1   Validity, Processes, Controls, and Verification Points for Interventional Research

Type of Validity	Underlying Process	Controlled for During	How Verified	Potential Pitfalls Later in the Process
Construct	Translation of concept to variable	Operational definition	Substruction	Treatment and measurement inconsistency Confounding variable identified
Internal	Minimizing intrusion of extraneous variables	Development of inclusion criteria Assignment to group Measurement of extraneous variable's effects	Confirmation of experimental and control group sameness by post hoc statistical analysis	Differential refusal rate or attrition rate, between groups after random assignment
External	Assuring sample representativeness	Sampling Site selection	Comparison of sample and population demographics	Large refusal or attrition rates
Statistical conclusion	Assuring a sufficient-sized sample Using correct statistical procedures Drawing appropriate conclusions	Power analysis Pilot testing Data analysis and data interpretation	Type II error avoided (sample size appropriate for effect size) Concordance with statistician	Effect size smaller than pilot predicted Faulty interpretation of statistical tests

operational definition for measurement of both independent and dependent variables. Rigorous research, throughout all of data collection, uses the same exact definitions, producing consistency over time. If the intervention is applied in a different way over the course of an experiment, or if its measurements of dependent variables vary, results can be invalid and the researcher will be unable to draw meaningful conclusions about the answer to the research question.

Another reason that the researcher must define the independent variable precisely is to make certain that it does not also contain a confounding variable. Especially in social science research, the research team delivering the independent variable possesses social skills. Interaction with them is pleasant for research subjects. When an intervention is to be enacted for members of the experimental group, sometimes a research design calls for a member of the research team to spend an equal amount of time with each member of the control group. This is a way to control for the confounding variable of positive social contact.

A **threat to construct validity** is a condition in which the measurement of a variable is not suitable for the concept it represents. Threats to construct validity are

many but, in general, they occur because of design flaws related to imprecise operational definitions or selected measurements, or to intra-study social considerations. Cook and Campbell (1979) identified many threats to construct validity, and many of these are listed in Table 11-2, with ways in which each threat is controlled. Those related to definition of variables include inadequate pre-operational clarification of constructs (roughly analogous to poor conceptual definition) and confounding constructs and levels of constructs (roughly equivalent to poor operational definitions, including definitions that specify degrees of measurement that are unlikely to produce effects). Threats relating to measurement are **mono-operational bias** (measuring the dependent variable only in one way, especially when it is a complex variable like task performance, pain, or life achievement) and **monomethod bias** (measuring the dependent variable in several similar ways, for instance, by using three self-assessment instruments that all measure life stress). Threats related to unintended interactions are **interaction of different treatments** (occurring when two or more independent variables are being tested) and interaction of testing and treatment (the pretest increases the posttest's measured effect).

TABLE 11-2 Threats to Construct Validity

Type of Validity	Name of Threat	Meaning	How to Control for It
Construct (design and measurement)	Inadequate preoperational clarification of constructs	Poor conceptual definition	Careful conceptual definition
Construct (design and measurement)	Confounding constructs and levels of constructs	Poor operational definitions, including definitions that specify degrees of measurement that are unlikely to produce effects	Thoughtful operational definition Pilot-testing of effects and measurement strategies Power analysis
Construct (design and measurement)	Mono-operational bias	Measuring the dependent variable only in one way, especially when it is complex	Measuring complex dependent variables with more than one strategy
Construct (design and measurement)	Mono-method bias	Measuring the dependent variable in several similar ways	Using different measurement approaches for the dependent variable
Construct (design and measurement)	Interaction of different treatments	The total effect is not the sum of the effects of each variable	Consideration of a design that tests both variables separately and in unison for each of the independent variables (like the factorial design)
Construct (design and measurement)	Interaction of testing and treatment	Pretesting causes an increase in scores on the posttest	Use of a design that controls for the effects of a pretest (like the Solomon four-group design) or one that does not utilize a pretest (posttest-only control group design)
Construct (social interplay)	Reactivity (the Hawthorne effect)	Subjects alter their normal behaviors because they are being scrutinized	Preceding data collection with other "tests" that are later discarded, to acclimatize subjects to being studied Considering several periods of data collection instead of one long period
Construct (social interplay)	Hypothesis guessing within experimental conditions	Subjects guess what the study hypothesis is and modify their behavior so as to support or undermine the hypothesis	Requesting that if subjects guess their group assignment, they do not modify their behavior (no known way to control)
Construct (social interplay)	Evaluation apprehension	Subjects demonstrate altered performance or responses on questions because of a desire to be perceived positively	Preceding data collection with other "tests" that are later discarded, to acclimatize subjects to being studied
Construct (social interplay)	Experimenter expectancies (the Rosenthal effect)	The beliefs of the person collecting the data may encourage responses from subjects that either support those beliefs or oppose them.	Using a double-blind strategy in which neither subjects nor data collectors are aware of subjects' group assignment

Continued

TABLE 11-2	Threats to Construct Validity—cont'd		
Type of Validity	**Name of Threat**	**Meaning**	**How to Control for It**
Construct (social interplay)	Novelty effect	Performance is better at the beginning of data collection because subjects are excited to be participating.	Preceding data collection with other "tests" that are later discarded, to acclimatize subjects to being studied
Construct (social interplay)	Compensatory rivalry	Control subjects who know they are in the control group try to demonstrate by trying extra hard that the treatment from which they were excluded is of no value.	Requesting that control group subjects not alter their behavior (no known way to control)
Construct (social interplay)	Compensatory equalization of treatment	Staff or family members try to compensate control group subjects for not having been included in an experimental group, providing what they perceive the experimental subjects are receiving.	Explaining to staff or family how important it is to learn exactly what differences are between treatment and nontreatment, and asking them not to interfere with the process (no known way to control)

Adapted from Cook, T. D., & Campbell, D. T. (1979). *Quasi-experimentation design and analysis issues for field settings.* Boston: Houghton Mifflin.

Cook and Campbell (1979) also identified threats to construct validity related to social interplay during the research process. In some social interplay threats, subjects independently modify their normal behaviors. Examples of these are reactivity, also called the **Hawthorne effect** (subjects alter their normal behaviors because they are being scrutinized), **hypothesis guessing within experimental conditions** (subjects guess what the study hypothesis is and modify their behavior so as to support or undermine the hypothesis), and evaluation apprehension (subjects want to be perceived positively and alter their performance or responses to questions). The latter is termed social desirability by some authors (Table 11-2).

Social interplay threats can be an outgrowth of the beliefs of the experimenter. One of these is the threat of **experimenter expectancies**, also called the Rosenthal effect (certain beliefs of the person collecting the data that may encourage responses from subjects that either support those beliefs or oppose them). Subjects can perform differently because of their emotional state, as well. Examples of this are the **novelty effect** (better performance at the beginning of data collection because subjects are excited to be participating) and compensatory rivalry (control subjects who know they are in the control group perform with additional effort to demonstrate that the treatment from which they were

excluded is of no value). Sometimes staff or family members try to compensate control group subjects for not having been included in an experimental group by giving them extra attention or advantages, providing what they perceive experimental subjects are receiving. This threat is termed **compensatory equalization of treatment**.

Reducing Threats to Construct Validity

The researcher can decrease design threats to construct validity (Table 11-2) by careful conceptual and operational definition of variables and by pilot-testing, followed by redefining variables. Measuring complex dependent variables with more than one strategy and using different measurement approaches can control for some threats to construct validity. Using a design that tests independent variables both separately and in unison, as does the factorial design, controls for the threat of interaction of different treatments. Selecting a design like the Solomon four-group design, presented later in this chapter, which controls for the effects of a pretest, can control for the interaction of testing and treatment.

Social interplay threats to construct validity are more difficult to control. Both reactivity (Hawthorne effect) and the novelty effect decrease if the researcher administers a pretest that will be discarded later, prior to administering the actual study instruments. Even when a sham pretest is not administered, reactivity and the novelty effect decrease over time, as subjects grow accustomed to being studied (Cook & Campbell, 1979).

One way to guard against the threat of experimenter expectancies is to use a double-blind strategy in which neither subjects nor data collectors are aware of subject assignment to group (Cook & Campbell, 1979). Subjects blinded to group assignment will not develop compensatory rivalry if they do not know their group membership, nor will family members and staff members be tempted to offer compensatory equalization if they are unaware of group membership.

Blinding or masking is the strategy of not revealing to subjects whether they are experimental or control subjects. They do not know their group assignment. **Double-blinding** is the strategy of withholding information about group assignment from both subjects and data collectors. This is a common practice in trials of new medications, in which subjects are administered either the experimental drug or a placebo. It is customary for one member of the research team, usually the pharmacist in medication studies, to know the group assignments of all subjects.

Internal Validity

Internal validity is the degree to which changes in the dependent variable occur as a result of the action of the independent variable (Campbell & Stanley, 1963). "Did in fact the experimental stimulus make some significant difference to this specific instance?" (Campbell, 1957, p. 297) is the question that inspires the researcher in the construction phase of a study to eliminate or control for variables that might produce rival hypotheses. Internal validity reflects design-embedded decisions that control for the effects of extraneous variables. An example of this type of decision in interventional research would be random assignment of a large sample to treatment and control groups, so that proportions of potentially extraneous variables would be similarly distributed between groups.

A **threat to internal validity** in interventional research is a factor that causes changes in the dependent variable, so that these do not occur solely as a result of the action of the independent variable. There exist many potential threats to internal validity. These are essential to consider when designing research. Although all threats to validity are important to understand, it would not be wrong to commit to memory the chief threats to internal validity. "Internal validity is the *sine qua non* for interventional research" (Campbell & Stanley, 1963, p. 5): it is essential to its logic. Quasi-experimental research

is especially prone to these threats, and reports of research that use interventional designs often mention one or more of the internal validity threats in their self-identified limitations to generalization.

Table 11-3 lists eight of the threats to internal validity, described by Campbell and Stanley (1963). The first is the **history threat**, often simply called history: an event external to the research occurs and affects the value of the dependent variable. An example of the history threat exists in a quasi-experimental study in which a researcher collects data about the effect of an in-hospital educational program on the quality and frequency of urinary catheter care and the related outcome of hospital-acquired urinary tract infection. The researcher collects data for 2 weeks. Then all nurses receive an educational intervention, emphasizing the importance of meticulous catheter care, following which the researcher collects data for 2 more weeks. At the beginning of the second data collection period, a coincidence occurs: all major news networks report a story regarding a famous film star's severe illness and partial loss of kidney function. The illness and kidney malfunction resulted from a urinary tract infection that occurred after a short-stay hospital procedure, after which the patient returned home with an indwelling catheter. If quality and frequency of catheter care improve in the second study phase, the researcher cannot be sure whether the extraneous variable of the breaking news story affected the dependent variables, or whether the educational program actually was effective. The researcher controls for the history threat by using a design that provides for a separate control group and concurrent data collection in both groups.

Another important threat to internal validity is **maturation**, which refers to normal changes like fatigue, hunger, growth, development, and aging that occur as a function of time, not because of the action of the independent variable. These normal changes may affect the value of the dependent variable (Table 11-3). An example of the threat of maturation would occur in research that measures 2- to 3-year-old children's ability to express their anger verbally instead of striking their playmates. The researcher's experimental intervention is to present a brief filmed dramatization in which characters strike their peers, who then exhibit distress, pain, and sadness. Young children see the film once a week at their day care center for 12 consecutive weeks. The dependent variable is the number of incidents of striking playmates that occur per child per week. The researcher tallies striking incidents for the 18 research subjects during the week before the intervention and again 4 weeks after the last film showing. If the incidence

TABLE 11-3   Threats to Internal Validity

Name of Threat	Meaning	How to Control for It
History	An event external to the research occurs and affects the value of the dependent variable	Data collection takes place in both intervention and control, or comparison, groups simultaneously
Maturation	Normal changes like fatigue, hunger, and aging that occur as a function of time, not as a result of the independent variable, affect the value of the dependent variable	Data collection takes place in both intervention and control, or comparison, groups simultaneously
Testing	Taking a pretest affects subsequent test scores	Use of a posttest-only with control group design or a Solomon four-group design Lengthening the period between tests, if possible, or using different forms of the same test
Instrumentation	Changes in the instrument used, or its calibration, occur during the course of the experiment	Consistent instruments, calibrated frequently and in the same manner each time
Statistical regression toward the mean	Subjects selected for extreme scores tend to have less extreme ones upon re-measurement, independent of intervention	Use of a control group, or a comparison group that demonstrates a similar amount of extreme scores
Selection	Subjects choose, or are chosen for, certain group membership, on a basis other than random assignment	Random assignment to group Selection of a design in which subjects are compared with themselves and a comparison group
Attrition (mortality)	Loss of subjects from the study after it is in progress	Large sample If differential (larger in one group than the other), perform subanalysis of attrition subjects (no known way to control)
Selection-maturation interaction	In nonrandomly assigned group assignment, the group's naturally occurring attributes change due to the passage of time, independently of the study treatment	Random assignment

of striking playmates decreases, the researcher will not be able to discern whether the film was effective, or whether the change was due to the effects of normal growth and development.

The **testing** threat refers to the effect of taking a pretest upon subsequent posttest scores (Table 11-3). If the same test serves as both pretest and posttest, subjects may purposely learn the answers in the interval between testing sessions. If a different test is used, subjects still may perform better on the posttest because they know what material is likely to be tested. The **instrumentation** threat refers to changes in the instrument used, or its calibration, that occur during the course of the experiment. An example of instrumentation could

be present in a study in which the researcher weighs hospitalized infants' diapers on a small portable scale, for the purpose of recording urine output, after the infants receive a diuretic. Failure to recalibrate the scale as recommended over the course of the study represents the instrumentation threat.

The threat of **statistical regression toward the mean** is present when subjects are selected for study participation because they display extreme scores of a screening variable (Table 11-3). An example would be a trial of a new medication for unusually high cholesterol readings. An inclusion criterion for the study is a low-density lipoprotein (LDL) cholesterol value of at least three times the norm. For some of the subjects, the cholesterol readings represent their normal values, but for others the cholesterol is unusually high, due to a transient cause, such as a new medication, an infection, or an illness. The latter subjects would be less likely to demonstrate extreme levels at their next lab draw, regardless of intervention: scores regress toward the mean value.

Two threats to internal validity can make experimental and control groups dissimilar. The first is the **selection threat**, in which subject assignment to group occurs in a nonrandom way (Table 11-3). Sometimes this occurs because of the manner in which the researcher makes group assignments. If the researcher assigns subjects to group based on the day of the week they first attend clinic, and the clinic has a policy that Wednesday appointments are reserved for Medicaid patients, a disproportionate number of clinic patients seen on Wednesday will be from lower-income strata and have poorer access to medical care. At other times, the selection threat is introduced when patients are allowed to choose whether to be members of the experimental group or the control group. Their decision as to group membership might represent a basic difference between types of subjects, which could affect the value of the dependent variable.

The second threat that can make experimental and control groups dissimilar is **attrition**, which is loss of subjects after a study has begun and before its completion, formerly referred to as **mortality**. When attrition is proportionately higher in one group than the other, randomly assigned groups become less alike. The difference in the value of the dependent variable may be due to the researcher's intervention, or to dissimilarity between the evolved groups.

Individual threats to internal validity can interact with one another, producing new threats. For instance, in a study with nonrandom group assignment, **selection-maturation interaction** can be a threat if the naturally occurring attributes in one group change due to the passage of time, independently of the study treatment.

An experimental design controls effectively for most or all of the threats to internal validity (Campbell & Stanley, 1963). Quasi-experimental designs that do not include a similar control or comparison group do not control as well for threats to internal validity.

For quasi-experimental research, in the worst-case scenario, there are so many threats to internal validity in a given study that no conclusions about causation can be made. However, this does not mean that the research has no value. A study with minimal control of extraneous variables functions like correlational or descriptive research and reveals information about the study variables and their relationships in that particular sample.

The study findings add to the body of descriptive knowledge. In recommendations for further research, which are based partially on limitations to validity, the researcher should include a recommendation for subsequent interventional research, using a design that controls more effectively for extraneous variables.

Reducing Threats to Internal Validity

Designs that use random assignment to group and concurrent data collection control for most threats to internal validity (Table 11-3). However, the testing threat results from pretesting or repeated testing, and it can be present even with some designs that use random assignment and concurrent data collection. Strategies that control effectively for the testing threat are discussed later in this chapter, in relation to individual designs. When repeated testing is necessary in a study, it is advantageous to attenuate the threat by collecting data over a long enough span of time so that subjects forget individual test items.

External Validity

External validity is the extent to which research results may be generalized back to the population: "To what populations, setting, and variables can this effect be generalized?" (Campbell, 1957, p. 297) is the underlying question. Campbell and Stanley (1963, p. 5) refer to "generalization to applied settings of known character" as "the *desideratum*," the essential goal of research. The external validity of a study is determined, to a great extent, by the representativeness and size of the sample, the number of study sites, and the findings of previous research in the same area. In the extreme case, external validity is so limited that generalization cannot be made beyond the study sample itself, reducing its usefulness to the level of descriptive research.

A **threat to external validity** is a factor that limits generalization, based on differences between the conditions of the study and the conditions of persons, settings, or treatments to which generalization is considered. Some threats to external validity (Table 11-4) reflect design-dependent decisions in sampling strategy that decrease the extent to which findings can be generalized. Subject refusal to participate and subject attrition also can affect external validity. Some of the threats to external validity are testing-intervention interaction (a pretest augments the effect of an intervention), selection-treatment interaction (an intervention is effective only in the accessible population), selection-testing interaction (a pretest augments the effect of an experimental treatment only in some groups), reactive arrangements (the effect of the intervention is modified by subjects'

TABLE 11-4   Threats to External Validity

Name of Threat	Meaning	How to Control for It
Testing-intervention interaction	Subjects score differently on the posttest because of a combination of the pretest and the intervention.	Use of a posttest-only design, or the Solomon four-group design
Selection-treatment interaction	Because the sample is not representative of the population, the intervention is effective only in the study sample.	Random selection or replication in different subpopulations
Selection-testing interaction	A pretest augments the effect of an experimental treatment only in some groups.	Random selection using a heterogeneous sample
Reactive arrangements	The effect of the intervention is modified by subjects' reactions to the study tests, measures, or setting.	Replicate often (no known way to control) If threat is present, results cannot be generalized to the "real world" setting
High refusal rate	Many potential subjects decline study participation	Check demographics to determine representativeness of the consented subjects Identify reasons for refusal Random assignment
High differential attrition rate	Many subjects in a study drop out of one of the groups, and fewer drop out of the other group	Check demographics to establish representativeness of the remaining subjects Identify reasons for attrition Very large samples

reactions to the study tests, measures, or setting), high refusal to participate, and high differential attrition (Campbell & Stanley, 1963). In general, external validity is greater with repeated replications of studies that use random selection of large representative samples from different parts of the population to which the researcher wishes to generalize. Low rates of refusal to participate and low differential attrition between groups also enhance external validity.

Cook and Campbell (1986) identified several threats to external validity, making a statement about them, as a group, "The threats to external validity are the factors that might limit the generalizability of causal relationships, making them specific to particular settings, kinds of people, or historical time settings" (p. 153). Threats to external validity sometimes have as their basis unusual ways in which an experimental treatment might interact with differences in groups of people, or with a certain setting or time, causing the researcher to draw conclusions that are not true for the general population. A high refusal rate for a study threatens external validity if the resultant sample is no longer representative of the population. Attrition of research subjects also threatens external validity, for the same reason. A researcher

controls for the effects of threats to external validity primarily through random selection, random assignment, large sample sizes, and replication (Table 11-4).

Statistical Conclusion Validity

Statistical conclusion validity refers to correctness of the decisions the researcher makes regarding statistical tests used in the study. Underlying all statistical testing is the principle of avoiding the threat to validity of violated assumptions of statistical tests (Table 11-5). Chapters 21 through 25 discuss the use of correct statistical tests, as well as the assumptions of each, related to levels of variables, distribution of values, and interaction with other variables.

A **threat to statistical conclusion validity** is a factor that produces a false data analysis conclusion. Assuming that assumptions of tests are not violated, the most pervasive threat to statistical conclusion validity is **low statistical power** (Cook & Campbell, 1986). This threat is present when a study sample is not large enough to detect statistically significant findings when they actually exist. Especially when the effect size of an intervention is small, a substantial sample may be required to generate power sufficient to demonstrate significance.

TABLE 11-5 Threats to Statistical Conclusion Validity

Type of Validity	Name of Threat	Meaning	How to Control for It
Statistical conclusion	Violated assumptions of statistical tests	Use of a test that cannot be used for a certain level of variable, distribution of values, or interaction with other variables	Consideration of the assumptions of all statistical tests Consultation with a statistician
Statistical conclusion	Low statistical power	Inadequate sample size for the amount of effect an intervention produces	Power analysis Pilot-testing Performance of a second power analysis, based on pilot data
Statistical conclusion	Fishing and the error rate problem	The researcher performs multiple statistical tests, fishing for statistically significant results	In the design phase, identify all statistical tests that will be analyzed

Low power is certainly the most common threat to statistical conclusion validity in nursing research. Using an inadequate-sized sample results in failure to reveal the true effect of the independent variable, and this is termed a **Type II error** (previously explained in Chapter 5). When the power of a study is low and there is the potential of a Type II error, the researcher cannot use negative results as evidence against causality. No conclusions about the interventional portion of the study can be made. Only the descriptive results of a study can be used, and the effort involved in conducting an interventional study is wasted.

To avoid the threat of low statistical power in interventional research, the researcher should perform a power analysis to estimate the number of subjects needed (Table 11-5). When the research employs a sample of sufficient size, if a difference really exists, it is very likely to be revealed through statistical testing. A power analysis estimates the sample size that will be required, based on the **effect size**, which is analogous to the percentage of change in the dependent variable, as well as to the strength of the relationship between variables. Almost invariably, the effect size of an intervention in a specific study is unknown until the researcher has collected data. For this reason, conducting a pilot-test to determine effect size is a wise prelude to performing a power analysis. This avoids the threat to statistical conclusion validity referred to by Shadish et al. (2002) as inaccurate effect size estimation. After an interventional study with a large enough sample, if the effect size remains as predicted and a statistical test fails to reject the null hypothesis, the researcher can be reasonably

certain that there was little real difference between the groups studied. If the sample is smaller than recommended and there is failure to reject the null hypothesis, the researcher cannot discern whether this was due to no real relationship between variables or to Type II error (failure to detect a difference due to small sample size). Consequently, it is impossible either to support or to reject the null hypothesis. There are online applications a researcher can use to estimate how large a sample is necessary for a research project when the researcher knows the approximate effect size (Lenth, 2006-2009). Chapters 15 and 21 discuss statistical power.

Another threat to statistical conclusion validity is **fishing and the error rate problem**, which refers to researchers performing multiple statistical tests, "fishing" for statistically significant results. Error rate is additive. For each inferential test conducted at the $p < 0.05$ level of significance, there is as great as a 5% chance of Type I error (previously explained in Chapter 5). Type I error means concluding that something is statistically significant when it is not. One can see that conducting 30 or 40 tests at the $p < 0.05$ level on the same data set would be likely to produce at least one false result that seemed promising but was merely a chance occurrence. Decisions as to which statistical tests the researcher will conduct and report should emanate from the research questions. The researcher should decide upon these tests before data are collected. Occasionally, an unanticipated finding will emerge, but the researcher should focus primarily on planned analyses and their meanings.

Inability of selected measurement strategies to detect differences has been described as a problem with statistical conclusion validity (Cook & Campbell, 1986). However, this text regards measurement difficulties as problems of construct validity. Unwise measurement choices fall under the rubric of confounding constructs and levels of constructs, because means of measurement are specified when variables are operationally defined. Failure to define variables clearly is a problem at the planning stage of design, rather than a fault in statistical conclusion. Basically, the threat relates more to the precision of data collection instruments than to the statistical tests themselves. In this case, study conclusions are faulty based on something other than the way in which statistical tests are employed.

The same is true for impaired intervention fidelity, random effects of the experimental setting, lack of treatment adherence, and random heterogeneity of respondents. Traditionally, these have been attributed to statistical conclusion validity (Campbell & Cook, 1986). The first three reflect on the suitability of operational definitions and their implementation. The latter threat is related to decisions regarding methods, not deficiencies at the statistical conclusion level.

CATEGORIZING AND NAMING RESEARCH DESIGNS

There is no universal standard for categorizing, or even naming, designs. Based on our review of 6 to 8 months of articles in three major U.S.-based nursing research journals, we found little standardization of design nomenclature for experimental and quasi-experimental designs. The pretest-posttest control group design, for instance, was variously referred to as a pretest-posttest experiment, a randomized controlled trial design, a randomized controlled trial, a repeat measurement with a randomized assignment and a controlled trial, a two-group pretest-posttest, a pre-test-post-test experimental randomized controlled design, and a controlled trial. A one-group pretest-posttest design was called a one-group pre and post quasi-experimental study design in one article, merely a quasi-experimental design in another, and was not named at all in a third. A nested strategy with a pretest-posttest control group design was variously termed a pre- and post-tested design and a two-arm cluster randomized experimental control trial. A posttest-only design with comparison group was termed a nonrandomized clinical trial. A time series design was termed a quasi-experimental interrupted timeseries. In short, the nomenclature used for interventional nursing research design varies both within and across journals. This brief review of the literature, however, did allow the establishment of the pretest-

posttest control group design as the most frequently used experimental strategy, and the one-group pretest-posttest design as the most frequently used quasi-experimental strategy.

The classification system used in this chapter (Tables 11-6 and 11-7) is based on Campbell and Stanley's (1963) general classifications, on Shadish et al.'s (2002) observations, and on current naming of research designs in the literature. Some designs retain Campbell and Stanley's original nomenclature and others have been modified in accordance with current usage. Two of Campbell and Stanley's so-called pre-experimental designs are included within the quasi-experimental group because they are used frequently in nursing and healthcare research and, under some circumstances, can provide some evidence of causation.

The effectiveness of a design in controlling for the effects of extraneous variables can only be approximated. Individual studies may be stronger or weaker, depending on factors internal to the design, specific to the site, and associated with decisions made about study methods. The relative strength of a design is most especially related to the representativeness of the control/comparison group. An unusually strong or weak control/comparison group affects both internal and external validity. Consequently, estimates of the strength of designs for internal validity must be taken judiciously.

EXPERIMENTAL DESIGNS

Many interventional designs are used in nursing and in other disciplines. Designs actually or potentially useful for nursing science are described fully. Examples from the literature are provided for designs that are currently used for nursing research. Illustrative structural models are provided for some of the most frequently used designs.

Sir Ronald A. Fisher (1935) developed the first experimental designs, and these were published in a book titled, *The Design of Experiments*. Experimental designs, as depicted in Figure 11-1, are the definitive way to establish evidence of causation. The reason researchers prefer these designs is that they assure a high degree of internal validity (Table 11-6), because random assignment creates experimental and control groups that are very similar. After assignment of subjects to groups, the researcher applies a treatment to the experimental group and measures the dependent variable in all subjects to determine its resultant difference in value between groups. The three essential elements of experimental research are (1) researcher-controlled manipulation of the independent variable, (2) the presence of a distinct

TABLE 11-6   Classification of Interventional Research Design Types: Experimental

In This Text	Campbell and Stanley (1963)	Other Designations in the Literature	Internal Validity
Pretest-posttest control group design (experimental design)	Pretest-posttest control group design	Pretest-posttest study, true experiment, classic experimental design	Very good
Randomized block design— subtype of experimental	*Blocking*	*Random block design; blocking; blocked sample*	*Very good*
Nested design—subtype of experimental	*Nested classification*	*Nested strategy; nested sample; nesting*	*Very good*
Posttest-only control group design	Posttest-only control group design	Posttest-only design	Excellent
Crossover design (counterbalanced design)	Counterbalanced or crossover design	Crossover strategy	Excellent
Wait-list strategy—subtype of crossover		*A wait-listed design; wait-listing*	*Excellent*
Solomon four-group design	Solomon four-group design	Solomon four-group	Excellent
Factorial design	Factorial designs	Factorial method, Fisher factorial design	Excellent

Note: Listings in italics represent subtypes of the designs that appear immediately above them.

TABLE 11-7   Classification of Interventional Research Design Types: Quasi-Experimental

In This Text	Campbell and Stanley (1963)	Other Designations in the Literature	Internal Validity
NO CONTROL GROUP OF ANY KIND			
One-group pretest-posttest design	One-group pretest-posttest design (pre-experimental)	One-group pretest-posttest strategy	Very poor
Posttest-only design with comparison with norms		Post-intervention study	Very poor
Pretest-posttest design with comparison with norms		Pre and post intervention study	Very poor
NONRANDOM CONTROL/COMPARISON GROUP			
Posttest-only with comparison group design	Static-group comparison (pre-experimental)	Posttest only design with nonequivalent controls	Very poor; Fair with concurrent comparison group
Pretest-posttest design with nonrandom control group	Nonequivalent control group design	Pretest-posttest design with nonequivalent controls	Very good
SUBJECTS AS THEIR OWN CONTROLS			
Time series design	Time-series design	Time-series design	Very good
Time series design with nonrandom control group	Multiple time-series design	Time series with nonequivalent controls	Excellent
Time series design with repeated reversal	Equivalent time samples design	Repeated reversal; withheld and reinstituted treatment; single subject research	Excellent

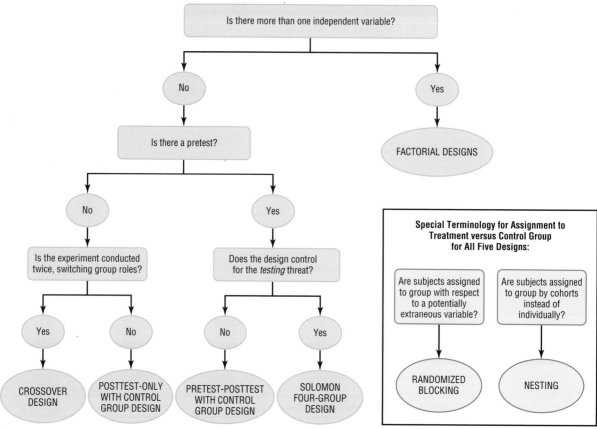

FIGURE 11-1 Algorithm for experimental designs.

control group, and (3) random assignment of subjects to either the experimental or the control condition.

Pretest-Posttest Control Group Design (True Experimental Design)

The **pretest-posttest control group design** (Figure 11-2) is also termed the experimental design or sometimes the true experimental design. It provides the simplest and most commonly used method of comparing treatment with absence of treatment. The researcher randomly assigns consented subjects to either treatment or control group and measures the dependent variable or variables in both groups. Then the researcher applies the intervention only to the treatment group and, after the intervention is complete, measures the dependent variable(s) again in both groups. The name for the design is the pretest-posttest control group design because there is both a pretest and a posttest of the dependent variable(s) in the experimental group, and

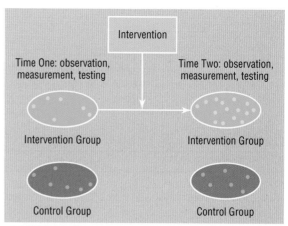

FIGURE 11-2 Pretest-posttest control group design.

there is a control group that is concurrently pretested and posttested. Randomized controlled trials use the pretest-posttest control group design or variations of it.

A very common variation of the pretest-posttest control group design is one in which the control group receives the "usual care," "usual treatment," or "standard protocol" and the experimental group receives the experimental treatment. This is the rule rather than the exception in most therapeutic research that trials a new therapy, because depriving half of the subjects of the usual treatment would be ethically unacceptable. In another variation used in trials of a new medication, experimental tests of its efficacy involve administration of a placebo to the control group. The placebo has the same appearance as the experimental medication, so that subjects do not know their group assignment.

Again, the features of a real experiment are present in this design: researcher intervention, a distinct control group, and random assignment to treatment or control group. The pretest-posttest control group design is the prototype for other experimental, and some quasi-experimental, designs.

An example of the pretest-posttest control group design is Kurdal, Tanriverdi, and Savaş's (2014) study of the effectiveness of a teaching intervention on functioning of patients with bipolar disorder. This excerpt from the abstract describes their design and findings:

"... This study was conducted as a two-group pretest–posttest design to determine the effect of psychoeducation on the functioning levels of patients with bipolar disorder. A total of 80 patients were assigned to either the experimental ($n = 40$) or the control group ($n = 40$). The data were collected using a questionnaire form, and the Bipolar Disorder Functioning Questionnaire. The experimental group scored significantly higher on the functioning levels (emotional functioning, intellectual functioning, feelings of stigmatization, social withdrawal, household relations, relations with friends, participating in social activities, daily activities and recreational activities, taking initiative and self-sufficiency, and occupation) ($p < .05$) compared with the control group after psychoeducation ..." (Kurdal, Tanriderdi, & Savaş, 2014, p. 312)

Common Variations of the Pretest-Posttest Control Group Design

Two common variations of the pretest-posttest control group design found in healthcare research are the randomized block design and the nested design. The subtypes do not differ in structure from the parent design, so we do not consider them separate designs as much as strategies. They differ from the parent design, and from

one another, only in the way in which subjects are randomly assigned to groups. The randomized block design is used to control for an identified extraneous variable. The nested design controls for the potential of several extraneous variables, which are often environmentally situated. Both blocking and nesting can be used to randomly assign groups in other experimental designs, described in the following sections.

The **randomized block design**, also called randomized blocking, uses the classic experimental design most frequently, but it adds the feature of making random assignment in two or more stages, so as to provide equal distribution of a potentially extraneous variable between or among groups. Values of the potentially extraneous variable are known before intervention occurs. Here, the word "block" denotes stratum or level. For instance, perhaps in previous research, results have been reported that indicate an interaction between gender and the dependent variable. Values of the dependent variable are likely to be higher in one gender. Blocking allows one stratum, for example all the women in the sample, to be assigned randomly to treatment or control group, and then the other stratum, all the men, to be assigned randomly to either group, providing similar proportions of men and women in each group. Computer-based subject-randomization programs can be used for this task of assigning.

Sometimes a researcher does not assign subjects to groups using blocking but realizes after data collection that a characteristic within the group seems to be associated with a higher value for the dependent variable. In this case, the statistical test analysis of covariance (ANCOVA) may be performed. The ANCOVA functions much like blocking by analyzing the subjects in groups to determine the degree of covariance between their characteristics and the dependent variable. The ANCOVA, however, requires several things: a normal distribution of the dependent variable, an extraneous variable that is at least at the continuous level of measurement, and a linear relationship between the dependent variable and the potentially extraneous variable (Plichta & Kelvin, 2012). Because two of these requisites usually are not confirmed until data collection is complete and statistical analysis has been performed, it is more practical to use random assignment by block. In a block design, the researcher must be clear that the blocked variable does not represent an important rival hypothesis, which in this case would be a different explanation of change in the dependent variable that occurs because of the blocked variable.

The **nested design** is the classic experimental design, in which random assignment is made by assigning groups of subjects instead of single subjects. Individual subjects are "nested" within a larger classification. In a healthcare institution, the researcher might use the strategy of nesting to randomly assign entire hospital units to one group or the other, instead of assigning the individuals within each unit. Nesting often is used when assigning individuals to group would prove unwieldy. Examples of three of these instances are (1) there is a possibility of attrition when subjects become aware that other subjects have been assigned to another group and object to their group assignment; (2) in an institutional setting, two different protocols will be used for the experimental and control conditions, and adherence to different protocols within the same unit would be confusing and potentially disruptive to care delivery; and (3) interactions between experimental and control group subjects might place the study at risk.

As an example, a researcher will test a new bar code identification system with half of the patients in a hospital. The other half of the patients will represent the control group. Patients in the treatment group will wear blue identification bands, and those in the control group will wear red identification bands. The healthcare team expresses concerns about mixing the two identification systems on one unit, creating an undue expenditure of time for nursing staff. Also, patients may have concerns if they become aware of the different bands, which could foster subject dissatisfaction with assignment. To avoid this issue, entire nursing units are assigned as large groups or "nests" to the experimental or the control condition. When using a nested design with a relatively small number of "nests," it is important to make certain that no group contains an undue amount of a potentially extraneous variable. With a large number of groups, this is a smaller concern, because random assignment should distribute extraneous variables rather evenly.

Experimental Posttest-Only Control Group Design

The experimental **posttest-only control group design** (Figure 11-3) is the classic experimental design without a pretest. Campbell and Stanley (1963) make a fine argument for the validity of the posttest-only control group design, pointing out that random assignment should serve to make the groups very similar before intervention occurs, making a pretest unnecessary. (Scores across groups should be similar.) For studies in which pre-measurement of one or more dependent variables is nonsensical, for instance when postoperative pain intensity is the dependent variable, it is sensible to use the posttest-only control group design. An example of this is Desmet et al.'s (2013) research testing two different methods of administering dexamethasone to

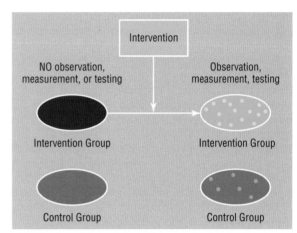

FIGURE 11-3 Posttest-only control group design.

increase the postoperative duration of ropivacaine for shoulder surgery.

In other studies, pretesting would change subjects' perceptions. For instance, in a study in which subjects complete an assessment of knowledge after they complete a learning activity, pretesting using an identical or similar instrument could introduce the testing threat. Subjects would learn from the first test, which would improve their scores on the second test. Consequently, it would be difficult to discern whether improvement in scores was due to the researcher's intervention or to the measurement administered before intervention. Here, the posttest-only control group design is reasonable to use, provided that random assignment occurs prior to treatment.

An example of the posttest-only control group design is Fredericks and Yau's (2013) study of the effects of an individualized education program delivered by telephone at two points in time after hospital discharge. Excerpts from the abstract describe their design and findings:

"... The purpose of this pilot study was to collect preliminary evidence to demonstrate the impact of an individualized education intervention given above and beyond usual care, delivered, at two points in time, following hospital discharge. A randomized controlled trial was used in which 34 patients were randomly assigned to one of two groups. Chi-square analyses to examine differences between groups on complications and hospital readmission rates were conducted.

Findings point to the impact of the intervention in reducing the number of hospital readmissions and complications at 3 months following hospital discharge." (Fredericks & Yau, 2013, p. 1251)

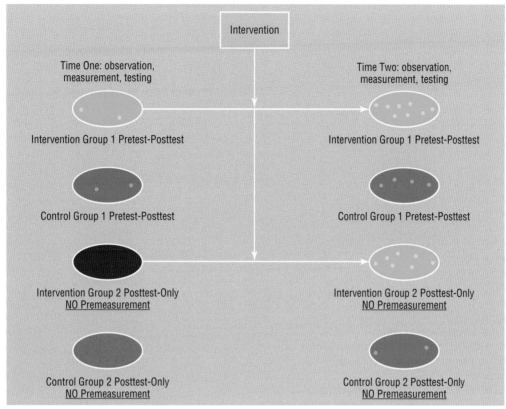

Intervention

Time One: observation, measurement, testing

Time Two: observation, measurement, testing

Intervention Group 1 Pretest-Posttest

Intervention Group 1 Pretest-Posttest

Control Group 1 Pretest-Posttest

Control Group 1 Pretest-Posttest

Intervention Group 2 Posttest-Only
NO Premeasurement

Intervention Group 2 Posttest-Only
NO Premeasurement

Control Group 2 Posttest-Only
NO Premeasurement

Control Group 2 Posttest-Only
NO Premeasurement

FIGURE 11-4 Solomon four-group design.

Solomon Four-Group Design

The Solomon four-group design (Figure 11-4) is an alternative to the posttest-only control group design and is used to control for the testing threat, not by eliminating testing from the design but by measuring the effect of testing on subsequent scores. Although this design is of some use in nursing education, it is rarely used in clinical settings because of most nurses' unfamiliarity with the design and with the complexity of its implementation.

The Solomon four-group design combines the groups of the classic experimental design and the posttest-only control group design. It consequently includes four groups, all randomly assigned, that receive pretest-treatment-posttest, pretest-no treatment-posttest, treatment-posttest only, and posttest only. The Solomon four-group design provides excellent control for the major threats to internal validity. As such, it is the polar opposite of the single group pretest-posttest quasi-experimental design, which has poor internal validity throughout.

Factorial Design

The **factorial design** also is called the Fisher factorial design after its inventor, Sir Ronald Fisher (Fisher, 1935). The factorial design is the classic experimental design with the addition of at least one independent variable that also is randomly assigned. In this way, the individual effect of either one of the variables, as well as the combined effect of the two independent variables, can be measured. A factorial design tests for multiple causality using two or more independent variables.

This is the way it works for two independent variables. Subjects are randomly assigned to one of four groups: A receives both variables, B receives one variable, C receives the other variable, and D is the control group and receives neither variable. This is a "2 × 2" design, referring to the diagram of the four groups, and is the simplest form. This design is illustrated in Figure 11-5, in which two independent variables are enacted. Here, Cell D subjects receive no treatment and serve as a control group. Cells B and C allow the researcher to examine the effect of each intervention separately. Cell

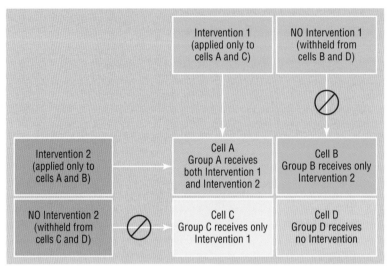

FIGURE 11-5 Factorial design.

A allows the researcher to examine the interaction between the two independent variables. Cells in a factorial design must contain approximately the same number of subjects.

More involved factorial experiments are possible. For instance, using three variables with two values each would produce eight different groups. The researcher also can examine an additional level of the independent variables, for instance using two variables with four values each, none-small-medium-large, yielding 16 different groups.

Good et al. (2012) used a factorial design in their research that examined the effect of two different interventions on postoperative salivary cortisol, which is a physiological marker of stress. The following excerpt from this study's abstract describes study design and outcomes.

"The present study was designed to determine whether two interventions, patient teaching (PT) for pain management and relaxation/music (RM), reduced cortisol levels, an indicator of stress, following abdominal surgery. Patients (18–75 years) were randomly assigned to receive PT, RM, a combination of the two, or usual care; the 205 patients with both pre-test and posttest cortisol values were analyzed. A 2 x 2 factorial design was used to compare groups for PT effects and RM effects. Stress was measured by salivary cortisol before and after 20-min tests of the interventions in the morning and afternoon of postoperative Day 2. ... Comparisons using analysis of covariance (ANCOVA), controlling for baseline levels, showed no PT effect or RM effect on cortisol in the morning or afternoon. Post hoc ANCOVA showed no significant effects when intervention groups were compared to the control group." (Good et al., 2012, p. 318)

Crossover or Counterbalanced Design

Rankin and Campbell (1955) discussed the counterbalanced design in its experimental form, using random assignment. Campbell and Stanley (1963) later described use of the design as a quasi-experimental method without random assignment, and its applications in the social science field. The design is conducted within health care as an experimental strategy, using random assignment, as the crossover design.

The **crossover design**, still occasionally called the counterbalanced design, is the classic experimental design with at least one additional period of data-collection, in which experimental and control conditions are reversed. In this design, all subjects receive the intervention once and the control condition once (Figure 11-6). Despite the fact that there is no permanent control group, each period of data collection has a control group and represents an independent experiment in itself. The design controls for threats to internal validity as well as a traditional experimental design does because of its random assignment of subjects to group.

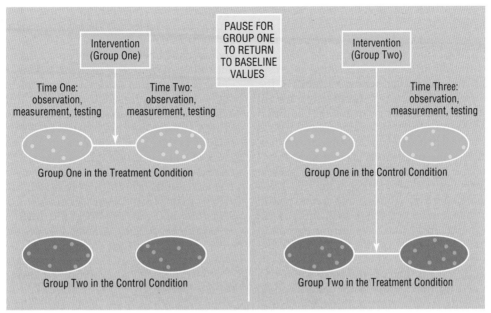

FIGURE 11-6 Crossover design.

The amount of time between data collection periods is set to allow the effects of the intervention to dissipate. In the most common form of the experiment, the subject is randomly assigned to treatment or control condition for the first data collection period; then for the second, each subject is placed into the opposite group. This strategy is ideal when a small pool of subjects is available, since each subject acts as its own control.

In crossover designs, the "usual treatment" frequently is used as the control condition, when the usual treatment and the experimental treatment are similar in both application and effects. As a caution, the researcher must be alert to the possibility that changes may be due to factors such as disease progression, the healing process, the normal growth process, the effects of aging, or the effects of treatment of the disease rather than the study treatment. These factors may represent the threat of maturation.

Crossover designs can involve more than two different interventions, so that each subject is tested more than twice. As testing periods increase in number, however, the length of the data collection process increases, with the attendant threat of subject attrition.

An example of this design is Liao et al.'s (2013) crossover study that tested the effect of a warm footbath on sleep and sleep quality. The following excerpts from the study abstract explain the design.

"Design: Two groups and an experimental crossover design was used ... Methods: All participants had body temperatures (core, abdomen, and foot) and polysomnography recorded for 3 consecutive nights. The first night was for adaptation and sleep apnea screening. Participants were then randomly assigned to either the structured foot bathing first (second night) and non-bathing second (third night) condition or the non-bathing first (second night) and foot bathing second (third night) condition. Results: A footbath before sleep significantly increased and retained foot temperatures in both good and poor sleepers. ... There were no significant changes in polysomnographic sleep and perceived sleep quality between non-bathing and bathing nights for both groups." (Liao et al., 2013, p. 1607)

When a large sample is available, a different method of assignment to group sometimes is performed, in which random assignment is used for both phases of the study. In this version of the experiment, some subjects are in the experimental group twice and some in the control group twice. In this variant of the design, not every subject would receive the experimental treatment. The variation yields a 2 × 2 analysis matrix, by which the researcher can make multiple comparisons as to efficacy of treatment, and also assess duration of effect by measuring whether washout is complete for early intervention groups. **Washout period** is the time that it takes for the effect of the first treatment to dissipate. This strategy is uncommon in health care but is used occasionally in education.

Another variation of the counterbalanced or crossover design is the strategy termed wait-listing. In the **wait-listed** variation, subjects in a therapeutic study are told that they will receive the new treatment but that if they are assigned to the control condition, there will be a delay and they will first act as control subjects and then receive the therapeutic intervention in the study's second phase. For new and promising medications, the guarantee of treatment assures low attrition in the wait-listed group. In addition, between the first and second phases of the study, there can be a period of evaluation, as the researchers analyze first-phase data before beginning the second phase. The primary difference between the crossover design and its wait-listed variation is that in wait-listed studies, the treatment group does not necessarily serve as a control group in the second phase because frequently an intervention is performed that affects measures permanently (a kidney transplant, for example). When this is the case, determination of sample size should be made as if there is only one study phase.

The wait-listed strategy is used infrequently by nurse researchers but is a rather common strategy for new and promising therapeutic research. Two advantages to the design are the ability to identify sudden changes, for good or ill, in the first experimental group, before applying the therapy to the other group, and the ability to offer a therapeutic intervention to all interested subjects. The design's disadvantage is that when the wait period is long, attrition rates rise.

QUASI-EXPERIMENTAL DESIGNS

Quasi-Experimental Designs and Internal Validity

Researchers use experimental designs because they assure a high level of internal validity. The way an experiment works is that it produces experimental and control groups that are very similar through random assignment. Then the researcher applies a treatment to the experimental group, and measures all subjects to determine how much difference occurs between groups. In a well-designed classic experiment, it is sometimes difficult even to imagine a rival hypothesis that might account for the change in the dependent variable.

A quasi-experimental design is used when a researcher decides that an experimental design cannot or should not be used for an interventional study. This means that when an experimental design can be used and is appropriate for considerations posed by control of extraneous variables, site limitations, subject availability, and time frame, it should be used. Quasi means "like," and so quasi-experimental designs are like experimental ones, but not equivalent to them, lacking one or more of the three essential elements of experimental research: (1) researcher-controlled manipulation of the independent variable, (2) the traditional type of control group instead of using either no control group at all or using subjects as their own controls, and (3) random assignment of subjects to groups (see Figure 11-7). Because these designs lack at least one of the elements of experimental research, many of them harbor threats to internal validity (Table 11-7). The reader of a research report can easily imagine rival hypotheses for many of the quasi-experimental designs. Among the dozens of quasi-experimental designs are some that are better and some that are worse at controlling for extraneous variables.

Sometimes a quasi-experimental design is chosen because a new researcher is unaware of the design's limitations related to issues of internal validity. At other times, choice of a quasi-experimental design is a fallback stance (Campbell & Stanley, 1963), made in response to disappointment or opportunity. In nursing, the disappointment may be site-associated barriers, or a shortage of potential subjects that would lengthen the period required for completion of an experimental study. Opportunity often takes the form of a newly imposed, untested hospital-wide protocol, a change in staffing ratios, adoption of a new product line for in-hospital oral care, a new classification system that affects intake of mental health clients, or a required training program that is intended to improve teamwork and morale. A quasi-experimental design is chosen because it is the only option available to test the effect of the emergent change.

Many threats to internal validity exist within the quasi-experimental group of studies and are described here for the actual studies that are used as exemplars, and for types of design that are known to predispose to certain threats to internal validity (Tables 11-3 and 11-7). The history threat, for instance, is present when data collection is not concurrent for intervention and control groups, and it is due to the possible existence of something other than the independent variable that occurs prior to or during data collection and causes the change in the dependent variable.

Two Pre-Experimental Designs

Campbell and Stanley (1963) identified several quasi-experimental designs that they designated pre-experimental. The designation was made because of

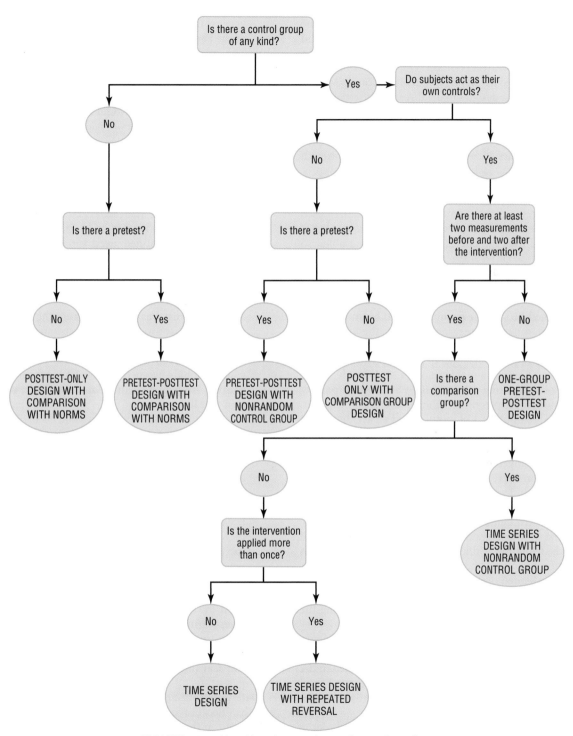

FIGURE 11-7 Algorithm for quasi-experimental studies.

the poor ability of the designs to control for any of the threats to internal validity. Thus, the designs usually did not produce meaningful information about causation related to a given intervention. One is described here, because it is used frequently in nursing research. A study exemplifying the design's many threats to internal validity is provided, with exemplars of all relevant threats along with a rival hypothesis for each threat that might explain the study results as well. The second pre-experimental design is described in a later section with other studies that lack random assignment to group.

The **one-group pretest-posttest**, a pre-experimental design named by Campbell & Stanley (1963) the single-group pretest-posttest, is the most common design used for quasi-experimental nursing research. It exerts almost no control over the effects of extraneous variables, so interpretation of results is difficult. Even in the face of statistically significant results, the reader can imagine many alternative hypotheses that might explain the reasons for the results. In this design, measurement is obtained for a single group, followed by an intervention and a second measurement of the dependent variable.

An example of single-group pretest-posttest research is Hooge, Benzies, and Mannion's (2014) study of the effect of a parenting program, *Baby and You*, on parenting knowledge, parenting morale, and social support. The study sample of 159 mothers had an average age of 31 years, and 94% were first-time mothers. Hooge et al. (2014) administered the Parenting Knowledge Scale (PKS), developed by the authors from the Reece Parent Expectation Survey (Reece, 1992), the Parenting Morale Index (PMI; Trute & Hiebert-Murphy, 2005), and the Family Support Scale (FSS; Dunst, Jenkins, & Trivette, 1984). Instruments were mailed to participants before the first of four classes. After attending three or four of the classes, subjects filled out the posttest instruments on-site or received them by mail. The course of four classes extended over a 4-week span. The findings were statistically significant only for the dependent variable of parenting knowledge, which did increase during the course of the study.

The study contained many threats to internal validity (Table 11-3), almost all arising from the fact that no control group or comparison group was included in the design. Reasons that various threats are present, and rival hypotheses that might explain the study's positive results, are detailed:

- The history threat was present because of the lapse of 4 weeks between pretest and posttest. During the 4 weeks, mothers could have sought knowledge independently, because of curiosity or because of the emergent health needs of their children. There was no control group.
- The maturation threat was present because mothers are in a continual "learning mode" when they have small children. Knowledge increases during the process of childrearing. It is not known how much knowledge would have been gained by the mothers during the 4-week period without the course.
- The testing threat was present because mothers might have engaged in focused learning based on what they did not know at the pretest.
- The threat of statistical regression toward the mean might have had an effect on the results because mothers chose to be in the course based on their self-identified need for knowledge, so their initial scores would have been toward the low end of the spectrum. The subsequent increase in scores might have been merely a statistical pattern of regression.
- Selection threat was present because the mothers may have chosen to take the course based on self-identified deficits. Also, transportation to the course and even a nominal course fee, if any, would exclude women of the lowest economic stratum from participation, also creating a selection threat.
- Experimental mortality, or attrition, occurred at a rate of 58% between initial course registration and completion of the requisite three out of four classes before completion of the posttest. The authors did not provide reasons that the mothers stopped attending the course. Perhaps the mothers who did not complete the course dropped out because they did not find the material helpful for increasing their knowledge. This would mean that the program would be effective only for women whose learning needs were extremely high.
- Selection-maturation interaction is possible as well. Women whose scores increased might have been low in knowledge but they may also have been learning at a rapid rate, on their own. Their gains in knowledge could have been due to the interaction of a low-knowledge state and the learning that normally takes place during parenting.

Data were collected for this study over a period of 4 months. Because advance registration was used for enrollment in the program, the researchers would have been able to constitute a comparison or control group, preferably the latter, in order to decrease threats to internal validity. For this study, some alternatives to the use of this very weak design might have been (1) the pretest-posttest with control group design, which controls for all threats to internal validity except testing; (2) the posttest-only control group design, which controls for all threats to internal validity; (3) the pretest-posttest design with a nonrandom control group, which controls for most threats to internal validity; and (4) the posttest-only nonrandom control group design, which also controls for most threats to internal validity.

Quasi-Experimental Studies and How They Deviate From Experimental Design, by Type

Three main categories of quasi-experimental research exist, and these are based on the three requisites for experimental studies. These categories are (1) those that lack researcher-controlled manipulation of the independent variable, (2) those that lack a separate control group, and (3) those that have two groups but lack random assignment to group.

Studies That Lack Researcher-Controlled Manipulation of the Independent Variable

For quasi-experimental studies that lack researcher-controlled manipulation of the independent variable, otherwise termed passive intervention studies, the independent variable occurs independently of the researcher's actions. Examples would be policy changes, trials of new in-agency protocols, mass inoculations required by a government or agency, sudden unavailability of a needed resource, or a group of procedures performed by someone other than the research team. The researcher, in this case, often takes advantage of the opportunity to obtain evidence, in a right-place-right-time sense, when outside forces create unique change. Although these designs do not control well for threats to internal validity, they provide some tentative answers about causation that can be tested later with more rigorous research, in order to provide stronger evidence.

The researcher who does not actually manipulate the independent variable must be very clear as to when the independent variable was enacted, the sequencing of the events of the change, the conditions under which the change occurred, and concurrent events that might affect the analysis. No real control group is possible because the "intervention" has already occurred. The comparison group the researcher chooses must be as much like the "experimental group" as possible. A comparison group that is quite similar to the intervention group improves internal validity.

To call these designs quasi-experimental may be, strictly speaking, a misnomer. Some are not experimental at all, but rather comparative descriptive or comparative correlational in nature. However, educational and, more recently, healthcare researchers have conducted studies about passively received changes and called them quasi-experimental, usually when measurement in the "experimental" group occurs in real time and the passive "intervention" also occurs in real time or in the not-too-distant past. The more time that lapses between intervention and measurement, the more occasions there are for threats to internal validity, especially the history threat, to arise (Campbell & Stanley, 1963). This kind of design uses comparison groups instead of control groups, making the studies somewhat suspect in terms of internal validity, especially when data collection for the comparison group occurs in the distant past. It is sometimes difficult to assure sameness of groups, based on what is available in existent databases.

Designs in the quasi-experimental group that are appropriate for passive intervention studies include several of the nonrandom comparison group designs (posttest-only design that uses either a comparison group or historical norms, and pretest-posttest design with a comparison group or historical norms), as well as the time series design and time series design with nonrandom control group. All of these are described in the following sections.

Studies That Lack the Traditional Type of Control Group (Subjects Used as Their Own Controls)

For studies that lack the traditional type of control group, and instead use subjects as their own controls, several of the available designs that use time series approaches present fewer threats to internal validity than would choosing a comparison group that has little, if any, similarity to the treatment group. Nurse researchers sometimes use designs that include subjects as their own controls when they are studying characteristics that differ considerably between individuals (inter-individual variation). Some people seem to have a different set-point of these characteristics, so standard comparison between individuals becomes problematic. However, these particular variables also can differ substantially within individuals (intra-individual variation), as a result of healthcare interventions. Using subjects as their own controls in a quasi-experimental design eliminates the problem of inter-individual variation. Some topics that have been studied using this group of designs have been pain, mood, anxiety, motivation, nausea, and fatigue.

The principal concern with these designs is that they involve measurement at two different points in time, at least, potentially introducing the history threat, and

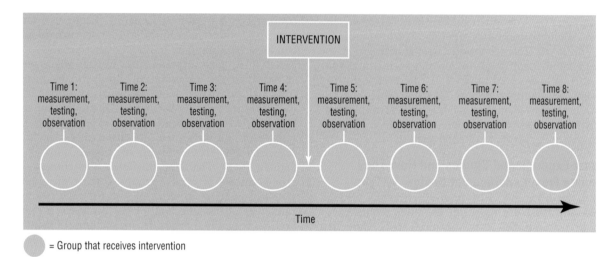

FIGURE 11-8 Time series design.

only one of the designs uses a control or comparison group. The one-group pretest-posttest design, described previously as a pre-experimental design is a generally unsuitable design, because of its many threats to internal validity. These threats stem principally from the fact that different values obtained at the second measurement are not clearly attributable to the independent variable but may be due to other factors. Other designs that use subjects as their own controls exist, however. They minimize threats by using multiple measurements. Two of them are the time series design and the time series design with repeated reversal, also called the repeated-reversal design. The time series design with nonrandom control group is an interesting variation of the time series design in that it provides an understanding of subjects' changes in the dependent variable over time and adds a nonrandom control group for further analysis, as well, to control for the history threat.

In both the time series design and the time series design with repeated reversal, changes over time may be due to maturation, which is sometimes present in clients whose condition is improving or deteriorating. A mathematical procedure called "de-trending the data" is used to remove the effect of directional change due to this threat of maturation when it is present.

The **time series design** (Figure 11-8) involves a single group and a series of measurements, preferably equally spaced over time. After several measurements are obtained, an intervention is performed, and several additional measurements are made. Research using the time series design may be conducted at least partially retrospectively. Sometimes the study uses a passive intervention, as do the studies without researcher-enacted interventions.

The time series design does not control for the threat of history, because some external event may cause change in the value of the dependent variable. It does, however, control for the selection threat, in that subjects are their own controls. It controls for maturation, because steady change over time would be noted before occurrence of the treatment and could be differentiated from change in response to the treatment, since subjects are their own controls. It controls for the testing threat and for statistical regression toward the mean for the same reason.

Addition of a comparison group to the time series design creates the **time series design with nonrandom control group** (Figure 11-9), which Campbell and Stanley (1963) called the multiple time-series design. This design succeeds in controlling for the threat of history. In most fields of inquiry, data collected for the time series design and the time series design with nonrandom control group are at least partially retrospective in nature. Studies using these designs provide evidence, indicating that causation might be present, but they do not establish it definitively.

An example of research that uses a time series design is Helder et al.'s (2014) study of temporal fluctuations in nosocomial infections in neonates. Excerpts from the study's abstract explain the research and its results:

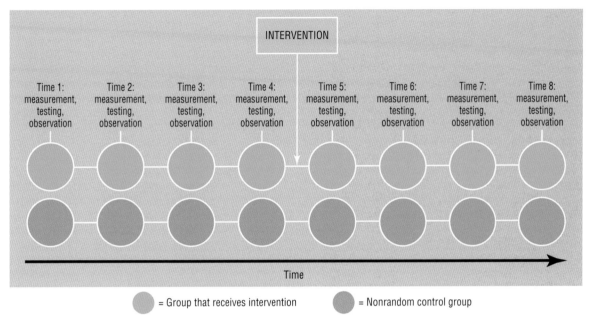

FIGURE 11-9 Time series design with nonrandom control group.

"… We studied the long-term effect of sequential HH [hand hygiene]-promoting interventions. … An observational study with an interrupted time series analysis of the occurrence of NBSI was performed in very low-birth weight (VLBW) infants. Interventions consisted of an education program, gain-framed screen saver messages, and an infection prevention week with an introduction on consistent glove use. … A total of 1,964 VLBW infants admitted between January 1, 2002, and December 31, 2011, were studied. … The first intervention was followed by a significantly declining trend in NBSIs [nosocomial bloodstream infections] of -1.27 per quartile (95% CI, -2.04 to -0.49). The next interventions were followed by a neutral trend change. The relative contributions of coagulase-negative staphylococci and Staphylococcus aureus as causative pathogens decreased significantly over time. Sequential HH promotion seems to contribute to a sustained low NBSI rate." (Helder et al., 2014, p. 718)

In its simplest form, **the time series with repeated reversal design**, called the equivalent time samples design by Campbell and Stanley (1963), involves subjects receiving an intervention followed by measurement. Then the intervention is removed, or it extinguishes, or the "usual treatment" is applied. Then dependent variables of the subjects are again measured. Then the treatment is applied again, and so forth, with treatment and removal of treatment continuing for two full cycles or more. It is useful for demonstrating the effect of a treatment, using subjects as their own controls (Figure 11-10).

The time series with repeated reversal design is just as successful as the time series design with nonrandom control group in controlling for threats to internal validity, because subjects are measured repeatedly over time, and they act as their own controls. In this design, data usually are interpreted within subjects, analyzing whether the treatment was effective at a statistically significant level for each single subject. For this reason, the time series with repeated reversal design also is termed single subject research. For obvious reasons, the researcher seeks a sample that is somewhat representative of the population but, more important, inclusive of major groups in terms of age, gender, race, and other demographics pertinent to the research. Generalization is limited, certainly, but the argument for use of the intervention in similar subjects is more compelling when based on a broad representation of many demographic factors. This design, although very desirable for small populations and limited access to subjects, is used seldom in nursing.

Studies That Lack Random Assignment to Group

For studies that lack random assignment to group, the researcher's choice of a comparison or control group is critical in decreasing threats to internal validity,

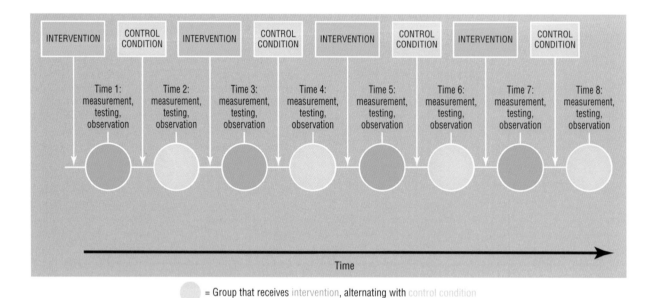

= Group that receives intervention, alternating with control condition

FIGURE 11-10 Time series design with repeated reversal.

especially the history threat. In the research report, the researcher should justify the reason that nonrandom assignment was selected for the study in terms of ethical concerns, study-specific considerations, or minimization of threats to validity. For instance, in studies in which a high refusal rate is expected, a researcher will sometimes allow subjects to self-select experimental or control group in order to have a reasonable-sized sample for proper statistical analysis. This tactic, of course, introduces the selection threat. However, having adequate numbers of subjects may be the researcher's primary concern.

The principal consideration of selecting a nonrandom control group is to simulate what Shadish et al. (2002) called a counterfactual, which literally means "something contrary to fact" and actually signifies the intervention group had it not received the intervention at all (p. 5). The implied question about the treatment group is, "What would have happened to those same people if they simultaneously had not received treatment?" (p. 5). The perfect control group is the counterfactual. Ideally, the control group is very similar to the treatment group in terms of distribution of age, gender, health, and other characteristics related to the concepts under investigation in the study.

Designs that lack random assignment to group are (1) the posttest-only design with a comparison group, (2) posttest-only design with comparison with norms,

(3) pretest-posttest design with a nonrandom control group, and (4) other pretest-posttest designs such as the reversed treatment or removed treatment that make comparisons with nonrandomly selected groups or with comparison norms. When comparison groups are very similar to treatment groups, and control for extraneous variables effectively minimizes threats to validity, the groups are sometimes termed control groups. If a comparison group does not control for threats to validity, it cannot be termed a control group.

The **pretest-posttest design with nonrandom control group**, also sometimes called the pretest-posttest design with comparison group, is used fairly often by healthcare researchers and social scientists. It has the same structure as the classic experimental design, except that its groups are not randomly assigned. The design's strengths are magnified when data are collected from the comparison group at the same time as from the experimental group, controlling for the history threat. Other threats are fairly well controlled for by this design, with the exception of the interaction between selection and maturation. When subject selection is based on the need to change and research subjects are aware of that need, the normal progress of maturation may account for the change in the value of the dependent variable.

An example of the pretest-posttest design with comparison group is Shah, Heylen, Srinivasan, Perumpil, and Ekstrand's (2014) study of reducing HIV stigma among nursing students. Excerpts from the study explain the rationale for using this design:

"The purpose of this project was to (a) assess the acceptability and feasibility of … delivering a brief stigma-reduction curriculum to Indian nursing students and (b) examine the preliminary effect of this curriculum on their knowledge, stigma attitudes, and intent to discriminate in a convenience sample of students. … A female U.S. medical student of Indian descent … recruited participants through an in-class announcement explaining the purpose and requirements of the project. … Due to pre-scheduled clinical placements following enrollment and because the timing of the intervention was pre-determined due to the availability of session facilitators, only 45 students were on-campus when the intervention was delivered. For this reason, the group available to receive the curriculum was designated the intervention group (n = 45), whereas the other served as the control group (n = 46)." (Shah et al., 2014, p. 1325-1326)

The **posttest-only design with comparison group**, known also as the posttest-only design with nonequivalent control group, is used in healthcare and occasionally nursing research. Campbell and Stanley (1963) called this design pre-experimental due to the many threats to internal validity that it harbors. In this design, an intervention is designed to produce values that are different from a certain range of values observed in similar populations. The values obtained for the intervention group are then compared with average values in a comparison group.

The rigor of the research is dependent on the comparison group that the researcher selects. In the following study, the comparison group was selectively matched with members of the total population not included in the 3-year treatment group, essentially creating the ideal control group, a near-perfect counterfactual. In contrast, consider the other pre-experimental study, the one-group pretest-posttest study by Hooge et al. (2014), in which the use of a comparison group essentially controlled for none of the threats to internal validity.

Kothari, Zielinski, James, Charoth, and Sweezy (2014) conducted research using the posttest-only design with comparison group, to determine whether mothers who had participated in "Healthy Babies Healthy Start, a maternal health program emphasizing racial equity and delivering services through case management home visitation" (p. S96), had better outcomes than did

mothers who did not participate. The researchers constructed their matched sample from an existent database, choosing it from the population of all mothers who met study inclusion criteria and whose babies were born during the 3-year span of the study but who did not participate in the program. The strategy of propensity score matching enabled selection of mothers who were demographically very similar to the subjects. The propensity strategy of purposeful matching selects individual comparison/control subjects because of demographic similarity to the experimental group. The resultant sample was the strongest comparison group able to be constituted for this particular study. Results showed that babies of participating mothers had better outcomes than those of women who did not participate.

Because of its extremely similar comparison group, the study contained only two identifiable threats to internal validity. The program's findings of significantly improved birth weights are discussed in relation to the threats that were potentially present, and rival hypotheses are provided below to explain the positive findings.

- Selection threat was present because the mothers who chose to become involved in the program might have differed from those who constituted the comparison group, especially in terms of motivation to learn.
- Selection-maturation interaction is possible, as well. Women who were enrolled in the program might have already been working to improve their healthcare practices prior to program participation, because of their pregnancies, which might have spurred them to participate. Their babies, consequently, might have been of a higher birth weight than average without the program.

The **posttest-only design with comparison with norms** is used infrequently in nursing but rather frequently in healthcare and pharmacology research. This design can be used to test the effectiveness of an intervention designed to produce a certain range of values, as compared with average population values. For instance, in northern climates in the winter months, use of a lamp to produce ultraviolet light might be trialed in its effectiveness to produce vitamin D values that are within normal range. This design could also be used to test the effect of an unwanted occurrence in producing out-of-range values, for instance renal function values after chemotherapy containing heavy metals.

The researcher can enhance internal validity in all of the studies that use a nonequivalent control group, or comparison group, through intelligent and creative choices. Sometimes it is possible to match experimental group subjects individually with controls, drawn from a database that spans a recent time period, as in Kothari et al.'s (2014) study. In this way, the researcher can control for extraneous variables identified as potentially important, such as age, marital status, and amount of education. At other times, choice of concurrent data collection in a group at a different site minimizes threats to validity more effectively. Sometimes it is most practical to strategize data collection at the same site. Choice of a same-size arbitrary on-site group, for instance the 42 consecutive patients seen in a clinic for pulmonary hypertension before data collection began with a convenience sample of 42 treatment group patients with pulmonary hypertension, controls for inter-site variability and probably socioeconomic status, but reintroduces the history threat.

MAINTAINING CONSISTENCY IN INTERVENTIONAL RESEARCH

The methods of an interventional study include all researcher-crafted decisions made after a design is formalized. They include strategies for subject recruitment, means of obtaining informed consent, selection and preparation of research sites, measurement modalities, pilot studies, assurance of consistency of research intervention and measurement, and analysis of data—essentially all the hard work of the study itself. There are no general rules that guide the new researcher in these tasks. However, faculty advisors, nurse researchers, and mentors can offer consultation and advice for specifics related to the research topic, design, and scope. In addition, review of the literature provides examples of research in the area and in related areas. Published reports often contain recommendations for further research that are both useful and practical.

Attention to the methods of the study has a detail-oriented focus. A few of the more common concerns for interventional researchers, related to enactment of independent and dependent variables, are described here. They are issues of consistency.

Precision of Delivery of the Independent Variable, and Measures of the Dependent Variable
Treatment Fidelity
Quasi-experimental and experimental studies examine the effect of an independent variable on a dependent variable or outcome. The study intervention, also called the treatment, must be chosen so that treatment fidelity can be maintained. The intervention must be able to be applied consistently, over time, without alteration. In many nursing studies, the researcher does not have complete control over the intervention. Whether the intervention is performed by research assistants or by agency staff, lack of treatment fidelity results in decreased internal validity.

Whatever the reason, the treatment must be described fully so that research assistants or agency personnel know exactly how it is to be applied. There should be a printed protocol available at all times when data collection is in progress. Everyone even remotely connected with performing the intervention must have a copy of the exact way the treatment is to be performed.

Assuring treatment fidelity is easier when data-collection occurs over a short period of time and the number of data collection persons is minimized. Shorter periods of time decrease the amount of drift, the gradual decrease in attention paid to consistent implementation. Strategies the researcher enacts to assure treatment fidelity are sometimes erroneously termed controls, but they are, more accurately, assurances of consistency to minimize error. If at all possible, researcher presence in the data collection area is a reminder of the importance of treatment fidelity, and allows observation of persons as they apply the treatment. This enables early correction of deviation from protocol, also presenting the opportunity for the researcher to create goodwill by expressing gratitude and showing patience with staff members who need a little more education and encouragement than do their peers.

Counterbalancing of Multiple Pieces of the Intervention

In perusing the literature, one occasionally finds a study in which the intervention has several steps or phases. If it is suspected that the application of one piece of the treatment can influence the response to later pieces, a phenomenon referred to as a **carryover effect** exists. For example, an adherence intervention may include a video, interactive computer game, and person-to-person teaching session. In some studies, the possibility of carryover is measured by **counterbalancing** pieces of the intervention, so that the various steps of the treatment are administered in random order rather than being provided consistently in the same order. In the example, some subjects would view the video at the first clinic visit, have the teaching session the next visit, and play the game at the next visit. Other subjects would play the game first, followed by the video, and then the teaching session. Other subjects would receive the interventions in a different order. The different orders of pieces of the intervention are then compared for total efficacy and for the carryover effects for each sequence.

For a new researcher, counterbalancing adds complexity and stress to the process. If this is your first study, interventional pieces should be enacted in the same order every time, much as a bundled intervention is enacted in a clinical setting. You keep the steps the same because this will control for variation in the strength of the intervention, just in case there is carryover.

Controlling Measurement

Reliability and validity of all measurement tools should be provided in the research report. This includes reported reliability and validity by the developers of the tools, reported values from studies focusing on the same concepts that you are researching, and also the reliability and validity demonstrated by the tools in your study (see Chapter 16). A statistician can assist you with the way these determinations are made.

Like treatments, measures of dependent variables must also be consistently implemented. This means that the timing of the measurements relative to the intervention and identification of the times of the day at which measurements are to be performed must be specified in advance. In addition, instructions given to the study subjects should be read to them from a standard set of printed instructions developed for the study (a protocol sheet), so that each research assistant delivers the same instructions in the same way.

Researchers concerned about the literacy of some potential subjects may decide to read the study questionnaires to all subjects to ensure understanding. This is a better approach than reading questionnaires to only those subjects who cannot read, because it affords consistency.

Randomized Controlled Trials

Randomized controlled trials (RCTs) use the pretest-posttest control group design, or one closely related to it. RCTs are conducted in order to produce definitive evidence for an intervention. In 1993, a panel of 30 experts met for the purpose of improving the quality of clinical trials and initiated the Standardized Reporting of Trials (SORT) statement (CONSORT, 2011). This

statement included a checklist and flow diagram that investigators were encouraged to follow when conducting and reporting RCTs. The initial work of this group was revised in 2001 and became the Consolidated Standards for Reporting Trials (CONSORT). This guideline was updated with the CONSORT 2010 Statement published by Schultz, Altman, and Moher (2010) as representatives of the CONSORT Group. Figure 11-11 provides a flow diagram of the progression through the phases of an RCT—enrollment, intervention allocation, follow-up, and data analysis—for two randomized parallel groups. This diagram was included in the CONSORT 2010 Statement to facilitate the conduct of quality RCTs nationally and internationally (Schulz et al., 2010). The CONSORT 2010 Statement also offers a checklist of information that researchers need to supply when reporting an RCT. It can be found in the Schulz et al. (2010) publication or online (http://www.consort-statement.org/consort-statement/) (CONSORT, 2012). Chapter 15, Figure 15-2 of this volume also includes an example from a published article related to CONSORT standards. In nursing, RCTs have been conducted over the past 15 years, conforming to the CONSORT standards.

Clinical trials may be carried out simultaneously in multiple geographical locations to increase sample size and resources and to obtain a more representative sample (Schulz et al., 2010). In this case, the primary researcher must coordinate activities at all study sites. Coordination and training at multiple sites can be difficult to achieve without grant funding.

ALGORITHMS OF RESEARCH DESIGN

Chapter 10 and this chapter contain several key algorithms. Figure 10-1 is an overview of the four major subdivisions of quantitative research design and may help you dentify the type of study you plan to conduct, or determine the type of study you find in a publication. Four algorithms display the major subdivisions of quantitative research: descriptive (see Figure 10-2), correlational (see Figure 10-6), experimental (see Figure 11-1), and quasi-experimental (see Figure 11-7). These algorithms will assist you in making decisions for study design in each of these four areas, and for identifying designs in published research. Most of the designs identified in these figures have been discussed in Chapter 10 or in this chapter.

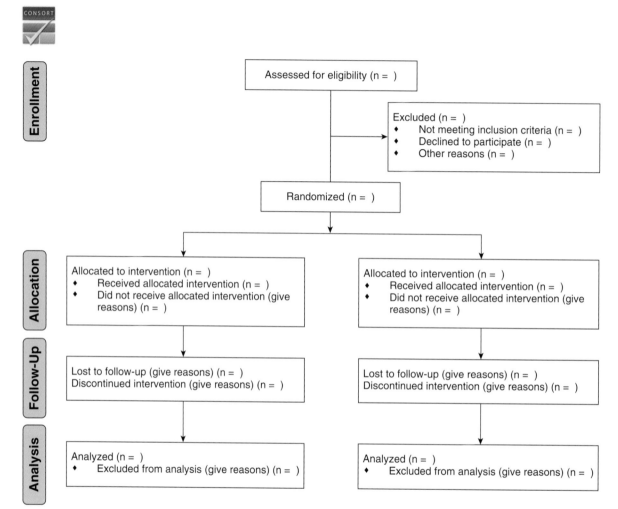

FIGURE 11-11 2010 Statement flow diagram of the progress through the phases of a parallel randomized trial of two groups (that is, enrollment, intervention allocation, follow-up, and data analysis). (From CONSORT. [2012]. The CONSORT Statement. Retrieved March 14, 2016 from http://www.consort-statement.org/consort-statement/; Schulz, K. F., Altman, D. G., Moher, D., for the CONSORT Group [2010]. CONSORT 2010 Statement: Updated guidelines for reporting parallel group randomised trials. *The BMJ, 340, c332.*)

KEY POINTS

- Selection of a research design depends upon both research question and feasibility.
- Even the weakest of research designs with the poorest control of potentially extraneous variables can provide preliminary information about causation that can be tested in subsequent research using designs with better internal validity.
- Simple studies without control groups can be implemented with less effort and expense but are highly likely to produce poorly generalizable results.
- Quasi-experimental and experimental designs examine causality.

- The three essential elements of experimental research are (1) researcher-controlled manipulation of the independent variable, (2) the presence of a distinct control group, and (3) random assignment of subjects to either the experimental or the control condition.
- The validity of findings from quasi-experimental research is dependent upon its basic design and the choices the researcher makes relative to methods, especially selection of control or comparison subjects.
- Design validity is an important concern that the researcher addresses by choices made during interventional study design. It has four major facets: construct validity, internal validity, external validity, and statistical conclusion validity.
- The four facets of validity are the basis for the "limitations" to generalization of the study, which appear in the Discussion section of a research report.
- A factor or condition that decreases the validity of research results is termed a threat to validity.
- Currently in medicine and nursing, the randomized controlled trial (RCT) generates valuable information for practice by testing the effectiveness of a treatment within a standardized structure. In many subdisciplines of medicine, the RCT is a multisite endeavor, pooling subjects to allow for stronger evidence. The CONSORT 2010 Statement clarifies the steps for conducting and reporting an RCT.
- Algorithms for design identification and selection are provided in Figures 10-1, 10-2, 10-6, 11-1, and 11-7.

REFERENCES

Campbell, D. T. (1957). Factors relevant to the validity of experiments in social settings. *Psychological Bulletin, 54*(4), 297–312.

Campbell, D. T., & Stanley, J. C. (1963). Experimental and quasi-experimental designs for research on teaching. In N. L. Gage (Ed.), *Handbook of research on teaching* (pp. 171–246). Chicago, IL: Rand McNally.

Cartwright, R. L. (1968). Some remarks on essentialism. *The Journal of Philosophy, 65*(20), 615–626.

CONSORT. (2011). *How CONSORT began.* Retrieved March 14, 2016 from http://www.consort-statement.org/about-consort/history/.

CONSORT. (2012). The *CONSORT* Statement. Retrieved March 14, 2016 from http://www.consort-statement.org/consort-statement/.

Cook, T. D., & Campbell, D. T. (1979). *Quasi-experimentation design and analysis issues for field settings.* Boston: Houghton Mifflin.

Cook, T. D., & Campbell, D. T. (1986). The causal assumptions of quasi-experimental practice. *Synthese, 68*(1), 141–180.

Desmet, M., Braems, H., Reynvoet, M., Plasschaert, S., Van Cauwelaert, J., Pottel, H., et al. (2013). I.V. and perineural dexamethasone are equivalent in increasing the analgesic duration of a single-shot interscalene block with ropivacaine for shoulder surgery: A prospective, randomized, placebo-controlled study. *British Journal of Anesthesia, 111*(3), 445–452.

Dunst, C. J., Jenkins, V. J., & Trivette, C. M. (1984). The Family Support Scale: Reliability and validity. *Journal of Individual, Family, and Community Wellness, 11*(4), 45–52.

Fisher, R. A. (1935). *The design of experiments.* Edinburgh, Scotland: Oliver & Boyd.

Fredericks, S., & Yau, T. (2013). Educational intervention reduces complications and rehospitalizations after heart surgery. *Western Journal of Nursing Research, 35*(10), 1251–1265.

Good, M., Albert, J. M., Arafah, B., Anderson, G. C., Wotman, S., Cong, X., et al. (2012). Effects on postoperative salivary cortisol of relaxation/music and patient teaching about pain management. *Biological Research for Nursing, 15*(3), 318–329.

Greene, D. E., Stanier, P., & Copp, A. J. (2009). Genetics of human neural tube defects. *Human Molecular Genetics, 18*(2), R113–R129. doi:10.1093/hmg/ddp347.

Helder, O. K., Brug, J., van Goudoever, J. B., Looman, C. W. N., Reiss, I. K. M., & Kornelisse, R. F. (2014). Sequential hand hygiene promotion contributes to a reduced nosocomial bloodstream infection rate among very low-birth weight infants: An interrupted time series over a 10-year period. *American Journal of Infection Control, 42*(7), 718–722.

Hooge, L. H., Benzies, K. M., & Mannion, C. A. (2014). Effects of a brief, prevention-focused parenting education program for new mothers. *Western Journal of Nursing Research, 36*(8), 957–974.

Hume, D. (1999). *A treatise of human nature: Being an attempt to introduce the experimental method of reasoning into moral subjects.* Kitchener, Ontario: Batoche.

Kothari, C. L., Zielinski, R., James, A., Charoth, R. M., & Sweezy, C. (2014). Improved birth weight for black infants: Outcomes of a Healthy Start program. *American Journal of Public Health, 104*(S1), S96–S104.

Kurdal, E., Tanriverdi, D. T., & Savaş, H. A. (2014). The effect of psychoeducation on the functioning level of patients with bipolar disorder. *Western Journal of Nursing Research, 36*(3), 312–328.

Lenth, R. V. (2006-2009). Java applets for power and sample size [Computer software]. Retrieved August 25, 2015 from http://www.stat.uiowa.edu/~rlenth/Power.

Liao, W.-C., Wang, L., Kuo, C.-P., Lo, C., Chiu, M.-J., & Ting, H. (2013). Effect of a warm footbath before bedtime on body temperature and sleep in older adults with good and poor sleep: An experimental crossover trial. *International Journal of Nursing Studies, 50*(12), 1607–1616.

Plichta, S. B., & Kelvin, E. (2012). *Munro's statistical methods for healthcare research* (6th ed.). Philadelphia: Wolters Kluwer Health.

Rankin, R. E., & Campbell, D. T. (1955). Galvanic skin response to Negro and white experimenters. *Journal of Abnormal and Social Psychology, 51*(1), 30–33.

Reece, S. (1992). The Parental Expectations Survey: A measure of perceived self-efficacy. *Clinical Nursing Research, 1*(4), 336–346.

Schulz, K. F., Altman, D. G., & Moher, D. (2010). CONSORT 2010 Statement: Updated guidelines for reporting parallel group randomized trials. *Annals of Internal Medicine, 152*(11), 726–733.

Shadish, S. R., Cook, T. D., & Campbell, D. T. (2002). *Experimental and quasi-experimental design for generalized causal inference.* Boston, MA: Houghton Mifflin Company.

Shah, S. M., Heylen, E., Srinivasan, K., Perumpil, S., & Ekstrand, M. L. (2014). Reducing HIV stigma among nursing students: A brief intervention. *Western Journal of Nursing Research, 36*(10), 1323–1337.

Trute, B., & Hiebert-Murphy, D. (2005). Predicting family adjustment and parenting stress in childhood: Disability services using brief assessment tools. *Journal of Intellectual & Developmental Disability, 30*(4), 217–225.

Qualitative Research Methods

Jennifer R. Gray

http://evolve.elsevier.com/Gray/practice/

During the process of identifying a research problem and developing a research question, the researcher considers the type of inquiry that best answers the question. When the qualitative methodology is the appropriate approach, the researcher determines the best qualitative design for the study (see Chapter 4). The early steps of the qualitative research process, which are similar to the early steps of the quantitative research process, are explored in Chapters 5 and 6. Other steps in the research process are implemented differently in, or are unique to, qualitative studies. In this chapter, information about the qualitative methodology will be provided so that you can understand the process and envision what the experience will be like if you conduct a qualitative study.

Qualitative analysis techniques use words rather than numbers as the basis of analysis. In qualitative analysis, reasoning flows from the images, documents, or words provided by the participant toward more abstract concepts and **themes**. Themes are patterns in the data, ideas that are repeated by more than one participant. This reasoning process, inductive thinking, guides the organizing, reducing, and clustering of data (Creswell, 2013; Maxwell, 2013). As themes are identified, the researcher uses deductive reasoning when considering the fit of the data to the themes (Creswell, 2013). To achieve the goal of describing and understanding participant perspectives, qualitative methods of sampling, data gathering, and analysis allow for more flexibility than the methods of the quantitative paradigm. Because data analysis in most qualitative designs begins as data are gathered, insights from early data may suggest additional questions that might be asked or other modifications to the study methods (Maxwell, 2013). For example, suppose a researcher conducts a grounded theory study about personal identity after losing a limb due to injuries from a motorcycle crash. During the interviews, a participant mentions feeling guilty because she was driving too fast and caused the crash by swerving in front of an automobile. Passengers in the automobile also were injured. Although the planned interview questions did not include a question about feelings of guilt and shame, the researcher may choose to ask an exploratory question on this topic during subsequent interviews. Although the researcher may adapt data collection or analysis strategies during a grounded theory study, changes are not impulsive and must be supported with clear rationale. These changes are documented in the study records as part of maintaining rigor of the study.

Maintaining rigor in the context of flexibility can be difficult. Therefore, a researcher new to qualitative methods should read primary sources related to the method being considered and seek guidance for understanding its philosophical base. A research mentor, especially a researcher with more experience with the specific methods or topic in which you are interested, can be invaluable (Corbin & Strauss, 2015). By sharing their personal experiences with the mentees, research mentors can guide less experienced researchers in planning the task and the study's timeline in a realistic manner (Marshall & Rossman, 2016).

This chapter provides examples of qualitative methods used to gather, analyze, and interpret data. Literature reviews, theoretical frameworks, study purposes, and research questions or objectives are described in the context of various qualitative approaches, because these are steps in the research process that are implemented somewhat differently in qualitative studies. The chapter also includes information relative to qualitative sampling and to the data collection methods of observation, interviews, focus groups, and electronically mediated data. Data analysis strategies are described, and examples are provided. The chapter ends with a presentation of methods specific to different philosophical approaches.

CLINICAL CONTEXT AND RESEARCH PROBLEMS

Qualitative researchers are motivated by the desire to know more about a phenomenon, a social process, or a culture from the perspectives of the people who are experiencing the phenomenon, involved in the social process, or living in the culture (Creswell, 2013). The motivation may be that nurses realize that patient teaching is not effective with a specific group. A new project may be planned for low-income teenage mothers, but all those implementing the project are more than 40 years of age and have above-average incomes. A hurricane ravages a community, and disaster relief efforts are not well received by the community. Persons with sickle cell anemia are living past age 60 years, and previous studies were focused on younger persons recently diagnosed with the disease. Any of these situations may indicate a need for understanding the insider's perspective that could be addressed by a qualitative study.

For example, Hyatt, Davis, and Barroso (2014) established the need for their grounded theory study by describing a frequently unrecognized and thus untreated problem among military veterans who served in Iraq and Afghanistan: mild traumatic brain injury (mTBI). The healthcare system and providers lacked an understanding of the effects of mTBI on post-deployment adjustment and mental health. The researchers identified the need for information from the perspective of veterans and their spouses.

"…little published research exists on rehabilitation, interventions, and health outcomes following mTBI. Therefore, the purpose of this study was to examine and describe post-mTBI recovery and rehabilitation from the perspective of soldiers and their spouses. Three research questions were asked: (1) How do soldiers and their spouses describe post-mTBI recovery and/or rehabilitation? (2) What difficulties, challenges, or problems do soldiers and their spouses experience during post-mTBI recovery? (3) What management strategies do soldiers and their spouses use to cope with the rehabilitation challenges?" (Hyatt et al., 2014, pp. 849–850)

LITERATURE REVIEW FOR QUALITATIVE STUDIES

Broome, Lutz, and Cook (2015) conducted a grounded theory study of parental responses to their children's severe food allergies and in the review of the literature presented the impact of the life-threatening condition upon family knowledge needs, adaptation strategies, emotional balance, and economics. They noted that parents may need support from healthcare professionals to develop and maintain a sense of being competent as parents. Their conclusion was that the lack of evidence about parental responses to children with severe food allergies supported the need for the study.

"Therefore, this study seeks to understand parents' perspectives about the impact of having a child with severe food allergies and adjustments required to effectively manage the condition." (Broome et al., 2015, p. 533)

Some qualitative researchers defer the literature review until after data collection and analysis to avoid biasing their analysis and interpretation of the data (Maxwell, 2013). Most often, qualitative researchers briefly review the literature at the beginning of the process to establish the need for the study and to provide guidance for the development of data collection methods. A more thorough review of published research findings and theories may occur during data analysis and interpretation to develop explanations in "studies that seek to explain, evaluate, and suggest linkages between events" (Marshall & Rossman, 2016, p. 91).

THEORETICAL FRAMEWORKS

Most qualitative researchers do not identify specific theoretical frameworks during the design of their studies, as is expected for quantitative studies. The concern is that designing a study in the context of a theory will influence the researcher's thinking and result in findings that are meaningful in the theoretical context, but may not be true to the participants' perspectives on the topic. However, the philosophical bases for the various approaches to qualitative studies provide theoretical grounding for qualitative studies without predisposing the data analysis to a single interpretation.

Theory is an explicit component in some qualitative research designs. The theory may be explicit in the findings of the study, such as a grounded theory study in which the inductive analysis allows an emerging theory to emerge (Corbin & Strauss, 2015). Other researchers identify their study's theoretical perspectives and describe their findings in the context of that perspective. Markle, Attell, and Treiber (2015) examined online blogs written by persons with multiple chronic illnesses in the context of the framework of chronic illness (Strauss & Glaser, 1975) and the concept of biographical disruption (Bury, 1982). The online blogs revealed an overarching process of "dual, yet dueling illnesses" (Markle et al., 2015, p. 1271). They discussed their findings in the context of these conceptual foundations, noting consistencies with the theoretical framework.

"… In addition to the problems identified by Strauss and Glaser (1975), the researchers noted additional problems that fall into the following categories: (a) diagnosis and management of multiple illnesses, (b) need for information, (c) identity dilemmas and threats to self-image, and (d) stigma and social rejection…Strauss and Glaser (1975) provided a foundation for understanding the labyrinthine quest for diagnosis, the complex process of illness management, the vital need for relevant information, and the ordeal of stigma and social rejection. Bury's (1982) concept of biographic disruption enabled us to appreciate the impact of the unexpected loss of the work identity and accelerated aging." (Markle et al. 2015, pp. 1277, 1279)

Exploratory qualitative study design may benefit from making explicit the researcher's theoretical perspective on the study problem. Mayer, Rosenfeld, and Gilbert (2013) identified the theoretical approach to their study of family bereavement following a sudden cardiac death.

"Symbolic interactionism and family systems theory provided the conceptual frameworks for this study … These complementary frameworks provide an understanding of family that recognizes both the individual family member and the larger family system in which individual family members interact with each other and have shared meaning…The sudden death of a family member disrupts the survivors' lives and drastically changes the family system. Family dynamics and family roles changed as college aged children provided care and support to grieving adults." (Mayer et al., 2013, pp. 168, 172)

Qualitative researchers who use frameworks during study development must maintain intellectual honesty to prevent the theoretical perspective from obscuring the perspectives of the participants. Your decision about whether to identify a theoretical perspective should be consistent with the research approach you have chosen. If a theoretical perspective has shaped your views of a research problem, you should acknowledge that influence and indicate explicitly the study components that were shaped by the theory.

Purposes should clearly identify the goal or aim of the study that has emerged from the research problem and literature review. The purposes of qualitative studies include the phenomenon of interest, the population, and often the setting (see Chapter 5). Ask yourself, "Can I achieve this purpose with a qualitative study?" Study purposes such as testing an intervention and measuring the effectiveness of a program are not consistent with qualitative approaches. To test interventions, a quasi-experimental or experimental design with a treatment group and a control group would be needed. A dependent variable would need to be measured (numbers as the data) in order to compare the effectiveness of the intervention or of a program. When the term measure is used, the data collected would be primarily numbers and the analysis would involve statistics. However, a qualitative researcher could address participants' experiences with the intervention or their perceptions about a program. The purpose of qualitative studies will vary slightly depending on the qualitative approach that is being used. For example, note in Table 12-1 that the phenomenological study focused on the lifeworld of the participants and the grounded theory study focused on the processes used to maintain hope. The studies used as examples in Table 12-1 have purposes consistent with each study's identified philosophical approach.

RESEARCH OBJECTIVES OR QUESTIONS

Hypotheses are not appropriate for qualitative studies because hypotheses specify outcomes of studies and variables that are to be manipulated or measured. This approach to a study is not consistent with the philosophical orientation of qualitative research. Qualitative researchers may identify research objectives or questions to connect the purpose of the study to the plan for data collection and analysis. Because qualitative research is more open-ended and the focus is on participants' perspectives, qualitative researchers may not specify research objectives or research questions in order to avoid prematurely narrowing the topic. It is unusual for a qualitative researcher to articulate the principal research question in a research report. On the other hand, Hatfield and Pearce (2014) did identify two research questions. Hatfield and Pearce recruited parents of newborns for a study of their decision making related to donating the baby's blood for genetic minimal risk research.

TABLE 12-1	Selected Examples of Purpose Statements in Qualitative Studies
Qualitative Approach	**Purpose Statement**
Phenomenological research	"The aim of this study is to illuminate the lived experience of adoptive parents who have been living with and caring for children with a diagnosis of RAD [reactive attachment disorder]" (Follan & McNamara, 2014, p. 1076).
Grounded theory research	"... developing a theory that better captures the healing process of non-Western torture survivors of various ethnic groups and genders" (Isakson, & Jurkovic, 2013, p. 750).
Ethnographic research	"... the purpose of this study was to describe generic (folk) and professional (nursing) factors that healthcare providers can apply to promote CCC [culture congruent care] for rural Appalachian people at EOL [end of life]" (Mixer, Fornehed, Varney, & Lindley, 2014, p. 526).
Exploratory qualitative research	"The purpose of study was to explore, from the patient perspective, the understanding of palliative care in African American heart failure patients in an ambulatory care setting" (Lem, & Schwartz, 2014, 536).
Historical research	"... examines how the Frontier Nursing Service (FNS) utilized nurse-midwives to respond to antepartum emergencies such as preterm birth, eclampsia, malpresentation and hemorrhage in the women of Appalachia in the years 1925 to 1939" (Schiminkey & Keeling, 2015, p. 48).

"What is the process parents utilized to arrive at a decision to enroll their healthy infant in minimal-risk genetic research? What do parents of newborn infants perceive as factors that influence their decision to donate their healthy infant's DNA for minimal-risk genetic research?" (Hatfield & Pearce, 2014, p, 399)

The research questions for the study were broad and still allowed thorough exploration of the topic. These questions were clearly written and did not limit what the researcher might find. Hatfield and Pearce (2014) interviewed 35 postpartum women and developed a model of the process involved in making these decisions. From the data emerged a "core category (benefit to the children in the present and the future) and three interacting components: the parents, the scientist, and the child's comfort" (Hatfield & Pearce, 2014, p. 401).

OBTAINING RESEARCH PARTICIPANTS

The goal of sampling for quantitative studies is to obtain data from a subgroup of a population that is statistically representative of the population, to allow the findings to be generalized to the population (see Chapter 15). Qualitative researchers seek participants who have experienced the phenomenon of interest (Streubert & Carpenter, 2011) and are able to share "information-rich accounts of their experiences" (Liamputtong, 2013a, p. 18). For ethnographic studies, participants may also include key informants who are knowledgeable about the culture being studied. The selection of participants is nonrandom and may not be totally specified in terms of number, group members, or characteristics before the study begins.

Depending on the research question and the aims of the study, the researcher may use more than one sampling strategy during the study. For example, a researcher who is studying the experience of reacting to a diagnosis of breast cancer may choose to select only women who have not previously been diagnosed with cancer, have not had a family member die from breast cancer, and have been diagnosed within the last six weeks. This approach to sampling is called **criterion sampling** (Liamputtong, 2013). Similar logic can be applied to identify participants for a focus group, when it is desirable to have participants who can identify with each other's experiences. Homogeneity of the group is a characteristic of focus groups (Krueger & Casey, 2015). Table 12-2 provides definitions and references for sampling strategies that are frequently used by qualitative researchers. These sampling strategies are not mutually exclusive, and one researcher may label the same strategy differently than another researcher does.

The sample for a rigorous qualitative study is not as large as the sample for a rigorous quantitative study. The researcher stops collecting data when enough rich, meaningful data have been obtained to achieve the study aims. For new researchers, this answer to "How big should my sample be?" is totally unsatisfactory. When applying for human subjects' approval, the researcher will be asked the maximum sample size. Giving a generous range of 12 to 25 participants can be a way to answer this question but will depend on the study design.

TABLE 12-2	Sampling Strategies Used by Qualitative Researchers
Sampling	**Definition**
Convenience sampling	Inviting participants from a location or group because of ease and efficiency (Liamputtong, 2013a).
Snowball sampling	After first participant is acquired, researcher asks participant to refer others who have had similar experiences for participation in the study (Howie, 2013); also called *chain sampling* or *network sampling*.
Historical sampling	Exhaustive search for all relevant, surviving primary and secondary sources about an event or phenomenon that occurred in the past (Lundy, 2012)
Purposive sampling	Recruitment of participants as sources of data because they can provide in-depth information needed to achieve the study aims (Howie, 2013)
Theoretical sampling*	Recruitment of participants who are considered to be best sources of data related to the study's generation of theory; additional participants may be recruited to validate or expand upon emerging concepts; associated with grounded theory approaches (Wuest, 2012)
Criterion sampling*	Recruitment of participants who do or do not have certain characteristics deemed to affect the phenomena being studied (Liamputtong, 2013)
Maximum variation sampling*	Recruitment of participants who represent potentially different experiences related to the domain of interest (Miles et al., 2014; Seidman, 2013)
Critical case sampling*	Recruitment of participants whose experiences with the research topic are expected to be very different and whose input may support or not support the emerging themes (Miles et al., 2014).
Deviant case sampling*	Recruitment of participants who may be outliers or represent extreme cases of the domain of interest (Liamputtong, 2013a; Miles et al., 2014).

*Considered by some authors to be subtypes of purposive sampling.

Researchers who use focus groups often have larger samples, usually comprising one or more groups of five to ten participants. The actual number of groups conducted may depend on how soon data saturation is achieved. **Data saturation** is the point at which new data begin to be redundant with what has already been found, and no new themes can be identified. Patterns emerge in the data. The researcher has the data needed to answer the research question and remain true to the principles of the study design. Marshall and Rossman (2016) indicate that a better term for data saturation is theoretical sufficiency, because one can never completely know all there is to know about a topic. In the study with parents about donating their newborns' DNA for genetic research, Hatfield and Pearce (2014) described their sample size in the following way:

"Each interview progressed at a comfortable pace, allowing the participants the opportunity for flexibility and expression, and lasted approximately 20 minutes...Data were theoretically saturated at 29 interviews. Six more interviews were conducted with no new comments, categories, or themes emerging." (Hatfield & Pearce, 2014, pp. 400, 401)

The interviews in the Hatfield and Pearce (2014) study were relatively short for qualitative interviews, so the amount of data per interview was small. In contrast, in a study of men with depression, each interview with the individual participants lasted 60 to 90 minutes (Ramirez & Badger, 2014, p. 22). Mayer et al. (2013) conducted seven family interviews followed by 17 interviews with members of the families in their study of bereavement following sudden cardiac death. Notice their discussion of the adequacy of their sample.

"Family interviews ranged from 90–150 minutes (mean 96 minutes), and individual interviews ranged from 45–90 minutes. Field notes were written after all interviews and the interviewer's thoughts recorded in a reflective journal. It was determined that we had an adequate sample size due to the breadth and depth of the qualitative data collected." (Mayer et al., 2013, p. 170)

Chapter 15 provides additional information about sampling methods and sample size in qualitative studies.

Researcher-Participant Relationships

One of the important differences between quantitative research and qualitative research is the nature of relationship between the researcher and the participant (Rubin & Rubin, 2012). The nature of this relationship has an impact on the quality of the data collected and the interpretation. In varying degrees, the researcher influences the individuals being studied and, in turn, is influenced by them. The mere presence of the researcher may alter behavior in the setting, because the researcher desires to connect at the human level with the participant (Marshall & Rossman, 2016; Rubin & Rubin, 2012). Although this involvement is considered a source of bias in quantitative research, qualitative researchers consider it to be a natural and necessary element of the research process. The researcher and the participant are answering the research question together through their interaction with each other (Rubin & Rubin, 2012).

The researcher's personality is a key factor in qualitative research, in which skills in empathy and intuition are cultivated. You will need to become closely involved in the subject's experience to interpret it. Participants need to feel safe and able to trust the researcher prior to sharing their deepest experiences with the researcher (Rubin & Rubin, 2012). It is necessary for you to be open to the perceptions of the participants rather than attaching your own meaning to the experience. To do this, you need to be aware of personal experiences and potential biases related to the phenomenon being studied (Creswell, 2013). It is helpful to document these experiences and potential biases before and during the study in a reflective journal, to be aware of them during the analysis phase of the study. For example, a researcher who plans to interview women undergoing irradiation for breast cancer would need to acknowledge that his/her own mother died from complications of breast cancer. This awareness and ability to be involved with the participants and yet be able to analyze the data abstractly with intellectual honesty is called **reflexivity**. Reflexivity consists of the ability to be aware of your biases and past experiences that might influence how you would respond to a participant or interpret the data (Creswell, 2013; Liamputtong, 2013a). This ability is critical in qualitative studies because data emerge from a relationship with the participant and are analyzed in the mind of the researcher, rather than through a statistical program (Wolf, 2012).

DATA COLLECTION METHODS

Because data collection occurs simultaneously with data analysis in most qualitative studies, the process is complex. Collecting data is not a mechanical process that can be completely planned before it is initiated. The researcher as a whole person is completely involved—perceiving, reacting, interacting, reflecting, attaching meaning, and recording (Marshall & Rossman, 2016). For a particular study, the researcher may need to address data collection issues related to relationships between the researcher and the participants, reflect on the meanings obtained from the data, and organize, manage and synthesize large volumes of data. Qualitative researchers are not limited to a single type of data or collection method during a study. For example, Martin and Yurkovich (2014) conducted 17 interviews with adults in their ethnography of Native American Indian families. In addition, their other data sources were 100 hours of participant observation, "several windshield surveys, fieldwork, and research team meetings" (Martin & Yurkovich, 2014, p. 55). Qualitative data collection may also be combined in a study with the collection of quantitative data. These mixed methods studies are described in detail in Chapter 14.

Observations, interviews, and focus groups are the most common methods of gathering qualitative data, and each is described here in detail, followed by an example from the literature. Electronic means of qualitative data collection, such as photographs, videos, and blogs, are described as well. Following the general types of data collection, methods specific to each qualitative approach are discussed.

Observations

In many qualitative studies, the researcher observes social behavior and may participate in social interactions with those being studied. **Observation** is the collecting of data through listening, smelling, touching, and seeing, with an emphasis on what is seen (Marshall & Rossman, 2016). Even when other data collection methods are being used, such as interviews, you must be aware of your surroundings and attend to the nonverbal communication that occurs between the participant and others in the immediate surroundings (Marshall & Rossman, 2016).

Unstructured observation involves spontaneously observing and recording what one sees. Although unstructured observations give the observer freedom, there is a risk that the observer may lose objectivity or may not remember all of the details of the event. Collecting data through unstructured observation may evolve later into structured observations. The researcher may begin with few predetermined ideas about what will be observed. As the study progresses, the researcher clarifies the situations or areas of focus that are most relevant to the research questions and begins to structure the observations. A researcher observing parent behavior in an ambulatory pediatric care clinic may initially focus on the interaction of parents with their children in the waiting area, and in the room with the provider. During data collection, the researcher begins to notice common nurturing behaviors of the parents and, from these observations, develops a checklist to use while observing. In this way, the researcher has structured the observations that might be the focus of this or of future studies. Other researchers may enter the setting with a checklist or tool for documenting observations, revising the tool as needed.

The most complete way to collect observational data is to video-record the situation being studied, but doing so may alter the behavior of those being observed or may not be possible because of confidentiality concerns (Tracy, 2013). If video recording is not possible, then the researcher may take notes during observation periods. If taking notes is a problem, the researcher needs to write down the observations made as soon as possible afterward. The notes made during and immediately following the observations are called **field notes** (Marshall & Rossman, 2016; Tracy, 2013) and can include content, metacommunication, and context, as well as the researcher's reactions, and immediate responses, to what has just transpired. Recording observations can be as simple as using a pad and writing utensil in a public place or as sophisticated as producing an electronic diagram of the locations of nurses by having them wear positioning devices. Observations may be supplemented by taking photographs in the setting (Tracy, 2013). After the observation, the diagrams of the participants' positions, the photographs, or the videos may serve to remind the observer of specific elements of the situation. In addition, the researcher may analyze a video by viewing short segments and making notes about each. By reflecting on photographs and videos, the researcher may identify details that were not captured during observation.

In an unusual study of experience, interruption management, and performance of scrub nurses, Koh, Park, and Wickens (2014) recruited ten nurses with 2 or more years of operating room (OR) experience (experienced nurses) and 10 with fewer than 2 years' experience (novices). The nurse, the patient, and the OR team members gave consent for their participation, including video recording. For one cesarean section operation, each participant wore a scene camera controlled by a visual tracker. The camera faced and recorded in the same direction that the nurse faced. The actions of the nurse were diagrammed, and the length of the interruptions measured. The field notes, notes about the electronic records made during the observation, and the

researcher's memories of and reflections about being in the setting were the data that were analyzed.

The researcher, by virtue of being in the setting, becomes a participant, to some degree. The balance between participation and observation has been described in four ways. The first is **complete participation**. The people in the situation may not be aware that the participant is a researcher (Streubert & Carpenter, 2011). In public settings, a researcher can ethically observe people and interactions without obtaining permission (Liamputtong, 2013b). In less public settings, the researcher may observe others who learn later that he or she is a researcher. When the researcher's role is unknown to the study participants, they need to have consented to incomplete disclosure before the study is conducted. After the study, they must be debriefed regarding the undisclosed aspects of the study (see Chapter 9). The participants have the option as to whether the data the researcher collected about them are included in the study. When the researcher is in the **participant as observer** role, participants usually are aware of the dual roles of the researcher from the beginning of the observation (Tracy, 2013).

Full engagement in the situation may interfere with the researcher's ability to note important details and move within the setting to follow an evolving situation. In these situations, the role of **observer as participant** may be more appropriate. As the term indicates, the researcher's observer role takes priority and is the focus of the data collection. **Complete observation** occurs when the researcher remains passive and has no direct social interaction in the situation (Streubert & Carpenter, 2011). Jessee and Mion (2013) conducted a study of adherence to contact precautions in two hospitals and noted the use of what they termed non-participant observation (complete observation) as one of the means of data collection.

"Surveillance of adherence was conducted by one nonparticipant observer using a standardized data collection tool to identify behaviors related to entering and exiting the rooms of patients requiring contact isolation precautions. Observable behaviors were noted on 10 separate days reflecting varying clinical times (i.e., morning, mid-afternoon, late afternoon). Observed behaviors were use of foam and/or hand washing just before entering rooms, isolation gown applied, gloves applied, gowns and gloves off in room, and foam and/or hand washing on exit from room. To the extent possible, actual type of personnel was noted." (Jessee & Mion, 2013, p. 967)

For both hospitals, the observed adherence to contact precautions was lower than the perceived adherence measured with an instrument. Hand hygiene prior to donning gloves was the behavior with the lowest adherence rate (Jessee & Mion, 2013).

Example Study Using Observation

An example of observation comes from the study conducted by Clissett, Porock, Harwood, and Gladman (2013) to explore care of persons with dementia, and their families, during hospitalization. They described the study's problem and purpose in regards to patient-centered care.

"However, although much work has considered person-centred care in long term settings, relatively little has focused on acute hospitals. This is important because there are factors in acute hospitals that might be expected to be make the delivery of person-centred care problematic because the priorities are rapid diagnosis and therapeutic intervention with short lengths of stay. As part of a wider study (Gladman et al., 2012a, b), this paper reports data focusing on the person-with-dementia using the five domains of Kitwood's model of personhood as an *a priori* framework for analysis with the aim of exploring the way in which current approaches to care in acute settings have potential to enhance personhood in older adults with dementia." (Clissett et al., 2013, p. 1496)

The family members were sources of information, but the researchers demonstrated their respect for the persons with dementia by including them as much as possible in the data collection process.

"Data collection involved observation and interview. 72 h of non-participant observations of care were conducted on 45 occasions on 11 wards of the study hospitals including orthopaedic, health care of older people and general medicine wards. Most observation periods lasted between 1 and 2 h, the shortest being 45 min and the longest 180 min. The observations were unstructured and conducted by two researchers. The aim of each observation was to produce a narrative account of the experiences of an identified individual with dementia. Field notes were maintained during the observation and were typed in detail as soon as the observation was concluded. The interviews were conducted by two researchers in patients' homes with family caregivers and with the patient present wherever possible." (Clissett et al., 2013, p. 1497)

The research team collected extensive data from the observations of care provided to 29 cognitively impaired persons and the 30 interviews with family members post hospitalization (Clissett et al., 2013). The robust data that the researchers generated allowed them to describe the core problem and process, as follows:

"The observation and interview study elaborated a 'core problem' and a 'core process.' The core problem was that admission to hospital of a confused older person was a disruption from normal routine for patients, their carers, staff and co-patients. The core process described was that patient, carer, staff and co-patient behaviours were often attempts to gain or give control to deal with the disruption (the core problem). Attempts to gain or give control could lead to good or poor outcomes for patients and their carers. Poor patient and carer outcomes were associated with staff not recognising the cognitive impairment which precipitated or complicated the admission and to diagnose its cause, and staff not recognising the importance of the relationship between the patient and their family carer. Better patient and carer outcomes were associated with a person-centred approach and early attention to good communication with carers." (Clissett et al., 2013, p.1497)

Interviews alone would not have provided the rich data that led to the study findings (Clissett et al., 2013). The researchers noted the study limitations to be data collection in one hospital, the possibility that being observed altered the healthcare professional's behaviors when interacting with patients, and the lack of documentation of specific interventions and whether they were patient-centered.

Interviews

Interviews are focused conversations between the participant and the qualitative researcher that produce data as words (Rubin & Rubin, 2012; Seidman, 2013). The researcher as an interviewer seeks information from a number of individuals, whereas the focus group strategy is designed to obtain the perspective of the normative group, not individual perspectives. Interviews may also be conducted in quantitative studies to assist subjects in the completion of a survey or questionnaire. This assistance may include reading the questions to subjects with limited literacy and documenting their responses to the questions in person or over the phone. The focus of this section is interviewing in qualitative studies.

Depending on the research question, the qualitative researcher conducts either a single interview or more than one. More than one interview may include multiple data collection interviews with each participant, or may entail following a single data collection interview with a second clarification interview, during which the participant can review the researcher's description of the first interview, confirming or correcting the researcher's perceptions and interpretations. A typewritten transcript of the first interview may be provided to the participant at the clarification interview.

Seidman (2013) recommends that the researcher interview each participant three times for phenomenological studies. The first interview is focused on a life history, the second on details of the phenomenon, and the third on reflection on the experience. Using multiple interviews allows the relationship between the researcher and the participant to develop. Over time, the participant may learn to trust the researcher more and reveal insights about his or her experiences that contribute to the study's findings. Follow-up interviews may be used to share the results of the ongoing data analysis with participants and ask additional questions for clarification. Multiple interviews also may be required to study an ongoing process. For a grounded theory study of younger adults who have experienced a stroke with subsequent challenges with eating, a research team conducted two to three interviews with five participants (Klinke Hafsteinsdóttir, Thorsteinsson, & Jónsdóttir, 2013). Studies with multiple interviews, however, are less common than studies during which the participant is interviewed one time.

In addition to determining how many times each participant will be interviewed, the researcher needs to plan the interview location, format, and method of documenting the interview. Interviews might be conducted in a room in a public library, a fast-food restaurant at an off-peak time, an exam room in a clinic, a public park or garden, or the participant's home. The location should be selected so as to be a neutral place that has private areas and is convenient for the participant (Seidman, 2013), with consideration for the safety of both participant and researcher. Accessibility and confidentiality should also be considerations. An exam room may not be a neutral site for a study exploring the patient-provider relationship. During a community-based study, the researcher's appearance may become associated with a stigmatized topic, such as HIV infection, substance use, or domestic violence. A public place may not protect the participant's identity and confidentiality. A participant's home may not be safe for the researcher to visit at certain times of day. A participant's home, however, can offer a sense of comfort and familiarity for the participant and provide the researcher

insight into the participant's experience. In the Klinke et al. (2013) study, researchers described the locations for their interviews as being the participants' homes or a "homey location at a rehabilitation centre" (p. 253).

The format of the interview can be unstructured, semistructured, or structured. **Unstructured interviews** are informal and conversational and may be useful during an ethnographical study or in the early stages of other qualitative studies. They are also the preferred interview method for phenomenology. Most other qualitative interviews are **semistructured**, or organized around a set of open-ended questions. Some experts call these topical or guided interviews (Marshall & Rossman, 2016). The degree of guidance may be as minimal as having a few initial questions or prompts or as structured as multiple predefined questions to narrow the interview to specific aspects of the phenomenon being studied. In either case, the researcher remains open to how the participant responds and carefully words follow-up questions or prompts to allow the **emic view**, the participant's perspective, to emerge. **Structured interviews** are organized with narrower questions in a specific order. The questions may be asked without follow-up questions, and the researcher responses may be scripted in a structured interview (Marshall & Rossman, 2016). Having this level of structure may decrease the anxiety of less experienced interviewers but may result in findings that reflect the **etic, or outsiders' view**, more than they reflect the emic view. As a best practice, consider testing your interview guide with one participant or, as in the case of the Mayer et al. (2013) study, one family.

"The interview guide was written, reviewed by content experts, and field tested with one family that experienced non-cardiac death of a family member prior to this study ... family interviews were done before individual interviews. This sequencing allowed the researcher to observe family dynamic and appreciate the families' collective understanding of the death, before collecting data from individuals within the family." (Mayer et al., 2013, p. 169)

The words spoken and the nonverbal communication during an interview are the data. Although most interviews are conducted face-to-face, interviews can be conducted by telephone or through Web-based meeting software. To explore distant caregiving for a parent with advanced cancer, Mazanec, Daly, Ferrell, and Prince-Paul (2011) conducted telephone interviews with caregivers residing in ten states. The travel to conduct face-to-face interviews would have been expensive, and most likely made the study unfeasible.

Most qualitative researchers audio-record or video-record the interview in order to be able to focus on the interaction and relationship with the participant during the interview (Maxwell, 2013). A recording of the interview results in a "transportable, repeatable resource that allows multiple hearings or viewings as well as access to other readers" (Nikander, 2008, p. 229). The participant must be aware that the interview is being electronically recorded, but the less obtrusive the equipment, the more quickly the participant will forget its presence, relax, and speak more freely. Logistically, the researcher needs to plan ahead to have the power cords or batteries needed for the recording device (Banner, 2010). Using batteries may make the device less obtrusive. A sensitive microphone will allow you to pick up even faint or distorted voices, thereby increasing your ability to make an accurate transcription later. Placing the microphone closer to the participant than to the researcher also may result in a better recording. The majority of recording devices are digital, but if using an older model that uses tapes, ensure that the lengths of the tapes are adequate to record the entire interview with few interruptions to change the tape. Recording with a digital device that can be saved on a computer can make transcription easier. Voice recognition software has become more sophisticated and may allow conversion of the audio recording directly to text. In some situations, recording devices may not be appropriate or the participant may prefer that the interview not be recorded. During the unrecorded interviews, the researcher may take notes and set aside time immediately following the interview to document the interview with as much detail as possible. Because life is uncertain, check all recordings as soon as possible after the interview, to confirm that they are completely audible. If a recording is not perfectly audible, make notes about the interview content immediately while the words are fresh in your memory. This is also a perfect time to make field notes about content, context, metacommunication, and one's initial reactions and responses.

Learning to Interview

Preparing to interview is critical because interviewing is a skill that directly affects the quality of the data produced (Marshall & Rossman, 2016). Interviewing skills can be learned (Seidman, 2013); however, researchers must give themselves the opportunity to develop this skill before they start interviewing study participants. A skilled interviewer can elicit higher-quality data than an inexperienced interviewer by allowing a silent pause, or asking a probing follow-up question without alienating the participant. Unskilled interviewers may not know

how or when to intervene, when to encourage the participant to continue to elaborate, or when to divert to another subject. The interviewer must know how to handle intrusive questions. For practice, conduct interviews with colleagues with experience in interviewing (Munhall, 2012). These rehearsals will help you identify problems before initiating the study (Rubin & Rubin 2012). You may want to conduct one or more trial interviews with individuals who meet the sampling criteria to allow you to try out the proposed questions. Practice sessions and pilot interviews also allow you to determine a realistic time estimate for the interviews. Researchers often underestimate the time needed for an interview. Allow yourself enough time so that you can conduct the interview without feeling rushed. Be sensitive to time-related concerns of the participants, however, and offer the option of stopping if an interview is going longer than expected. Participants may need to catch a bus to get home, pick up children from childcare, or stop to take a dose of medication.

On the whole, qualitative researchers need to learn to be perfectly quiet: to be still, without moving, and to make no sound while the participant speaks. An interview, although interactive, is not a social conversation. The focus is not on the researcher. Rather the focus is on the participant and the participant's experience. Before beginning data collection, practice interviewing a friend or colleague, possibly about grocery shopping or other noncontroversial or unemotional topic. Record the conversation. Listen to it, and listen to the total number of words you say, and how many the interviewee says. Try to limit what you say to phrases or questions that facilitate the interviewee's story. About 90% of the words on the tape should be the interviewee's. Practice looking empathetic and communicating without words. For example, nod instead of saying "Yes," and chuckle without laughing aloud at humor. More neutral responses allow the interviewee to share good and bad information and events, including socially undesirable feelings and thoughts.

Establishing a Positive Environment for an Interview

When preparing for an interview, establish an environment that encourages an open, relaxed conversation (Seidman, 2013). Be sensitive to the physical surroundings. Sit in comfortable chairs, and orient the chairs so that neither you nor the participant is facing windows with direct sunlight. Sitting at a table may be more comfortable and provides a surface for the participant to sign the consent form or complete a demographic form. You may want to offer water or other beverage as a way to provide time for a social connection prior to beginning the interview. When dressing for an interview, the researcher needs to consider how the participant is likely to be dressed. Dressing in formal business attire or a nursing uniform may emphasize the power differences in the relationship. Dressing too casually may be viewed as an indication that the interaction is not important to the researcher. Power issues may affect the effectiveness of the interview. Visual neutrality is important, as well, in clothing colors. Remember, *it is not about you; it is about the participant.* Emphasize that by de-emphasizing yourself. Olfactory neutrality is important, for the same reason. As nurses do for patient care, researchers should avoid cologne, perfume, and other strong smells.

Conducting an Effective Interview

As the researcher, you have the power to shape the interview agenda. Participants have the power to choose the level of responses they will provide. You might begin the interview with a broad request such as "Describe for me your experience with …" or "Tell me about …" Ideally, the participant will respond as though she or he is telling a story. You respond nonverbally with a nod or eye contact to convey your interest in what is being said. Try to avoid agreeing or disagreeing with what the participant is saying (Seidman, 2013). Being nonjudgmental allows the participants to share their experiences more freely. When it seems appropriate, encourage your subject to elaborate further on a particular dimension of the topic. Use of nonthreatening but thought-provoking questions is often called **probing**. Seidman (2013) notes that "probing" sounds intrusive. He prefers the word "exploring" for the process of asking thoughtful questions to gain additional insights into what the participant is sharing. Participants may need validation that they are providing the needed information. Some participants may give short answers, so you may have to encourage them to elaborate. When the participant stops talking, ask a follow-up question that reflects back on what you have heard. Interviewer responses should be encouraging and supportive without being leading. Listening more and talking less is a key principle of effective interviews (Seidman, 2013). That includes tolerating silence. If the participant is not talking but seems to be thinking or considering the topic, stay quiet. Silence can be a powerful invitation that allows the participant to show deeper emotions and thoughts.

Problems During Interviews

Difficulties can occur during interviews. Common problems include interruptions such as telephone calls or text messages, "stage fright" that often arises when the participant realizes he or she is being recorded, failure to establish a rapport with your subject, verbose participants, and those who tend to wander off the subject. Turn off or silence your cell phone at the beginning of the interview, and ask the participant to do the same. If a participant seems paralyzed by the presence of the recording device, move the device out of his or her line of sight if possible. Ask demographic questions or factual questions to ease into the interview. When the participant moves to a subject that you think is unrelated to the focus of the study, you may want to ask how this new subject is related to previous comments on the topic of interest (Seidman, 2013). You may be surprised to learn that what you perceived to be unrelated is associated with the topic, from the participant's perspective. You may also need to tactfully guide the interview back to the topic. Remind participants that they can decline to answer any question and can end the interview at any time.

When using a series of interview questions, let the participant answer the first question fully. If the topic is an emotional one, the participant will almost always provide a story or example. This sometimes answers one or more of the subsequent interview questions on your list. If this happens, as you proceed down the question list, you can say, "The next question is . . . and you have already told me some things about that. Is there anything else you want to add?"

The physical, mental, and emotional condition of the participant may cause difficulties during the interview. The data obtained are affected by characteristics of the person being interviewed (Rubin & Rubin, 2012). These include age, ethnicity, gender, professional background, educational level, and relative status of interviewer and interviewee, as well as impairments in vision or hearing, speech impediments, fatigue, pain, poor memory, disorientation, emotional state, and language difficulties. Although institutional review boards tend to view interviews as noninvasive, interviews are an invasion of the psyche. An interview is capable of producing risks to the health of the participant. Therefore, the interviewer must always avoid inflicting unnecessary harm upon the participant. Participants with fatigue or pain related to illness or treatments should be offered the opportunity to stop, take a break, or schedule a second interview for another day.

For some participants, the experience may be therapeutic but that is not the purpose of the interview (Seidman, 2013). Nevertheless, participants in qualitative interviews are often glad for the ability to express their feelings to an interested listener. It is common for participants to say, after a lengthy interview, "Thank you so much for listening to my story. It's not something I can tell everyone."

In an exploratory-descriptive qualitative study, Alexis (2012) interviewed internationally educated nurses who were employed in a hospital in England. The participating nurses were "made aware of the purpose of the study, and they were free to divulge as much information or as little information as they wished" (Alexis, 2012, p. 963). Furthermore, the researcher told the participants they could ask to have the audio recording turned off at any time and "their wish would be respected" (p. 973). Jones (2015) interviewed African American women with breast cancer but carefully selected the participants to minimize risks. Each woman had to have survived breast cancer for one year and completed the prescribed treatments. "These preferences were put in place so that the individuals would be stabilized medically and free from any discomfort that might occur as a result of cancer care" (Jones, 2015, p. 5).

Emotional expression during an interview may be expected, depending on the topic. Participants who become visibly upset while telling their story should be asked, "Do you want to pause the interview for awhile while you take a deep breath and compose yourself?" or even, "You seem upset. Do you want to end this interview, or do you want to proceed?" When the participant becomes distressed or overcome with emotion, however, you may choose to turn off the recording device and stop the interview completely for a few minutes. You may be able to continue if the participant is able to become composed. Stay with the individual. Offer a tissue. Recognize topics that are more likely to be distressing, and have a plan developed for emergency assistance, if needed, or a list of mental health professionals available if support or a referral is needed. For example, you might schedule interviews in collaboration with a hospital chaplain or psychiatric mental health nurse practitioner to ensure that one of them is available for consultation when you will be interviewing family members whose spouses are receiving hospice care. Recognize that you, the researcher, may also need emotional and psychological support. The researcher may be strongly affected by the stories of the participants. Arrange to have a mentor or trusted friend available to talk with before or after interviews. The researcher may need to rest following an interview, because the experience of conducting good interviews is tiring (Creswell, 2013).

Example Study Using Interviews

When one child in a family experiences a traumatic injury, the family's focus is rightfully shifted to the child,

at the possible expense of other children in the family. Bugel (2014) interviewed the siblings of children who had experienced a traumatic injury. The research problem and purpose are clearly stated.

> "Understanding what it is like to be a well school-age sibling of a child with a traumatic injury is largely unknown ... This unique age group of siblings is experiencing crisis at a personal level, as well as at a family systems level. Their lives are in turmoil, yet the experience of these children has not been studied as a distinct phenomenon. This research study examines the lived experience of well school-age siblings of children who have sustained a serious traumatic injury from the perspective of the siblings." (Bugel, 2014, p. 179)

Bugel (2014) indicated that she used van Manen's (1984, 1990) method of phenomenology and interviewed seven siblings. The children ranged in age from 8 to 18 years.

> "Data were collected through interviews with research participants conducted over a period of 13 months. The interviews were semi-structured individual conversations with the school-age siblings and the researcher. The siblings spoke for themselves, using their own words, based on their own perspective and perceptions. Only the researcher and the sibling informants were present at the private interviews. All interviews were conducted in a conference room or office at the pediatric hospital. Each interview was audio-recorded on a small digital recorder, positioned inconspicuously in the room. Code numbers were assigned to each interview, and no real names were used. Privacy during the interviews was never breached, nor did any of the siblings have a serious or upsetting reaction during the interview. All siblings showed a favorable response to the interviews, and many displayed noticeable enthusiasm, as shown when one sibling spontaneously hugged the researcher and said 'Can we talk again!?'" (Bugel, 2014, p. 180)

The siblings described the aspects of their lives that had changed, such as sleeping arrangements, daily routines, and other adults who were assisting with their care (Bugel, 2014). The children also noted changes in their relationships with their injured sibling. School routines and their ability to have fun had not changed, as well as the presence of sibling rivalry. When asked what they wanted adults to know, the siblings described their need to be noticed and validated. Nurses had communicated with them very little and had not inquired about their needs. Consequently, the siblings knew very little about the injured child's condition. When visiting the injured child, siblings needed information about what to expect and what they could do, such as touching the child.

Focus Groups

Focus groups were designed to obtain the participants' perceptions in a focused topic in a setting that is permissive and nonthreatening (Krueger & Casey, 2015). One of the assumptions underlying the use of focus groups is that interactions among people can help them express and clarify their views in ways that are less likely to occur in a one-on-one interview (Gray, 2009). People in a focus group are selected because they are alike in some characteristic (Krueger & Casey, 2015). Many different communication forms occur in focus groups, including teasing, arguing, joking, anecdotes, and nonverbal clues, such as gesturing, facial expressions, and other body language.

Focus groups as a means of data collection serve a variety of purposes in nursing research. Focus groups have been used to understand the experiences of people who are receiving care or may need care. Researchers have used focus groups to explore adolescent mothers' preferences for recruitment materials (Logsdon et al., 2015), describe the perceptions of Nigerian immigrants of healthy eating and physical activity (Turk, Fapohunda, & Zoucha, 2015), inform the development of an intervention to address depression and anxiety during pregnancy (Stewart, Umar, Gleadow-Ware, Creed, & Bristow, 2015), and develop a list of safety and quality issues, thereby generating themes (Marck, Molzahn, Berry-Hauf, Hutchings, & Hughes, 2014).

Instrument development and refinement are frequently based on the data collected during focus groups. An example of instrument development was the study conducted by Yan et al. (2015). They conducted a focus group with physicians to refine items generated through a review of the literature for a tool to measure postpartum depression. Widger, Tourangeau, Steele, and Streiner (2015) also began their instrument development with a literature review and developed a list of indicators of quality care surrounding the death of a child. Parents who had lost a child participated in the three focus groups and were asked to list indicators of quality care, review the researchers' list, compare the two lists, and assist with determining the final list of quality care indicators. Widger et al. (2015) developed at least one item to measure each of the indicators on the final list. These items became the first version of an instrument to assess the "quality of end of life care for

children" from the perspective of the bereaved parent (Widger et al., 2015, p. 7).

The effective use of focus groups requires careful planning. The location needs to be carefully selected to ensure privacy, comfort, and safety. Meeting rooms in public facilities such as schools, libraries, or churches may be appropriate community locations for focus groups, depending on the research question and the study aims. For focus groups with specific populations, the facility used for support services may have a quiet room that is accessible and familiar to participants. Nurses or other health professionals may participate in focus groups in a healthcare facility but might be more forthcoming in a location away from the facility. If a focus group is planned for a sensitive topic, indicate on the invitation and on any materials the name by which the group will be identified. For example, instead of identifying the group as the "Testicular Cancer Study," a better name might be the "Men's Health Study."

Other logistics include the expected length of the meeting, recruiting subjects, and recording the group interactions. Focus groups typically last from 45 minutes to 2 hours. A 2-hour focus group usually has about 10 questions (Krueger & Casey, 2015). As an extreme example, Krueger and Casey (2015) provided an example of "focus groups in Inuit villages…that last most of the afternoon and into the evening" (p. 202). This length of meeting is consistent with local culture in remote villages of northern Canada. In contrast, focus groups with younger participants should be shorter in order to keep the participants engaged (Krueger & Casey, 2015). Be clear on the recruitment materials about the expected duration of the focus group. Allow for the time it will take to complete consent and demographic forms in determining the length of the data collection process. Provide a reasonable estimate of the time needed, recognizing that whether people attend may be affected by how long the group meeting is expected to last.

Recruiting appropriate participants for each of the focus groups is critical, because recruitment is the most common source of failure. Each focus group should consist of 4 to 12 participants (Marshall & Rossman, 2016). If there are fewer participants, the discussion tends to be inadequate. In most cases, participants are expected to be unknown to one another. However, for a focus group targeting professional groups such as clinical nurses or nurse educators, such anonymity usually is not possible. You may use purposive sampling to seek out individuals known to have the desired expertise (see Chapter 15). In other cases, you may look for participants through the media, posters, or advertisements. A single contact with an individual who agrees to attend a focus group does not ensure that this person will attend the group session. You will need to make repeated phone calls and remind the candidates by mail or email. You may need to offer compensation for their time and effort in the form of cash, phone card, gift card, or bus tokens. Cash payments are, of course, the most effective if the resources are available through funding. Other incentives include offering refreshments at the focus group meeting, T-shirts, coffee mugs, gift certificates, and coupons (Krueger & Casey, 2015). Over-recruiting may be necessary; a good rule is to invite two more potential participants than you need for the group.

Recruiting participants with common social and cultural experiences creates more homogeneous groups (Liamputtong, 2013a). Selecting participants who are similar to one another in lifestyle or experiences, views, and characteristics is believed to facilitate open discussion and interaction. These characteristics might be age, gender, social class, income level, ethnicity, culture, lifestyle, or health status. For example, for a study of barriers to implementing HIV/AIDS clinical trials in low-income minority communities, focus groups might be organized by race/ethnicity and gender. In heterogeneous groups, communication patterns, roles, relationships, and traditions might interfere with the interactions within the focus group. Be cautious about bringing together participants with considerable variation in social standing, education, or authority (Liamputtong, 2013a), because some group members may hesitate to participate fully, whereas others may discount the input of those with perceived lower standing. If a fairly heterogeneous sample is desired, in order to provide a variety of responses, participants may be selected somewhat randomly from a large group. Although qualitative researchers typically use nonrandom sampling, it is not wrong to use random sampling for focus group research when there is a rationale for doing so.

The setting for focus groups should be a relaxed atmosphere with space for participants to sit comfortably in a circle or U shape and maintain eye contact with one another. Ensure that the acoustics of the room will allow you to obtain a quality audio-recording of the sessions. As with the one-on-one interview discussed earlier, place your audio or video recorders unobtrusively. Use a highly sensitive microphone. Hiring a court reporter to do a real-time transcription may have advantages over recording the interaction for transcription later (Scott et al., 2009). Inaudible voices on the recording or overlapping voices can pose challenges to later transcription.

The facilitator, also called a **moderator**, is critical to the success of a focus group. Select a facilitator when possible who reflects the age, gender, and race/ethnicity of the group. In contrast, having a facilitator who does not share the same "culture, role, or behavior" may elicit more "amplification and examples" (Krueger & Casey, 2015, p. 106). The researcher may be the facilitator of the group or may train another person for the role. Training of the facilitator should be thorough and allow time for practice (Gray, 2009). The facilitator needs to understand the aims of the focus groups and to communicate these aims to the participants before the group session. Instruct participants that all points of view are valid and helpful and that speakers should not be asked to defend their positions. Make clear to the group that the moderator's role is to facilitate the discussion, not to contribute. In addition to the moderator, you may want to have an observer or assistant moderator who takes field notes (Krueger & Casey, 2015), especially of facial expressions or interactions not captured by an audio recording (Liamputtong, 2013a). Making notes on the dynamics of the group is also useful, including how group members interact with one another.

Carefully plan the questions that are to be asked during the focus group and, if time permits, pilot-test them (Krueger & Casey, 2015). Limit the number of questions to those most essential to allow adequate time for discussion. You may elect to give participants some of the questions before the group meeting to enable them to give careful thought to their responses. Questions should be posed in such a way that group members can build on the responses of others in the group, raise their own questions, and question one another. Probes can be used to elicit richer details, by means of questions such as "How would that make a difference?" or responses such as "Tell us more about that situation." Avoid pushing participants toward taking a stand and defending it. Once rapport has been established, you may be able to question or challenge ideas and increase group interaction.

The researcher and/or moderator may come to the focus groups with preconceived ideas about the topic. Early in the session, provide opportunities for participants to express their views on the topic of discussion. Use probes or questions if the discussion wanders too far from the focus of the study. A good moderator weaves questions into the discussion naturally and clarifies, paraphrases, and reflects back what group members have said. These discussions tend to express group norms, or the majority voice, and individual voices of contrasting viewpoints may be stifled. A participant may be uncomfortable sharing a less acceptable viewpoint, because those with opposing views are listening. However, when a sensitive topic is being discussed, the group format may actively facilitate the discussion because less inhibited members break the ice for those who are more reticent. Participants may also provide group support for expressing feelings, opinions, or experiences. Late in the session, the facilitator may encourage group members to go beyond the current discussion or debate and reflect on differences among the views of participants and inconsistencies within their own thinking.

Example Study Using Focus Groups

Cancer prevalence rates vary among Native American nations. Eschiti et al. (2014) used focus groups as part of a community-based participatory research project to develop cancer education modules acceptable to members of the Comanche Nation. The Native American Cancer Research Corporation (NACR) developed cancer education modules for Native Americans, in general, but no specific education interventions were available for the Comanche people. Eschiti et al. (2014) identified two research questions in collaboration with a team that included Native American navigators and researchers. The questions addressed how to modify available cancer-related education materials so that the content would be "culturally and geographically appropriate" for the community members of the Comanche Nation (Eschiti et al., 2014, p. E27).

The researchers recruited 23 key informants of the Comanche Nation to participate in focus groups during which the cancer education modules were reviewed, for the purpose of evaluating the content and cultural congruence of workshop materials. The key informants who participated in the focus groups were "selected for their knowledge and insights of the Comanche culture, health education needs, and age-related considerations" (Eschiti et al., 2014, p. E28).

The researchers provided a rich description of the focus groups and their implementation. They gave the potential focus group participants the informed consent document a week in advance so the participants could make a thoughtful decision about being part of the study. The study was implemented with cultural sensitivity, including sharing a meal before the focus group started. The researchers also considered the work schedules of potential participants and scheduled two focus groups in the daytime and two in the evening. Moderators were members of the Comanche Nation who were known in their community. The moderators' use of colloquial language and their

experiences in the Comanche Nation contributed to their effectiveness.

Each focus group reviewed the modules and made recommendations for changes to make the words and graphics of the content more acceptable to the community. The main points identified by the participants were recorded on a large pad of paper on an easel "so participants could view ideas presented and comment on them" (Eschiti et al., 2014, p. E28). Transcripts were prepared for each focus group, along with field notes and observations. The data were analyzed, and five major themes emerged that reflected cultural perspectives, such as "Nourishing Body, Mind, and Spirit: Connecting With the Past" (Eschiti et al., 2014, p. E28).

The focus groups were modified to be culturally appropriate and were a critical element in the community-based participatory research project (Eschiti et al., 2014). The study findings enforced the importance of nurses being aware of cultural differences between the Indian nations.

ELECTRONICALLY MEDIATED DATA

Images created by still and video photography and Internet communication are newer methods of qualitative data collection that are being used by nurse researchers. Each is described briefly, and an example provided. Prior to using one of these forms of data, the reader is encouraged to study in greater depth the technology used and the ethical issues due to potential loss of confidentiality and breach of the privacy of participants' protected health information (see Chapter 9).

Photographs and Video

Anthropologists and historical researchers have included photographs as data in their studies for many years. However, creating photographic images as part of data collection is a viable scientific method in different types of qualitative and quantitative studies. The ubiquitous nature of digital photography is likely to speed the acceptance of the method. When used as research data, participants, researchers, or a combination of the two may have taken the photographs or recorded the videos. **Photovoice** is the idea of participants using photographs to describe aspects of their communities and their lives, "recording and reflecting on the strengths and concerns," and is most often used in participatory research studies (Findholt, Michael, & Davis, 2011, p. 186). Wang and Burris (1994) are credited with guiding the first health-related study during which rural Chinese women were given cameras to photograph their lives and especially their health needs. Wang called this practice photo novella, but others since have used the term **photovoice**.

Nurse researchers have used photovoice to gain insights into different cultures, even within the United States. Turk et al. (2015) used photovoice to study the eating habits and physical activity of Nigerians who had immigrated to the United States. The study's design was identified as a "qualitative visual ethnography" (p. 17). The participants were provided with a digital camera and instructed to "take photos of what they considered unhealthy and healthy eating and activity" (p. 18). The participants had two weeks to take photos of unhealthy behaviors followed by a focus group to discuss each participant's top four photos. Following the focus groups, participants were asked to take photos of healthy behaviors. A second focus group was held to discuss the photos of healthy behaviors. Analysis revealed four themes about healthy and unhealthy behaviors. Traditional eating and activity patterns were deemed to be healthier than American eating and activity patterns. Turk et al. (2015) demonstrated that photovoice is a versatile tool and can be combined with other data collection methods, such as interviews and focus groups.

Marck et al. (2014) used photographs as a source of data in a participatory study with hemodialysis nurses concerned about the quality and safety of their work environment. The research team began the data collection with a focus group. The focus group was used to generate an initial list of quality and safety concerns followed by "a digitally recorded photographic walk-about in the unit" (Marck et al., 2014, p. 28).

> "During this practitioner-led data collection, team members collected digital photographs, and the participating nurses' narratives of the safety and quality concerns were identified, both on the initial validated list, as well as additional issues identified throughout the walk-about. The nurse educator and nurse participants narrated each photographic subject as it was captured, providing detail about the subject area was seen as relevant to safety and quality issues in renal care." (Marck et al., 2014, p. 28)

The researchers coded the visual and textual data, identifying themes that were represented by specific photographs. The themes and photographs were shared with a second focus group of the patient care team. The major themes (Box 12-1) were presented in the research report along with representative photographs. Human subject protection is frequently a concern when using

---

BOX 12-1   Major Themes From a Study Using Participatory Photographic Methods

- Areas of **clutter** are apparent throughout the unit.
- There are multiple environmental challenges in maintaining **infection control**.
- The **unit design** leads to problematic arrangement of patient care areas.
- There are ongoing safety concerns related to **chemical fumes and air quality**.
- A **lack of storage space** leads to crowding of equipment and blocking of exits.
- There is a variety of other **health and safety hazards**, such as tripping hazards.

Adapted from Marck, P., Molzahn, A., Berry-Hauf, R., Hutchings, L., & Hughes, S. (2014). Exploring safety and quality in a hemodialysis environment with participatory photographic methods: A restorative approach. *Nephrology Nursing Journal*, *41*(1), 29.

---

photovoice, a concern addressed by Marck et al. (2014) in the study methods section of their report.

> "The study received institutional and administrative approval from the hospital and ethical approval from the university employing the investigators. Written informed consent forms were signed by all participants. Confidentiality of participants was assured. No photographs were taken that could identify any individual patient or nurse." (Marck et al., 2014, p. 28)

Photographs were identified as playing a major role in the findings of the study and as a means for continued improvement of the work environment.

> "A wide range of issues was identified, and participants were able to readily recognize and freely discuss areas of concern that may not have been as visible or noteworthy without the visual prompts to their imaginations. The digital photo walkabout approach was user-friendly and the nurse educator was confident that she could use it on an ongoing basis independent of the researchers to monitor, document, and address both safety issues and concrete improvements in collaboration with the dialysis team." (Marck et al., 2014, p. 33)

Photovoice can often generate a deeper understanding of stigmatizing conditions. Photovoice may pose unique ethical considerations because people in photographs can be identified and may not have consented to participation in the study (Marshall & Rossman,

2016). Researchers who are considering photovoice as a research methodology are urged to read primary sources and consult with researchers experienced in the methodology. The rights of the research participants must be protected during the conduct and reporting of the research.

Internet-Based Data

Internet communication provides a way to collect data from persons separated by distance. Quantitative researchers are regularly using Internet-based surveys and instruments to gather data, but qualitative researchers are also using Web-based communities such as online forums and blogs for research purposes. The number of participants available for Internet-based research is extensive but does have the limitation that samples include only those who can read and write, are comfortable using a computer, and have access to the Internet (Marshall & Rossman, 2016). A nurse leader using Internet communication for data collection is Eun-Ok Im. Im has used mixed methods study designs with quantitative and qualitative phases. The focus here is on the qualitative phases. Im, Chee, Lim, Liu, and Kim (2008) used an online forum created for their study to gather data about physical activity of middle-aged women. The month-long online forum was completed by 15 of the 30 women who started. The researchers posted 17 topics for discussion with three or four topics introduced each week. The topics were about physical activity and cultural influences on physical activity. The participants used pseudonyms when posting to the forum to protect anonymity. The text of the discussions was converted into transcripts for analysis.

As themes were identified, the researchers shared them with participants and asked for feedback. Im has used online forums for data collection to develop a robust program of research. As examples, her team has completed studies on ethnic differences in cancer pain (Im et al., 2009) and Asian Americans' perspectives on Internet cancer support groups (Im, Lee, & Chee, 2010). Since 2008, she has been studying midlife women with a focus on physical activity and menopausal symptoms. Table 12-3 identifies her studies using online forums by the sample and topic. Table 12-4 describes the two papers the research team has published comparing menopausal symptoms and physical activity across ethnic groups. Im and other colleagues noted in these studies that one of the limitations was that the data represent only those who have Internet access and are comfortable describing personal experiences in the online forum.

TABLE 12-3   Studies Using Online Forums With Women of Different Ethnicities: Publications by Dr. Eun-Ok Im and Team

Researchers (Year)	Sample	Topic
Im, Chee, Lim, Liu, & Kim (2008)	Midlife women	Physical activity
Im, Lim, Lee, Dormire, Chee, & Kresta (2009)	Hispanic midlife women in the U.S.	Menopausal symptoms
Im, Lee, & Chee (2010)	Asian American women with cancer	Perspectives on online cancer support group
Im, Seoung Hee Lee, & Chee (2010)	Black women	Menopausal transition
Im, Lee, Chee, Stuifbergen, and the eMAPA Research Team (2011)	White women	Physical activity
Im, Ko, Hwang, Chee, Stuifbergen, Lee, & Chee (2012)	Asian American midlife women	Physical activity

TABLE 12-4   Secondary Analyses of Physical Activity and Menopause: Publications by Dr. Eun-Ok Im and Team

Researchers (Year)	Sample	Topic
Im, Lee, Chee, Dormire, & Brown (2010)	Multiethnic midlife women	Menopausal symptom experience
Im, Ko, Hwang, Chee, Stuifbergen, Walker, & Brown (2013)	Multiethnic midlife women	Attitudes toward physical activity

The number of studies using Internet communication for collecting data, or Internet-mediated research, is growing. Whitehead (2007) produced an integrated review of the literature on issues of quantitative and qualitative Internet-mediated research. On the basis of her review of 46 papers, she concluded that three major themes affect the credibility of the findings of Internet-mediated studies. The first is sample bias. This concern is diminishing as access to the Internet continues to increase, but bias still exists relative to frequency of use throughout the age spectrum. A researcher could assess the reality of sample bias, and its various types, by comparing demographic characteristics of an online sample with those of samples in traditional studies on the same topic. Whitehead (2007) identified the second concern to be ethical issues such as seeking consent, assuring anonymity of the participants, and protecting the security of the site. The third concern was the reliability and validity of the data collected because the researcher cannot verify whether participants meet the inclusion criteria for the study and has no control over distractions that may occur during data collection. Despite these issues, studies will continue to be conducted using the Internet, because researchers aware of these issues can develop studies to minimize the concerns. Researchers considering this methodology may benefit from reading the research reports of Im's teams, which contain details of how they addressed issues of confidentiality and security.

TRANSCRIBING RECORDED DATA

Transcription of verbal data into written data is a routine component of qualitative studies. Transcripts present data in a form that allows the researcher to review the data visually, and to share it with team members for analysis and validation. Data collected during a qualitative study may be narrative descriptions of observations, transcripts from audio recordings of interviews, entries in the researcher's diary reflecting on the dynamics of the setting, or notes taken while reading and reflecting on written documents.

Transcription may require 3 to 8 hours for each hour of interview or focus group time, depending on the equipment used and the transcriber's skill (Marshall & Rossman, 2016). Audio-recorded interviews are generally transcribed verbatim with different punctuation marks used to indicate laughter, changes in voice tone, or other nuances. Hiring a professional transcriptionist may decrease the time but may be too expensive, depending on the study's budget. When hiring a transcriptionist, be clear about the details, such as whether to correct grammar and how to indicate pauses or laughter. Although some researchers allow for general transcription, nurse researchers most frequently report verbatim transcription and link the accuracy of the transcript to the rigor of the study (Rubin & Rubin, 2012).

Transcribing the recordings yourself has the advantage of immediately immersing you in the data. If using tapes, a pedal-operated recorder allows you to listen, stop, and start the recording without removing your hands from the keyboard. With digitalized data, you can start and stop the recording with a click. Even when you hire another person to transcribe the recordings, you will check the transcription by listening to the recording while reviewing the transcript. Voice recognition programs can be of significant benefit as the capacity of the software to "learn" the voice of the interviewee continues to improve with new versions or updates. For transcription of focus group recordings, voice recognition software may not be as effective. To overcome the challenges of multiple voices on the recording, Krueger and Casey (2015) suggest the transcriber listen to the recording and repeat aloud what is heard to allow the voice recognition software to learn only one voice. Other software may allow conversion of audio recording to digital formats ready for analysis within computer analysis software. You also may code the actual recording, negating the need for a word transcription.

Video recordings are maintained in their original format. However, the researcher may make notes on sequential segments of the recording, creating a type of field notes. The researcher may also code the recordings directly. When video recordings are used for quantitative studies, the recordings are coded by time lapses or some other quantifiable variable and assigned a numerical value. For example, the researcher will watch 15 seconds of the recording and note whether a specific behavior occurred.

DATA MANAGEMENT

Because data are frequently collected simultaneously with data analysis, the study manager, who may be the researcher, needs to have a plan developed for how to organize and store data. Label electronic files consistently. For example, the digital files from recordings can be labeled with the date and the code number or pseudonym of the participant. Make copies of all original files on a second computer or external storage device. Similarly, scan or copy all handwritten notes, field notes, or memos and, if possible, store originals in a waterproof and fireproof storage box. Any electronic files containing personally identifiable information (family member, hospital name, addresses, doctor's name) should be encrypted prior to being sent electronically to a transcriptionist or team member. Because of the risk of unauthorized persons accessing documents and recordings sent through the Internet, best practice is to electronically transmit only de-identified files. You may want to keep a Word document or Excel file listing all files by date, file name, and type of document, such as observational memo, transcript, analysis record, or field note. The study manager may also want to keep records of who is currently working on that file and whether it is being transcribed, analyzed, or reviewed by a team member. With Internet-based storage systems (Google drive, cloud storage), researchers can simultaneously analyze files with all input saved quickly and attributed to the contributor.

Some researchers may prefer to make notes, mark text, and label (code) sections of data on a hard copy of a transcript or field note using colored markers, pencil, or pen. If hard copy is used, ensure that each page is clearly identified with the file name in the header or footer of the document. You may want to format the document with large right-hand margins to allow more space for coding and notes. It is recommended that you also include line numbers, not for each page, but for the entire document continuously. Having line numbers allows the researcher to note the source of a code by line number within a specific document.

Other researchers prefer to work on electronic files within a software program, using tools ranging from as simple as the highlight or comment functions in a document within a word processing file to as complex as analysis of visual images, transcripts, field notes, and memos within one of several specialized computer programs, called computer-assisted qualitative data analysis software (CAQDAS). The program does not analyze the data but allows the researcher to makes notes about tentative themes and record decisions made during the analysis (Krueger & Casey, 2015; Liamputtong, 2013a). CAQDAS can maintain a file directory, allow for annotation of coding decisions, produce diagrams of relationships among codes, and retrieve sections of text that the researcher has identified with the same code (Creswell, 2013; Hoover & Koerber, 2011; Liamputtong, 2013a). Box 12-2 provides a list of the advantages and disadvantages of CAQDAS, extracted from Creswell (2013) and Hoover and Koerber (2011). Table 12-5 contains descriptions and online suppliers of a selected group of CAQDAS programs.

DATA ANALYSIS

Qualitative data analysis is "both the code and the thought processes that go behind assigning meaning to data" (Corbin & Strauss, 2015, p. 58). Qualitative data analysis is creative, challenging, time-consuming, and, consequently, expensive (Jirwe, 2011). Less experienced researchers may feel uncertain about how to proceed because the process feels ambiguous (Streubert & Carpenter, 2011). Data analysis in grounded theory research

---

BOX 12-2   Advantages and Disadvantages of Computer-Assisted Qualitative Data Analysis Software (CAQDAS)

Advantages

Store and organize data files
Provide means for line-by-line analysis
Provide documentation of coding and analysis
Click and drag to merge codes
Have concept-mapping features
Search for related codes and quotations efficiently
Send coded data files to others
Link memos to text
Generate a list of all codes
Retrieve memos related to specific codes
Minimize clerical tasks to allow focus on actual analysis
Support and integrate the work of multiple team members
Decrease paper usage

Disadvantages

Cost of software
Need to allow time and expend energy to learn the software and its functions
Unavailability of understandable instructions for use of the software
Potential that technical/functional aspects will overwhelm thinking about the analysis
Potential for computer problems interfering with the software and causing data and analysis to be lost

Data from Creswell, J. W. (2013). *Qualitative inquiry and research design: Choosing among five approaches* (3rd ed.). Thousand Oaks, CA: Sage; and Hoover, R. S., & Koerber, A. L. (2011). Using NVivo to answer the challenges of qualitative research in professional communication: Benefits and best practices. *IEEE Transactions on Professional Communication, 54*(1), 68–82.

---

and ethnographic research occurs concurrently with data collection. Analysis of data from an interview may result in the researcher asking an additional question in subsequent interviews to confirm or disconfirm an initial interpretation of the data. The process of interpretation occurs in the mind of the researcher. Corbin and Strauss (2015) describe **interpretation** as translating the words and actions of participants into meanings that readers and consumers can understand. The virtual text grows in size and complexity as the researcher reads and rereads the transcripts. Throughout the process of analysis, the virtual text develops and evolves. Although

TABLE 12-5   Examples of Computer-Assisted Qualitative Data Analysis Software (CAQDAS)

Software	Description	Website
ATLAS/ti 8.0	Robust CAQDAS functions; large searchable data storage including media files; multiple users allowed; facilitates theory building; flexible; supports use of PDF files.	http://www.atlasti.com/
Ethnograph v6	Originally developed for use by ethnographers; import and code data files; sort and sift codes; retrieve data and files.	http://www.qualisresearch.com/
HyperRESEARCH	Code and retrieval functions; theory building features added on; handles media files.	http://www.researchware.com/
MAXQDA 10	Robust CAQDAS functions, but less powerful search tool; allows integration of quantitative and qualitative analysis; color-based filing; supports different types of text analysis.	http://www.maxqda.com/products
NVivo 10	Robust CAQDAS functions including several types of queries; familiar format of file organization system; handles multimedia files; latest version includes compatibility with quantitative analysis and bibliographic software.	http://www.qsrinternational.com/-tab_you/

Synthesized from Hoover and Koerber (2011), Streubert and Carpenter (2011), and websites of suppliers and professional organizations.

multiple valid interpretations may occur if different researchers examine the text, all findings must remain trustworthy to the data. Interpretations should be data-based: in the words of grounded theory, *grounded in the data*. This trustworthiness applies to the unspoken meanings emerging from the totality of the data, not just the written words of the text. The first step in data analysis is to be familiar with the data.

Immersion in the Data

Becoming familiar with the data involves reading and rereading notes and transcripts, recalling observations and experiences, listening to audio recordings and viewing videotapes until you have become **immersed in the data** (Patton, 2015). Being immersed means that you are fully invested in the data and are spending extensive amounts of time reading and thinking about the data. Recordings contain more than words; they contain feeling, emphasis, and nonverbal communications. These aspects are at least as important to the communication as the words are. As you listen to recordings, look at photographs, or read transcripts, you relive the experiences described and become very familiar with the phrases that different participants used or the images that were especially poignant. In phenomenology, this immersion in the data has been referred to as

dwelling with the data (Munhall, 2012). Earlier in the chapter, Bugel's (2014) phenomenological study with siblings of children with traumatic brain injury was used as an example. Continuing with the example, Bugel (2014) described dwelling with the data in the following excerpt:

"The written transcriptions of the interviews were read and re-read so that patterns and themes common to the experience of the school-age siblings became manifest. Much time was spent reflecting upon the data ... in such as way that a deeper understanding of the meaning of the experience was uncovered." (Bugel, 2014, p. 181)

Other qualitative methods also rely on dwelling with the data, although researchers may describe the process as spending extensive time thinking about the data or rereading transcripts repeatedly.

Coding

Because of the volumes of data acquired in a qualitative study, initial efforts at analysis focus on reducing the volume of data so that the researcher can more effectively examine them. The reduction of the data occurs as you attach meaning to elements in your data and document that meaning with a word, symbol, or phrase.

TABLE 12-6   Types of Coding for Qualitative Data Analysis*

Type	Description
Axial coding	Finding and labeling connections between concepts; assigning codes to categories (Liamputtong, 2013a); also may be called Level II coding in grounded theory studies
Descriptive coding	Classifying elements of data using terms that are close to the participant's words, also called first-level and primary cycle coding (Tracy, 2013)
Explanatory coding	Connecting coded data to an emerging theory; describing coded data as patterns (Miles et al., 2014)
Interpretive coding	Labeling coded data into more abstract terms that represent merged codes; interpretations may be checked with participants; participants may contribute to the actual interpretation (Munhall, 2012).
In-vivo coding	"Concepts using actual words of research participants" (Corbin & Strauss, 2015, p. 85), instead of words selected by the researcher
Open coding	"Breaking down data into manageable analytic pieces" (Corbin & Strauss, 2015, p. 221); also called Level I coding in grounded theory studies
Selective coding	"Building a 'story' that connects the categories" (Creswell, 2007). Categories are compared and a core category is identified (Liamputtong, 2013a). The researcher may generate propositions or statements that bridge the categories.
Substantive coding	Using in-vivo coding (using words of participants) and implicit coding to put terms on similar groups of raw data (Streubert & Carpenter, 2011)

*These terms are not mutually exclusive, because different writers have used different labels for similar analytical processes.

In grounded theory research, this is known as a code. **Coding** is a means of naming, labeling, and later sorting data elements, which allows the researcher to find themes and patterns.

A **code** is a symbol or abbreviation used to label words or phrases in the data. Through coding, the researcher explores the phenomenon of the study. Miles et al. (2014, p. 72) state, "coding *is* analysis." Coding is more than "technical, preparatory work for higher level thinking about the study … coding is deep reflection about and, thus, deep analysis and interpretation of the data's meanings" (Miles et al., 2014, p. 72). Therefore, it is important that the codes be consistent with the philosophical base of the study. Organization of data, selection of specific elements of the data for categories, and naming of these categories all reflect the philosophical basis of the study. The type and level of coding vary somewhat according to the qualitative approach being used. Table 12-6 displays types of codes described in the social science literature and used primarily in grounded theory analysis. The terms can be confusing because different writers have given different names to similar types of codes.

As data analysis continues, coding may progress to the development of a taxonomy, the emergence of codes into patterns, or, in grounded theory research, to the description of a theoretical framework. For example, you might develop a classification of types of pain, types of patients, or types of patient education. Initial categories should be as broad as possible with minimal overlap. As data analysis proceeds, the codes may be merged and relabeled at a higher level of abstraction. In a study of medication adherence, the initial codes might be "paying attention to time," "counting and recounting," and "remembering to get prescriptions." These codes might be grouped later into the more abstract code "attending to logistics." The first level of coding is descriptive and uses participant phrases as the label for the code, also called in vivo coding. The label for the merged codes is interpretive and might be called a **theme** if repeatedly identified in the data.

Isakson and Jurkovic (2013) studied the experiences of 11 adults from Asia and Africa who survived torture and came to the United States as refugees. The researchers interviewed each participant twice to allow clarification and additional questions, which resulted in 21 hours of interviews to analyze.

"Using the grounded theory methodology of Strauss & Corbin (1990), we analyzed the transcripts using several operational procedures: open, axial, and selective coding." (Isakson & Jurkovic, 2013, p. 752)

Isakson and Jurkovic (2013) trained a team of graduate students and colleagues to work independently to accomplish open coding, and then to negotiate agreement. Throughout this time, codes were defined and redefined until the team achieved a high degree of consensus on the open codes. Then they moved into axial and selective coding.

"Next, using axial coding through NVivo (QSR International, 2008), we linked themes, categories, and subcategories and organized them systematically according to context, conditions, and strategies that enabled or hindered the healing process. Then, as a part of selective coding, we developed a model in which these enabling factors were systematically related to healing. To facilitate this process, we constructed a storyline that provided a descriptive overview of the data. "Moving on" emerged as the core variable that best captured the process of healing and recovery after torture, and we linked enabling conditions and strategies to moving on." (Isakson & Jurkovic, 2013, p. 752)

Content Analysis

Content analysis is designed to classify the words in a text into categories. The researcher is looking for repeated ideas or patterns of thought. In exploratory-descriptive qualitative studies, researchers may analyze the content of the text using concepts from a guiding theory, if one was selected during study development. During historical studies, the researcher analyzes documents and photographs to describe their content related to the focus of the study.

Eschiti et al. (2014) conducted focus groups with members of the Comanche Nation during their study to develop educational materials related to cancer. True to the community-based design of the study, participants were involved in reviewing the results of the team's content analysis.

"Content analysis of the data from focus group responses, field notes, and observations were recorded (Morse, 1993). All data were reviewed by the PI, the qualitative project consultant, and native navigators. Research team members developed consensus on code categories and emerging themes. Once completed, the themes and supportive quotes were shared with select participants to ensure accuracy and validation. Clarifications were noted; however, no theme modifications were required." (Eschiti et al., 2014, p. E28)

Eschiti et al. (2014) provided a thorough description of measures taken to enhance the rigor of the study.

"Credibility was achieved through validation from focus group data, audio recordings, field notes, and observations. Credibility was enhanced by participation of the PI who is experienced in culturally sensitive research methods, as well as the Comanche native navigators and the Comanche qualitative analyst who were familiar with the culture. Trustworthiness was confirmed when the findings provided rich descriptions of experiences that were substantiated by participants (Morse, 1993). Transferability was enhanced by including men and women of varied ages, education, and life experiences. That allowed for a broad understanding of the topic under investigation, making the findings representative of the data from which they originated (Morse, 1993)." (Eschiti et al., 2014, pp. E28-E29)

The measures the researchers used to enhance rigor are applicable to more than content analysis, and can be used in qualitative studies in data collected through interviews and focus groups. Content analysis is one of several types of qualitative data analyses. Table 12-7 includes several additional types of data analysis.

Narrative Analysis

Narrative inquiry is a qualitative approach that uses stories as its data (Duffy, 2012). Through a series of life experiences, people create their identities in the historical and social context in which they live. As a philosophical approach to qualitative research, narrative inquiry is not included in this textbook (see Duffy, 2012, for additional information on the method). Data analysis, however, may yield new stories, and researchers using other philosophical approaches may tell a participant's story in their analysis and presentation of findings. In addition to being organized chronologically, you might analyze a story as one would a published novel during a literature course, looking for characters, setting, plot, conflict, and resolution. Historical researchers may compare participants' stories to present a broader picture of an event.

Mayer et al. (2013), in their exploratory-descriptive qualitative study of families after the sudden cardiac death (SCD) of a loved one, chose narrative analysis to "analyze family stories of bereavement" (p. 166). They stated their rationale for using narrative analysis with both structural and thematic analysis.

TABLE 12-7 Types of Qualitative Data Analysis

Data Analysis	Description
Chronological analysis	Identifying and organizing major elements in a time-ordered description as events and epiphanies
Componential analysis	Identifying units of meaning that are cultural attributes; process allows ethnographer to identify gaps in observations and selectively collect additional data
Constant comparison	Analyzing new data for similarities to and differences from existing data
Direct interpretation	Identifying a single instance of the phenomenon or topic and drawing out its meaning without comparing to other instances
Domain analysis	Focusing on specific aspects of a social situation such as people involved; used in ethnography
Narrative analysis	Looking for the story in the data; identifying the characters, setting, plot, conflict, and resolution as an exemplar of the phenomenon being studied
Taxonomic analysis	Identifying categories with a domain (see domain analysis); used in ethnography
Thematic analysis	Finding within the data three to six overriding abstract ideas that summarize the phenomenon of interest
Theoretical comparison	Thinking about the properties and characteristics of categories; linking to existing theories and models
Three-dimensional analysis	Thinking about and identifying continuity, interactions, and situations within a story

Synthesized from Corbin and Strauss (2008) and Creswell (2007).

"Narrative analysis (Riessman, 2008) was chosen because it allowed us to describe how the same event, the SCD of a family member, may have different meanings. Structural analysis focused on how the stories were organized and structured, while thematic techniques focused on content, or what was included in the stories (Riessman, 2008). The use of structural and thematic techniques allowed us to describe patterns across the shared experience of family bereavement while also identifying differences in individual meanings (Riessman, 2008)." (Mayer et al., 2013, p. 170)

For the first four themes identified, Mayer et al. (2013) relayed a story to support the theme. For the fifth theme, they provided a contrasting story. Here is the story supporting the theme of "sudden cardiac death... boom" (p. 170).

"A story of questions: why did the death occur?
Janet and Kim (family 3) had questions after Dick's death. Janet was aware of her brother's recent visits to the doctor; she knew that his medications were changed. Even with this knowledge, Janet was shocked when Dick died. Janet's initial questions were related to the cause of Dick's death: What happened to his heart? When did he die? Why didn't Dick's doctor 'do something

different?' An autopsy was done and Janet and her daughter Kim talked with the medical examiner, who explained the cause of death as cardiac rupture. Over time additional questions arose...." (Mayer et al., 2013, p. 170)

Jane went on to say how patient and empathetic the medical examiner who did the autopsy was, responding to additional questions over time. His explanations helped the family come to terms with Dick's death. These stories allow nurses to connect with the participants' experiences and feelings, increasing nurses' capacity to empathize with families in similar situations.

Memoing

The researcher develops a memo to record insights or ideas related to notes, transcripts, or codes. **Memos** move the researcher toward theorizing and are conceptual rather than factual. Marshall and Rossman (2016) indicate that memos may be about the methods, the emerging themes, or the links between the data, the literature, and existing theories. They may link pieces of data together or use a specific piece of data as an example of a conceptual idea. The memo may be written to someone else involved in the study or may be just a note to yourself. The important thing is to value your ideas and document them quickly. Initially you might feel that the idea is so clear in your mind that you can write or record it later. However, you may soon forget the thought and be unable to retrieve it. As you become immersed in the data, these ideas will occur at odd times, such as when you are sleeping, walking, or driving. Whenever an idea emerges, even if it is vague and not well thought out, develop the habit of writing it down immediately or recording it on a hand-held device such as a cell phone.

Audit Trail

Qualitative researchers create an audit trail as a key element of enhancing the rigor of a study. Marshall and Rossman (2016, p. 230) describe audit trails as a transparent way to provide "evidence and trace the logic leading to the representation and interpretation of findings." The audit trail may include, but is not limited to, the date and location of data collection episodes (interviews, observations, focus groups), location of original recordings and electronic transcription files, team meeting minutes, journals, memos, and decisions about code definitions and analyses. Coty, McCammon, Lehna, Twyman, and Fahey (2015) used focused ethnography to gain understanding of the fire prevention beliefs and actions of older adults living in their homes. Through participant observation and interviews, the researchers found two themes related to fire safety: the risks of the living environment and the journey to maintain independence. In addition to transcriptions of interviews, the data included photos of fire hazards, information about medical conditions, and the participants' ability to perform activities of daily living. They describe their audit trail in this excerpt:

"Consistency was supported through the use of an audit trail which was implemented with data assessment. Descriptions of procedures implemented, rationale for decision making, and dense description of people in their home and community further supported consistency (Lincoln & Guba, 1985; Sandelowski, 1986). Data analysis began with first transcription as cases were summarized and ongoing peer debriefing promoted dependability of findings." (Coty et al., 2015, p. 179)

Findings and Conclusions

Qualitative findings reflect the study's philosophical roots and the data that were collected. Unlike quantitative research, conclusions are formed throughout the data analysis process in qualitative research. Conclusions are intertwined with the findings in a qualitative study. For a phenomenological study, the findings are presented as an exhaustive description (Streubert & Carpenter, 2011). The findings of a focused ethnographic study may include a description of the culture that achieved the study objectives or answered the research questions. In grounded theory studies, the researcher's aim is to produce a text or graphic description of social processes. As the description is refined, a theoretical structure or framework emerges that might be considered a tentative theory (Corbin & Strauss, 2015; Fawcett & Garity, 2009; Marshall & Rossman, 2016; Munhall, 2012). Conclusions in qualitative research are not generalizable. They describe a culture, a social process, a personal journey, or a situation as perceived by the participants, interpreted by the researcher, and then (often) verified with the participants. The findings are specific to the sample. Generalization is not the goal for qualitative research as it is for quantitative research.

Even though conclusions in qualitative nursing research apply only to the sample, they may be transferable to another group. Grounded theory research involves theorizing and serves to inform the reader. This informing is tantamount to educating the reader or perhaps inspiring the reader, relative to culturally appropriate behaviors, social forces in play, the experience of a given diagnosis, or common challenges to wellness. In a parallel way, however, qualitative research findings that describe social pressures on a child with spina bifida in Atlanta, Georgia, might resonate, or ring true, with a nurse who works in Tokyo, Japan, with young adult survivors of stroke secondary to aneurism. The nurse may be more sensitive to the clients' needs and concerns and more aware of factors that impact their quality of life, after reading the report on children in Atlanta.

Reporting Results

In any qualitative study, the first section of a research report should be a detailed description of the participants. The ethnography report also includes details about the setting and the environment in which the data were gathered. The results of data analysis may be displayed in the form of a table with the themes in the first column of a table and exemplar quotations in the second column. In phenomenological studies, a table may be accompanied by a **paradigm case.** The paradigm case may be a quotation that best encapsulates a theme or an example that best depicts the study's findings (Givens, 2008). Using tables in this way increases the transparency of the analysis and interpretation. Other writers, using other methods, may incorporate supporting or disconfirming evidence from the literature within the results section of the report. The report may include quotations for each theme or pattern that was identified.

How the results are presented depends on the philosophical approach upon which the study was developed. As previously mentioned, phenomenologists provide a thick, rich, and exhaustive description of the phenomenon that was studied. Grounded theorists present their findings and whatever tentative theory was generated by the study. Ethnographers present findings within the context of culture, its leaders, normative behaviors, relationships, and other interactive exchanges. Findings of exploratory-descriptive qualitative studies are reported by addressing each research question and providing the pertinent findings. The report of a historical study may have limited information about the methods; rather, the report is the story of the events or series of events that were studied.

METHODS SPECIFIC TO QUALITATIVE APPROACHES

Phenomenological Research Methods

Phenomenological researchers have several choices about methods that are related to their specific philosophical views on phenomenology. In Chapter 4, differences in Husserl's and Heidegger's views on phenomenology were described. Researchers subscribing to Husserl's views would use **bracketing**, which is consciously identifying, documenting, and choosing to set aside one's own views on the phenomenon (Dowling, 2007). Heidegger's (1962) view was that researchers could not separate their own perspectives from that of the participants' during the collection, analysis, and interpretation of the data. In phenomenology, additional philosophical approaches to the analysis and interpretation of data are available, such as those advocated by van Kaam (1966), Giorgi (1970), Colaizzi (1978), and van Manen (1984). Munhall (2012) calls these men "second-generation phenomenologists" (p. 126). Prior to selecting an approach, you are encouraged to read the primary sources listed in the references. Shorter and Stayt (2010) conducted a phenomenology study according to Heidegger's philosophy. They emphasized the importance of co-creating the data, as follows:

"A key tenet of Heideggerian phenomenology is co-construction of knowledge between researcher and participant, which assumes that both contribute to understanding the topic. Adequate participant contribution to the construction of knowledge was ensured in the present study by providing each participant with an annotated version of their interview transcription, detailing subject themes that had been identified. They were offered the opportunity to clarify meaning and comment on identified themes." (Shorter & Stayt, 2010, p. 161)

Shorter and Stayt (2010) concluded with the following paragraph:

"Confronting death and dying is unavoidable in critical care settings. End-of-life care is therefore an important aspect of critical care nursing. This study has revealed a complex web of predisposing factors and occurrences that can shape both the nature of care for the dying and critical care nurses' subsequent grief experiences." (Shorter & Stayt, 2010, p. 165)

This study was congruent with the Heideggerian philosophy, as evidenced by the validation of the analysis with the participants. From their findings, the researchers indicated several areas needing additional study, such as the informal support structures that allow critical care nurses to deal with patient deaths. The inferred clinical implication is that nurses involved in end-of-life care in acute care settings experience patients' deaths in complex ways and use multiple ways to deal with their grief. Nurses and managers in critical care units need to be aware of the diversity of grief responses and coping methods.

Grounded Theory Methodology

Philosophical discussions of grounded theory methodology center on the nuances of the different approaches (Cooney, 2010). Sociologists Glaser and Strauss (1967) worked together during their early years, but eventually their philosophies resulted in at least two variations of grounded theory. The original works provided little detail on data analysis methods, so Corbin and Strauss (2008) described a structured method of data analysis (Cooney, 2010). In Table 12-6, substantive and theoretical codes are attributed to Glaser, and open, axial, and selective are attributed to Strauss (Cooney, 2010). Researchers considering grounded theory methodology will want to read the primary sources on the different methods and choose the one that is most compatible with the researchers' philosophy. During grounded theory studies, data analysis formally begins with the first interview or focus group. The researchers review the transcript and code each line, constantly comparing the meaning of one line with the meanings in the lines that preceded it. Concepts as abstract representations of processes or entities are named. As the data analysis continues, relationships between concepts are hypothesized and then examined for validity by looking for additional examples within the data (Charmaz, 2014; Wuest, 2012). Researchers look for a core category that explains the underlying social process in the experience. Finally, existing theory and literature are reviewed, for similarities and parallels to the emergent theory and study findings, including the core category. Isakson and Jurkovic (2013) described the knowledge gap that resulted in their grounded theory study of torture survivors.

"The current research fills a gap in the growing literature by developing a theory that better captures the healing process of non-Western torture survivors of various ethnic groups and genders." (Isakson & Jurkovic, 2013, p. 750)

The researchers interviewed 11 torture survivors from Asian and African countries (Isakson & Jurkovic, 2013). Isakson and Jurkovic (2013) discussed their reasons for selecting grounded theory as their method.

"Grounded theory was chosen as the methodology to address this topic because it enabled us to construct a substantive theory regarding the process being studied. Grounded theory also allowed us to develop this theory from the perspective of the survivor, which is essential to begin to help survivors of torture, because the survivors have identified how the process works, what aspects of their lives need to be impacted, and how these aspects are prioritized... A comprehensive theory will help treatment providers and policy makers decide how to best support torture survivors in the healing process." (Isakson & Jurkovic, 2013, p. 751)

Consistent with grounded theory methods, Isakson and Jurkovic (2013) identified the core variable or process that is the social process in the phenomenon of interest.

"The core variable that emerged through the process of data analysis in this study was the torture survivors' relentless determination and struggles to move on, which included aspects of cognitive reframing and empowerment. Participants described a complex process involving invocation of beliefs and values, restoration of safety and stability, and reestablishment of emotional support and sociofamilial connection." (Isakson & Jurkovic, 2013, p. 753)

The study by Isakson and Jurkovic (2013) had its strengths and limitations, as noted by the researchers. Approaching the research problem from the qualitative perspective was identified as a strength, as was the diversity of the participants. Limitations were the need to use interpreters for eight of the interviews and the researchers' training as Western psychologists. Isakson and Jurkovic (2013) proposed that their training may have biased their perspectives of the data and the emerging theory. Despite the limitations, the researchers made a significant contribution to understanding a vulnerable population that needs healthcare support during the transition into a new country.

Ethnographical Methodology

Ethnography is unique among the qualitative approaches because of its cultural focus. Thus, ethnography requires **fieldwork**, which is spending time in the selected culture to learn by being present, observing, and asking questions. Wolf (2012, p. 302) defines fieldwork as a "disciplined mode of inquiry that engages the ethnographer firsthand in data collection over extended periods of time." Fieldwork allows the researcher to participate in a wide range of activities. The observations of the researcher typically focus on objects, communication patterns, and behaviors to understand how values are socially constructed and transmitted (Wolf, 2012). The researcher looks below the surface to identify the shared meaning and values expressed through everyday actions, language, and rituals (Creswell, 2013). Meanings and values may reveal power differences, gender issues, optimism, or views of diversity.

One difficulty in planning an ethnographic study is not knowing in advance how much time will be needed and actually what will be observed. Enough time in the field is needed to achieve some degree of cultural immersion (Patton, 2015; Streubert & Carpenter, 2011). The resources—money and time—that the researcher has allotted for the project usually limit the length of an ethnographic study. When one is studying a different culture, the time might extend to months or even a year. When studying the culture of a nursing unit or waiting area, the researcher will not live on the unit, but would identify a tentative plan for observing on the unit at different times during the day and night and on different days of the week. The researcher may want to observe unit meetings, change-of-shift reports, or other unit rituals, such as holiday meals. Initial acceptance into a culture may lead to resistance later if the researcher's presence extends beyond the community's expectations or the ethnographer is perceived as prying or violating the community's privacy. The researcher needs to blend into the culture but remain in an outsider role. A researcher who over-identifies with the culture being studied and becomes an insider is said to be going native. In **going native**, the researcher becomes a part of the culture and loses all objectivity—and with it the ability to observe clearly (Creswell, 2013). Negotiating relationships and roles is a critical skill for ethnographers, who must possess self-awareness and social acumen.

Ethnographic research allows researchers to be participant observers. Graduate students and other nurse researchers may select ethnography about social cultures and work cultures of which the nurse is a part. If graduate students choose ethnographic research situated in their own social culture or work culture, they must employ reactivity on an ongoing basis, in order to be clear about what ideas belong to the culture and what notions are theirs. One's advisors and mentors can be very useful in clarifying these matters.

Gatekeepers and Informants

Gatekeepers are people who can provide access to the culture, facilitate the collection of data, and increase the legitimacy of the researcher (Creswell, 2013; Wolf, 2012). A gatekeeper may be a formal leader, such as a mayor, village leader, or nurse manager, or an informal leader, such as the head of the women's club, the village midwife, or the nurse who is considered the unit's clinical expert. The support of people who are accepted in the culture is key to gaining the access needed to understand that culture. In addition to gatekeepers, you may seek out other individuals who are willing to interpret the culture for you. These other individuals may be informants, insiders in the community who can provide their perspective on what the researcher has observed (Wolf, 2012). Not only will the informants answer questions, they may help you formulate questions because they understand the culture better than you do.

Gathering and Analyzing Data

During fieldwork, the researcher makes extensive notes about what is observed and thoughts on possible interpretations. The researcher may seek input on possible interpretations with an informant or a person being interviewed. Data analysis consists of analyzing field notes and interviews for common ideas, and allowing patterns to emerge. Data may also be subjected to content analysis. The notes themselves may be superficial. However, during the process of analysis, you will clarify, extend, and interpret those notes. Interview data are compared to observational field notes (Patton, 2015); perspectives of different people within the culture

are compared as well. Abstract thought processes such as intuition and reasoning are involved in analysis. The data are then formed into categories and relationships developed between categories. From these categories and relationships, the ethnographer describes patterns of behavior and supports the patterns with specific examples.

The analysis process in ethnography produces detailed descriptions of cultures. The descriptions may be presented as cultural themes or a cultural inventory (Streubert & Carpenter, 2011). These descriptions may be applied to existing theories of cultures. Although the goal of ethnographic research is not theory, in some cases the findings may lead to the later development of hypotheses, theories, or both. The results may be useful to nurses when members of the community that was described interact with the health system. If the results include generalizations about the culture, those results may be tested by the degree to which another ethnographer, using the findings of the first ethnographical study, can accurately anticipate human behavior in the studied culture.

Martin and Yurkovich (2014) conducted a focused ethnography of Native American Indian (NAI) families. They describe this design and its fit with their study purpose in the following excerpt:

"A qualitative design called focused ethnography was used for this study. This methodology provided the core principles for conducting a valid study about the cultural experiences and processes of a healthy NAI family ... Focused ethnography is a process of inquiry that provides an accurate account of how people organize their cultural existence. It assumes that any cultural group is able to comment on and analyze itself. This method of inquiry fits with the purpose of our study: to define healthy NAI families living in the context of a single reservation by interviewing adult tribal members. Without a discernible definition of a healthy NAI family, health promotion and illness prevention programs may be incongruent with NAI families' perceptions and practices of health." (Martin & Yurkovich, 2014, p. 54)

The researchers collected and analyzed data from numerous sources, as described here:

"Data sources were the transcripts and field notes generated primarily from interviews, participant observation, several windshield surveys, fieldwork, and research team meetings. Also, a focus group consisting of four key informants was carried out for the purposes of sharing, verifying, and refuting the preliminary findings as well as determining cultural congruency. This 'member check' meeting was audiotaped and transcribed verbatim, and its analysis was included in the data analysis to document penultimate findings." (Martin & Yurkovich, 2014, pp. 55–56)

The data were collected during 100 hours of fieldwork with the families on the reservation (Martin & Yurkovich, 2014). The close partnership with the community and incorporation of a cultural liaison ensured accountability to the Native American Indian families that were the subject of the ethnography. The analysis went through several phases to produce descriptions of healthy and unhealthy families.

"After we identified 'a healthy family is close-knit' as the largest domain, we explored the field notes and transcripts for further characteristics that explicated the domain. For example, connectedness, commitment, balance, stability, adaptability, and resourcefulness were other terms used to describe a healthy family." (Martin & Yurkovich, 2014, p. 58)

The researchers affirmed that close-knit was the most pervasive description of healthy families. The religious and cultural ceremonies were identified as one of several protective buffers of families. Martin and Yurkovich (2014) continued by identifying community factors that support healthy families.

"Informants related freely that traditional spiritual practices supported the characteristics of a close-knit, healthy family…Influential community factors affect the buffers that support maintenance of a healthy NAI family. These factors were identified via windshield survey reports, interview transcripts, and researchers' field notes and were validated by the focus group as well as by members at a Tribal Council meeting while sharing the study's findings." (Martin & Yurkovich, 2014, pp. 63–64)

Through the focused ethnography, Martin and Yurkovich (2014) concluded that understanding the tribal views of families allowed service providers to revise how care was delivered and to mobilize community assets.

Exploratory-Descriptive Qualitative Methodology

Researchers often design exploratory-descriptive qualitative studies to address a specific research question and may or may not use a theoretical framework to structure the study design. As mentioned earlier in the chapter, Jones (2015) studied the perspectives of African American women who had breast cancer by interviewing them and their biological mothers.

"A naturalistic inquiry design was the type of qualitative research approach used and 14 African American women were interviewed using a semi-structured interview guide. The data were analyzed using a qualitative content analysis." (Jones, 2015, p. 5)

The data analysis revealed beliefs about breast cancer that included distrust and disrespect.

"The women … reported many incidents by the medical community of receiving degrading and humiliating care. Lack of privacy and embarrassment were major concerns … Two of the women reported that they did not want to take off their clothes in front of the male doctors." (Jones, 2015, p. 6)

Several other themes emerged from the data such as "limited treatment options" and "it's a death sentence" (Jones, 2015, p. 7). The women's vicarious experiences due to the breast cancer of friends and family members had been the primary influence on their beliefs about breast cancer. Jones (2015) concluded the report with practical application to the education of African American women.

"Education about breast cancer must focus … on an exchange of ideas and the richness of the human experience of one living with breast cancer … culturally based testimonies from African American women and their experiences." (Jones, 2015, p. 10)

Historical Research Methodology

The methodology of **historical research** consists of (1) identifying a question or study topic; (2) identifying, inventorying, and evaluating sources; and (3) writing the historical narrative. Whether motivated by curiosity, personal factors, or professional reasons, the researcher's interest in a specific topic needs to be explainable to others (Lundy, 2012). One way to explain is for the researcher to develop a clear, concise statement of the topic. The topic may be narrowed to be manageable with available resources. Although the historical researcher may be interested in the effect of World War

II on nursing science, the researcher may need to narrow the study to one or a few nurse theorists who were nurses during the war or the nurse scientists educated at one university. The statement of the topic may evolve into a title for the study, which includes the period being addressed. Prior to determining the years to be studied, you must have knowledge of the broader social, political, and economic factors that would have an impact on the topic. Using this knowledge, you can identify the questions you will examine during the research process.

Sources

Sources in a historical study may be documents such as books, letters, newspaper clippings, professional journals, and diaries (Lundy, 2012). Sources may also be people who were alive during the time being studied or who heard stories from older relatives. Review the literature that is available on the topic you have selected, and start a bibliography or inventory of materials you want to review. Library searches identify published materials and may maintain some archives pertinent to your topic, such as unpublished materials purchased or donated for their historical value (Streubert & Carpenter, 2011). Pay attention to the organizations and institutions with which the person was affiliated. These organizations and affiliations provide clues to the location of primary sources (Lundy, 2012). **Primary sources** are "firsthand accounts of the person's experience, an institution, or an event and may lack critical analysis" (Streubert & Carpenter, 2011, p. 237). For example, historical researchers interested in Martha Rogers and the effect of World War II on her theory would note that Rogers was the Dean of New York University, increasing the likelihood that the university has documents written by her. In the case of Rogers, however, an Internet search reveals that many of her materials are housed in Boston University's Howard Gotlieb Archival Research Center. Accessing these documents would include obtaining permission to review the documents, traveling to Boston, and making notes about or taking photographs of the documents.

Secondary sources are those written about the time or the people involved, but not by the person of interest. Secondary sources also are examined because they may validate or corroborate primary sources or present additional information or opinions (Lundy, 2012; Streubert & Carpenter, 2011). In fact, validation and corroboration are important for determining whether sources are genuine and authentic. **External criticism** determines the "genuineness of primary sources" (Lundy, 2012, p. 265). The researcher needs to know where, when, why, and by whom a document was written, which may involve verifying the handwriting or determining the age of the paper on which it was written. **Internal criticism** involves establishing the authenticity of the document. The researcher may ask whether the document's content is consistent with what was known at the time the document was written. Are dates, locations, and other details consistent across sources? The researcher is open to the views presented in the documents or other sources, but remains somewhat skeptical until sources are verified.

Historical Data Analysis

Data gathering and analysis occur simultaneously (Streubert & Carpenter, 2011) as the researcher samples documents, seeking descriptions, conflicting records, or contextual details. As with other qualitative approaches, historical researchers become immersed in the data. Content analysis and narrative analysis yield data that the researcher uses to develop a description of the topic. The connections made among documents, opinions, and stories constitute the interpretation of the data that are essential to an unfolding, deep understanding of the topic. Determining when to stop examining sources may be one of the major challenges faced by historical researchers. Like grounded theory researchers, who stop interviewing participants when redundancy in the data is confirmed, historical researchers decide to stop gathering data when new data are no longer being found. The researcher may return to data gathering if gaps or questions emerge as the findings are being written.

Writing the Historical Narrative

The historical researcher keeps extensive records of the source of each fact, event, and story that is extracted. The extracted data may be organized as a chronology or attached to an outline. The chronology or outline will become the skeleton of the narrative that will be written. The historical narrative may take the form of a case study, a rich narrative, or a biography. The links made by the historical researcher from the past to the present give historical research its significance to nursing (Lundy, 2012).

DeGuzman, Schminkey, and Koyen (2014) conducted a historical study of women's health services in a Detroit neighborhood in the 1960s. A nurse who had come from the neighborhood, Nancy Milio, established a clinic to provide family planning and prenatal services. The primary figure and the context are stated early in the paper, along with the purpose and method.

"... Nancy Milio, a young public health nurse, established the *Mom and Tots Center*, a community-based center housing a prenatal and family planning clinic ... during the tumultuous civil rights era ... The purpose of this article is to describe and analyze Milio's role in the provision of women's health services in this at-risk, inner city population in the context of the social and political environment of the 1960s, using historical research methods." (DeGuzman et al., 2014, pp.199–200)

DeGuzman et al. (2014) described the primary sources that were used in this historical study. The researchers used a variety of sources to construct a multifaceted description of Nurse Milio's accomplishments, such as "the Nancy Milio Papers housed at the Center for Nursing Historical Inquiry at the University of Virginia," newspaper articles, and a book that Milio wrote about her experiences (DeGuzman et al., 2014, p. 200).

At the time, public health nursing had shifted to a professionalism model that elevated the nurse above the community. In contrast, DeGuzman et al. (2014) recognized the strengths of the community, despite the unrest that characterized that era. They also noted that the availability of birth control pills allowed women a more reasonable option for contraception.

"The Feminist Movement was concurrent with ... the Civil Rights and Antiwar Movements ... The first commercially available oral contraceptive pill (referred to as *the pill*) was approved by the Food and Drug Administration ... marking a significant change in the delivery of women's health care...." (DeGuzman et al., 2014, p. 204)

Into this place, at this time, came Nancy Milio, who knew the neighborhood from her childhood and also had learned much more about it while working in the community as a visiting nurse. Her appreciation and connection with the community prompted a new approach to prenatal care, named by the women in the community as the Neighborhood-Oriented Approach. The women received all clinic visits at the Mom and Tots Center after the initial visit at the hospital (DeGuzman et al., 2014).

DeGuzman et al. (2014) indicated how the social environment and Milio's history in the community converged to support her approach to care.

"Milio's genuine respect for ... the Kerchevel Street community women may have been directly related to the social reform ... during the 1960s ... Nancy ... encouraged and authorized them to dictate their vision of how their health care should be provided." (DeGuzman et al., 2014, pp. 208–209)

DeGuzman et al. (2014) explicitly stated the application of Nancy Milio's work to the health disparities that continue today. They advocate for using her grass roots approach to provide culturally acceptable care in the United States and other countries.

DeGuzman et al. (2014) conducted a rigorous historical study with extensive use of government documents, newspapers, peer-reviewed articles, and Nancy Milio's personal and professional papers. One of the reasons her work is well known is that Milio published 12 books and two articles, one in the *American Journal of Nursing* and the other in the *American Journal of Public Health*. The most famous of her publications is *9226 Kercheval: The Storefront That Did Not Burn* (Milio, 1970). Historical research requires a combination of attention to detail and the ability to tell a persuasive story.

▮ KEY POINTS

- Qualitative methods are more flexible than quantitative methods to ensure the process of discovery and that, within the story, the participant's voice is heard.
- Qualitative data collection and data analysis occur simultaneously in some methods.
- Researchers and participants in qualitative studies work together to generate the findings specific to the research question.
- Qualitative methods of data collection include observation, interviews, focus groups, images, and electronically mediated communication.
- Recordings and notes are transcribed into data files prior to analysis.
- Qualitative researchers select coding and analysis strategies consistent with the philosophical approach of their studies.
- Data analysis begins by immersing oneself in the data and coding the transcripts, field notes, and other data.
- Coding is identifying key ideas and phrases in the data. As analysis continues, the codes may be merged into themes, incorporated into a narrative, or organized into a taxonomy.
- Qualitative findings are not generalized: they are used to inform the reader and inspire thoughts and actions leading to improvements in care.
- Phenomenological methods may include bracketing and interviewing to elicit rich descriptions of lived experiences.
- Methods specific to grounded theory studies are coding, describing concepts, and identifying links

between the concepts for the purpose of developing a theory.

- Ethnographic methods are characterized by extensive fieldwork that includes observations and interviews for the purpose of describing aspects of the culture being studied.
- Exploratory-descriptive qualitative studies may use a theoretical perspective relevant to the research topic as an organizing structure for data analysis.
- Historical researchers extract the meaning from primary and secondary source documents to describe and analyze the context and chronology of past events, often in the light of what is known at the present time. This perspective gives historical research its own particular flavor.
- Rigorous qualitative researchers are reflexive, a characteristic that requires the ability to be aware of nuances of the research situation and one's own biases.

REFERENCES

Alexis, O. (2012). Internationally educated nurses' experiences in a hospital in England: An exploratory design. *Scandinavian Journal of Caring Sciences, 27*(4), 962–968.

Banner, D. (2010). Qualitative interviewing: Preparation for practice. *Canadian Journal of Cardiovascular Nursing, 20*(2), 27–30.

Broome, S., Lutz, B., & Cook, C. (2015). Becoming the parent of a child with life-threatening food allergies. *Journal of Pediatric Nursing, 30*(4), 532–542.

Bugel, M. (2014). Experiences of school-age siblings of children with a traumatic injury: Changes, constants, and needs. *Pediatric Nursing, 40*(4), 179–186.

Bury, M. (1982). Chronic illness as biographical disruption. *Sociology of Health & Illness, 4*(2), 167–182.

Charmaz, K. (2014). *Constructing grounded theory* (2nd ed.). Los Angeles, CA: Sage.

Clissett, P., Porock, D., Harwood, R., & Gladman, J. (2013). The challenges of achieving person-centred care in acute hospitals: A qualitative study of people with dementias and their families. *International Journal of Nursing Studies, 50*(11), 1495–1503.

Colaizzi, P. (1978). Psychological research as the phenomenologist views it. In R. S. Valle & M. King (Eds.), *Existential phenomenological alternatives for psychology* (pp. 48–71). New York, NY: Oxford University Press.

Cooney, A. (2010). Choosing between Glaser and Strauss: An example. *Nurse Researcher, 77*(4), 18–28.

Corbin, J., & Strauss, A. (2008). *Basics of qualitative research: Techniques and procedures for developing grounded theory* (3rd ed.). Thousand Oaks, CA: Sage.

Corbin, J., & Strauss, A. (2015). *Basics of qualitative research: Techniques and procedures for developing grounded theory* (4th ed.). Thousand Oaks, CA: Sage.

Coty, M.-B., McCammon, C., Lehna, C., Twyman, S., & Fahey, E. (2015). Home fire safety beliefs and practices in homes of urban older adults. *Geriatric Nursing, 36*(3), 177–181.

Creswell, J. W. (2013). *Qualitative inquiry and research design: Choosing among five approaches* (3rd ed.). Thousand Oaks, CA: Sage.

DeGuzman, P., Schminkey, D., & Koyen, E. (2014). "Civil unrest does not stop ovulation:" Women's prenatal and family planning services in a 1960s Detroit neighborhood clinic. *Journal of Family and Community Health, 37*(3), 199–211.

Dowling, M. (2007). From Husserl to van Manen: A review of different phenomenological approaches. *International Journal of Nursing Studies, 44*(1), 131–142.

Duffy, M. (2012). Narrative inquiry: The method. In P. L. Munhall (Ed.), *Nursing research: A qualitative perspective* (5th ed., pp. 421–440). Sudbury, MA: Jones & Bartlett.

Eschiti, V., Lauderdale, J., Burhansstipanov, L., Weryackwe-Sanford, S., Weryackwe, L., & Flores, Y. (2014). Developing cancer-related educational content and goals tailored to the Comanche Nation. *Clinical Journal of Oncology Nursing, 18*(2), E26–E31.

Fawcett, J., & Garity, J. (2009). *Evaluating research for evidence-based nursing practice.* Philadelphia, PA: F. A. Davis.

Findholt, N. E., Michael, Y. L., & Davis, M. M. (2011). Photovoice engages rural youth in childhood obesity prevention. *Public Health Nursing, 28*(2), 186–192.

Follan, M., & McNamara, M. (2013). A fragile bond: Adoptive parents' experiences caring for children with a diagnosis of reactive attachment disorder. *Journal of Clinical Nursing, 23*(7–8), 1076–1085.

Giorgi, A. (1970). *Psychology as a human science: A phenomenologically based approach.* New York, NY: Harper & Row.

Given, L. (Ed.), (2008). *The Sage encyclopedia of qualitative research methods: Volume 1.* Thousand Oaks, CA: Sage.

Gladman, J., Harwood, R., Jones, R., Porock, D., Griffiths, A., Schneider, J., et al. (2012a). *Medical and mental health/ Better mental health development study protocol.* Retrieved March 26, 2016 from https://www.nottingham.ac.uk/mcop/documents/papers/issue10-mcop-issn2044-4230.pdf.

Gladman, J., Porock, D., Griffiths, A., Clissett, P., Harwood, R., Knight, A., et al. (2012b). *Care of older people with cognitive impairment in general hospitals.* SDO funded project. Retrieved March 26, 2016 from http://www.netscc.ac.uk/hsdr/files/project/SDO_FR_08-1809-227_V01.pdf.

Glaser, B. G., & Strauss, A. (1967). *The discovery of grounded theory: Strategies for qualitative research.* Chicago, IL: Aldine.

Gray, J. (2009). Rooms, recording, and responsibilities: The logistics of focus groups. *Southern Online Journal of Nursing Research, 9*(1), Article 5. Retrieved March 26, 2016 from http://www.resourcenter.net/images/snrs/files/sojnr_articles2/Vol09Num01Art05.html.

Hatfield, L., & Pearce, M. (2014). Factors influencing parents' decision to donate their healthy infant's DNA for minimal-risk genetic research. *Journal of Nursing Scholarship, 46*(6), 398–407.

Heidegger, M. (1962). *Being and time.* (J. Macquarrie & E. Robinson, Trans). New York, NY: Harper Perennial Modern Thought.

Hoover, R. S., & Koerber, A. L. (2011). Using NVivo to answer the challenges of qualitative research in professional communication: Benefits and best practices. *IEEE Transactions on Professional Communication, 54*(1), 68–82.

Howie, L. (2013). Narrative enquiry and health research. In P. Liamputtong (Ed.), *Research methods in health: Foundations for evidence-based practice* (2nd ed., pp. 72–84). South Melbourne, Australia: Oxford University Press.

Hyatt, K., Davis, L., & Barroso, J. (2014). Chasing the care: Soldiers experience following combat-related mild traumatic brain injury. *Military Medicine, 179*(8), 849–855.

Im, E.-O., Chee, W., Lim, H.-J., Liu, Y., & Kim, H. K. (2008). Midlife women's attitudes toward physical activity. *Journal of Obstetric, Gynecologic, and Neonatal Nursing, 37*(2), 203–213.

Im, E.-O., Ko, Y., Hwang, H., Chee, W., Stuifbergen, A., Lee, H., et al. (2012). Asian American midlife women's attitudes toward physical activity. *Journal of Gynecological and Neonatal Nursing, 41*(5), 650–658.

Im, E.-O., Ko, Y., Hwang, H., Chee, W., Stuifbergen, A., Walker, L., et al. (2013). Racial/ethnic differences in midlife women's attitudes toward physical activity. *Journal of Midwifery & Women's Health, 58*(4), 440–450.

Im, E.-O., Lee, B., & Chee, W. (2010). Shielded from the real world: Perspectives on Internet cancer support groups by Asian Americans. *Cancer Nursing, 33*(3), E10–E20.

Im, E.-O., Lee, S.-H., & Chee, W. (2010). Black women in menopausal transition. *Journal of Gynecological and Neonatal Nursing, 39*(4), 435–443.

Im, E.-O., Lee, B., Chee, W., Domire, S., & Brown, A. (2010). A national multiethnic online forum study on menopausal symptom experience. *Nursing Research, 59*(1), 26–33.

Im, E.-O., Lee, B., Chee, W., Stuifbergen, A., & the eMAPA Research Team. (2011). Attitudes toward physical activity of white midlife women. *Journal of Obstetric, Gynecologic, and Neonatal Nursing, 40*(3), 312–321.

Im, E.-O., Lee, S. H., Liu, Y., Lim, H.-J., Guevara, E., & Chee, W. (2009). A national online forum on ethnic differences in cancer pain experiences. *Nursing Research, 58*(2), 86–91.

Im, E.-O., Lim, H.-J., Lee, S., Dormire, S., Chee, W., & Kresta, K. (2009). Menopausal symptom experience of Hispanic midlife women in the United States. *Health Care for Women International, 30*(10), 919–934.

Isakson, B., & Jurkovic, G. (2013). Healing after torture: The role of moving on. *Qualitative Health Research, 23*(6), 749–761.

Jessee, M., & Mion, L. (2013). Is evidence guiding practice? Reported versus observed adherence to contact precautions. *American Journal of Infection Control, 41*(11), 965–970.

Jirwe, M. (2011). Analysing qualitative data. *Nurse Researcher, 18*(3), 4–5.

Jones, D. (2015). Knowledge, beliefs, and feelings about breast cancer: The perspective of African American women. *ABNF Journal, 26*(1), 5–10.

Klinke, M., Hafsteinsdóttir, T., Thorsteinsson, B., & Jónsdóttir, H. (2013). Living at home with eating difficulties following stroke: A phenomenological study of younger people's experiences. *Journal of Clinical Nursing, 23*(1/2), 250–260.

Koh, R., Park, T., & Wickens, C. (2014). An investigation of differing levels of experience and indices of task management in relation to scrub nurses' performance in the operating theatre: Analysis of video-taped caesarean section surgeries. *International Journal of Nursing Studies, 51*(9), 1230–1240.

Krueger, R., & Casey, M. (2015). *Focus group: A practical guide for applied research* (5th ed.). Los Angeles, CA: Sage.

Lem, A., & Schwartz, M. (2014). African American heart failure patients' perspectives on palliative care in the outpatient setting. *Journal of Hospice & Palliative Nursing, 16*(8).

Liamputtong, P. (2013a). *Qualitative research methods* (4th ed.). Victoria, Australia: Oxford University Press.

Liamputtong, P. (2013b). *Research methods in health: Foundations for evidence-based practice* (2nd ed.). South Melbourne, Australia: Oxford University Press.

Lincoln, Y., & Guba, E. (1985). *Naturalistic inquiry.* Newbury Park, CA: Sage.

Logsdon, M., Martin, V., Stikes, R., Davis, D., Ryan, L., Yang, I., et al. (2015). Lessons learned from adolescent mothers: Advice on recruitment. *Journal of Nursing Scholarship, 47*(4), 294–299.

Lundy, K. S. (2012). Historical research. In P. L. Munhall (Ed.), *Nursing research: A qualitative perspective* (5th ed., pp. 381–397). Sudbury, MA: Jones & Bartlett.

Marck, P., Molzahn, A., Berry-Hauf, R., Hutchings, L., & Hughes, S. (2014). Exploring safety and quality in a hemodialysis environment with participatory photographic methods: A restorative approach. *Nephrology Nursing Journal, 41*(1), 25–35.

Markle, G., Attell, B., & Treiber, L. (2015). Dual, yet dueling illnesses: Multiple chronic illness experience at midlife. *Qualitative Health Research, 25*(9), 1271–1282.

Marshall, C., & Rossman, G. B. (2016). *Designing qualitative research* (6th ed.). Los Angeles, CA: Sage.

Martin, D., & Yurkovich, E. (2014). "Close knit" defines a healthy Native American Indian family. *Journal of Family Nursing, 20*(1), 51–72.

Maxwell, J. (2013). *Qualitative research design: An interactive design* (3rd ed.).

Mayer, D., Rosenfeld, A., & Gilbert, K. (2013). Lives forever changed: Family bereavement experiences after sudden cardiac death. *Applied Nursing Research, 26*(4), 168–173.

Mazanec, P., Daly, B., Ferrell, B., & Prince-Paul, M. (2011). Lack of communication and control: Experiences distance caregivers of parents with advanced cancer. *Oncology Nursing Forum, 38*(3), 307–313.

Milio, N. (1970). *9226 Kercheval: The storefront that did not burn.* Ann Arbor, MI: University of Michigan Press.

Miles, M., Huberman, A., & Saldaña, J. (2014). *Qualitative data analysis: A methods sourcebook* (3rd ed.). Los Angeles, CA: Sage.

Mixer, S., Fornehed, M., Varney, J., & Lindley, L. (2014). Culturally-congruent end-of-life care for rural Appalachian people and their families. *Journal of Hospice & Palliative Nursing, 16*(8), 526–535.

Morse, J. M. (Ed.), (1993). *Critical issues in qualitative research methods.* Thousand Oaks, CA: Sage.

Munhall, P. L. (2012). *Nursing research: A qualitative perspective* (5th ed.). Sudbury, MA: Jones & Bartlett.

Nikander, P. (2008). Working with transcripts and translated data. *Qualitative Research in Psychology, 5*(3), 225–231.

Patton, M. (2015). *Qualitative research & evaluation methods* (4th ed.). Thousand Oaks, CA: Sage.

QRS International Pty Ltd (2008). *NVivo (Version 8)*. Doncaster, Australia: Author.

Ramirez, J., & Badger, T. (2014). Men navigating inward and outward through depression. *Archives of Psychiatric Nursing, 28*(1), 21–28.

Riessman, C. K. (2008). *Narrative methods for the human sciences.* Thousand Oaks, CA: Sage.

Rubin, H., & Rubin, I. (2012). *Qualitative interviewing: The art of hearing data* (3rd ed.). Los Angeles, CA: Sage.

Sandelowski, M. (1986). The problem of rigor in qualitative research. *Advances in Nursing Science, 8*(3), 27–37.

Schiminkey, D., & Keeling, A. (2015). Frontier nurse-midwives and antepartum emergencies. *Journal of Midwifery & Women's Health, 60*(1), 48–55.

Scott, D., Sharpe, H., O'Leary, K., Dehaeck, U., Hindmarsh, K., Moore, J. G., et al. (2009). Court reporters: A viable solution for the challenges of focus group data collection? *Qualitative Health Research, 19*(1), 140–146.

Seidman, I. (2013). *Interviewing as qualitative research: A guide for researchers in education and the social sciences* (4th ed.). New York City, NY: Teachers College Press.

Shorter, M., & Stayt, L. C. (2010). Critical care nurses' experiences of grief in an adult intensive care unit. *Journal of Advanced Nursing, 66*(1), 159–167.

Stewart, R., Umar, E., Gleadow-Ware, S., Creed, F., & Bristow, K. (2015). Perinatal distress and depression in Malawi: An exploratory qualitative study of stressors, supports and symptoms. *Archives of Women's Mental Health, 18*(2), 177–185.

Strauss, A., & Corbin, J. (1990). *Basics of qualitative research: Grounded theory procedures and techniques.* London: Sage.

Strauss, A., & Glaser, B. (1975). *Chronic illness and the quality of life.* St. Louis, MO: C.V. Mosby.

Streubert, H., & Carpenter, D. (2011). *Qualitative research in nursing: Advancing the humanistic imperative* (5th ed.).

Philadelphia, PA: Wolters Kluwer/Lippincott Williams & Wilkins.

Tracy, S. (2013). *Qualitative research methods: Collecting evidence, crafting analysis, communicating impact.* Malden, MA: Wiley Blackwell.

Turk, M., Fapohunda, A., & Zoucha, R. (2015). Using photovoice to explore Nigerian immigrants' eating and physical activity in the United States. *Journal of Nursing Scholarship, 47*(1), 16–24.

van Kaam, A. (1966). *Existential foundations of psychology.* Pittsburgh, PA: Duquesne University Press.

van Manen, M. (1984). *"Doing" phenomenological research and writing.* Alberta, Canada: University of Alberta Press.

van Manen, M. (1990). *Researching lived experience: Human science for an action sensitive pedagogy.* London, Ontario, Canada: The State University of New York.

Wang, C., & Burris, M. (1994). Empowerment through photo novella: Portraits of participation. *Health Participation & Behavior, 21*(2), 171–186.

Whitehead, L. C. (2007). Methodological and ethical issues in Internet-mediated research in the field of health: An integrated review of the literature. *Social Science & Medicine, 65*(4), 782–791.

Widger, K., Tourangeau, A., Steele, R., & Streiner, D. (2015). Initial development and psychometric testing of an instrument to measure the quality of children's end-of-life care. *BMC Palliative Care, 14*, Article 1. Retrieved March 26, 2016 from http://www.biomedcentral.com/1472-684X/14/1.

Wolf, Z. E. (2012). Ethnography: The method. In P. L. Munhall (Ed.), *Nursing research: A qualitative perspective* (5th ed., pp. 285–338). Sudbury, MA: Jones & Bartlett.

Wuest, J. (2012). Grounded theory: The method. In P. L. Munhall (Ed.), *Nursing research: A qualitative perspective* (5th ed., pp. 225–256). Sudbury, MA: Jones & Bartlett.

Yan, X., Lu, J., Shi, S., Wang, X., Zhao, R., Yan, Y., et al. (2015). Development and psychometric testing of the Chinese Postnatal Risk Factors Questionnaire (CPRFQ) for postpartum depression. *Archives of Women's Mental Health, 18*(2), 229–237.

Outcomes Research

Suzanne Sutherland

http://evolve.elsevier.com/Gray/practice/

Outcomes research is globally defined as research that investigates the outcomes of care, relating them to attributes of care delivery. It is now an established focus within health care. Its research setting may be an individual physician's practice, an agency providing direct care, or the community as a whole. Its research sample is an accessible population, small or large. Its research methodology is overwhelmingly quantitative, and its designs include a variety of established strategies that establish prevalence, investigate correlates of various outcomes, and occasionally test strategies to change outcomes. Correlational designs predominate. Although from time to time outcomes research employs qualitative strategies within mixed methods studies, the qualitative findings are subordinate in importance to the quantitative, serving to explain the latter's results and sometimes to suggest ensuing quantitative investigation.

The bulk of the data for outcomes research is obtained from preexistent sources such as clinical and administrative databases, and analyzed in the aggregate, and its application level is to an undefined future population of clients within hospitals, communities, caseloads or practices, rather than to specific clients. Its typical research questions address outcomes in terms of practice patterns, attributes of clients, attributes of caregivers, health, efficiency, economics, geography, and other aspects of care delivery. Within nursing, changes based on findings are not implemented without further testing but, rather, scrutinized again in subsequent outcomes studies. The outcomes research process is, optimally, a series of loops, centering on the elusive goal of the best possible outcomes.

The roots of outcomes research have existed informally as long as health care has existed, and persons delivering health care have been curious enough to count, to measure, and to hypothesize. More formal inquiry began in the 19th and 20th centuries. In nursing, Florence Nightingale conducted descriptive longitudinal and trend research in Crimea in the 19th century, documenting morbidity and mortality among the soldiers. She later utilized the data and analyses to argue successfully for reforms in hospitals and hospital barracks, which proved effective in decreasing morbidity and mortality in those settings (Kopf, 1916). Within medicine, in 1910 the Carnegie Foundation chose Flexner (2002) to conduct an evaluation study of the quality of United States (U.S.) medical schools. The report made recommendations for medical school control of hospitals in which teaching occurred, use of full-time faculty who did not maintain a separate practice, and increased education for physicians prior to medical school. Better academic and hospital-based preparation for physicians ensued, with better patient outcomes.

Avedis Donabedian developed the theoretical basis for outcomes research, including its core components and primary elements, 60 years ago (Donabedian, 1980). Concepts foundational to outcomes research overlap those that underlie professional accountability, quality of life, intervention research, prevention, competence, patient satisfaction, self-determination, cost effectiveness, and evidence-based practice (EBP).

This chapter presents the current status of outcomes research, its theoretical basis, its three primary elements, current federal agencies involved in outcomes research, its relationship to practice, and the research designs and statistical approaches it most commonly uses.

CURRENT STATUS OF OUTCOMES RESEARCH

Researchers conducting outcomes studies do not always state, "This is outcomes research." Although many studies that can be considered outcomes research do not contain the word outcomes in their titles, most of these can be accessed using the word outcomes as a search term.

Although most outcomes studies represent isolated research projects, several authors are notable for their sustained research trajectories on various topics focusing on patients and nurse outcomes in hospitals and subacute settings. Linda Aiken and Douglas Sloane have coauthored dozens of outcomes research publications (Aiken et al., 2012; Kutney-Lee et al., 2009; Lasater, Sloane, & Aiken, 2015) over the past decade on the topic of patient outcomes, including investigations of associations between patient mortality rates and nurse characteristics. Their geographical focus has been primarily within the U.S., but they have collaborated with authors from 12 European countries, China, and South Korea over the past few years, extending their findings.

In Belgium, Koen Van den Heede has conducted many outcomes research studies (Bruyneel et al., 2013; Li et al., 2013; Van den Heede et al., 2009a), some in collaboration with Aiken, examining hospital mortality rates, staffing ratios, nurse burnout, and readmissions. Ann Tourangeau in Toronto, Canada, has conducted many outcomes research studies (Carter & Tourangeau, 2012; Tourangeau et al., 2014; Tourangeau, Widger, Cranley, Bookey-Bassett, & Pachis, 2009) on the topics of nurse and faculty retention, and nurse staffing mix.

The uptrend in outcomes publications has continued within the current climate of EBP. The momentum propelling outcomes research arises from healthcare workers themselves, policymakers, public agencies, and the public. On a more tangible level, insurers and individual healthcare agencies add impetus because of heightened competition for the healthcare dollar, as well as do changes in Medicare reimbursement (Centers for Medicare and Medicaid Services (CMS), 2015). The CMS require healthcare agencies to maintain outcome data, with the intent of reimbursing only for care that did not result in negative outcomes such as hospital-acquired infections and decubitus ulcers. Whatever the cause, everyone is invested in better outcomes.

THEORETICAL BASIS OF OUTCOMES RESEARCH

Avedis Donabedian was a physician, born in Beirut and educated there at the American University, where he completed medical school in 1944. He then completed a postgraduate fellowship at University of London in pediatrics and public health. He was a university physician at the American University and taught there, as well, until migrating to America in 1953 and receiving his master's degree in public health from Harvard University in 1955. He taught at Harvard, New York Medical College, and University of Michigan, the latter for over 30 years (Frenk, 2000).

Donabedian developed a theory, often called the Donabedian paradigm. It focuses on how to assess the quality of health care by examining its structures, processes, and outcomes, each component of which is multifaceted (2003). He envisioned structure as preceding processes and processes as preceding outcomes (Figure 13-1).

As structures, Donabedian (2003) listed essential equipment of care and qualified healthcare personnel. The processes he identified included expert execution of technical care, "an empathetic, participatory patient-practitioner interaction, prompt institution of care, active patient participation in the process," and standards of care (p. 50). Outcomes were defined as improvement in health and satisfied clients, and described in Donabedian's (1980, 1987, 2003, 2005) various publications as clinical endpoints, satisfaction with care, and general well-being. He theorized that the dimensions of health are defined by the subjects of care, not by the providers of care, and are based on "what consumers expect, want, or are willing to accept" (Donabedian, 1987, p. 5).

Donabedian's definition of quality of care was that it was "the balance of health benefits and harm" (1980,

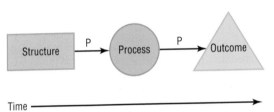

FIGURE 13-1 *P*, precedes. Donabedian's theory of quality. (Adapted from Donabedian, A. [2003]. *An introduction to quality assurance in health care*. Oxford, UK: Oxford University Press.)

BOX 13-1   The Seven Pillars of Quality

"Seven attributes of health care define its [health care] quality: (1) efficacy: the ability of care, at its best, to improve health; (2) effectiveness: the degree to which attainable health improvements are realized; (3) efficiency: the ability to obtain the greatest health improvement at the lowest cost; (4) optimality: the most advantageous balancing of costs and benefits; (5) acceptability: conformity to patient preferences regarding accessibility, the patient-practitioner relation, the amenities, the effects of care, and the cost of care; (6) legitimacy: conformity to social preferences concerning all of the above; and (7) equity: fairness in the distribution of care and its effects on health. Consequently, healthcare professionals must take into account patient preferences as well as social preferences in assessing and assuring quality. When the two sets of preference disagree the physician faces the challenge of reconciling them."

Reprinted from Donabedian, A. (1990). The seven pillars of quality. *Archives of Pathology and Laboratory Medicine,* *114*(11), 1115–1118, with permission from *Archives of Pathology and Laboratory Medicine.* Copyright 1990. College of American Pathologists.

p. 27), and that there were many attributes of health care that contributed to quality (Box 13-1).

Underlying Donabedian's theory are a sense of fairness and honesty; firm linkage of cause and effect; placing the responsibility for a deficit in structures, processes, or outcomes where it truly belongs; commitment to openly studying healthcare quality and making findings known; and personal accountability. After lifelong pursuit of quality in health care, and his background in epidemiology and systems design, he still maintained that "to love your profession" was essential to the delivery of high-quality care (Mullan, 2001, p. 140)

Donabedian (1980) presented what he called a "schematic representation of a framework for identifying scope and level of concern as factors in defining the quality of medical care" (p. 17). This appears as Figure 13-2. This cubic diagram is *not* a conceptual map of Donabedian's theory or an explanation of the elements of quality. It is, rather, a graphic demonstration of the interactions among human functional levels, care provider levels, and size of consumer network, displaying their interactive breadth and depth. The human functional levels represented are the physical, psychological, and social. Provider levels range from individual through systems. Recipients of care range from the individual

through the target population. Essentially, the schematic means that there are several levels of each entity, and that analysis can reflect any combination. It is multiplicative: there are 48 possible levels of analysis in the $4 \times 4 \times 3$ cube.

Donabedian's initial work focused on the quality of the physician's practice, using data gained through evaluation of a surgeon's technique and judgment of its outcomes revealed by records review, observations, documented behaviors, and opinions (Donabedian, 2005). However, his expanded focus also included care that patients receive within healthcare agencies and contributing factors that are external to the physician's control.

Patterns of Data Collection

Early in his work, Donabedian stressed the importance of periodic review of data and of paying attention to patterns within the data set (1980). He described this as a continuous loop using the review process, which later evolved into continuous quality improvement (CQI). This type of periodic review presupposes that agencies, provider groups, and individual providers are motivated to seek CQI, which is now a mainstay of practice in many hospitals. On the practical level, Donabedian encouraged measurement of short-term goals when long-term goals were years in the future, using tracking strategies like critical pathways and care maps to determine proximate outcomes.

Attribution

Donabedian also emphasized that in the process of evaluation, outcomes must be linked with their true causes, which in medicine is especially challenging because so many health-illness problems are multifactorial. For this reason, a healthcare system may not be able to attribute causation to the agency or to the physician unilaterally in all instances in which the patient's condition worsens or new morbidity arises (Donabedian, 1980). Clearly, his public health education had broadened Donabedian's view to include the patient, the environment, cultural systems, social conventions, employers, the government, and even insurers as various causes of illness and death.

Figure 13-3 depicts the typical interplay among structures, processes, and outcomes, supporting the difficulty of attributing definitive cause to any given outcome. Structures of care may have a direct impact on outcomes and also may foster certain processes that impact those same outcomes, for a synergistic effect. It is the usual pattern that many different structures and processes affect one outcome, to a greater or lesser degree, because they are so very interrelated.

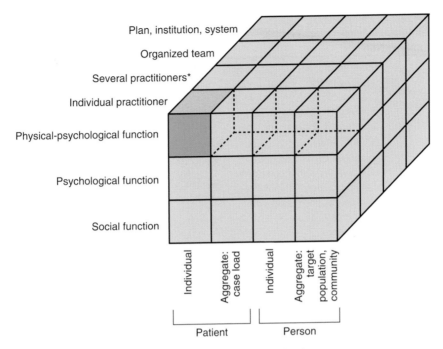

FIGURE 13-2 Levels of complexity for provider, recipient of care, and aspect of health.

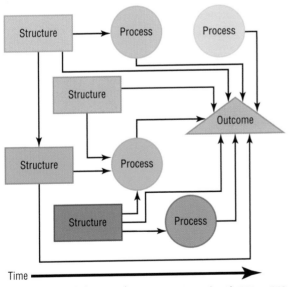

FIGURE 13-3 Interactions among structures, processes, and outcomes.

STRUCTURE AND PROCESS VERSUS OUTCOME IN TODAY'S HEALTHCARE AND OUTCOMES RESEARCH

Structures have come to be viewed in an expanded way, over the years, because it has been found that many do make a difference in outcomes. Recent research focusing on the association between outcomes and various structural elements has included not only the essential equipment of care and qualified healthcare personnel but also educational preparation / skill mix of healthcare workers (Kutney-Lee, Sloane, & Aiken, 2013; Trinkoff et al., 2013), care protocols (Asher et al., 2015; Hirashima et al., 2012), staffing (Brennan, Daly, & Jones, 2013), and size of the workforce (West et al., 2014), among many other topics. Table 13-1 lists 25 recent studies investigating outcomes in relation to various structures of care.

Processes address the actual care delivered by healthcare persons both in a technical sense, as reflected by standards of care and individual performance, and in relation to interactions with patients. Although technical care is measurable, patient-practitioner interactions are more difficult to evaluate. Processes also address the promptness with which care is instituted, as well as patient inclusion in decision making and choices.

TABLE 13-1	Recent Outcomes Research Focusing Primarily on Structures of Care		
Researcher (Year)	**Title**	**Outcomes**	**Structures**
Aiken et al. (2012)	Patient safety, satisfaction, and quality of hospital care: Cross-sectional surveys of nurses and patients in 12 countries in Europe and the United States	Patient safety, satisfaction, and quality of hospital care	Nurse staffing and work environment
Asher et al. (2015)	Clinical outcomes and cost effectiveness of accelerated diagnostic protocol in a chest pain center compared with routine care of patients with chest pain	Clinical outcomes and cost effectiveness	Accelerated diagnostic protocol in a chest pain center
Baoyue et al. (2013)	Group-level impact of work environment dimensions on burnout experiences among nurses: A multivariate multilevel probit model	Burnout experiences among nurses	Work environment dimensions
Bednarczyk, Curran, Orenstein, & Omer (2014)	Health disparities in human papillomavirus vaccine coverage: Trends analysis from the National Immunization Survey-Teen, 2008–2011	HPV vaccine coverage	Race, poverty level
Brennan, Daly, & Jones (2013)	State of the science: The relationship between nurse staffing and patient outcomes	Patient outcomes	Nurse staffing
Carter & Tourangeau (2012)	Staying in nursing: What factors determine whether nurses intend to remain employed	Staying in nursing	Factors that determine whether nurses intend to remain employed
Chen, Lin, Ho, Chen, & Kao (2015)	Risk of coronary artery disease in transfusion-naive thalassemia populations: A nationwide population-based retrospective cohort study	Coronary artery disease	Carrier state thalassemia
Fenton, Jerant, Bertakis, & Franks (2012)	The cost of satisfaction: A national study of patient satisfaction, healthcare utilization, expenditures, and mortality	Expenditures, healthcare utilization, mortality, patient satisfaction	
Hirashima et al. (2012)	Use of a postoperative insulin protocol decreases wound infection in diabetics undergoing lower extremity bypass	Wound infection in diabetics after lower extremity bypass	Postoperative insulin protocol

TABLE 13-1   Recent Outcomes Research Focusing Primarily on Structures of Care—cont'd

Researcher (Year)	Title	Outcomes	Structures
Kutney-Lee, Sloane, & Aiken, 2013	An increase in the number of nurses with baccalaureate degrees is linked to lower rates of postsurgery mortality	Postsurgery mortality	The number of nurses with baccalaureate degrees
Lasater, Sloane, & Aiken (2015)	Hospital employment of supplemental registered nurses and patients' satisfaction with care	Patient satisfaction with care	Hospital employment of supplemental registered nurses
Li et al. (2013)	Group-level impact of work environment dimensions on burnout experiences among nurses: A multivariate multilevel probit model	Burnout experiences among nurses	Work environment dimensions
Palacios et al. (2014)	A prospective analysis of airborne metal exposures and risk of Parkinson disease in the Nurses' Health Study cohort	Parkinson disease	Airborne metal exposure
Pape (2013)	The effect of a five-part intervention to decrease omitted medications	Omitted medications	Designated quiet zone for medication preparation
Pyenson, Sander, Jiang, Kahn, & Mulshine (2012)	An actuarial analysis shows that offering lung cancer screening as an insurance benefit would save lives at relatively low cost	Projected lives saved	Lung cancer screening by tomography as an insurance benefit
Ramis et al. (2012)	Analysis of matched geographical areas to study potential links between environmental exposure to oil refineries and non-Hodgkin lymphoma mortality in Spain	Mortality due to non-Hodgkin lymphoma	Exposure to oil refineries
Reistetter et al. (2015)	Geographical and facility variation in inpatient stroke rehabilitation: Multilevel analysis of functional status	Quality of inpatient stroke rehabilitation	Geographical location, facility variation
Tourangeau, Widger, Cranley, Bookey-Bassett, & Pachis (2009)	Work environments and staff responses to work environments in institutional long-term care	Staff responses to work environments	Work environments
Tourangeau et al. (2014)	Work, work environments, and other factors influencing nurse faculty intention to remain employed: A cross-sectional study	Nurse faculty intention to remain employed	Work, work environments, other factors

Continued

TABLE 13-1   Recent Outcomes Research Focusing Primarily on Structures of Care—cont'd

Researcher (Year)	Title	Outcomes	Structures
Trinkoff et al. (2013)	Turnover, staffing, skill mix, and resident outcomes in a national sample of U.S. nursing homes	Nursing home resident outcomes	Nurse turnover, staffing, skill mix
Van Bogaert et al. (2014)	Nursing unit teams matter: Impact of unit-level nurse practice environment, nurse work characteristics, and burnout on nurse reported job outcomes, and quality of care, and patient adverse events: A cross-sectional survey.	Nurse-reported job outcomes, quality of care, patient adverse events	Unit-level nurse practice environment, nurse work characteristics, burnout
Van den Heede et al. (2009a)	The relationship between inpatient cardiac surgery mortality and nurse numbers and educational level: Analysis of administrative data	Inpatient cardiac surgery mortality	Staffing and educational level
Van den Heede et al. (2009b)	Nurse staffing and patient outcomes in Belgian acute hospitals: Cross-sectional analysis of administrative data	Patient outcomes	Nurse staffing
West et al. (2014)	Nurse staffing, medical staffing, and mortality in intensive care: An observational study. International Journal of Nursing Studies	Mortality in Intensive Care	Nurse staffing, medical staffing
Zivin et al. (2015)	Associations between depression and all-cause and cause-specific risk of death: A retrospective cohort study in the Veterans Health Administration	All-cause and cause-specific risk of death in veterans	Depression

Several of the seven attributes of health care (Box 13-1) are considered process-based: efficacy and effectiveness, surely, but also cost-effectiveness (efficiency) and optimality (balancing of costs and benefits). Recent literature has focused less on processes than structures, but there is some recent work exploring associations between outcomes and processes of care (Table 13-2), such as different surgeons performing the same procedure (Martin et al., 2013), a different way to teach behavioral skills for managing depression and anxiety (Mazurek Melnyk, Kelly, & Lusk, 2014), "rationing" or prioritizing nursing care in response to overwork (Schubert, Clarke, Aiken, & De Geest, 2012), and the patient's and family's interpersonal interactions with healthcare workers and hospital employees (Mishra & Gupta, 2012).

Burnout: Structure of Care or Process of Care?

Sometimes outcomes research that is primarily focused on structures also includes a variable or two that might also be considered processual, such as nurse burnout. Burnout can contribute to patient outcomes as a process, of course, by its effect on the interpersonal dimension of patient care. However, burnout also can contribute in a structural sense through increased absenteeism, thereby increasing workload for other nurses.

TABLE 13-2	**Recent Outcomes Research Focusing Primarily on Processes of Care**				
Researcher (Year)	**Title**	**Outcomes**	**Associated Structures Examined**	**Processes**
Martin et al. (2013)	Hospital and surgeon variation in complications and repeat surgery following incident lumbar fusion for common degenerative diagnoses	Complications and repeat surgery following incident lumbar fusion for common degenerative diagnoses	Hospital variation	Surgeon variation
Mazurek Melnyk, Kelly, & Lusk (2014)	Outcomes and feasibility of a manualized cognitive-behavioral skills building intervention: Group COPE for depressed and anxious adolescents in school settings.	Depression and anxiety in adolescents	—	Manualized cognitive-behavioral skills building intervention: Group COPE
Mishra & Gupta (2012)	Study of patient satisfaction in a surgical unit of a tertiary teaching hospital	Patient satisfaction	Clean rooms, food quality	Behavior of doctors and non-professional workers Explanation about disease and treatment
Schubert, Clarke, Aiken, & De Geest (2012)	Association between rationing of nursing care and inpatient mortality in Swiss hospitals	Inpatient mortality	Patient-nurse ratios, patient acuity	"Rationing" of nursing care—omitting some care

COPE, Creating Opportunities for Personal Empowerment.

Outcomes are results, and they are the direct results of health care received. Not all occurrences are necessarily outcomes, even if we name them as such. For example, the birth of a healthy full-term infant is usually not the result of a healthcare intervention but a passive and expected occurrence.

Outcomes are clinical endpoints, satisfaction with care, functional status, and general well-being. They are results of treatment, such as level of rehabilitation; continued or subsequent morbidity; mortality; and total days of hospitalization. It is important to be aware that not every freestanding outcome is necessarily credible. For instance, patient satisfaction may not be the best isolated measurement of quality of care. Fenton, Jerant, Bertakis, and Franks (2012) reported that in a 7-year cohort study, "higher patient satisfaction was associated with less emergency department use but with greater inpatient use, higher overall healthcare and prescription drug expenditures, and increased mortality" (p. 405). It is important to devise multiple ways to measure outcomes, for improved validity.

Like outcomes, functional status can be measured in several ways. For instance, rehabilitation therapists measure the amount of extension at the elbow joint in degrees, as a quantification of recovery of function after surgery, illness, or injury. This provides a numerical rating: fewer degrees, poorer functional status. However, for patients who have sustained traumatic injury and may not elect to undergo further surgeries, what a physical therapist might deem a "poor" ability to extend the arm may be quite acceptable to the patient. As cited previously, it is important to determine "what

BOX 13-2 Proximate Point Versus Endpoint Outcome Measurement

Strict adherence to diabetes management results in more years of good vision, functional kidneys, patent coronary arteries, and healthy retinal vasculature. Most persons with adult-onset diabetes who maintain only moderately good management enjoy 10 to 20 years before they suffer consequences of hyperglycemic episodes. Because the elapsed time from disease diagnosis until first negative consequence may be so extended, primary healthcare providers concentrate instead on the proximate outcome measure of glycosylated hemoglobin (HbA1c) levels, by which average blood sugar over the past 3 to 4 months is tracked in an indirect way.

consumers expect, want, or are willing to accept" (Donabedian, 1987, p. 5).

Because endpoints are often extremely distant, setting proximate points is recommended for quality assessment purposes, allowing some evaluation of a treatment program after a reasonable increment of time. It is difficult to remain focused on a goal that will not be measured until decades later (Box 13-2).

Evaluating Structures

Structures of care are the elements of organization and administration, as well as provider and patient characteristics, that exist prior to care and may affect outcomes. The first step in evaluating structure is to identify and describe the elements of the structure. Various administration and management theories can be used to identify structural elements within a healthcare agency. Some of these are leadership, tolerance of innovativeness, organizational hierarchy, power distribution, financial management, and administrative decision-making patterns. Nurse researchers investigating the influence of structural variables on quality of care and outcomes have studied factors such as nurse staffing, nursing education, nursing work environment, hospital characteristics, and organization of care delivery.

The second step in evaluation is to determine the strength and direction of relationships between one or more structures and selected outcomes. This evaluation requires comparing different structures that provide the same types of care. In evaluating structures, the unit of measurement is the structure. The evaluation requires access to a sufficiently large sample of similar structures with similar functions, which then can be contrasted with a sample of other structures providing the same functions, so as to compare outcomes. An example is a comparison among a metropolitan primary healthcare practice, a primary healthcare practice maintained through a full-service health maintenance organization (HMO), a rural health clinic, a community-oriented primary care clinic, and a nurse-managed center, with respect to an identified outcome. The focus of the study is calculation of the differing outcome values in different venues.

Federal and state governments require nursing homes, home healthcare agencies, and hospitals to collect and report specifically measured quality variables at periodic intervals (AHRQ, 2015a; CMS, 2014; Kleib, Sales, Doran, Malette, & White, 2011). Mandates for reporting were established because of considerable variation in quality of care across facilities (Kleib et al., 2011). Various governmental agencies analyze care provided by healthcare facilities so that they can oversee quality of care provided to the American public. These data are available also to the general public, so that individuals can make their own determination of the quality of care provided by various nursing homes, home healthcare agencies, or hospitals. Researchers also can access these data for studies of the quality of various structures, through a computer search using the phrases *nursing home compare*, *home health compare*, and *hospital compare*. A specific facility can be selected and considerable general information about outcomes of care accessed. The American Nurses Credentialing Center (ANCC, 2015) provides the current status of individual hospitals in their quest for magnet status certification based on excellence in nursing care. (For further information about magnet status, refer to Chapter 19.)

Processes of Care and Their Relationship to Outcomes
Standards of Care

A **standard of care** is a norm on which quality of care is judged. According to Donabedian (1987), a practitioner has legitimate responsibility to apply available knowledge when managing a dysfunction or disease state. This management consists of (1) identifying or diagnosing the dysfunction, (2) deciding whether to intervene, (3) choosing intervention objectives, (4) selecting methods and techniques to achieve the objectives, and (5) skillfully executing the selected techniques or interventions.

Donabedian (1987) recommended the development of criteria to be used as a basis for judging quality of care. These criteria may take the form of clinical guidelines, critical paths, or care maps based on prior validation that the care contributed to the desired outcomes. The clinical guidelines published by the Agency for Healthcare Research and Quality (AHRQ, 2015b) establish norms or standards against which the adequacy of clinical management can be judged. However, the core of the problem, from Donabedian's perspective, is **clinical judgment**, which is the quality of reasoned decision making in healthcare practice. Analysis of the physician's process of making diagnoses and therapeutic decisions is critical to the evaluation of quality of care. The emergence of decision trees and algorithms is partially attributable to Donabedian's work on clinical judgment as it impacts quality.

Practice Styles

The style of a practitioner's practice is another dimension of the process of care that influences quality; however, it is problematic to judge what constitutes "goodness" in style in interpersonal relationships. The Medical Outcomes Study (MOS), described later in this chapter, was designed to determine whether variations in patient outcomes are explained by differences in system of care, clinician specialty, and clinicians' technical and interpersonal styles (Tarlov et al., 1989).

Practice pattern is a concept closely related to practice style. Although **practice style** represents variation in *how* care is provided, **practice pattern** represents variation in *what* care is provided. Researchers of variations in practice patterns have found that such variation is not wholly explained by patients' clinical conditions. For example, researchers have found that prescribing practices differ by region of the country (McDonald, Carlson, & Izrael, 2012) and are influenced, in part, by drug company resources and marketing practices (Zerzan et al., 2006). Because of this, small area analysis is suitable for comparisons of practice patterns; it is described later in this chapter, in the section on geographical analyses.

Costs of Care

Donabedian's **costs of care** (1990) refer to costs to the individual or the family. These can be divided into direct and indirect costs. **Direct costs** are those the patient incurs for direct payment for health care, as well as insurance payments and copayments. Direct costs of hospitalization for surgery, for instance, include insurance payments, copayments for the hospitalization or take-home medications not covered by insurance, and "supercharges" made by the hospital for certain amenities, such as television and newspaper. Direct costs also include the small portion of a publicly funded hospital's

budget arising from the tax base in support of a public institution that provides health care. This public funding applies also to university hospitals and healthcare practices associated with the university system. In comparison with other costs, the latter are almost negligible. **Indirect costs** are "hidden" costs the patient incurs. Indirect costs for surgery include transportation to the facility for the patient and family members, overnight accommodations for the family, parking fees, food purchased at the hospital by the family, and loss of pay for work missed by the patient and family members.

Critical Paths or Pathways

Critical pathways are linear displays, along which common markers of clinical progress are situated, and the anticipated temporal norms for their achievement. They also are known as **clinical guidelines** or **care maps**. Critical pathways were developed to allow practitioners to identify a number of proximate outcomes or proximate endpoints, which are a series of clinical goals occurring earlier in the process of treatment, instead of using only the endpoint to assess quality (Pearson, Goulart-Fisher, & Lee, 1995). Critical pathways may be useful on a shift-to-shift basis for fast-moving inpatient processes, such as recovery from knee replacement surgery, and on a week-to-week basis for slower-moving rehabilitative processes, such as stroke recovery. In unknown outcome scenarios, such as recovery from an untimed hypoxic event, use of a critical pathway allows an eventual diagnosis to be made as well, based on the patient's ability or inability to achieve proximate outcomes (Box 13-3).

FEDERAL GOVERNMENT INVOLVEMENT IN OUTCOMES RESEARCH

Agency for Healthcare Research and Quality

Nurses participated in the initial federal study of the quality of health care. In 1959, two National Institutes of Health (NIH) study sections, the Hospital and Medical Facilities Study Section and the Nursing Study Section, met to discuss concerns about the adequacy and appropriateness of medical care, patient care, and hospital and medical facilities. As a result of their dialogue, a Health Services Research Study Section was initiated. This study section eventually became the Association for Health Services Research (AHSR) and, subsequently, the Agency for Health Care Policy and Research (AHCPR). A reauthorization act changed the name of the AHCPR to the Agency for Healthcare Research and Quality (AHRQ). The AHRQ is designated as a scientific research agency. The new legislation

---

BOX 13-3   Example of Critical Pathways and Proximate Endpoints

The film *Regarding Henry* (Nichols, Abrams, Greenhut, Rudin, & MacNair, 1991) depicts the lead character after he suffers massive blood loss in an accident, resulting in tissue hypoxia. He eventually regains only some of his personality and some of his mental quickness, most of his ability to walk, and his full ability to speak, but his outcomes cannot be predicted at the onset of his hospitalization. His intensive care unit (ICU) course focuses on Henry's achievement of two event-markers on the critical pathway for ICU patients: the proximate endpoints of physical stabilization of oxygenation and perfusion, first, and then ability to exist without mechanical support. His acute care after the ICU focuses on gaining the endpoints of having Henry drink enough fluids to go without an IV and eat well enough to obtain nourishment independently, establishing his readiness to be discharged to rehabilitation. Henry's brain is essentially a black box—determination of final outcome is impossible, so the endpoints of circulatory and respiratory stability for exiting the ICU, and independent hydration and nutrition for exiting acute care, are fairly good proximate endpoints for assessment of quality, as well as very good markers of his progress. Achievement of proximate endpoints does not represent only quality of care. As with all outcomes, achievement of proximate endpoints is multifactorial and can be dependent on structures and even processes

outside the scope of healthcare provision, as well as on the pathophysiology of the individual patient. In addition, failure to achieve proximate endpoints does not imply that care was deficient. The inability to achieve the ability to eat and drink independently may be due solely to hypoxic damage and not attributable to less than perfect care delivery.

Henry's final functional outcome represents confirmation of the extent of his original hypoxia and hypoperfusion. This is modified by structural variables, such as the time of response of the ambulance and the distance from the hospital; how long it takes to begin stabilization procedures in the ambulance and in the emergency department; the educational levels of physicians and nurses; how mentally adept his healthcare workers are at 4:00 AM, as a function of the length of the shift they work; the fact that he has a family; and his general health, intelligence, determination, abilities, and status in the community prior to his accident. It is also modified by process variables, such as the attentiveness of individual nurses and respiratory therapists to his pulmonary status; the technical skill of his diagnosticians; standards of care for weaning from mechanical ventilation; the willingness of doctors and nurses to teach and support his wife; and the availability of rehabilitation to him, based on insurance coverage.

---

of 1999 also eliminated the requirement that the AHRQ develop clinical practice guidelines. However, the AHRQ (2015b) continues support of these efforts through evidence-based practice centers (EPCs) and the dissemination of evidence-based guidelines through its National Guideline Clearinghouse (see Chapter 19 for a more detailed discussion of EPC guidelines).

The AHRQ, as a part of the U.S. Department of Health and Human Services (DHHS), supports research designed to improve outcomes and quality of health care, reduce its costs, address patient safety and medical errors, and broaden access to effective services (AHRQ, 2015b). The AHRQ website contains information about outcomes research, funding opportunities, and results of recently completed research, including nursing research. In 2015 AHRQ committed $52 million to be spent over a 5-year period, "to study how complex delivery systems disseminate and apply evidence from patient-centered outcomes research" (AHRQ, 2015a). In addition, AHRQ invested $17 million to expand projects to help prevent healthcare-associated infections, the

most common complication of hospital care. The AHRQ has initiated several major research efforts to examine medical outcomes and improve quality of care.

American Recovery and Reinvestment Act

Funding from the American Recovery and Reinvestment Act (Recovery Act), signed into law in February 2009, allowed AHRQ to expand its work in support of comparative effectiveness research, including enhancing the Effective Health Care Program. A total of $473 million was awarded to AHRQ by DHHS in 2012 and disbursed over a 5-year period, beginning in 2013 for the purpose of funding patient-centered outcomes research (AHRQ, 2015a). This AHRQ program provides patients, clinicians, and others with evidence-based information to make informed decisions about health care, through activities such as comparative effectiveness reviews conducted through the AHRQ's EPCs (see Chapter 19). **Comparative effectiveness research** is descriptive or correlational research that compares different treatment options for their risks and benefits

(AHRQ, 2015c). The AHRQ's broad research portfolio touches on nearly every aspect of health care, including clinical practice, outcomes and effectiveness of care, EBP, primary care and care for priority populations, healthcare quality, patient safety/medical errors, organization and delivery of care and use of healthcare resources, healthcare costs and financing, health information technology, and knowledge transfer.

The U.S. is not the only country demanding improvements in quality of care and reductions in healthcare costs. Many countries are experiencing similar concerns and addressing them in relation to their particular government structures. Thus, the movement into outcomes research and the approaches described in this chapter are a worldwide phenomenon.

NONGOVERNMENTAL INVOLVEMENT IN OUTCOMES RESEARCH

Medical Outcomes Study

The MOS was conducted almost 30 years ago, representing the first large-scale study in the U.S. to examine factors influencing patient outcomes. The study was designed to identify elements of physician care associated with favorable patient outcomes, using a three-city sample of 1681 chronically ill ambulatory patients in 367 medical practices.

The MOS did not control for the effects of nursing interventions, staffing patterns, and nursing practice delivery models on medical outcomes. Consequently, coordination of care, counseling, and referral activities, which are areas of overlapping responsibility for physicians and nurses, were included as components of medical practice. Kelly, Huber, Johnson, McCloskey, and Maas (1994) suggested modifications to the MOS framework that would represent the collaboration among physicians, nurses, and allied health practitioners and allow analysis of the influence of their separate interactions on patient outcomes. These researchers also suggested adding the domain of societal outcomes to include such outcome variables as cost. They noted that "the MOS outcomes framework incorporated areas in which nursing science contributed to health and medical care effectiveness. It also includes structure, process, and outcome variables in which nursing practice overlaps with that of other health professionals" (p. 213). Kelly et al. (1994) further observed that "client outcome categories of the MOS framework that go beyond the scope of physician treatment and intervention alone include functional status, general well-being, and satisfaction with care" (p. 213). A review of the state of the science

on nursing-sensitive outcomes published in 2011 confirmed the relevance of these outcomes to nursing practice and suggested several more, including self-care; therapeutic self-care, defined as patients' ability to manage their disease and its treatment; symptom control; psychosocial functioning; healthcare utilization; and mortality (Doran, 2011).

Origins of Outcomes/Performance Monitoring

Efforts to collect data systematically did not gain widespread attention in the U.S. until the late 1970s. At that time, concerns about quality of hospital care prompted the development of the Universal Minimum Health Data Set, which established the minimum data that could be recorded for any patient's hospital stay (Kleib et al., 2011). The Uniform Hospital Discharge Data Set followed. These data sets prescribed the elements to be gathered, providing a database that could be used for assessment of quality of care in hospitals and at the point of discharge. Other countries developed similar data sets. In Canada, the Standards for Management Information Systems (MIS) were developed in the 1980s. Upon the establishment of the Canadian Institute for Health Information (CIHI) in 1994, the MIS designations became a set of national standards used to collect and report financial and statistical data from health service organizations' daily operations. As in the U.S., these data sets did not include data distinct to nursing care (Kleib et al., 2011).

OUTCOMES RESEARCH AND EVIDENCE-BASED PRACTICE

Evidence-based practice presupposes evidence, a substantial amount of which emanates from outcomes research. Evidence-based care is based on information that is utilized, sometimes as processes of care, sometimes as structures, to enhance outcomes. Reports of empirical studies explicating the impact of various interventions upon nursing practice and consequently on patient outcomes usually name one or the other of the terms, evidence-based practice or outcome. However, some explicate both. For example, Mazurek Melnyk, Kelly, and Lusk (2014) reported the feasibility and effects of using the COPE (Creating Opportunities for Personal Empowerment) focused manual for a group therapy intervention with 16 depressed adolescents. The intervention consisted of seven weeks of cognitive-behavioral therapy delivered once weekly as group sessions, followed by homework from a printed manual. The intervention was effective in decreasing depression and anxiety. The authors identified their intervention as evidence-based, adding to the body of knowledge in nursing, and also contributory to better outcomes.

Although most research self-identifies as being outcomes research or contributing to EBP, but not both, research that measures outcomes using a strategy confirmed by prior research is clearly evidence-based and contributes to further evidence for practice. Conversely, it can be argued that research that is evidence-based and designed for application to practice affects outcomes. Trajectories of evidence, some of which emanate from outcomes research, and various paths to the creation of EBP are detailed in Figure 13-4. As pictured, outcomes research often provides initial evidence of incidence or association through descriptive and correlational research. As Donabedian (1980) recommended, periodic review of data and of paying attention to patterns within the data set reveal incidence and association. After initial evidence is established through either focused outcomes studies or routine data review, if the findings are reproducible, then theoretical modeling may occur, and finally theory testing follows through descriptive, correlational, or interventional research. Multiple replications ensue, eventually contributing to evidence for practice, producing the ability to anticipate incidence, to predict, or to intervene.

Nursing-Sensitive Patient Outcomes

Very large studies about the work of individual nurses would be impractical. Such research would be inordinately time-consuming, and would involve scrutiny that might be construed as workplace harassment. Methodologically, designing such studies would be prohibitive, because patients are cared for by a variety of nurses over a typical hospital stay, compromising the ability to attribute outcomes to any one of them. Consequently, for outcomes research in which nurses and their characteristics function as structures (nursing educational preparation, for example) or as processes (technical capability), aggregates must be used in data analysis.

Although formal published outcomes research in which nurses themselves function as processes or structures has been modest in quantity, there is a wealth of ongoing agency-generated quality improvement research that uses data generated from nurses' charting, reflecting task completion relative to nursing-sensitive indicators, using the medical record as data. As Donabedian (1980) recommended, formal quality improvement functions as an ongoing process, in which outcomes are scrutinized so as to reveal connections with structures or processes. Hypotheses are formed. Changes in structures and processes are tracked, so as to demonstrate trends. Ultimately, changes in processes

are mandated, and the results measured. Sometimes structural modifications take place if enough evidence is accrued. Then the results are measured. For instance, research examining correlations between patient outcomes and percentage of BSN nurses has been replicated so often that many hospitals aware of the body of research offer preferential hiring to BSN graduates. Another example is the process of ongoing revision for standards of care, instituted in response to the body of evidence.

In current hospital quality improvement research, a **nursing-sensitive patient outcome** (**NSPO**) is one influenced by nursing care decisions, actions, or attributes. It may not be caused by nursing but is associated with nursing. In various situations, "nursing" might signify the actions of one nurse, nurses as a working group, an approach to nursing practice, the nursing unit, or the institution. The institution determines numbers of nurses, salaries, educational levels of nurses, assignments of nurses, workload of nurses, management of nurses, and policies related to nurses and nursing practice. It might even include the structural variable of the physical plant of the nursing unit, in respect to whether there is a sequestered area on a nursing unit, in which nurses can prepare medications. In Pape's (2013) study describing an intervention to decrease interruptions and distractions during medication preparation, which prior research had linked to errors of medication administration, the hospital unit studied had a medication area that was open, without a door or well-defined perimeter. Prior research has linked the nursing-sensitive patient outcome of administration errors to interruptions and distractions during medication preparation. As the intervention, the researcher used yellow duct tape to mark off the medication area as a quiet zone, and posted signs, "STOP. Quiet Zone. Do not interrupt nurses during medication administration. Avoid conversation in this area." The researcher could not create a closed room but could artificially create the impression of a physical area for medication administration. Results indicated that the structure of a dedicated quiet zone medication area was effective in decreasing interruptions and distractions by 84%.

Professional accountability dictates that nurses identify and document outcomes influenced by care they provide. Efforts to study nursing-sensitive outcomes were initiated by the American Nurses Association (ANA). In 1994, the ANA, in collaboration with the American Academy of Nursing Expert Panel on Quality Health Care, launched a plan to identify indicators of quality nursing practice and to collect and analyze data

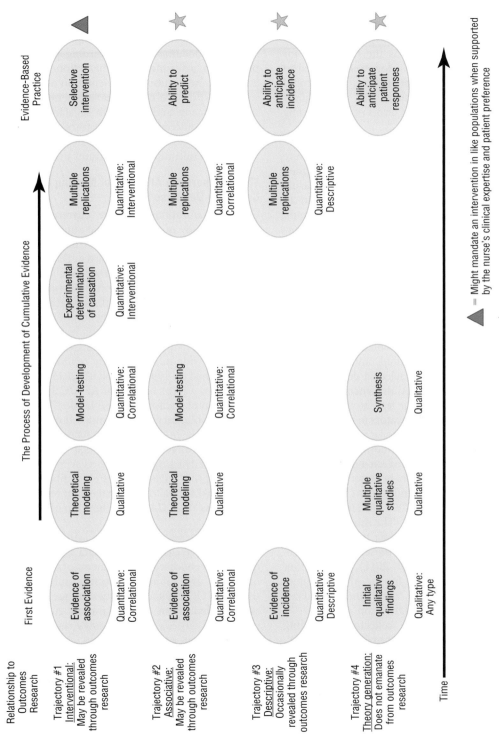

FIGURE 13-4 Outcomes research and evidence-based practice.

using these indicators throughout the U.S. (Mitchell, Ferketich, & Jennings, 1998). The goal was to identify and/or develop nursing-sensitive quality measures. Donabedian's theory was used as the framework for the project. Together, these indicators were referred to as the ANA **Nursing Care Report Card**, which could facilitate setting a desired standard that would allow comparisons among hospitals in terms of their nursing care quality.

At the outset, it was not known which indicators were sensitive to patient outcomes or what outcomes were associated with nurse characteristics and care provided by nurses. Hospitals chose their own ways of measuring the ANA-selected indicators but were persuaded to change to a standardized measure for each indicator. Nurse researchers within cooperating hospitals conducted multiple pilot studies, tested consistent mechanisms for data collection, resolved problems, agreed on consistent measurement strategies, and continued to amplify indicators and test them (Jennings, Loan, DePaul, Brosch, & Hildreth, 2001).

The ANA proposed that all hospitals collect and report data based on nursing-sensitive quality indicators. To encourage researchers to collect these indicators, ANA-accredited organizations and the federal government helped by sharing selected data and findings with key groups. The ANA also encouraged state nurses' associations to lobby state legislatures to include the nursing-sensitive quality indicators in regulations or state law.

In 1998, the ANA provided funding to develop a national database to house data collected using nursing-sensitive quality indicators. This became the National Database of Nursing Quality Indicators (NDNQI). In 2015 NDNQI had more than 2000 participating organizations (Press Ganey, 2015). The purpose of the NDNQI is to provide unit-level data for participating organizations, so that they can use those data in quality-improvement activities (NDNQI, 2011). Participation in NDNQI meets requirements for the ANCC Magnet Recognition Program® (ANCC, 2015), and some database members participate for that reason.

Detailed guidelines for data collection, including definitions and decision guides, are provided by NDNQI. Healthcare organizations submit data electronically. Quarterly and annual reports of structure, process, and outcome indicators are available to participants after each analysis is complete. The database is funded by the ANA, housed at the Kansas University Medical Center School of Nursing, and managed by Press Ganey (2015). The NDNQI nursing sensitive indicators related to structure include items such as hours of nursing care per patient day, skill mix of nursing providers, nurse turnover rate, registered nurse (RN) education, and certification. Indicators pertaining to process include items related to documentation regarding patient falls and prevention, assessment documentation related to pediatric pain medication, documentation of care provided related to pressure ulcers, nurse practice environment self-assessment, and nurse job satisfaction. Indicators related to outcomes include nosocomial infections, patient falls, pressure ulcer, pediatric peripheral intravenous (IV) infiltration, and restraint use.

The Collaborative Alliance for Nursing Outcomes California Database Project

Other organizations that are currently involved in efforts to study nursing-sensitive outcomes include the National Quality Forum (NQF), Collaborative Alliance for Nursing Outcomes California Database, Veterans Affairs Nursing Outcomes Database, the Center for Medicare and Medicaid Services' Hospital Quality Initiative, the American Hospital Association, the Federation of American Hospitals, The Joint Commission, and the AHRQ.

California Nursing Outcomes Coalition (CalNOC) was a statewide nursing quality report card pilot project launched in 1996 (CALNOC, 2015). ANA funded CalNOC as a joint venture of ANA/California and the Association of California Nurse Leaders (ACNL). Membership is voluntary and is composed of approximately 300 hospitals in the U.S. As its membership grew nationally, CalNOC was renamed the Collaborative Alliance for Nursing Outcomes (CALNOC, 2015). It is a not-for-profit corporation, and member hospitals pay a size-based annual data management fee to participate and access the CALNOC benchmarking reporting system.

Hospital-generated unit-level acute care nurse staffing, workforce characteristics, data related to processes of care, and endorsed measurements of nursing-sensitive outcomes are submitted electronically. In addition, the CALNOC database includes unique measures such as the Medication Administration Accuracy metric (CALNOC, 2015), which assesses actual occurrences of medication errors and tracks changes over time. CALNOC data are stratified by unit type and hospital characteristics, and reports can be aggregated by division, hospital, system/group, and geographical location. CALNOC's nursing-sensitive indicators overlap with those of NDNQI, with the addition of utilization of registry personnel, workload intensity, medication administration accuracy, process of insertion of peripherally inserted central catheters, and restraint use.

National Quality Forum

The National Quality Forum (NQF) was created in 1999 for the purpose of setting national standards for healthcare performance. It "leads national collaboration to improve health and healthcare quality through measurement" (NQF, 2015). Its goals include establishment of its endorsed standards as "the primary standards used to measure and report on the quality and efficiency of healthcare in the United States," and "to be a major driving force for and facilitator of continuous quality improvement of American healthcare quality" (NQF, 2015). A complete list of measures included in the NQF portfolio can be found on the NQF (2015) website. Approximately one third of the measures in NQF's portfolio are measures of patient outcomes. Examples are mortality, readmissions, depression, and experience of care (NQF, 2015). The NQF includes in their performance measurement portfolio several nursing-sensitive measures, which are similar to those of the agencies described previously.

Oncology Nursing Society

The Oncology Nursing Society (ONS) is a professional organization of more than 35,000 RNs and other healthcare providers dedicated to excellence in patient care, education, research, and administration in oncology nursing (ONS, 2015). The ONS has taken a leadership role among specialty nursing organizations in maintaining an EBP resource, Putting Evidence into Practice, on its website. The site provides nurses with a guide to identify, critically appraise, and use evidence to solve clinical problems. It also provides outcome measures, best-practice summaries, and evidence tables related to care of patients with cancer, maintaining an ongoing role in both EBP and outcomes research.

METHODOLOGICAL CONSIDERATIONS FOR OUTCOMES STUDIES

Methodology and Design

We consider outcomes research a distinct methodology because of three attributes: its unique focus upon quality as described by Donabedian (1980), its theoretical framework, and its shared dependent variable (various markers of quality). These and other aspects that distinguish outcomes research are presented here.

Unlike the qualitative and mixed-methods methodologies, the outcomes research methodology does not possess its own exclusive array of distinct designs. In terms of methodology and design, outcomes research uses the quantitative methodology and some of the quantitative designs. Within this design cluster, most of its designs are correlational and descriptive. The vast majority of data for outcomes research are obtained retrospectively because of reliance on preexistent databases.

We conducted a focused literature search with keywords *outcomes research, qualitative,* and *nursing.* This revealed no published qualitative studies that were outcomes research for the period 2012 through 2015. Surely, there is qualitative inquiry that contributes preliminary impressions, so that subsequent outcomes research can be generated, but this may not be formalized. Keeley, West, Tutt, and Nutting (2014), for example, identified implications for further research on the topic of the discrepancy between physicians' and clients' perceptions of their depression as, "Future research would investigate a potential mismatch between clinicians' and patients' perceptions of the effects of stigma on achieving care for depression, and on whether time spent discussing depression during the clinical visit improves outcomes" (p. 13), which could be either quantitative or qualitative in design. However, unless qualitative research's data can be reanalyzed quantitatively, for instance as "Care was acceptable" versus "Care was not acceptable," they are of no direct use in modern outcomes research, other than to indicate direction for subsequent inquiry or to explain quantitative results.

Philosophical Origins, Theoretical Framework, Overriding Purpose

Like quantitative research, the distant philosophical origin of outcomes research is logical positivism. It relies on what can be measured, and it relies on observed measurements and statistics to identify differences and patterns. Unlike quantitative research as a whole, it also reflects the more recent influence of Donabedian's public health-rooted beliefs of fairness and social justice (Mullan, 2001): there is an underlying implication that the recipients of health care deserve quality care. Quantitative research in health care shares that same goal of quality care—sometimes from a humanistic point of view, sometimes from an economic one—but it is clearly implied in problem statements, in purpose statements, and in recommendations for subsequent research.

The overarching theoretical framework for all outcomes research is Donabedian's paradigm (Lawson & Yazdany, 2012) or a derivative of it. Occasional outcomes studies use a secondary framework, especially when examining a common phenomenon like pain.

In terms of its general purpose, outcomes research is a type of evaluation research (Dawson & Tilley,

1997), just as public health research tends to be, focusing on evaluation of quality/delivery of human health care. Outcomes research shares its focus with public health research; considering Donabedian's background, this is not surprising. Outcomes research overlaps epidemiologic research as well, when the focus of epidemiologic research is humans (Petitti, 1998). Economic research has some overlap with outcomes research, when the latter focuses on economic resources and outcomes in the context of healthcare delivery (Chelimsky, 1997).

Methods

The overall focus of analysis for outcomes research is quality of care, reflected as safety, effectiveness, efficiency, system responsiveness, equity of care, and timeliness or access to care. Consequently, the dependent variable cluster in outcomes research is quality of care, operationalized as some tangible outcome such as clinical endpoint of care, proximate clinical endpoint, patient satisfaction, functional status, length of hospital stay, incidence of rehospitalization, cost, resource utilization, prevention, or response time to emergencies. The predictor variables are structures and processes of care. For interventional testing, the independent variable is a structure or process.

Samples and Sampling

Donabedian (1980) recommended use of huge databases in outcomes research so that, at the analysis level, connections among variables would be apparent. In contrast to the type of sampling usually found in the quantitative methodology, descriptive or correlational outcomes research tends to use an entire data set for establishment of basic measured values, as well as examination of trends over time. In this case, the sample includes the entire accessible population. Random sampling is used infrequently, primarily for initial testing of interventions designed to impact outcomes. When using an entire database, heterogeneous samples result, enabling generalization to that same accessible population (Kerlinger & Lee, 2000).

Outcomes research is unusual in that when whole databases are used, information emanates retrospectively from the past, and generalization is made to the future situation or population represented by the sample. Because of temporal drift, generalizations are more accurate when recent data are used.

Large Databases as Sample Sources

Two broad categories of databases are used as sources for outcomes research: clinical databases and administrative databases. **Clinical databases** are created by providers such as hospitals, HMOs, and healthcare professionals. Clinical data are generated either as a result of routine documentation of care or in relation to data-collection for research purposes. Some databases are data registries that have been developed to gather data related to a particular disease, such as heart disease or cancer (Lee & Goldman, 1989). For instance, the Centers for Disease Control and Prevention (CDC) report information about diseases, treatment, and injuries on the CDC A-Z Index page of their website (CDC, 2015). A clinical database allows longitudinal analysis, by practitioner, by disease process, or by treatment modality. At this time, because of minimum data set regulations for both inpatients and outpatients, clinical data continue to accrue rapidly.

Administrative databases are created by insurance companies, government agencies, and others not directly involved in providing patient care. Administrative databases maintain standardized sets of data for enormous numbers of patients and providers, as part of analyses they perform, relative to cost and expenditures. An example is the Medicare database managed by the CMS. These databases can be used to determine incidence or prevalence of disease, demographic profiles of persons using different types of care, geographical variations in medical care utilization, characteristics of medical care by provider, and outcomes of care. For instance, Riley, Levy, and Montgomery (2009) used part of the Medicare database for their descriptive study of patients' selections of the various Medicare drug programs and the costs and benefits associated with each.

THE SPECIFIC DESIGNS OF OUTCOMES RESEARCH

Designs

"Outcomes research uses observational study designs that are the same as the observational designs used in traditional epidemiology" (Petitti, 1998, p. 269). Those noninterventional designs used in outcomes research are what nursing research terms descriptive and correlational. The few interventional outcomes research designs are experimental and quasi-experimental.

The noninterventional designs for outcomes research were originally developed by many different disciplines: epidemiology, population studies, medicine, economics, and statistics. Some of these designs are practice pattern profiling (epidemiology and medicine), prospective and retrospective cohort studies (epidemiology), trend studies (epidemiology), geographic designs (epidemiology, surveying, and cartography), meta-analyses (medicine and statistics), and cost-benefit analyses (epidemiology and economics).

Practice Pattern Profiling

Practice pattern profiling is an epidemiological technique that focuses on patterns of care. It was used originally in healthcare research to compare the outcomes of one physician's practice with norms or averages among other physicians. Now researchers use large database analyses to identify the practice pattern of an individual physician, a physician practice group, a combined practice including NPs and physician's assistants (PAs), or a given HMO or hospital, comparing outcomes with those of similar providers or with accepted standards of practice. The technique has been used to determine overutilization and underutilization of services, to examine costs associated with a particular provider's care, to uncover problems related to efficiency and quality of care, and to assess provider performance (Flexner, 2002; Martin et al., 2013). An example of practice profiling is Martin et al.'s (2013) research, with the stated purpose "to identify factors that account for variation in complication rates across hospitals and surgeons performing lumbar spinal fusion surgery" (p. 1). Using 6091 patients from an inpatient discharge database in Washington State, the authors retrospectively analyzed 4 years of consecutive data, deriving conclusions predominantly from correlational analyses. This is typical of outcomes research: a huge sample retrospectively obtained and analyzed with tests of correlation. Martin et al.'s (2013) findings identified patient characteristics and operative features as explanatory of complication rates and need for repeat surgery, across the country.

Profiling does not address methods of improving outcomes, merely identifying the range of performance and outliers. Given existent databases in nursing, profiling nursing care by institution is possible and is now performed by groups such as NDNQI that track nursing-sensitive indicators for purposes of providing benchmarking data to participating database members. Other than tracking by such groups, profiling of nurses' practice patterns has not yet been undertaken.

Prospective Cohort Studies

Prospective cohort studies, which originated in the field of epidemiology, use a descriptive, or occasionally correlational, longitudinal design. The researcher identifies a group of persons at risk for experiencing a particular event, and follows that same group over time, collecting data at intervals (Kelsey, Petitti, & King, 1998). Sample sizes for these studies must be large when only a small portion of the at-risk group will experience the event. The entire group is followed and multiple measurements obtained, often using dichotomous variables. Gradations of outcomes, both before and after confirmation of event occurrence, also can be determined (Kelsey et al., 1998).

The Harvard Nurses' Health Study is an example of a prospective cohort study. In the initial phase, the researchers recruited 100,000 nurses, so as to investigate the long-term consequences of the use of birth control pills, smoking, and alcohol use in relation to health outcomes such as cancer, cognitive status, and cardiovascular disease (Nurses' Health Study 3, 2013). The study has been in progress for more than 40 years. Multiple studies reported in the literature have used the same large data set yielded by the study. Palacios et al. (2014) used existing data from the Nurses' Health Study to examine the relationship between airborne metal exposures and the subsequent development of Parkinson disease.

"Background: Exposure to metals has been implicated in the pathogenesis of Parkinson disease (PD). Objectives: We sought to examine in a large prospective study of female nurses whether exposure to airborne metals was associated with risk of PD. Methods: We linked the U.S. Environmental Protection Agency (EPA)'s Air Toxics tract-level data with the Nurses' Health Study, a prospective cohort of female nurses. Over the course of 18 years of follow-up from 1990 through 2008, we identified 425 incident cases of PD. We examined the association of risk of PD with the following metals that were part of the first U.S. EPA collections in 1990, 1996, and 1999: arsenic, antimony, cadmium, chromium, lead, manganese, mercury, and nickel. To estimate hazard ratios (HRs) and 95% CIs, we used the Cox proportional hazards model, adjusting for age, smoking, and population density. Results: In adjusted models, the HR for the highest compared with the lowest quartile of each metal ranged from 0.78 (95% CI: 0.59, 1.04) for chromium to 1.33 (95% CI: 0.98, 1.79) for mercury. Conclusions: Overall, we found limited evidence for the association between adulthood ambient exposure to metals and risk of PD. The results for mercury need to be confirmed in future studies." (Palacios et al., 2014, p. 933)

Retrospective Cohort Studies

A **retrospective cohort study** is also an epidemiological design, in which the researcher identifies a group of people who have experienced a particular event or outcome in the present or the recent past (Kelsey et al., 1998). Data are obtained from existent records or other previously collected data, predating the occurrence of the event. In this way, researchers can establish possible causal relationships for further investigation.

In addition to use of a database, researchers can ask patients to recall information relevant to their previous health status. Because some research subjects are quite poor historians, corroboration of the information using records review, or verification by relatives or close friends, is preferable.

Zivin et al.'s (2015) study of depression and death in veterans cared for through the Veterans Health Administration used data collected from patient records, including demographics. Excerpts from their abstract explain the study findings.

"… We used Cox regression models to estimate hazard ratios associated with baseline depression diagnosis (N = 849,474) and three-year mortality among 5,078,082 patients treated in Veterans Health Administration (VHA) settings in fiscal year (FY) 2006. Cause of death was obtained from the National Death Index (NDI) … Baseline depression was associated with 17% greater hazard of all-cause three-year mortality (95% CI hazard ratio [HR]: 1.15, 1.18) after adjusting for baseline patient demographic and clinical characteristics and VHA facility characteristics. Depression was associated with a higher hazard of three-year mortality from heart disease, respiratory illness, cerebrovascular disease, accidents, diabetes, nephritis, influenza, Alzheimer's disease, septicemia, suicide, Parkinson's disease, and hypertension. Depression was associated with a lower hazard of death from malignant neoplasm and liver disease. Depression was not associated with mortality due to assault … In addition to being associated with suicide and injury-related causes of death, depression is associated with increased risk of death from nearly all major medical causes, independent of multiple major risk factors. Findings highlight the need to better understand and prevent mortality seen with multiple medical disorders associated with depression." (Zivin et al., 2015, p. 324)

Population-Based Studies

Some **population-based studies** are cohort studies, either prospective or retrospective, undertaken so as to discover information about a population, usually after an event occurs, such as a treatment or an exposure. The sample is derived exclusively from that population, probabilistically whenever possible, allowing generalization of the findings to that specific population. This method enables researchers to understand the natural history of a condition or of the long-term risks and benefits of a particular intervention (Guess et al., 1995). In outcomes research using an entire administrative database like Medicare that spans an entire state or country, the yield is a population-based data set, because it is presumed to include the entire population that is 65 years and older (Petitti, 1998).

Chen, Lin, Ho, Chen, and Kao (2015) studied the risk of heart disease in heterozygotic carriers of thalassemia who had not received transfusions. Their abstract explains the study.

"Objective: Few studies have focused on the association between coronary artery disease (CAD) and transfusion naïve thalassemia populations (this term means silent carrier, thalassemia minor or intermedia), who usually had less clinical manifestations and didn't require frequently blood transfusion.

Design, setting and patients: This nationwide population-based cohort study involved analyzing data obtained between 1998 and 2010 from the Taiwanese National Health Insurance Research Database, with a follow-up period extending to the end of 2011. We identified patients with thalassemia and selected a comparison cohort that was frequency matched with the patients with thalassemia according to age, sex, and diagnosis year at a ratio of 1 patient with thalassemia to 4 control patients. We analyzed the risks of thalassemia and CAD by using Cox proportional hazard regression models.

Measurements and main results: In this study, 1537 patients with thalassemia and 6418 controls were included. The overall risks of developing CAD were 1.5-fold in patients with thalassemia compared with those in the comparison cohort after adjustment for age, sex, and comorbidities. Patients with thalassemia and with comorbidities, including hypertension, diabetes, hyperlipidemia, and chronic obstructive pulmonary disease, were 3.73-fold more likely to develop CAD than those without thalassemia and comorbidity (95% confidence interval = 2.41–5.79).

Conclusion: This is the first large long-term cohort study of which the results showed that transfusion-naïve thalassemia populations should be considered a crucial risk factor for CAD, even in patients with relatively mild clinical manifestations of thalassemia." (Chen et al., 2015, p. 250)

Some population-based research is longitudinal and its data collection extends over a period of months or years. A study of this type usually is referred to as having a **trend analysis** design. In addition to trend analysis, population studies are sometimes termed **trend studies.** Trend research measures the prevalence of a variable, and its value, over time within an entire population, often examining relationships with other variables as well. Because this group of designs uses a whole population instead of a defined cohort, data collected over time do not reflect individual changes, and sequential determination of variable values are based on whichever individuals comprise the population at the time of measurement.

Prevention studies often use trend designs, measuring the occurrence of a disease over time, in response to various interventions. Bednarczyk, Curran, Orenstein, and Omer (2014) studied trends in the U.S. in adolescent vaccination with human papillomavirus; their abstract summarizes the study.

"Adolescent uptake of human papillomavirus (HPV) vaccine remains low. We evaluated HPV vaccine uptake patterns over 2008–2011 by race/ethnicity, poverty status, and the combination of race/ethnicity and poverty status, utilizing National Immunization Survey—Teen data. Minority and below-poverty adolescents consistently had higher series initiation than white and above-poverty adolescents." (Bednarczyk et al., 2014, p. 238)

Geographical Analyses

Another epidemiological strategy is the **geographical analysis**, which examines variations in health status, health services, patterns of care, or patterns of use by geographical area. Geographical analyses are sometimes referred to as **small area analyses**. Variations may be associated with sociodemographic, economic, medical, cultural, or behavioral characteristics. Locality-specific factors of a healthcare system, such as capacity, access, and convenience, may play a role in explaining variations. The social setting, environment, living conditions, and community also may be important factors. For instance, the use of breast-conserving surgery (BCS) with radiation for women with breast cancer was found to differ significantly by region within the Canadian province of Alberta (Fisher, Gao, Yasui, Dabbs, & Winget, 2015). BCS was more prevalent in the major city of Calgary than elsewhere in the province.

Regression analyses are used to develop models using risk factors and the characteristics of the community. Results often are displayed through the use of maps (Kieffer, Alexander, & Mor, 1992). From a more theoretical perspective, the researcher must then explain the geographical variation uncovered by the analysis (Volinn, Diehr, Ciol, & Loeser, 1994).

Geographical information systems (GISs) are important tools for performing geographical analyses. The GIS is a computer-based modality that supports methodologies for geographical analyses. Interfacing with Internet resources, GIS also can collect information, provide visual arrays, analyze data, and support the various methodologies for geographical healthcare analysis (Ramani, Mavalankar, Patel, & Mehandiratta, 2007). Relational databases facilitate processing of spatial information. Potential output from GIS-based research includes mapping, summarizing data, and analyzing spatial relationships among datasets. For instance, map-embedded data, such as distance from health care and travel conditions, can be included in a program, allowing an instantaneous calculation of access to care (Ramani et al., 2007). In addition, GISs can provide animated models showing change over time, as well as projected change reflecting proposed interventions. This makes GISs especially attractive for presentation of proposals, as well as interim results.

Ramis et al. (2012) studied the relationship between environmental exposure to oil refineries and non-Hodgkin lymphoma (NHL) in Spain. Excerpts from their abstract describe the study methods, results, and conclusions.

"… We designed an analysis of matched geographical areas to examine non-Hodgkin lymphoma mortality in the vicinity of the 10 refineries sited in Spain over the period 1997–2006. Population exposure to refineries was estimated on the basis of distance from town of residence to the facility in a 10 km buffer. We defined 10 km radius areas to perform the matching, accounting for population density, level of industrialization and socio-demographic factors of the area using principal components analysis. For the matched towns we evaluated the risk of NHL mortality associated with residence in the vicinity of the refineries and with different regions using mixed Poisson models. Then we study the residuals to assess a possible risk trend with distance. … Relative risks (RRs) associated with exposure showed similar values for women and for men, 1.09 (0.97–1.24) and 1.12 (0.99–1.27). RRs for two regions were statistically significant: Canary Islands showed an excess of risk of 1.35 (1.05–1.72) for women and 1.50 (1.18–1.92) for men, whilst Galicia showed an excess of risk of 1.35 (1.04–1.75) for men, but not significant excess for women. … The results suggest a possible increased risk of NHL mortality among populations residing in the vicinity of refineries; however, a potential distance trend has not been shown. Regional effects in the Canary Islands and Galicia are significantly greater than the regional average." (Ramis et al., 2012 para. 1)

Economic Studies

Donabedian (1980) described efficiency as the "ability to obtain the greatest health improvement at the lowest cost" and optimality as the "most advantageous balancing of costs and benefits" (p. 27). In the field of outcomes research, economic studies often focus on outcomes as they relate to efficiency. The cost here is the cost to the institution, not the cost passed on to the insurance company and consumer. The total cost for health care is the unit of analysis in economic studies, rather than the welfare of the individual.

The most widely used term in the discussion of cost is the cost-benefit analysis. In general, cost-benefit analysis is analogous to Donabedian's concept of optimality, in that it involves comparison of costs and increased benefits, in terms of some single unit of analysis. In financial systems, the unit is money. However, in medical epidemiology, various other units of analysis may be selected, as well as cost, such as lives, disability, missed workdays, number of vials of vaccine used, or extent of visible scarring. When a cost-benefit analysis uses money for the unit of analysis, it is often referred to as a cost-effectiveness analysis.

Pyenson, Sander, Jiang, Kahn, and Mulshine (2012) performed a cost-benefit analysis to determine whether offering annual screening chest tomography to high-risk smokers ages 50 through 64 years would represent a net benefit. Using actuarial models, the authors estimated that the cost would be approximately $1 per commercially insured member, and that the "cost per life-year saved would be below $19,000, an amount that compares favorably with screening for cervical, breast, and colorectal cancers" (Pyenson et al., 2012, p. 770). The authors' conclusion was that "commercial insurers should consider lung cancer screening of high-risk individuals to be high-value coverage and provide it as a benefit to people who are at least fifty years old and have a smoking history of thirty pack-years or more" (p. 770). They referred to this initiation of high-quality screening from low-cost providers as an "efficient system innovation" (p. 770).

In economics, efficiency refers to the most benefit with the least possible cost. In public health, efficiency has two meanings: technical efficiency and allocative efficiency. **Technical efficiency** refers to whether there is waste-minimum utilization of precious resources, which are usually inadequate for serving an entire population and can be scarce. Technical efficiency is critical for issues such as storage and transportation of scarce vaccines and use of expiration-sensitive items before they are obsolete. **Allocative efficiency** refers to whether resources go to the area in which they will do the most good in terms of delivery of services: effectiveness, usefulness to persons served, number of persons actually reached, and adherence rates (McQuestion et al., 2011). Allocative efficiency addresses such issues as nurse staffing during a shortage and scheduling in clinic settings.

Cost-efficiency is merely the cheapest way of delivering a commodity or service. In all business endeavors, cost-efficiency means paying the lowest price for an acceptable product or worker. A cost-effectiveness analysis essentially provides an assessment of how much was purchased for a given sum, determining cost per unit of commodity. As noted earlier, cost-effectiveness analysis is a subtype of cost-benefit analysis, using money as the unit of analysis. It is currently used within healthcare outcomes research to make decisions based on dollar power. Goossens et al.'s (2013) research of criteria for early discharge from the hospital after exacerbations of chronic lung disease is an example of a cost-effectiveness analysis. The study findings revealed that neither the early discharge program nor the usual seven-day hospitalization was more effective or less costly.

Measurement Problems and Methods

The selection of appropriate outcome variables is critical to the success of a study (Bernstein & Hilborne, 1993), but the method of measurement of those variables is just as important. As in any study, the researcher must evaluate the evidence of validity and the reliability of the measurement methods. However, because so much of the data used for outcomes research is drawn from existent data sources, the researcher often has no control over the method of measurement or its accuracy (see Chapter 17 for discussion of the quality of databases).

As previously discussed, rather than selecting the final outcome of care, which may not occur for months or years, researchers use measures of proximate outcomes, sometimes those that are available in existent databases. It is important for the researcher to make a logical argument as to the validity of the proximate outcomes in predicting the final outcome (Freedman & Schatzkin, 1992). Analyses of the degree of correlation between the proximate outcome and the final outcome of care should be included, whenever possible.

In most population-based or other large-sample outcome studies, researchers select outcome measures so that they can utilize secondary data sources (e.g., Lasater, Sloane, & Aiken, 2015). Secondary analysis is "any reanalysis of data or information collected by another researcher or organization, including analysis of data sets collected from a variety of sources to create time-series or area-based data sets" (Shi, 2008, p. 129). Data collected through NDNQI or CALNOC can be used in nursing outcomes research. Secondary analysis poses problems because, in most cases, data cannot be verified.

In evaluating a particular outcome measure, the researcher should consult the literature for previous studies that have used that same method of measurement, including the publication describing development of the method of measurement. Sensitivity to change is an important measurement property to consider in outcomes research because researchers often are interested in evaluating how outcomes change in response to healthcare interventions. As the sensitivity of a measure increases, statistical power increases, allowing smaller sample sizes to detect significant differences. Chapter 16 provides a more complete discussion of reliability and validity of scales and questionnaires, precision and accuracy of physiological measures, and sensitivity and specificity of diagnostic tools.

Statistical Methods for Outcomes Studies

On a methodological level, Donabedian (1980) stressed that when performing research on healthcare quality, Type I error should be preferred to Type II error: in other words, sample sizes should not be small, and level of significance should be set high enough (0.05 to 0.10) to achieve possibly erroneous positive results with moderate samples. This was quite divergent from the medical research practices of the time, in which levels of significance were set at 0.01 to 0.05.

Because of the huge samples utilized for much of outcomes research, mastery of statistical methods or employment of a statistician is mandatory. In addition, some databases are compiled using weighted sampling, in which persons of minority groups are oversampled. When studies are conducted using these weighted databases, sophisticated statistical methods are needed to report the results for a corresponding unweighted sample. Multiple regression analysis is just as much an art as a science, and a good statistician develops an eye for best methods of analysis. Some effects discerned in large-sample database data are subtle, so it is essential to calculate the needed sample size for a given effect size, using power analysis (Grove & Cipher, 2017).

Analysis of Change and Analysis of Improvement

Analysis of change is used in trend analysis studies. Analysis of change can be determined by using *t*-tests, percentage comparison, ANOVA (analysis of variance), ANCOVA (analysis of covariance), correlational analyses, and chi-square analyses. However, the interpretation of the test must be appropriate, and the test must fit the level of measurement and the research question. To reiterate, careful operationalization of variables is essential. There is much benefit in performing multiple measures and tracking an indicator and an outcome over time. With analysis of change, more data are better than not enough.

Analysis of improvement is a directional version of analysis of change. Because statistical tests for analysis of improvement focus on one direction only, statistical significance may be reached with smaller samples than for analysis of change. Whenever possible, quantification of improvement is preferable to a binary "did improve versus did not improve" measure.

Measures of Outcomes That May Be Used Non-Numerically

Variance analysis in outcomes research, in practice, is a lot less like arithmetic than it sounds. It is merely a strategy that defines expected outcomes, and the times they are expected to occur, based on population means, and then tracks delay or non-achievement of these outcomes. Delays and non-achievements are called variances. A critical pathway is a listing of expected short-term and long-term outcomes within a specific problem focus. When a patient fails to achieve an intermediate outcome by the expected time, a variance is said to have occurred. Variance analysis can also be used to identify at-risk patients who might benefit from the services of a case manager. Variance analysis tracking is sometimes expressed through the use of graphics, with the expected pathway plotted on a graph. The care providers plot deviations (negative variances) on the graph.

Longitudinal modeling is a method for analysis of data collected over time (Pretz et al., 2013). Data are obtained from population means and reflect achievement of anticipated outcomes. As with variance analysis, longitudinal models are useful for tracking outcomes that have an indefinite time of appearance because they reflect repeated measures.

Latent transition analyses (Scorza, Masyn, Salomon, & Betancourt, 2015) are projected probabilities or proportions of expected outcomes, and they track movement over a series of outcomes. They are helpful in keeping perspective about a patient's recovery or progress during an attenuated treatment, providing an idea of how an individual patient responds over time. Because they are based on an average of actual patient progress within the population, they allow simple quantification of the concept of outcome variance.

Multilevel Analysis

Multilevel analysis is merely use of more than one way to analyze a data set. In outcomes research, an unexpectedly positive outcome may be associated with increases or decreases in certain structural or process variables. Multilevel analysis uses statistical techniques, allowing the researcher to "tease out" various different factors that seem promising in predicting an outcome using multiple regression analysis. In outcomes research, multilevel analysis is useful for assigning attribution when many factors are involved. It also may be used to determine major predictors of an outcome and to predict the proposed effect of planned changes.

Reistetter et al. (2015) used multilevel analysis in their research examining functional status with inpatient stroke recovery treatment, from standpoints of both geography and facility variation. Excerpts from their abstract explain their study and its findings.

"Objective: To examine geographic and facility variation in cognitive and motor functional outcomes after post-acute inpatient rehabilitation in patients with stroke.

Design: Retrospective cohort design using Centers for Medicare and Medicaid Services (CMS) claims files. Records from 1209 rehabilitation facilities in 298 hospital referral regions (HRRs) were examined … Multilevel models were used to calculate the variation in outcomes attributable to facilities and geographic regions …

Participants: Patients (N = 145,460) with stroke discharged from inpatient rehabilitation from 2006 through 2009 …

Main Outcome Measures: Cognitive and motor functional status at discharge measured by items in the CMS Inpatient Rehabilitation Facility—Patient Assessment Instrument.

Results: Variation profiles indicated that 19.1% of rehabilitation facilities were significantly below the mean functional status rating (mean SD, 81.58 22.30), with 221 facilities (18.3%) above the mean. Total discharge functional status ratings varied by 3.57 points across regions. Across facilities, functional status values varied by 29.2 points, with a 9.1-point difference between the top and bottom deciles. Variation in discharge motor function attributable to HRR was reduced by 82% after controlling for cluster effects at the facility level.

Conclusions: Our findings suggest that variation in motor and cognitive function at discharge after post-acute rehabilitation in patients with stroke is accounted for more by facility than geographic location." (Reistetter et al. 2015, p. 1248)

In this example, the multilevel analysis was a useful technique for determining that differences in facilities were more important to stroke rehabilitation than geographical location.

KEY POINTS

- Outcomes research is quantitative. Qualitative methods may inform the direction and interpretation of outcomes research.
- Donabedian developed the theory on which outcomes research is based.
- Quality is the overriding construct of Donabedian's theory, which he defined as "the balance of health benefits and harm" (1980, p. 27).
- The three major concepts of the theory are structures, processes, and outcomes.
- Some structural variables are attributes of a healthcare facility, such as equipment of care, educational preparation/skill mix of healthcare workers, care protocols, staffing, and workforce size.
- Some process variables are standards of care, individual technical expertise, professional judgment, degree of patient participation, and patient-practitioner interactions.
- Donabedian defined outcomes as clinical endpoints, satisfaction with care, functional status and general well-being. He emphasized that outcome was determined by "what consumers expect, want, or are willing to accept" (1987, p. 5).
- Outcomes, whenever possible, should be clearly linked with the processes and structures with which they are associated.
- An NSPO is an outcome influenced by nursing care decisions, actions, or attributes.
- Organizations currently involved in efforts to study nursing-sensitive outcomes include the American Nurses Association, the National Quality Forum, the Collaborative Alliance for Nursing Outcomes, the Veterans Affairs Nursing Outcomes Database, the Center for Medicare and Medicaid Services' Hospital Quality Initiative, the American Hospital Association, the Federation of American Hospitals, The Joint Commission, and the Agency of Healthcare Research and Quality.
- Most measurements obtained for outcomes research are retrospective and obtained from existent data sources, such as clinical and administrative databases.
- Statistical approaches used in outcomes studies are usually descriptive or correlational, using very large samples. Levels of significance are usually $p < 0.05$ or occasionally even less stringent. In outcomes research, Type I error is preferred to Type II error.

REFERENCES

Agency for Healthcare Research and Quality (AHRQ). (2015a). *Agency for Health Research and Quality. PCOR Grant* Awards.

Retrieved August 29, 2015 from http://www.ahrq.gov/news/newsroom/press-releases/2015/pcorawards.html.

Agency for Healthcare Research and Quality (AHRQ). (2015b). *Agency for Healthcare Research and Quality. Clinical guidelines and recommendations.* Retrieved August 29, 2015 from http://www.ahrq.gov/professionals/clinicians-providers/guidelines-recommendations/index.html.

Agency for Healthcare Research and Quality (AHRQ). (2015c). *Agency for Healthcare Research and Quality. What is comparative effectiveness research.* Retrieved March 17, 2016 from http://effectivehealthcare.ahrq.gov/index.cfm/what-is-comparative-effectiveness-research1/.

Aiken, L. H., Sermeus, W., Van den Heede, K., Sloane, D. M., Busse, R., McKee, M., et al. (2012). Patient safety, satisfaction, and quality of hospital care: Cross-sectional surveys of nurses and patients in 12 countries in Europe and the United States. *British Medical Journal, 2012*(344), 1–14. doi:10.1136/bmj.e1717. Retrieved March 19, 2016 from http://www.bmj.com/content/344/bmj.e1717.

American Nurses Credentialing Center (ANCC). (2015). *ANCC Magnet Recognition Program.* Retrieved March 19, 2016 from http://nursecredentialing.org/Magnet.aspx.

Asher, E., Reuveni, H., Shlomo, N., Gerber, Y., Beigel, R., Narodetski, M., et al. (2015). Clinical outcomes and cost effectiveness of accelerated diagnostic protocol in a chest pain center compared with routine care of patients with chest pain. *PLoS ONE, 10*(1), e0117287.

Baoyue, L., Bruyneel, L., Sermeus, W., Van den Heede, K., Matawie, K., Aiken, L. H., et al. (2013). Group-level impact of work environment dimensions on burnout experiences among nurses: A multivariate multilevel probit model. *International Journal of Nursing Studies, 50*(2), 281–291.

Bednarczyk, R. A., Curran, E. A., Orenstein, W. A., & Omer, S. B. (2014). Health disparities in human papillomavirus vaccine coverage: Trends analysis from the National Immunization Survey-Teen, 2008–2011. *Clinical Infectious Diseases, 58*(2), 238–241.

Bernstein, S. J., & Hilborne, L. H. (1993). Clinical indicators: The road to quality care? *Joint Commission Journal on Quality Improvement, 19*(11), 501–509.

Brennan, C. W., Daly, B. J., & Jones, K. R. (2013). State of the science: The relationship between nurse staffing and patient outcomes. *Western Journal of Nursing Research, 35*(6), 760–794.

Bruyneel, L., Baoyue, L., Aiken, L., Lesaffre, E., Van den Heede, K., & Sermeus, W. (2013). A multi-country perspective on nurses' tasks below their skill level: Reports from domestically trained nurses and foreign trained nurses from developing countries. *International Journal of Nursing Studies, 50*(2), 202–209.

Carter, M., & Tourangeau, A. E. (2012). Staying in nursing: What factors determine whether nurses intend to remain employed. *Journal of Advanced Nursing, 68*(7), 1589–1600.

Centers for Disease Control and Prevention (CDC). (2015). *CDC A-Z Index.* Retrieved March 19, 2016 from http://www.cdc.gov/az/c.html.

Centers for Medicare and Medicaid Services (CMS). (2015). *Hospital-acquired conditions.* Retrieved March 19, 2016 from https://www.cms.gov/medicare/medicare-fee-for-service-payment/hospitalacqcond/hospital-acquired_conditions.html.

Centers for Medicare and Medicaid Services (CMS). (2014). *IRFS (Inpatient Rehabilitation Facilities) quality reporting program (QRP).* Retrieved March 19, 2016 from https://www.cms.gov/medicare/quality-initiatives-patient-assessment-instruments/irf-quality-reporting/index.html.

Chelimsky, E. (1997). The political environment of evaluation and what it means for the development of the field. In E. Chelimski & W. R. Shadish (Eds.), *Evaluation for the 21st century: A handbook* (pp. 53–68). Thousand Oaks, CA: Sage Publications.

Chen, Y.-G., Lin, C.-L., Ho, C. L., Chen, Y.-C., & Kao, C.-H. (2015). Risk of coronary artery disease in transfusion-naïve thalassemia populations: A nationwide population-based retrospective cohort study. *European Journal of Internal Medicine, 26*(4), 250–254.

Collaborative Alliance for Nursing Outcomes (CALNOC). (2015). *CALNOC. About.* Retrieved March 19, 2016 from http://www.calnoc.org/?page=A1.

Dawson, R., & Tilley, N. (1997). An introduction to scientific realist evaluation. In E. Chelimski & W. R. Shadish (Eds.), *Evaluation for the 21st century: A handbook* (pp. 405–418). Thousand Oaks, CA: Sage Publications.

Donabedian, A. (1980). *Explorations in quality assessment and monitoring. Volume I. The definition of quality and approaches to its assessment.* Ann Arbor, MI: Health Administration Press.

Donabedian, A. (1987). Some basic issues in evaluating the quality of health care. In L. T. Rinke (Ed.), *Outcome measures in home care* (Vol. I, p. 338). New York, NY: National League for Nursing. (Original work published 1976.).

Donabedian, A. (1990). The seven pillars of quality. *Archives of Pathology and Laboratory Medicine, 114*(11), 1115–1118.

Donabedian, A. (2003). *An introduction to quality assurance in health care.* Oxford, UK: Oxford University Press.

Donabedian, A. (2005). Evaluating the quality of medical care. *Milbank Quarterly, 83*(4), 691–729.

Doran, D. M. (Ed.), (2011). *Nursing outcomes: The state of the science* (2nd ed.). Sudbury, MA: Jones & Bartlett.

Fenton, J. J., Jerant, A. F., Bertakis, K. D., & Franks, P. (2012). The cost of satisfaction: A national study of patient satisfaction, health care utilization, expenditures, and mortality. *JAMA Internal Medicine, 172*(5), 405–411.

Fisher, S., Gao, H., Yasui, Y., Dabbs, K., & Winget, M. (2015). Treatment variation in patients diagnosed with early stage breast cancer in Alberta from 2002 to 2010: A population-based study. *BMC Health Services Research, 15*, 35. Retrieved March 19, 2016 from http://www.ncbi.nlm.nih.gov/pmc/articles/PMC4308832/?report=classic.

Flexner, A. (2002). Medical education in the United States and Canada: A report to the Carnegie Foundation for the Advancement of Teaching. *World Health Organization. Bulletin of the World Health Organization, 80*(7), 594–602. Retrieved March 18, 2016 from http://www.ncbi.nlm.nih.gov/pmc/articles/PMC2567554/.

Freedman, L. S., & Schatzkin, A. (1992). Sample size for studying intermediate endpoints within intervention trials or observational studies. *American Journal of Epidemiology, 136*(9), 1148–1159.

Frenk, J. (2000). Obituary: Avedis Donabedian. *World Health Organization. Bulletin of the World Health Organization, 78*(12), 1475.

Goossens, L. M. A., Utens, C., Smeenk, F., Van Schayck, O. C. P., Van Vliet, M., Van Litsenburg, W., et al. (2013). Cost-effectiveness of early assisted discharge for COPD exacerbations in the Netherlands. *Value in Health: The Journal of the International Society for Pharmacoeconomics and Outcomes Research, 16*(4), 517–528.

Grove, S. K., & Cipher, D. J. (2017). *Statistics for nursing research: A workbook for evidence-based practice* (2nd ed.). St. Louis, MO: Elsevier.

Guess, H. A., Jacobsen, S. J., Girman, C. J., Oesterling, J. E., Chute, C. G., Panser, L. A., et al. (1995). The role of community-based longitudinal studies in evaluating treatment effects. Example: Benign prostatic hyperplasia. *Medical Care, 33*(Suppl. 4), AS26–AS35.

Hirashima, F., Patel, R. B., Adams, J. E., Bertges, D. J., Callas, P. W., Steinthorsson, G., et al. (2012). Use of a postoperative insulin protocol decreases wound infection in diabetics undergoing lower extremity bypass. *Journal of Vascular Surgery, 56*(2), 396–402.

Jennings, B. M., Loan, L. A., DePaul, D., Brosch, L. R., & Hildreth, P. (2001). Lessons learned while collecting ANA indicator data. *Journal of Nursing Administration, 31*(3), 121–129.

Keeley, R. D., West, D. R., Tutt, B., & Nutting, P. A. (2014). A qualitative comparison of primary care clinicians' and their patients' perspectives on achieving depression care: Implications for improving outcomes. *BMC Family Practice, 15*(1), 13–36. Retrieved March 19, 2016 from http://www.ncbi.nlm.nih.gov/pmc/articles/PMC3907132/?report=classic.

Kelly, K. C., Huber, D. G., Johnson, M., McCloskey, J. C., & Maas, M. (1994). The Medical Outcomes Study: A nursing perspective. *Journal of Professional Nursing, 10*(4), 209–216.

Kelsey, J. L., Petitti, D. B., & King, A. C. (1998). Key methodologic concepts and issues. In R. C. Brownson & D. B. Petitti (Eds.), *Applied epidemiology: Theory to practice* (pp. 35–69). Cary, NC: Oxford University Press.

Kerlinger, F. N., & Lee, H. B. (2000). *Foundations of behavioral research* (4th ed.). Fort Worth, TX: Harcourt College Publishers.

Kieffer, E., Alexander, G. R., & Mor, J. (1992). Area-level predictors of use of prenatal care in diverse populations. *Public Health Reports, 107*(6), 653–658.

Kleib, M., Sales, A., Doran, D. M., Malette, C., & White, D. (2011). Nursing minimum data sets. In D. M. Doran (Ed.), *Nursing outcomes: The state of the science* (2nd ed., pp. 487–512). Sudbury, MA: Jones & Bartlett.

Kopf, E. W. (1916). Florence Nightingale as statistician. *Publications of the American Statistical Association, 15*(116), 388–404.

Kutney-Lee, A., McHugh, M. D., Sloane, D. M., Cimiotti, J. P., Flynn, L., Neff, D. F., et al. (2009). Nursing: A key to patient satisfaction. *Health Affairs, 28*(4), W669–W677.

Kutney-Lee, A., Sloane, D. M., & Aiken, L. H. (2013). An increase in the number of nurses with baccalaureate degrees is linked to lower rates of postsurgery mortality. *Health Affairs, 32*(3), 579–586.

Lasater, K. B., Sloane, D. M., & Aiken, L. H. (2015). Hospital employment of supplemental registered nurses and patients' satisfaction with care. *Journal of Nursing Care Quality, 45*(3), 145–151.

Lawson, E. F., & Yazdany, J. (2012). Healthcare quality in systemic lupus erythematosus: Using Donabedian's conceptual framework to understand what we know. *International Journal of Clinical Rheumatology, 7*(1), 95–107.

Lee, T. H., & Goldman, L. (1989). Development and analysis of observational data bases. *Journal of the American College of Cardiology, 14*(Suppl. 3A), 44A–47A.

Li, B., Bruyneel, L., Sermeus, W., Van den Heede, K., Matawie, K., Aiken, L., et al. (2013). Group-level impact of work environment dimensions on burnout experiences among nurses: A multivariate multilevel probit model. *International Journal of Nursing Studies, 50*(2), 281–291.

Martin, B. I., Mirza, S. K., Franklin, G. M., Lurie, J. D., MacKenzie, T. A., & Deyo, R. A. (2013). Hospital and surgeon variation in complications and repeat surgery following incident lumbar fusion for common degenerative diagnoses. *Health Services Research, 48*(1), 1–25.

Mazurek Melnyk, B., Kelly, S., & Lusk, P. (2014). Outcomes and feasibility of a manualized cognitive-behavioral skills building intervention: Group cope for depressed and anxious adolescents in school settings. *Journal of Child and Adolescent Psychiatric Nursing, 27*(1), 3–13.

McDonald, D. C., Carlson, K., & Izrael, D. (2012). Geographic variation in opioid prescribing in the U.S. *The Journal of Pain, 13*(10), 988–996.

McQuestion, M., Gnawali, D., Kamara, C., Kizza, D., Mambu-Ma-Disu, H., Mbwangue, J., et al. (2011). Creating sustainable financing and support for immunization programs in fifteen developing countries. *Health Affairs, 30*(6), 1134–1140.

Mishra, P. H., & Gupta, S. (2012). Study of patient satisfaction in a surgical unit of a tertiary teaching hospital. *Journal of Clinical Orthopaedics and Trauma, 3*(1), 43–47.

Mitchell, P. H., Ferketich, S., Jennings, B. M., & American Academy of Nursing Expert Panel on Quality Health Care. (1998). Quality Health Outcomes Model. *Image: Journal of Nursing Scholarship, 30*(1), 43–46.

Mullan, F. (2001). A founder of quality assessment encounters a troubled system firsthand. *Health Affairs, 20*(1), 137–141.

National Database of Nursing Quality Indicators (NDNQI). (2011). *National database of nursing quality indicators. What is NDNQI?* Retrieved March 19, 2016 from http://nursingandndnqi.weebly.com/what-is-ndnqi.html.

National Quality Forum. (NQF). (2015). *National Quality Forum.* Retrieved March 19, 2016 from http://www.qualityforum.org/Home.aspx.

Nichols, M., Abrams, J. J., Greenhut, R., Rudin, S., MacNair (Producers), & Nichols, M. (Director) (1991). *Regarding Henry* [film]. Los Angeles, CA: Paramount.

Nurses' Health Study 3. (2013). *Nurses' Health Study 3 Our Story.* Retrieved March 18, 2016 from http://www.nhs3.org/index.php/our-story.

Oncology Nursing Society (ONS). (2015). *Oncology Nursing Society. Putting evidence into practice.* Retrieved March 19, 2016 from https://www.ons.org.

Palacios, N., Fitzgerald, K., Roberts, A. L., Hart, J. E., Weisskopf, M. G., Schwarzschild, M. A., et al. (2014). A prospective analysis of airborne metal exposures and risk of Parkinson disease in the Nurses' Health Study cohort. *Environmental Health Perspectives, 122*(9), 933–938.

Pape, T. (2013). The effect of a five-part intervention to decrease omitted medications. *Nursing Forum, 48*(3), 211–222.

Pearson, S. D., Goulart-Fisher, D., & Lee, T. H. (1995). Critical pathways as a strategy for improving care: Problems and potential. *Annals of Internal Medicine, 123*(12), 941–948.

Petitti, D. B. (1998). Epidemiologic issues in outcomes research. In R. C. Brownson & D. B. Petitti (Eds.), *Applied epidemiology: Theory to practice* (pp. 177–211). Cary, NC: Oxford University Press.

Press Ganey. (2015). *Press Ganey performance and advanced analytics. Quality and clinical outcomes. Nursing quality: NDNQI.* Retrieved March 19, 2016 from http://www.pressganey.com/oursolutions/performance-and-advanced-analytics/clinical-business-performance/nursing-quality-ndnqi.

Pretz, C. R., Kozlowski, A. J., Dams-O'Connor, K., Kreider, S., Cuthbert, J. P., Corrigan, J. D., et al. (2013). Descriptive modeling of longitudinal outcomes measures in traumatic brain injury: A National Institute on Disability and Rehabilitation Research Traumatic Brain Injury Model Systems study. *Archives of Physical Medicine and Rehabilitation, 94*(3), 579–588.

Pyenson, B., Sander, M., Jiang, Y., Kahn, H., & Mulshine, J. (2012). An actuarial analysis shows that offering lung cancer screening as an insurance benefit would save lives at relatively low cost. *Health Affairs, 31*(4), 770–779.

Ramani, K. V., Mavalankar, D., Patel, A., & Mehandiratta, S. (2007). A GIS approach to plan and deliver healthcare services to urban poor: A public private partnership model for Ahmedabad City, India. *International Journal of Pharmaceutical and Healthcare Marketing, 1*(2), 159–173.

Ramis, R., Diggle, P., Boldo, E., Garcia-Perez, J., Fernandez-Navarro, P., & Lopez-Abente, G. (2012). Analysis of matched geographical areas to study potential links between environmental exposure to oil refineries and non-Hodgkin lymphoma mortality in Spain. *International Journal of Health Geographics, 11*, 4. Retrieved March 18, 2016 from http://www.ij-healthgeographics.com/content/11/1/4.

Reistetter, T. A., Kuo, Y.-F., Karmarkar, A. M., Eschbach, K., Teppala, S., Freeman, J. L., et al. (2015). Geographic and facility variation in inpatient stroke rehabilitation: Multilevel analysis of functional status. *Archives of Physical Medicine and Rehabilitation, 96*(7), 1248–1254.

Riley, G. F., Levy, J. M., & Montgomery, M. A. (2009). Adverse selection in the Medicare prescription drug program. *Health Affairs, 28*(6), 1826–1837.

Schubert, M., Clarke, S., Aiken, L. H., & De Geest, S. (2012). Association between rationing of nursing care and inpatient mortality in Swiss hospitals. *International Journal for Quality in Health Care, 24*(3), 230–238. doi:10.1093/intqhc/mzs009.

Scorza, P., Masyn, K. E., Salomon, J. A., & Betancourt, T. S. (2015). A latent transition analysis for the assessment of structured diagnostic interviews. *Psychological Assessment, 27*(3), 975–984.

Shi, L. (2008). *Health services research methods* (2nd ed.). Clifton Park, NY: Delmar Cengage Learning.

Tarlov, A. R., Ware, J. E., Jr., Greenfield, S., Nelson, E. C., Perrin, E., & Zubkoff, M. (1989). The Medical Outcomes Study: An application of methods for monitoring the results of medical care. *JAMA: The Journal of the American Medical Association, 262*(7), 925–930.

Tourangeau, A. E., Saari, M., Patterson, E., Themson, H., Ferron, E. M., Widger, K., et al. (2014). Work, work environments and other factors influencing nurse faculty intention to remain employed: A cross-sectional study. *Nurse Education Today, 34*(6), 940–947.

Tourangeau, A. E., Widger, K., Cranley, L., Bookey-Bassett, S., & Pachis, J. (2009). Work environments and staff responses to work environments in institutional long-term care. *Health Care Management Review, 34*(2), 171–181.

Trinkoff, A. M., Han, K., Storr, C. L., Lerner, N., Johantjen, M., & Gartrell, K. (2013). Turnover, staffing, skill mix, and resident outcomes in a national sample of U.S. nursing homes. *Journal of Nursing Administration, 43*(12), 630–636.

Van Bogaert, P., Timmermans, O., Weeks, S. M., van Heusden, D., Wouters, K., & Franck, E. (2014). Nursing unit teams matter: Impact of unit-level nurse practice environment, nurse work characteristics, and burnout on nurse reported job outcomes, and quality of care, and patient adverse events—A cross-sectional survey. *International Journal of Nursing Studies, 51*(8), 1123–1134.

Van den Heede, K., Lasaffre, E., Diya, L., Vleugels, A., Clarke, S. P., Aiken, L. H., et al. (2009a). The relationship between inpatient cardiac surgery mortality and nurse numbers and educational level: Analysis of administrative data. *International Journal of Nursing Studies, 46*(6), 796–803.

Van den Heede, K., Sermeus, W., Diya, L., Clarke, S. P., Lesaffre, E., Vleugels, A., et al. (2009b). Nurse staffing and patient outcomes in Belgian acute hospitals: Cross-sectional analysis of administrative data. *International Journal of Nursing Studies, 46*(7), 928–939.

Volinn, E., Diehr, P., Ciol, M. A., & Loeser, J. D. (1994). Why does geographic variation in health care practices matter (and seven questions to ask in evaluating studies on geographic variation)? *Spine, 19*(18S), 2092S–2100S.

West, E., Barron, D. N., Harrison, D., Rafferty, A. M., Rowan, K., & Sanderson, C. (2014). Nurse staffing, medical staffing and mortality in intensive care: An observational study. *International Journal of Nursing Studies, 51*(5), 781–794.

Zerzan, J. T., Morden, N. E., Soumerai, S., Ross-Degnan, D., Roughhead, E., Zhang, F., et al. (2006). Trends and geographic variation of opiate medication use in state Medicaid fee-for-service programs, 1996-2002. *Medical Care, 44*(11), 1005–1010.

Zivin, K., Yosef, M., Miller, E. M., Valenstein, M., Duffy, S., Kales, H. C., et al. (2015). Associations between depression and all-cause and cause-specific risk of death: A retrospective cohort study in the Veterans Health Administration. *Journal of Psychosomatic Research, 78*(4), 324–331.

Mixed Methods Research

Jennifer R. Gray

ⓔ http://evolve.elsevier.com/Gray/practice/

Quantitative research and qualitative research have different philosophical foundations. Because of these differences in philosophy, researchers do not always agree on the best approach with which to address a research problem. The convergence of technology with health disparities and the complexity of the healthcare system have given rise to several research problems that cannot be answered completely with either type of research (Morgan, 2014; Sadan, 2014; Shneerson & Gale, 2015; van Griensven, Moore, & Hall, 2014). As a result, researchers combine quantitative and qualitative designs into one study, with increasing frequency, using the methodology called **mixed methods research** (Creswell, 2014; 2015). Using mixed methods offers researchers the ability to use the strengths of both qualitative and quantitative research designs (Creswell, 2015) to answer different stages or parts of a complex research question. Although some research experts (Munhall, 2012) have argued that using two qualitative methodologies in a single study is mixed methods research, for this chapter we will be describing only designs in which quantitative and qualitative methods are combined.

This chapter begins with a description of the philosophical foundation of mixed methods research and continues with descriptions of three mixed methods study designs, with an example of a published study for each type. The challenges of conducting a mixed methods enquiry will be discussed, followed by criteria by which mixed methods studies can be evaluated.

PHILOSOPHICAL FOUNDATIONS

The philosophical underpinnings of mixed methods research and the paradigms that best fit these methods continue to evolve. At the foundation of the differences between qualitative and quantitative studies are philosophical differences regarding the question, "What is truth?" A philosophy's ontology (What is? or What is true?) shapes the epistemology (how we can know the truth), that then influences the methodology (research design) (Morgan, 2014). Over the last few years, many researchers have departed from the idea that one paradigm or one research strategy is superior, and instead have taken the position that the search for knowledge requires the use of all available strategies. Researchers who hold these views and seek answers using mixed methods may have exchanged the dichotomy of positivism and constructivism for the "epistemological middle ground" of pragmatism (Yardley & Bishop, 2015, p. 1). However, the interpretations of what pragmatism is, as applied to mixed methods research, have differed (Bishop, 2015). For our purposes, pragmatism refers to the researcher's consideration of the research question and the knowledge needed for the discipline (desired outcome) before selecting a methodology. The desired outcome guides the selection of a methodology that is most likely to address questions within a problem area (Florczak, 2014; Morgan, 2014). As discussed in previous chapters, the process of developing a study design is iterative and reflexive. Decisions are made tentatively about the question and the design and then reconsidered as each phase is developed. Because an in-depth analysis of pragmatism as a philosophy is beyond the scope of this chapter, we are basing our discussion on the goal of pragmatism, which is solving the problem by "choosing the appropriate design for the research aim" (Yardley & Bishop, 2015, p. 2). With mixed methods designs, the researcher can allow the strengths of one method to compensate for the possible limitations of the other (Creswell, 2015). Stated in a more positive way, mixed methods research allows the strengths of each method to interact in a complementary way with the other.

OVERVIEW OF MIXED METHODS DESIGNS

The focus on problem-solving or answering the research question means that a mixed methods research design is selected based on study purpose, timing of the quantitative and qualitative elements, and emphasis on one element over the other. Table 14-1 provides a description of mixed methods designs classified by the research-er's reason for combining methods. The purpose of combining two methods may result in a classification based on the order in which quantitative and qualitative elements of the study are implemented (Table 14-2). Another way to label mixed methods designs is according to which element is emphasized. In this classification, the emphasized element is noted in uppercase letters (QUANT or QUAL) and the other element in lowercase font (quant or qual). Table 14-3 provides an overview of this classification.

Creswell (2014) presented three basic designs that are a combination of the other classifications: convergent parallel mixed methods, explanatory sequential mixed methods, and exploratory sequential mixed methods. Three advanced designs, according to Creswell (2014, 2015), are: (1) embedded mixed methods designs, also called intervention designs; (2) transformative mixed methods, also called social justice methods; and (3) multiphase mixed methods, also called multistage evaluation designs. Morgan (2014) described using the initial method (quantitative or qualitative) as prelude to the second, or using the initial method as the priority and using the second to clarify or follow up on the first phase's results.

From this discussion, you can see that there are multiple perspectives from which you can describe mixed methods designs. For simplicity, we are limiting our discussion to the three approaches usually implemented in nursing and health research and consistent with

TABLE 14-1 Mixed Methods Classified by Purpose

Label	Description
Exploratory	Qualitative methods are used to explore a new topic, followed by quantitative methods that measure aspects of what was learned qualitatively
Explanatory	Quantitative methods are used to establish evidence related to incidence, relationship, or causation. Then qualitative methods provide a more robust explanatory description of the human experience aspect of the quantitative results.
Transformative	Quantitative and qualitative methods are used with a community-based research team to address a social problem in the community.
Advocacy	Quantitative and qualitative methods are used, guided by feminism, disability theory, race/ethnicity theory, or other approach to providing information to raise awareness of the needs of a specific group; aspects of advocacy research may overlap with transformative designs.

Data from Creswell, J. W. (2015). *A concise introduction to mixed methods research.* Los Angeles, CA: Sage; and Bishop, F. (2015). Using mixed methods research designs in health psychology: An illustrative discussion from a pragmatist perspective. *British Journal of Health Psychology,* 20(1), 5–20.

TABLE 14-2 Typology of Mixed Methods Designs Based on Timing of Quantitative and Qualitative Elements

Label	Description
Sequential	Either the quantitative or the qualitative phase may be implemented first. Results from the first phase of the study are used to inform the specific methods of the second phase.
Concurrent	Qualitative and quantitative elements are implemented at the same time through the study. Findings are integrated at interpretation.

Data from Creswell, J. W. (2015). *A concise introduction to mixed methods research.* Los Angeles, CA: Sage; and Bishop, F. (2015). Using mixed methods research designs in health psychology: An illustrative discussion from a pragmatist perspective. *British Journal of Health Psychology,* 20(1), 5–20.

TABLE 14-3 Typology of Mixed Methods Designs by Emphasis, Sequence, and Integration

Label	Description
QUANT + qual	Quantitative elements are the primary methods used to answer the research question; at the same time, a supplementary aim or secondary question may be addressed by using qualitative methods.
QUANT → qual	Quantitative methods are implemented first, chronologically, and are emphasized in the analysis and in the reporting of findings.
QUAL + quant	Qualitative elements are the primary methods used to answer the research question; at the same time, a supplementary aim or secondary question may be addressed by using quantitative methods.
QUAL → quant	Qualitative methods are implemented first, chronologically, and are emphasized in the analysis and in the reporting of findings.
quant → QUAL	Quantitative methods are implemented first, chronologically, but qualitative methods are emphasized in the analysis and in the reporting of findings.
qual → QUANT	Qualitative methods are implemented first, chronologically, but quantitative methods are emphasized in the analysis and in the reporting of findings.

Note: Uppercase font indicates the study element that is emphasized with lowercase font indicating the less emphasized element; + indicates concurrent implementation; → indicates sequential implementation.
Data from Creswell, J. W. (2015). *A concise introduction to mixed methods research*. Los Angeles, CA: Sage; Bishop, F. (2015). Using mixed methods research designs in health psychology: An illustrative discussion from a pragmatist perspective. *British Journal of Health Psychology*, 20(1), 5–20; and Morse, J., & Nierhaus, L. (2009). *Mixed method design: Principles and procedures*. Walnut Creek, CA: Left Coast Press.

Creswell's (2014) three basic designs: (1) exploratory sequential strategy, (2) explanatory sequential strategy, and (3) convergent concurrent strategy.

To decide which design is appropriate, you should begin by contemplating the purpose for combining the methods. This decision will shape the study. A researcher may implement a sequential study design in which the results of the first phase, either quantitative or qualitative, will determine the specific methods for the second phase. To accomplish this, the findings of the first phase must be completed prior to beginning the second phase. When this is the goal of using the two methods, the design will be sequential (Morgan, 2014), but sequential studies can also be performed to expand findings by using two types of data, providing a more robust view of the phenomenon of interest. In additive studies, data may be collected sequentially but could just as easily be collected concurrently, because integration of all data occurs during analysis.

Mixed methods studies in which data are collected concurrently are called **parallel designs** by some research experts (Creswell, 2014, 2015), because convergence does not occur until interpretation. When convergence occurs at interpretation, each phase could stand alone as a separate study and may be published separately (Morgan, 2014). Concurrent mixed methods designs can also have multiple points of convergence

with both types of data being examined throughout data collection and analysis. In this chapter, models of the three mixed methods approaches and examples of each are provided to expand your understanding of these designs.

Exploratory Sequential Designs

The **exploratory sequential design** begins with collection and analysis of qualitative data, followed by collection of quantitative data. Often, findings of the qualitative data analysis are used to design the quantitative phase (Figure 14-1). This approach may be used to design a quantitative tool (Morgan, 2014). For example, focus groups may be conducted with members of a target population and items for the quantitative tool developed using phrases and content generated qualitatively. Another reason to use this strategy is to collect data about patients' perspectives concerning an issue or problem, so that their point of view is represented. With this input, an intervention can be developed or refined, incorporating the patients' perspectives about the intervention. An example would be a research team planning to implement an educational intervention and seeking input from members of the target population to gain the patient's perspective concerning the content to be taught. Morgan (2014) noted also that qualitative findings may generate hypotheses for the quantitative phase.

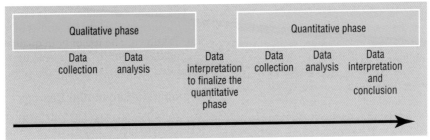

FIGURE 14-1 Exploratory sequential mixed methods.

Exploratory sequential designs may be selected for reasons other than shaping of quantitative methods by qualitative findings. Exploratory sequential strategies also may be indicated when a topic has not been studied previously, and qualitative data are collected first so that participants will not be biased by the content of the quantitative instruments. Ladegard and Gjerde (2014) provide an example of an exploratory sequential study in which the qualitative findings along with the literature were used to determine the hypotheses and outcomes of a theory-based leadership coaching intervention.

"A two-phase exploratory sequential design (Creswell & Clark, 2011) was chosen to address different research questions: What generic outcome criteria should be used to assess the effect of leadership coaching? Does leadership coaching have a positive effect on these outcome criteria? To what extent do differences in facilitative coach behavior influence this effect? An additional reason for choosing this research design was that it enables a more comprehensive account of leadership as a leadership development tool." (Ladegard & Gjerde, 2014, pp. 632, 635)

The qualitative phase of the study was a focus group to address the first research question. Through the focus group with five experienced leadership coaches, Lardegard and Gjerde (2014) identified the outcome to be assessed for the quantitative phase of the study. From the qualitative findings, the researchers integrated existing theory into two hypotheses.

"Two valuable and appropriate outcome criteria for evaluating coaching effectiveness stood out from the focus group discussion: confidence in one's ability to be an effective leader, and confidence in subordinates' ability to take on responsibility." (Ladegard & Gjerde, 2014, pp. 632, 635)

Ladegard and Gjerde (2014) placed their qualitative findings into a theoretical context and recognized that confidence in one's ability to be an effective leader was the same concept as self-efficacy. The researchers examined the literature related to self-efficacy in leadership roles and, based on their review, hypothesized that leadership coaching would "positively influence leader role-efficacy" (Ladegard & Gjerde, 2014, p. 636). The relational aspects of the leadership role had been articulated clearly in the literature, allowing the researchers to identify the concept to be measured as "trust in subordinates" (p. 636). The second hypothesis was that leadership coaching would positively "influence leaders' trust in subordinates" (p. 636). Based on their qualitative findings and examination of the literature, Ladegard and Gjerde (2014) proposed three additional hypotheses.

"**Hypothesis 3**. A leader's increased trust in his/her subordinates is associated with (a) an increase in the subordinates' psychological empowerment and (b) a decrease in their turnover intentions ... **Hypothesis 4**. Facilitative coach behavior will affect leader role-efficacy positively... **Hypothesis 5**. Facilitative coach behavior will affect trust in subordinates positively." (Ladegard & Gjerde, 2014, pp. 637–638)

Ladegard and Gjerde (2014) described the quantitative portion of their study as a field experiment. They described the sampling and the intervention given to the treatment group.

"The second part of this study was a field experiment chosen to test the propositions and hypotheses developed in the first part of the study. The objective was to reveal the effect of coaching on LRE [leadership role-efficacy] and LTS [leader's trust in subordinates] compared with a control group (between-group analysis) and whether changes in trust had any effect on subordinates, and to test whether facilitative coach behavior would predict variation in the two leader outcome variables (within-group analysis). We collaborated with a small coaching company that invited coaches from their network into the project ... The leader questionnaire developed during the first part of the study was distributed to the 34 participants one week before the coaching sessions started ... a follow-up questionnaire was sent to the 30 participants who replied in the first round. Of these, six did not respond, and the final sample included 24 participating leaders, which represents a response rate of 73% ... From the participating organizations, we received 192 email addresses to subordinates, to which we distributed a questionnaire at the same points of time as we did to the leaders. We then matched the subordinates to their leaders, a process that shrank the sample considerably ... The resulting final sample of subordinates comprised 80 respondents, of which 63 belonged to the coaching group of leaders. The number of subordinates per leader in the final sample ranged from two to seven, with an average of 2.7 per leader." (Ladegard & Gjerde, 2014, p. 638)

The results of the quantitative data analysis supported all five hypotheses. Ladegard and Gjerde (2014) noted the practical and theoretical implications of their findings, as well as the study limitations.

"Our study adds to the knowledge base of both formative and summative evaluation, and argues that leadership coaching is a valuable leadership development tool. The strength of our study lies in our use of a mixed methods design combining qualitative and quantitative methods, providing us with opportunities for expansion and development. Our combination of methods and data sources should give a more complete picture of the effects of leadership coaching as a leadership development tool than any one of these alone." (Ladegard & Gjerde, 2014, p. 644)

The study exemplifies the benefits of using exploratory sequential designs for studies of topics about which little is known. The use of both qualitative and quantitative methods allowed the researchers to develop well-grounded hypotheses and test them in the same study.

Explanatory Sequential Designs

When using an **explanatory sequential design**, the researcher collects and analyzes quantitative data, and then collects and analyzes qualitative data to explain the quantitative findings (Figure 14-2). The findings represent integration of the data. Qualitative examination of the phenomenon facilitates a fuller understanding and is well suited to explaining and interpreting relationships.

Explanatory sequential designs are easier to implement than are designs in which quantitative and qualitative data are collected at the same time. This type of approach shares the disadvantage of other sequential designs in that it also requires a longer period of time and more resources than would be needed for one single-method study. Published studies using this strategy are more difficult to identify in the literature because the two phases sometimes are published separately, as was the case for Lam, Twinn, and Chan's (2010) study of dietary adherence in patients with renal failure. Lam et al. (2010) reported the findings from the quantitative phase of a study of self-reported adherence with dialysis, medications, diet, and fluid restriction in a sample of 173 persons who were on a regimen of continuous peritoneal dialysis. The participants were asked if they would be willing to participate in a follow-up qualitative interview if selected. The patients reported being more adherent with medications and dialysis than with diet and fluid restrictions. Lam et al. (2010) also found relationships between adherence and gender, age, and the patients' length of time since beginning dialysis.

Based on these findings, Lam, Lee, and Shiu (2014) designed the qualitative methods to include maximum

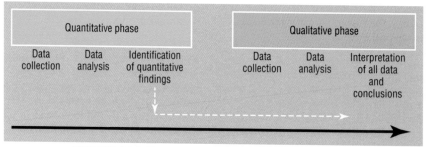

FIGURE 14-2 Explanatory sequential mixed methods.

variation sampling, selecting participants who exemplified different ages, genders, and time since dialysis treatment had begun. Lam et al.(2014) explored patients' perspectives on living with continuous ambulatory peritoneal dialysis. The researchers interviewed 36 persons (18 female, 18 male), analyzing data qualitatively as they continued their interviews with subsequent participants. One of the categories identified, the process of adherence, was the focus of the Lam et al. (2014) study report. The authors found that participants adjusted their adherence over time to fit with their lives. During the first 2 to 6 months of dialysis, participants followed instructions carefully for all aspects of the regimen. Most were completely adherent; however, some did not achieve strict adherence with respect to diet and fluids because of knowledge deficits about what they needed to do and how diet and fluid restrictions were related to the dialysis (Lam et al. 2014). Others attributed their partial adherence to an "inability to abstain from their desires to eat or drink" (Lam et al. 2014, p. 911).

During these first few months, participants became increasingly aware of the restrictions imposed by their regimen and the requirements of adherence (Lam et al. 2014). Travel was difficult because of having to sequester time for three dialysate exchange periods every day. Favorite, easily available foods were not allowed. Participants began to adjust the regimen to be more manageable and less restrictive. The consequences of less than strict adherence caused uncomfortable symptoms and complications, some resulting in hospitalizations.

After the first 6 months, "participants began to secretly experiment with an easy-going approach to adherence" (Lam et al. 2014, p. 912) and developed their own adherence profile, which the researchers labeled as sustained adherence. As they experimented, the participants worked through a process of letting some aspects of the regimen "slip" followed by monitoring the effects of the change. The participants made "continuous adjustments to live as normal a life as possible" (Lam et al., 2014, p. 912). This phase lasted 3 to 5 years.

Long-term adherence emerged as the participants assimilated to a new way of life that became normal (Lam et al., 2014, p. 914). They selectively made modifications that had fewer negative consequences by knowing their physiological limits. The dynamic process of adherence emerged from the qualitative data because the selected participants had been maximally diverse: male and female, different ages, and on dialysis for different lengths of time. The researchers selected this type of sample because of the results of the quantitative phase of the overall study.

Convergent Concurrent Designs

The **convergent concurrent design** is a more familiar approach to researchers. This type of design is selected when a researcher wishes to use quantitative and qualitative methods in an attempt to confirm, cross-validate, or corroborate findings within a single study, using a single sample. Convergent concurrent designs generally use separate quantitative and qualitative methods as a mechanism to allow the strengths of the two methods to complement each other. Therefore, quantitative and qualitative data collection processes are conducted concurrently. This strategy usually integrates the results of the two methods during the interpretation phase, and convergence strengthens the knowledge claims, whereas the lack of convergence identifies areas for future studies or theory development (Figure 14-3). Great researcher effort and expertise are needed to study a phenomenon with two methods. Because two different methods are employed, researchers are challenged with the difficulty of comparing the study results from each arm of the study and determining the overriding findings. It is still unclear how to best resolve discrepancies in findings between methods (Creswell, 2014).

Njie-Carr (2014) conducted a convergent concurrent study on the topic of interpersonal violence (IPV) with African American (AA) male perpetrators and AA women who were HIV-infected and had experienced or been threatened with IPV in the past 12 months. Njie-Carr described the research problem as being the need for gender-specific interventions to decrease women's vulnerability to IPV and the lack of research on "men's perceptions of their roles in violence against women" (p. 376). Especially noted was the lack of a concurrent approach to study this common problem. The researcher argued that female and male perspectives were needed to develop "effective and sustainable prevention interventions tailored to the unique needs of AA women who are survivors of IPV" (Njie-Carr, 2014, p. 377). To obtain a multifaceted view of IPV, Njie-Carr identified one study purpose related to factors of IPV in HIV-infected women, another purpose to explore the self-perceptions of abusers' roles as perpetrators of IPV, and a final purpose to determine the implications of triangulating the data.

"... IPV is a critical component of HIV risk and infection ... integrating information gained from understanding male perpetrators' roles in propagating violence against women is critically needed to ensure effective, culturally relevant, and sustainable interventions." (Njie-Carr, 2014, p. 378)

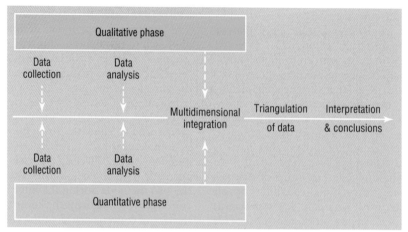

FIGURE 14-3 Convergent concurrent mixed methods.

Njie-Carr (2014) used Fishbein's (2000) integrative model as a conceptual framework for the study. The integrative model combines concepts of the theories of planned behavior, health belief, and social cognitive theory. The integrative model itself offered multiple perspectives that supported the various aspects of the study design.

Figure 14-4 is a diagram of the study design that Njie-Carr (2014) provided in the article. In the diagram, the quantitative and qualitative arms of the study are identified as remaining separate until results were obtained from each, followed by triangulation of the integrated results and finally critical interpretation of those triangulated results. Triangulation is a metaphor taken from navigating ships and surveying land. In these fields, a location is determined by obtaining measurements from two perspectives. The point of intersection between the two perspectives determines the location of a distant object. In this study, triangulation was the process used to integrate data from two samples (men and women) and two methodologies (quantitative and qualitative).

"A concurrent Mixed Method study design was used ... to adequately capture multiple dimensions of male and female participant experiences by comparing and contrasting qualitative and quantitative results. The qualitative component was guided by Giorgi's method. This phenomenological descriptive approach was thought to be appropriate because it would help gain a better understanding of AA women's lived experiences of abuse and AA men's perceptions of their roles as perpetrators of violence

(Dowling & Cooney, 2012) ... In this study, it was important to capture unique contributions of each methodological approach in the context of the participants' cultural and social relationship experiences in order to triangulate the findings." (Njie-Carr, 2014, p. 378)

Njie-Carr (2014) specified inclusion and exclusion criteria for study participants. Quantitative and qualitative data were collected from "15 AA male and 15 AA female participants" who were recruited from different sites (Njie-Carr, 2014, p. 377). The women were recruited from the clinic where they received HIV care. The men had been arrested for domestic abuse and mandated by the court to attend a rehabilitation program that focused on developing their skills in anger management and in conflict management. The men in the study were in a situation in which signing an informed consent for a study on this topic could be viewed as an admission of guilt, so they provided verbal consent. The women signed consent forms.

"To ensure consistency across the research team (project investigator and research assistants), a data collection guide was included as a cover sheet that itemized the sequence of activities during the data collection process: (a) introductions and brief overview of the study, (b) consent with either a signed form (female) or verbal agreement (male), (c) personal data form/review of medical records, (d) interview using interview guide, (e) completion of eight survey instruments, and (f) provision of health information brochure." (Njie-Carr, 2014, pp. 379–380)

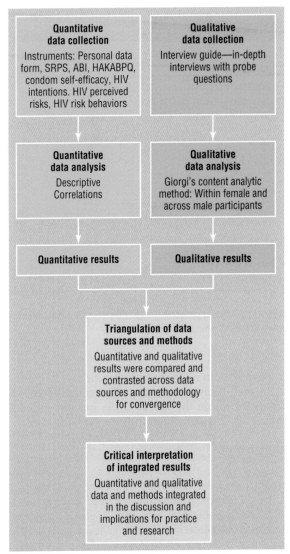

FIGURE 14-4 *SRPS*, Sexual Relationships Power Scale; *ABI*, Abusive Behaviors Inventory; *HAKABPQ*, HIV/AIDS Knowledge, Attitudes, and Beliefs Patient Questionnaire. Study design. (Adapted from Njie-Carr, V. [2014]. Violence experiences among HIV-infected women and perceptions of male perpetrators' roles: A concurrent mixed method study. *Journal of the Association of Nurses in AIDS Care, 25*[5], 379.)

Giorgi's phenomenological techniques for analysis (Sandelowski, 2000) were used, which are consistent with Husserl's views of phenomenology. Integration of data collected from the men and the women occurred first during the qualitative analysis, as noted in the study

excerpt about clustering quotes with similar meanings into themes.

"… similar patterns of meanings from each source (male or female) were identified and clustered into categories related to the emerging themes … meanings related to women's abuse experiences as well as perceptions of men's roles in perpetrating violence. Themes were also compared across male and female responses to determine convergence … themes were synthesized and conceptualized within the context of the participants' experiences. Analyses were conducted in an iterative process to ensure that themes were consistent with the raw data and could be identified across samples." (Njie-Carr, 2014, p. 381)

Njie-Carr (2014) articulated the steps taken to ensure auditability, credibility, and confirmability of the qualitative phase of the study. The quantitative component involved administration of eight instruments (Table 14-4). The Decision-Making Dominance subscale of the Power Scale had much lower reliability in the male group (0.21) than in the female group (0.89). Both groups were small for quantitative research, a factor that decreases the internal consistency of instruments. However, only one other subscale, HIV/AIDS Knowledge, had an internal consistency reliability coefficient lower than 0.7 and only in the male group.

Njie-Carr's (2014) quantitative findings revealed that the men in the sample engaged in more unprotected oral, vaginal, and anal sexual intercourse than did the women. Among the women, as expected, statistically significant positive relationships were found between age and education ($r = .743$, $p \leq 0.001$), physical abuse and social beliefs ($r = .718$, $p = 0.003$), and psychological and physical abuse ($r = .845$, $p \leq 0.001$). Expected negative relationships were also found in that higher levels of psychological abuse were linked to lower levels of control in their dyadic relationships ($r = -.750$, $p \leq 0.001$). An unexpected finding was that strong social support had a statistically significant positive relationship with high incidence of psychological abuse ($r = .718$, $p = 0.003$) and high incidence of physical abuse ($r = .718$, $p = 0.003$). Njie-Carr (2014) explained this by noting that women who are being abused may be more likely to seek support from their networks.

The triangulation of Njie-Carr's (2014) quantitative and qualitative data did not occur until both sets of data were analyzed and interpreted. The researchers first triangulated the qualitative results for the women and men and provided a side-by-side table with themes and exemplars from either group.

TABLE 14-4   Instruments Used in a Convergent Concurrent Mixed Methods Study of Interpersonal Violence in the Context of HIV Infection

Instrument	Variables	Number of Items
Personal Data Form	Age, education, employment, mean income per week, current and past substance use, medical information (not specified)	22
Sexual Relationship Power Scale (Pulerwitz et al., 2000)	Relationship control, decision making	23
HIV and AIDS Questionnaire (Njie-Carr, 2005)	Knowledge of HIV, attitudes, social beliefs, spiritual beliefs, cultural beliefs	60
Condom Self-Efficacy Scale (Hanna, 1999)	Effective communication related to condoms, safe application of condoms	14
Abusive Behavior Inventory (Shepard & Campbell, 1992)	Dimensions of abuse: psychological, sexual, emotional, physical	29
HIV Intentions Scale (Melendez et al., 2003)	Intentions to use a condom	9
Perceived HIV Risk Scale (Harlow, 1989)	Perception of HIV risk	
HIV Risk Behavior Inventory (Gerbert et al., 1998)	Specific risk behaviors	12*

*Based on possible maximum score of 12.
Data from Njie-Carr, V. (2014). Violence experiences among HIV-infected women and perceptions of male perpetrators' roles: A concurrent mixed method study. *Journal of the Association of Nurses in AIDS Care, 25*(5), 376–391.

"When female and male data sources were triangulated, data convergence was noted, with similar themes expressed by male and female participants. Both groups shared the perception that males dominated relationships, resulting in power imbalances … a similar theme was patriarchal ideology and the need to control and institute power … most of the male and female participants reported childhood abuse. When asked how their experiences as children impacted adulthood, participants reported that negative childhood experiences might have resulted in the use of substances and alcohol, and for males being abusive to their female partners." (Njie-Carr, 2014, pp. 384, 386)

Both groups also identified what they believed could be done to prevent abuse in the future. Men and women provided different views, however, of the motivations for abusing women.

"Female participants noted that a partner's level of education, inability to deal with stress, and drugs may have contributed to her vulnerability to abusive experiences. Male participants reported that they were stressed and frustrated in their efforts to make a living, which resulted in abusive tendencies." (Njie-Carr, 2014, p. 386)

Triangulation resulted in convergence across quantitative and qualitative results. The convergence was expected because the items on the quantitative tools guided the development of the interview questions.

"Specifically, the contribution of relationship power on the psychological and physical abuse experiences of female participants, as noted in the quantitative analyses, were significant. Furthermore, similar findings were found with substance and alcohol abuse, childhood abuse, and increased risk for HIV infection from abusive experiences. These results demonstrated that variables and themes were cross-validated by using two data sources and two methodological approaches." (Njie-Carr, 2014, p. 386)

One limitation of the study noted by the researcher was "the small sample size for the quantitative component" (Njie-Carr, 2014, p. 389). Njie-Carr (2014, p. 389) did make the case that her study generated "important preliminary evidence." The researcher was committed to triangulating the results in parallel, thus requiring use of the same sample for both arms of the study. Although the modest sample size increased the risk of Type II error due to low power, conducting the qualitative analysis with data from a larger sample would have made the study unwieldy and likely unfeasible. Nonetheless, statistical significance was achieved for the quantitative tests, implying that the small sample size, despite the author's observation, was not a true limitation and not representative of Type II error. Other limitations were the use of self-report instruments and the researcher's lack of access to the male participants' medical records to ascertain their HIV status. The low reliability of the Power Scale for the men's group indicated an unacceptable level of measurement error, making these data uninterpretable. Self-report instruments may produce inaccurate data due to social desirability, but self-report may be the only way to operationalize the relevant concepts. Implications for future research and health services were identified.

"Interviewing females and their partners as a dyad may have provided a stronger methodological approach, but concerns for the women's safety precluded undertaking such a design in this study ... additional research studies identifying contextual and structural causal pathways are needed to clarify critical factors that substantially contribute to HIV infection in the context of IPV ... AA female participants reported their hesitancy to access medical care and treatment as a result of negative experiences with healthcare providers. This finding shows the need to educate healthcare workers about effective approaches to care for women survivors of violence." (Njie-Carr, 2014, p. 389)

The extensive data collected from each person, the triangulation of findings across the different groups, and the types of data obtained resulted in a robust study. As noted, the sample size was small, but the findings represent a solid foundation for additional studies by this researcher and others interested in the topic of IPV. The study involved concurrent data collection, but integration across data did not occur until the analysis and interpretation of each type of data were completed. Other concurrent convergence studies may show more evidence of data integration during the data collection and analysis such as Goldman and Little's (2015) study of Maasai women's empowerment in Northern Tanzania.

CHALLENGES OF MIXED METHODS DESIGNS

Combining Quantitative and Qualitative Data

Limited guidance is available concerning how to combine data that are collected using two different research approaches (Östlund, Kidd, Wengström, & Rowa-Dewar, 2011). Historically, methodological

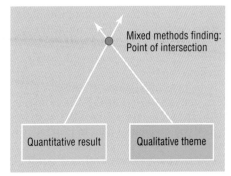

FIGURE 14-5 Triangulation with convergence.

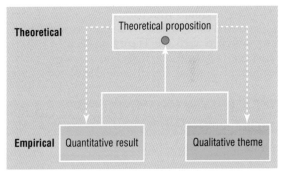

FIGURE 14-6 Empirical and theoretical triangulation.

triangulation (Denzin, 1970) was what mixed methods studies were first called. However, the process whereby integration of findings occurred was not well defined. In research, triangulation may be the use of more than one research design or multiple sources of data, to allow the researcher to approximate "truth" more precisely.

Figure 14-5 displays triangulation as simple convergence. Östlund et al. (2011) describe triangulation as empirical findings integrated into one theoretical proposition, with the triangulation occurring between the grounded or empirical findings and the more abstract or theoretical implications. Figure 14-6 is a visual representation of empirical-theoretical triangulation. The authors also provided diagrams of other types of integration of data between the empirical findings and theoretical propositions. Östlund et al. (2011) describe using theoretical propositions to guide the development of mixed methods studies and seeking convergence between the empirical findings and the theory. In Figure 14-6, the arrows down from the theoretical level toward the empirical indicate theory concepts and propositions guiding the study design. The arrows from the empirical to the theoretical indicate the findings being integrated at the theory level.

In keeping with pragmatism, the motivation for the study and the desired outcome determine the best way to integrate the data of a mixed methods study (Morgan, 2014). Depending on the purposes of the study, presentation of findings can be accomplished using various types of graphs, tables, and figures (Creswell, 2015). Some researchers support converting the data from one arm of the study to the same type as the other arm: essentially, this means using qualitative data to generate (quantitative) counts of frequency with which various codes or themes occurred. For example, DuBay et al. (2014) quantified their qualitative data, so as to make confirmatory comparisons with their quantitative data. They studied organ donation registration of African Americans by conducting focus groups with participants, some of whom had registered as organ donors and others who had not. The researchers used the Theory of Planned Behavior (Ajzen, 1991) to guide the study and provided a table of the theory's concepts linked with related focus group questions. For themes that emerged related to each concept, the percent of responses to the specific focus group question that was related to each concept was determined. The display and the analysis required to create that display reflected the point of integration.

Whether you build one phase of a study on the previous one, expanding the view of a phenomenon, or strengthen support for the findings by producing both quantitative and qualitative results that are interpreted together, articulate your plans to integrate the data in the study proposal. It is critical to make at least tentative decisions about integrating the data as you plan the study. The plans may need to be adjusted during the study, but they provide the structure needed to successfully complete the study.

Table 14-5 provides possible ways to display the findings of studies with different motivations and strategies. Tables 14-6, 14-7, 14-8, 14-9, and 14-10 are examples of each type of display using mythical data.

TABLE 14-5 **Exploratory Sequential: Integration and Display of Quantitative and Qualitative**

Strategy	Study Goal	Type of Display	Description
Exploratory sequential	Use qualitative findings to develop a quantitative instrument or intervention	Construction of instrument display	Table: First column with quote or theme; second column has the item or items developed from the specific finding.
Exploratory sequential	Add quantitative findings to the qualitative findings	Expanding perspective display	Table: First column with qualitative study finding; second column has supportive evidence that may be numerical or textual.
Explanatory sequential	Explain the quantitative results using qualitative results	Follow-up results joint display	Table: First column with quantitative findings; second column has the corresponding additional information from the qualitative component; third column has information articulating the links between the two types of data.
Convergent concurrent	Display findings that converge between the components	Matrix of interpretation of convergence and divergence	Matrix: First column of each row is filled with the qualitative results (themes or patterns); columns are labeled with quantitative variables; cells contain findings that result from the integration of that theme and variable. Not all cells will be filled.
Convergent concurrent	Identify similarities (convergence) and difference (divergence) between the two types of data	Matrix/graph of points of convergence and divergence	Matrix/graph: x-axis is the quantitative findings by question or variable; y-axis is the themes or qualitative findings. Where findings converged, mark the point with a plus sign; where findings diverged, mark the point with a negative sign.

Adapted from Creswell, J. W. (2015). *A concise introduction to mixed methods research.* Los Angeles, CA: Sage.

TABLE 14-6 Example Display for an Exploratory Sequential Study: Developing an Instrument

Quotation from a Participant	Resulting Item on Instrument (Respondents Select Five Options from *Strongly Disagree* [1] to *Strongly Agree* [5])
"When I looked in the mirror and saw how fat I looked, I knew I had to stop eating junk food and eat healthy food."	My appearance motivates me to eat healthier.
"Some of my friends are real health nuts and it is easier to exercise and eat right around them. Other of my friends think exercising is texting their friends."	My health-related behaviors are influenced by whom I hang out with.
"I tried going to the gym and there wasn't anyone my age who was there. The music they used during classes was really old-school."	I want to exercise in a safe place with other people my age. When I exercise, I want to listen to my favorite music.
"I have a job at a fast-food restaurant. I can eat for free, but there isn't much on the menu that is healthy. I can't afford to bring fruit and healthier snacks."	I eat healthier when in a place with many healthy foods on the menu. The cost influences my food choices.

Data from a mythical study to develop an instrument to measure "Intent to Change Health Behaviors among Adolescents."

TABLE 14-7 Example Display for an Exploratory Sequential Study: Expanding Perspectives

Quotation From a Participant	Related Quantitative Finding
"When I looked in the mirror and saw how fat I looked, I knew I had to stop eating junk food and eat healthy food."	$M = 4.5$ ($SD = 0.8$) on the Body Image Scale $r = 0.4$ ($p = 0.001$) between body image and healthy food choices
"Some of my friends are real health nuts and it is easier to exercise and eat right around them. Other of my friends think exercising is texting their friends."	$r = -0.28$ ($p = 0.01$) between sensitivity to peer pressure and healthy food choices
"I tried going to the gym and there wasn't anyone my age who was there. The music they used during classes was really old-school."	Response to open-ended question about reasons for not exercising: "No gyms where my age goes"
"I have a job at a fast-food restaurant. I can eat for free, but there isn't much on the menu that is healthy. I can't afford to bring fruit and healthier snacks."	Subjects with lower incomes scored lower on Healthy Food Choice Scale than subjects with higher incomes did ($t = 8.3$, $df = 1$, $p = 0.05$).

Data from a mythical study to provide an expanded perspective on the intent of adolescents to change their health behaviors.

TABLE 14-8 Example Display for an Explanatory Sequential Study: Follow-Up Results Joint Display

Quantitative Results	Qualitative Results	Integration
Low scores on self-efficacy related to healthy eating	"I never know what to eat at a party." "I usually eat what everyone else is eating."	Lack of knowledge may contribute to low self-efficacy related to healthy eating.
Significant difference in knowledge of healthy foods between adolescents with higher incomes and adolescents with lower incomes	"There is no grocery store in my neighborhood, only a convenience store on the corner." "I've read about nutritious fruits like kiwi and cantaloupe but I don't even know what they are. No one eats that kind of thing where I live."	Adolescents living in lower income neighborhoods may have limited access and exposure to healthy foods.

Integration of data from a mythical study to explain adolescents' intent to change their health behaviors using a mixed methods study.

TABLE 14-9 Example Display for a Convergent Concurrent Study: Matrix of Interpretation of Convergence and Divergence

Qualitative Themes	QUANTITATIVE FINDINGS				
	Body Image	Self-Efficacy	Knowledge	Environment	Behaviors
Desire to fit in				Being accepted in my neighborhood	
Inner beauty	Positive view of self				
Knowing I can do it		Strong belief in self			Healthy behaviors require commitment
Access to healthy foods			Without access, hard to know	Neighborhood makes a difference	
"Cool" place to exercise	No mirrors but great music				Easier to exercise in an adolescent-friendly place

Note: Cells contain findings that result from the integration of that theme and variable.
Integration of data from a mythical study to explain adolescents' intent to change their health behaviors using a mixed methods study.

TABLE 14-10 Example Display for a Convergent Concurrent Study: Matrix Graph of Points of Convergence and Divergence

Qualitative Themes	Body image	Self-efficacy	Knowledge	Environment	Behaviors
Desire to fit in		(−)			
Inner beauty	+			(−)	+
Knowing I can do it		+	+		+
Access to healthy foods	(−)		(−)	+	+
"Cool" place to exercise			(−)	+	
	Quantitative Results				

Note: Convergence noted by plus sign. Divergence noted by negative sign.
Integration of data from a mythical study to explain adolescents' intent to change their health behaviors using a mixed methods study.

Use of Resources

As you can surmise from the examples provided in the chapter, mixed methods studies require time commitment that may exceed that required for single method studies. Goldman and Little (2015) collected data over a 4-year period for their mixed methods study of Maasai women's empowerment in Northern Tanzania. Qualitative data were generated through 47 individual interviews, 11 group interviews, and 150 hours of ethnographic observation. The authors' time commitment and extensive data collection resulted in a rigorous study. Studies with an advocacy focus or ethnographic data collection, such as the Goldman and Little (2015) study, require longer periods of time than many other designs because researchers must spend extensive time becoming accepted in the community. Sequential designs require collection and analysis of data amassed during the first phase of the study before moving to the second phase. Phased data collection also lengthens the time required to complete the study. Sequential methods are not recommended when the researcher has limited time to complete a degree or establish a trajectory of research for advancement on tenure track at a university (Creswell, 2015).

Additional time also may mean that additional financial resources are needed (van Griensven et al., 2014). Because of the complexity of concurrent designs, funding may be needed to ensure that the study is completed. It is sometimes possible to assemble a research team of health professionals with different education and experiences, each one of which is responsible for a portion of a study. Individual researchers may hire a consultant to provide guidance for the component of the study with which the researcher is less familiar. Either approach can result in additional funding needs. Extra time may be required for research teams to come to agreement on the study purpose, design, and methods. Points of disagreement among team members may become a deterrent to study completion.

Functioning of the Research Team

Mixed methods studies require a team of researchers with skills in different methods (Creswell, 2015). A single researcher who is expert in all of the skills needed for a mixed methods study is rare (van Griensven et al., 2014; Yardley & Bishop, 2015). When members of different professions comprise a team, disagreements may arise when each member is biased as to the superiority of his or her preferred method, leading to minimization or negation of the findings of the other method (Morgan, 2014; Wisdom & Creswell, 2013). The means of integration can be a particularly difficult issue unless the team's philosophical foundation was discussed during the design phase (van Griensven et al., 2014). Quantitative researchers on a team may be skeptical about the value of the qualitative findings (van Griensven et al., 2014) or require that qualitative data be analyzed by frequencies of the quotes linked to each theme. Qualitative researchers on a team may lack the knowledge of quantitative methods required to assess the data and the methods for rigor or may resist presentation of findings they perceive to be disrespectful of the perspectives of the participants. When working with a team, a well-planned study allows such issues to be addressed early in project development.

CRITICALLY APPRAISING MIXED METHODS DESIGNS

The quality standards by which to appraise mixed methods designs continue to evolve (Creswell, 2015). Pluye, Gagnon, Griffiths, and Johnson-Lafleur (2009) conducted a systematic review of the literature to identify or develop quality standards for mixed methods reviews. Their conclusion was that each component of a mixed methods study could be appraised separately followed by a three-question assessment of the quality of the data integration. The Office of Behavioral and Social Science Research at the National Institutes of Health (NIH) convened a panel of experts to develop best practices for mixed methods research (Creswell, Klassen, Clark, & Smith, 2011). Part of the panel's charge was to identify criteria by which applications for NIH funding could be evaluated. For this text, we have synthesized standards across sources, resulting in a concise set of quality standards for mixed methods research (Table 14-11).

Building on your knowledge of quantitative and qualitative methods, learning how to critique mixed methods studies extends your capacity as a scholar. These standards of quality displayed in Table 14-11 provide a systematic method for critically appraising mixed methods studies. Using the quality standards proposed, a critical appraisal of a mixed methods study conducted by DuBay et al. (2014) is provided as an example.

Summary of the Study

DuBay et al. (2014), a team of 13 researchers, examined decisions by African Americans (AA) to become organ donors. The convergent concurrent mixed methods design included qualitative data that were collected through six focus groups and quantitative data that were collected through a survey administered to focus group participants. The Theory of Planned Behavior (Azjen, 1991) guided both components of the study. During the integration and interpretation of the findings, qualitative data were quantified using frequency of responses and were displayed side-by-side with the quantitative findings for comparison and confirmation.

Significance

AAs are underrepresented among registered organ donors and overrepresented among persons on waiting lists for transplants (DuBay et al., 2014). The study was socially and clinically relevant because the need for organ donors is increasing and the number of persons registered to donate organs is inadequate to meet current needs. The only reason that DuBay et al. (2014, p. 274) gave for using a mixed methods design was that the design had been "previously used in community health research to address health disparities" (Kawamura, Ivankova, Kohler, Perumean-Chaney, 2009; Ruffin et al., 2009). A more compelling reason for using mixed methods would have strengthened the study description.

Expertise

The research team was comprised of three physicians, two of whom also held master's degrees in public health; nine PhD-prepared researchers; and a baccalaureate-prepared employee of an organ center. The first author and the majority of the team were affiliated with the Division of Transplantation at the University of Alabama at Birmingham. DuBay reported the funding received from NIH that supported implementation of the study. The clinical expertise of team members and their educational preparation in research were noted, indicating the team's ability to implement a rigorous study. Two team members coded transcripts because of their experience in qualitative research; information about the

TABLE 14-11	Criteria for Critically Appraising Mixed Methods Studies
Study Characteristic	**Questions Used to Guide the Appraisal**
Significance	1. Was the relevance of the research question convincingly described?
	2. Was the need to use mixed methods established?
Expertise	3. Did the researcher or research team possess the necessary skills and experience to rigorously implement the study?
	4. Were the contributions or expertise of each team member noted?
Appropriateness	5. Were the study purposes aligned with the mixed methods strategy that was used?
	6. Did the mixed methods strategy fulfill the purpose or purposes of the study?
Sampling	7. Was the rationale for selecting the samples for each component of the study provided?
	8. Were study participants selected who were able to provide data needed to address the research question?
Methods	9. Were the methods for each component of the study described in detail?
	10. Were the data collection methods for each study component appropriate to the philosophical foundation of that component?
	11. Was protection of human subjects addressed in the study?
	12. Were the reliability and validity of quantitative methods described?
	13. Were the trustworthiness, dependability, and credibility of qualitative methods described?
	14. Were the timing of data collection, analysis, interpretation, and integration of the data specified?
Findings	15. Was the integration of quantitative and qualitative findings presented visually in a table, graph, or matrix?
	16. Was the integration presented as a narrative?
	17. Were the study limitations noted?
	18. Were the findings consistent with the analysis, interpretation, and integration of the qualitative and quantitative data?
Conclusions and implications	19. Were the conclusions and implications congruent with the findings of the study?
Contribution to knowledge	20. Was the study's contribution to knowledge worth the time and resources of a mixed methods study?

Synthesized from Creswell, J. W. (2015). *A concise introduction to mixed methods research.* Los Angeles, CA: Sage; Creswell, J. W. (2014). *Research design: Qualitative, quantitative, and mixed methods approaches* (4th ed.). Los Angeles, CA: Sage; and Creswell, J., Klassen, A., Plano Clark, V., & Smith, K. (2011). *Best practices for mixed methods research in health sciences.* Retrieved from http://obssr.od.nih.gov/mixed_methods_research.

specific contributions of other team members was not provided.

Appropriateness

The study purpose was stated to be identifying "factors (beyond those already identified) associated with AAs choosing to become a registered organ donor" (DuBay et al., p. 274). Guided by the Theory of Planned Behavior (Azjen, 1991), the qualitative data provided a deeper, contextual description of barriers and facilitators related to organ donation. The quantitative data provided the opportunity to compare and contrast the barriers and facilitators described by participants who were regis-

tered organ donors with those identified by the participants who were not registered organ donors. Qualitative and quantitative study components were simultaneously implemented and were analyzed separately and then combined in a table displaying frequency statistics for qualitative themes, matched with odds ratios for quantitative items, for an expanded understanding of the phenomenon of organ donation. The methods fulfilled the purpose of the study.

Sampling

The sample, used for both study components, was recruited through existing partnerships and networks between the university and the community. To provide a more comprehensive description of the phenomenon, three focus groups were conducted in an urban area and three in a rural area (DuBay et al., 2014). The recruited participants were able to provide data needed to answer the research question because both registered organ donors and those not registered were included.

Methods

For the qualitative component, the stated methods of the study included the protocol for the focus groups and the focus group questions, framed to be consistent with the major constructs of the guiding theory.

"Using the constructs of the Theory of Planned Behavior and the procedures outlined by Morgan (1988) and Kreuger and Casey (2008), members of the investigative team developed the qualitative research protocol to guide focus group discussions … The digitally recorded focus group discussions were transcribed verbatim and analyzed inductively in 2 stages … a standard thematic analysis was conducted to search for common categories and themes in the data. Two qualitative investigators (N.I. and I.H.) independently coded the original transcripts by identifying key points and recurring categories and themes that were central to areas of discussion both within and across focus groups… Particular emphasis in the analysis was placed on how the themes interacted with others to explain intentions to become a registered organ donor within the study's theoretical framework, the Theory of Planned Behavior." (DuBay et al., 2014, pp. 274, 275)

The authors described the development of the survey used to collect the quantitative data. The process was described with adequate detail to convince the reader of its rigor. A preliminary focus group provided input for the survey and assisted in refining the survey down to 31 items (DuBay et al, 2014). To maintain consistency with the Theory of Planned Behavior (Azjen, 1991), questions for the quantitative survey were developed to address the theory's major constructs. Data collected from the preliminary group were not combined with the data collected from study participants. The reading level of the survey was assessed to be at the seventh-grade level. Parametric and non-parametric analyses used were appropriate for data that compared groups.

"Questionnaire results were compared between registered organ donors and nonregistered participants. The primary analytic approaches for dichotomous variables used Pearson χ^2 and Fisher exact test analyses. To summarize the strength and direction of associations, odds ratios and their respective 95% confidence intervals were calculated. Data were expressed as means and standard deviations. The Student t test was used to compare means and the Wilcoxon Rank-Sum test was used to compare median values between registered organ donors and nonregistered participants. Analyses were conducted by using SAS 9.2 software." (DuBay et al., 2014, p. 275)

Qualitative data and quantitative data were collected in a manner congruent with their respective philosophical foundations. Human subjects protection was not described thoroughly, but the researchers indicated that the study was approved by the institutional review board (IRB) of University of Alabama at Birmingham (DuBay et al., 2014). IRB approval is an indicator that the study followed the standards of ethical research.

The content and construct validity of the quantitative instruments were established by the researchers' report of the iterative process used to develop items consistent with the theory that served as the study framework. No information was provided about assessment of the reliability of the survey or its subsections. Although not identified by the researchers as indicators of rigor, the description provided of qualitative data collection, and analysis included measures used to increase credibility, specifically the level of agreement between the independent coding done by two researchers, use of a qualitative software program that included an audit trail for the process, and the inclusion of quotations in the research report that were consistent with identified themes. The NVivo 10 software used for coding allows researchers to explore various combinations of codes, in their search for themes. The software created an audit trail that documented and provided the rationale for the researchers' decision-making process. Evidence to support the credibility and dependability of the qualitative data collection and analysis was documented using these methods. The researchers specified the timing of the data collection and analysis for each phase.

"Mixed methods data analysis and integration of the quantitative and qualitative results were performed at the completion of the separate analyses of the survey and focus group discussion data." (DuBay et al., 2014, p. 275)

Findings

The integration of DuBay et al.'s (2014) quantitative and qualitative results was described and displayed in a table.

"Qualitative themes and categories, organized according to the constructs of the Theory of Planned Behavior, were compared with quantitative survey items in a joint display matrix...the number of text references for qualitative categories were compared with the statistical test probability values for quantitative survey items to identify consistency in the participants' viewpoints about becoming a registered organ donor." (DuBay et al., 2014, p. 275)

The sample consisted of 87 AAs, 22 of whom were registered organ donors. With a mean age of 50 years, the participants were primarily female (DuBay et al., 2014). Study limitations were specified.

"Underrepresentation of males may be especially important, as studies have demonstrated that non-donation attitudes are more likely to be related to medical mistrust in African American males than in African American females (Boulware et al., 2002)...The self-developed items on the questionnaire were not subjected to construct validity testing because of the small sample size... despite attempts to (prospectively) include items on the questionnaire that would measure each qualitative theme discussed during the mock focus group, some new themes emerged during the focus groups (and thus after the questionnaire was developed) for which there were no matching quantitative items. This situation is consistent with the inductive nature of qualitative research and its ability to yield more in-depth exploration of the phenomenon of interest and thus may also be a strength of the study (Lincoln & Guba, 1985)." (DuBay et al., 2014, p. 282)

Because of the matrix display and the description of the methods, the reader can feel confident that the findings were consistent with the collection, analysis, and integration of the data.

Conclusions and Implications

DuBay et al. (2014) identified a previously undocumented finding, which was the "emergence of a self-perception that organs from AAs are often unusable because of the higher prevalence of health issues compared with the prevalence in other races" (p. 281, 282). The implication for practice is that there is a need to include facts related to the usability of organs in community education programs. The findings validated common barriers to organ donation found in the literature such as fear, financial impact on the donor's family, the lack of a proper burial for the donor, and disfigura-

tion of the donor's body. In keeping with AA culture, potential donors would benefit from discussing their decision with family and friends. Familial notification should be incorporated into donor registration, so as to increase the likelihood that a donor's wishes are supported at the time of death (DuBay et al., 2014). Conclusions and implications were congruent with findings.

Contributions to Knowledge

The convergent concurrent mixed methods study conducted by DuBay et al. (2014) uncovered novel insights about organ donation decisions of AAs. Critical appraisal of this mixed methods study supports its rigor and contribution to knowledge.

"Using a mixed methods approach helped not only produce more rigorous conclusions, but allowed better capturing of the nuances that may account for differences in the intentions to become or not to become a registered organ donor. Results from this study suggest new content and motivational messages to include in campaigns to increase African American donor registration." (DuBay et al., 2014, p. 282)

▌ KEY POINTS

- Mixed methods approaches most commonly combine quantitative and qualitative research methods. Data are collected either sequentially or concurrently.
- The philosophical motivation for many mixed methods studies is pragmatism.
- The three mixed methods approaches usually implemented in nursing research are (1) exploratory sequential designs, (2) explanatory sequential designs, and (3) convergent concurrent designs.
- Exploratory sequential designs may be used when the researcher wants to expand on what is known about a phenomenon and the researcher does not want the content of the quantitative instruments to bias data collected qualitatively. These designs are used when the researcher needs insight into participants' perspectives prior to finalizing the quantitative component: they represent explanation of a phenomenon, followed by quantification.
- When using an exploratory sequential strategy, the researcher collects and analyzes qualitative data before beginning the quantitative component of the study. Results from the qualitative component are used to plan or refine the methods of the quantitative phase.

- Explanatory sequential strategies are used to provide additional insight into the topic being studied by providing multiple viewpoints.
- When using the explanatory sequential strategy, the researcher conducts the quantitative component of the study before beginning the qualitative component. After the quantitative data are analyzed, the researcher finalizes the questions for the qualitative phase for the purpose of explaining the quantitative findings. These studies are most useful in providing answers to "why" and "how" questions that arise from quantitative findings.
- Convergent concurrent strategies are used when the research question can be addressed using quantitative and qualitative methods, with one method weighted more heavily. When using convergent concurrent strategies, the researcher collects quantitative and qualitative data at the same time, analyzes each set of data, and integrates the findings. Quantitative and qualitative methods each offer a unique perspective.
- Quantitative and qualitative data usually are combined during analysis or interpretation.
- Mixed methods research strategies require a depth and breadth of research knowledge, as well as a significant commitment of time for completion.
- It is critical to determine the method of integration prior to beginning the study. Integration of the data can be displayed in tables, graphs, or matrices.

REFERENCES

Azjen, I. (1991). The theory of planned behavior. *Organizational Behavior and Human Decisions Processes*, 50(2), 179–211.

Bishop, F. (2015). Using mixed methods research designs in health psychology: An illustrative discussion from a pragmatist perspective. *British Journal of Health Psychology*, 20(1), 5–20.

Boulware, L., Ratner, L., Cooper, L., Sosa, J., LaVeist, T., & Powe, N. (2002). Understanding disparities in donor behavior: Race and gender differences in willingness to donate blood and cadaveric organs. *Medical Care*, 40(2), 85–95.

Creswell, J. W. (2014). *Research design: Qualitative, quantitative, and mixed methods approaches* (4th ed.). Los Angeles, CA: Sage.

Creswell, J. W. (2015). *A concise introduction to mixed methods research*. Los Angeles, CA: Sage.

Creswell, J. W., & Clark, P. (2011). *Designing and conducting mixed methods research* (2nd ed.). Thousand Oaks, CA: Sage.

Creswell, J., Klassen, A., Plano Clark, V., & Smith, K. (2011). *Best practices for mixed methods research in health sciences*. Retrieved March 27, 2016 from https://obssr-archive.od.nih.gov/mixed_methods_research/.

Denzin, N. K. (1970). *The research act*. Chicago, IL: Aldine Publishing.

Dowling, M., & Cooney, A. (2012). Research approaches related to phenomenology: Negotiating a complex landscape. *Nurse Researcher*, 20(2), 21–27.

DuBay, D., Ivankova, N., Herby, I., Wynn, T., Kohler, C., Berry, B., et al. (2014). African American organ donor registration: A mixed methods design using the theory of planned behavior. *Progress in Transplantation*, 24(3), 273–283.

Fishbein, M. (2000). The role of theory in HIV prevention. *AIDS Care*, 12(3), 273–278.

Florczak, K. (2014). Purists need not apply: The case for pragmatism in mixed methods research. *Nursing Science Quarterly*, 27(4), 278–282.

Gerbert, B., Bronstone, A., McPhee, S., Pantilat, S., & Allerton, M. (1998). Development and testing of an HIV-risk screening instrument for use in health care settings. *American Journal of Preventive Medicine*, 15(103), 103–113.

Goldman, M., & Little, J. (2015). Innovative grassroots NGOs and the complex processes of women's empowerment: An empirical investigation from northern Tanzania. *World Development*, 66(2), 762–777.

Hanna, K. (1999). An adolescent and young adult condom self-efficacy scale. *Journal of Pediatric Nursing*, 14(1), 59–66.

Harlow, L. (1989). *Young adult life expectancy survey*. Unpublished manuscript.

Kawamura, Y., Ivankova, N., Kohler, C., & Perumean-Chaney, S. (2009). Utilizing mixed methods to assess parasocial interaction of an entertainment-education program audience. *International Journal of Multiple Research Approaches*, 3(1), 88–104.

Kreuger, R., & Casey, M. (2008). *Focus groups: A practical guide for applied research* (4th ed.). Thousand Oaks, CA: Sage.

Ladegard, G., & Gjerde, S. (2014). Leadership coaching, leader role-efficacy, and trust in subordinates: A mixed methods study assessing leadership coaching as a leadership development tool. *The Leadership Quarterly*, 25(4), 631–646.

Lam, L., Lee, D., & Shiu, A. (2014). The dynamic process of adherence to a renal therapeutic regimen: Perspectives of patients undergoing continuous ambulatory peritoneal dialysis. *International Journal of Nursing Studies*, 51(6), 908–916.

Lam, L., Twinn, S., & Chan, S. (2010). Self-reported adherence to a therapeutic regimen among patients undergoing continuous ambulatory peritoneal dialysis. *Journal of Advanced Nursing*, 66(4), 7763–7773.

Lincoln, Y., & Guba, E. (1985). *Naturalistic inquiry*. Beverly Hills, CA: Sage.

Melendez, R., Hoffman, S., Exner, T., Leu, C., & Ehrhardt, A. (2003). Intimate partner violence and safer sex negotiation: Effects of a gender-specific intervention. *Archives of Sexual Behavior*, 32(6), 499–511.

Morgan, D. (1988). *Focus groups as qualitative research*. Thousand Oaks, CA: Sage.

Morgan, D. (2014). *Integrating qualitative & quantitative methods: A pragmatic approach*. Los Angeles, CA: Sage.

Morse, J., & Nierhaus, L. (2009). *Mixed method design: Principles and procedures*. Walnut Creek, CA: Left Coast Press.

Munhall, P. L. (2012). *Nursing research: A qualitative perspective* (5th ed.). Sudbury, MA: Jones & Bartlett.

Njie-Carr, V. P. (2005). *The HIV/AIDS Knowledge, Attitudes, and Beliefs Patient Questionnaire (HAKABQ)*. Unpublished manuscript. Washington, DC: The Catholic University of America.

Njie-Carr, V. (2014). Violence experiences among HIV-infected women and perceptions of male perpetrators' roles: A concurrent mixed method study. *Journal of the Association of Nurses in AIDS Care, 25*(5), 376–391.

Östlund, U., Kidd, L., Wengström, Y., & Rowa-Dewar, N. (2011). Combining qualitative and quantitative research within mixed method research designs: A methodological review. *International Journal of Nursing Studies, 48*(3), 369–383.

Pluye, P., Gagnon, M. P., Griffiths, F., & Johnson-Lafleur, J. (2009). A scoring system for appraising mixed methods research, and concomitantly appraising qualitative, quantitative and mixed methods primary studies in mixed studies reviews. *International Journal of Nursing Studies, 46*(4), 529–546.

Pulerwitz, J., Gortmaker, S. L., & DeJong, W. (2000). Measuring sexual relationship power in HIV/STD research. *Sex Roles, 42*(7/8), 637–660.

Ruffin, M., Creswell, J., Jimbo, M., & Fetters, M. (2009). Factors influencing choices for colorectal cancer screening among previously unscreened African and Caucasian Americans: Findings from a triangulation mixed methods investigation. *Journal of Community Health, 34*(2), 79–89.

Sadan, V. (2014). Mixed methods research: A new approach. *International Journal of Nursing Education, 6*(1), 254–260.

Sandelowski, M. (2000). Combining qualitative and quantitative sampling, data collection, and analysis techniques in mixed methods. *Research in Nursing & Health, 23*(3), 246–255.

Shepard, M., & Campbell, J. (1992). The Abusive Behavior Inventory—a measure of psychological and physical abuse. *Journal of Interpersonal Violence, 7*(3), 291–305.

Shneerson, C., & Gale, N. (2015). Using mixed-methods to identify and answer clinically relevant research questions. *Qualitative Health Research, 25*(6), 845–856.

van Griensven, H., Moore, A., & Hall, V. (2014). Mixed methods research—The best of both worlds? *Manual Therapy, 19*(5), 367–371.

Wisdom, J., & Creswell, J. (2013). *Mixed methods: Integrating quantitative and qualitative data collection and analysis while studying patient-centered medical home models*. Rockville, MD: Agency for Healthcare Research and Quality. AHRQ Publication No. 13-0028-EF.

Yardley, L., & Bishop, F. (2015). Using mixed methods in health research: Benefits and challenges. *British Journal of Health Psychology, 20*(1), 1–4.

Sampling

Susan K. Grove

ⓔ http://evolve.elsevier.com/Gray/practice/

Many of us have preconceived notions about samples and sampling, acquired from television commercials, polls of public opinion, online surveys, and reports of research findings. The advertiser boasts that four of five doctors recommend its product; the newscaster announces that John Jones is predicted to win the senate election by a margin of 3 to 1; an online survey identifies the jobs with the highest satisfaction rate; and researchers in multiple studies conclude that taking a statin drug, such as atorvastatin (Lipitor), significantly reduces the risk of coronary artery disease.

All of these examples use sampling techniques. However, some of the outcomes are more valid than others, partly because of the sampling techniques used. In most instances, television, news reports, and advertisements do not explain their sampling techniques. You may hold opinions about the adequacy of these techniques, but there is not enough information to make a judgment about the quality of these samples. Published studies usually include a detailed description of the sampling process because the nature of the sample is critical to the credibility of the study findings.

The sampling component is an important part of the research process that needs to be carefully thought out and clearly described. To accomplish this, you need to understand the techniques of sampling and the reasoning behind them. With this knowledge, you can make intelligent judgments about sampling when you are critically appraising studies or developing a sampling plan for your own study. This chapter examines sampling theory and concepts; sampling plans; probability and nonprobability sampling methods for quantitative, qualitative, mixed methods, and outcomes research; sample size; and settings for conducting studies. The chapter concludes with a discussion of the process for

recruiting and retaining participants for study samples in various settings.

SAMPLING THEORY

Sampling theory was developed to determine mathematically the most effective way to acquire a sample that would accurately reflect the population under study. The theoretical, mathematical rationale for decisions related to sampling emerged from survey research, although the techniques were first applied to experimental research by agricultural scientists. Some important concepts of sampling theory include sampling, sampling plan, and sample. **Sampling** involves selecting a group of people, events, behaviors, or other elements with which to conduct a study. A **sampling plan** defines the process of making the sample selections; **sample** denotes the selected group of people or elements included in a study. One of the most important surveys that stimulated improvements in sampling techniques was the United States (U.S.) Census. Researchers have adopted the assumptions of sampling theory identified for census surveys and incorporated them within the research process (Thompson, 2002; Yates, 1981).

Key concepts of sampling theory included in the following sections are: (1) populations, (2) elements, (3) sampling criteria, (4) representativeness, (5) sampling errors, (6) randomization, (7) sampling frames, and (8) sampling plans. The following sections explain these concepts; later in the chapter, these concepts are used to critically appraise various sampling methods.

Populations and Elements

The **population** is a particular group of people, such as people who have had a myocardial infarction, or type of

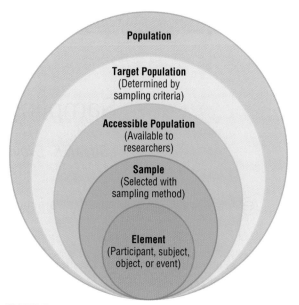

Population

Target Population
(Determined by
sampling criteria)

Accessible Population
(Available to
researchers)

Sample
(Selected with
sampling method)

Element
(Participant, subject,
object, or event)

FIGURE 15-1 Linking populations, sample, and element in research.

element, such as nasogastric tubes, that is the focus of the research. The **target population** is the entire set of individuals or elements meeting the sampling criteria, such as women who have experienced their first myocardial infarction in the past 12 months. Figure 15-1 shows the relationships among the population, target population, and accessible population. An **accessible population** is the portion of the target population to which researchers have reasonable access. The accessible population might be elements within a country, state, city, hospital, nursing unit, or clinic, such as the adults with diabetes in a primary care clinic in Fort Worth, Texas. The sample is obtained from the accessible population by a particular sampling method, such as simple random sampling. The individual units of the population and sample are called **elements**. An element can be a person, event, behavior, or any other single unit of study. When elements are persons, they are usually referred to as **subjects, participants,** or **informants** (see Figure 15-1). The term used by researchers depends on the philosophical paradigm that is reflected in the study and the design. The term "subject," and sometimes "research participant," is used within the context of the positivist or postpositivist paradigm of quantitative research (Shadish, Cook, & Campbell, 2002). The terms "study" or "research participant" and "informant" are used in the context of the naturalistic paradigm of qualitative and often mixed methods research (Creswell,

2014; Munhall, 2012). In quantitative and outcomes research, the findings from a study are generalized first to the accessible population and then, if appropriate, more abstractly to the target population (Doran, 2011; Kerlinger & Lee, 2000).

Generalizing means that the findings can be applied to more than just the sample under study because the sample is representative of the target population (see Figure 15-1). Because generalizing is important, there are risks to defining the accessible population too narrowly. A narrow definition of the accessible population reduces the ability to generalize from the study sample to the target population and diminishes the meaningfulness of the findings. Biases may be introduced with a narrowly defined accessible population that makes generalization to the broader target population difficult to defend. If the accessible population is defined as individuals in a white, upper-middle-class setting, one cannot generalize to nonwhite or lower-income populations. These biases are similar to those that may be encountered in a nonrandom sample and are threats to external validity (Borglin & Richards, 2010).

In some studies, the entire population is the target of the study. These studies are referred to as **population studies**. Many of these studies use data available in large databases, such as the census data or other government-maintained databases. Epidemiologists sometimes use entire populations for their large database studies. In other studies, the entire population of interest might be small and well defined. For example, one could conduct a study in which the target population was all living recipients of heart and lung transplants.

In some cases, a hypothetical population is defined for a study. A **hypothetical population** assumes the presence of a population that cannot be defined according to sampling theory rules, which require a list of all members of the population. For example, individuals who successfully lose weight would be a hypothetical population. The number of individuals in the population, who they are, how much weight they have lost, how long they have kept the weight off, and how they achieved the weight loss are unknown. Some populations are elusive and constantly changing. For example, identifying all women in active labor in the U.S., all people grieving the loss of a loved one, or all people coming into an emergency department would be impossible.

Sampling or Eligibility Criteria

Sampling criteria, also referred to as **eligibility criteria**, include a list of characteristics essential for membership or eligibility in the target population. The criteria are developed from the research problem, the purpose, a review of literature, the conceptual and operational definitions of study variables, and the design. The sampling criteria determine the target population, and the sample is selected from the accessible population within the target population (see Figure 15-1). When the study is complete, the findings are generalized from the sample to the accessible population and then to the target population if the study has a representative sample (see the next section).

You might identify broad sampling criteria for a study, such as all adults older than 18 years of age able to read and write English. These criteria ensure a large target population of **heterogeneous** or diverse potential subjects. A heterogeneous sample increases your ability to generalize the findings to the target population. In descriptive or correlational studies, the sampling criteria may be defined to ensure a heterogeneous population with a broad range of values for the variables being studied. However, in quasi-experimental or experimental studies, the primary purpose of sampling criteria is to limit the effect of extraneous variables on the particular interaction between the independent and dependent variables. In these types of studies, sampling criteria need to be specific and designed to make the population as **homogeneous** or similar as possible to control for the extraneous variables (Shadish et al., 2002). Subjects are selected to maximize the effects of the independent variable and minimize the effects of variation in other extraneous variables so that they have a limited impact on the dependent variable scores or values.

Sampling criteria may include characteristics such as the ability to read, to write responses on the data collection instruments or forms, and to comprehend and communicate using the English language. Age limitations are often specified, such as adults 18 years and older. Subjects may be limited to individuals who are not participating in any other study. Persons who are able to participate fully in the procedure for obtaining informed consent are often selected as subjects. If potential subjects have diminished autonomy or are unable to give informed consent, consent must be obtained from their legal representatives. Thus, persons who are legally or mentally incompetent, terminally ill, or confined to an institution are more difficult to access as subjects and may require additional ethical precautions since they are considered vulnerable populations (see Chapter 9). Sampling criteria should be appropriate for a study but not so restrictive that researchers cannot find an adequate number of study participants.

A study report should specify the inclusion or exclusion sampling criteria (or both). **Inclusion sampling criteria** are characteristics that a subject or element must possess to be part of the target population. **Exclusion sampling criteria** are characteristics that can cause a person or element to be eliminated or excluded from the target population. Individuals with these characteristics would be excluded from a study even if they met all the inclusion criteria. For example, when studying patients with heart failure (HF), you might exclude all patients with HF who are acutely ill due to their increased risk of harm. The inclusion and exclusion sampling criteria for a study should be different and not repetitive. For example, you should not have inclusion criteria of individuals 18 years of age and older and exclusion criteria of individuals less than 18 years of age because these criteria are repetitive. Researchers need to provide logical reasons for their inclusion and exclusion sampling criteria, and certain groups should not be excluded without justification. In the past, some groups, such as women, ethnic minorities, elderly adults, and economically disadvantaged people, were unnecessarily excluded from studies (Larson, 1994). Today, federal funding for research is strongly linked to including these populations in studies. Exclusion criteria limit the generalization of the study findings and should be carefully considered before being used in a study.

Newnam et al. (2015) implemented a randomized experimental study design to identify differences in frequency and severity of nasal injuries in extremely low birth weight (BW) neonates receiving nasal continuous positive airway pressure (CPAP) treatments. The study included 78 neonates in a 70-bed level III neonatal intensive care unit (NICU) receiving nasal CPAP who were "randomized into three groups: continuous nasal prong, continuous nasal mask, or alternating mask/prongs every 4 hours" (Newnam et al., 2015, p. 37). The inclusion and exclusion sampling criteria implemented in this study were described as follows.

"Each infant admitted to the NICU between April, 2012 and January, 2013 was screened for inclusion criteria. Inclusion criteria included preterm infants with birth weight (BW) 500 to 1500 grams that required nasal CPAP treatment. Exclusion criteria included infants born with airway or physical anomalies that influenced their ability to extubate to nasal CPAP, infants not consented within 8 hours of nasal CPAP initiation, infants not treated with nasal CPAP or infants who had nasal skin breakdown at enrollment." (Newnam et al., 2015, p. 37)

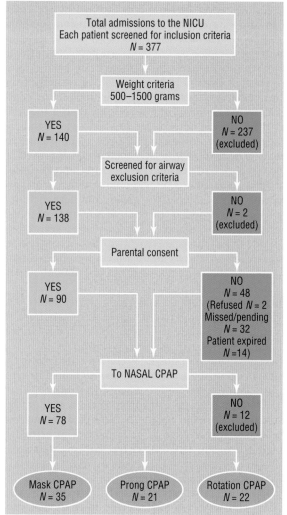

FIGURE 15-2 Consort table for study screening and enrollment. (Adapted from Newnam, K. M., McGrath, J. M., Salyer, J., Estes, T., Jallo, N., & Bass, T. (2015). A comparative effectiveness study of continuous positive airway pressure-related skin breakdown when using different nasal interfaces in the extremely low birth weight neonate. *Applied Nursing Research, 28*(1), 37.)

Newnam et al. (2015) clearly identified the inclusion and exclusion sampling criteria implemented to designate the potential subjects in the target population. The screening of the neonates with these sampling criteria is detailed in Figure 15-2. The accessible population included the neonates admitted to the NICU during the study, who were then screened. Of the 377 neonates screened, 140 met the inclusion sampling criteria and 78 of these neonates remained after the exclusion criteria and consent process were applied. The 78 neonates were randomized into the mask group ($N = 35$), prong group ($N = 21$), and rotation mask/prong group ($N = 22$) (see Figure 15-2). The sampling criteria were appropriate for this study to reduce the effect of possible extraneous variables that might have an impact on the CPAP treatment delivery methods (nasal mask or prong) and the measurement of the dependent variables (frequency and severity of nasal injuries). The increased controls imposed by the sampling criteria strengthened the likelihood that the study outcomes were caused by the treatment and not by extraneous variables or sampling errors. Newnam and colleagues (2015) found that the neonates in the group with alternating CPAP by nasal mask and prongs had significantly less skin injury than those receiving CPAP by mask or prongs only.

Sample Representativeness

For a sample to be **representative**, it must be similar to the target population in as many ways as possible. It is especially important that the sample be representative in relation to the variables you are studying and to other factors that may influence the study variables. For example, if you examine attitudes toward acquired immunodeficiency syndrome (AIDS), the sample should represent the distribution of attitudes toward AIDS that exists in the specified population. You may want the sample to include persons who are friends or a family member of a person with AIDS as well as those who do not know a person with AIDS, if these characteristics have been shown to influence attitudes. In addition, a sample must represent the demographic characteristics of the target population, such as age, gender, ethnicity, income, and education, which often influence study variables.

The accessible population must be representative of the target population. If the accessible population is limited to a particular setting or type of setting, the individuals seeking care at that setting may be different from the individuals who would seek care for the same problem in other settings or from individuals who self-manage their problems. Studies conducted in private hospitals usually exclude economically disadvantaged patients, and other settings could exclude elderly or undereducated patients. People who do not have access to care are usually excluded from health-focused studies. Study participants and the care they receive in research centers are different from patients and the care they receive in community clinics, public hospitals, veterans' hospitals, and rural health clinics. Obese individuals who choose to enter a program to lose weight may differ from obese individuals who do not enter a program. All of these factors limit representativeness and limit our understanding of the phenomena important in practice.

Representativeness is usually evaluated by comparing the numerical values of the sample (a **statistic** such as the mean) with the same values from the target population. A numerical value of a population is called a **parameter**. We can estimate the **population parameter** by identifying the values obtained in previous studies examining the same variables. The accuracy with which the population parameters have been estimated within a study is referred to as **precision**. Precision in estimating parameters requires well-developed methods of measurement that are used repeatedly in several studies (Waltz, Strickland, & Lenz, 2010). You can define parameters by conducting a series of descriptive and correlational studies, each of which examines a different segment of the target population; then you perform a meta-analysis to estimate the population parameter (Kerlinger & Lee, 2000).

Sampling Error

The **sampling error** is the difference between a sample statistic and the estimated population parameter that is actual but unknown (Figure 15-3). A large sampling error means that the sample statistic does not provide a precise estimate of the population parameter; it is not representative. Sampling error is usually larger with small samples and decreases as the sample size increases. Sampling error reduces the **power** of a study, or the ability of the statistical analyses conducted to detect differences between groups or to describe the relationships among variables (Aberson, 2010; Cohen, 1988). Sam-

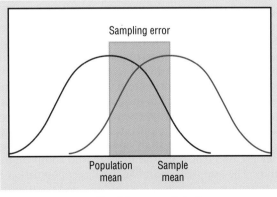

FIGURE 15-3 Sampling error.

pling error occurs as a result of random variation and systematic variation.

Random Variation

Random variation is the expected difference in values that occurs when one examines different subjects from the same sample. If the mean is used to describe the sample, the values of individuals in that sample will not all be exactly the same as the sample mean. Values of individual subjects vary from the value of the sample mean. The difference is random because the value of each subject is likely to vary in value and direction from the previously-measured one. Some values are higher and others are lower than the sample mean. The values are randomly scattered around the mean. As the sample size becomes larger, overall variation in sample values decreases, with more values being close to the sample mean. As the sample size increases, the sample mean is also more likely to have a value similar to that of the population mean.

Systematic Variation

Systematic variation, or **systematic bias**, is a consequence of selecting subjects whose measurement values are different, or vary, in some specific way from the population. Because the subjects have something in common, their values tend to be similar to the values of others in the sample but different in some way from the values of the population as a whole. These values do not vary randomly around the population mean. Most of the variation from the mean is in the same direction; it is systematic. All the values in the sample may tend to be higher or lower than the mean of the population (Thompson, 2002). For example, if all the subjects in a study examining some type of healthcare knowledge have an intelligence quotient (IQ) higher than 120, many of their scores will likely be higher than the mean of a population that includes individuals with a wide variation in IQ, such as IQs that range from 90 to 130. The IQs of the subjects have introduced a systematic bias. This situation could occur, for example, if all the subjects were college students, which has been the case in the development of many measurement methods in psychology.

Because of systematic variance, the sample mean is different from the population mean. The extent of the difference is the sampling error (see Figure 15-3). Exclusion criteria tend to increase the systematic bias in the sample and increase the sampling error, but it may be necessary to exclude persons who could be harmed by participating. An extreme example of this problem is the highly restrictive sampling criteria used in some experimental studies that result in a large sampling error that diminishes representativeness.

If the method of selecting subjects produces a sample with a systematic bias, increasing the sample size does not decrease the sampling error. When systematic bias occurs in an experimental study, researchers may conclude that the treatment has made a difference when, in actuality, the values would be different even without the treatment. This situation usually occurs because of an interaction of the systematic bias with the treatment.

Refusal and acceptance rates in studies. Sampling error from systematic variation or bias is most likely to occur when the sampling process is not random. However, even in a random sample, systematic variation can occur if potential subjects decline participation. Systematic bias increases as the subjects' refusal rate increases. A **refusal rate** is the number and percentage of subjects who decline to participate in the study. High refusal rates to participate in a study have been linked to individuals with serious physical and emotional illnesses, low socioeconomic status, and weak social networks (Bryant, Wicks, & Willis, 2014; Neumark, Stommel, Given, & Given, 2001). The higher the refusal rate, the less representative the sample is of the target population.

In the Newnam et al. (2015) study presented earlier, only two parents, of the 138 neonates meeting sampling criteria, refused to allow their neonates to be in the study (see Figure 15-2). The refusal rate is calculated by dividing the number of potential subjects refusing to participate by the number of potential subjects meeting sampling criteria and multiplying the results by 100%. The refusal rate for the Newnam et al. (2015) study was very small at 1.45% ([2 ÷ 138] × 100% = 0.0145 × 100% = 1.45%), which supports the representativeness of the sample.

Refusal rate formula

= (number potential subjects refusing

to participate ÷ number potential subjects

meeting sample criteria) × 100%

For example, if 200 potential subjects met the sampling criteria and 40 refused to participate in the study, the refusal rate would be 20%.

Refusal rate = (40 [number refusing]

÷ 200 [number meeting sampling criteria])

× 100% = 0.2 × 100% = 20%

Sometimes researchers provide an **acceptance rate**, or the number and percentage of the subjects who agree to participate in a study, rather than a refusal rate. The acceptance rate is calculated by dividing the number of potential subjects who agree to participate in a study by the number of potential subjects who meet sampling criteria and multiplying the result by 100%.

Acceptance rate formula

= (number potential subjects agreeing

to participate ÷ number potential subjects

meeting sample criteria) × 100%

If you know the refusal rate, you can also subtract the refusal rate from 100% to obtain the acceptance rate. Usually researchers report either the acceptance rate or the refusal rate but not both. In the example mentioned earlier, 200 potential subjects met the sampling criteria; 160 agreed to participate in the study, and 40 refused.

Acceptance rate

= (160 [number accepting] ÷ 200 [number

meeting sampling criteria]) × 100%

= 0.8 × 100% = 80%

Acceptance rate = 100% − refusal rate

or 100% − 20% = 80%

Sample attrition and retention rates in studies. Sampling error can also occur in studies with large sample attrition. **Sample attrition** is the withdrawal or loss of subjects or study participants from a study before its completion. Systematic variation tends to increase when a high number of subjects withdraw from the study before the data have been collected or when a large number of subjects withdraw from one group but not the other in the study (Kerlinger & Lee, 2000; Thompson, 2002). In studies involving a treatment, subjects in the control group who do not receive the treatment may be more likely to withdraw from the study. Sample attrition should be reported in the published study to determine if the final sample represents the target population. Researchers also need to provide a rationale for subjects withdrawing from the study and to determine whether they are different from the subjects who complete the study. The sample is most like the target population if the attrition rate is low (< 10% to 15%) and the subjects withdrawing from the study are similar to the subjects completing the study. Sample attrition rate is calculated by dividing the number of subjects withdrawing from a study by the sample size and multiplying the results by 100%.

Sample attrition rate formula

= (number subjects withdrawing

÷ sample size) × 100%

For example, if a study had a sample size of 160 and 40 people withdrew from the study, the attrition rate would be 25%.

Attrition rate = (40 [number withdrawing]

÷ 160 [sample size]) × 100%

= 0.25 × 100% = 25%

The opposite of the attrition rate is the **retention rate**, or the number and percentage of subjects completing the study. The higher the retention rate, the more representative the sample is of the target population, and the more likely the study results are an accurate reflection of reality. Often researchers identify either the attrition rate or the retention rate but not both. It is better to provide a rate in addition to the number of subjects withdrawing or completing a study. In the example just presented with a sample size of 160, if 40 subjects withdrew from the study, then 120 subjects were retained or completed the study. The retention rate is calculated by dividing the number of subjects completing the study by the initial sample size and multiplying by 100%.

Sample retention rate formula

= (number subjects completing study

÷ sample size) × 100%

Retention rate = (120 [number retained]

÷ 160 [sample size]) × 100%

= 0.75 × 100% = 75%

Researchers need to report both refusal and attrition rates in their studies to clarify for the reader the representativeness of the sample and the potential for sampling error. Raurell-Torredà et al. (2015) conducted a quasi-experimental study to determine the effectiveness of a case-based learning program with human patient simulator (intervention) versus traditional lecture and discussion (control) on the clinical assessment skills of undergraduate nursing students. A total of 123 students were enrolled in a medical-surgical course, and five students did not meet sample inclusion criteria. The following excerpt presents the sample attrition for this study.

"Of the 123 possible undergraduates, 118 were included in the study, 43 in the intervention group and 75 in the control group. In each group, there were students who did not take the course examination or failed the course (8 and 9, respectively) and therefore did not participate in the OSCE [objective structured clinical examination]. Thus, the participants in the study included in the analysis were 101 undergraduates (35 in the intervention, 66 controls)." (Raurell-Torredà et al., 2015, p. 38)

Raurell-Torredà and colleagues (2015) indicated that 118 undergraduate students met the sampling criteria and were enrolled in the study indicating a 100% acceptance rate for the study (0% refusal rate). The sample retention number was 101 undergraduate nursing students with a retention rate of 85.6% ([101 ÷ 118] × 100% = 0.8559 × 100% = 85.6%). The sample attrition number was 17 students (8 from the intervention group and 9 from the control group) for an attrition rate of 14.4% (100% − 85.6% = 14.4%). The group assignment of the students was based on their course schedule (the control group included students in the morning class and the intervention group included students in the afternoon class), which resulted in unequal groups sizes. The attrition from the intervention group was 8 students because 5 did not present for the course examination and 3 failed the course. The attrition rate for the intervention group was 18.6% ([8 ÷ 43] × 100% = 18.6%). The control group attrition was 9 students because 7 did not present for the course examination and 2 failed the course. The attrition rate for the control group was 12% ([9 ÷ 75] × 100% = 12%). This study has a very strong acceptance rate (100%) and an adequate sample retention rate of 85.6% for a semester-long study. The researchers provided rationale for the study attrition, which was typical and appropriate for a university course. However, the intervention and control groups were not randomly assigned and there might have been a difference in the students enrolled in a morning versus an afternoon class. The intervention group attrition rate (18.6%) was higher than that of the control group (12%); and the final control group (n = 66) was much larger than the intervention group (n = 35). These weaknesses increase the potential for sampling error and decrease the representativeness of the sample. Raurell-Torredà et al. (2015) found that the case-based learning intervention significantly improved the students' patient assessment skills. Additional research is needed to determine the credibility of the findings for generalization to the target population.

Randomization

From a sampling theory point of view, **randomization** means that each individual in the population should have a greater than zero opportunity to be selected for the sample. The method of achieving this opportunity is referred to as **random sampling**. In experimental studies, participants are sometimes randomly selected and randomly assigned to either the control group or the experimental group. The use of the term **control group**—the group not receiving the treatment or intervention—is used when study participants are possibly randomly selected and are randomly assigned to either the intervention group or control group. If nonrandom sampling methods are used for sample selection, the group not receiving the intervention receives usual or standard care and is generally referred to as a **comparison group**. With a comparison group, there is an increase in the possibility of preexisting differences between that group and the intervention group.

Random sampling increases the extent to which the sample is representative of the target population. However, random sampling must take place in an accessible population that is representative of the target population (see Figure 15-1). Exclusion criteria limit true randomness. Thus, a study that uses random sampling techniques may have such restrictive sampling criteria that the sample is not truly a random sample of the population. In any case, it is rarely possible to obtain a purely random sample for nursing studies because of informed consent requirements. Even if the original sample is random, persons who volunteer or consent to participate in a study may differ in important ways from persons who are unwilling to participate. All samples with human subjects must be **volunteer samples**, which includes individuals willing to participate in the study, to protect the rights of the individuals (Fawcett & Garity, 2009). Methods of achieving random sampling are described later in the chapter.

Sampling Frame

For each person in the target population to have an opportunity to be selected for the sample, each person in the population must be identified. To accomplish this goal, the researcher must acquire a list of every member of the target population through the use of the sampling criteria to define membership. This listing of members of the population is referred to as the **sampling frame**. The researcher selects subjects from the sampling frame using a sampling plan. In the Raurell-Torredà et al. (2015, p. 37) study identified earlier, the sampling frame was identified as "all students enrolled in the 'Adult Patients 1' course in 2011-2012." The sampling frame in this study included the names of 123 undergraduate nursing students, and 118 met the sampling criteria for inclusion in the study.

Sampling Plan

A **sampling plan** describes the strategies that will be used to obtain a sample for a study. The plan is developed to enhance representativeness, reduce systematic bias, and decrease sampling error. Sampling strategies have been devised to accomplish these three tasks and to optimize sample selection. The sampling plan may use probability (random) sampling methods or nonprobability (nonrandom) sampling methods.

A **sampling method** is the process of selecting a group of people, events, behaviors, or other elements that represent the population being studied. A sampling method is similar to a design; it is not specific to a study. The sampling plan provides detail about the application of a sampling method in a specific study. The sampling plan must be described in depth for purposes of critical appraisal, replication, and future meta-analysis. The sampling method implemented in a study varies with the type of research being conducted. Quantitative and outcomes studies apply a variety of probability and nonprobability sampling methods. Qualitative and mixed methods studies usually include nonprobability sampling methods (Charmaz, 2014; Creswell, 2013, 2014; Shadish et al., 2002). The sampling methods included in this text are identified in Table 15-1 and are linked to the types of research that most commonly incorporate them. The representativeness of the sample obtained is discussed for each of the sampling methods (Marshall & Rossman, 2016; Miles, Huberman, & Saldaña, 2014). The following sections describe the types of probability and nonprobability sampling methods most commonly used in quantitative, qualitative, mixed methods, and outcomes research in nursing.

PROBABILITY (RANDOM) SAMPLING METHODS

Probability sampling methods have been developed to ensure some degree of precision in estimations of the population parameters. The term **probability sampling method** means that every member (element) of the population has a greater than zero opportunity to be selected for the sample. Inferential statistical analyses are based on the assumption that the sample from which data were derived has been obtained randomly. Thus, probability sampling methods are often referred to as **random sampling methods**. These samples are more likely to represent the population and minimize

TABLE 15-1   Probability and Nonprobability Sampling Methods Commonly Applied in Nursing Research

Sampling Method	Common Application(s)	Representativeness
Probability		
Simple random sampling	Quantitative and outcomes research	Strong representativeness of the target population that increases with sample size.
Stratified random sampling	Quantitative and outcomes research	Strong representativeness of the target population that increases with control of stratified variable(s).
Cluster sampling	Quantitative and outcomes research	Less representative of the target population than simple random sampling and stratified random sampling.
Systematic sampling	Quantitative and outcomes research	Less representative of the target population than simple random sampling and stratified random sampling methods.
Nonprobability		
Convenience sampling	Quantitative, qualitative, mixed methods, and outcomes research	Questionable representativeness of the target population that improves with increasing sample size in quantitative and outcomes research. May be representative of the phenomenon, process, or cultural elements in qualitative or mixed methods research.
Quota sampling	Quantitative and outcomes research and rarely qualitative or mixed methods research	Use of stratification for selected variables in quantitative and outcomes research makes the sample more representative than convenience sampling. In qualitative and mixed methods research, stratification might be used to provide greater understanding of the subgroups of the populations to increase the representativeness of the phenomenon, processes, or cultural elements studied (Marshal & Rossman, 2016; Miles, Huberman, & Saldaña, 2014).
Purposeful or purposive sampling	Qualitative and mixed methods research and sometimes quantitative research	Focus is on insight, description, and understanding of a phenomenon, cultural event, situation, or process with specially selected study participants who are representative of the area of study (Miles et al., 2014).
Snowball or network sampling	Qualitative and mixed methods research and sometimes quantitative research	Focus is on insight, description, and understanding of a phenomenon, cultural element, situation, or process in a difficult to access population. Intent is to identify participants who are representative of the study focus (Munhall, 2012; Miles et al., 2014).
Theoretical sampling	Qualitative and mixed methods research	Focus is on obtaining quality participants of an adequate number for developing a relevant theory or model for a selected area of study.

sampling error than are samples obtained with non-probability sampling methods. All subsets of the population, which may differ from one another but contribute to the parameters of the population, have a chance to be represented in the sample. Probability sampling methods are most commonly applied in quantitative and outcomes studies (see Table 15-1).

There is less opportunity for systematic bias or error when subjects are selected randomly. Using random sampling, the researcher cannot decide that person X would be a better subject for the study than person Y. In addition, a researcher cannot exclude a subset of people from selection as subjects because he or she does not agree with them, does not like them, or finds them hard to deal with. Potential subjects cannot be excluded just because they are too sick, not sick enough, coping too well, or not coping adequately. The researcher, who has a vested interest in the study, could (consciously or unconsciously) select subjects whose conditions or behaviors are consistent with the study hypothesis. Because random sampling leaves the selection to chance and decreases sampling error, the validity of the study is increased (Kandola, Banner, Okeefe-McCarthy, & Jassal, 2014; Thompson, 2002).

Theoretically, to obtain a probability sample, the researcher must develop a sampling frame that includes every element in the population. The sample must be randomly selected from the sampling frame. According to sampling theory, it is impossible to select a sample randomly from a population that cannot be clearly defined. Four commonly implemented probability sampling designs are included in this text: simple random sampling, stratified random sampling, cluster sampling, and systematic sampling (see Table 15-1).

Simple Random Sampling

Simple random sampling is the most basic of the probability sampling methods. To achieve simple random sampling, elements are selected at random from the sampling frame. This goal can be accomplished in various ways, limited only by the imagination of the researcher. If the sampling frame is small, the researcher can write names on slips of paper, place the names in a container, mix well, and draw out one at a time until the desired sample size has been reached. Another technique is to assign a number to each name in the sampling frame. In large population sets, elements may already have assigned numbers. For example, numbers are assigned to medical records, organizational memberships, and professional licenses. The researcher can use a computer to select these numbers randomly to obtain a sample.

There can be some differences in the probability for the selection of each element, depending on whether the name or number of the selected element is replaced before the next name or number is selected. Selection with replacement, the most conservative random sampling approach, provides exactly equal opportunities for each element to be selected. For example, if the researcher draws names out of a hat to obtain a sample, each name must be replaced before the next name is drawn to ensure equal opportunity for each subject.

Selection without replacement gives each element different levels of probability for selection. For example, if the researcher is selecting 10 subjects from a population of 50, the first name has a 1 in 5 chance (10 draws, 50 names), or a 0.2 probability, of being selected. If the first name is not replaced, the remaining 49 names have a 9 in 49 chance, or a 0.18 probability, of being selected. As further names are drawn, the probability of being selected decreases.

Random selection of a sample can also be achieved using a computer, a random numbers table, or a roulette wheel. The most common method of random selection is the computer, which can be programmed to select a sample randomly from the sampling frame with replacement. However, some researchers still use a table of random numbers to select a random sample. Table 15-2 shows a section from a random numbers table. To use a table of random numbers, the researcher places a pencil or a finger on the table with the eyes closed. The number touched is the starting place. Moving the pencil or finger up, down, right, or left, the researcher identifies the next element to be included and uses the numbers in order until the desired sample size is obtained. For example, the researcher places a pencil on 58 in Table 15-2, which is in the fourth column from the left and fourth row down. If five subjects are to be selected from a population of 100 and the researcher decides to go across the column to the right, the subject numbers chosen are 58, 25, 15, 55, and 38. Table 15-2 is useful only if the population number is less than 100. However, tables are available for larger populations, such as the random numbers

TABLE 15-2	**Section From a Random Numbers Table**								
06	84	10	22	56	72	25	70	69	43
07	63	10	34	66	39	54	02	33	85
03	19	63	93	72	52	13	30	44	40
77	32	69	58	25	15	55	38	19	62
20	01	94	54	66	88	43	91	34	28

table provided in the Thompson (2002, pp. 14–15) sampling text.

Lee, Faucett, Gillen, Krause, and Landry (2013, p. 36) conducted a predictive correlational study to determine critical care nurses' perception of "the risk of musculoskeletal (MSK) injury from work and to identify factors associated with their risk perception." The simple random sampling method implemented in this study is described in the following excerpt with the key sampling concepts identified in [brackets].

> "The study population consisted of 1,000 critical care nurses randomly selected [sampling method] from a 2005 American Association of Critical Care Nurses (AACN) membership list [sampling frame]… A total of 412 nurses returned completed questionnaires (response rate = 41.5%), excluding eight for whom mailing addresses were incorrect). Of these, 47 nurses who did not meet the inclusion criteria were excluded: not currently employed ($n = 5$); not employed in a hospital ($n = 1$); not employed in critical care ($n = 8$); not a staff or charge nurse ($n = 28$); or not performing patient-handling tasks ($n = 5$). In addition, four nurses employed in a neonatal ICU were excluded because of the different nature of their physical workload. The final sample for data analysis comprised 361 [sample size] critical care nurses." (Lee et al., 2013, p. 38)

Lee and colleagues (2013) clearly identified that a random sampling method was used to select study participants from a population of critical care nurses. The 41.5% response rate for mailed questionnaires is considered adequate, because the response rate to questionnaires averages 25% to 50% (Kerlinger & Lee, 2000). The 47 nurses who did not meet sample criteria and the four nurses working in a NICU were excluded, ensuring a more homogeneous sample and decreasing the potential effects of extraneous variables. These sampling activities limit the potential for systematic variation or bias and increase the likelihood that the study sample is representative of the accessible and target populations. The study would have been strengthened if the researchers had indicated how the nurses were randomly selected from the AACN membership list, which was probably a random selection by computer.

Lee et al. (2013, p. 43) identified the following findings from their study: "Improving the physical and psychosocial work environment may make nursing jobs safer, reduce the risk of MSK injury, and improve nurses' perceptions of job safety. Ultimately, these efforts would contribute to enhancing safety in nursing settings and to maintaining a healthy nursing workforce. Future research is needed to determine the role of risk perception in preventing MSK injury."

Stratified Random Sampling

Stratified random sampling is used when the researcher knows some of the variables in the population that are critical to achieving representativeness. Variables commonly used for stratification are age, gender, ethnicity, socioeconomic status, diagnosis, geographical region, type of institution, type of care, care provider, and site of care. The variable or variables chosen for stratification are those found in previous studies to be correlated with the dependent variables being examined in the study. Subjects within each stratum are expected to be more similar (homogeneous) in relation to the study variables than they are to be similar to subjects in other strata or the total sample. In stratified random sampling, the subjects are randomly selected on the basis of their classification into the selected strata.

For example, you want to select a stratified random sample of 100 adult subjects using age as the variable for stratification. The sample might include 25 subjects in the age range 18 to 39 years, 25 subjects in the age range 40 to 59 years, 25 subjects in the age range 60 to 79 years, and 25 subjects 80 years or older. Stratification ensures that all levels of the identified variable, in this example age, are adequately represented in the sample. With a stratified random sample, you could use a smaller sample size to achieve the same degree of representativeness as that provided by a large sample acquired through simple random sampling. Sampling error decreases, power increases, data collection time is reduced, and the cost of the study is lower if stratification is used (Fawcett & Garity, 2009; Thompson, 2002).

One question that arises in relation to stratification is whether each stratum should have equivalent numbers of subjects in the sample (termed **disproportionate sampling**) or whether the numbers of subjects should be selected in proportion to their occurrence in the population (termed **proportionate sampling**). For example, if stratification is being achieved by ethnicity and the population is 45% white non-Hispanic, 25% Hispanic nonwhite, 25% African American, and 5% Asian, your research team would have to decide whether to select equal numbers of each ethnic group or to calculate a proportion of the sample. Good arguments exist for both approaches. Stratification is not as useful if one stratum contains only a small number of subjects. In the aforementioned situation, if proportions are used and the sample size is 100, the study would include only five Asians, hardly enough to be representative or to identify statistical significance. If equal numbers of each group are used, each group would contain at least 25 subjects; however, the white non-Hispanic group would be underrepresented. In this case, mathematically weighting the findings from each stratum can equalize the representation to ensure proportional contributions of each stratum to the total score of the sample. Most textbooks on sampling describe this procedure. Alternatively, the researcher can seek the assistance of a statistician for this process (Levy & Lemsbow, 1980; Thompson, 2002; Yates, 1981).

Sezgin and Esin (2015) used a stratified random sampling method to investigate the prevalence of musculoskeletal symptoms and associated risk factors in a population of intensive care unit (ICU) nurses from Turkey. This study is similar to the Lee et al. (2013) investigation previously discussed. Sezgin and Esin (2015) provided the following description of their sampling process.

"... There were 281 hospitals (public, private, and university hospitals) in Istanbul during the period when this study was conducted. Data for this study were obtained from 51 adult ICUs (general, coronary, cardiovascular surgery, and reanimation) in 17 hospitals, where ergonomic risks, such as weight-lifting, are considered to be high.

Sample
A total of 1515 nurses [population] work at these 51 ICUs... When data loss was taken into consideration; the final sample size was set at 350 nurses [sample size]. The nurses were selected by stratified random sampling [sampling method]. As the working conditions of the strata are different, the nurses were stratified according to public, private, and university hospitals. The procedure was to select a sample randomly from each stratum that was proportional to the stratum's size in relation to the

population. The strata weights and the number of nurses from each stratum are shown in Table 15-3. Sample selection was performed using a simple random sampling method. The lists of nurses working at each hospital [sampling frame] were obtained from the respective hospitals. Thirty-three ICU nurses from the first stratum and one ICU nurse from the second stratum could not be reached during the study. All the nurses intended for selection from the third stratum were reached, and an additional seven nurses were included in the sample. Thus, 323 ICU nurses [sample size] comprised the sample." (Sezgin & Esin, 2015, pp. 93–94)

The study sampling frame for ICU nurses was representative of the nurses working in public, university, and private hospitals in Istanbul, Turkey. Proportionate stratified random sampling was implemented in this study and the proportions and numbers of ICU nurses from public, private, and university hospitals are detailed in Table 15-3. The sampling method (proportionate stratified random sampling) and sample size ($N = 323$) are strengths in this study, which increase the representativeness of the sample and reduce the potential for sampling error. Sezgin and Esin (2015, p. 92) found that "musculoskeletal symptoms... are mainly associated with organizational factors, such as type of hospital, type of shift work, and frequency of changes in work schedule, rather than with personal factors." They recommended that nursing administrators assess the risks for musculoskeletal injuries in ICU nurses, provide risk prevention programs, and make policy changes to decrease these risks.

Cluster Sampling

Cluster sampling is a probability sampling method that is similar to stratified random sampling but takes advantage of the natural clusters or groups of population units that have similar characteristics. Cluster sampling is used in two situations. The first situation is one in which

TABLE 15-3	**Number of Selected Nurses With Stratified Random Sampling**				
Stratum No.	Hospital Type (number)	Number of Nurses	Strata Weights	Number of Nurses to Be Selected	Number of Selected Nurses
1	Public hospital (9)	950	950/1515 = 0.62	0.62 × 350 = 217	184
2	University hospital (2)	265	265/1515 = 0.18	0.18 × 350 = 63	62
3	Private hospital (6)	300	300/1515 = 0.20	0.20 × 350 = 70	77
Total	17	1515	1.00	350	323

From Sezgin, D., & Esin, M. N. (2015). Predisposing factors for musculoskeletal symptoms in intensive care unit nurses. *International Nursing Review, 62*(1), 94.

a simple random sample would be prohibitive in terms of travel time and cost. Imagine trying to arrange personal meetings with 100 people, each in a different part of the U.S. The second situation exists in cases in which the individual elements making up the population are unknown, preventing the development of a sampling frame (Kandola et al., 2014). For example, there is no list of all the heart surgery patients who complete rehabilitation programs in the U.S. In these cases, it is often possible to obtain lists of institutions or organizations with which the elements of interest are associated.

In cluster sampling, the researcher develops a sampling frame that includes a list of all the states, cities, institutions, or organizations with which elements of the identified population would be linked. States, cities, institutions, or organizations are selected randomly as units from which to obtain elements for the sample. In some cases, this random selection continues through several stages and is referred to as **multistage cluster sampling**. For example, the researcher might first randomly select states and next randomly select cities within the sampled states. Hospitals within the randomly selected cities might then be randomly selected. Within the hospitals, nursing units might be randomly selected. At this level, either all of the patients on the nursing unit who fit the criteria for the study might be included, or patients could be randomly selected.

Cluster sampling provides a means for obtaining a larger sample at a lower cost than simple random sampling. However, it has some disadvantages. Data from subjects associated with the same institution are likely to be correlated and not completely independent. This correlation can cause a decrease in precision and an increase in sampling error. However, such disadvantages can be offset to some extent by the use of a larger sample.

Subaiya, Moussavi, Velasquez, and Stillman (2014, p. 632) conducted a "rapid needs assessment of the Rockaway Peninsula in New York City (NYC) after hurricane Sandy and examined the relationship of socioeconomic status to recovery." These researchers described their cluster sampling method in the following excerpt from their study.

"The Rockaway Peninsula is on the southern coast of the borough of Queens, within NYC, and it extends into the Atlantic Ocean... A modified cluster approach [sampling method] was utilized to select households within a central, highly populated portion of the Rockaway Peninsula. Each cluster was defined as a 10-block region between Beach 50th street to Beach 150th street,

covering roughly half of the peninsula, including 7 of its 11 neighborhoods. Teams were assigned to 10-block clusters with a goal of completing 7 to 10 well-spaced, random household interviews per cluster. Each team began at a randomly selected location within their 10-block radius. They were instructed to select every fifth to seventh household for an interview. When an apartment complex or housing project was encountered, the team selected 1 building and a random floor was selected. Every fifth to seventh apartment was selected until a total of 2 surveys were completed within that complex. The CDC's [Centers for Disease Control] Community Assessment for Public Health Emergency Response (CASPER) recommends selecting 30 clusters and completing 7 interviews per cluster; however, CASPER typically covers multiple census blocks. Given the size of the Rockaway Peninsula, approximately 2 census blocks, we chose to cover a smaller area, surveying 7 of 10 neighborhoods in entirety...

Enumerators visited a total of 208 households on the Rockaway Peninsula. Approximately 40% of households approached did not answer the door, of which 25% appeared vacant. Ten percent of households refused to participate in the study. Information was collected on 105 households with an overall response rate of 51%. Fourteen surveys were excluded from final analysis because of incorrect acquisition and recording of location data, leaving 91 households [sample size] for inclusion in the final analysis." (Subaiya et al., 2014, pp. 632–633)

These researchers detailed their use of cluster sampling with random selection of the households within the clusters for interviews. The probability cluster sampling method used in this study has a potential to provide a representative sample. However, the number of households surveyed was only 91 (51%) of those identified for surveying, which is a small number for this type of study and decreases the representativeness of the sample.

The findings reported by Subaiya et al. (2014, p. 632) indicated that "Storm preparation should include disseminating information regarding carbon monoxide and proper generator use, considerations for prescription refills, neighborhood security, and location of food distribution centers. Lower-income individuals may have greater difficulty meeting their needs following a natural disaster." Additional research is needed to explore relationships between socioeconomic status and long-term recovery, as well as the development of interventions to improve outcomes following hurricanes.

Systematic Sampling

Systematic sampling can be conducted when an ordered list of all members of the population is available. The process involves selecting every *k*th individual on the list, using a starting point selected randomly. If the initial starting point is not random, the sample is not a probability sample. To use this design in your research, you must know the number of elements in the population and the size of the sample desired. Divide the population size by the desired sample size, giving *k,* the size of the gap between elements selected from the list. For example, if the population size is $N = 1200$ and the desired sample size is $n = 100$, then you could calculate the value of *k*:

$$k = \text{population size} \div \text{sample size desired}$$

$$\text{Example: } k = 1200 \text{ (population size)}$$
$$\div 100 \text{ (sample size desired)} = 12$$

Thus, $k = 12$, which means that every 12th person on the list would be included in the sample. Some authors argue that this procedure does not truly give each element an opportunity to be included in the sample; it provides a random but unequal chance for inclusion (Thompson, 2002).

Researchers must be careful to determine that the original list has not been set up with any ordering that could be meaningful in relation to the study. The process is based on the assumption that the order of the list is random in relation to the variables being studied. If the order of the list is related to the study, systematic bias is introduced. In addition to this risk, it is difficult to compute sampling error with the use of this design (Floyd, 1993).

De Silva, Hanwella, and de Silva (2012) used systematic sampling in their outcomes study of the direct and indirect costs of care incurred by patients with schizophrenia (population) in a tertiary care psychiatric unit. Their sampling method is described in the following excerpt from the study.

"Systematic sampling [sampling method] selected every second patient with an ICD-10 clinical diagnosis of schizophrenia [target population] presenting to the clinic during a two month period [sampling frame]… The sample consisted of 91 patients [sample size]. Direct cost was defined as cost incurred by the patient (out-of-pocket expenditure) for outpatient care." (De Silva et al. 2012, p. 14)

De Silva et al. (2012) clearly identified that systematic sampling was used in their study. The population and target population identified seem appropriate for this study. Using systematic sampling increased the representativeness of the sample and the sample size of 91 schizophrenic patients seems adequate for the focus of this study. However, the sampling frame was identified as only the patients presenting over two months and *k* was small (every second patient) in this study. The researchers might have provided more details on how they implemented the systematic sampling method to ensure the start of the sampling process was random (Thompson, 2002). De Silva et al. (2012, p. 14) concluded that "Despite low direct cost of care, indirect cost and cost of informal treatment results in substantial economic impact on patients and their families. It is recommended that economic support should be provided for patients with disabling illnesses such schizophrenia, especially when patients are unable to engage in full-time employment."

NONPROBABILITY (NONRANDOM) SAMPLING METHODS COMMONLY APPLIED IN QUANTITATIVE AND OUTCOMES RESEARCH

In **nonprobability sampling**, not every element of the population has an opportunity to be included in the sample. Nonprobability sampling methods increase the likelihood of obtaining samples that are not representative of their target populations. In conducting studies in nursing and other health disciplines, limited subjects are available, and it is often impossible to obtain a random sample. Thus, most nursing studies use nonprobability sampling, especially convenience sampling, to select study samples. Researchers often include any subjects willing to participate who meet the eligibility criteria.

There are several types of nonprobability (nonrandom) sampling designs. Each addresses a different research need. The five nonprobability sampling designs described in this textbook are (1) convenience sampling, (2) quota sampling, (3) purposive or purposeful sampling, (4) network or snowball sampling, and (5) theoretical sampling. These sampling methods are applied in both quantitative and qualitative research. Convenience sampling and quota sampling are applied more often in quantitative, outcomes, and mixed methods research than in qualitative studies and are discussed in this section (see Table 15-1). Purposive sampling, network sampling, and theoretical sampling are more commonly applied in qualitative studies and are discussed later in this chapter and in Chapter 12.

Convenience Sampling

In **convenience sampling**, subjects are included in the study because they happen to be in the right place at the right time. Researchers simply enter available subjects into the study until they have reached the desired sample size. Convenience sampling, also called **accidental sampling**, is not considered a strong approach to sampling for interventional studies because it provides little opportunity to control for biases. Multiple biases may exist in convenience sampling; these biases range from minimal to serious. Researchers need to identify and describe known biases in their samples. You can identify biases by carefully thinking through the sample criteria used to determine the target population and taking steps to improve the representativeness of the sample. For example, in a study of home care management of patients with complex healthcare needs, educational level would be an important extraneous variable. One solution for controlling this extraneous variable would be to redefine the sampling criteria to include only patients with a high school education. Doing so would limit the extent of generalization but decrease the bias created by educational level. Another option would be to select a population known to include individuals with a wide variety of educational levels. Data could be collected on educational level so that the description of the sample would include information on educational level. With this information, one could judge the extent to which the sample was representative with respect to educational level (Thompson, 2002).

Decisions related to sample selection must be carefully described to enable others to evaluate the possibility of biases. In addition, data should be gathered to allow a thorough description of the sample that can also be used to evaluate for possible biases. Data on the sample can be used to compare the sample with other samples and to estimate the parameters of populations through meta-analyses.

Many strategies are available for selecting a convenience sample. A classroom of students might be used. Patients who attend a clinic on a specific day, subjects who attend a support group, patients currently admitted to a hospital with a specific diagnosis, and every person who enters the emergency department on a given day are examples of types of commonly selected convenience samples.

Convenience samples are inexpensive and accessible, and they usually require less time to acquire than other types of samples. This sampling method allows the conduct of studies on topics that could not be examined through the use of probability sampling. Convenience sampling also enables researchers to acquire information in unexplored areas. According to Kerlinger and Lee (2000), a convenience sample is probably adequate when used with reasonable knowledge and care in implementing a study. Healthcare studies are usually conducted with particular types of patients experiencing varying numbers of health problems; these patients often are reluctant to participate in research. Thus, nurse researchers often find it very difficult to recruit subjects for their studies and frequently must use convenience sampling to obtain their sample.

Wang and colleagues (2015) conducted a quasi-experimental study to determine the effectiveness of a biofeedback relaxation intervention on the pain experienced by patients following total knee replacement. The following excerpt describes their population, sampling method, and sample size.

"A convenience sample [sampling method] of 66 patients undergoing primary total knee replacement [population] were recruited and randomly assigned to the intervention or control groups.... The 69 potentially eligible patients were approached; three refused to participate, and 66 were recruited and randomized to groups. All 66 participants [sample size], with 33 in each group, completed the study." (Wang et al., 2015, p. 41)

Wang et al. (2015) clearly identified their sampling method, population, and sample size. The refusal rate for the study was small at 4.3% ([$3 \div 69$] $\times 100\% = 0.043 \times 100\% = 4.3\%$). The attrition rate was 0% because all 66 participants admitted to the study completed it. A power analysis reported in the study identified 30 participants per group as adequate to determine significant differences between the intervention and control groups. Power analysis is discussed in more detail later in this chapter. The convenience sampling method decreased the representativeness of the sample, but the 4.3% refusal rate and 0% attrition rate increased its representativeness. The groups were equal size ($n = 33$) and had an adequate number of participants, based on the power analysis, both of which decreased the potential for sampling error.

Wang et al. (2015, p. 39) study "results provided preliminary support for biofeedback relaxation, a non-invasive and non-pharmacological intervention, as a complementary treatment option for pain management in this population." These researchers recommended using this intervention in the management of patients' pain following a total knee replacement but noted that "more studies are required to define the role of the biofeedback relaxation intervention in managing post-operative pain" (Wang et al., 2015, p. 48).

Quota Sampling

Quota sampling is a nonprobability convenience sampling technique in which the proportion of identified groups is predetermined by the researchers. Quota sampling may be used to ensure the inclusion of subject types or strata in a population that are likely to be underrepresented in the convenience sample, such as women, minority groups, elderly adults, poor people, rich people, and undereducated adults. This method may also be used to mimic the known characteristics of the target population or to ensure adequate numbers of subjects in each stratum for the planned statistical analyses. The technique is similar to the one used in stratified random sampling, but the initial sample is not random. If necessary, mathematical weighting can be used to adjust sample values so that they are consistent with the proportion of subgroups found in the population. Quota sampling offers an improvement over convenience sampling and tends to decrease potential biases. In most studies in which convenience samples are used, quota sampling could be used and should be considered (Thompson, 2002).

Newnam et al.'s (2015) study purpose and sampling criteria were introduced earlier in this chapter. The original study sample was one of convenience and the neonates were stratified by birth weight (BW). The stratification by BW might have been accomplished using quota sampling or implemented as part of the study design. The following excerpt describes their sampling process.

"The study was conducted in a 70 bed level III neonatal intensive care unit (NICU) in the southeastern United States. The study was approved by the Institutional Review Board (IRB), and parents provided informed consent for infant participation. A flow diagram described the process of screening through completion of data collection (see Figure 15-2)...

The neonates [population] were extubated to nasal CPAP [continuous positive airway pressure]. They were randomized into one of the three groups, (1) continuous nasal prongs, (2) continuous nasal mask, or (3) alternating mask/prongs every 4 hours. The specific timing of extubation was based on demonstrated clinical readiness... Participants were block stratified according to BW into four categories: <750 g; 750–1000 g; 1001–1250 g; and 1251–1500 g. Known differences in skin integrity have been demonstrated with the lowest BW infants considered the most vulnerable; thus, stratification was used to keep the groups more homogeneous since it was expected that the <750 g group would contain the fewest patients." (Newnam et al., pp. 37–38)

The population was neonates in the NICU and the accessible population was those in a 70 bed level III NICU. The neonates admitted to this unit were screened and those meeting sampling criteria were admitted with parental consent, which is convenience sampling. The quota sampling involved stratification of the sample based on BW. The stratification of neonates by BW was used to make the groups more homogeneous and reduce the potential for error from extraneous variables, since skin integrity had been demonstrated to be poorer in the smallest neonates. The limited refusal and attrition rates increased the sample's representativeness of the target population. However, the sample was selected from only one NICU and the group sizes were small ($n = 21, 22,$ and 35), which decreased the representativeness of the sample and increased the potential for sampling error.

NONPROBABILITY SAMPLING METHODS COMMONLY APPLIED IN QUALITATIVE AND MIXED METHODS RESEARCH

Qualitative research is conducted to gain insights and discover meaning about a particular experience, situation, cultural element, or historical event. The intent is an in-depth understanding of a selected sample and not the generalization of the findings from a randomly selected sample to a target population, as in quantitative and outcomes research. In qualitative and some mixed methods research, experiences, events, and incidents are more the focus of sampling than people (Charmaz, 2014; Marshall & Rossman, 2016; Munhall, 2012). Researchers attempt to select participants or informants who can provide extensive information about the experience or event being studied. For example, if the goal of your study was to describe the phenomenon of living with chronic pain, you would purposefully select participants who were articulate and reflective, had a history of chronic pain, and were willing to share details of their chronic pain experiences.

The three common sampling methods applied in qualitative nursing research are purposive or purposeful sampling, network or snowball sampling, and theoretical sampling (see Table 15-1). These sampling methods enable the researcher to select the specific participants who would provide the most extensive information about the phenomenon, event, or situation being studied (Marshall & Rossman, 2016). The sample selection process can have a profound effect on the quality of the research. Because of this, it should be representative of both the area of study and the philosophy underlying the study design, and described in enough depth to promote the interpretation of the findings and the replication of the study (Miles et al., 2014; Munhall, 2012).

Purposive Sampling

In **purposive sampling**, sometimes referred to as *purposeful, judgmental,* or *selective sampling,* the researcher consciously selects certain participants, elements, events, or incidents to include in the study. In purposive sampling, qualitative researchers select **information-rich cases**, or cases that can teach them a great deal about the central focus or purpose of the study (Marshall & Rossman, 2016). Efforts might be made to include typical and atypical participants or situations representative of the area of study. Researchers also seek **critical cases**, or cases that make a point clearly or are extremely important in understanding the purpose of the study (Miles et al., 2014; Munhall, 2012). The researcher might select participants or informants of various ages, participants with differing diagnoses or illness severity, or participants who received an ineffective treatment versus an effective treatment for their illness.

This sampling plan has been criticized because it is difficult to evaluate the precision of the researcher's judgment. How does one determine that the patient or element was typical or atypical, good or bad, effective or ineffective? Researchers must indicate the characteristics that they desire in participants and provide a rationale for selecting these types of participants to obtain essential data for their study. Purposive sampling method is used in qualitative research to gain insight into a new area of study or to obtain in-depth understanding of a complex experience or event (Munhall, 2012).

Andersen and Owen (2014, p. 252) conducted a grounded theory study to "explain the process of quitting smoking cigarettes, with specific attention to the question of whether the help of another person was important." The population included individuals from a large academic institution. Purposeful and theoretical sampling methods were used to obtain the sample for this study. The purposeful sampling method used in this study is discussed in the following excerpt.

"A purposeful sampling strategy was used, whereby new study participants were sought out based on questions arising from the ongoing analysis of the data... The sampling strategy led to inclusion of participants from a variety of work backgrounds, ages, ethnicities, and marital statuses...

An intensive qualitative interviewing approach was used to engage participants individually in a directed and focused conversation about quitting, staying abstinent from smoking, and the identification and use of helpers... Additional questions were a part of the purposive interviewing. One interviewer conducted and audiotaped all sessions. Transcripts were created verbatim. Each participant was interviewed once...

Key constructs and relationships were identified during the analysis. Participants were asked whether the 'help' of another person was important and whether the role of the helper mattered." (Andersen & Owen, 2014, p. 253)

Andersen and Owen (2014) clearly detailed their use of purposive sampling in their study, which seemed appropriate for the investigation of smoking cessation. A stratified purposive sampling was used to ensure that study participants had a variety of work backgrounds, ages, ethnicities, and marital statuses, which increased the sample's representativeness through inclusion of the actual subgroups in the population (Marshall & Rossman, 2016; Miles et al., 2014). The authors also included a list of their interview questions in their research report and indicated how purposive sampling was used to obtain essential data. The final sample size was 16 participants, who provided the essential data to address the study focus. Additional data were gathered using theoretical sampling that is discussed later in this chapter. Andersen and Owen (2014) concluded that a formal helping relationship in an environment that was supportive of smoking cessation was important. They recommend future studies focus on the use of informal helpers in promoting smoking cessation.

Network (Snowball) Sampling

Network sampling, sometimes referred to as *snowball* or *chain sampling*, holds promise for locating samples difficult or impossible to obtain in other ways or that had not been previously identified for study. Network sampling takes advantage of social networks and the fact that friends tend to have characteristics in common. When you have found a few participants with the necessary criteria, you can ask for their assistance in getting in touch with others with similar characteristics. The first few participants are often obtained through convenience or purposive sampling methods, and the sample size is expanded using network or snowball sampling. This sampling method is rarely used in quantitative studies, but it is commonly used in qualitative studies. In qualitative research, network sampling is an effective strategy for identifying participants who know other potential participants who can provide the greatest insight and essential information about an experience or event that is identified for study (Marshall & Rossman, 2016; Munhall, 2012).

This strategy is also particularly useful for finding participants in socially devalued populations, such as alcoholics, child abusers, sex offenders, drug addicts, and criminals. These individuals are seldom willing to identify themselves as fitting these categories. Other groups, such as widows, grieving siblings, or individuals successful at lifestyle changes, can be located using this strategy. These individuals are outside the existing healthcare system and are difficult to find. Biases are built into the sampling process because the participants are not independent of one another. However, the participants selected have the expertise to provide the essential information needed to address the study purpose.

Milroy, Wyrick, Bibeau, Strack, and Davis (2012) conducted an exploratory-descriptive qualitative study to investigate student physical activity promotion on college campuses. The study included 14 of the 15 (93%) universities recruited, and 22 employees from these universities participated in the study interviews. Milroy et al. (2012) implemented purposive and snowball (network) sampling methods to recruit individuals into their study. Their sampling process is described in the following study excerpt.

"Participants were recruited from a southeastern state university system... Initially, nonprobabilistic purposive sampling [sampling method] was used to identify one potential participant from each university. Individuals selected for recruitment were identified to be most likely responsible for student physical activity promotion [study participants]... Snowball sampling [sampling method] followed the nonprobabilistic purposive sampling to identify additional individuals on each campus who were engaged in promoting physical activity to students. Guidelines of snowball sampling prescribe that each interview participant be asked to identify any other individuals on their campus who are also responsible for promoting physical activity to students. Using snowball sampling helps to reduce the likelihood of omitting key participants. This technique was initiated during each interview until all those responsible for student physical activity promotion on each campus were identified and interviewed." (Milroy et al., 2012, p. 306)

Milroy and colleagues (2012) clearly identified the focus of their purposive sample and their rationale for using snowball sampling. The study was conducted in multiple settings with knowledgeable participants who provided in-depth information about the health promotion physical activities on university campuses. This study demonstrated a quality sampling process for addressing the study purpose. Milroy et al. (2012) concluded that great efforts were put forth to encourage students to attend fitness classes or to join incentive programs but the students' involvement in physical activities was limited. Thus, the researchers concluded that new methods were needed to promote physical activity on college campuses and that the administration was important in creating a culture that supported and valued these activities. Milroy et al. (2012, p. 305) recommended "Replication of this study is needed to compare these findings with other types of universities, and to investigate the relationship between promotion of activities (type and exposure) and physical activity behaviors of college students."

Theoretical Sampling

Theoretical sampling is usually applied in grounded theory research to advance the development of a selected theory or model throughout the research process (Charmaz, 2014). The researcher gathers data from any individual or group that can provide relevant data for theory generation. The data are considered relevant if they include information that generates, delimits, and saturates the theoretical codes in the study needed for theory or model generation. A code is saturated if new participants present similar ideas or concepts and the researcher can see how it fits into the emerging theory. The researcher continues to seek sources likely to advance the theoretical knowledge in progress and to gather data until the codes are saturated and the theory or model evolves from the codes and the data. Diversity or heterogeneity in the sample is encouraged so that the theory developed represents a wide range of behavior in varied situations (Miles et al., 2014).

The Andersen and Owen (2014) study of the helping relationships for smoking cessation was introduced earlier in this chapter with the discussion of purposive sampling. This study also included theoretical sampling, which is commonly used in grounded theory studies for the development of theories or models. The theoretical sampling method in this study is presented in the following excerpt.

"Key constructs and relationships were identified during the analysis. Participants were asked whether the 'help' of another person was important and whether the role of the helper mattered... Subsequent discussions led to the formation and refinement of categories. Relationships between categories promoted reexamination of transcripts to ground the developing theory in the data.

In keeping with the intent of theoretical sampling, as data analysis was engaged, additional participants were sought in an attempt to better understand emerging categories and the relationship between categories... A rich diversity of individual experiences with smoking cessation and use of helpers emerged. When new interviews ceased to provide new insights into the theoretical meaning of categories and the building of a model, participant accrual ceased...

Throughout the sampling process, conduct of interviews, data coding, and data analysis, we engaged in thoughtful approaches to enhance the trustworthiness of study findings... Confirmability was addressed by creating a detailed account of the methods used to collect and analyze data (Miles et al., 2014). Dependability was addressed by the use of a single interviewer using a written protocol with each participant... Transferability was addressed through the use of thorough descriptions of participant characteristics." (Andersen & Owen, 2014, pp. 253–254)

Andersen and Owen (2014) provided extensive coverage of the theoretical sampling process implemented in their study. The additional sampling of participants to ground the developing theory in data and to build a model is discussed. However, the researchers did not discuss the numbers of additional participants interviewed and only indicated that the total sample size was 16. The greatest strength in this study's sampling process is the discussion of how trustworthiness, confirmabiltiy, dependability, and transferability of the findings were achieved (Charmaz, 2014; Miles et al., 2014).

SAMPLE SIZE IN QUANTITATIVE RESEARCH

One of the questions beginning researchers commonly ask is, "What size sample should I use?" Historically, the response to this question has been that a sample should contain at least 30 subjects for each study variable measured. Statisticians consider 30 subjects the minimum number for data on a single variable to approach a normal distribution. So if a study includes four variables, researchers would need at least 120 subjects in their final sample. Researchers are encouraged to determine the probable attrition rate for their study to ensure an adequate sample size at the completion of their study. For example, researchers might anticipate a 10%–15% attrition rate in their study and need to obtain a sample of 132 to 138 subjects to ensure the final sample size after attrition is 120. The best method of determining sample size is a power analysis, but if information is not available to conduct a power analysis, this recommendation of 30 subjects per study variable might be used.

The deciding factor in determining an adequate sample size for correlational, quasi-experimental, and experimental studies is power. **Power** is the capacity of the study to detect differences or relationships that actually exist in the population. Expressed another way, power is the capacity to reject a null hypothesis correctly. The minimum acceptable power for a study is commonly recommended to be 0.80 (80%) (Aberson, 2010; Cohen, 1988; Kraemer & Thiemann, 1987). If you do not have sufficient power to detect differences or relationships that exist in the population, you might question the advisability of conducting the study. You determine the sample size needed to obtain sufficient power by performing a **power analysis**. Power analysis includes the standard power of 80%, level of significance (usually set at 0.05 in nursing studies), effect size (discussed in the next section), and sample size (Grove & Cipher, 2017).

An increasing number of nurse researchers are using power analysis to determine sample size, but it is essential that the results of the power analyses be included in the published studies. Not conducting a power analysis for a study or omitting the power analysis results in a published study are significant problems if the study failed to detect significant differences or relationships. Without this information, you do not know whether the results are due to an inadequate sample size or to a true absence of a difference or relationship. The calculation for power analysis varies with the types of statistical analyses conducted to determine study results. Statistical programs are available to conduct a power analysis for a study (see Chapter 21). Grove and Cipher (2017) detail the process for conducting a power analysis in their text.

The adequacy of sample sizes must be evaluated more carefully in future nursing studies prior to data collection. Studies with inadequate sample sizes should not be approved for data collection unless they are preliminary pilot studies conducted before a planned larger study. If it is impossible for you to obtain a larger sample because of time or numbers of available subjects, you should redesign your study so that the available sample is adequate for the planned analyses. If you cannot obtain a sufficient sample size, you should not conduct the proposed study.

Large sample sizes may be costly and difficult to obtain in nursing studies, resulting in long data collection periods. In developing the methodology for a study, you must evaluate the elements of the methodology that affect the required sample size. Kraemer and Thiemann (1987) identified the following factors that must be taken into consideration in determining sample size:

1. The more stringent the significance level (e.g., 0.001 versus 0.05), the greater the necessary sample size. Most nursing studies include a level of significance or alpha (α) = 0.05.
2. Two-tailed statistical tests require larger sample sizes than one-tailed tests. (Tailedness of statistical tests is explained in Chapters 21 and 25.)
3. The smaller the effect size (*ES*), the larger the necessary sample size. The *ES* is a determination of the effectiveness of a treatment on the outcome (dependent) variable or the strength of the relationship between two variables.
4. The larger the power required, the larger the necessary sample size. Thus, a study requiring a power of 90% requires a much larger sample than a study with power set at 80%.
5. The smaller the sample size, the smaller the power of the study.
6. The factors that must be considered in decisions about sample size (because they affect power) are *ES*, type of study, number of variables, sensitivity of the measurement methods, and data analysis techniques. These factors are discussed in the following sections.

Effect Size

Effect is the presence of a phenomenon. If a phenomenon exists, it is not absent, and the null hypothesis is in error. However, effect is best understood when not considered in a dichotomous way—that is, as either present or absent. If a phenomenon exists, it exists to some degree. **Effect size** (*ES*) is the extent to which a phenomenon is present in a population. In this case, the term effect is used in a broader sense than the term cause and effect. For example, you might examine the impact of distraction on the experience of pain during an injection. To examine this question, you might obtain a sample of participants receiving injections and measure the perception of pain in the group that was distracted during the injection and the group that was not distracted. The null hypothesis would be: "There is no difference in the level of pain perceived by the

treatment group receiving distraction when compared with that of the comparison group receiving no distraction." If this were so, you would say that the effect of distraction on the perception of pain was zero, and the null hypothesis would be accepted. In another study, the Pearson product moment correlation *r* could be conducted to examine the relationship between coping and anxiety. Your null hypothesis would be that the population *r* would be zero, meaning that coping is not related to anxiety (Cohen, 1988).

In a study, it is easier to detect large differences between groups than to detect small differences. Strong relationships between variables in a study are easier to detect than weak relationships. Thus, smaller samples can detect large *ESs*; smaller *ESs* require larger samples. *ESs* can be positive or negative because variables can be either positively or negatively correlated. A negative *ES* exists when a treatment causes a decrease in the study mean, such as an exercise program that decreases the weight of subjects. Broadly speaking, the definitions for *ES* strengths might be as follows:

Small *ES* would be < 0.3 or < −0.3
Medium *ES* would be about 0.3 to 0.5 or −0.3 to −0.5
Large *ES* would be > 0.5 or > −0.5

These broad ranges are provided because the *ES* definitions of small, medium, and large vary based on the analysis being conducted. For example, the *ESs* for comparing two means, such as the treatment group mean and the comparison group mean (expressed as *d*), are small = 0.2 or −0.2, medium = 0.5 or −0.5, and large = 0.8 or −0.8. The *ESs* for relationships (expressed as *r*) might be defined as small = 0.1 or −0.1, medium = 0.3 or −0.3, and large = 0.5 or −0.5 (Aberson, 2010; Cohen, 1988).

Extremely small *ESs* (e.g., < 0.1) may not be clinically important because the relationships between the variables are small or the differences between the treatment and comparison groups are limited. Knowing the *ES* that would be regarded as clinically important allows us to limit the sample to the size needed to detect that level of *ES* (Kraemer & Thiemann, 1987). A result is clinically important if the effect is large enough to alter clinical decisions. For example, in comparing glass thermometers with electronic thermometers, an *ES* = 0.1° F in oral temperature is probably not important enough to influence selection of a particular type of thermometer in clinical practice. The clinical importance of an *ES* varies on the basis of the variables being studied and the population. For example, a decrease in average ambulance transfer time to a trauma center from 22 minutes to 21 minutes may have clinical significance for unstable patients. Researchers must determine the *ES* for the particular relationship or effect being studied in a population. The most desirable source of this information is evidence from previous studies (Aberson, 2010; Melnyk & Fineout-Overholt, 2015).

A correlation value (r) is equal to the *ES* for the relationship between two variables. For example, if depression is correlated with anxiety at $r = 0.45$, the $ES = r = 0.45$, a medium *ES*.

$$ES \text{ formula for relationships} = r$$

$$\text{Example: } ES = r = 0.45$$

Most *ESs* are calculated using a computer program (Grove & Cipher, 2017). However, in published studies with treatments, means and standard deviations can be used to calculate the *ES*. For example, if the mean weight loss for the treatment or intervention group is 5 pounds per month with a standard deviation (SD) = 4.5, and the mean weight loss of the comparison group is 1 pound per month with $SD = 6.5$, you can calculate the *ES*, which is usually expressed as *d*.

ES formula for group differences = d = (mean of the treatment group − mean of the control group) ÷ standard deviation of the control group

$$\text{Example: } ES = d = (5 - 1) \div 6.5 = 4 \div 6.5$$

$$= 0.615 = 0.62$$

This calculation can be used only as an estimate of *ES* for a specific study. If the researcher changes the measurement method used, the design of the study, or the population being studied, the *ES* will be altered. When estimating *ES* based on previous studies, you might note the *ESs* vary from 0.33 to 0.45; it is best to choose the lower *ES* of 0.33 to calculate a sample size for a study. As the *ES* decreases, the sample size needed to obtain statistical significance in a study increases. The best estimate of a population parameter of *ES* is obtained from a meta-analysis in which an estimated population *ES* is calculated through the use of statistical values from all studies included in the analysis (Aberson, 2010; Cohen, 1988; Grove & Cipher, 2017).

If few relevant studies have been conducted in the area of interest, a small pilot study can be performed, and data analysis results can be used to calculate the *ES*. If pilot studies are not feasible, a dummy power table analysis can be used to calculate the smallest *ES* with clinical or theoretical value. Yarandi (1991) described the process of calculating a dummy power table. If all else fails, *ES* can be estimated as small, medium, or large. Numerical values would be assigned to these

estimates and the power analysis performed. As mentioned earlier, Cohen (1988) and Aberson (2010) indicated the numerical values for small, medium, and large effects on the basis of specific statistical procedures. In new areas of research, *ESs* for studies are usually set as small (< 0.3). Gaskin and Happell (2014) conducted a study of the statistical practices in nursing research and noted inconsistent reporting and infrequent interpretation of *ESs*, which require attention by nurse researchers.

Newnam and colleagues (2015, p. 36) conducted a power analysis to determine the sample size needed for study of the effectiveness of "continuous positive airway pressure [CPAP]-related skin breakdown when using different nasal interfaces in the extremely low birth weight [BW] neonate." The sample criteria and sampling methods for this study were discussed earlier and the power analysis and sample size are described in the following excerpt.

"An a priori sample size estimation was calculated using 80% power, $\alpha = 0.05$ with F tests as the statistical basis of the calculation using G*Power 3.0™. The calculated group size of 72 total subjects, 24 subjects in each of the three groups was deemed adequate to determine significant difference between groups." (Newnam et al., 2015, p. 37)

Newnam et al. (2015) conducted a power analysis to determine an adequate sample size for their study. The standard power of 80% was used, and alpha was set at 0.05. The statistical basis for the power analysis was identified as the F test or analysis of variance (ANOVA). However, the researchers did not provide the *ES* used in the calculation. The focus of the study was determining differences among the three groups of neonates receiving CPAP by the following methods: mask CPAP, $n = 35$; prong CPAP, $n = 21$; and rotation of mask/prong CPAP, $n = 22$ (see Figure 15-2). The total sample size was 78, which is larger than the 72 participants recommended by power analysis. However, the study would have been stronger if the group sizes had been more equal and each group had included at least 24 neonates. Newnam et al. (2015) did find significantly less skin injury in the group treated with the rotation of mask and prongs. The significant results indicate the study had an adequate sample size to determine differences among the three groups using ANOVA with a Bonferroni correction (see Chapter 25). If the study findings had been nonsignificant, the researchers would need to have determined whether adequate power had been achieved in the study.

Type of Study

Descriptive case studies tend to use small samples. Groups are not compared, and problems related to sampling error and generalization have little relevance for such studies. A small sample size may better serve the researcher who is interested in examining a situation in depth from various perspectives. Other descriptive studies, particularly studies using survey questionnaires, and correlational studies often require large samples. In these studies, multiple variables may be examined, and extraneous variables are likely to affect subject responses to the variables under study. Statistical comparisons are often made among multiple subgroups in the sample, requiring that an adequate sample be available for each subgroup being analyzed. In addition, subjects are likely to be heterogeneous in terms of demographic variables, and measurement tools are sometimes not adequately refined. Although target populations may have been identified, sampling frames may be unavailable, and parameters have not usually been well defined by previous studies. All of these factors decrease the power of the study and require increases in sample size (Aberson, 2010; Kraemer & Thiemann, 1987).

In the past, quasi-experimental and experimental studies often have used smaller samples than descriptive and correlational studies. As control in the study increases, the sample size can decrease and still approximate the population. Instruments in these studies tend to be refined, improving precision. However, sample size must be sufficient to achieve an acceptable level of power (0.8) and reduce the risk of a type II error (indicating the study findings are nonsignificant, when they really are significant) (Aberson, 2010; Kraemer & Thiemann, 1987).

The study design influences power, but the design with the greatest power may not always be the most valid design to use. The experimental design with the greatest power is the pretest-posttest design with a historical control or comparison group. However, this design may have questionable validity because of the historical control group. Can the researcher demonstrate that the historical control group is comparable to the experimental group? The repeated measures design increases power if the trait being assessed is relatively stable over time. Designs that use blocking or stratification usually require an increase in the total sample size. The sample size increases in proportion to the number of cells included in the data analysis. Designs that use matched pairs of subjects have greater power and require a smaller sample (see Chapter 11 for a discussion of these designs). The higher the degree of correlation between subjects on the variable on which the subjects

are matched, the greater the power (Kraemer & Thiemann, 1987).

Kraemer and Thiemann (1987) classified studies as *exploratory* or *confirmatory*. According to their approach, confirmatory studies should be conducted only after a large body of knowledge has been gathered through exploratory studies. **Confirmatory studies** are expected to have large samples and to use random sampling techniques. These expectations are less stringent for exploratory studies. **Exploratory studies** are not intended for generalization to large populations. They are designed to increase the knowledge in the field of study. For example, pilot or preliminary studies to test a methodology or provide estimates of an *ES* often are conducted before a larger study. In other studies, the variables, not the subjects, are the primary area of concern. Several studies may examine the same variables using different populations. In these types of studies, the specific population used may be incidental. Data from these studies may be used to define population parameters. This information can be used to conduct confirmatory studies using large, randomly selected samples.

Confirmatory studies, such as studies testing the effects of nursing interventions on patient outcomes or studies testing the fit of a theoretical model, require large sample sizes. Clinical trials are conducted in nursing for these purposes. The power of these large, complex studies must be carefully analyzed (Leidy & Weissfeld, 1991). For the large sample sizes to be obtained, subjects are acquired in numerous clinical settings, sometimes in different parts of the U.S. Kraemer and Thiemann (1987) believed that these studies should not be performed until extensive information is available from exploratory studies. This information should include a meta-analysis and the definition of a population *ES*.

Number of Variables

As the number of variables under study grows, the needed sample size may also increase. Adding variables such as age, gender, ethnicity, and education to the analysis plan (just to be on the safe side) can increase the sample size by a factor of 5 to 10 if the selected variables are uncorrelated with the dependent variable. In this case, instead of a sample of 50, you may need a sample of 250 to 500 if you plan to include the variables in the statistical analyses. (Using them only to describe the sample does not cause a problem in terms of power.) If the variables are highly correlated with the dependent variable, however, the *ES* will increase, and the sample size can be reduced.

Variables included in the data analysis must be carefully selected. They should be essential to the research purpose or should have a documented strong relationship with the dependent variable (Kraemer & Thiemann, 1987). Sometimes researchers have obtained sufficient sample size for the primary analyses but failed to plan for analyses involving subgroups, such as analyzing the data by age categories or by ethnic groups, which require a larger sample size. A larger sample size is also needed if multiple dependent variables have been measured in the study.

Measurement Sensitivity

Well-developed instruments measure phenomena with precision. For example, a thermometer measures body temperature precisely, usually to one-tenth of a degree. Instruments measuring psychosocial variables tend to be less precise. However, a scale with strong reliability and validity tends to measure more precisely than an instrument that is not as well developed. Variance tends to be higher in a less well-developed tool than in one that is well developed. An instrument with a smaller variance is preferred because the power of a test always decreases when within-group variance increases (Kraemer & Thiemann, 1987). If you were measuring the phenomenon of anxiety and the actual anxiety score for several subjects was 80, the subjects' scores on a less well-developed scale might range from 70 to 90, whereas a well-developed scale would tend to show a score closer to the actual score of 80 for each subject. As variance in instrument scores increases, the sample size needed to gain an accurate understanding of the phenomenon increases (Waltz et al., 2010).

The range of measured values influences power. For example, a variable might be measured in 10 equally spaced values, ranging from 0 to 9. *ESs* vary according to how near the value is to the population mean. If the mean value is 5, *ESs* are much larger in the extreme values and lower for values near the mean. If you decided to use only subjects with values of 0 and 9, the *ES* would be large, and the sample could be small. The credibility of the study might be questionable, however, because the values of most individuals would not be 0 or 9 but rather would tend to be in the middle range of values. If you decided to include subjects who have values in the range of 3 to 6, excluding the extreme scores, the *ES* would be small, and you would require a much larger sample. The wider the range of values sampled, the larger the *ES* (Kraemer & Thiemann, 1987). In a heterogeneous group of study participants, you would expect them to have a wide range of scores on a depression scale, which would increase the *ES*. A strong

measurement method has validity and reliability, and measures variables at the interval or ratio level (see Chapter 16). The stronger the measurement methods used in a study, the smaller the sample that is needed to identify significant relationships among variables and differences between groups.

Data Analysis Techniques

Data analysis techniques vary in their ability to detect differences in the data. Statisticians refer to this as the power of the statistical analysis. For your data analysis, choose the most powerful statistical test appropriate to the data. Overall, parametric statistical analyses are more powerful than nonparametric techniques in detecting differences and should be used if the data meet criteria for parametric analysis. However, in many cases, nonparametric techniques are more powerful if your data do not meet the assumptions of parametric techniques. Parametric techniques vary widely in their capacity to distinguish fine differences and relationships in the data. Parametric and nonparametric analyses are discussed in Chapter 21.

There is also an interaction between the measurement sensitivity and the power of the data analysis technique. The power of the analysis technique increases as precision in measurement increases. Larger samples must be used when the power of the planned statistical analysis is low (Gaskin & Happell, 2014).

For some statistical procedures, such as the *t*-test and ANOVA, having equal group sizes increases power because the *ES* is maximized. The more unequal the group sizes are, the smaller the *ES*. In unequal groups, the total sample size must be larger (Kraemer & Thiemann, 1987).

The chi-square (χ^2) test is the weakest of the statistical tests and requires very large sample sizes to achieve acceptable levels of power. As the number of categories (cells in the chi-square analysis) in a study grows, the sample size needed increases. Also, if there are small numbers in some of the categories, you must increase the sample size. Kraemer and Thiemann (1987) recommended that the chi-square test be used only when no other options are available. In addition, the categories should be limited to those essential to the study.

SAMPLE SIZE IN QUALITATIVE RESEARCH

In quantitative research, the sample size must be large enough to describe variables, identify relationships among variables, or determine differences between groups. However, in qualitative research, the focus is on the quality of information obtained from the person, situation, event, or documents sampled versus the size of the sample (Marshall & Rossman, 2016; Munhall, 2012; Sandelowski, 1995). The sample size and sampling plan are determined by the purpose and philosophical basis of the study. In addition, the sample size varies with the depth of information needed to gain insight into a phenomenon, explore and describe a concept, describe a cultural element, develop a theory, or describe a historical event (Miles et al., 2014; Munhall, 2012). The sample size can be too small when the data collected lack adequate depth or richness. An inadequate sample size can reduce the quality and credibility of the research findings. Many qualitative researchers use purposive or purposeful sampling methods to select the specific participants, events, or situations that they believe would provide them the rich data needed to gain insights and discover new meaning in an area of study.

The researchers should justify the adequacy of the sample size in a qualitative study. Often the number of participants in a qualitative study is adequate when saturation of information is achieved in the study area. **Saturation of data**, also referred to as informational redundancy, occurs when additional sampling provides no new information, only redundancy of previously collected data. Important factors that must be considered in determining sample size to achieve saturation of data are (1) scope of the study, (2) nature of the topic, (3) quality of the data, and (4) study design (Charmaz, 2014; Marshall & Rossman, 2016; Morse, 2000, 2012; Munhall, 2012).

Scope of the Study

If the scope of a study is broad, researchers need extensive data to address the study purpose, and it takes longer to reach data saturation. A study with a broad scope requires more sampling of participants, events, or documents than a study with a narrow scope (Morse, 2000, 2012). A study that has a clear focus and employs focused data collection usually has richer, more credible findings. For example, fewer participants would be needed to detail the phenomenon of chronic pain in adults with rheumatoid arthritis than would be needed to describe the phenomenon of chronic pain in elderly adults. A study of chronic pain experienced by elderly adults has a much broader focus, with less clarity, than a study of chronic pain experienced by adults with a specific medical diagnosis of rheumatoid arthritis.

Nature of the Topic

If the topic of your study is clear and the participants can easily discuss it, fewer individuals are needed to obtain the essential, rich data. If the topic is difficult to define and awkward for people to discuss, you will probably need a larger number of participants or informants to reach the point of data saturation (Marshall & Rossman, 2016; Miles et al., 2014). For example, a phenomenological study of the experience of an adult living with a history of childhood sexual abuse is a sensitive, complex topic to investigate. This type of topic would probably require a greater number of participants and increased interview time to collect the essential data.

Quality of the Data

The quality of information obtained from an interview, observation, focus group, or document review influences the sample size. The higher the quality and richness of the data, the fewer research participants needed to saturate data in the area of study. Quality data are best obtained from articulate, well-informed, and communicative participants. These participants are able to share richer and often more data in a clear and concise manner. In addition, participants who have more time to be interviewed usually provide data with greater depth and breadth. Qualitative studies require that you critically appraise the quality of the richness of communication elicited from the participants, the degree of access provided to events in a culture, or the number and quality of documents studied. These characteristics directly affect the richness of the data collected and influence the sample size needed to achieve quality study findings (Miles et al., 2014).

Study Design

Some studies are designed to conduct more than a single interview with each participant. The more interviews conducted with a participant, the greater the quantity and probably the quality of the data collected. For example, a study design that includes an interview both before and after an event would produce more data than a single interview. Designs that involve interviewing a family or a group of individuals produce more data than an interview with a single study participant. In grounded theory studies, participants are interviewed until a model or theory is developed for the area of study. Theoretical sampling is usually implemented to achieve theoretical clarity in a grounded theory study (Charmaz, 2014). In critically appraising a qualitative study, determine whether the sample size is adequate for the design of the study.

Sun, Long, Tsao, and Huang (2014) conducted a grounded theory study to develop a theory to assist suicidal individuals in healing after their suicide attempt. The sample was obtained with theoretical sampling, and the following study excerpt provides the researchers' rationale for the final sample size of 20 participants.

"Theoretical sampling was used because it helped to integrate the concepts and to clarify the relationship between one concept and another. Accordingly, each interview guide was modified before the next interview in harmony with concepts that emerged during the previous interview; for instance, when the patient participants expressed that psychiatric consultants had helped cure them from their depression and prevented suicide attempts, an additional four psychiatric professionals were selected for interview to reach saturation for the data. Moreover, when this study achieved data saturation, the researcher, added three more participants to confirm that this study had really achieved saturation. That is, no new concept was elicited in the three participants. The total number of participants in this study was 20 participants including patients who were healing from suicide attempts ($n = 14$) and their caregivers ($n = 6$)." (Sun et al., 2014, p. 56)

The study by Sun et al. (2014) has many strengths in the area of sampling, including quality of the theoretical sampling method that resulted in a robust sample size of 20 conscientious participants. The investigators provide extensive details of the theoretical sampling conducted to ensure saturation was achieved with no new categories emerging when interviewing the last three study participants. Sun et al. (2014) identified that caring family and friends, treatment by mental health professionals, support from society, religious support, and decreased stress were important for healing following a suicide attempt. The healing journey was impeded by received negative aspects of self, family predicaments, environmental difficulties, and escalation of stress. These healing and impeding circumstances were incorporated into a model that might be used in suicide prevention centers.

RESEARCH SETTINGS

The **setting** is the location where a study is conducted. There are three common settings for conducting nursing research: natural, partially controlled, and highly controlled. A **natural setting**, or *field setting*, is an uncontrolled, real-life situation or environment (Kerlinger & Lee, 2000). Conducting a study in a natural setting means that the researcher does not manipulate or change the environment for the study. Descriptive and correlational quantitative studies, qualitative, mixed methods, and outcomes studies often are conducted in

natural settings. Subaiya and colleagues (2014) conducted their study of a needs assessment after Hurricane Sandy in a natural setting. This study was discussed earlier in this chapter in the section on cluster sampling. The study setting was "the Rockaway Peninsula on the southern coast of the borough of Queens, within NYC, and it extends to the Atlantic Ocean" (Subaiya et al., 2014, p. 623). This setting was selected because it is highly populated and one of the areas hardest hit by Hurricane Sandy. Data were collected by interviewing participants in their homes.

A **partially controlled setting** is an environment that the researcher manipulates or modifies in some way while conducting a study. An increasing number of nursing studies are being conducted in partially controlled settings. Wang et al. (2015) conducted their quasi-experimental study of the effects of biofeedback relaxation on the pain associated with a total knee arthroplasty (TKA) in a partially controlled setting. This study was introduced previously in the section on convenience sampling. The setting for the implementation of the intervention and data collection is described in the following study excerpt.

"The typical length of stay for TKA in Taiwan is 5–7 days. All participants were prescribed the standard of care for the study hospital of two 30-minute daily sessions of CPM [continuous passive motion] therapy, beginning the first postoperative day until the discharge day." (Wang et al., 2015, p. 41)

"The study intervention consisted of a 30-minute biofeedback-assisted progressive muscle relaxation training session during the CPM sessions twice daily for 5 days... Then in each CPM treatment session, the patients practiced progressive muscle relaxation while observing how the computerized images changed to indicate successful muscle tension and muscle relaxation. An interventionist guided the patient through the biofeedback intervention in each session...The data were collected during 2010. At baseline, each participant completed a demographics questionnaire. A research nurse also collected data on disease variables, including diagnosis, surgical procedures, CPM, and analgesic prescriptions, from the patients' charts... Data on pain intensity were collected before and after each CPM therapy from postoperative days one through five in both groups." (Wang et al, 2015, pp. 42–43)

The setting for the Wang et al. (2015) study was partially controlled because it was conducted in a hospital setting, where the intervention and data collection processes were controlled. All subjects received standard care during their hospitalization, and the patients in the intervention group received the biofeedback intervention guided by an interventionist. The data were collected by a research nurse. The hospital setting was appropriate for this study and provided a controlled environment for the manipulation of the intervention and collection of essential data.

A **highly controlled setting** is a structured environment that often is artificially developed for the purpose of conducting research. Laboratories, research or experimental centers, and test or highly structured units in hospitals or other healthcare agencies are highly controlled settings. Often experimental and sometimes quasi-experimental studies are conducted in these types of settings. A highly controlled setting reduces the influence of extraneous variables, which enables researchers to examine accurately the effect of an intervention on an outcome. Newnam et al. (2015) conducted an experimental study to determine the effectiveness of CPAP on related skin breakdown when using different nasal interfaces in extremely low BW neonates. This study, introduced earlier, had strong inclusion and exclusion sampling criteria to ensure a homogenous sample was selected (see Figure 15-2). The highly controlled setting used in this study is described in the following excerpt.

"A three group prospective randomized experimental study design was conducted in a 70 bed level III neonatal intensive care unit (NICU) in the southeastern United States... A team of skin experts, described as the Core Research Team (CRT) was made up of the principal investigator and three advanced practice nurses. The CRT was responsible for obtaining parental consent and conducting serial skin care evaluations on enrolled subjects during routine care in an effort to protect the infant's quiet environment. The initial skin assessment was completed within 8 hours of extubation and at intervals of every 10–12 hours while receiving nasal CPAP." (Newnam et al., 2015, pp. 37–38)

The setting for Newnam et al. (2015) study was highly controlled due to the structure of the NICU and the organization and type of care delivered in this setting. The researchers also ensured that the CPAP treatments were continuously implemented with a selected nasal device (mask, prongs, or mask/prongs). The nasal skin evaluations were done in a precise and accurate way by experts, the CRT. This controlled setting is appropriate for this study to reduce the effects of extraneous variables and increase the credibility of the findings.

RECRUITING AND RETAINING RESEARCH PARTICIPANTS

After a research team makes a decision about the size of the sample, the next step is to develop a plan for **recruiting research participants**, which involves identifying, accessing, and communicating with potential study participants who are representative of the target population. Recruitment strategies differ, depending on the type of study, population, and setting. Special attention must focus on recruiting subjects who tend to be underrepresented in studies, such as minorities, women, children, elderly adults, the critically ill, the economically disadvantaged, and the incarcerated (Bryant et al., 2014; Goshin & Byrne, 2012; Hines-Martin, Speck, Stetson, & Looney, 2009). The sampling plan, initiated at the beginning of data collection, is almost always more difficult than expected. In addition to participant recruitment, retaining acquired participants is critical to achieve an acceptable sample size and requires researchers to consider the effects of the data collection strategies on sample attrition. **Retaining research participants** involves the participants completing the required behaviors of a study to its conclusion. The problems with retaining participants increase as the data collection period lengthens. Some researchers never obtain their planned sample size, which could decrease the power of the study and potentially produce nonsignificant results (Aberson, 2010; Gul & Ali, 2010). With an increasing number of studies being conducted in health care, recruiting and retaining subjects have become more complex issues for researchers to manage (Irani & Richmond, 2015; McGregor, Parker, LeBlanc, & King, 2010; Reifsnider et al., 2014).

Recruiting Research Participants

The effective recruitment of subjects is crucial to the success of a study. An increasing number of studies examining the effectiveness of various strategies of participant recruitment and retention have appeared in the recent professional literature (Bryant et al., 2014; Davidson, Cronk, Harrar, Catley, & Good, 2010; Engstrom, Tappen, & Ouslander, 2014; Reifsnider et al., 2014; Whitebird, Bliss, Savik, Lowry, & Jung, 2010). Irani and Richmond (2015, p. 161) conducted an exploratory-descriptive study to identify the reasons "adult patients seeking emergency department care for minor injuries agreed to participate in clinical research." They identified the themes and subthemes for the adults

TABLE 15-4 Reasons for Participation in Clinical Research After Minor Physical Injury

Themes	Subthemes
1. Being asked	Recruiter's approach
	Setting and circumstances
2. Altruism	Helping other injured individuals
	Contributing to knowledge development
3. Potential for personal benefit	Sharing concerns
	Practicing self-reflection
	Being regularly monitored
4. Financial gain	
5. Curiosity	Interest in the study
6. Valuing knowledge of research	Personal experience with being part of a research study/team

From Irani, E., & Richmond, T. S. (2015). Reasons for and reservations about research participation in acutely injured adults. *Journal of Nursing Scholarship, 47*(2), 164.

participating in their study in Table 15-4. These themes provide direction to researchers in recruiting study participants.

The researcher's initial communication with a potential subject usually strongly affects the subject's decision about participating in the study. Therefore, the approach must be pleasant, positive, informative, culturally sensitive, and nonaggressive. The researcher needs to explain the importance of the study and clarify exactly what the subject will be asked to do, how much of the subject's time will be involved, and what the duration of the study will be. Study participants are valuable resources, and researchers must communicate this value to the potential participant. High-pressure techniques, such as insisting that the potential subject make an instant decision to participate in a study, usually lead to resistance and a higher rate of refusals. If the study involves minorities, researchers must be culturally competent or knowledgeable and skilled in relating to the particular ethnic group being studied (Hines-Martin et al., 2009; Papadopoulos & Lees, 2002). If the researcher is not of the same culture as the potential subjects, he or she may employ a data collector who is of the same culture. Hendrickson (2007) used a video for recruiting

Hispanic women for her study, and she provided all the details related to the study in the subjects' own language in the video. This approach greatly improved the subjects' understanding of the study and their desire to participate.

If a potential subject refuses to participate in a study, you must accept the refusal gracefully—in terms of body language as well as words. Your actions can influence the decision of other potential participants who observe or hear about the encounter. Studies in which a high proportion of individuals refuse to participate have a serious validity problem (see the earlier discussion of acceptance and refusal rates). The sample is likely to be biased because often only a certain type of individual has agreed to participate. You should keep records of the numbers of persons who refuse and, if possible, their reasons for refusal. With this information, you can include the refusal rate in the published research report with the reasons for refusal. It would also be helpful if you could determine whether the potential subjects who refused to participate differed from the individuals who agreed to participate in the study, in terms of demographics, reasons for seeking health care, course of medical treatment, or other pertinent factors. This information will help you determine the representativeness of your sample.

Recruiting minority subjects for a study can be particularly problematic. Minority individuals may be difficult to locate and are often reluctant to participate in studies because of feelings of being *used* while receiving no personal benefit from their involvement or because of their distrust of the medical community. Effective strategies for recruiting minorities include developing partnerships with target groups, community leaders, and potential participants in the community; using active face-to-face recruitment in nonthreatening settings; and using appropriate language to communicate clearly the purpose, benefits, and risks of the study (Alvarez, Vasquez, Mayorga, Feaster, & Mitrani, 2006; Bryant et al., 2014). Hines-Martin et al. (2009) studied the recruitment and retention process for intervention research conducted with a sample of primarily low-income African American women. Their complex, multistage recruitment strategies are introduced in the following excerpt.

"Phase 1 involved the development of a recruitment team, composed of a co-investigator, in addition to an African American nurse familiar with the target population, and two women who were long-standing community members.

Phase 1 activities began with periods of observation in the community setting and discussions with community center personnel to improve the investigators' understanding of who used the community center services and when. It became increasingly clear that only two of the three communities felt a connection with or used the community center routinely.... Therefore, the recruitment team, with the assistance from nursing graduate students, walked every block of the two relevant communities at different times of the day and different days of the week to better understand when and where community women could be found in their daily lives.... Community women were informed of new initiatives at the center and were provided with recruitment flyers including pictures of the research team. The recruitment team then undertook usual recruitment activities, such as meeting with women's groups in the communities and recruitment at community fairs." (Hines-Martin et al., 2009, pp. 665–666)

Hines-Martin and colleagues (2009) stressed the benefit from the endorsement of community leaders, such as city officials, key civic leaders, and leaders of social, educational, religious, or labor groups. In some cases, these groups may be involved in planning the study, leading to a sense of community ownership of the project. Community groups may also help researchers to recruit subjects for the study. Subjects who meet the sampling criteria sometimes are found in the groups assisting with the study. These activities can add legitimacy to the study and make involvement in the study more attractive to potential subjects (Davidson et al., 2010; Engstrom et al., 2014).

If researchers use data collectors in their studies, they need to verify that the data collectors are following the sampling plan, especially in studies using random samples. For instance, when data collectors encounter difficult subjects or are unable to make contact easily, they may simply shift to the next available person without informing the principal investigator. This behavior could violate the rules of random sampling and bias the sample. If data collectors do not understand, or do not believe in, the importance of randomization, their decisions and actions can undermine the intent of the sampling plan. Thus, data collectors must be carefully selected and thoroughly trained. A plan for the supervision and follow-up of data collectors to increase their accountability should be developed (see Chapter 20).

If you conduct a survey as part of your study, you may never have personal contact with the subjects. To recruit such subjects, you must rely on the use of attention-getting techniques, persuasively written materials, and strategies for following up on individuals who do not respond to the initial written or email communication. The strategies need to be appropriate to the potential participants; mailed surveys are probably still the best way to obtain information from elderly adults. Because of the serious problems of analysis and interpretation posed by low response rates with survey research, using strategies to increase the response rate is critical. Creativity is required in the use of such strategies because they tend to lose their effect on groups who receive questionnaires frequently. In some cases, small amounts of money ($1.00 to $5.00) are enclosed with the letter, which may suggest that the recipient buy a soft drink or that the money is a small offering for completing the questionnaire. This strategy imposes some sense of obligation on the recipient to complete the questionnaire, but it is not thought to be coercive. Also, you should plan emailing or mailings to avoid holidays or times of the year when activities are high for potential subjects, possibly reducing the return rate. For example, if you were conducting a study with mothers of school-age children, you would want to avoid the beginning of a new school term.

Researchers frequently use the Internet to recruit participants and to collect survey data. This method makes it easier for you to contact potential participants and for them to provide the requested data. However, an increased number of surveys are being sent by the Internet, which can decrease the response rate of potential participants who are frequently surveyed, but increase the participation of potential participants not accessible by traditional recruitment measures. Most Internet questionnaires or scales are going to an email list of potential study participants or are posted on a website. The letter encouraging potential participants to take part in the study must be carefully composed. It may be your only chance to persuade them to invest the time needed to complete the study questionnaire or scale. You must sell the reader on the importance of both your study and his or her response. The tone of your letter will be the potential subject's only image of you as a person; yet, for many subjects, their response to the perception of you as a person most influences their decision about completing the questionnaire. Seek examples of letters sent by researchers who have had high response rates, and save letters you received to which you responded positively. You also might pilot-test your letter on potential research participants who can give you feedback about their reactions to the letter's tone.

The use of follow-up emails, letters, or cards has been repeatedly shown to raise response rates to surveys. The timing is important. If too long a period has lapsed, the potential subject may have deleted the questionnaire from his or her email inbox or discarded the mailed copy. However, sending the follow-up too soon could be offensive. A bar graph could be developed to record the return of the questionnaires as a means of suggesting when the follow-up mailing or emailing should occur. The cumulative number and percentage of responses over time would be logged on the graph to reflect the overall data collection process. When the daily or weekly responses decline, a follow-up email or first-class letter could be sent encouraging individuals to complete the study questionnaire. Often a third follow-up, with a modified cover letter, is emailed or mailed to participants with a final request that they complete the study questionnaires or scales.

The factors involved in the decision of whether to respond to a questionnaire are not well understood. One factor is the time required to respond; this includes the time needed to orient oneself to the directions and the emotional energy necessary to deal with any threats or anxieties generated by the questions. There is also a cognitive demand for making decisions. Subjects seem to make a judgment about the relevance of the research topic and the potential for personal application of findings. Previous experience with questionnaires is also a deciding factor.

Traditionally, subjects for physiological nursing studies have been sought in the hospital setting. However, access to these subjects is becoming more difficult—in part because of the larger numbers of nurses and other healthcare professionals now conducting research. The largest involvement of research subjects within a healthcare agency usually occurs in the field of medical research, and is primarily associated with clinical trials that include large samples (Gul & Ali, 2010). Whitebird et al. (2010) identified three successful recruitment methods to use in healthcare agencies: (1) identifying potential participants using administrative databases, (2) obtaining referrals of potential participants through healthcare providers and other sources, and (3) approaching directly a known potential subject. An initial phase of recruitment may involve obtaining community and institutional support for the study. Support from other healthcare professionals, such as nurses, physicians, and clinical agency staff, is usually crucial for the successful recruitment of study participants.

Recruitment of subjects for clinical trials requires a different set of strategies because the recruitment may occur simultaneously in several sites (perhaps in different cities). Many of these multisite clinical trials never achieve their planned sample size. The number of participants meeting the sampling criteria who are available in the selected clinical sites may not be as large as anticipated. Researchers must often screen twice as many patients as are required for a study in order to obtain a sufficient sample size. Screening logs must be kept during the recruiting period to record data on patients who met the criteria but were not entered into the study. Researchers commonly underestimate the amount of time required to recruit study participants for a clinical trial. In addition to defining the number of participants and the time set aside for recruitment, it may be helpful to develop short-term or interim recruitment goals designed to maintain a constant rate of patient entry (Gul & Ali, 2010). Hellard, Sinclair, Forbes, and Fairley (2001) studied methods to improve the recruitment and retention of subjects in clinical trials and found that the four most important strategies were to (1) use nonaggressive recruitment methods, (2) maintain regular contact with the participants, (3) ensure that the participants are kept well informed of the progress of the study, and (4) provide constant encouragement to subjects to continue participation. Sullivan-Bolyai et al. (2007) detailed the barriers to recruiting study participants from clinical settings in their article. Table 15-5 identifies these common barriers to research participant recruitment and provides possible strategies to manage them.

Media support can be helpful in recruiting subjects. Researchers can place advertisements in local newspapers and church and neighborhood bulletins. Radio stations can make public service announcements. Members of the research team can speak to groups relevant to the study population. Your team can place posters in public places, such as supermarkets, drugstores, and public laundries. With permission, you can set up tables in shopping malls with a member of the research team present to recruit subjects. Plan for possible challenges in recruitment and include multiple methods and two to three locations in your application for human subject approval for your study. Otherwise, you would need to submit a modified protocol to the institutional review board (IRB) when you add a method or site for recruitment. However, obtaining access to additional locations is time-consuming due to the IRB process.

Davidson et al. (2010) used multiple strategies to recruit and retain college smokers in a cessation clinical trial. Their four-phase recruitment process is presented in the following study excerpt.

TABLE 15-5   Barriers to Recruitment with Actions and Strategies for Engaging Healthcare Providers in the Referral Process

Barriers and Actions	Strategies
HIPAA* Create alternative recruitment methods	Ask clinicians to distribute letters to potential study participants Obtain institutional review board waiver of authorization requirement for the use or disclosure of personal health information Work with clinics to secure a consent that meets HIPAA* regulations and allows the staff to provide names and contact information of patients with specific conditions that may be of interest to researchers Recognize and acknowledge the burden that recruitment places on healthcare providers
Work burden Create compensations	Provide salary support Provide educational incentives (e.g., purchase laptop, journals, books, pay for conference attendance in the field under study) for healthcare providers who do not normally have access to such opportunities as part of their job Assess administrative or managerial perceptions of healthcare providers' recruitment-related responsibilities, and if salary support is given, how that money will be used Discuss the designated recruitment tasks and responsibilities with the assigned staff to determine their perceptions and expectations
Financial disincentives Recognize that patient numbers or productivity may be linked to the clinic's livelihood	Assess the clinic's financial situation and determine if it is realistic, pragmatic, or feasible to use that site, especially if its funding depends on patient numbers Help keep participants linked to the clinical site while they are participating in the study
Provider competition Create a partnership with healthcare providers involved in recruitment so that they are rewarded and acknowledged for their participation in the research process	Develop a research proposal that reflects the clinical site's philosophical and policy perspectives and priorities Include healthcare providers in the development of a study Hire and pay a clinical staff member to be responsible for introducing the study to potential participants Link recruitment activities to nursing clinical ladder or organization values Maintain open communication between the clinical and research teams regarding the workings of the study
Provider concerns Demystify research process Develop a team atmosphere and a spirit of "we're all in this together"	Assess healthcare providers' perceptions of research Encourage healthcare providers to participate in developing the research proposal Include healthcare providers in developing study-related manuscripts Include healthcare providers in research team meetings at a mutually convenient time Express appreciation in an ongoing basis for healthcare providers' involvement in recruitment process Share recruitment status information on a monthly basis with healthcare providers Share pilot or feasibility data with healthcare providers to support the study rationale and choice of specific methods

TABLE 15-5 Barriers to Recruitment with Actions and Strategies for Engaging Healthcare Providers in the Referral Process—cont'd	
Barriers and Actions	**Strategies**
Desire to protect patients	Acknowledge responsibility of healthcare providers to protect patients from harm
Work with healthcare providers to acknowledge and respect patient decision-making abilities	Address concerns of healthcare providers by emphasizing the pilot data that support the protocol
Encourage healthy partnerships between patients and healthcare providers	Model respectful partnerships with study participants

HIPAA, Health Insurance Portability and Accountability Act.
From Sullivan-Bolyai, S., Bova, C., Deatrick, J. A., Knafl, K., Grey, M., Leung, K., et al. (2007). Barriers and strategies for recruiting study participants in clinical settings. *Western Journal of Nursing Research, 29*(4), 498–499.

"Participants in this study were members of Greek fraternities and sororities enrolled at a large Midwestern university, and data were collected from 2006 to 2009.... The clinical trial involved testing a four-session, MI [motivational interviewing] counseling intervention on smoking cessation. Participants were recruited from college fraternity and sorority chapters regardless of their interest in quitting smoking. Recruitment involved four phases. First, out of 41 fraternity and sorority chapters from a large Midwestern university, the 30 chapters with the larger memberships were invited to participate. Second, within these invited chapters, individuals were recruited to participate in an initial, 5-minute, 8-item screening survey (i.e., Screener).

Third, individual members of these 30 chapters who met the inclusion criteria based on the Screener and who were interested in participating in the study were recruited to participate in a more extensive (30–45 minute) computerized baseline assessment approximately 1–4 days following the Screener.... Fourthly, eligible individuals who completed the baseline assessment were recruited for enrollment in the clinical trial." (Davidson et al., 2010, pp. 146–147)

The recruitment for this smoking cessation clinical trial was accomplished by using the Greek chapters. Davidson et al. (2010) developed relationships with these Greek organizations by meeting with leaders and members and attending special events. To accomplish phases two and three, the researchers met with the participants at convenient times and in accessible locations. The participants were also provided incentives of food (cookies and pizza), small cash gifts, and raffles for iPods. These creative strategies increased the recruitment and retention of the study participants.

Retaining Participants in a Study

A serious problem in many studies is participant retention, and sometimes participant attrition cannot be avoided. Subjects move, die, or withdraw from a treatment. If you must collect data at several points, over time, subject attrition can become a problem. Study participants who move frequently or are without phones pose particular problems. Numerous strategies have been found to be effective in maintaining the sample. It is a good idea to obtain the names, email addresses, and phone numbers (cell and home numbers if possible) of at least two family members or friends when you enroll the participant in the study. Ask whether the participant would agree to give you access to unlisted phone numbers in the event of changes in his or her number.

In some studies, subjects are reimbursed for time and expenses related to participation. A bonus payment may be included for completing a certain phase of the study. Gifts can be used in place of money. Sending greeting cards for birthdays and holidays helps maintain contact. Researchers have found that money was more effective than gifts in retaining subjects in longitudinal studies. However, some people think this strategy can compromise the voluntariness of participation in a study and particularly has the potential of exploiting low-income persons. When the monetary gift is small ($5.00 to $20.00) and consistent with the responsibilities of the participants, most consider these acceptable (Engstrom et al., 2014). It is important that the incentives used to recruit and retain research participants be documented in the published study.

Collecting data takes time. The participant's time is valuable and should be used frugally. During data collection, it is easy to begin taking the participant for granted. Taking time for social amenities with participants may also pay off. However, take care that these interactions do not influence the data being collected. Beyond that, nurturing subjects participating in the study is critical. In some situations, providing refreshments and pleasant surroundings are helpful. During the data collection phase, you also may need to nurture others who interact with the participants; these may be volunteers, family, staff, students, or other professionals. It is important to maintain a pleasant climate for the data collection process, which pays off in the quality of data collected and the retention of study participants (Bryant et al., 2014; Davidson et al., 2010; Gul & Ali, 2010; McGregor et al., 2010).

Qualitative studies with more than one data collection point and longitudinal quantitative studies require extensive time commitments from participants. They are asked to participate in detailed interviews or to complete numerous forms at various intervals during a study (Marshall & Rossman, 2016; Munhall, 2012). Sometimes data are collected with diaries that require daily entries over a set period of time. These studies face the greatest risk of participant attrition. Chapters 4 and 12 provide more details on the recruitment and retention of research participants for qualitative studies.

Davidson et al. (2010), whose recruitment strategies were introduced earlier, describe their success with retention in their smoking cessation clinical trial in the following excerpt.

"A very high proportion of participants (89%) completed at least one session (90% treatment; 87% comparison). The majority (73%) were retained, completing three or more sessions (75% treatment; 70% comparison), and over half completed the maximum of four sessions (63% treatment; 61% comparison). At the follow-up assessment occurring 6 months after the baseline assessment, 79% of the participants (n = 357) were retained (80% treatment; 78% comparison)." (Davidson et al., 2010, p. 150)

In summary, research participants who have a personal investment in a study are more likely to complete the study. This investment occurs through interactions with and nurturing by the researcher. A combination of the participant's personal belief in the significance of the study, the perceived altruistic motives of the researcher in conducting the study, the ethical actions of the researcher, and the nurturing support provided by the researcher during data collection can greatly diminish subject attrition (Irani & Richmond, 2015). Recruit-

ment and retention of study participants will continue to be significant challenges for researchers, and creative strategies are needed to manage these challenges.

KEY POINTS

- Sampling involves selecting a group of people, events, behaviors, or other elements with which to conduct a study. Sampling denotes the process of making the selections; sample denotes the selected group of elements.
- A sampling plan is developed to increase representativeness, decrease systematic bias, and decrease the sampling error; there are two main types of sampling plans—probability and nonprobability.
- Sampling error includes random variation and systematic variation. Refusal and attrition rates are important to calculate in a study to determine potential systematic variation or bias.
- The probability or random sampling designs commonly used in nursing studies include simple random sampling, stratified random sampling, cluster sampling, and systematic sampling (see Table 15-1).
- In nonprobability (nonrandom) sampling, not every element of the population has an opportunity for selection in the sample. The five nonprobability sampling designs described in this textbook are (1) convenience sampling, (2) quota sampling, (3) purposive or purposeful sampling, (4) network or snowball sampling, and (5) theoretical sampling.
- In quantitative studies, sample size is best determined by a power analysis, which is calculated using the level of significance (usually $\alpha = 0.05$), standard power of 0.80 (80%), and ES. Factors important to sample size in quantitative research include (1) type of study, (2) number of variables studied, (3) measurement sensitivity, and (4) data analysis techniques.
- The number of participants in a qualitative study is adequate when saturation of information is achieved in the study area, which occurs when additional sampling provides no new information, only redundancy of previously collected data. Important factors that must be considered in determining sample size needed to achieve saturation of data are (1) scope of the study, (2) nature of the topic, (3) quality of the data, and (4) study design.
- The three common settings for conducting nursing research are natural, partially controlled, and highly controlled. A natural setting, or field setting, is an uncontrolled, real-life situation or environment. A partially controlled setting is an environment that

the researcher has manipulated or modified in some way. A highly controlled setting is often an artificially constructed environment, such as a laboratory or research unit in a hospital, developed for the sole purpose of conducting research.

- Recruiting and retaining research participants have become significant challenges in research; some strategies to assist researchers with these challenges are provided so that their samples might be more representative of their target population.

REFERENCES

Aberson, C. L. (2010). *Applied power analysis for the behavioral sciences.* New York, NY: Routledge Taylor & Francis Group.

Alvarez, R. A., Vasquez, E., Mayorga, C. C., Feaster, D. J., & Mitrani, V. B. (2006). Increasing minority research participation through community organization outreach. *Western Journal of Nursing Research, 28*(5), 541–560.

Andersen, J. S., & Owen, D. C. (2014). Helping relationships for smoking cessation: Grounded theory development of the process of finding help to quit. *Nursing Research, 63*(4), 252–259.

Borglin, G., & Richards, D. A. (2010). Bias in experimental nursing research: Strategies to improve the quality and explanatory power of nursing science. *International Journal of Nursing Studies, 47*(1), 123–128.

Bryant, K., Wicks, M. N., & Willis, N. (2014). Recruitment of older African American males for depression research: Lessons learned. *Archives of Psychiatric Nursing, 28*(1), 17–20.

Charmaz, K. (2014). *Constructing grounded theory: A practical guide through qualitative analysis* (2nd ed.). Thousand Oaks, CA: Sage.

Cohen, J. (1988). *Statistical power analysis for the behavioral sciences* (2nd ed.). New York, NY: Academic Press.

Creswell, J. W. (2013). *Qualitative inquiry & research design: Choosing among five approaches* (3rd ed.). Thousand Oaks, CA: Sage.

Creswell, J. W. (2014). *Research design: Qualitative, quantitative and mixed methods approaches* (4th ed.). Thousand Oaks, CA: Sage.

Davidson, M. M., Cronk, N. J., Harrar, S., Catley, D., & Good, G. E. (2010). Strategies to recruit and retain college smokers in cessation trials. *Research in Nursing & Health, 33*(2), 144–155.

De Silva, J., Hanwella, R., & de Silva, V. A. (2012). Direct and indirect cost of schizophrenia in outpatients treated in a tertiary care psychiatry unit. *Ceylon Medical Journal, 57*(1), 14–18.

Doran, D. M. (2011). *Nursing outcomes: The state of the science.* Sudbury, MA: Jones & Bartlett Learning.

Engstrom, G. A., Tappen, R. M., & Ouslander, J. (2014). Brief report: Costs associated with recruitment and interviewing of study participants in a diverse population of community-dwelling older adults. *Nursing Research, 63*(1), 63–67.

Fawcett, J., & Garity, J. (2009). *Evaluating research for evidence-based nursing practice.* Philadelphia, PA: F. A. Davis.

Floyd, J. A. (1993). Systematic sampling: Theory and clinical methods. *Nursing Research, 42*(5), 290–293.

Gaskin, C. J., & Happell, B. (2014). Power, effects, confidence, and significance: An investigation of statistical practices in nursing research. *International Journal of Nursing Studies, 51*(5), 795–806.

Goshin, L. S., & Byrne, M. W. (2012). Predictors of post-release research retention and subsequent reenrollment for women recruited while incarcerated. *Research in Nursing & Health, 35*(1), 94–104.

Grove, S. K., & Cipher, D. (2017). *Statistics for nursing research: A workbook for evidence-based practice.* St. Louis, MO: Saunders.

Gul, R. B., & Ali, P. A. (2010). Clinical trials: The challenge of recruitment and retention of participants. *Journal of Clinical Nursing, 19*(1–2), 227–233.

Hellard, M. E., Sinclair, M. I., Forbes, A. B., & Fairley, C. K. (2001). Methods used to maintain a high level of participant involvement in a clinical trial. *Journal of Epidemiology & Community Health, 55*(5), 348–351.

Hendrickson, S. G. (2007). Video recruitment of non-English-speaking participants. *Western Journal of Nursing Research, 29*(2), 232–242.

Hines-Martin, V., Speck, B. J., Stetson, B., & Looney, S. W. (2009). Understanding systems and rhythms for minority recruitment in intervention research. *Research in Nursing & Health, 32*(6), 657–670.

Irani, E., & Richmond, T. S. (2015). Reasons for and reservations about research participation in acutely injured adults. *Journal of Nursing Scholarship, 47*(2), 161–169.

Kandola, D., Banner, D., Okeefe-McCarthy, S., & Jassal, D. (2014). Sampling methods in cardiovascular nursing research: An overview. *Canadian Journal of Cardiovascular Nursing, 24*(3), 15–18.

Kerlinger, F. N., & Lee, H. B. (2000). *Foundations of behavioral research* (4th ed.). Fort Worth, TX: Harcourt College Publishers.

Kraemer, H. C., & Thiemann, S. (1987). *How many subjects? Statistical power analysis in research.* Newbury Park, CA: Sage.

Larson, E. (1994). Exclusion of certain groups from clinical research. *Image: Journal of Nursing Scholarship, 26*(3), 185–190.

Lee, S., Faucett, J., Gillen, M., Krause, N., & Landry, L. (2013). Risk perception of musculoskeletal injury among critical care nurses. *Nursing Research, 62*(1), 36–44.

Leidy, N. K., & Weissfeld, L. A. (1991). Sample sizes and power computation for clinical intervention trials. *Western Journal of Nursing Research, 13*(1), 138–144.

Levy, P. S., & Lemsbow, S. (1980). *Sampling for health professionals.* Belmont, CA: Lifetime Learning.

Marshall, C., & Rossman, G. B. (2016). *Designing qualitative research* (6th ed.). Los Angeles, CA: Sage.

McGregor, L., Parker, K., LeBlanc, P., & King, K. M. (2010). Using social exchange theory to guide successful study recruitment and retention. *Nurse Researcher, 17*(2), 74–82.

Melnyk, B. M., & Fineout-Overholt, E. (2015). *Evidence-based practice in nursing & healthcare: A guide to best practice* (3rd ed.). Philadelphia, PA: Lippincott Williams & Wilkins.

Miles, M. B., Huberman, A. M., & Saldaña, J. (2014). *Qualitative data analysis: A methods sourcebook* (3rd ed.). Los Angeles, CA: Sage.

Milroy, J. H., Wyrick, D. L., Bibeau, D. L., Strack, R. W., & Davis, P. G. (2012). A university system-wide qualitative investigation into student physical activity promotion conducted on college campuses. *American Journal of Health Promotion, 26*(5), 305–312.

Morse, J. M. (2000). Determining sample size. *Qualitative Health Research, 10*(1), 3–5.

Morse, J. M. (2012). *Qualitative health research: Creating a new discipline.* Walnut Creek, CA: Left Coast Press.

Munhall, P. L. (2012). *Nursing research: A qualitative perspective* (5th ed.). Sudbury, MA: Jones & Bartlett.

Neumark, D. E., Stommel, M., Given, C. W., & Given, B. A. (2001). Brief report: Research design and subject characteristics predicting nonparticipation in panel survey of older families with cancer. *Nursing Research, 50*(6), 363–368.

Newnam, K. M., McGrath, J. M., Salyer, J., Estes, T., Jallo, N., & Bass, T. (2015). A comparative effectiveness study of continuous positive airway pressure-related skin breakdown when using different nasal interfaces in the extremely low birth weight neonate. *Applied Nursing Research, 28*(1), 36–41.

Papadopoulos, I., & Lees, S. (2002). Developing culturally competent researchers. *Journal of Advanced Nursing, 37*(3), 258–264.

Raurell-Torredà, M., Olivet-Pujol, J., Romero-Collado, À., Malagon-Aguilera, M. C., Patiño-Masó, J., & Baltasar-Bagué, A. (2015). Case-based learning and simulation: Useful tools to enhance nurses' education? Nonrandomized controlled trial. *Journal of Nursing Scholarship, 47*(1), 34–42.

Reifsnider, E., Bishop, S. L., An, K., Mendias, E., Welker-Hood, K., Moramarco, M. W., et al. (2014). We stop for no storm: Coping with an environmental disaster and public health research. *Public Health Nursing, 31*(6), 500–507.

Sandelowski, M. (1995). Sample size in qualitative research. *Research in Nursing & Health, 18*(2), 179–183.

Sezgin, D., & Esin, M. N. (2015). Predisposing factors for musculoskeletal symptoms in intensive care unit nurses. *International Nursing Review, 62*(1), 92–101.

Shadish, W. R., Cook, T. D., & Campbell, D. T. (2002). *Experimental and quasi-experimental designs for generalized causal inference.* Chicago, IL: Rand McNally.

Subaiya, S., Moussavi, C., Velasquez, A., & Stillman, J. (2014). A rapid needs assessment of the Rockaway Peninsula in New York after hurricane Sandy and the relationship of socioeconomic status to recovery. *American Journal of Public Health, 104*(4), 632–638.

Sullivan-Bolyai, S., Bova, C., Deatrick, J. A., Knafl, K., Grey, M., Leung, K., et al. (2007). Barriers and strategies for recruiting study participants in clinical settings. *Western Journal of Nursing Research, 29*(4), 486–500.

Sun, F., Long, A., Tsao, L., & Huang, H. (2014). The healing process following a suicide attempt: Context and intervening conditions. *Archives of Psychiatric Nursing, 28*(1), 55–61.

Thompson, S. K. (2002). *Sampling* (2nd ed.). New York, NY: John Wiley & Sons.

Waltz, C. F., Strickland, O. L., & Lenz, E. R. (2010). *Measurement in nursing and health research* (4th ed.). New York, NY: Springer Publishing Company.

Wang, T., Chang, C., Lou, M., Ao, M., Liu, C., Liang, S., et al. (2015). Biofeedback relaxation for pain associated with continuous passive motion in Taiwanese patients after total knee arthroplasty. *Research in Nursing & Health, 38*(1), 39–50.

Whitebird, R. R., Bliss, D. Z., Savik, K., Lowry, A., & Jung, H. G. (2010). Comparing community and specialty provider-based recruitment in a randomized clinical trial: Clinical trial in fecal incontinence. *Research in Nursing & Health, 33*(6), 500–511.

Yarandi, H. N. (1991). Planning sample sizes: Comparison of factor level means. *Nursing Research, 40*(1), 57–58.

Yates, F. (1981). *Sampling methods for censuses and surveys.* New York, NY: MacMillan.

Measurement Concepts

Susan K. Grove

e http://evolve.elsevier.com/Gray/practice/

Measurement is the process of assigning numbers to objects, events, or situations in accord with some rule (Kaplan, 1963). The numbers assigned can indicate numerical values or categories for the objects being measured for research or practice. **Instrumentation**, a component of measurement, is the application of specific rules to develop a measurement device such as a scale or questionnaire. Quality instruments are essential for obtaining trustworthy data when measuring outcomes for research and practice (Melnyk & Fineout-Overholt, 2015; Streiner, Norman, & Cairney, 2015; Waltz, Strickland, & Lenz, 2010).

The rules of measurement were developed so that the assigning of values or categories might be done consistently from one subject (or event) to another and eventually, if the measurement method is found to be meaningful, from one study to another. The rules of measurement established for research are similar to the rules of measurement implemented in nursing practice. For example, when nurses measure the urine output from patients, they use an accurate measurement device, observe the amount of urine in the device or container in a consistent way, and precisely record the urine output in the medical record. This practice promotes accuracy and precision and reduces the amount of error in measuring physiological variables such as urine output.

When measuring a subjective concept such as pain experienced by a child, researchers and nurses in practice need to use an instrument that captures the pain the child is experiencing. A commonly used scale to measure a child's pain is the Wong-Baker FACES Pain Rating Scale (Wong-Baker FACES Foundation, 2015). By using this valid and reliable rating scale to measure the child's pain, the change in the measured value can be attributed to a change in the child's pain rather than measurement error (see Chapter 17 for a copy of the Wong-Baker FACES Pain Rating Scale).

Researchers need to understand the logic within measurement theory so they can select and use existing instruments or develop new quality measurement methods for their studies. Measurement theory, as with most theories, uses terms with meanings that can be best understood within the context of the theory. The following explanation of the logic of measurement theory includes definitions of directness of measurement, measurement error, levels of measurement, and reference of measurement. The reliability and validity of measurement methods, such as scales and questionnaires, are detailed. Some of the sources in this chapter were developed more than 10 years ago but are included here because it takes extensive time to develop a quality scale. The accuracy, precision, and error of physiological measures are described. The chapter concludes with a discussion of sensitivity, specificity, and likelihood ratios (LRs) examined to determine the quality of diagnostic tests and instruments used in healthcare research and practice.

DIRECTNESS OF MEASUREMENT

Measurement begins by clarifying the object, characteristic, or element to be measured. Only then can one identify or develop strategies or methods to measure it. In some cases, identification of the measurement object and measurement strategies can be objective, specific, and straightforward, as when we are measuring concrete factors, such as a person's weight or waist circumference; this is referred to as **direct measurement**. Healthcare technology has made direct measures of objective elements—such as height, weight, vital signs, and oxygen saturation—familiar to us. Technology is also available to measure many biological and chemical characteristics, such as laboratory values, pulmonary functions, and sleep patterns (Ryan-Wenger, 2010). Nurses are also experienced in gathering direct measures of demographic variables, such as age, gender, ethnicity, diagnosis, marital status, income, and education.

However, in nursing, the characteristic we want to measure often is an abstract idea or concept, such as pain, stress, depression, anxiety, caring, or coping. If the element to be measured is abstract, it is best clarified through a conceptual definition (see Chapter 6). The conceptual definition can be used to select or develop appropriate means of measuring the concept. The instrument or measurement strategy used in the study must match the conceptual definition. An abstract concept is not measured directly; instead, indicators or attributes of the concept are used to represent the abstraction. This is referred to as **indirect measurement**. For example, the complex concept of coping might be defined by the frequency or accuracy of identifying problems, the creativity in selecting solutions, and the speed or effectiveness in resolving the problem. A single measurement strategy rarely, if ever, can completely measure all aspects of an abstract concept. Multi-item scales have been developed to measure abstract concepts, such as the Spielberger State-Trait Anxiety Inventory developed to measure individuals' innate anxiety trait and their anxiety in a specific situation (Spielberger, Gorsuch, & Lushene, 1970).

MEASUREMENT ERROR

There is no perfect measure. Error is inherent in any measurement strategy. **Measurement error** is the difference between what exists in reality and what is measured by an instrument. Measurement error exists in both direct and indirect measures and can be random or systematic. Direct measures, which are considered to be highly accurate, are subject to error. For example, the weight scale may not be accurate, laboratory equipment may be precisely calibrated but may change with use, or the tape measure may not be placed in the same location or held at the same tension for each measurement of a patient's waist.

There is also error in indirect measures. Efforts to measure concepts usually result in capturing only part of the concept but also contain other elements that are not part of the concept. Figure 16-1 shows a Venn diagram of the concept *A* measured by instrument *A-1*.

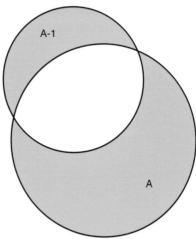

FIGURE 16-1 Measurement error when measuring a concept.

In this figure, *A-1* does not measure all of concept *A*. In addition, some of what *A-1* measures is outside the concept of *A*. Both of these situations are examples of errors in measurement and are shaded in Figure 16-1.

Types of Measurement Errors

Two types of errors are of concern in measurement: random error and systematic error. To understand these types of errors, we must first understand the elements of a score on an instrument or an observation. According to measurement theory, there are three components to a measurement score: true score, observed score, and error score (Cappelleri , Lundy, & Hays, 2014). The **true score** (T) is what we would obtain if there was no error in measurement. Because there is always some measurement error, the true score is never known. The **observed score** (O) is the measure obtained for a subject using a selected instrument during a study. The **error score** (E) is the amount of random error in the measurement process. The theoretical equation of these three measures is as follows:

Observed score (O) = true score (T) + error score (E)

This equation is a means of conceptualizing random error and not a basis for calculating it. Because the true score is never known, the random error is never known but only estimated. Theoretically, the smaller the error score, the more closely the observed score reflects the true score. Therefore, using instruments that reduce error improves the accuracy of measurement (Cappelleri et al., 2014; Waltz et al., 2010).

Several factors can occur during the measurement process that can increase random error. Transient personal factors, such as fatigue, hunger, attention span, health, mood, mental status, and motivation; and situational factors, such as a hot stuffy room, distractions, the presence of significant others, rapport with the researcher, and the playfulness or seriousness of the situation, can increase random error. Factors on the part of the researcher that can increase random error include: variations in the administration of the measurement procedure, such as interviews in which wording or sequence of questions is varied; questions are added or deleted; or researchers code responses differently. During data processing, errors in accidentally marking the wrong column, hitting the wrong key when entering data into the computer, or incorrectly totaling instrument scores will increase random error (Devon et al., 2007; Waltz et al., 2010).

Random error causes individuals' observed scores to vary in no particular direction around their true score. For example, with random error, one subject's observed score may be higher than his or her true score, whereas another subject's observed score may be lower than his or her true score. According to measurement theory, the sum of random errors is expected to be zero, and the random error score (E) is not expected to correlate with the true score (T) (Waltz et al., 2010). Random error does not influence the mean to be higher or lower but rather increases the amount of unexplained variance around the mean. When this occurs, estimation of the true score is less precise.

If you were to measure a variable for three study participants and diagram the random error, it might appear as shown in Figure 16-2. The difference between the true score of participant one (T_1) and the observed score (O_1) is two positive measurement intervals. The difference between the true score (T_2) and observed score (O_2) for participant two is two negative measurement intervals. The difference between the true score (T_3) and observed score (O_3) for participant three is zero. The random error for these study participants is zero ($+2 - 2 + 0 = 0$). In viewing this example, one must remember this is only a means of conceptualizing random error.

Measurement error that is not random is referred to as *systematic error*. A scale that measures all study participants as weighing three more pounds than their true weights is an example of systematic error. All the measurements of body weights would be higher than the true scores and, as a result, the mean based on these measurements would be higher than the true mean. **Systematic error** occurs because something else is being measured in addition to the concept. A conceptualization of systematic error is presented in Figure 16-3. Systematic error (represented by the shaded area in the figure) is due to the part of *A-1* that is outside of *A*. This part of *A-1* measures factors other than *A* and biases scores in a particular direction.

Systematic error is considered part of T (true score) and reflects the true measure of *A-1*, not *A*. Adding the true score (with systematic error) to the random error (which is 0) yields the observed score, as shown by the following equations:

T (true score with systematic error)
+ E (random error of 0) = O (observed score)

or

$$T + E = O$$

Some systematic error is incurred in almost any measure; however, a close link between the abstract theoretical concept and the development of the instrument that measures it can greatly decrease systematic error. Because of the importance of this factor in a study, researchers spend considerable time and effort in

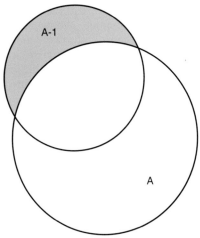

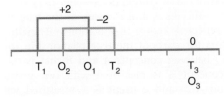

FIGURE 16-2 Conceptualization of random error.

FIGURE 16-3 Conceptualization of a systematic error.

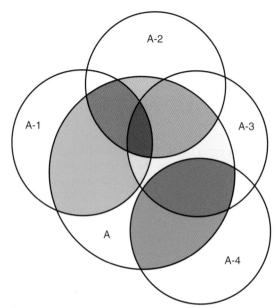

FIGURE 16-4 Multiple measures of an abstract concept.

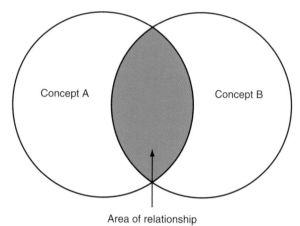

Area of relationship

FIGURE 16-5 True relationship of concepts *A* and *B*.

selecting and developing quality measurement methods to decrease systematic error (Cappelleri et al., 2014).

Another effective means of diminishing systematic error is to use more than one measure of an attribute or a concept and to compare the measures. To make this comparison, researchers use various data collection methods, such as scale, interview, and observation. Campbell and Fiske (1959) developed a technique of using more than one method to measure a concept, referred to as the **multimethod-multitrait technique**. More recently, the technique has been described as a measurement version of mixed methodology (Creswell, 2014). This technique allows researchers to measure more dimensions of abstract concepts, which decreases the effect of the systematic error on the composite observed score. Figure 16-4 illustrates how various dimensions of concept *A* are captured through the use of four instruments, designated *A-1, A-2, A-3,* and *A-4*.

For example, a researcher could decrease systematic error in measures of anxiety by (1) administering the Spielberger State-Trait Anxiety Inventory (Spielberger et al., 1970), (2) recording blood pressure (BP) readings, (3) asking the subject about anxious feelings, and (4) observing the subject's behavior. Multimethod measurement strategies decrease systematic error by combining the values in some way to give a single observed score of anxiety for each subject. However, sometimes it

may be difficult logically to justify combining scores from various measures, and a mixed-methods research design might be the most appropriate to use in the study (see Chapter 14). A mixed-methods study, previously referred to as *triangulation*, uses two research designs to better represent truth. The vast majority of mixed methods studies use one quantitative and one qualitative design (Creswell, 2014).

In some studies, researchers use instruments to examine relationships. Consider a hypothesis that tests the relationship between concept *A* and concept *B*. In Figure 16-5, the shaded area enclosed in the dark lines represents the true relationship between concepts *A* and *B*, such as the relationship between anxiety and depression. For example, two instruments, *A-1* (Spielberger State-Trait Anxiety Inventory; Spielberger et al., 1970) and *B-1* (Center for Epidemiological Studies Depression Scale; Radloff, 1977), are used to examine the relationship between concepts *A* and *B*. The part of the true relationship actually reflected by *A-1* and *B-1* measurement methods is represented by the colored areas in Figure 16-6.

Because two instruments provide a more accurate measure of concepts *A* and *B*, more of the true relationship between concepts *A* and *B* can be measured. So if additional instruments (*A-2* and *B-2*) are used to measure concepts *A* and *B*, more of the true relationship is reflected. Figure 16-7 demonstrates with different colors the parts of the true relationship (outlined in blue) between concepts *A* and *B* that is measured when concept *A* is measured with two instruments (*A-1* and *A-2*) and concept *B* is measured with two instruments (*B-1* and *B-2*).

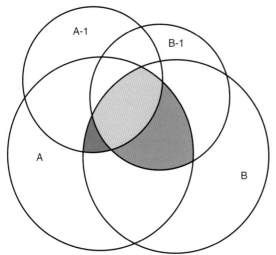

FIGURE 16-6 Examining a relationship using one measure of each concept.

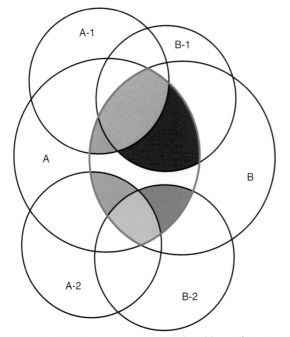

FIGURE 16-7 Examining a relationship using two measures of each concept.

LEVELS OF MEASUREMENT

In 1946, Stevens organized the rules for assigning numbers to objects so that a hierarchy in measurement was established called the **levels of measurement**. The levels of measurement, from lower to higher, are

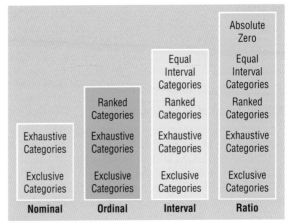

FIGURE 16-8 Summary of the rules for levels of measurement.

nominal, ordinal, interval, and ratio and are described in the following sections.

Nominal Level of Measurement

Nominal level of measurement is the lowest of the four measurement levels or categories. It is used when data can be organized into categories of a defined property but the categories cannot be ordered. For example, diagnoses of chronic diseases are nominal data with categories such as hypertension, type 2 diabetes, and dyslipidemia. One cannot say that one category is higher than another or that category A (hypertension) is closer to category B (diabetes) than to category C (dyslipidemia). The categories differ in quality but not quantity. One cannot say that subject A possesses more of the property being categorized than does subject B. (**Rule: The categories must be unorderable.**) Categories must be established so that each datum fits into only one of the categories. (**Rule: The categories must be exclusive.**) For example, you would not want a category of cardiovascular disease and another of heart failure because the datum for a person with heart failure could fit in either category. All the data must fit into the established categories. (**Rule: The categories must be exhaustive.**) For example, the datum for a person with chronic obstructive pulmonary disease would not be included if the categories were cardiovascular disease, metabolic disease, and neurological disease. A category for respiratory disease would be needed to include the person's datum. Figure 16-8 provides a summary for the rules for the levels of measurement—nominal, ordinal, interval, and ratio.

Data such as ethnicity, gender, marital status, religion, and diagnoses are examples of nominal data.

When data are coded for entry into the computer, the categories are assigned numbers. For example, gender may be classified as 1 = male and 2 = female. The numbers assigned to categories in nominal measurement are used only as labels and cannot be used for mathematical calculations.

Ordinal Level of Measurement

Data that can be measured at the **ordinal level of measurement** can be assigned to categories of an attribute that can be ranked. As with nominal-scale data, the categories must be exclusive and exhaustive. With ordinal level data, the ranking an attribute possesses can be identified. However, it cannot be shown that the intervals between the ranked categories are equal (see Figure 16-8). Ordinal data are considered to have unequal intervals. Scales with unequal intervals are referred to as **metric ordinal scales** or **ordered metric scales**.

Many scales used in nursing research are ordinal levels of measure. For example, one could rank intensity of pain, degree of coping, level of mobility, ability to provide self-care, or daily amount of exercise on an ordinal scale. There are rules for how one ranks data. For daily exercise, the scale could be 0 = no exercise; 1 = moderate exercise, no sweating; 2 = exercise to the point of sweating; 3 = strenuous exercise with sweating for at least 30 minutes per day; 4 = strenuous exercise with sweating for at least 1 hour per day. This type of scale is an example of a metric ordinal scale because the different levels for measuring exercise are numbered in order from a low of 0 to a high of 4.

Interval Level of Measurement

In **interval level of measurement**, distances between intervals of the scale are numerically equal. Such measurements also follow the previously mentioned rules: mutually exclusive categories, exhaustive categories, and rank ordering. Interval scales are assumed to represent a continuum of values (see Figure 16-8). The researcher can identify the magnitude of the attribute much more precisely. However, it is impossible to provide the absolute amount of the attribute because of the absence of a zero point on the interval scale that actually signifies an absence of the concept being measured.

Fahrenheit and Celsius temperatures are commonly used as examples of interval scales. A difference between a temperature of 70° F and one of 80° F is the same as the difference between a temperature of 30° F and one of 40° F. We can measure changes in temperature precisely. However, it is impossible to say that a temperature of 0° C or 0° F means the absence of temperature because, although these indicate very cold temperatures, they still contain energy and so do not signify the absolute absence of heat and energy.

All interval scales like the Spielberger State-Trait Anxiety Inventory (Spielberger et al., 1970) are artificial. They have been created by humans for indirect measurement of complex concepts and are considered by most researchers to be interval level measurement (Grove & Cipher, 2017).

Ratio Level of Measurement

Ratio level of measurement is the highest form of measurement and meets all the rules of the lower forms of measures: mutually exclusive categories, exhaustive categories, rank ordering, equal spacing between intervals, and continuous values. In addition, ratio level measures have absolute zero points (see Figure 16-8). Weight, length, and volume are common examples of ratio scales. Each has an **absolute zero point**, at which a value of zero indicates the absence of the property being measured: Zero weight means the absence of weight. In addition, because of the absolute zero point, one can justifiably say that object A weighs twice as much as object B, or that container A holds three times as much as container B. Laboratory values are also an example of ratio level of measurement where the individual with a fasting blood sugar (FBS) of 180 has an FBS twice that of an individual with a normal FBS of 90. To help expand understanding of levels of measurement (nominal, ordinal, interval, and ratio) and to apply this knowledge, Grove and Cipher (2017) developed a statistical workbook focused on examining levels of measurement, reliability, and validity of measurement methods in published studies.

Importance of Level of Measurement for Statistical Analyses

An important rule of measurement is that one should use the highest level of measurement possible. For example, you can collect data on age measured in a variety of ways: (1) you can obtain the actual age of each subject based on year, month, or day of birth (ratio level of measurement); (2) you can ask subjects to indicate their age by selecting from a group of categories, such as 20 to 29, 30 to 39, and so on (ordinal level of measurement); or (3) you can sort subjects into two categories of younger than 65 years of age and 65 years of age and older (nominal level of measurement). The highest level of measurement in this case is the actual age of each subject, which is the preferred way to collect these data (Grove & Cipher, 2017). If age categories are to be used for specific analyses in your study, the computer can be instructed to create age categories from the initial age data. However researchers need a compelling reason for categorizing a continuous variable like age, because this limits the statistical techniques that can be conducted on the data (Knapp & Brown, 2014; Waltz et al., 2010).

The level of measurement is associated with the types of statistical analyses that can be performed on the data. Mathematical operations are limited in the lower levels of measurement. With nominal levels of measurement, only summary statistics, such as frequencies, percentages, and contingency correlation procedures, can be conducted. Variables measured at the interval or ratio level can be analyzed with the most powerful statistical techniques available, which are more effective in identifying relationships among variables and determining differences between groups (see Chapters 21–25; Plichta & Kelvin, 2013).

Controversy Over Measurement Levels

Controversy exists over the system that is used to categorize measurement levels, dividing researchers into two factions: fundamentalists and pragmatists. Pragmatists regard measurement as occurring on a continuum rather than by discrete categories, whereas fundamentalists adhere rigidly to the original system of categorization (Nunnally & Bernstein, 1994; Stevens, 1946).

The primary focus of the controversy relates to the practice of classifying data into the categories ordinal and interval. This controversy developed because, according to the fundamentalists, many of the current statistical analysis techniques can be conducted only with interval and ratio data. Many pragmatists believe that if researchers rigidly adhered to rules developed by Stevens (1946), few, if any, measures in the social sciences would meet the criteria to be considered interval-level data. They also believe that violating Stevens' criteria does not lead to serious consequences for the outcomes of data analysis. Pragmatists often treat summed ordinal data from multi-item scales as interval data, using statistical methods (parametric analysis techniques) to analyze them, such as Pearson's product-moment correlation coefficient, t-test, and analysis of variance (ANOVA). These analyses are traditionally reserved for interval or ratio level data (Armstrong, 1981; Knapp, 1990). Fundamentalists insist that the analysis of ordinal data be limited to statistical procedures designed for ordinal data, such as nonparametric techniques. Parametric analysis techniques were developed to analyze interval and ratio level data (see Chapter 21).

The Likert scale uses scale points such as *strongly disagree, disagree, uncertain, agree,* and *strongly agree.* Numerical values (e.g., 1, 2, 3, 4, and 5) are assigned to these categories. Fundamentalists claim that equal

intervals do not exist between these categories. It is impossible to prove that there is the same magnitude of feeling between *uncertain* and *agree* as there is between *agree* and *strongly agree.* Therefore, they hold that this is ordinal level data, and parametric analyses cannot be used. Pragmatists believe that with many measures taken at the ordinal level, such as scaling procedures, an underlying interval continuum is present that justifies the use of parametric statistics (Knapp, 1990; Nunnally & Bernstein, 1994).

Our position agrees more with the pragmatists than with the fundamentalists. Many nurse researchers analyze data from Likert scales and other rating scales as though the data were interval level (Grove & Cipher, 2017; Waltz et al., 2010). However, some of the data in nursing research are obtained through the use of crude measurement methods that can be classified only into the lower levels of measurement (ordinal or nominal). Therefore, we have included the nonparametric statistical procedures needed for analyses at those levels in Chapters 22 to 25.

REFERENCE TESTING MEASUREMENT

Reference testing involves comparing a subject's score against a standard. Norm-referenced testing and criterion-referenced testing are two common types of testing that involve referencing. **Norm-referenced testing** is a type of evaluation that yields an estimate of the performance of the tested individual in comparison to the performance of others in a well-defined population. This testing involves standardization of scores for an instrument that is accomplished by data collection over several years, with extensive reliability and validity information available on the instrument. Standardization involves collecting data from thousands of subjects expected to have a broad range of scores on the instrument. From these scores, population parameters such as the mean and standard deviation (described in Chapter 22) can be developed. Evidence of the reliability and validity of the instrument can also be evaluated through the use of methods described later in this chapter.

Many college entrance exams and national school tests use norm-referenced tests. For example, the Graduate Record Examination (GRE) compares an individual's performance to the performances of a normative sample of potential graduate students. Over many decades GRE scores have been standardized and used as an admission criterion by some graduate programs. Norm-referenced tests can also be used in research and clinical practice (see Waltz et al. [2010] for a detailed discussion of norm-referenced and criterion-referenced testing).

Criterion-referenced testing involves making a decision about whether or not an individual or research participant has demonstrated mastery in an area of content and competencies. It involves comparing an individual's score with a criterion of achievement that includes the definition of target behaviors. When individuals master these behaviors, they are considered proficient in the behaviors (Waltz et al., 2010). The criterion might be a level of knowledge and clinical performance required of students in a course. For example, a criterion-referenced clinical evaluation form would include the critical behaviors the nurse practitioner student is expected to demonstrate in a pediatric course in order to be considered clinically competent to care for pediatric patients at the end of the course. Many certification and licensure exams are criterion-referenced tests.

Criterion-referenced measures have been used for years to examine the outcomes of healthcare agencies, nurse providers, and patients. For example, Magnet status for hospitals is achieved when agencies and personnel have accomplished the criteria designated by the American Nurses Credentialing Center (ANCC, 2016) for the Magnet Recognition Program®. Criterion-referenced measures are also used in nursing research, such as tests to measure the clinical expertise of a nurse or the self-care of a cardiac patient after cardiac rehabilitation (see Waltz et al., 2010, for additional details).

RELIABILITY

The **reliability** of an instrument denotes the consistency of the measures obtained of an attribute, concept, or situation in a study or in clinical practice. Reliability is concerned with the precision, reproducibility, and comparability of a measurement method (Bartlett & Frost, 2008). An instrument with strong reliability demonstrates consistency in the participant scores obtained, resulting in less measurement error (Bannigan & Watson, 2009; Waltz et al., 2010). For example, if you use a scale to measure depression levels of 10 individuals at two points in time one day apart, you would expect the individuals' depression levels to be relatively unchanged from one measurement to the next if the scale is reliable. If two data collectors observe the same event and record their observations on a carefully designed data collection instrument, the measurement would be reliable if the recordings from the two data collectors were comparable. The equivalence of their results would indicate the reliability of the measurement technique. If responses vary each time a measure is performed, there is a chance that the instrument is unreliable, meaning that it yields data with a large random

error. Reliability also includes the validity or accuracy of measurement methods. An instrument is valid to the extent that it accurately measures what it was developed to measure. Thus, an instrument must be both reliable and valid to limit measurement error. (Validity is discussed in detail later in this chapter).

Reliability Testing

Reliability testing examines the amount of measurement error in the instrument being used in a study. All measurement techniques contain some random error, and the error might be due to the measurement method used, the study participants, or the researchers gathering the data. Reliability exists in degrees and is usually expressed as a correlation coefficient, with 1.00 indicating perfect reliability and 0.00 indicating no reliability (Bialocerkowski, Klupp, & Bragge, 2010; see Chapter 23). Reliability coefficients of 0.80 or higher would indicate strong reliability for a psychosocial scale such as the State-Trait Anxiety Inventory by Spielberger et al. (1970). With test-retest, the closer that a reliability coefficient is to 1.00, the more stable the measurement method is over time. Reliability coefficients vary based on the aspect of reliability being examined. The three main aspects of reliability are: (1) stability, (2) equivalence, and (3) internal consistency (Bialocerkowski et al., 2010; DeVon et al., 2007; Waltz et al., 2010). Table 16-1 summarizes the common types of reliability included in nursing research reports.

Stability Reliability

Stability reliability is concerned with the consistency of repeated measures over time of the same attribute with a given instrument. **Test-retest reliability** is conducted to examine instrument stability, which reflects the reproducibility of a scale's scores on repeated administration over time when a subject's condition has not changed (Cappelleri et al., 2014). This measure of reliability is generally used with physical measures, technological measures, and psychosocial scales. Test-retest reliability of scales can be applied to both single-item and multi-item scales. The technique requires an assumption that the factor to be measured remains essentially the same at the two testing times and that change in the value or score is a consequence of measurement error.

The optimal time period between test-retest measurements depends on the variability of the variable being measured, complexity of the measurement process, and characteristics of the participants (Bialocerkowski et al., 2010). Physical measures can be tested and then immediately retested to determine reliability. For example, in measuring BP, researchers often take two to

TABLE 16-1   Determining the Quality of Measurement Methods

Quality Indicator	Description
Reliability	**Stability reliability:** Consistency of repeated measures of the same concept or attribute with an instrument or scale over time. Stability is usually examined with **test-retest reliability.**
	Equivalence reliability: Includes interrater reliability and alternate forms reliability.
	Interrater reliability: Comparison of two observers or judges in a study to determine their equivalence in making observations or judging events.
	Alternate forms reliability: Comparison of two paper-and-pencil instruments to determine their equivalence in measuring a concept.
	Internal consistency: Also known as homogeneity reliability testing used primarily with multi-item scales where each item on the scale is correlated with all other items to determine the consistency of the scale in measuring a concept.
Validity	**Face validity:** Verifies that an instrument looks like it is valid or gives the appearance of measuring the construct it is to measure.
	Content validity: Examines the extent to which a measurement method includes all the major elements relevant to the construct being measured.
	Construct validity: Focuses on determining whether the instrument actually measures the theoretical construct that it purports to measure, which involves examining the fit between the conceptual and operational definitions of a variable.
	Validity from factor analysis: Focuses on the various dimensions or subconcepts of the construct being measured that are represented as subscales in a newly developed scale or instrument.
	Convergent validity: Two scales measuring the same concept are administered to a group at the same time and the subjects' scores on the scales should be positively correlated. For example, subjects completing two scales to measure depression should have positively correlated scores.
	Divergent validity: Two scales that measure opposite concepts, such as hope and hopelessness, administered to subjects at the same time should result in negatively correlated scores on the scales.
	Validity from contrasting (known) groups: An instrument or scale is given to two groups that are expected to have opposite or contrasting scores; one group scores high on the scale and the other scores low.
	Validity from discriminant analysis: Used to test the discrimination achieved by simultaneously administering two instruments to a sample, to measure similar concepts.
	Successive verification of validity: Developed when an instrument is used over time in a variety of studies with different populations and settings.
	Criterion-related validity: Validity that is strengthened when a study participant's score on an instrument can be used to infer his or her performance on another variable or criterion.
	Predictive validity: The extent to which an individual's score on a scale or instrument can be used to predict future performance or behavior on a criterion.
	Concurrent validity: Focuses on the extent to which an individual's score on an instrument or scale can be used to estimate his or her present or concurrent performance on another variable or criterion.
Readability	**Readability level:** The approximate level of educational mastery required to comprehend a given piece of text. Researchers need to report the level of education subjects need to read the instrument. Readability must be appropriate to promote reliability and validity of an instrument.

Continued

TABLE 16-1	Determining the Quality of Measurement Methods—cont'd
Quality Indicator	**Description**
Accuracy	**Accuracy of physiological measure:** Addresses the extent to which the physiological instrument or equipment measures what it is supposed to in a study; comparable to validity for scales.
Precision	**Precision of physiological measure:** Degree of consistency or reproducibility of the measurements made with physiological instruments or equipment; comparable to reliability for scales.
Error	**Error:** Sources of error in physiological measures can be grouped into the following five categories: (1) environment, (2) user, (3) study participant, (4) machine, and (5) interpretation.

three BP readings five minutes apart and average the readings to obtain a reliable or precise measure of BP (Weber et al., 2014). The test-retest of a measurement method might involve a longer period of time between measurements if the variable being measured changes slowly. For example, the diagnosis of osteoporosis is made by a bone mineral density (BMD) study of the hip and spine. BMD scores are determined with a dual energy X-ray absorptiometry (DEXA) scan. Because the BMD does not change rapidly in people, even with treatment, test-retest over a 1- to 2-month time period could be used to show reliable or consistent DEXA scan scores for patients. With educational tests, a period of two to four weeks is recommended between the two testing times (Waltz et al., 2010).

For some tests or scales, test-retest reliability has not been as effective as originally anticipated. The procedure presents numerous problems. Subjects may remember their responses from the first testing time, leading to overestimation of the reliability. Subjects may be changed by the first testing and may respond to the second test differently, leading to underestimation of the reliability (Bialocerkowski et al., 2010). Many of the phenomena studied in nursing, such as hope, coping, pain, and anxiety, do change over short intervals. Thus, the assumption that if the instrument is reliable, values will not change between the two measurement periods may not be justifiable. If the factor being measured does change, then the value obtained is a measure of change and not a measure of reliability. If the measures stay the same even though the factor being measured has changed, the instrument may lack reliability. If researchers are going to examine the reliability of an instrument with test-retest, they need to determine the optimum time between administrations of the instrument based on the variable being measured and the study participants (Cappelleri et al., 2014).

Stability of a measurement method needs to be examined as part of instrument development and discussed when the instrument is used in a study. When describing test-retest results, researchers need to discuss the process and the time period between administering an instrument and the rationale for this time frame (Bannigan & Watson, 2009; Bialocerkowski et al., 2010; Waltz et al., 2010). After the study participants have been retested with the same instrument, researchers perform a correlational analysis on the scores from the two measurement times. This correlation is called the **coefficient of stability**, and the closer the coefficient is to 1.00, the more stable the instrument (Waltz et al., 2010).

Equivalence Reliability

Equivalence reliability involves examining the consistency of scores between two versions of the same paper-and-pencil instrument or two observers measuring the same event. Comparison of the equivalence of the judging or rating of two observers is referred to as **inter-rater reliability** (see Table 16-1). Comparison of two paper-and-pencil instruments to determine their equivalence in measuring a concept is referred to as **alternate-forms reliability** or **parallel-forms reliability**. Alternate forms of instruments are complicated in the development of normative knowledge testing. However, when repeated measures are part of the design, alternative forms of measurement, although not commonly used, would improve the design. Demonstrating that one is actually testing the same content in both tests is extremely complex; thus, the procedure is rarely used in clinical research (Bialocerkowski et al., 2010).

The procedure for developing parallel forms involves using the same objectives and procedures for both forms, in order to develop two similar instruments. These two instruments when completed by the same group of study participants on the same occasion, or on two different occasions, should have approximately equal means and standard deviations. In addition, these two instruments should correlate equally with a related variable. For example, if two instruments were developed to measure pain, the scores from these two scales should correlate equally with perceived anxiety score. If both forms of the instrument are administered on the same occasion, a reliability coefficient can be calculated to determine equivalence. A coefficient of 0.80 or higher indicates strong equivalence (Waltz et al., 2010).

Determining interrater reliability is important when observational measurement is used in quantitative, mixed-methods, and ethnographic studies. Interrater reliability values need to be reported when observational data are collected or judgments are made by two or more data gatherers. Two techniques determine interrater reliability. Both techniques require that two or more raters independently observe and record the same event using the protocol developed for the study or that the same rater observes and records an event on two occasions. To judge interrater reliability adequately, the raters need to observe at least 10 subjects or events (DeVon et al., 2007; Waltz et al., 2010). A digital recorder can be used to record the raters to determine their consistency in recording essential study information. Every data collector used in the study must be tested for interrater reliability and trained until they are consistent in rating and recording information related to data collection.

One procedure for calculating interrater reliability requires a simple computation involving a comparison of the agreements obtained between raters on the coding form with the number of possible agreements. This calculation is performed using the following equation:

$$\text{Number of agreements} \div \text{number of possible agreements} = \text{interrater reliability}$$

This formula tends to overestimate reliability, a particularly serious problem if the rating requires only a dichotomous judgment, such as present or absent. In this case, there is a 50% probability that the raters will agree on a particular item through chance alone. If more than two raters are involved, a statistical procedure to calculate coefficient alpha (discussed later in this chapter) may be used. ANOVA may also be used to test for differences among raters.

There is no absolute value below which interrater reliability is unacceptable. However, any value less than 0.80 (80%) raises concern about the reliability of the

data because there is 20% chance of error. The more ideal interrater reliability value is 0.90, which means 90% reliability and 10% error. Researchers are expected to include the process for determining interrater reliability and the value achieved in the report of the study (DeVon et al., 2007).

When raters know they are being watched, their accuracy and consistency are usually better than when they believe they are not being watched. Interrater reliability declines (sometimes dramatically) when the raters are assessed covertly (Topf, 1988). You can develop strategies to monitor and reduce the decline in interrater reliability, but they may entail considerable time and expense.

Internal Consistency

Tests of instrument **internal consistency** or **homogeneity**, used primarily with paper-and-pencil tests or scales, address the intercorrelation of various items within the instrument. The original approach to determining internal consistency was **split-half reliability**. This strategy was a way of obtaining test-retest reliability without administering the test twice. The instrument items were split in odd-even or first-last halves, and a correlational procedure was performed between the two halves. In the past, researchers generally reported the Spearman-Brown correlation coefficient in their studies (Nunnally & Bernstein, 1994). One of the problems with the procedure was that although items were usually split into odd-even items, it was possible to split them in a variety of ways. Each approach to splitting the items would yield a different reliability coefficient. The researcher could continue to split the items in various ways until a satisfactorily high coefficient was obtained.

More recently, testing the internal consistency of all the items in the instrument has been developed, resulting in a better approach to determining reliability. Although the mathematics of the procedure are complex, the logic is simple. One way to view it is as though one conducted split-half reliabilities in all the ways possible and then averaged the scores to obtain one reliability score. Internal consistency testing examines the extent to which all the items in the instrument consistently measure a concept. **Cronbach's alpha coefficient** is the statistical procedure used for calculating internal consistency for interval and ratio level data. This reliability coefficient is essentially the mean of the inter-item correlations and can be calculated using most data analysis programs such as the Statistical Program for the Social Sciences (SPSS). If the data are dichotomous, such as a symptom list that has responses of present or absent, the Kuder-Richardson formulas (*KR 20* or *KR 21*) can be used to calculate the internal consistency of the instrument (DeVon et al., 2007). The *KR 21* assumes that all the items on a scale or test are equally difficult; the *KR 20* is not based on this assumption. Waltz et al. (2010) provided the formulas for calculating both *KR 20* and *KR 21*.

Cronbach's alpha coefficients can range from 0.00, indicating no internal consistency or reliability, to 1.00, indicating perfect internal reliability with no measurement error. Alpha coefficients of 1.00 are not obtained in study results because all instruments have some measurement error. However, many respected psychosocial scales used for 15 to 30 years to measure study variables in a variety of populations have strong 0.8 or greater internal reliability coefficients. The coefficient of 0.80 (or 80%) is determined by calculating Cronbach's alpha and the percentage of error is calculated by (1 − coefficient squared) × 100%. Thus, the error for this scale would be $(1 - 0.8^2) \times 100\% = (1 - 0.64) \times 100\% = 0.36 \times 100\% = 36\%$ (Cappelleri et al., 2014; DeVon et al., 2007; Waltz et al., 2010). Scales with 20 or more items usually have stronger internal consistency coefficients than scales with 10 to 15 items or less. Often scales that measure complex constructs such as quality of life (QOL) have subscales that measure different aspects of QOL, such as health, mental health, physical functioning, and spirituality. Some of these complex scales with distinct subscales, such as the QOL scale, have somewhat lower Cronbach's alpha coefficients because the scale is measuring different aspects of an overall concept. Subscales usually have lower Cronbach's alpha coefficients than does the total scale but they must demonstrate internal consistency in measuring the identified subconcepts (Bialocerkowski et al., 2010; Waltz et al., 2010).

Newer instruments, such as those developed in the last five years, initially show only limited to moderate internal reliability (0.70 to 0.79) when used in measuring concepts in a variety of samples. The subscales of these new instruments may have internal reliability ranging from 0.60 to 0.69. However, when the authors of these scales continue to refine them based on available reliability and validity information, the reliability of both the total scale and the subscales will improve. Reliability coefficients less than 0.60 are considered low and indicate limited instrument reliability or consistency in measurement with high random error. Higher levels of reliability or precision (0.90 to 0.99) are important for physiological measures that are used to determine critical physiological functions that are used to guide treatment decisions, such as arterial pressure and oxygen saturation (Bialocerkowski et al., 2010; DeVon et al., 2007).

The quality of an instrument's reliability must be examined in terms of the type of study, measurement method, and population (DeVon et al., 2007; Kerlinger & Lee, 2000). In published studies, researchers need to identify the reliability coefficients of an instrument from both previous research and for their particular study. Because the reliability of an instrument can vary from one population or sample to another, it is important that the reliability of the scale and subscales be determined and reported for the sample in each study (Bialocerkowski et al., 2010).

Reliability plays an important role in the selection of measurement methods for use in a study. Researchers need instruments that are reliable and provide values with limited amounts of error. Reliable instruments enhance the power of a study to detect significant differences or relationships actually occurring in the population under study (Waltz et al., 2010). The strongest measure of reliability is obtained from heterogeneous samples versus homogeneous samples. Heterogeneous samples have more between-participant variability, and this is a stronger evaluation of reliability than homogeneous samples with limited between-participant variation (Bialocerkowski et al., 2010). Researchers need to perform reliability testing for each instrument used in their study before performing other statistical analyses, to ensure that the reliability is at least 0.70.

Smith, Theeke, Culp, Clark, and Pinto (2014) conducted a correlational study to examine the relationships among selected psychosocial variables (self-esteem, sleep quality, loneliness, and perceived stress) and self-rated health in obese young adult women. The following study excerpt includes the reliability information for the scales used to measure loneliness, self-esteem, and sleep quality.

"Loneliness

Loneliness was measured using the Revised UCLA Loneliness Scale (Russell, Peplau, & Cutrona, 1980). Scores range from 20 to 80 and a higher score indicates increased loneliness. The scale has high internal consistency ($\alpha = 0.89–0.94$) and adequate test–retest reliability ($r = 0.73$)…

Self-esteem

Self-esteem was measured using the Rosenberg Self-esteem Scale (Rosenberg, 1979). He describes adequate reliability and validity of a global measure of self-esteem for both adult men and women. Test-retests using the scale over 2 weeks demonstrated correlations of 0.85 and 0.88 demonstrating very good reliability … The score range on the 10 item scale is 0–30 where higher scores indicate higher self-esteem (Rosenberg, 1979).

Sleep Quality

Sleep was determined using the Pittsburgh Sleep Quality Index which assesses sleep over a 1 month interval (Buysse, Reynolds, Monk, Berman, & Kupfer, 1989). It consists of 19 self-rated items. The global score has a range of 0–21 where higher scores indicate poorer sleep quality. In a study of sleep quality with in-patients and outpatients in a psychiatric clinic, the global score had an overall reliability coefficient (Cronbach's alpha) of 0.83 indicating a high degree of reliability (Buysse et al., 1989)…

[Table 16-2] reports the psychometric properties of the study instruments. The reliability coefficients as determined by Cronbach's alpha are 0.90 or better for stress, loneliness, and self-esteem. The reliability coefficient for the Pittsburgh Sleep Quality Index was 0.70 demonstrating minimally acceptable reliability." (Smith et al., 2014, pp. 68–69)

Based on previous research, Smith and colleagues (2014) used reliable scales to measure their study variables and documented this in their article. Both the loneliness and self-esteem scales had demonstrated adequate test-retest or stability reliability in previous studies. Also in previous studies, the self-esteem scale and Sleep Quality Index had demonstrated strong internal consistency. The Cronbach's alphas for the scales used in this study were strong, except for the Sleep Quality Index, which demonstrated minimal acceptable reliability (see Table 16-2). Additional research is needed to ensure that these scales (especially the Sleep Quality Index) are reliable for this population. Based on their study results, Smith et al. (2014, p. 67) concluded that "assessing and addressing stress, loneliness, sleep quality,

and self-esteem could lead to improved health outcomes in obese young women."

It is essential that an instrument be both reliable and valid for measuring a study variable in a population. If the instrument has low reliability values, it cannot be valid because its measurement is inconsistent and has high measurement error (DeVon et al., 2007; Waltz et al., 2010). An instrument with strong reliability cannot be assumed to be valid for a particular study or population. You need to examine the validity of the instrument you are using for your study.

VALIDITY

The **validity** of an instrument indicates the extent to which it actually reflects or is able to measure the construct being examined. The *Standards for Educational and Psychological Testing* were revised in 1999 to operationalize measurement validity in terms of five types of evidence (American Psychological Association, 1999; Goodwin, 2002). When investigating validity, the types of evidence examined include: (1) evidence based on test or instrument content, (2) evidence based on response processes, (3) evidence based on internal structure, (4) evidence based on relations to other variables, and (5) evidence based on consequences of testing (Goodwin, 2002). These types of evidence are often examined using several validity procedures. The validity procedures conducted to determine the accuracy of instruments or scales are usually reported in articles focused on instrument development or psychometric sources. The development of an instrument's validity is complex, includes several validity procedures, and develops over years with the use of the instrument in studies. The multiple types of validity discussed in the literature are confusing, especially because the types are not discrete but are interrelated (Bannigan & Watson, 2009; DeVon et al., 2007). In this text, three main categories of validity (content validity, construct validity,

TABLE 16-2   Psychometric Properties of Major Study Instruments

Instrument	Cronbach's Alpha	*M (SD)*	Study Range	Scale Range
Perceived stress scale (10-item)	0.91	19.13 (7.53)	4–36	0–44
Sleep Quality Index (7-item)	0.70	6.56 (3.70)	1–19	0–21
Loneliness scale (20-item)	0.92	40.07 (10.66)	24–66	20–80
Self-esteem scale (10-item)	0.94	20.65 (7.03)	3–30	0–30

M, mean; *SD*, standard deviation.
From Smith, M. J., Theeke, L., Culp, S., Clark, K., & Pinto, S. (2014). Psychosocial variables and self-rated health in young adult obese women. *Applied Nursing Research, 27*(1), 69.

and criterion-related validity) are presented and linked to the five types of evidence previously identified. The readability of an instrument is also discussed because this affects the validity and reliability of an instrument in a study.

Validity, similar to reliability, is not an all-or-nothing phenomenon but rather a matter of degree. No instrument is completely valid. One determines the degree of validity of a measure rather than whether or not it has validity. Determining the validity of an instrument often requires years of work. Many authors equate the validity of the instrument with the rigorousness of the researcher. The assumption is that because the researcher develops the instrument, the researcher also establishes the validity. However, this is an erroneous assumption because validity is not a commodity that researchers can purchase with techniques. Validity is an ideal state—to be pursued, but not to be attained. As the roots of the word imply, *validity* includes truth, strength, and value. Some authors might believe that validity is a tangible "resource," which can be acquired by applying enough appropriate techniques. However, we reject this view and believe measurement validity is similar to integrity, character, or quality, to be assessed relative to purposes and circumstances and built over time by researchers conducting a variety of studies (Brinberg & McGrath, 1985).

Figure 16-9 illustrates validity (the shaded area) by the extent to which the instrument *A-1* reflects concept *A*. As measurement of the concept improves, validity improves. The extent to which the instrument *A-1* measures items other than the concept is referred to as *systematic error* (identified as the unshaded area of *A-1* in Figure 16-9). As systematic error decreases, validity increases.

Validity varies from one sample to another and from one situation to another; therefore, validity testing affirms the appropriateness of an instrument for a specific group or purpose rather than establishing validity of the instrument itself (DeVon et al., 2007; Waltz et al., 2010). An instrument may be valid in one situation but not valid in another. Instruments used in nursing studies that were developed for use in other disciplines need to be examined for validity in terms of nursing knowledge. An instrument developed to measure cognitive function in educational studies might not capture the cognitive function level of elderly adults measured in a nursing study. Nurse researchers are encouraged to reexamine their instruments' validity in each of their study situations. However, researchers often indicate that their measurement methods have good validity but do not describe the specific validity results from previous research or the current study. An enhanced discussion of the instruments' validity would improve the quality of such research reports. The following sections include the common types of content, construct, and criterion-related validity reported in nursing studies (see Table 16-1).

Content Validity

The discussion of content validity also includes face validity and the content validity index. In the 1960s and 1970s, the only type of validity that most studies addressed was referred to as **face validity**, which verified basically that the instrument looked as if it was valid or gave the appearance of measuring the construct it was supposed to measure. Face validity is a subjective assessment that might be made by researchers, expert clinicians, or even potential subjects. Because this is a subjective judgment with no clear guidelines for making the judgment, face validity is considered the weakest form of validity (DeVon et al., 2007). However, it is still an important aspect of the usefulness of the instrument because the willingness of subjects to complete the instrument relates to their perception that the instrument measures the construct about which they agreed to provide information (Thomas, 1992). Face validity is often considered a precursor of or an aspect of content validity.

Content validity examines the extent to which the measurement method includes all major elements relevant to the construct being measured. For an instrument or scale, content evidence is obtained from the following three sources: the literature, representatives of the relevant population, and content experts (DeVon

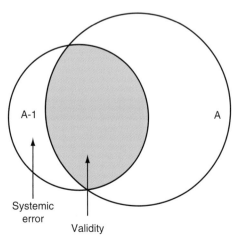

FIGURE 16-9 Representation of instrument validity.

et al., 2007; Goodwin, 2002; Waltz et al., 2010). Documentation of content validity begins with development of the instrument. The first step of instrument development is to identify *what* is to be measured; this is referred to as the *universe* or *domain* of the construct. You can determine the domain through a concept analysis or an extensive literature search. Qualitative research methods can also be used for this purpose.

Jansson and colleagues (2015) developed a Patient Advocacy Engagement Scale (Patient-AES) for health professionals. Nurses and other health professionals are required by accreditation guidelines and their codes of ethics to engage in patient advocacy in the course of their work. However, Jansson et al. (2015, p. 162) noted that no scale "had been developed to measure the extent to which specific health professionals engage in patient advocacy in the course of their work in acute care hospitals." Examples of the different types of validity for the Patient-AES are provided throughout this section. In the following study excerpt, Jansson et al. (2015) described the initial development of the Patient-AES and its content validity.

"A definition of patient advocacy developed by Jansson (2011) was adapted for this project:... An intervention to help patients obtain services and rights and benefits that would (likely) not otherwise be received by them and that would advance their well-being...

To identify appropriate patient problems, we began with Jansson's (2011) typology of 118 patient problems in seven categories. This list represented an array of problems beyond the biological or physiological, consonant with a biopsychosocial framework that considers the impact of the social and cultural environment as well as psychological factors upon individuals' well-being...

Jansson's (2011) seven categories of patient problems were: (1) ethical problems; (2) problems related to quality of care; (3) lack of culturally responsive care; (4) lack of preventive care; (5) lack of affordable or accessible care; (6) lack of care for mental health issues and distress; and (7) lack of care that addresses household and community barriers to care. A review of 800 sources confirmed that specific problems in these categories often adversely affect patient health outcomes." (Jansson et al., 2015, pp. 163–164)

"The Patient Advocacy Engagement Scale (Patient-AES) was constructed using an applied mode of classical test theory (Nunnally & Bernstein, 1994). The stages... included instrument development and instrument validation. The instrument development stage included three steps: (1) preliminary planning; (2) generating an initial item pool; and (3) refining the scale. The instrument validation stage included four steps: (1) data collection; (2) estimation of content validity; (3) estimation of construct validity; and (4) estimation of reliability." (Jansson et al., 2015, p. 164)

"Instrument Development
Step 1: Preliminary planning. We assembled a stakeholder panel in fall 2012 whose nine members had expertise in patient advocacy...

Step 2: Generating an item pool. We identified 44 specific patient problems from the list of 118 (Jansson, 2011) by excluding problems not likely to be seen by health professionals during a 2-month period. Items were developed and grouped in the seven categories developed by Jansson (2011)... Participants were asked, "During the last 2 months, how often have you engaged in patient advocacy to address a patient's problem related to each of these numbered issues below?" After reading the definition of patient advocacy, respondents were asked to report on the five-point frequency [with the anchors 1 (never), 2 (seldom), 3 (sometimes), 4 (frequently), and 5 (always)] how often they engaged in advocacy with regard to each of the 44 problems during the prior 2 months." (Jansson et al., 2015, pp. 165–166)

Jansson et al. (2015) provided a detailed description of the development and selection of items for their Patient-AES. These researchers, building on Jansson's (2011) previous work, conducted an extensive review of the literature (800 sources) to define patient advocacy and determine potential items for their scale. A helpful strategy commonly used in determining items for a scale is to develop a blueprint or matrix, which was done by Jansson et al. (2015) using the seven categories of patient problems. The blueprint specifications should be submitted to an expert panel to validate that they are appropriate, accurate, and representative. At least five experts are recommended, although a minimum of three experts is acceptable if you cannot locate additional individuals with expertise in the area. Researchers might seek out individuals with expertise in various fields—for example, one individual with knowledge of instrument development, a second with clinical expertise in an appropriate field of practice, and a third with expertise in another discipline relevant to the content area. Jansson et al. (2015) assembled a stakeholder panel that included nine members with expertise in patient advocacy.

The experts need specific guidelines for judging the appropriateness, accuracy, and representativeness of the specifications. Berk (1990) recommended that the experts first make independent assessments and then meet for a group discussion of the specifications. The instrument specifications then can be revised and resubmitted to the experts for a final independent assessment. Davis (1992) recommended that researchers provide expert reviewers with theoretical definitions of concepts and a list of which instrument items are expected to measure each of the concepts, which was done by Jansson et al. (2015).

Researchers need to determine how to measure the domain. The item format, item content, and procedures for generating items must be carefully described. Items are then constructed for each cell in the matrix, or observational methods are designated to gather data related to a specific cell. Researchers are expected to describe the specifications used in constructing items or selecting observations. Sources of content for items must be documented. Then researchers can assemble, refine, and arrange the items in a suitable order before submitting them to the content experts for evaluation. Specific instructions for evaluating each item and the total instrument must be given to the experts. Jansson et al. (2015) described in detail their process for refining the scale.

"**Step 3: Refining the scale**. These 44 items were reduced to 33 by a panel of three experts, selected from among the project's stakeholders: the associate professor of social work who pioneered research on advocacy related to ethical issues in hospitals, the clinical associate professor with expertise in advocacy for senior citizens, and the professor of nursing who had done extensive research on advocacy for persons with HIV/AIDS. These experts were asked to eliminate any items that they viewed as repetitive, poorly worded, confusing, or not essential.

The experts also slightly reworded some items... The 33 items in seven categories are listed in [Table 16-3]." (Jansson et al., 2015, p. 166)

Content Validity Ratio and Index

In developing content validity for an instrument, researchers can calculate a **content validity ratio** (CVR) for each item on a scale by rating it 0 (not necessary), 1 (useful), or 3 (essential). A method for calculating the CVR was developed by Lawshe (1975) and is presented in Table 16-4 (DeVon et al., 2007). Minimum CVR

TABLE 16-3   Item Content Validity Based on Proportion of Ratings of Relevant or Very Relevant by Seven Experts

Dimension	Item	I-CVI
Patient advocacy for patient rights	1. Informed consent to a medical intervention	0.86
	2. Accurate medical information	0.86
	3. Confidential medical information	0.71
	4. Advanced directives	0.86
	5. Competence to make medical decisions	0.86
Patient advocacy for quality care	6. Lack of evidence-based health care	0.71
	7. Medical errors	1.00
	8. Whether to take specific diagnostic tests	1.00
	9. Fragmented care[a]	1.00
	10. Non-beneficial treatment	1.00
Patient advocacy for culturally competent care	11. Information in patients' preferred language	1.00
	12. Communication with persons with limited literacy or health knowledge	1.00
	13. Religious, spiritual, and cultural practices[a]	0.86
	14. Use of complementary and alternative medicine[a]	0.57
Patient advocacy for preventive care	15. Wellness exams	0.86
	16. At-risk factors[a]	1.00
	17. Chronic disease care	1.00
	18. Immunizations[a]	1.00
Patient advocacy for affordable care	19. Financing medications and healthcare needs	1.00
	20. Use of publicly funded programs	1.00
	21. Coverage from private insurance companies	0.71

TABLE 16-3 Item Content Validity Based on Proportion of Ratings of Relevant or Very Relevant by Seven Experts—cont'd

Dimension	Item	I-CVI
Patient advocacy for mental health care	22. Screening for specific mental health conditions	1.00
	23. Treatment of mental health conditions while hospitalized	1.00
	24. Follow-up treatment for mental health conditions after discharge	1.00
	25. Medications for mental health conditions	1.00
	26. Mental distress stemming from health conditions	1.00
	27. Availability of individual counseling and or group therapy[a]	1.00
	28. Availability of support groups[a]	0.86
Patient advocacy for community-based care	29. Discharge planning	0.86
	30. Transitions between community-based levels of care	1.00
	31. Referrals to services in communities	1.00
	32. Reaching out to referral sources on behalf of the patient	0.71
	33. Assessment of home, community, and work environments	1.00

Note: I-CVI = item content validity index. The overall scale CVI (S-CVI) was 0.92.
[a]Item excluded from calculation of S-CVI and final scale based on I-CVI and confirmatory factor analysis.
From Jansson, B. S., Nyamathi, A., Duan, L., Kaplan, C., Heidemann, G., & Ananias, D. (2015). Validation of the Patient Advocacy Engagement Scale for health professionals. *Research in Nursing & Health, 38*(2), 169.

TABLE 16-4 Two Methods of Calculating the Content Validity Ratio (CVR) and the Content Validity Index (CVI)

Rating Scale	Lawshe (1975) Scale Used for Rating Items			Lynn (1986) Scale Used for Rating Items			
	0	1	3	1	2	3	4
	Not Necessary	Useful	Essential	Irrelevant			Extremely Relevant
Calculations	To calculate CVR (a score for individual scale items)			CVI for each scale item is the proportion of experts who rate the item as a 3 or 4 on a 4-point scale. *Example:* If 4 of 6 content experts rated an item as relevant (3 or 4), CVI would be 4/6 = 0.67.			
	$CVR = (n_e - N/2)/(N/2)$			This item would not meet the 0.83 level of endorsement required to establish content validity using a panel of 6 experts at the 0.05 level of significance. Therefore, it would be dropped.			
	Note: n_e = The number of experts who rated an item as "essential"			CVI for the entire scale is the proportion of the total number of items deemed content valid. *Example:* If 77 of 80 items were deemed content valid, CVI would be 77/80 = 0.96.			
	N = the total number of experts. *Example:* If 8 of 10 experts rated an item as essential, CVR would be (8 − 5/5) = 0.60						
Acceptable range	Depends on number of reviewers			Depends on number of reviewers			

From DeVon, H. A., Block, M. E., Moyle-Wright, P., Ernst, D. M., Hayden, S. J., Lazzara, D. J., et al. (2007). A psychometric toolbox for testing validity and reliability. *Journal of Nursing Scholarship, 39*(2), 158.

scores for including items in an instrument can be based on a one-tailed test with a 0.05 level of significance.

The content validity score calculated for the complete instrument is called the **content validity index** (CVI). The CVI was developed to obtain a numerical value that reflects the level of content-related validity evidence for a measurement method. In calculating CVI, experts rate the content relevance of each item in an instrument using a 4-point rating scale. Lynn (1986, p. 384) recommended standardizing the options on this scale to read as follows: "1 = not relevant; 2 = unable to assess relevance without item revision or item is in need of such revision that it would no longer be relevant; 3 = relevant but needs minor alteration; 4 = very relevant and succinct." In addition to evaluating existing items, the experts were asked to identify important areas not included in the instrument. The calculation for the CVI is presented in Table 16-4 using the format developed by Lynn (1986). Complete agreement needs to exist among the expert reviewers to retain an item, when there are seven or fewer reviewers. If few reviewers are used and many of the experts support most of the items on an instrument, this often results in an inflated CVI and an inflation in the evidence for the instrument's content validity (DeVon et al., 2007; Waltz et al., 2010). Before sending the instrument to experts for evaluation, researchers need to decide how many experts must agree on each item and on the total instrument for the content to be considered valid. Items that do not achieve minimum agreement by the expert panel must be eliminated from the instrument, revised, or retained based on a clear rationale (DeVon et al., 2007; Lynn, 1986).

Jansson et al. (2015) developed the Patient-AES to measure health professions' provision of patient advocacy care and described their content validity testing process and outcomes as follows.

"Estimation of content validity is a process in which the appropriateness, quality, and representativeness of each item is evaluated to determine the degree to which the items, taken together, constitute an adequate operational definition of a construct... A panel of seven experts (five members of the project stakeholder group and two recruited from participating hospitals) who had not reviewed the instrument in the refinement stage were asked to rank the 33 items in the Patient-AES as: (1) not relevant, (2) somewhat relevant, (3) relevant, or (4) very relevant. Using these ratings, the item-level content validity index (I-CVI) and scale-level content validity (S-CVI) were determined. I-CVI was defined as the proportion of items that achieved a rating of 3 or 4 by the panel of expert reviewers. Polit, Beck, and Owen (2007) recommended that when there are seven experts, an I-CVI score above 0.71 can be considered good, and a score above 0.86 can be considered excellent. We follow this criterion of 0.71 as the minimally acceptable standard for I-CVI. As shown in [Table 16-3], the I-CVI of the Patient-AES items ranged from 0.57 to 1.00, with 28 items scoring 0.86 or higher, four items scoring between 0.71 and 0.86, and one item scoring 0.57. In general, these results showed good to excellent content validity, with the exception of the item measuring advocacy to address unresolved problems related to complementary and alternative medicine. This item was discussed in a subsequent meeting of the stakeholders and the research team and retained because it measures an aspect of patient care that they viewed as important and is often overlooked in traditional medical settings, and therefore one with a high need for advocacy. The overall S-CVI for patient advocacy, calculated using the average agreement approach (Polit et al., 2007), was 0.92, suggesting good overall content validity." (Jansson et al., 2015, p. 168)

Jansson and colleagues (2015) provided excellent detail about the development of the Patient-AES and the process for determining the scale's content validity. They also provided extensive information about the expert review panel for conducting the content validity testing. The strength of the review panel is their research and clinical expertise in determining patient advocacy needs.

With some modifications, the content validity procedure previously described can be used with existing instruments, many of which have never been evaluated for content-related validity. With the permission of the author or researcher who developed the instrument, you could revise the instrument to improve its content-related validity (Lynn, 1986). In addition, the panel of experts or reviewers evaluating the items of the instrument for content validity might also examine it for readability and language acceptability from the perspective of possible study participants and data collectors (Berk, 1990; DeVon et al., 2007).

Readability of an Instrument

Readability is an essential element of the validity and reliability of an instrument. Assessing the level of readability of an instrument is simple and takes only seconds with the use of a computer. There are more than 30 readability formulas. These formulas count language elements in the document and use this information to estimate the degree of difficulty a reader may have in comprehending the text. Readability formulas are now a standard part of word-processing software.

Although readability has never been formally identified as a component of content validity, it is essential that subjects be able to comprehend the items of an instrument. Jansson et al. (2015) could have strengthened the measurement section of their research report by including the readability level of the Patient-AES, even though the study participants were professional nurses.

Construct Validity

Construct validity focuses on determining whether the instrument actually measures the theoretical construct that it purports to measure, which involves examining the fit between the conceptual and operational definitions of a variable (see Chapter 6). Thus, construct validity testing attempts to validate the theory (concepts and relationships) supporting the instrument. The instrument's evidence based on content, response processes, and internal structure is examined to determine construct validity (Goodwin, 2002; Waltz et al., 2010). Construct validity is developed using a variety of techniques and the ones included in this text are: validity from factor analysis, convergent validity, divergent validity, validity from contrasting groups, and validity from discriminant analysis (see Table 16-1).

Validity From Factor Analysis

Factor analysis is a valuable approach for determining evidence of an instrument's construct validity. This analysis technique is used to determine the various dimensions or subcomponents of a phenomenon of interest. To employ factor analysis, the instrument must be administered to a large, representative sample of participants at one time. Usually the data are initially analyzed with **exploratory factor analysis** (EFA) to examine relationships among the various items of the instrument. Items that are closely related are clustered into a factor. The researcher needs to preset the minimum loading for an item to be included in a factor. The minimum loading is usually set at 0.30 but might be as high as 0.50 (Waltz et al., 2010). Determining and naming the factors identified through EFA require detailed work on the part of the researcher. Researchers can validate the number of factors or subcomponents in the instrument and measurement equivalence among comparison groups through the use of **confirmatory factor analysis** (CFA). Items that do not fall into a factor (because they do not correlate with other items) may be deleted (DeVon et al., 2007; Plichta & Kelvin, 2013; Stommel, Wang, Given, & Given, 1992; Waltz et al., 2010). A more extensive discussion of EFA and CFA is presented in Chapter 23.

Jansson and colleagues (2015) conducted a CFA to determine the factor structure for their Patient-AES.

The scale had 33 items that were sorted into seven subscales (patient advocacy for patient rights, patient advocacy for quality care, patient advocacy for culturally competent care, patient advocacy for preventive care, patient advocacy for affordable care, patient advocacy for mental health care, and patient advocacy for community-based care) that are identified in Table 16-3. The results of the CFA are presented in the following study excerpt.

"Confirmatory factor analysis was conducted to verify the latent structure of the hypothesized seven-factor model. Seven cross loading items had factor loadings ≥ 0.32 and were removed...: items 9, 13, 14, 16, 18, 27, and 28 [Table 16-3]. The final CFA model was composed of seven latent factors and 26 items... There were no double-loading items or correlated errors in the final CFA... Consistent with theory, the measure captured the seven aforementioned domains of patient advocacy, with five items loading on the latent factor of patients' ethical rights, four items loading on quality care, two items loading on culturally competent care, two items loading on preventive care, three items loading on affordable care, five items loading on mental health care, and five items loading on community-based care. The factor loadings from the CFA of all 26 items ranged from 0.53 to 0.96, and the interfactor correlations ranged from 0.2 to 0.8 [Table 16-5]." (Jansson et al., 2015, pp. 168–169)

Jansson et al. (2015) CFA results supported the conceptual structure of the Patient-AES and added to the construct validity of the scale. The Patient-AES and the seven subscales had strong reliability as indicated in the following study excerpt and Table 16-5. Because the Patient-AES is a new scale, additional research is essential to expand the validity and reliability of this scale.

"Reliability
The test–retest Pearson correlation coefficients for seven subscales were all statistically significant and ranged from 0.57 to 0.83 [Table 16-5]. The test–retest r for entire scale was 0.81, indicating adequate stability of the overall scale and its subscales. Cronbach α for the seven subscales ranged from 0.55 to 0.94. The Patient Advocacy for Preventive Care subscale had the lowest α of 0.55 but contains only two items. Given the large impact of number of items on the Cronbach α value, we judged the relatively low value as an acceptable level of internal consistency. The Cronbach α value for overall scale was 0.94, supporting the internal consistency of the Patient-AES [Table 16-5]." (Jansson et al., 2015, p. 169)

TABLE 16-5   Means, Standard Deviations, Test-Retest Stability, and Intercorrelations of Items in the Seven-Factor Final Patient Advocacy Engagement Scale (N = 295)

Dimension	Number of Items	Mean (SD)	Test–Retest Reliability (r)	Cronbach α	INTERFACTOR CORRELATION (R)					
					1	2	3	4	5	6
Patient advocacy for patient rights	5	14.8 (4.9)	0.62	0.82						
Patient advocacy for quality care	4	9.5 (3.7)	0.68	0.83	0.7					
Patient advocacy for culturally competent care	2	6.7 (2.2)	0.62	0.87	0.5	0.4				
Patient advocacy for preventive care	2	5.9 (2.1)	0.73	0.55	0.8	0.8	0.7			
Patient advocacy for affordable care	3	9.1 (3.5)	0.56	0.85	0.5	0.2	0.6	0.6		
Patient advocacy for mental health care	5	13.6 (5.7)	0.83	0.91	0.6	0.3	0.5	0.6	0.7	
Patient advocacy for community-based care	5	15.6 (5.6)	0.57	0.89	0.6	0.3	0.5	0.7	0.8	0.7

AES, Advocacy Engagement Scale; SD, standard deviation.
Note: The 26-item scale as a whole had a mean score of 75.3 (SD 20.6), test–retest r = 0.78, and Cronbach α = 0.94.
From Jansson, B. S., Nyamathi, A., Duan, L., Kaplan, C., Heidemann, G., & Ananias, D. (2015). Validation of the Patient Advocacy Engagement Scale for health professionals. *Research in Nursing & Health, 38*(2), 170.

Convergent Validity

In examining the construct validity of a new instrument, it is important to determine how closely an existing instrument measures the same construct as a newly developed instrument (**convergent validity**). For example, different instruments are available to measure the construct depression. However, for many possible reasons, the existing instruments may be unsatisfactory for a particular purpose or a particular population, such as measuring major depression in young children, and the researcher may choose to develop a new instrument for a study. Another instance might be the case in which an existing instrument takes 20 minutes to administer, and the researcher develops a new scale that takes only four minutes. One can administer all of the instruments (the new one and the existing ones) to a sample concurrently and evaluate the results using correlational analyses. If the measures are highly positively correlated, the construct validity of each instrument is strengthened.

Jansson et al. (2015, p. 162) stated that the Patient-AES "was the first scale that measures patient advocacy engagement by healthcare professionals in acute-care settings related to a broad range of specific patient problems." At this time, they did not identify other scales that measured advocacy and convergent validity information was not provided. Construct validity of an instrument is a complex process that is developed over years. In the future, Jansson and colleagues (2015) can examine the Patient-AES for convergent and divergent validity.

However, convergent validity was addressed for the loneliness scale introduced earlier in a study by Smith et al. (2014) that examined the relationships among the concepts of loneliness, self-esteem, and sleep quality in a population of young obese women. The convergent validity of the loneliness scale was confirmed with significant positive correlations between it and the Beck Depression Inventory ($r = 0.62$), and the Costello-Comrey Anxiety Scale ($r = 0.32$).

Divergent Validity

Divergent validity can be examined when an instrument is available that measures the construct opposite to the construct measured by the newly developed instrument. For example, if the newly developed instrument measures hope, you could search for an instrument that measures hopelessness or despair. Ideally, scores on the hope instrument would be negatively correlated with the sores on the hopelessness or despair instrument to provide evidence of divergent validity. If possible, you could administer this instrument and the instruments used to test convergent validity at the same time. This approach of combining convergent and divergent validity testing of instruments is called **multitrait-multimethod** (MT-MM).

The MT-MM approach can be used when researchers are examining two or more constructs being measured by two or more measurement methods (DeVon et al., 2007). Correlational procedures are conducted with the different scales and subscales. If the convergent measures positively correlate and the divergent measures negatively correlate with other measures, validity for each of the instruments is strengthened

Validity From Contrasting (or Known) Groups

To test the validity of an instrument, identify groups that are expected (or known) to have contrasting scores on the instrument and generate hypotheses about the expected response of each of these known groups to the construct. Next, select samples from at least two groups that are expected to have opposing responses to the items in the instrument. Smith et al.'s (2014) study, previously discussed, reported validity from contrasting groups of good and poor sleepers. The following study excerpt presents the validity discussion for the Sleep Quality Index from previous research.

"Sleep was determined using the Pittsburgh Sleep Quality Index... It consists of 19 self-rated items. The global score has a range of 0-21 where higher scores indicate poorer sleep quality. In a study of sleep quality with in-patients and outpatients in a psychiatric clinic, the global score had an overall reliability coefficient (Cronbach's alpha) of 0.83 indicating a high degree of reliability... Validity was determined by identifying good and poor sleepers in a group of healthy subjects and sleep disturbed subjects. A global sleep score of ≥ 5 offered a sensitive and specific measure of poor sleep quality." (Smith et al., 2014, p. 69)

The identified good and poor sleepers had appropriate scores on the Sleep Quality Index. Thus, the construct validity of the instrument is strengthened in that the scores of the good and poor sleeper groups were as anticipated.

Evidence of Validity From Discriminant Analysis

Instruments sometimes have been developed to measure constructs closely related to the construct measured by a newly developed instrument. For example, an instrument might exist to measure patient advocacy in another work environment that is similar to the Patient-AES that Jansson et al. (2015) developed for professionals working in acute care hospitals. If such an instrument

can be located, you can strengthen the validity of the Patient-AES by testing the extent to which the two instruments can finely discriminate between these related concepts. Testing of this discrimination involves administering the two instruments simultaneously to a sample and performing a discriminant analysis (see Kerlinger & Lee, 2000, for a discussion of discriminant analysis).

Successive Verification of Validity

After the initial development of an instrument, it is hoped that other researchers would begin using the instrument in additional studies. In each of these studies, researchers make a validity determination of the instrument in their research. Every time this happens, the validity and reliability information on the instrument increases. An instrument's **successive verification of validity** develops over time when the instrument is used in a variety of studies with different populations and settings. For example, when additional researchers use the Patient-AES to measure health professionals' patient advocacy in different studies, this will add to the successive verification validity of the scale. Because the Patient-AES Scale is newly developed and published, no additional studies were found that have used it.

Criterion-Related Validity

Criterion-related validity is strengthened when a study participant's score on an instrument can be used to infer his or her performance on another variable or criterion. The two types of criterion-related validity are predictive validity and concurrent validity. **Predictive validity** is the extent to which an individual's score on a scale or instrument can be used to predict future performance or behavior on a criterion (Waltz et al., 2010). For example, nurse researchers often want to determine the ability of scales developed to measure selected health behaviors to predict the future health status of individuals. One approach might be to examine reported stress levels of selected individuals in highly stressful careers such as nursing and see whether stress is linked to the nurses' future incidence of hypertension. French, Lenton, Walters, and Eyles (2000) completed an expanded evaluation of the reliability and validity of the Nursing Stress Scale (NSS) with a random sample of 2280 nurses working in a wide range of healthcare settings. They noted that the NSS included nine subscales, originally developed as factors through factor analysis: death and dying, conflict with physicians, inadequate preparation, problems with supervisors, workload, problems with peers, uncertainty concerning treatment, patients and their families, and discrimination (construct validity). CFA supported the factor structure. Cronbach alpha coefficients of eight of the subscales were 0.70 or higher. Hypothetically, predictive validity could be examined if the nurses' scores on the NNS scale were correlated with their BP readings at one, three, and five years. The predictive validity of the NNS would be strengthened if the nurses with high NNS scores had higher incidences of hypertension at one, three, or five years. The accuracy of predictive validity is determined through regression analysis (Waltz et al., 2010).

Concurrent validity focuses on the extent to which an individual's score on an instrument or scale can be used to estimate his or her present or concurrent performance on another variable or criterion. Thus, the difference between concurrent validity and predictive validity is the timing of the measurement of the other criterion. Concurrent validity is examined within a short period of time and predictive validity is examined in the future, as previously discussed (Waltz et al., 2010). For example, concurrent validly could be examined if you measured individuals' self-esteem and use these scores to estimate their scores on a coping with illness scale. Individuals with high scores on self-esteem would be expected also to have high coping scores. If these results held true in a study in which both measures were obtained concurrently, the two instruments would have evidence of concurrent validity.

ACCURACY, PRECISION, AND ERROR OF PHYSIOLOGICAL MEASURES

Accuracy and precision of physiological and biochemical measures tend not to be reported in published studies. These routine physiological measures are assumed to be accurate and precise, an assumption that is not always correct. The most common physiological measures used in nursing studies are blood pressure, heart rate, temperature, height, and weight. These measures often are obtained from the patient's record with no consideration given to their accuracy. It is important to consider the possibility of differences between the obtained value and the true value of physiological measures. Thus, researchers using physiological measures need to provide evidence of the accuracy and precision of their measures (Ryan-Wenger, 2010).

The evaluation of physiological measures may require a slightly different perspective from that applied to behavioral measures, in that standards for most biophysical measures are defined by national and international organizations such as the International Organization for Standardization (ISO, 2015a) and the Clinical Laboratory Standards Institute (CLSI, 2015).

CLSI develops standards for laboratory and other healthcare-related biophysical measures. The ISO is the world's largest developer and publisher of international standards and includes a network of 160 countries (see ISO website for details at http://www.iso.org/iso/home.htm). The ISO standards were developed for a broad mission, but the goals specific to research include the following:

- Make the development, manufacturing, and supply of products and services more efficient, safer, and cleaner
- Share technological advances and good management practice
- Disseminate innovations
- Safeguard consumers and users in general of products and services
- Make life simpler by providing solutions to common problems (ISO, 2015b)

Another measurement resource is the Bureau International des Poids et Measures (BIPM, 2015). The unique role of the BIPM is to:

"(1) Coordinate the realization and improvement of the world-wide measurement system to ensure it delivers accurate and comparable measurement results;

(2) Undertake selected scientific and technical activities that are more efficiently carried out in its own laboratories on behalf of member states; and

(3) Promote the importance of metrology to science, industry, and society, in particular through collaboration with other intergovernmental organizations and international bodies and in international forums" (BIPM, 2015; http://www.bipm.org/en/about-us/role.html).

Using these resources, you can locate the standards for different biophysical equipment, products, or services that you might use in a study or in clinical practice. When discussing a physiological measure in a study, researchers need to address the accuracy, precision, and error rate of the measurement method (see Table 16-1).

Accuracy

Accuracy involves determining the closeness of the agreement between the measured value and the true value of the quantity being measured. Accuracy is similar to validity, in which evidence of content-related validity addresses the extent to which the instrument measured the construct or domain defined in the study. New measurement devices are compared with existing standardized methods of measuring a biophysical property or concept (Ryan-Wenger, 2010). For example, measures of oxygen saturation with a pulse oximeter were strongly correlated with arterial blood gas measures of oxygen saturation, which supports the accuracy of the pulse oximeter. Thus, there should be a very strong, positive correlation (≥ 0.95) between pulse oximeter and blood gas measures of oxygen saturation to support the accuracy of the pulse oximeter.

Accuracy of physiological measures depends on the (1) quality of the measurement equipment or device, (2) detail of the data collection plan, and (3) expertise of the data collector (Ryan-Wenger, 2010). The data collector or person conducting the biophysical measures must conduct the measurements in a standardized way that is usually directed by a measurement protocol. For example, the measurement protocol for obtaining BP readings in a study need to include the following steps:

1. Calibrate the BP equipment for accuracy according to equipment guidelines.
2. Have the subject empty his or her bladder.
3. Place the subject in a chair with back support and allow five minutes of rest.
4. Remove restrictive clothing from the subject's arm.
5. Measure the subject's upper arm and select the appropriate cuff size.
6. Instruct the subject to place his or her feet flat on the floor.
7. Place the subject's arm on a table at heart level when taking the BP reading.
8. Take two to three BP readings each five minutes apart.
9. Calculate an average of BP readings.
10. Enter the averaged BP reading into a computer. (Weber et al., 2014)

This protocol was developed by the American Society of Hypertension and the International Society of Hypertension for their clinical practice guidelines for the management of hypertension in the community (Weber et al., 2014). Using a standardized, detailed protocol greatly increases the accuracy and precision of physiological measures.

Some measurements, such as arterial pressure, can be obtained by the biomedical device producing the reading and automatically recorded in a computerized database. This type of data collection greatly reduces the potential for error and increases accuracy and precision.

The biomedical device or equipment used to measure a study variable must be examined for accuracy. Researchers should document the extent to which the biophysical measure is an accurate measurement of a study variable and the level of error expected. Reviewing the ISO (2015b) and CLSI (2015) standards could provide essential accuracy data and information about the company that developed the device or equipment. Contact the company that developed the physiological

equipment to obtain recalibration and maintenance recommendations.

Selectivity, an element of accuracy, is "the ability to identify correctly the signal under study and to distinguish it from other signals" (Gift & Soeken, 1988, p. 129). Because body systems interact, the researcher must choose instruments that have selectivity for the dimension being studied. For example, electrocardiographic readings allow one to differentiate electrical signals coming from the myocardium from similar signals coming from skeletal muscles.

To determine the accuracy of biochemical measures, review the standards set by CLSI (2015) and determine whether the laboratory where the measures are going to be obtained is certified. Most laboratories are certified, so researchers could contact experts in the agency about the laboratory procedure and ask them to describe the process for data collection and analysis, and the typical values obtained for specimens. You might also ask these experts to judge the appropriateness of the biophysical device for the construct being measured in the study. Use contrasted groups' techniques by selecting a group of subjects known to have high values on the biochemical measures and comparing them with a group of subjects known to have low values on the same measure. In addition, to obtain concurrent validity, compare the results of the test with results from the use of a known standard, such as the example of the comparison of pulse oximeter values with blood gas values for oxygen saturation.

Precision

Precision is the degree of consistency or reproducibility of measurements made with physiological instruments or devices. There should be close agreement in the replicated measures of the same variable or object under specified conditions (Ryan-Wenger, 2010). Precision is similar to reliability. The precision of most physiological devices or equipment is determined by the manufacturer and is part of quality control testing done in the agency using the device. Similar to accuracy, precision depends on the collector of the biophysical measures and the consistency of the measurement equipment. The protocol for collecting the biophysical measures improves precision and accuracy (see the previous example of protocol to measure BP readings).

The data collectors need to be trained to ensure consistency, which is documented with intrarater (within a single data collector) and interrater (among data collectors) percentages of agreements (see the earlier discussion of interrater reliability). The kappa coefficient of agreement is one of the most common and simplest statistics conducted to determine intrarater and interrater accuracy and precision for nominal level data (Cohen, 1960; Ryan-Wenger, 2010). The equipment used to measure physiological variables needs to be maintained according to the standards set by ISO and the manufacturers of the devices. Many devices need to be recalibrated according to set criteria to ensure consistency in measurements. Because of fluctuations in some physiological measures, test-retest reliability might be inappropriate.

Two procedures are commonly used to determine the precision of biochemical measures. One is the Levy-Jennings chart. For each analysis method, a control sample is analyzed daily for 20 to 30 days. The control sample contains a known amount of the substance being tested. The mean, the standard deviation, and the known value of the sample are used to prepare a graph of the daily test results. Only one value of 22 is expected to be greater than or less than two standard deviations from the mean. If two or more values are more than two standard deviations from the mean, the method is unreliable in that laboratory. Another method of determining the precision of biochemical measures is the duplicate measurement method. The same technician performs duplicate measures on randomly selected specimens for a specific number of days. The results are essentially the same each day if there is high precision. Results are plotted on a graph, and the standard deviation is calculated on the basis of difference scores. The use of correlation coefficients is not recommended (DeKeyser & Pugh, 1990).

Sensitivity

Sensitivity of physiological measures relates to "the amount of change of a parameter that can be measured correctly" (Gift & Soeken, 1988, p. 130). If changes are expected to be small, the instrument must be very sensitive to detect the changes. For example, a glucometer that could detect incremental changes of five points in a patient's blood sugar would not be sensitive enough to use when adjusting regular insulin doses. Sensitivity is associated with effect size (see Chapter 15). With some instruments, sensitivity may vary at the ends of the spectrum, which is referred to as the frequency response. The stability of an instrument is also related to sensitivity, which may be judged in terms of the ability of the system to resume a steady state after a disturbance in input. For electrical systems, this feature is referred to as freedom from drift (Gift & Soeken, 1988).

Error

Sources of **error in physiological measures** can be grouped into the following five categories: (1) environment, (2) user, (3) study participant, (4) machine, and (5) interpretation. The environment affects both the machine and the subject. Environmental factors include temperature, barometric pressure, and static electricity. User errors are caused by the person using the instrument and may be associated with variations by the same user, different users, changes in supplies, or procedures used to operate the equipment. Study participant errors occur when the person alters the machine or the machine alters the person. In some cases, the machine may not be used to its full capacity. Machine error may be related to calibration or to the stability of the machine. Signals transmitted from the machine are also a source of error and can cause misinterpretation (Ryan-Wenger, 2010).

Sources of error in biochemical measures are biological, pre-analytical, analytical, and post-analytical. Biological variability in biochemical measures is due to factors such as age, gender, and body size. Variability in the same individual is due to factors such as diurnal rhythms, seasonal cycles, and aging. Pre-analytical variability is due to errors in collecting and handling of specimens. These errors include sampling the wrong patients; using an incorrect container, preservative, or label; lysis of cells; and evaporation. Pre-analytical variability may also be due to patient intake of food or drugs, exercise, or emotional stress. Analytical variability is associated with the method used for analysis and may be due to materials, equipment, procedures, and personnel used. The major source of post-analytical variability is transcription error. This source of error can be greatly reduced by entering data into the computer directly (DeKeyser & Pugh, 1990).

When the scores obtained in a study are at the interval or ratio level, a commonly used method of analyzing the agreement between two different measurement strategies is the Bland-Altman chart (Bland & Altman, 1986, 2010). This chart is a scatter plot of the differences between observed scores on the y-axis and the combined mean of the two methods on the x-axis. The distribution of the difference scores is examined in context of the limits of agreement that are drawn as a horizontal line across the chart or scatter plot (see Chapter 23). The limits are set by the researchers and might include 1 or 2 standard deviations from the mean or might be the clinical standards of the maximum amount of error that is safe. The data points are examined for level of agreement (congruence) and for level of bias (systematic error). Outliers are readily visible from the chart, and each outlier case should be examined to identify the cause of such a large discrepancy. Clinical laboratory standards indicate that "more than three outliers per 100 observations suggest there are major flaws in the measurement system" (Ryan-Wenger, 2010, p. 381).

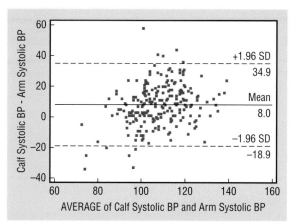

FIGURE 16-10 Bland-Altman plot of systolic BP. (Adapted from Schell, K., Briening, E., Lebet, R., Pruden, K., Rawheiser, S., & Jackson, B. [2011]. Comparison of arm and calf automatic noninvasive blood pressures in pediatric intensive care patients. *Journal of Pediatric Nursing, 26*[1], 9.)

Schell et al. (2011) conducted a study to compare upper arm and calf automatic noninvasive BPs in children in a pediatric intensive care unit (PICU). The researchers documented the accuracy of their BP monitoring equipment, the training of their data collectors, and the procedures for taking the BPs in their study. The errors in precision and accuracy are documented with Bland-Altman charts for systolic BP, diastolic BP, and mean arterial pressure readings. The chart of the systolic BP is included as an example in Figure 16-10. This study was conducted to determine an alternative method of obtaining BP when the injuries of the child prevent BP readings using the upper arm.

"BP Monitor
BP was obtained using a Spacelabs Ultraview SL monitoring system (Spacelabs Healthcare, Issaquah, WA), which consists of hemodynamic parameter modules that can be inserted into stationary bedside and portable monitor housings. All monitoring functions were controlled through the modules. During data collection, each set of arm and calf BP measurements was obtained simultaneously using two identical parameter modules: one inserted into the subject's stationary bedside housing and the other inserted into a portable monitor housing brought to the subject's bedside. Modules and housings are inspected and tested annually by Biomedical Support Services to ensure accurate functioning. The accuracy of these monitors for arm BPs meets or exceeds SP10-1992

Association for the Advancement of Medical Instrumentation standards (mean error = ±4.5 mm Hg, *SD* = ±7.3 mm Hg) for arm measurements (White et al., 1993). Spacelabs Healthcare did not report data regarding accuracy of calf BPs.

Training of Data Collectors
Data were collected by five pediatric intensive care nurses who attended a data training session that addressed location of arm and calf sites, measurement of limb circumference, and use of the RASS [Richmond Agitation Sedation Scale]. The nurses also attended a BP monitor in-service offered by the Spacelab representative when the monitors were adopted in the PICU in January 2006....

Procedure
Subjects were placed in a supine position with the head of bed elevated 30° as determined by a handheld protractor or the degree indicator incorporated into the bed frame. Subjects remained in this position for at least 5 minutes prior to data collection. Cuff sizes were selected based on limb circumferences measured to the nearest 0.5 cm. Spacelabs cuff sizes were as follows: neonate, 6–11 cm; infant, 8–11 cm; child, 12–19 cm; small adult, 17–26 cm; and adult, 24–32 cm. Per manufacturer's recommendations, if circumference overlapped two categories of cuff size, the larger cuff was selected. Using a paper tape measure, arm circumference was obtained at the point halfway between the elbow and the shoulder. Calf circumference was measured at the point midway between the ankle and the knee. The BP cuffs were applied to the arm and calf on the same side. Subjects' extremities were positioned at the side of their bodies, resting on the bed, for all measurements.... Systolic, diastolic, and mean BP values for the arm and calf as well as a simultaneous heart rate were documented. Data collectors notified the child's nurse or physician if an abnormal arm reading was obtained." (Schell et al., 2011, pp. 6–7)

"To promote best practice, clinicians should base treatment choices on individual patient data, not group data. Therefore, Bland-Altman analyses were used to determine agreement between arm and calf oscillometric BPs for individual subjects. Perfect agreement occurs when all data points lie on the line of equality of the x-axis. The bias (mean difference between arm and calf pressures) systolic BP was 8.0 mm Hg with the limits of agreement −18.9 and 34.9 mm Hg. Limits of agreement indicated that 95% of the sample falls between these values [see Figure 16-10]. The limits of agreement for diastolic BP were −22.7 and 25.0 mm Hg with a bias of 1.1 mm Hg." (Schell et al., 2011, p. 9)

Schell et al. (2011) provided evidence of the accuracy, precision, and error of the BP monitoring equipment used in their study. They also provided a detailed discussion of the procedures for data collection that followed a rigorous protocol to ensure that accurate and precise BP readings were obtained for children of all ages based on their measured arm and calf sizes. The data collectors were trained in BP monitoring by the Spacelab representative, which would increase their expertise in the use of the equipment. However, the study would have been strengthened by a discussion of the intrarater and interrater percentage of agreement for the data collectors. The credibility of the findings was enhanced by the use of the Bland-Altman plot to identify the error in precision and accuracy for systolic BPs, diastolic BPs, and mean arterial pressures. The researchers found that arm and calf BPs were not interchangeable for many of the children 1 to 8 years old. "Clinical BP differences were the greatest in children between ages 2 and less than 5 years. Calf BPs are not recommended for this population. If the calf is unavoidable due to medical reasons, trending of BP from this site should remain consistent during the child's stay" (Schell et al., 2011, p. 10).

SENSITIVITY, SPECIFICITY, AND LIKELIHOOD RATIOS

An important part of building evidence-based practice is the development, refinement, and use of quality diagnostic tests and measures in research and practice. Researchers want to use the most accurate and precise measure or test in their study to promote quality outcomes. If a quality diagnostic test does not exist, some nurses have participated in the development and refinement of new biophysical tests. Clinicians want to know what diagnostic test to order, such as a laboratory or imaging study, to help screen for and accurately determine the absence or presence of an illness (Sackett, Straus, Richardson, Rosenberg, & Haynes, 2000). When you order a diagnostic test, how can you be sure that the results are valid or accurate? This question is best answered by current, quality research to determine the sensitivity and specificity of the test.

Sensitivity and Specificity

The **accuracy of a screening test** or a test used to confirm a diagnosis is evaluated in terms of its ability to assess correctly the presence or absence of a disease or condition as compared with a gold standard. The **gold standard** is the most accurate means of currently diagnosing a particular disease and serves as a basis for comparison with newly developed diagnostic or screening tests (Campo , Shiyko, & Lichtman, 2010). If the test is positive, what is the probability that the disease is present? If the test is negative, what is the probability that the disease is not present? When you talk to the patient about the results of their tests, how sure are you that the patient does or does not have the disease? **Sensitivity** and **specificity** are the terms used to describe the accuracy of a screening or diagnostic test (Table 16-6). There are four possible outcomes of a screening test for a disease: (a) **true positive**, which accurately identifies the presence of a disease; (b) **false positive**, which indicates a disease is present when it is not; (c) **false negative**, which indicates that a disease is not present when it is; or (d) **true negative**, which indicates accurately that a disease is not present) (Campo et al., 2010; Grove & Cipher, 2017). The 2 × 2 contingency table shown in Table 16-6 should help you visualize sensitivity and specificity and these four outcomes (Craig & Smyth, 2012; Sackett et al., 2000).

Sensitivity and specificity can be calculated based on research findings and clinical practice outcomes to determine the most accurate diagnostic or screening tool to use in identifying the presence or absence of a disease for a population of patients. The

TABLE 16-6   Results of Sensitivity and Specificity of Screening Tests

Diagnostic Test Result	Disease Present	Disease Not Present or Absent	Total
Positive test	a (true positive)	b (false positive)	a + b
Negative test	c (false negative)	d (true negative)	c + d
Total	a + c	b + d	a + b + c + d

a = The number of people who have the disease and the test is positive (true positive).
b = The number of people who do not have the disease and the test is positive (false positive).
c = The number of people who have the disease and the test is negative (false negative).
d = The number of people who do not have the disease and the test is negative (true negative).
From Grove, S. K., & Cipher, D. (2017). *Statistics for nursing research: A workbook for evidence-based practice* (2nd ed.). St. Louis, MO: Saunders.

calculations for sensitivity and specificity are provided as follows:

Sensitivity calculation = proportion of patients with disease who have a positive test result

= a/(a + c)

= ability of the instrumer to correctly detect the presence of a disease

Specificity calculation = proportion of patients without disease who have a negative test result

= d/(b + d)

= ability of the instrument to correctly detect the absence of a disease

Sensitivity is the proportion of patients with the disease who have a positive test result or true positive rate. The ways the researcher or clinician might refer to the test sensitivity include the following:

- *Highly sensitive test* is very good at identifying the patient with a disease.
- If a test is highly sensitive, it has a low percentage of false negatives.
- *Low sensitivity test* is limited in identifying the patient with a disease.
- If a test has low sensitivity, it has a high percentage of false negatives.
- If a sensitive test has negative results, the patient is less likely to have the disease.
- Use the acronym *SnNout:* High sensitivity (*Sn*), test is negative (*N*), rules the disease out (*out*). (Campo et al., 2010; Grove & Cipher, 2017)

Specificity of a screening or diagnostic test is the proportion of patients without the disease who have a negative test result or true negative rate. The ways the researcher or clinician might refer to the test specificity include the following:

- Highly specific test is very good at identifying patients without a disease.
- If a test is very specific, it has a low percentage of false positives.
- Low specificity test is limited in identifying patients without a disease.
- If a test has low specificity, it has a high percentage of false positives.

- If a specific test has positive results, the patient is more likely to have the disease.
- Use the acronym *SpPin:* High specificity (*Sp*), test is positive (*P*), rules the disease in (*in*) (Grove & Cipher, 2017).

Sarikaya, Aktas, Ay, Cetin, and Celikmen (2010) conducted a study to determine the sensitivity and specificity of rapid antigen diagnostic testing (RADT) for diagnosing pharyngitis in patients in the emergency department. Acute pharyngitis is primarily a viral infection, but in 10% of the cases it is caused by bacteria. Most cases of bacterial pharyngitis are caused by group A beta-hemolytic streptococci (GABHS). One laboratory method for diagnosing GABHS is RADT, which has become more popular than a throat culture because it can be processed rapidly during an emergency department and primary care visit.

"We conducted a study to define the sensitivity and specificity of RADT, using throat culture results as the gold standard, in 100 emergency department patients who presented with symptoms consistent with streptococcal pharyngitis. We found that RADT had a sensitivity of 68.2% (15 of 22), a specificity of 89.7% (70 of 78), a positive predictive value of 65.2% (15 of 23), and a negative predictive value of 90.9% (70 of 77). We conclude that RADT is useful in the emergency department when the clinical suspicion is GABHS, but results should be confirmed with a throat culture in patients whose RADT results are negative." (Sarikaya et al., 2010, p. 180)

The results of the study by Sarikaya et al. (2010) were put into Table 16-7 so that you might see how the sensitivity and specificity were calculated in this study.

Sensitivity calculation = a/(a + c)

Sensitivity = proportion of patients with GABHS pharyngitis who had a positive RADT

= 15/(15 + 7) = 15/22 = 68.18% = 68.2%

Specificity calculation = d/(b + d)

Specificity = proportion of patients without GABHS pharyngitis who had a negative RADT

= 70/(8 + 70) = 70/78 = 89.74% = 89.7%

The sensitivity of 68.2% indicates the percentage of patients with a positive RADT who had GABHS pharyngitis (true positive rate). The specificity of 89.7% indicates the percentage of patients with a negative

TABLE 16-7 Results of Sensitivity and Specificity of Rapid Antigen Diagnostic Testing (RADT)

RADT Result	GABHS Disease Present	GABHS Disease Absent	Total
Positive test	a (true positive) = 15	b (false positive) = 8	a + b = 15 + 8 = 23
Negative test	c (false negative) = 7	d (true negative) = 70	c + d = 7 + 70 = 77
Total	a + c = 15 + 7 = 22	b + d = 8 + 70 = 78	a + b + c + d = 100

GABHS, Group A beta-hemolytic streptococci.
a = The number of people who have GABHS pharyngitis disease and the test is positive (true positive).
b = The number of people who do not have GABHS pharyngitis disease and the test is positive (false positive).
c = The number of people who have GABHS pharyngitis disease and the test is negative (false negative).
d = The number of people who do not have GABHS pharyngitis disease and the test is negative (true negative).

RADT who did not have GABHS pharyngitis (true negative rate). In developing a diagnostic or screening test, researchers need to achieve the highest sensitivity and specificity possible. In selecting screening tests to diagnose illnesses, clinicians need to determine the most sensitive and specific screening test but also examine cost and ease of access to these tests in making their final decision (Craig & Smyth, 2012; Grove & Cipher, 2017).

Likelihood Ratios

Likelihood ratios (LRs) are additional calculations that can help researchers to determine the accuracy of diagnostic or screening tests, which are based on the sensitivity and specificity results. LRs are calculated to determine the likelihood that a positive test result is a true positive and a negative test result is a true negative. The ratio of the true positive results to false positive results is known as the **positive LR** (Campo et al., 2010). The positive LR is calculated as follows using the data from the study by Sarikaya et al. (2010):

Positive LR = sensitivity ÷ (100% − specificity)

$$\text{Positive LR for GABHS pharyngitis}$$
$$= 68.2\% \div (100\% - 89.7\%)$$
$$= 68.2\% \div 10.3\% = 6.62$$

The **negative LR** is the ratio of true negative results to false negative results, and it is calculated as follows:

Negative LR = (100% − sensitivity) ÷ specificity

$$\text{Negative LR for GABHS pharyngitis}$$
$$= (100\% - 68.2\%) \div 89.7\%$$
$$= 31.8\% \div 89.7\% = 0.35$$

The very high positive LRs (or LRs that are > 10) rule in the disease or indicate that the patient has the disease. The very low negative LRs (or LRs that are < 0.1) virtually rule out the chance that the patient has the disease (Campo et al., 2010; Craig & Smyth, 2012; Melnyk & Fineout-Overholt, 2015). Understanding sensitivity, specificity, and LRs increases your ability to read clinical studies and to determine the most accurate diagnostic test to use in research and clinical practice.

▌KEY POINTS

- Measurement is the process of assigning numbers to objects, events, or situations in accord with some rule.
- Instrumentation is the application of specific rules to develop a measurement device or instrument.
- Measurement theory and the rules within this theory have been developed to direct the measurement of abstract and concrete concepts.
- There are two types of measurement: direct and indirect.
- Healthcare technology has made researchers familiar with direct measures of concrete elements, such as height, weight, heart rate, temperature, and blood pressure.
- Indirect measurement is used with abstract concepts, when the concepts are not measured directly, but when the indicators or attributes of the concepts are used to represent the abstractions. Common abstract concepts measured in nursing include anxiety, stress, coping, quality of life, and pain.
- Measurement error is the difference between what exists in reality and what is measured by a research instrument.
- The levels of measurement, from lower to higher, are nominal, ordinal, interval, and ratio.
- Reliability refers to how consistently the measurement technique measures the concept of interest and includes stability reliability, equivalence reliability, and internal consistency.

- Stability reliability is concerned with the consistency of repeated measures of the same concept or attribute with an instrument or scale over time.
- Equivalence reliability includes interrater and alternate forms reliability.
- Internal consistency is used primarily with multi-item scales in which each item on the scale is correlated with all other items to determine the consistency of the scale in measuring a concept.
- The validity of an instrument is determined by the extent to which the instrument actually reflects the abstract construct being examined. Content, construct, and criterion-related validity are covered in this text.
- Content validity examines the extent to which the measurement method includes all major elements relevant to the construct being measured.
- Construct validity focuses on determining whether the instrument actually measures the theoretical construct that it purports to measure, which involves examining the fit between the conceptual and operational definitions of a variable.
- Construct validity is developed using a variety of techniques such as: validity from factor analysis, convergent validity, divergent validity, validity from contrasting groups, validity from discriminant analysis, and successive verification of validity.
- Criterion-related validity is strengthened when a study participant's score on an instrument can be used to infer his or her performance on another variable or criterion. The two types of criterion-related validity are predictive validity and concurrent validity.
- Evaluation of physiological measures requires a different perspective from that of psychosocial measures and requires evaluation for accuracy, precision, and error.
- Accuracy involves determining the closeness of the agreement between the measured value and the true value of the quantity being measured.
- Precision is the degree of consistency or reproducibility of measurements made with physiological instruments or devices.
- Sources of error in physiological measures can be grouped into the following five categories: (1) environment, (2) user, (3) study participant, (4) machine, and (5) interpretation.
- The accuracy of screening or diagnostic tests is determined by calculating the sensitivity, specificity, and LRs for the test.
- Sensitivity is the proportion of patients with the disease who have a positive test result or true positive rate.

- Specificity is the proportion of patients without the disease who have a negative test result or true negative rate.
- LRs are additional calculations that can help researchers to determine the accuracy of diagnostic or screening tests, which are based on the sensitivity and specificity results. The ratio of the true positive results to false positive results is known as the positive LR. The negative LR is the ratio of true negative results to false negative results.

REFERENCES

American Nurses Credentialing Center (ANCC). (2016). *Magnet program overview*. Retrieved March 14, 2016 from www.nursecredentialing.org/Magnet/ProgramOverview.

American Psychological Association's (APA) Committee to Develop Standards. (1999). *Standards for educational and psychological testing*. Washington, DC: American Psychological Association.

Armstrong, G. D. (1981). Parametric statistics and ordinal data: A pervasive misconception. *Nursing Research*, 30(1), 60–62.

Bannigan, K., & Watson, R. (2009). Reliability and validity in a nutshell. *Journal of Clinical Nursing*, 18(23), 3237–3243.

Bartlett, J. W., & Frost, C. (2008). Reliability, repeatability and reproducibility: Analysis of measurement errors in continuous variables. *Ultrasound Obstetric Gynecology*, 31(4), 466–475.

Berk, R. A. (1990). Importance of expert judgment in content-related validity evidence. *Western Journal of Nursing Research*, 12(5), 659–671.

Bialocerkowski, A., Klupp, N., & Bragge, P. (2010). Research methodology series: How to read and critically appraise a reliability article. *International Journal of Therapy & Rehabilitation*, 17(3), 114–120.

Bland, J. M., & Altman, D. G. (1986). Statistical methods for assessing agreement between two methods of clinical measurement. *Lancet*, 1(8476), 307–310.

Bland, J. M., & Altman, D. M. (2010). Statistical methods for assessing agreement between two methods of clinical measurement. *International Journal of Nursing Studies*, 47(8), 931–936.

Brinberg, D., & McGrath, J. E. (1985). *Validity and the research process*. Beverly Hills, CA: Sage.

Bureau International des Poids et Measures (BIPM). (2015). *About the BIPM*. Retrieved June 15, 2015 from http://www.bipm.org/en/about-us/.

Buysse, D. J., Reynolds, C. F., Monk, T. H., Berman, S. R., & Kupfer, D. J. (1989). The Pittsburgh Sleep Quality Index: A new instrument for psychiatric practice and research. *Psychiatry Research*, 28(2), 193–213.

Campbell, D. T., & Fiske, D. W. (1959). Convergent and discriminant validation by the multitrait-multimethod matrix. *Psychological Bulletin*, 56(2), 81–105.

Campo, M., Shiyko, M. P., & Lichtman, S. W. (2010). Sensitivity and specificity: A review of related statistics and controversies in the context of physical therapist education. *Journal of Physical Therapy Education*, 24(3), 69–78.

Cappelleri, J. C., Lundy, J. J., & Hays, R. D. (2014). Overview of classical test theory and item response theory for the quantitative assessment of items in developing patient-reported outcomes measures. *Clinical Therapeutics, 36*(5), 648–662.

Clinical and Laboratory Standards Institute (CLSI). (2015). *About CLSI: Committed to continually advancing laboratory practice.* Retrieved July 15, 2015 from http://clsi.org/about-clsi/.

Cohen, J. A. (1960). A coefficient of agreement for nominal scales. *Education & Psychological Measurement, 20*(1), 37–46.

Craig, J. V., & Smyth, R. L. (2012). *The evidence-base practice manual for nurses* (3rd ed.). Edinburgh, Scotland: Churchill Livingstone.

Creswell, J. W. (2014). *Research design: Qualitative, quantitative, and mixed methods approaches* (4th ed.). Thousand Oaks, CA: Sage.

Davis, L. L. (1992). Instrument review: Getting the most from a panel of experts. *Applied Nursing Research, 5*(4), 194–197.

DeKeyser, F. G., & Pugh, L. C. (1990). Assessment of the reliability and validity of biochemical measures. *Nursing Research, 39*(5), 314–317.

DeVon, H. A., Block, M. E., Moyle-Wright, P., Ernst, D. M., Hayden, S. J., Lazzara, D. J., et al. (2007). A psychometric toolbox for testing validity and reliability. *Journal of Nursing Scholarship, 39*(2), 155–164.

French, S. E., Lenton, R., Walters, V., & Eyles, J. (2000). An empirical evaluation of an expanded nursing stress scale. *Journal of Nursing Measurement, 8*(2), 161–178.

Gift, A. G., & Soeken, K. L. (1988). Assessment of physiologic instruments. *Heart and Lung: The Journal of Critical Care, 17*(2), 128–133.

Goodwin, L. D. (2002). Changing conceptions of measurement validity: An update on the new standards. *Journal of Nursing Education, 41*(3), 100–106.

Grove, S. K., & Cipher, D. (2017). *Statistics for nursing research: A workbook for evidence-based practice* (2nd ed.). St. Louis, MO: Saunders.

International Organization for Standardization (ISO). (2015a). *About IOS.* Retrieved July 15, 2015 from http://www.iso.org/iso/home/about.htm.

International Organization for Standardization (ISO). (2015b). *Standards: Benefits of International Standards.* Retrieved July 15, 2015 from http://www.iso.org/iso/home/standards/benefitsofstandards.htm.

Jansson, B. S. (2011). *Improving healthcare through advocacy: A guide for the health and helping professions.* Hoboken, NJ: John Wiley & Sons.

Jansson, B. S., Nyamathi, A., Duan, L., Kaplan, C., Heidemann, G., & Ananias, D. (2015). Validation of the Patient Advocacy Engagement Scale for health professionals. *Research in Nursing & Health, 38*(2), 162–172.

Kaplan, A. (1963). *The conduct of inquiry: Methodology for behavioral science.* New York, NY: Harper & Row.

Kerlinger, F. N., & Lee, H. B. (2000). *Foundations of behavioral research* (4th ed.). Fort Worth, TX: Harcourt College Publishers.

Knapp, T. R. (1990). Treating ordinal scales as interval scales: An attempt to resolve the controversy. *Nursing Research, 39*(2), 121–123.

Knapp, T. R., & Brown, J. K. (2014). Ten statistics commandments that almost never should be broken. *Research in Nursing & Health, 37*(4), 347–351.

Lawshe, C. H. (1975). A quantitative approach to content validity. *Personnel Psychology, 28*(4), 563–575.

Lynn, M. R. (1986). Determination and quantification of content validity. *Nursing Research, 35*(6), 382–385.

Melnyk, B. M., & Fineout-Overholt, E. (2015). *Evidence-based practice in nursing & healthcare: A guide to best practice* (3rd ed.). Philadelphia, PA: Lippincott Williams & Wilkins.

Nunnally, J. C., & Bernstein, I. H. (1994). *Psychometric theory* (3rd ed.). New York, NY: McGraw-Hill.

Plichta, S. B., & Kelvin, E. (2013). *Munro's statistical methods for health care research* (6th ed.). Philadelphia, PA: Lippincott Williams & Wilkins.

Polit, D. F., Beck, C. T., & Owen, S. V. (2007). Is the CVI an acceptable indicator of content validity? Appraisal and recommendations. *Research in Nursing & Health, 30*(4), 459–467.

Radloff, L. S. (1977). The CES-D scale: A self-report depression scale for research in the general population. *Applied Psychological Measures, 1*(3), 385–394.

Rosenberg, M. (1979). *Conceiving self.* New York, NY: Basic Books.

Russell, D., Peplau, L. A., & Cutrona, C. E. (1980). The revised UCLA Loneliness Scale: Concurrent and discriminant validity evidence. *Journal of Personality and Social Psychology, 39*(3), 472–480.

Ryan-Wenger, N. A. (2010). Evaluation of measurement precision, accuracy, and error in biophysical data for clinical research and practice. In C. F. Waltz, O. L. Strickland, & E. R. Lenz (Eds.), *Measurement in nursing and health research* (4th ed., pp. 371–383). New York, NY: Springer.

Sackett, D. L., Straus, S. E., Richardson, W. S., Rosenberg, W., & Haynes, R. B. (2000). *Evidence-based medicine: How to practice and teach EBM* (2nd ed.). Edinburgh: Churchill Livingstone.

Sarikaya, S., Aktas, C., Ay, D., Cetin, A., & Celikmen, F. (2010). Sensitivity and specificity of rapid antigen detection testing for diagnosing pharyngitis in emergency department. *Ear Nose & Throat Journal, 89*(4), 180–182.

Schell, K., Briening, E., Lebet, R., Pruden, K., Rawheiser, S., & Jackson, B. (2011). Comparison of arm and calf automatic noninvasive blood pressures in pediatric intensive care patients. *Journal of Pediatric Nursing, 26*(1), 3–12.

Smith, M. J., Theeke, L., Culp, S., Clark, K., & Pinto, S. (2014). Psychosocial variables and self-rated health in young adult obese women. *Applied Nursing Research, 27*(1), 67–71.

Spielberger, C. D., Gorsuch, R. L., & Lushene, P. R. (1970). *Manual for the State-Trait Anxiety Inventory (Form Y).* Palo Alto, CA: Consulting Psychologists Press.

Stevens, S. S. (1946). On the theory of scales of measurement. *Science, 103*, 677–680.

Stommel, M., Wang, S., Given, C. W., & Given, B. (1992). Confirmatory factor analysis (CFA) as a method to assess measurement equivalence. *Research in Nursing & Health, 15*(5), 399–405.

Streiner, D. L., Norman, G. R., & Cairney, J. (2015). *Health measurement scales: A practical guide to their development and use* (5th ed.). Oxford, UK: University Press.

Thomas, S. (1992). Face validity. *Western Journal of Nursing Research*, *14*(1), 109–112.

Topf, M. (1988). Interrater reliability decline under covert assessment. *Nursing Research*, *37*(1), 47–49.

Waltz, C. F., Strickland, O. L., & Lenz, E. R. (2010). *Measurement in nursing and health research* (4th ed.). New York, NY: Springer.

Weber, M. A., Schiffrin, E. L., White, W. B., Mann, S., Lindholm, L. H., Kenerson, J. G., et al. (2014). Clinical practice guidelines for the management of hypertension in the community: A statement by the American Society of Hypertension and the International Society of Hypertension. *Journal of Clinical Hypertension*, *16*(1), 14–26.

White, W. B., Berson, A. S., Robbins, C., Jamieson, M. J., Prisant, L. M., Roccella, E., et al. (1993). National standard for measurement of resting and ambulatory blood pressures with automated sphygmomanometers. *Hypertension*, *21*(4), 504–509.

Wong-Baker FACES Foundation. (2015). *Wong-Baker FACES® Pain Rating Scale*. Retrieved May 22, 2015 with permission from http://www.wongbakerfaces.org/.

Measurement Methods Used in Developing Evidence-Based Practice

Susan K. Grove

ⓔ http://evolve.elsevier.com/Gray/practice/

Nursing research examines a wide variety of phenomena, requiring an extensive array of measurement methods. However, nurse researchers have sometimes found limited instruments available to measure phenomena central to the studies essential for generating evidence-based practice (Melnyk & Fineout-Overholt, 2015; Polit & Yang, 2016). Thus, for the last 30 years, nurse researchers have made it a priority to develop valid and reliable instruments to measure phenomena of concern to nursing. As a result, the number and quality of measurement methods have greatly increased (Waltz, Strickland, & Lenz, 2010).

Knowledge of measurement methods is important to all aspects of nursing. For critical appraisal of a study, nurses must grasp measurement theory and understand the state of the science for instrument development, relative to a phenomenon of interest. For example, when evaluating someone else's research, you might want to know whether the researcher was using an older tool that has been surpassed by more precise and accurate physiological measures. It might help you to know that measuring a particular phenomenon has been a problem with which nurse researchers have struggled for many years. Your understanding of the successes and struggles in measuring nursing phenomena may stimulate your creative thinking and lead you to contribute your own research to developing measurement approaches.

This chapter describes common measurement approaches used in nursing research, including physiological measures, observations, interviews, questionnaires, and scales. Other measurement methods discussed include Q-sort methodology, the Delphi technique, diaries, and use of existing databases. The chapter

also describes the process for locating existing instruments, determining their reliability and validity, and assessing their readability. Directions are provided for describing an instrument in a research report. The chapter concludes with a brief description of the process of scale construction and issues related to translating an instrument into another language.

PHYSIOLOGICAL MEASUREMENT

Much of nursing practice is oriented toward physiological dimensions of health. Therefore, many of our questions require us to be able to measure these dimensions. Of particular importance are studies linking physiological, psychological, and social variables. The need for physiological research reached national attention in 1993 when the National Institute of Nursing Research (NINR) recommended an increase in physiologically based nursing studies because 85% of NINR-funded studies involved nonphysiological variables (Cowan, Heinrich, Lucas, Sigmon, & Hinshaw, 1993). Over the last 20 years, a group of nurse researchers have focused their careers on the conduct of biological and pathological studies and expanded their use and development of precise and accurate physiological measures (Rudy & Gray, 2005). The current NINR (2011) Strategic Plan emphasizes the conduct of biological research to provide a foundation for understanding and managing diseases and to test preventative care and self-management strategies. NINR (2016) is expanding the training of nurse scientists and promoting the conduct of genomic research with the implementation of a yearly Summer Genetics Institute (SGI). An increased number of biological researchers and the expanded funding for biological research have increased both quality and quantity of physiological measures used in nursing studies.

Physiological measures include two categories, biophysical and biochemical. Biophysical measures might include the use of the stethoscope and sphygmomanometer to measure blood pressure, and a biochemical measure might include the laboratory value for total cholesterol. Biophysical measures can be acquired in a variety of ways from instruments within the body (in vivo), such as a reading from an arterial line, or from application of an instrument on the outside of a subject (in vitro), such as a blood pressure cuff (Stone & Frazier, 2010).

Physiological variables can be measured either directly or indirectly. **Direct measures** are measurements that count and quantify the variable itself. They are objective, and consequently not subjective to judgment issues. They are also specific to that particular variable. **Indirect measures** are measurements that are obtained to represent count or quantity of a variable by measuring one or more characteristics or properties that are related to it. They are often more subjective than are direct measures, and may be affected by judgment or experience in administration. For example, patients might be asked to report any irregular heartbeats during waking hours over a 24-hour period (an indirect measurement of heart rhythm), or each patient's heart could be monitored with a Holter monitor over the same 24-hour time frame (direct measure of heart rhythm). Whenever possible, researchers usually select direct measures of study variables because of the accuracy and precision of these measurement methods. However, if a direct measurement method does not exist, an indirect measure could be used in the initial investigation of a physiological variable. Sometimes researchers use both direct and indirect measurement methods to expand the understanding of a physiological variable. The following sections describe how to obtain physiological measures by self-report, observation, laboratory tests, and electronic monitoring. The measurement of physiological variables across time is also addressed. This section concludes with a discussion of how to select physiological measures for a particular study.

Obtaining Physiological Measures by Self-Report

Self-report has been used effectively in research to obtain physiological information and may be particularly useful when subjects are not in closely monitored settings such as hospitals, clinics, or research facilities. Physiological phenomena that have been or could be measured by self-report include hours of sleep, patterns of daily activities, eating patterns, stool frequency and consistency, patterns of joint stiffness, variations in degree of mobility, and exercise patterns. For some variables, self-report may be the only means of obtaining the information. Such may be the case when study participants experience a physiological phenomenon that cannot be observed or measured by others. Nonobservable physiological phenomena include pain, nausea, dizziness, indigestion, hot flashes, tinnitus, fatigue, and dyspnea (DeVon et al., 2007; Waltz et al., 2010).

Moon, Phelan, Lauver, and Bratzke (2015) examined the relationship between sleep quality and cognitive function in individuals with heart failure (HF). Sleep quality was measured using a self-report instrument that is described in the following study excerpt.

> **"Sleep Quality**
>
> Sleep quality was measured using the PSQI [Pittsburg Sleep Quality Index]. The PSQI is a self-report measure of global sleep quality. The instrument consists of 19 items that are grouped into seven subscales reflecting different dimensions of sleep, such as sleep quality, sleep latency, sleep duration, sleep efficiency, sleep disturbances, use of sleep medication, and daytime dysfunction. Each subscale was weighted equally on a 0 to 3 scale, yielding a global score from 0 to 21. Poor sleep quality is defined as a global PSQI score $\geq$ 5. The measure has adequate internal consistency among adults (Cronbach's alpha = 0.83). We reported the raw scores for sleep duration, sleep latency, sleep efficiency, and use of sleep medications subscales because they are meaningful descriptions of different dimensions of sleep quality." (Moon et al., 2015, p. 213)

Moon and colleagues (2015) identified that the Pittsburgh Sleep Quality Index (PSQI) included 19 items and seven subscales reflecting the dimensions of sleep, which supports the content and construct validity of the scale (see Chapter 16). The PSQI had strong reliability in this study but the reliabilities for the subscales were not discussed. Researchers should discuss the reliability and validity of all scales and subscales used in a study, based on previous research. Moon et al. (2015) found that sleep quality as measured by the PSQI was not associated with cognitive decline in patients with HF.

Using self-report measures may enable nurses to study research questions that were not previously considered, which could be an important means to build knowledge in areas not yet explored. The insight gained could alter the way nurses manage patient situations that are now considered problematic and improve patient outcomes (Doran, 2011). However, self-report is a subjective way to measure physiological variables, and studies are strengthened by having both subjective and objective measurements of physiological variables.

Obtaining Physiological Measures by Observation

Researchers sometimes obtain data about physiological parameters by using observational data collection measures. These measures provide criteria for quantifying various levels or states of physiological functioning. In addition to collecting clinical data, this method provides a means to gather data from the observations of caregivers. This source of data has been particularly useful in studies involving critically ill patients in intensive care units (ICUs) and patients with Alzheimer's disease, advanced cancer, and severe mental illness. Observation is also an effective way to gather data on frail elderly adults, infants, and young children. Studies involving home health agencies and hospices often use observation tools to record physiological dimensions of patient status. These data sometimes are stored electronically and are available to researchers for large database analysis. Measuring physiological variables using observation requires a quality tool for data collection and consistent use of this tool by data collectors. If the observations in a study are being conducted using multiple data collectors, it is essential that the consistency or interrater reliability of the data collectors be determined at the start of the study and periodically during data collection (see Chapter 16; Bialocerkowski, Klupp, & Bragge, 2010; Waltz et al., 2010).

Klein, Dumpe, Katz, and Bena (2010) developed a Nonverbal Pain Assessment Tool (NPAT) to measure the pain experience by nonverbal adult patients in the ICU. Testing of the tool occurred in three phases that focused on the internal reliability, content validity, and criterion validity of the tool and the interrater reliability of the data collectors. The following excerpt describes development of the NPAT and its demonstrated reliability and validity.

"Content validity examines the extent of the tool's ability to measure the construct under consideration (in this study, pain). Construction of the scale began with an in-depth review of the literature to determine commonly accepted signs and behaviors of pain. Three nurse experts, including 2 clinical nurse specialists and a nurse from the Pain Management Service, reviewed the tool and selected behaviors.

Criterion-related validity compares the new tool to a 'gold standard.'... We hypothesized that a significant correlation would be found between the NPAT score and the patient's self-report of pain, the 'gold standard' for pain assessment." (Klein et al., 2010, p. 523)

"The internal reliability for the entire scale was 0.82 (Cronbach's alpha) ... Subscale internal reliability scores comprised: emotion, 0.77; movement, 0.78; verbal, 0.79; facial, 0.77; and position, 0.78. ... To determine the interrater reliability of the revised NPAT, a convenience sampling included all patients more than 16 years old and admitted to any of the 4 ICUs during the data collection period. The same teams of nurses were used. Data were collected for 50 patients, although data from only 39 patients were useable. The concordance correlation coefficient was 0.72 (95% confidence interval), demonstrating strong interrater reliability. ... The criterion validity of the revised NPAT was again tested. ... The concordance correlation coefficient was 0.66 (95% confidence interval), indicating moderate to strong validity." (Klein et al., 2010, pp. 525–526)

Klein et al. (2010) found the NPAT had moderately strong validity and strong internal reliability for both the total scale (Cronbach's alpha = 0.82) and the subscales (Cronbach's alpha ranging from 0.77 to 0.79). Because the NPAT is a new tool, these researchers described the content and criterion validity of the tool and recognized the need for additional research to determine the reliability and validity of the tool with different samples. The researchers concluded that the NPAT was "easy to use and provided a standard approach to assessing pain in the nonverbal adult patient" (Klein et al., 2010, p. 521). The final copy of this tool is presented later in this chapter.

Obtaining Physiological Measures From Laboratory Tests

Laboratory tests are usually very precise and accurate and provide direct measures of many physiological variables. Biochemical measures, such as total cholesterol, triglycerides, hemoglobin, and hematocrit, must be obtained through invasive procedures. Sometimes these invasive procedures are part of routine patient care, and researchers, with institutional review board (IRB) approval, can obtain the results from the patient's record. Although nurses perform some biochemical measures in the nursing unit, these measures often require laboratory analysis. When invasive procedures are not part of routine care but are instead performed specifically for a study, great care must be taken to protect the subjects and to follow guidelines for informed consent and IRB approval (see Chapter 9). Neither the patients nor their insurers can be billed for invasive procedures that are not part of routine care. Thus, to obtain data for the procedures performed strictly for research, investigators need to seek external funding or obtain support from the institution in which the patient is receiving care.

Researchers need to ensure the accuracy and precision of laboratory measures and the methods of collecting specimens for their studies. The laboratory performing the analyses must be certified and in compliance with national standards developed by the Clinical and Laboratory Standards Institute (CLSI, 2015). Data collectors need to be trained to ensure that intrarater reliability and interrater reliability are maintained during the data collection process (see Chapter 16; Bialocerkowski et al., 2010). Ancheta et al. (2015) examined the cardiovascular disease (CVD) risk factors in Asian American women to determine whether a disparity exists as a function of ethnicity. This study was conducted in Florida and included 147 participants (Cambodians, Chinese, Filipinos, and Vietnamese). Various measures were obtained to examine cardiovascular health (blood pressure, weight, height, abdominal circumference, and cholesterol), but the following study excerpt is focused on laboratory tests for measuring cholesterol levels.

"Participants were asked to fast for 12 hours prior to the study. Blood was obtained from a finger stick and analyzed by the Cardio Check P.A. Lipid Analyzer for total cholesterol, low-density lipoprotein (LDL), high-density lipoprotein (HDL), and triglycerides. Participants were immediately notified of all body measurements and laboratory results. Instruments that were used to determine blood pressure, weight, height, and cholesterol levels were calibrated and the use of quality control measures was performed prior to each use. Trained and licensed volunteer registered nurses collected the demographics and physiological measurements with the use of a local translator for those that did not understand English. Every 10th participant and random selection of blood sample was tested twice in order to ensure reliability." (Ancheta et al., 2015, p. 100)

Ancheta et al. (2015) provided a detailed description of the physiological measures obtained from laboratory testing. To promote precision and accuracy in the cholesterol values, the participants were instructed to fast and trained nurses drew the blood. The blood samples were analyzed in a certified laboratory (Cardio Check

P.A.). Laboratory equipment was calibrated and quality control measures were implemented to ensure accuracy in the lipid values obtained. The random retesting of selected blood samples was used to document the precision and accuracy of the results. The blood was drawn in a physician's office and transferred to the laboratory for analysis. The study report would have been strengthened by a discussion of the consistency achieved by the nurses collecting the blood, the storage method for the blood specimens prior to transfer to the lab, and the transfer process for the specimens. Ancheta et al. (2015, p. 99) concluded that the "modifiable CVD risk factor profiles significantly differed as a function of ethnicity supporting the premise that Asian-American women cannot be categorized as one group and the traditional 'one size fits all' prevention or treatment of CVD risk factors should be reconsidered."

Obtaining Physiological Measures Through Electronic Monitoring

The availability of electronic monitoring equipment has greatly increased the possibilities for both the number and type of physiological measurements useful in nursing studies, particularly in critical care environments. Understanding the processes of electronic monitoring can make procedures less formidable to individuals critically appraising published studies and individuals considering using electronic monitoring methods for measurement.

To use electronic monitoring, usually sensors are placed on or within study participants. The sensors measure changes in body functions such as electrical energy. Figure 17-1 shows the process of electronic measurement. Many sensors need an external stimulus to trigger the measurement process. Transducers convert an electrical signal to numerical data. Electrical signals often include interference signals as well as the desired signal, so you may choose to use an amplifier to decrease interference and amplify the desired signal. The electrical signal is digitized (converted to numerical digits or values) and stored in a computer. In addition, it is immediately displayed on a monitor. The display equipment may be visual or auditory or both. One type of display equipment is an oscilloscope that displays the data as a waveform; it may provide information such as time, phase, voltage, or frequency of the target event or behavior. The final phase is the recording, data processing, and transmission that might be done through computer, camera, graphic recorder, or digital audio recorder (Stone & Frazier, 2010). A graphic recorder provides a printed version of the data. Some electronic equipment simultaneously records multiple physiological measures

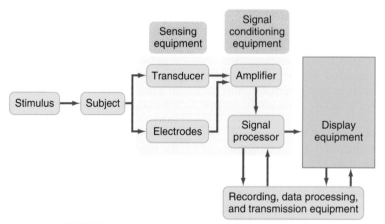

FIGURE 17-1 Process of electronic measurement.

that are displayed on a monitor. The equipment is often linked to a computer or might be wireless, which allows the researcher to store, review, and retrieve the data for analysis. Computers often contain complex software for detailed analysis of data and provide a printed report of the analysis results (Stone & Frazier, 2010).

The advantages of using electronic monitoring equipment are the collection of accurate and precise data, recording of data accurately within a computerized system, potential for collection of large amounts of data frequently over time, and transmission of data electronically for analysis. One disadvantage of using certain sensors to measure physiological variables is that the presence of a transducer within the body can alter the actual physiological value. For example, the presence of a flow transducer in a blood vessel can partially block the vessel and alter blood flow, resulting in an inaccurate reflection of the flow (Ryan-Wenger, 2010).

Ng, Wong, Lim, and Goh (2010) compared the Cadi ThermoSENSOR wireless skin-contact thermometer readings with ear and axillary temperatures in children on a general pediatric medical unit in a Singapore hospital. The ThermoSENSOR thermometer (Figure 17-2) provides a continuous measurement of body temperature and transmits the readings wirelessly to a central server. The measurement with the Thermo-SENSOR thermometer is described in the following excerpt.

"Developed by Cadi Scientific in Singapore as part of an integrated wireless system for temperature monitoring and location tracking, this system uses a reusable skin-contact thermometer or sensor called the *ThermoSEN-SOR*. This thermometer takes the form of a small disc

that can be easily adhered to the patient's skin, and each disc is assigned a unique radio frequency identification (RFID) number [see Figure 17-2]. The thermometer measures body temperature continuously and transmits a temperature reading and the RFID number approximately every 30 seconds to a computer or server through one or more signal receivers (nodes) installed in the vicinity of the patient [Figure 17-3]." (Ng et al., 2010, pp. 176–177)

"Before the study, a ThermoSENSOR wireless temperature monitoring system was installed in the ward. A wireless signal receiver (node) was installed in the ceiling of each of the five-bedded rooms.... These receivers were connected to the hospital's local area network (LAN) ... Web-based application software designed for use with the wireless system and installed on the computer was used to configure the computer to receive, store, and display the temperature and RFID data. A total of 32 sensors were used for the study.

The ThermoSENSOR uses a thermistor as the sensing element. When in use, the sensor is attached to the patient using a two-layer dressing system that prevents the sensor from coming in direct contact with the skin [see Figure 17-2]... The manufacturer provided the following specifications for the sensor: operating ambient temperature range, 10°C to 50°C; thermistor accuracy, ± 0.2°C for temperature range of 32.0°C to 42.0°C; data transmission rate, every 30 seconds on average; radio frequency, 868.4 MHz; typical transmission range, 10 m (unblocked); power source, internal 3-V lithium coin-cell battery; battery life, 12 months (continuous operation); dimensions, diameter of 36 mm, height of 11.6 mm; weight, 10 g without battery; applicable radio equipment standards, ETSI 300 220, ETSI EN 301 489." (Ng et al., 2010, pp. 177–178)

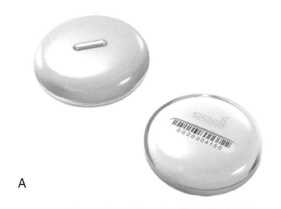

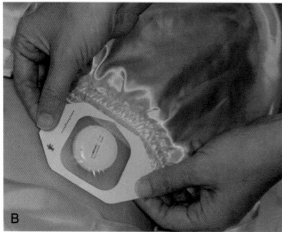

FIGURE 17-2 A, OR wireless thermometer. The disc has an elliptical cross section, and the sensing element consists of a metal strip located at the center of the skin-contact side. **B,** ThermoSENSOR. The device has been placed over the first piece of hypoallergenic adhesive film dressing on the lower abdomen and is about to be secured to the lower abdomen by a second piece of the same dressing. (From Ng, K., Wong, S., Lim, S., & Goh, Z. [2010]. Evaluation of the Cadi ThermoSENSOR wireless skin-contact thermometer against ear and axillary temperatures in children. *Journal of Pediatric Nursing, 25*[3], 177.)

Ng et al. (2010) provided detailed descriptions and pictures of both the ThermoSENSOR thermometer and the wireless setup by which signals were captured and transmitted. The thermometer was consistently applied to the abdomen of each child. The manufacturer specifications of the thermometer documented that it was an accurate device to measure temperature. The wireless system was described in detail with documentation of its precision and accuracy in obtaining and

transferring the children's temperatures to a computer for recording, display, and analysis of the data. The findings of the study indicated that ThermoSENSOR wireless skin-contact thermometer readings were comparable to both ear and axillary temperature readings and would be an accurate way to measure temperature in research and clinical practice.

Genetic Advancements in Measuring Nucleic Acids

The Human Genome Project has greatly expanded the understanding of deoxyribonucleic acid (DNA) that contains the code for controlling human development. The U.S. Human Genome Project was begun in 1990 by the Department of Energy and the National Institutes of Health and was completed in 2003. The genome is the entire DNA sequence in an organism, which includes the genes. The genes carry information for making all the proteins required by the organism that are used to determine how the body looks, functions, and behaves. The DNA is a double-stranded helix and serves as the code for the production of the single-stranded messenger ribonucleic acid (RNA) (Stone & Frazier, 2010).

"The project goals related to research were to:
- Identify all the approximately 20,000–25,000 genes in human DNA.
- Determine the sequences of the 3 billion chemical base pairs that make up human DNA.
- Store this information in databases.
- Improve tools for data analysis.
- Transfer related technologies to the private sector.
- Address the ethical, legal, and social issues (ELSI) that may arise from the project." (Department of Education Genomic Science, 2014)

Advancements in genetics have facilitated the development of new technologies that have permitted the analysis of normal and abnormal genes for the detection and diagnosis of genetic diseases. Through the use of molecular cloning, sufficient quantities of DNA and RNA have been produced to permit analysis in research. The Southern blotting technique is the standard way for analyzing the structure of DNA. The Northern blotting technique is used for RNA analysis. Analyses of both normal and mutant genes are of interest, and the Western blotting technique is used to examine mutant proteins in cells obtained from patients with diseases. In addition, polymerase chain reaction (PCR) can selectively amplify DNA and RNA molecules for study (Stone & Frazier, 2010). It is important that nurses be aware of the advances in technologies to measure nucleic acids and use them in their programs of research. Nurses are becoming more aware of the conduct of genetic research

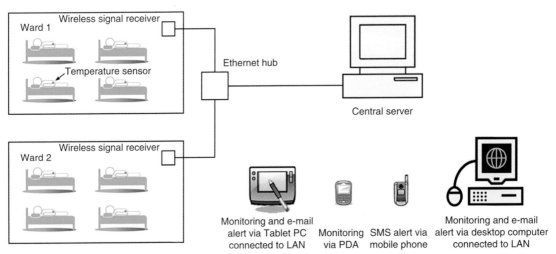

FIGURE 17-3 Setup of the ThermoSENSOR wireless temperature monitoring system. Each sensor transmits data wirelessly to a signal receiver (node) that is within the prescribed transmission range. The signal receiver uploads the data to a central server through the local area network (LAN), through which the data can be accessed from computers and other devices that are connected, wirelessly or by wired means, to the LAN. The server can be configured to send out e-mail and short message service (SMS) alerts. (From Ng, K., Wong, S., Lim, S., & Goh, Z. [2010]. Evaluation of the Cadi ThermoSENSOR wireless skin-contact thermometer against ear and axillary temperatures in children. *Journal of Pediatric Nursing, 25*[3], 177.)

through doctoral and postdoctoral programs specialized in this area.

Kubik, Permenter, and Saremain (2015) conducted a comparative descriptive study to determine the stability of the human papillomavirus (HPV) DNA when retested 21 days after the collection date. The sample included 50 BD SurePath specimens that initially tested positive for high-risk HPV using the Roche Cobas 4800 assay. The BD SurePath liquid-based Papanicolaou (Pap) test is approved for only Pap testing by the U.S. Food and Drug Administration (FDA); but these specimens are often used for HPV testing. In the Kubik et al. (2015) study, initial and repeat testing for HPV were performed per manufacturer instructions using 1 mL of SurePath specimen. When the specimens were retested 21 days after their collection date, eight tested negative (false-negative rate of 16%). False-negative occurs when the test results are negative for a disease but the individual has the disease (see Chapter 16). The genetic testing used for HPV DNA is discussed in the following study excerpt.

"The Roche Cobas 4800 assay is a fully automated, in vitro test for detection of HPV that uses amplification of target DNA via PCR [polymerase chain reaction] and nucleic acid hybridization for the detection of 14 HR-HPV types in a single analysis" (Kubik et al., 2015, p. 52). The

PCR assay provides specific genotyping for HPV 16 and 18 types, (which account for approximately 70% of the cervical cancers worldwide) and pools the results of all the other high risk "HPV types (31, 33, 35, 39, 45, 51, 52, 56, 58, 59, 66, and 68). The system uses β-globin as an internal control to assess specimen quality and potential inhibitors of the amplification process." (Kubik et al., 2015, p. 52)

Kubik and colleagues (2015) described the accuracy and precision of the Roche Cobas 4800 assay for genotyping many types of high-risk HPV. The researchers also documented the accuracy and precision of the SurePath Pap specimens that were collected according to manufacturers' specifications. Kubik et al. (2015, p. 51) concluded: "Aged BD SurePath–preserved Pap test specimens older than 21 days from collection date may produce false-negative HPV DNA testing results when testing with assays such as Roche Cobas 4800, most likely due to degradation of DNA." The researchers recommended additional large sample studies to facilitate the development of guidelines "to limit the age of the specimen to less than two weeks to prevent false-negative test results and improve diagnostic accuracy and patient care" (Kubik et al., 2015, p. 51).

Obtaining Physiological Measures Across Time

Many nursing studies use physiological measures that focus on a single point in time. Thus, there is insufficient information on normal variations in physiological measures across time and much less information on changes in physiological measures across time in individuals with abnormal physiological states. Circadian rhythms, activities, emotions, dietary intake, or posture can also affect physiological measures. Researchers need to determine to what extent these factors affect the ability to interpret measurement outcomes. An important question to ask is "How labile is the measure?" Some measures vary within the individual from time to time, even when conditions are similar. When a clinician observes variation in a physiological value, it is important to know whether the variation is within the normal range or signals a change in the patient's condition.

Some of the specimens collected from patients and research subjects can vary with the passage of time and researchers need to determine when the analysis of the specimen is most accurate. For example, Kubik et al. (2015) retested 50 SurePath Pap specimens 21 days after their initial collection. The Pap specimens that were 21 days or older had a 16% false-negative result (indicating that eight women did not have HPV when they did). The repeat testing of the Pap specimens indicated that the DNA tested had degraded over time and should be examined within two weeks of collection.

Selecting a Physiological Measure

Researchers designing a physiological study have fewer printed resources for selecting methods of measurement than do researchers conducting studies using psychosocial variables. Multiple books and electronic sources are available that discuss various methods for measuring psychosocial variables. In addition, numerous articles in nursing journals describe the development of psychosocial scales or discuss various means of measuring a particular psychosocial variable. However, literature guiding the selection of physiological measures in nursing is still sparse. You might consider the following factors when selecting a physiological measure for a study:

1. What physiological variables are relevant to the study?
2. Will the variables need to be measured continuously or at a particular point in time?
3. Will repeated measures be needed?
4. Do certain characteristics of the population under study place limits on the measurement approaches that can be used?
5. How has the variable been measured in previous research?
6. Is more than one measurement method available to measure the physiological variable being studied (Stone & Frazier, 2010)?
7. Which measurement method is the most accurate and precise for the population you are studying (Ryan-Wenger, 2010)?
8. Could the study be designed to include more than one measurement method for the variable being studied (Waltz et al., 2010)?
9. Where can the measurement device or devices be obtained that will measure the physiological variable being studied?
10. Can the measurement device be obtained from the manufacturer for use in the study, or must it be purchased?
11. What are the national and international standards for the measurement device or equipment that has been designated (International Organization for Standardization [ISO], 2015)?

The sources most commonly used to identify physiological measurement methods are previous studies that have measured a particular physiological variable. Literature reviews or meta-analyses can provide reference lists of relevant studies. Because the measure you select might have been used in studies unrelated to the current research topic, it is usually important to examine the research literature broadly. Other disciplines, such as engineering and biomedical science, have technology and other devices for measuring physiological and pathological variables.

Physiological measures must be linked conceptually with the framework of the study. The link of the physiological variable to the concept in the framework must be made explicit in the published report of your study. The logic of operationalizing the concept in a particular way must be well thought out and expressed clearly (see Chapter 6). It is often a good idea to use diverse physiological measures of a single concept, which reduces the impact of extraneous variables that might affect measurement. The operationalization of a physiological variable in a study should clearly indicate the physiological measure(s) to be used.

You also need to evaluate the accuracy and precision of physiological measures. Until recently, researchers commonly used information from the equipment manufacturer to describe the accuracy of measurement. This information is useful, but it is insufficient to evaluate accuracy and precision. The accuracy and precision of physiological measures are discussed in Chapter 16 (CLSI, 2015; ISO, 2015; Ryan-Wenger, 2010).

You need to consider problems you might encounter when using various approaches to physiological measurement. One factor of concern is the sensitivity of the measure. Will the measure detect differences finely enough to avoid a Type II error—known as a false negative—that occurs when the investigator claims there is no difference between groups or relationships among variables when one really exists (see Chapter 21)? Physiological measures are usually norm referenced (see Chapter 16). Data obtained from a study participant are compared with a norm as well as with other participants. You need to determine whether the norm used for comparison is relevant for the population you are studying. Laboratories are certified by ensuring that the analyses conducted in the laboratory meet a national standard (CLSI, 2015). New physiological measures are compared with the "gold standard" or the current best measurement method for a physiological variable.

Many measurement strategies require the use of specialized equipment. Often the equipment is available in the patient care area and is part of routine patient care in that unit. Otherwise, the researcher may need to purchase, rent, or borrow the equipment specifically for the study. You need to be skilled in operating the equipment or obtain the assistance of someone who has these skills. You need to ensure that the equipment is operated in an optimal fashion and is used in a consistent manner. Sometimes equipment must be recalibrated, or reset, regularly to ensure consistent readings. For example, weight scales are recalibrated periodically to ensure that the weight indicated is accurate and precise. According to federal guidelines, recalibration must be performed as follows:

- In accordance with the manufacturers' instructions
- In accordance with national and international standards (ISO, 2015)
- In accordance with criteria set up by the laboratory (CLSI, 2015)
- At least every 6 months
- After major preventive maintenance or replacement of a critical part
- When quality control indicates a need for recalibration

Reporting Physiological Measures in Studies

When the results of a physiological study are published, researchers must describe the measurement technique in considerable detail to allow an adequate critical appraisal of the study, enable others to replicate the study, and promote clinical application of the results. A detailed description of physiological measures in a research report includes the following:

1. Description of the equipment or device used in performing the measurement
2. Identification of the name of the equipment manufacturer
3. Account of the accuracy and precision of the equipment or device based on previous research, the manufacturers' specifications, and national and international standards
4. Explanation of the exact procedure followed to measure the physiological variable
5. Overview of the process used to record, retrieve, and store data

The examples discussed in the previous sections can be used as models for describing the process for obtaining and implementing physiological measures in studies to ensure quality outcomes.

OBSERVATIONAL MEASUREMENT

Observational measurement is the use of unstructured and structured inspection to gauge a study variable. This section focuses on structured observational measurement; unstructured observation is described in Chapter 12. Although data collection by observation is most common in qualitative research, it is used to some extent in all types of studies (Creswell, 2014; Marshall & Rossman, 2016). First, you must decide what you want to observe, and then you need to determine how to ensure that every variable is observed in a similar manner in each instance. Much attention must be given to training data collectors, especially when the observations are complex and examined over time (Waltz et al., 2010). You must create opportunities for the observational technique to be pilot-tested and for generation of data on interrater reliability (see Chapter 16). Observational measurement tends to be more subjective than other types of measurement and often is perceived as less credible. However, in many cases, observation is the only possible way to obtain important evidence for practice.

Structured Observations

The first step in a **structured observation** is to define carefully what specific behaviors or events are to be inspected or observed in a study. From that point, researchers determine how the observations are to be made, recorded, and coded. In most cases, the research team develops an observational checklist or category system to direct collecting, organizing, and sorting of the specific behaviors or events being observed (Polit & Yang, 2016). The extent to which these categories are exhaustive varies with the study.

Category Systems

Observational categories should be mutually exclusive. If categories overlap, the observer will be faced with making judgments regarding which category should contain each observed behavior, and data collection and recording may be inconsistent. In some category systems, only the behavior that is of interest is recorded. Most category systems require the observer to make some inference from the observed event to the category. The greater the degree of inference required, the more difficult the category system is to use. Some systems are applicable in a wide variety of studies, whereas others are specific to the study for which they were designed. The number of categories used varies considerably with the study. An optimal number for ease of use and therefore effectiveness of observation is 15 to 20 categories.

Klein et al. (2010) developed the NPAT that was introduced earlier in this chapter. The NPAT included categories of behaviors that were to be observed to determine the pain level for nonverbal adults in the ICU (Figure 17-4). The interrater reliability of the tool in this study was ensured when "Two RNs, trained in the use and scoring of the NPAT, simultaneously observed a patient unable to verbalize his or her pain" (Klein et al., 2010, p. 523).

Another type of category system used to direct the collection of observational data is a checklist. **Observational checklists** are techniques used to establish whether a behavior occurred. The observer places a tally mark on a data collection form each time he or she witnesses the behavior. Behavior other than that on the checklist is ignored. In some studies, the observer may place multiple tally marks in various categories while witnessing a particular event. However, in other studies, the observer is required to select a single category in which to place the tally mark.

Rating Scales

Rating scales (discussed in detail later in this chapter) can be used for observation and for self-reporting. A rating scale allows the observer to rate the behavior or event on a scale. This method provides more information for analysis than the use of dichotomous data, which indicate only that the behavior either occurred or did not occur. The NPAT also included a rating scale in which each observational category was scored on a scale of 0 to 2 or 0 to 3 (see Figure 17-4). The tool resulted in a total score between 0 and 10, with 0 indicating no pain and 10 indicating the worst pain ever experienced by the patient (Klein et al., 2010). The number of marks, or tallies, serves as the operational definition for each behavior.

INTERVIEWS

Interviews involve verbal communication during which the subject provides information to the researcher. Although this data collection strategy is used most commonly in qualitative, mixed-methods, and descriptive studies, it is also used in other types of studies. The various approaches for conducting interviews range from unstructured interviews in which study participants are asked broad questions (see Chapter 12) to interviews in which the participants respond to a questionnaire, selecting from a set of specific responses (Waltz et al., 2010). Although most interviews are conducted face to face or by telephone, computer-based interviews are also commonly used (Streiner, Norman, & Cairney, 2015).

Using the interview method for measurement requires carefully detailed work with a scientific approach. Excellent books are available on the techniques of developing interview questions (Dillman, Smyth, & Christian, 2009; Gorden, 1998; Streiner et al., 2015). If you plan to use this strategy, consult a text on interview methodology before designing your instrument. Because nurses frequently use interview techniques in nursing assessment, the dynamics of interviewing are familiar; however, using this technique for measurement in research requires greater sophistication.

Structured Interviews

Structured interviews are verbal interactions with subjects that allow the researcher to exercise increasing amounts of control over the content of the interview, for the purpose of obtaining essential data. The researcher designs the questions before data collection begins, and the order of the questions is specified. In some cases, the interviewer is allowed to explain the meaning of the question further or modify the way in which the question is asked so that the subject can understand it better. In more structured interviews, the interviewer is required to ask each question precisely as it has been designed. If the study participant does not understand the question, the interviewer can only repeat it. The participant may be limited to a range of responses previously developed by the researcher, similar to those in a questionnaire. For example, the interviewer may ask participants to select from the responses weak, average, or strong in describing their functioning level. If the possible responses are lengthy or complex, they

Is patient able to make vocalizations or sound cues? Score under the yes **or** no column; add scores for total score (range 0–10)				
YES				**NO**
SCORE	**EMOTION**	**An affective response to a situation**	**EMOTION**	SCORE
0		Smiling; calm; relaxed or none due to coma state or analgesia		0
1		Anxious; irritable; withdrawn; closes eyes; does not engage with physical environment		1
2		Tearful/crying **or** uncooperative		2
	MOVEMENT	**Change in placement and positioning of the body and extremities when not engaged in any care activities**	**MOVEMENT**	
0		None; sleeping comfortable; no unusual movements; **or** none due to coma state or analgesia		0
1		Restless **or** slow, decreased movement; reluctant to move; muscle tenseness		2
2		Rigidity; increasing motion; stiffening; tossing; turning; flapping of arms; stiffening		3
	VERBAL CUES	**Sound cues or vocalizations other than speech**		
0		No vocalization		
1		Whimpering; moaning; sighing		n/a
2		Screaming; crying out		
	FACIAL CUES	**Expressions on face**	**FACIAL CUES**	
0		Relaxed, calm expression **or** none due to coma state or analgesia		0
1		Drawn around the mouth and eyes; narrowed eyes		1
2		Wincing; grimacing; clenched teeth; furrowed brows; tightened lips		2
	POSITIONING/GUARDING	**Body responses that imply a protection of the body from contact with external touch**	**POSITIONING/GUARDING**	
0		Relaxed body **or** none due to coma state or analgesia		0
1		Guarding/tense		2
2		Jumpy when touched; clutching of siderails; withdraws when touched		3
TOTAL				

Choose only one behavior per category

FIGURE 17-4 Nonverbal Pain Assessment Tool—final. (Adapted from Klein, D. G., Dumpe, M., Katz, E., & Bena, J. [2010]. Pain assessment in the intensive care unit: Development and psychometric testing of the nonverbal pain assessment tool. *Heart & Lung, 39*[6], 527.)

may be printed on a card so that study participants can review them visually before selecting a response.

Designing Interview Questions

The process for developing and sequencing interview questions progresses from broad and general to narrow and specific. Questions are grouped by topic, with fairly *safe* topics being addressed first and sensitive topics reserved until late in the interview process to make participants feel more comfortable in responding. Demographic information, such as age, educational level, usually are collected last. These data are best obtained from other sources, such as patient records, to allow more time for the primary interview questions. The wording of questions in an interview is crafted toward the minimum expected educational level of study participants. Participants may interpret the wording of certain questions in a variety of ways, and researchers must anticipate this possibility. After the interview protocol has been developed, it is wise to seek feedback from an expert on interview technique and from a content expert.

Pilot-Testing the Interview Protocol

After the research team has satisfactorily developed the interview protocol, team members need to pretest or pilot-test it on subjects similar to the individuals who will be included in their study. Pilot-testing allows the research team to identify problems in the design of questions, sequencing of questions, and procedure for recording responses. The time required for the informed consent and interviewing processes also needs to be determined. Pilot-testing also provides an opportunity to assess the reliability and validity of the interview instrument (Streiner et al., 2015; Waltz et al., 2010).

Training Interviewers

Skilled interviewing requires practice, and interviewers must be familiar with the content of the interview. They need to anticipate situations that might occur during the interview and develop strategies for dealing with them. One of the most effective methods of developing a polished approach is role-playing. Playing the role of the subject can give the interviewer insight into the experience and facilitate an effective response to unscripted situations.

The interviewer should establish a permissive atmosphere in which the subject is encouraged to respond to sensitive topics. He or she also must develop an unbiased verbal and nonverbal manner. The wording of a question, the tone of voice, a raised eyebrow, or a shifting body position can communicate a positive or negative reaction to the subject's responses—either of which can alter subsequent data.

Preparing for an Interview

If you are serving as an interviewer in person, on the telephone, or by real-time computer communication, you need to make an appointment. For face-to-face interviews, choose a site for the interview that is quiet, private, and provides a pleasant environment. Before the appointment, carefully plan and develop a script for the instructions you will give the subject. For example, you might say, "I am going to ask you a series of questions about. … Before you answer each question you need to. … Select your answer from the following … , and then you may elaborate on your response. I will record your answer and then, if it is not clear, I may ask you to further explain some aspects."

Probing

Interviewers use **probing** to obtain more information in a specific area of the interview. In some cases, you may have to repeat a question. If your subject answers, "I don't know," you may have to press for a response. In other situations, you may have to explain the question further or ask the subject to explain statements that he or she has made. At a deeper level, you may pick up on a comment the participant made and begin asking questions to understand better what the subject meant. Probes should be neutral to avoid biasing participants' responses.

Recording Interview Data

Qualitative data obtained from interviews are recorded, either during the interview or immediately afterward. The recording may be in the form of handwritten notes, video recordings, or audio recordings. If you hand-record your notes, you must have the skill to identify key ideas (or capture essential data) in an interview and concisely record this information. With a structured interview, often an interview form is developed and researchers can record responses directly on the form. Data must be recorded without distracting the interviewee. Some interviewees have difficulty responding if it is obvious that the interviewer is taking notes or recording the conversation. In such a case, the interviewer may need to record data *after* completing the interview. If you wish to record the interview, you first must obtain IRB approval and then obtain the participant's permission. Plan to prepare verbatim transcriptions of the recordings before data analysis. In some studies, researchers use content analysis to capture the meaning within the data (see Chapter 12).

Advantages and Disadvantages of Interviews

Interviewing is a flexible technique that can allow researchers to explore greater depth of meaning than they can obtain with other techniques. Use your interpersonal skills to encourage your subject's cooperation and elicit more information. The response rate to interviews is higher than the response rate to questionnaires; thus, collecting data through interview instead of questionnaire yields a more representative sample. Interviews allow researchers to collect data from participants who are unable or unlikely to complete questionnaires, such as very ill subjects or those whose reading, writing, and ability to express their thoughts are marginal. Interviews are a form of self-report, and the researcher must assume that the information provided is accurate. Interviewing requires much more time than do questionnaires and scales, and it is more costly. Because of time and cost, sample size usually is limited. Subject bias is always a threat to the validity of the findings, as is inconsistency in data collection from one subject to another (Doody & Noonan, 2013; Dillman et al., 2009).

Interviewing children requires a special understanding of the art of asking children questions. The interviewer must use words that children tend to use to define situations and events. Interviewers also must be familiar with the language skills that exist at different stages of development. Children view topics differently than adults do. Children's perception of time, and the concepts of past, and present are also different.

Kim, Harrison, Godecker, and Muzyka (2014) conducted two structured interviews to examine posttraumatic stress disorder (PTSD) in women receiving prenatal care in federally qualified health centers. One interview involved using the prenatal risk overview (PRO) instrument to conduct a comprehensive prenatal psychosocial risk screening. The second interview was conducted using the Structured Clinical Interview for DSM-IV (SCID) to validate the "depression, alcohol use, and drug use domains against the diagnoses of major depressive episode, alcohol use disorder, and drug use disorder" (Kim et al., 2014, p. 1057). The following excerpt describes the interviews conducted in this study.

"This study was an additional component to a research project to validate the PRO, a structured and standardized psychosocial screening interview developed to identify women in need of enhanced case management services ... At local Healthy Start sites, a prenatal care staff member administered the PRO, which took an average of 10–15 min to complete, to all clinic prenatal care patients at their intake appointment ... A Research Assis-

tant later called participants to schedule the interview, and to ease participant burden, the SCID was conducted in conjunction with a scheduled medical or laboratory visit whenever possible. The SCID interview took approximately 30–45 min to complete and all interviews were conducted by the same Research Assistant. Interview completers were provided with a grocery or discount store gift card with a cash value of $50." (Kim et al., 2014, p. 1057)

"Study Instruments
The Structured Clinical Interview for DSM-IV (SCID)
Selected modules (alcohol use disorders, drug use disorders, major depressive episodes, and PTSD) of the SCID research version were used in this study. The PTSD module was introduced with a statement that 'Sometimes things happen to people that are extremely upsetting,' and giving some examples, such as being in a life-threatening situation, being assaulted or raped, seeing another person killed or badly hurt, or hearing about something horrible to someone close to the respondent. This was followed by the question, 'At any time during your life, have any of these kinds of things happened to you?' If the respondent identified one or more such experiences, each was recorded, and the interviewer asked how long ago that event occurred. If any event was recorded, the interviewer asked about the occurrences of 'nightmares, flashbacks, or thoughts you can't get rid of' ... A 'Yes' response to either of these questions was followed by a question to determine which traumatic event (if more than one) affected the respondent the most and an item to ascertain whether the trauma elicited intense fear, horror, or helplessness ...

Prenatal Risk Overview (PRO)
The PRO consisted of 58 questions that addressed 13 psychosocial domains: Telephone Access, Transportation Access, Food Security, Housing Stability, Social Support, Partner Violence, Physical/Sexual Abuse by a Non-partner, Depression, Cigarette Smoking, Alcohol Use, Drug Use, Legal Problems, and Child Protection Involvement. Domains were scored high, moderate or low risk based on participant responses." (Kim et al., 2014, p. 1058)

Kim and colleagues (2014) detailed the implementation of their structured interviews. The SCID-directed interviews were implemented consistently by one research assistant. The PRO-directed interviews were administered by a prenatal care staff member; it is unclear if one or more staff members collected the data and what training they received. The PRO and SCID are standardized forms that have been used in federal healthcare agencies over time, which supports their validity and reliability. However, the researchers might have provided more details from previous studies on the PRO and SCID development, validity, and reliability. The structure of the SCID did involve probing by the interviewer to gather additional, relevant data. The study participants were treated with respect, as demonstrated by interviews being scheduled on the same day as other healthcare appointments and a gift card being provided to thank them for study participation. Kim et al. (2014) found that PTSD was common in this population of women receiving prenatal care in federal healthcare centers. The women with PTSD were four times more likely to be depressed and two times as likely to be at risk for drug abuse. These study results support the need for psychosocial risk screening and enhanced management services in this population.

QUESTIONNAIRES

A **questionnaire** is a written self-report form designed to elicit information that can be obtained from a subject's written responses. Information derived through questionnaires is similar to information obtained by interview, but the questions tend to have less depth. The subject is unable to elaborate on responses or ask for questions to be clarified, and the data collector cannot use probing strategies. However, questions are presented in a consistent manner, and there is less opportunity for bias than in an interview.

Questionnaires can be designed to determine facts about the study participants or persons known by the participants; facts about events or situations known by the participants; or beliefs, attitudes, opinions, levels of knowledge, or intentions of the participants. Questionnaires can be distributed to large samples directly, or indirectly through the mail or by computer. The design, development, and administration of questionnaires have been addressed in many excellent books that focus on survey techniques (Saris & Gallhofer, 2007; Streiner et al., 2015; Thomas, 2004; Waltz et al., 2010).

Although items on a questionnaire appear easy to design, a well-designed item requires considerable effort. Similar to interviews, questionnaires can have varying degrees of structure. Some questionnaires ask open-ended questions that require written responses. Others ask closed-ended questions with options selected by the researcher. Data from open-ended questions are often difficult to interpret, and content analysis may be used to extract meaning. Open-ended questionnaire items are not advised if data are obtained from large samples.

Researchers frequently use computers to gather questionnaire data (Harris, 2014; McPeake, Bateson, & O'Neill, 2014). Computers are made available at the data collection site, such as a clinic or hospital; the questionnaire is presented on the screen; and subjects respond by using the keyboard or mouse. Data are stored in a computer file and are immediately available for analysis. Data entry errors are greatly reduced. Most researchers email subjects and direct them to a website where they can complete the questionnaire online, allowing the data to be stored securely and analyzed immediately. Thus, researchers can keep track of the number of subjects completing their questionnaire and the evolving results.

Development of Questionnaires

The first step in either selecting or developing a questionnaire is to identify the information desired. The research team develops a blueprint or table of specifications for the questionnaire. The blueprint identifies the essential content to be covered by the questionnaire; the content must be at the educational level of the potential subjects. It is difficult to stick to the blueprint when designing the questionnaire because it is tempting to add "just one more question" that seems to be a "neat idea" or a question that someone insists "really should be included." However, as a questionnaire lengthens, fewer subjects are willing to respond, and more questions are left blank.

The second step is to search the literature for questionnaires or items in questionnaires that match the blueprint criteria. Sometimes published studies include questionnaires, but, frequently, you must contact the authors of a study to request a copy of their questionnaire and obtain their permission to use the questionnaire. Researchers are encouraged to use questions in exactly the same form as questionnaires in previous studies to examine the questionnaire validity for new samples. However, questions that are poorly written need to be modified, even if rewriting makes it more difficult to compare the validity results of the questionnaire directly with those from previous studies.

In some cases, you may find a questionnaire in the literature that matches the questionnaire blueprint that you have developed for your study. However, you may have to add items to or delete items from an existing questionnaire to accommodate your blueprint. In some situations, items from several questionnaires are combined to develop an appropriate questionnaire. In all situations, you must obtain permission to use a questionnaire or the items from different questionnaires from the authors of these questionnaires.

An item on a questionnaire has two parts: a question (or stem) and a response set. Each question must be carefully designed and clearly expressed (Polit & Yang, 2016). Problems include ambiguous or vague language, leading questions that influence the response, questions that assume a preexistent state of affairs, and double questions.

In some cases, respondents interpret terms used in the question in one way when the researcher intended a different meaning. For example, the researcher might ask how heavy the traffic is in the neighborhood in which the family lives. The researcher might be asking about automobile traffic, but the respondent interprets the question in relation to drug traffic. The researcher might define neighborhood as a region composed of a three-block area, whereas the respondent considers a neighborhood to be a much larger area. Family could be defined as people living in one house or as all close blood relations. If a question includes a term that is unfamiliar to the respondent or for which several meanings are possible, the term must be defined (Harris, 2014; Waltz et al., 2010).

Leading questions suggest to the respondent the answer the researcher desires. These types of questions often include value-laden words and indicate the researcher's bias. For example, a researcher might ask, "Do you believe physicians should be catered to on the nursing unit?" or "All hospitals are stressful places to work, aren't they?" These examples are extreme, and leading questions are usually constructed more subtly. The degree of formality and permissive tone with which the question is expressed, in many cases, are important for obtaining a true measure. A permissive tone suggests that any of the possible responses are acceptable. Questions implying a preexisting state of affairs often lead respondents to admit to a previous behavior regardless of how they answer. Examples are "How long has it been since you used drugs?" or, to an adolescent, "Do you use a condom when you have sex?"

Double questions ask for more than one bit of information: "Do you like critical care nursing and working closely with physicians?" It would be possible for the respondent to like working in critical care settings but dislike working closely with physicians. In this case, the question would be impossible to answer accurately. A similar question is, "Was the in-service program educational and interesting?" Questions with double negatives are often difficult for study participants to interpret. For example, one might ask, "Do you believe nurses should not question doctors' orders? Yes or No." In this case, the

wording of this question can be easily misinterpreted and the word "not" possibly overlooked. This situation can lead participants to respond in a way contrary to how they actually think or feel.

Each item in a questionnaire has a **response set** that provides the parameters within which the respondent can answer. This response set can be open and flexible, as it is with open-ended questions, or it can be narrow and directive, as it is with closed-ended questions (Polit & Yang, 2016). For example, an open-ended question might have a response set of three blank lines. With closed-ended questions, the response set includes a specific list of alternatives from which to select.

Response sets can be constructed in various ways. The cardinal rule is that every possible answer must have a response category. If the sample includes respondents who might not have an answer, a response category of "don't know" or "uncertain" should be included. If the information sought is factual, include "other" as one of the possible responses. However, recognize that the item "other" is essentially lost data. Even if the response is followed by a statement such as "Please explain," it is rarely possible to analyze the data meaningfully. If a large number of study participants (> 10%) select the alternative "other," the alternatives included in the response set might not be appropriate for the population studied (Harris, 2014).

The simplest response set is the dichotomous *yes/no* option. Arranging responses vertically preceded by a blank reduces errors. For example,

_____ Yes
_____ No

is better than

_____ Yes _____ No

because in the latter example, the respondent might not be sure whether to indicate yes by placing a response before or after the "Yes."

Response sets must be mutually exclusive, which might not be the case in the following response set because a respondent might legitimately need to select two responses:

_____ Working full-time
_____ Full-time graduate student
_____ Working part-time
_____ Part-time graduate student

Mary Cazzell, a pediatric nurse practitioner at Cook's Children's Hospital in Fort Worth, TX, developed the Self-Report College Student Risk Behavior Questionnaire, an eight-item questionnaire with a response set of yes and no possible answers. This questionnaire was developed and refined as part of her dissertation at The University of Texas at Arlington. Cazzell's (2010)

Self-Report College Student Risk Behavior Measure

Unique ID:

Shade Circles Like This --> ●
Not Like This --> ⊗ ☑

Answer YES or NO based on your participation in these behaviors over the <u>past 30 days.</u>

1. I smoked a cigarette (even a puff).	○ Yes	○ No
2. I drank alcohol (even one drink). <u>If you answered YES to Question #2:</u>	○ Yes	○ No
a. If you are a female, did you have 4 or more drinks on one occasion?	○ Yes	○ No
b. If you are a male, did you have 5 or more drinks on one occasion?	○ Yes	○ No
3. I used an illegal drug (even once).	○ Yes	○ No
4. I had sexual intercourse without a condom.	○ Yes	○ No
5. I rode in a car without wearing my seatbelt (even once).	○ Yes	○ No
6. I drove a car without wearing my seatbelt (even once).	○ Yes	○ No
7. I rode in a car with a person driving under the influence (even once).	○ Yes	○ No
8. I drove a car while under the influence (even once).	○ Yes	○ No

FIGURE 17-5 Self-Report College Student Risk Behavior Questionnaire. (Adapted from Cazzell, M. (2010). College student risk behavior: The implications of religiosity and impulsivity. Ph.D. dissertation, The University of Texas at Arlington, United States: Texas. Proquest Dissertations & Theses. (Publication No. AAT 3391108.)

questionnaire was developed based on the 87 risk behaviors identified in a national survey conducted by the U.S. Centers for Disease Control and Prevention (CDC) on the *Youth Risk Behavior Surveillance System* (Brener et al., 2004). Cazzell included the most commonly identified adolescent risk behaviors from the CDC survey. Content validity of the questionnaire was developed by having a doctorally prepared social worker and a pediatric clinical nurse specialist, both risk behavior experts, evaluate the items. The content validity index calculated for the questionnaire was 0.88, supporting the inclusion of these eight items in the questionnaire. Cazzell (personal communication, 2015) presented her questionnaire at three national conferences and expanded question #2 on use of alcohol to target binge drinking (Figure 17-5).

Questionnaire instructions should be pilot-tested on naïve subjects who are willing and able to express their reactions to the instructions. Each question should clearly instruct the subject how to respond (i.e., *Choose one, Mark all that apply*), or instructions should be included at the beginning of the questionnaire. The subject must know whether to circle, underline, or fill in a circle as he or she responds to items. Clear instructions are difficult to construct and usually require several attempts. Cazzell (2010) provided clear directions and an example of how to complete her questionnaire and directed the students to report their participation in these risk behaviors over the past 30 days (see Figure 17-5).

After the questionnaire items have been developed, you need to plan carefully how they will be ordered. Questions related to a specific topic must be grouped together. General items are included first, with progression to more specific items. More important items might be included first, with subsequent progression to items of lesser importance. Questions of a sensitive nature or questions that might be threatening should appear near the end of the questionnaire. In some cases, the response to one item may influence the response to another. If so, the order of such items must be carefully considered. The general trend is to ask for demographic data about the subject at the end of the questionnaire.

An introductory page in the computer or a cover letter for a mailed questionnaire is needed to explain the purpose of the study and identify the researchers, the approximate amount of time required to complete the form, and organizations or institutions supporting the study. Because researchers indicate that completion of the questionnaire implies informed consent, researchers need to obtain a waiver of consent from the IRB. Returning mailed questionnaires is much more complex. The instructions need to include an address to which the questionnaire can be returned. This address must be at the end of the questionnaire and on the cover letter and envelope. Respondents often discard both the envelope and the cover letter and do not know where to send the questionnaire after completing it. It is also wise to provide a stamped, addressed envelope for the subject to return the questionnaire. If possible, the best way to provide questionnaires to potential subjects is by emailing a Web address so that participants can easily complete the questionnaire at their leisure, and their responses are automatically submitted at the end of the questionnaire. Sending questionnaires by email has many advantages, but one disadvantage is being able to access only individuals with email. Researchers need to determine whether the population they are studying has email access and, if they have email, whether the addresses are available to the researchers.

Your questionnaire must be pilot-tested to determine clarity of questions, effectiveness of instructions, completeness of response sets, time required to complete the questionnaire, and success of data collection techniques. As with any pilot test, the subjects and techniques must be as similar as possible to those planned for the main study. In some cases, the open-ended questions are included in a pilot test to obtain information for the development of closed-ended response sets for the main study.

Questionnaire Validity

One of the greatest risks in developing response sets is leaving out an important alternative or response. For example, if the questionnaire item addressed the job position of nurses working in a hospital and the sample included nursing students, a category representing the student role would be necessary. When seeking opinions, there is a risk of obtaining a response from an individual who actually has no opinion on the research topic. When an item requests knowledge that the respondent does not possess, the subject's guessing interferes with obtaining a true measure of the study variable.

The response rate to questionnaires is generally lower than that with other forms of self-reporting, particularly if the questionnaires are sent out by mail. If the response rate is less than 50%, the representativeness of the sample is seriously in question. The response rate for mailed questionnaires is usually small (25% to 35%), so researchers are frequently unable to obtain a representative sample, even with randomization. There seems to be a stronger response rate for questionnaires that are sent by email, but the response is still usually less than 50%. Strategies that can increase the response rate for an emailed or mailed questionnaire are discussed in Chapter 20.

Study participants commonly fail to respond to all the questions on a questionnaire. This problem, especially with long questionnaires, can threaten the validity of the instrument. In some cases, study participants may write in an answer if they do not agree with the available choices, or they might write comments in the margin. Generally, these responses cannot be included in the analysis; however, you should keep a record of such responses. These responses might be used later to refine the questionnaire questions and responses.

Consistency in the way the questionnaire is administered is important to validity. Variability that could confound the interpretation of the data reported by the study participants is introduced by administering some questionnaires in a group setting, mailing some questionnaires, and emailing some questionnaires. There should not be a mix of mailing or emailing to business addresses and to home addresses. If questionnaires are administered in person, the administration needs to be consistent. Several problems in consistency can occur: (1) Some subjects may ask to take the form home to complete it and return it later, whereas others will complete it in the presence of the data collector; (2) some subjects may complete the form themselves, whereas others may ask a family member to write the responses that the respondent dictates; and (3) in some cases, a secretary or colleague may complete the form, rather than the individual whose response you are seeking. These situations may lead to biases in responses that are unknown to the researcher and can alter the true measure of the variables.

Analysis of Questionnaire Data

Data from questionnaires are often at the nominal or ordinal level of measurement that limit analyses, for the most part, to descriptive statistics, such as frequencies and percentages, and nonparametric inferential statistics, such as chi square, Spearman rank-order correlation, and Mann-Whitney U (see Chapters 22 through 25). However, in certain cases, ordinal data from questionnaires are treated as interval data, and t-tests and analysis of variance are used to test for differences between responses of various subsets of the sample (Grove & Cipher, 2017). Discriminant analysis may be used to determine the ability to predict membership in various groups from responses to particular questions.

SCALES

Scales, a form of self-report, are a more precise means of measuring phenomena than questionnaires. Most scales have been developed to measure psychosocial variables. However, self-reports can be obtained on physiological variables such as pain, nausea, or functional capacity by using scaling techniques, as discussed earlier in this chapter. Scaling is based on mathematical theory, and there is a branch of science whose primary concern is the development of measurement scales. From the point of view of scaling theory, considerable measurement error, both random and systematic error, is expected in a single item (Spector, 1992; Waltz et al., 2010). Therefore, in most scales, the various items on the scale are summed to obtain a single score, and these scales are referred to as **summated scales**. Less random and systematic error exists when using the total score of a scale in conducting data analyses,

although subscale comparisons are usually of interest and are conducted. Using several items in a scale to measure a concept is comparable to using several instruments to measure a concept (see Figure 16-4 in Chapter 16). The various items in a scale increase the dimensions of the concept that are reflected in the instrument. The types of scales commonly used in nursing studies include rating scale, Likert scale, and visual analog scale (VAS).

Rating Scale

A **rating scale** lists an ordered series of categories of a variable that are assumed to be based on an underlying continuum. A numerical value is assigned to each category, and the fineness of the distinctions between categories varies with the scale, making this one of the crudest forms of scaling technique. The general public commonly uses rating scales. In conversations, one can hear statements such as "On a scale of 1 to 10, I would rank that …" Rating scales are easy to develop; however, one must be careful to avoid end statements that are so extreme that no subject would select them. A rating scale could be used to rate the degree of cooperativeness of the patient or the value placed by the subject on nurse-patient interactions. This type of scale is often used in observational measurement to guide data collection.

The Wong-Baker FACES® Pain Rating Scale is commonly used to assess the pain of children in clinical practice and has been shown to be valid and reliable over the years (Figure 17-6; Wong-Baker FACES Foundation, 2015). Pain in adults is often assessed with a numeric rating scale such as the one presented in Figure 17-7. Klein et al. (2010) developed the NPAT rating scale, which was introduced earlier in this chapter to determine the pain level for nonverbal adults in the ICU (see Figure 17-4).

Likert Scale

The **Likert scale** determines the opinion or attitude of a subject and contains a number of declarative statements with a scale after each statement. The Likert scale is the most commonly used of the scaling techniques in nursing and healthcare studies. The original version of the scale included five response categories. Each response category was assigned a value, with a value of 1 given to the most negative response and a value of 5 given to the most positive response (Nunnally & Bernstein, 1994).

Response choices in a Likert scale most commonly address agreement, evaluation, or frequency. Agreement options may include statements such as *strongly disagree, disagree, uncertain, agree,* and *strongly agree*. Evaluation

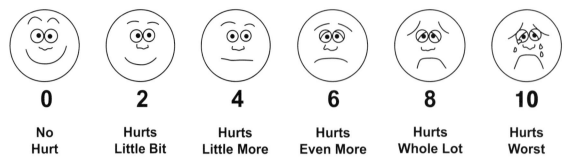

FIGURE 17-6 Wong-Baker FACES® Pain Rating Scale. (From Wong-Baker FACES Foundation [2015]. *Wong-Baker FACES® Pain Rating Scale.* Retrieved October 12, 2015 from http://www.wongbakerfaces.org/.)

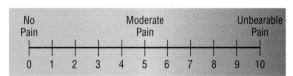

FIGURE 17-7 Numeric Rating Scale (NRS).

responses ask the respondent for an evaluative rating along a good/bad continuum, such as *very negative, negative, positive,* and *very positive.* Frequency responses may include statements such as *never, rarely, sometimes, frequently,* and *all the time.* The terms used are versatile and must be selected for their appropriateness to the stem (Spector, 1992). Likert scale responses often contain four to seven options. If the scale has an odd number of response options, then it includes a neutral or uncertain option. Use of the uncertain or neutral category is controversial because it allows the subject to avoid making a clear choice of positive or negative statements. Thus, sometimes only four or six options are offered, with the uncertain category omitted. This type of scale is referred to as a **forced choice** version. Researchers who use the forced choice version consider an item that is left blank as a response of "uncertain." However, responses of "uncertain" are difficult to interpret, and if a large number of respondents select that option or leave the question blank, the data may be of little value (Froman, 2014). In addition, some computer-administered programs do not allow a subject to progress to the next item or section of an instrument if an item is left blank. In this instance, subjects either arbitrarily select an answer or close the program and never complete the instrument.

How the researcher phrases the stem of an item depends on the type of judgment that the respondent is being asked to make. Agreement item stems are declarative statements such as "Nurses should be held accountable for managing a patient's pain." Frequency item stems can be behaviors, events, or circumstances to which the respondent can indicate how often they occur. A frequency stem might be "You read research articles in nursing journals." An evaluation stem could be "The effectiveness of 'X' drug for relief of nausea after chemotherapy." Items must be clear, concise, and concrete (Streiner et al., 2015).

An instrument using a Likert scale usually consists of 15 to 30 items, each addressing an element of the concept being measured. Response-set bias tends to occur when participants anticipate that either the positive or the negative (*agree* or *disagree*) response is consistently provided either in the right or left hand columns of the scale. Participants might note a pattern that agreeing with scale items consistently falls to the right and disagreeing to the left. Thus, they might fail to read all questions carefully and just mark the right or left column based on whether they agree or disagree with scale items. Thus, half the statements should be expressed positively and half should be expressed negatively, termed *counterbalancing,* to avoid inserting response-set bias into the participants' responses. Participants would need to mark some agreement items in the right column and others in the left column of the scale, based on the direction in which each item is printed.

Scale values of negatively worded items require reverse-coding prior to analysis. For example, if a scale had a set of four responses, 1—strongly disagree, 2—disagree, 3—agree, and 4—strongly agree, and a study participant strongly disagreed with a negatively worded item, the score of 1 would be reverse-coded to a score of 4. Thus, the scores for participants' agreement with certain positively worded items and, accordingly, their disagreement with negatively worded items (reverse-coded) could be interpreted in a meaningful way. Usually, the values obtained from each item in the instrument are summed to obtain a single score for each subject. Although the values of each item are technically ordinal-level data, the summed score is often analyzed as interval-level data, allowing more powerful parametric statistical analyses to be conducted (Grove & Cipher, 2017; Nunnally & Bernstein, 1994).

The Center for Epidemiological Studies Depression Scale (CES-D) is an example of a 4-point Likert scale that is commonly used to measure depression in nursing studies (Figure 17-8). The CES-D was developed by Radloff in 1977 and has shown to be a reliable and valid

Center for Epidemiologic Studies Depression Scale
DEPA

THESE QUESTIONS ARE ABOUT HOW YOU HAVE BEEN FEELING LATELY.
AS I READ THE FOLLOWING STATEMENTS, PLEASE TELL ME HOW OFTEN YOU FELT OR BEHAVED THIS WAY IN THE <u>LAST WEEK</u>. [*Hand card*]. FOR EACH STATEMENT, DID YOU FEEL THIS WAY:
[Interviewer: You may help respondent focus on the whichever "style" answer is easier]

          0 = **R**arely or none of the time (or less than 1 day)?
          1 = **S**ome or a little of the time (or 1–2 days)?
          2 = **O**ccasionally or a moderate amount of time (or 3–4 days)?
          3 = **M**ost or all of the time (or 5–7 days)?

	R	S	O	M	NR
1. I WAS BOTHERED BY THINGS THAT USUALLY DON'T BOTHER ME.	0	1	2	3	--
2. I DID NOT FEEL LIKE EATING; MY APPETITE WAS POOR.	0	1	2	3	--
3. I FELT THAT I COULD NOT SHAKE OFF THE BLUES EVEN WITH HELP FROM MY FAMILY AND FRIENDS.	0	1	2	3	--
4. I FELT THAT I WAS JUST AS GOOD AS OTHER PEOPLE.	0	1	2	3	--
5. I HAD TROUBLE KEEPING MY MIND ON WHAT I WAS DOING.	0	1	2	3	--
6. I FELT DEPRESSED.	0	1	2	3	--
7. I FELT THAT EVERYTHING I DID WAS AN EFFORT.	0	1	2	3	--
8. I FELT HOPEFUL ABOUT THE FUTURE.	0	1	2	3	--
9. I THOUGHT MY LIFE HAD BEEN A FAILURE.	0	1	2	3	--
10. I FELT FEARFUL.	0	1	2	3	--
11. MY SLEEP WAS RESTLESS.	0	1	2	3	--
12. I WAS HAPPY.	0	1	2	3	--
13. I TALKED LESS THAN USUAL.	0	1	2	3	--
14. I FELT LONELY.	0	1	2	3	--
15. PEOPLE WERE UNFRIENDLY.	0	1	2	3	--
16. I ENJOYED LIFE.	0	1	2	3	--
17. I HAD CRYING SPELLS.	0	1	2	3	--
18. I FELT SAD.	0	1	2	3	--
19. I FELT PEOPLE DISLIKED ME.	0	1	2	3	--
20. I COULD NOT GET GOING.	0	1	2	3	--

FIGURE 17-8 Center for Epidemiologic Studies Depression Scale (CES-D). (Adapted from Radloff, L. S. [1977]. The CES-D scale: A self-report depression scale for research in the general population. *Applied Psychological Measurement, 1*[3], 385–394.)

measure of depression for over 35 years. Holden, Ramirez, and Gallion (2014) studied the depressive symptoms in Latina breast cancer survivors to determine whether their symptoms were a barrier to obtaining colorectal and ovarian cancer screenings. The implementation of the CES-D is described by the researchers in the following study excerpt.

"Depressive symptoms were assessed using the 20-item Center for Epidemiological Studies Depression Scale (CES-D), an instrument designed for diverse samples (Radloff, 1977). It is a screening tool recommended by the U.S. Preventive Services Task Force (U.S. Preventative Task Force, 2002) and has been widely used with diverse populations of varying socioeconomic and demographic characteristics (Finch, Kolody, & Vega, 2000; ...; Radloff, 1991). Item responses range from 0 (*never or rarely*) to 3 (*most of the time or all of the time*). Four items assessing positive symptoms are reverse-coded. Summed-item scale scores range from 0–60 with higher scores representing higher levels of depressive symptoms experienced over the past week. We identified persons below the cutoff for significant symptomatology (0–15) and above the cutoff for significant symptomatology (16+) using established and validated criteria (Coyne et al., 2001; Radloff, 1991). In this study, statistical reliability for the CES-D was α = 0.93." (Holden et al., 2014, p. 244)

Holden and colleagues (2014) clearly described the CES-D used to measure depression in their study. The item response range (0–3) and scoring of the scale were discussed, with a score of 16+ indicating elevated depressive symptoms in Latina women surviving breast cancer. The U.S. Preventive Services Task Force recommended this scale, and it has been used with diverse populations that add to the reliability and validity of this scale for use in this population of breast cancer survivors. The reliability of the scale for this study was strong: r = 0.93. The discussion of the scale would have been strengthened by expanding the validity and reliability information from previous research. Holden et al. (2014) found that the CES-D scores for their study participants were three times those of the general population. These Latina women "demonstrated high rates of depressive symptoms and low rates of cancer screening compliance" indicating that depressive symptoms may be a barrier to cancer screening in this population (Holden et al., 2014, p. 246). Preventative strategies need to be developed to promote cancer screening behaviors in Latina breast cancer survivors.

Visual Analog Scale

One of the problems with scaling procedures is the difficulty of obtaining a fine discrimination of values. In an effort to resolve this problem, the **visual analog scale** (VAS) was developed to measure magnitude, strength, and intensity of an individual's sensations or feelings (Wewers & Lowe, 1990). The VAS is referred to as *magnitude scaling* (Gift, 1989). This technique seems to provide interval-level data, and some researchers argue that it provides ratio-level data (Sennott-Miller, Murdaugh, & Hinshaw, 1988). It is particularly useful in scaling stimuli. This scaling technique has been used to measure pain, mood, anxiety, alertness, craving for cigarettes, quality of sleep, attitudes toward environmental conditions, functional abilities, and severity of clinical symptoms (Waltz et al., 2010; Wewers & Lowe, 1990).

The stimuli must be defined in a way that the subject clearly understands. Only one major cue should appear for each scale. The scale is a line 100 mm (or 10 cm) in length with right-angle stops at each end. The line may be horizontal or vertical as shown in Figure 17-9. Bipolar anchors are placed beyond each end of the line. The anchors should *not* be placed underneath or above the line before the stop. These end anchors should include the entire range of sensations possible in the phenomenon being measured. Examples include *all* and *none*, *best* and *worst*, and *no pain* and *worst pain imaginable*.

The VAS is frequently used in healthcare research because it is easy to construct, administer, and score. A VAS can be administered using a drawn, printed, or computer-generated 100-mm line (Raven et al., 2008; Waltz et al., 2010). The research participant is asked to place a mark through the line to indicate the intensity of the sensation or stimulus. A ruler is used to measure the distance between the left end of the line and the mark placed by the subject. This measure is the value of the subject's sensation. With a computer-generated VAS, research participants can touch the VAS line on the computer screen to indicate the degree of their sensations, such as pain. The computer can determine

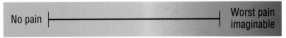

FIGURE 17-9 Example of a visual analog scale to measure pain.

the value of the sensation for each subject and store it in a database (Raven et al., 2008). The scale is designed to be used while the subject is seated. Whether use of the scale from the supine position influences the results by altering perception of the length of the line has yet to be determined (Gift, 1989). A VAS can be developed for children by using pictorial anchors at each end of the line rather than words (Lee & Kieckhefer, 1989).

Wewers and Lowe (1990) published an extensive evaluation of the reliability and validity of VAS, although reliability is difficult to determine. Reliability of the VAS is most often determined with the test-retest method (see Chapter 16), which is effective if the variable being measured is fairly stable, such as chronic pain. Because most of the variables measured with the VAS are labile, test-retest consistency might not be applicable, and because a single measure is obtained, internal consistency cannot be examined. The VAS is more sensitive to small changes than are numerical and rating scales and it can discriminate between two dimensions of pain. Validity of the VAS has most commonly been determined by comparing VAS scores with other measures of a concept.

Liu and Chiu (2015, p. 182) conducted a randomized controlled trial (RCT) to determine the effectiveness of vitamin B_{12} in relieving the pain of aphthous ulcers. The mouth ulcers are the most common mucosal lesions seen in primary care. The sample included 42 patients suffering from aphthous ulcers with 22 in the intervention group and 20 in the control group. The ulcer pain was measured using a VAS and is described in the following study excerpt.

"The VAS is an extensively used self-reporting device for pain measurement. The VAS in this study comprised a 10-cm horizontal line between poles connoting no pain (origin) to unbearable pain. Although the VAS adopted for this study was horizontal, some VAS scales are blank on one side and numerically labeled on the other side, with 'no pain = 0' on one end and 'unbearable pain = 10' on the other end. The VAS represents a continuum of pain intensity and is used to assess the level of pain at the time of reporting. The patient only sees the side with the single horizontal line with a no pain label at one end and an unbearable label at the other end. Subjects were told to mark a vertical line at the point that best represented the present pain level of the ulcer. The research assistant recorded their baseline pain score using a VAS before patients were randomly assigned to the groups and after 2 days of treatment." (Liu & Chiu, 2015, p. 184)

Liu and Chiu (2015) clearly described the VAS used in their study and how the scale was administered and scored. These researchers found that the VAS was easy to use and an effective way to assess the pain from the mouth ulcers. The measurement discussion would have been strengthened by a discussion of the reliability and validity of the VAS based on previous research. Additional research is needed with the VAS to ensure that it is a reliable and valid measure of certain patients' sensations (Waltz et al., 2010). Liu and Chiu (2015, p. 182) concluded "that vitamin B_{12} is an effective analgesic treatment for aphthous ulcers" and healthcare providers could use this vitamin as an adjunctive therapy for their treatment.

Q-SORT METHODOLOGY

Q-sort methodology is a technique of comparative rating that preserves the subjective point of view of the individual (McKeown & Thomas, 1988). Cards are used to categorize the importance placed on various words or phrases in relation to the other words or phrases in the list. Each phrase is placed on a separate card. The number of cards should range from 40 to 100 (Tetting, 1988). The subject is instructed to sort the cards into a designated number of piles, usually 7 to 10 piles ranging from the most to the least important or from the most to least agreement (Tetting, 1988; van Hooft, Dwarswaard, Jedeloo, Bal, & van Staa, 2015). However, the subject is limited in the number of cards that may be placed in each pile. If the subject must sort 60 cards, Category One (of greatest importance) may allow only 2 cards; Category Two, 5 cards; Category Three, 10 cards; Category Four, 26 cards; Category Five, 10 cards; Category Six, 5 cards; and Category Seven (the least important), 2 cards. Placement of the cards fits the pattern of a normal curve. Study participants are usually advised to select first the cards they wish to place in the two extreme categories and then work toward the middle category, which contains the largest number of cards, rearranging the cards until they are satisfied with the results. When sorting the cards, subjects might be encouraged to make comments about the statements on the cards and provide a rationale for the categories into which they placed the cards (Akhtar-Danesh, Baumann, & Cordingley, 2008).

Q-sort methodology also can be used to determine the priority of items or the most important items to include in the development of a scale. In the previously mentioned example, the behaviors sorted into Categories One, Two, and Three might be organized into a 17-item scale. Correlational or factor analysis is used to analyze the data (Akhtar-Danesh et al., 2008; van Hooft

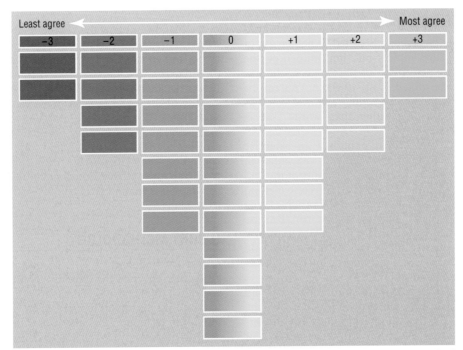

FIGURE 17-10 Forced-choice frequency distribution in Q-sort. (Adapted from Van Hooft, S. M., Dwarswaard, J., Jedeloo, S., Bal, R, & van Staa, A. [2015]. Four perspectives on self-management support by nurses for people with chronic conditions: A Q-methodological study. *International Journal of Nursing Studies, 52*[1], 161.)

et al., 2015). Simpson (1989) suggested using the Q-sort method for cross-cultural research, with pictures used rather than words for non-literate groups.

Van Hooft and colleagues (2015) used Q-sort methodology to examine nurses' perspectives on self-management support for people with chronic conditions. In this study, 49 registered nurses were asked to sort 37 statements into 7 categories. Their use of Q-sort methodology is presented in the following study excerpt.

"The first step of a Q-methodological study is the design of the collection of representative statements. These statements should cover all the relevant ground on a subject ... The purpose of a Q-methodological study is to identify different opinions on a topic, instead of generalization (Akhtar-Danesh et al., 2008). A limited sample is sufficient, therefore, as long as this sample holds a maximum variation of opinions ...

The statements are printed on separate cards with random numbers. The participants were asked to read the statements carefully and then sort them in three piles: agree, disagree, or neutral. Thereafter, they sorted the statements even more precisely on a Q-sort table with a forced-choice frequency distributions [Figure 17-10] on a range from '-3 least agree' to '+3 most agree.' This forced participants to make choices about which statement was more and which was less important to them. Next, participants in face-to-face interviews explained their motivations for the choice of the statements sorted on -3 and +3, and at random about other statements. The interviews lasted between 10 and 65 min and were recorded and transcribed ad verbatim." (van Hooft et al., 2015, p. 159)

Van Hooft et al. (2015, p. 165) conducted factor analysis on their data and identified "four distinct nurses' perspectives toward self-management support: the Coach, the Clinician, the Gatekeeper, and the Educator." Nurses in a Coach role focus on promoting patients' activities of daily living, and nurse Clinicians help patients adhere to their treatment regimes. Support from nurses in the Gatekeeper role helps reduce healthcare costs. Educator nurses focus on instructing patients and families in the management of the illness. Each perspective requires distinct competencies from nurses; and they need specific education to fulfill these roles of supporting patients in their management of chronic illnesses.

DELPHI TECHNIQUE

The **Delphi technique** measures the judgments of a group of experts for the purpose of making decisions, assessing priorities, or making forecasts (Vernon, 2009). Using this technique allows a wide variety of experts to express opinions and provide feedback, nationally and internationally, without meeting together. When the Delphi technique is used, the opinions of individuals cannot be altered by the persuasive behavior of a few people at a meeting. Three types of Delphi techniques have been identified: classic or consensus Delphi, dialectic Delphi, and decision Delphi. In classic Delphi, the focus is on reaching consensus. Dialectic Delphi is sometimes called *policy Delphi,* and the aim is not consensus but rather to identify and understand a variety of viewpoints and resolve disagreements. In decision Delphi, the panel consists of individuals in decision-making positions and the purpose is to come to a decision (Waltz et al., 2010).

To implement the Delphi technique, researchers identify a panel of experts, who have a variety of perceptions, personalities, interests, and demographics to reduce biases in the process. Members of the panel usually remain anonymous to one another. A questionnaire is developed that addresses the topics of concern. Although most questions call for closed-ended responses, the questionnaire usually contains opportunities for open-ended responses by each expert. Once they have completed the questionnaires, the respondents return them to the researcher, who then analyzes and summarizes the results. The statistical analyses usually include measures of central tendency and measures of dispersion. The role of the researcher is to maintain objectivity. The numerical outcomes of the most frequently selected items are returned to the panel of experts, along with a second questionnaire. Respondents with extreme responses to the first round of questions may be asked to justify their responses. The respondents return the second round of questionnaires to the researcher for analysis. This procedure is repeated until the data reflect consensus among the panel. Limiting the process to two or three rounds is not a good idea if consensus is the goal. In some studies, true consensus is reached, whereas in others, "majority rules." Some authors question whether the agreement reached is genuine (Vernon, 2009; Waltz et al., 2010). Couper (1984) developed a

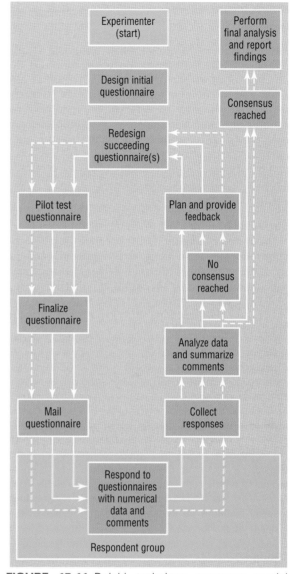

FIGURE 17-11 Delphi technique sequence model. Multiple arrows indicate repeated cycles of review by experts.

model of the Delphi technique, which is presented in Figure 17-11. This model might assist you in implementing a Delphi technique in a study.

Vernon (2009) identified benefits and limitations of the Delphi technique. The benefits include increased access to experts and usually good response rates. The Delphi design has simplicity and flexibility in its use; it is easily understood and implemented by researchers.

Because the participants are anonymous, views can be expressed freely without direct persuasion from others.

There are also several potential problems that researchers could encounter when using the Delphi technique. There has been no documentation that the responses of *experts* are different from responses one would receive from a random sample of subjects. Because the panelists are anonymous, they have no accountability for their responses. Respondents could make hasty, ill-considered judgments because they know that no negative feedback would result. Feedback on the consensus of the group tends to centralize opinion, and traditional analysis with the use of means and medians may mask the responses of individuals who are resistant to the consensus sentiment. Conclusions could be misleading (Vernon, 2009).

Green and colleagues (2014) used the Delphi technique to identify the nursing research priorities and the key challenges facing pediatric nursing. The study participants are members of the Society of Pediatric Nursing (SPN) and are recognized as experts in pediatric care and practice. The following study excerpt describes the Delphi methodology they used.

"The Delphi technique is a process that begins with an initial round of open-ended questions (Round 1), which acts as an idea-generating strategy for identifying issues pertinent to the topic of interest. These responses are used as a springboard for the follow up phases of the study. In a classical Delphi study, three or more rounds are conducted to identify group consensus (Keeney, Hasson, & McKenna, 2011). A Delphi study using 3 rounds of on-line surveys was conducted to identify consensus on the challenges facing pediatric nursing and research priorities for the next 10 years." (Green et al., 2014, p. 403)

"Round 1
The Round 1 survey contained two broad open-ended questions designed to elicit qualitative responses from the SPN members: 1) "In pediatric nursing practice what are 3 problems that need to be studied through nursing research?" and 2) "What do you see as the 3 greatest challenges to pediatric nursing in the next 10 years?" … The 2 open-ended questions generated 1,644 responses from 274 pediatric nurse participants (8.25% response rate) … During multiple conference calls over a one month period the team reached 100% agreement on the list of mutually exclusive items for Round 2. The 1,644 responses were collapsed into 49 items on the research needs list and 56 on the challenges list.

Round 2
Respondents to the Round 1 survey were invited to participate in the second round electronically. The second round survey consisted of the two lists generated in Round 1 organized alphabetically. Subjects were asked to rank the lists in order of priority using a Likert scale with response options ranging from extreme importance to lowest importance. The Round 2 response rate was 141 participants representing 51.5% of the original sample …

Round 3
Previous respondents from Round 1 were asked to select the top 10 research priorities and top 10 practice challenges from the alphabetized lists generated in Round 2. The response rate for round three was 38% of the Round 1 sample with 104 SPN members participating. The research team used average ranking and number and percent of respondents indicating the item was ranked in the top 3 to generate the lists of 10 research priorities and 10 practice challenges." (Green et al., 2014, p. 404)

Green et al. (2014) provided a detailed description of the Delphi technique and how it was implemented in their study. The response rate for Round 1 was very low (8.25%) for the members of SPN ($N = 3321$), decreasing the representativeness of the sample. The response rates for Round 2 (51.5%) and Round 3 (38%) were limited when compared to the initial sample size. Green et al. (2014, p. 401) concluded that the top 10 research priorities and challenges were identified by conducting this Delphi study and "would serve as a valuable guide for pediatric nursing practice, education, policy, and administration over the coming decade."

DIARIES

A **diary** is a recording of events over time by an individual to document experiences, feelings, or behavior patterns. Diaries are also called *logs* or *journals* and have been used since the 1950s to collect data for research from various populations including children, patients with acute and chronic illness, pregnant women, and elderly adults (Aroian & Wal, 2007; Nicholl, 2010). A diary, which allows recording shortly after an event, is thought to be more accurate than obtaining the information through recall during an interview. In addition, the reporting level of incidents is higher, and one tends to capture the participant's immediate perception of situations.

The diary technique gives nurse researchers a means to obtain data on topics of particular interest within nursing that have not been accessible by other means. Some potential topics for diary collection include expenses related to a healthcare event (particularly out-of-pocket expenses), self-care activities (frequency and time required), symptoms of disease, eating behavior, exercise behavior, sexual activities, the child development process, and care provided by family members in a home care situation. Although diaries have been used primarily with adults, they are also an effective means of collecting data from school-age children.

Diaries may also be used to determine how people spend their days; this information could be particularly useful in managing the care needs of individuals with chronic illnesses. In experimental studies, diaries may be used to determine responses of subjects to experimental treatments. Diaries can take a variety of forms and might include filling in blanks, selecting the best response from a list of options, or checking a column. Figure 17-12 shows a page from a diary for patients to record their symptoms and how they were managed. This diary includes blanks to identify the symptoms and an option to check how the symptoms were managed. This type of diary is used to collect numerical data for a quantitative study. Validity and reliability of diaries have been examined by comparing the results with data obtained through interviews and have been found to be acceptable. Participation in studies using health diaries has been good, and attrition rates are reported as low. Some diaries include the collection of narrative data and are more common in qualitative studies (Alaszewski, 2006).

Nicholl (2010) and Burman (1995) provided some key points to consider when selecting a diary for collecting data in a study:
1. Analyze the phenomenon of interest to determine whether it can be adequately captured using a diary.
2. Determine whether a diary is the best data collection approach when compared with interviews, questionnaires, and scales.
3. Decide whether the diary will be used alone or with other measurement methods.
4. Determine which format of the diary to use so that the most valid information can be obtained to address the study purpose without burdening the study participants. Diaries can be paper, online, phone text-messaging formats, or apps on the iPad or smartphone. Some researchers are using blogs as a way to collect diary data (Lim, Sacks-Davis, Aitken, Hocking, & Hellard, 2010). The format of the questions in diaries can also vary based on the purpose of the study. Diaries with closed-ended questions are usually used in quantitative research, and participants are provided specific direction on the data to be recorded. Diaries with open-ended questions are more common in qualitative research with the narrative data requiring content analysis (Alaszewski, 2006; Nicholl, 2010).
5. Pilot-test any new or refined diary with the target population of interest to identify possible problems, determine whether the instructions and terminology are clear, ensure that the data can be recorded

Date	What symptom did you have?	Did you talk with a family member or friend about the symptom?		Did you talk with a health professional about it?		Did you take any pills or treatments for the symptom?	
		No	Yes	No	Yes	No	Yes, Specify

FIGURE 17-12 Sample diary page.

with this approach, and examine the ability of participants to complete diaries.

6. Determine the period of time that the diary will be completed to accomplish the purpose of the study, taking into consideration the burden on the participants. Typical diary periods are 2 to 8 weeks.

7. Provide clear instructions to participants on the use of a diary before the study begins to enhance the quality of data collected. Participants need to know how to use the diaries, what types of events are to be reported, and how to contact the researcher with questions.

8. Use follow-up procedures, such as phone calls or emails, during data collection to enhance completion rates.

9. Diaries might be emailed, mailed, or picked up by the researchers. Picking up the diary in person promotes a higher completion rate than mailing.

10. Plan data analysis procedures during diary development and refine these plans to ensure that the most appropriate analyses are used. Diary data are very dense and rich, and carefully prepared analysis plans can minimize problems.

The use of diaries has some disadvantages. In some cases, keeping the diary may alter the behavior or events under study. For example, if a person were keeping a diary of the nursing care that he or she was providing to patients, the insight that the person gained from recording the information in the diary might lead to changes in care. In addition, patients can become more sensitive to items (e.g., symptoms or problems) reported in the diary, which could result in overreporting. Subjects may also become bored with keeping the diary and become less thorough in recording items, which could result in underreporting (Aroian & Wal, 2007; Nicholl, 2010).

Lim et al. (2010) conducted an RCT to determine the best diary format for collecting sexual behavior information from adolescents. The three formats for the diaries were paper, online, and phone text messaging, short message service (SMS). These formats were compared for response rate, timeliness, completeness of data, and acceptability. The following excerpt describes the use of the diaries for data collection and the outcomes.

"Participants were recruited by telephone and randomized into one of three groups. They completed weekly sexual behavior diaries for 3 months by SMS, online, or paper (by post). An online survey was conducted at the end of 3 months to compare retrospective reports with the diaries and assess opinions on the diary collection method. ... Conclusions were that the SMS is a convenient and timely method of collecting brief behavioral data, but online data collection was preferable to most participants and more likely to be completed. Data collected in retrospective sexual behavior questionnaires were found to agree substantially with data collected through weekly self-report diaries." (Lim et al., 2010, p. 885)

Lim et al. (2010) provided some valuable information about the formats for collecting data with diaries. Researchers might want to consider using online or phone text messaging to collect diary data from younger populations. These formats could significantly increase the response rate and the completeness of the data collected. The paper format for collecting diary data also provides quality information and might be better used for populations with limited access to technology.

MEASUREMENT USING EXISTING DATABASES

Nurse researchers are increasing their use of existing databases to address the research problems they have identified as relevant for practice. The reasons for using these databases in studies are varied. With the computerization of healthcare information, more large data sets have been developed internationally, nationally, regionally, at the state level, and within clinical agencies. These databases include large amounts of information that have relevance in developing research evidence needed for practice (Brown, 2014; Melnyk & Fineout-Overholt, 2015). The costs and technology for secure storage of data have improved over the last 10 years, making these large data sets more reliable and accessible. Outcomes studies often are conducted using existing databases to expand understanding of patient, provider, and health agency outcomes (Doran, 2011). Another reason for the increased use of preexistent databases is that primary collection of data in a study is limited by the availability of participants and the expense of the data collection process. By using existing databases, researchers are able to have larger samples, conduct more longitudinal studies, experience lower costs during the data collection process, and limit the burdens placed on study participants (Johantgen, 2010).

There are also problems with using data from existing databases. The data in the database might not clearly address the researchers' study purpose. Most researchers identify a study problem and purpose and then develop a methodology to address these. The data collected are specific to the study and clearly focused on answering the research questions or testing the study hypotheses. However, with existing databases, researchers need to ensure that the data they require for their study are in the database that they are planning to use. Sometimes researchers must revise their study questions and variables based on what data exist in the database. The level of measurement of the study variables might limit the analysis techniques that can be conducted. There is also the question of the validity and reliability of the data in existing databases; unless these are specifically reported, researchers using these data files need to be cautious in their interpretation of findings.

Existing Healthcare Data

Existing healthcare data consist of two types: secondary and administrative. Data collected for a particular study are considered primary data. Data collected from previous research and stored in databases are considered secondary data when used by other researchers to address their study purposes. Because these data were collected as part of research, details can be obtained about the data collection and storage processes. Researchers should clearly indicate in the methodology section of a research report when secondary data analyses represent all or part of their total study data (Johantgen, 2010).

Data collected for reasons other than research are considered administrative data. Administrative data are collected within clinical agencies; obtained by national, state, and local professional organizations; and collected by federal, state, and local agencies. The processes for collection and storage of administrative data are more complex and often more unclear than the data collection process for research (Johantgen, 2010). The data in administrative databases are collected by different people in different sites using different methods. However, the data elements collected for most administrative databases include demographics, organizational characteristics, clinical diagnosis and treatment, and geographical information. These database elements were standardized by the Health Insurance Portability and Accountability Act (HIPAA) of 1996 to improve the quality of databases. The HIPAA regulations can be viewed online at http://www.hhs.gov/ocr/privacy/ (U.S. Department of Health and Human Services, 2015).

Ahn, Stechmiller, Fillingim, Lyon, and Garvan (2015) conducted a secondary data analysis of the national Minimum Data Set 3.0 (MDS 3.0) to determine the relationship between pressure ulcer stage and bodily pain intensity in nursing home (NH) residents. "Data were examined from residents with pressure ulcers who completed a bodily pain intensity interview between January and March 2012 ($N = 41,680$) as part of the MDS comprehensive assessment" (Ahn et al., 2015, p. 207). The residents were from 10,550 NHs over 53 U.S. states and territories. The following study excerpt describes the quality of the data obtained from the MDS 3.0 database.

> **"Measurements**
>
> All the measures were collected from the MDS 3.0 data set. Either a numeric rating scale (NRS) or verbal descriptor scale (VDS), which allow residents to self-report symptoms, was used to measure the worst bodily pain intensity of residents over the previous 5 days. The scores of NRS and VDS were summarized in a 4-point ordinal scale, 1 (*mild or no pain*), 2 (*moderate pain*), 3 (*severe pain*), and 4 (*excruciating pain*). NRS and VDS have been validated to measure bodily pain intensity in many different contexts and patient populations (AGS Panel on Persistent Pain on Older Persons, 2002; Edelen & Saliba, 2010; Herr, 2011). In the MDS 3.0 validation study, the average kappa for the interrater agreement on bodily pain intensity was 0.97 (Saliba & Buchanan, 2008).
>
> The pressure ulcer items in the MDS 3.0, indicated by the MDS coordinator in each NH, were used to indicate the stages of pressure ulcers. The pressure ulcer stages were categorized as Stages I, II, III, IV, and SDTI [suspected deep tissue injury]. In the MDS 3.0 validation study, the average kappa for the interrater agreement on pressure ulcers was 0.94 (Saliba & Buchanan, 2008)." (Ahn et al., 2015, p. 208)

Ahn et al. (2015) provided a detailed description of the national database (MDS 3.0) that they used in their study. This database was selected because it included essential data about pressure ulcer pain and staging needed to address the study purpose. The NH residents' pressure ulcer pain was measured with reliable and valid scales (numeric rating scale [NRS] and verbal descriptor scale [VDS]) used in many different contexts and patient populations. The staging of pressure of ulcers was made in a consistent way as indicated by the interrater agreement of 0.97, which indicates 97% consistency in staging ulcers and 3% error. The analysis of quality data from the MDS 3.0 greatly strengthened the credibility of these study findings that are representative of the U.S. population of NH residents with pressure ulcers. Ahn et al. (2015, p. 207) concluded that "greater bodily pain intensity was associated with an advanced stage of pressure ulcer, healthcare providers should assess bodily pain intensity and order appropriate pain management for nursing home residents with pressure ulcers, particularly for those with advanced pressure ulcers who are vulnerable to greater bodily pain intensity."

SELECTION OF AN EXISTING INSTRUMENT

Selecting an instrument to measure the variables in a study is a critical process in research. The method of measurement selected must fit closely the conceptual definition of the variable. Researchers must conduct an extensive search of the literature to identify appropriate methods of measurement. In many cases, they find instruments that measure some of the needed elements but not all, or the content may be related to but somehow different from what is needed for the planned study. Instruments found in the literature may have little or no documentation of their validity and reliability. Beginning researchers often conclude that no appropriate method of measurement exists and that they must develop a tool. At the time, this solution seems to be the most simple because the researcher has a clear idea of what needs to be measured. *This solution is not recommended unless all else fails.* This is because tool development is a lengthy process and requires sophisticated research. Using a new instrument in a study without first evaluating its validity and reliability can be problematic and leads to questionable findings.

For novice researchers developing their first study, it is essential to identify existing instruments to measure study variables. Jones (2004) developed a flow chart that might help you to select an existing instrument for your study (Figure 17-13). The major steps include (1) identifying an instrument from the literature; (2) determining whether the instrument is appropriate for measuring a study variable; and (3) examining the performance of the measurement method in research, such as identifying the reliability and validity of psychosocial instruments and the accuracy and precision of physiological measures. These steps are detailed in the following sections.

Locating Existing Instruments

Locating existing measurement methods has become easier in recent years. A computer database, the Health and Psychological Instruments Online (HAPI), is available in many libraries and can be used to search for instruments that measure a particular concept or for information on a particular instrument. Sometimes a search on Medline or CINAHL might uncover an instrument that is useful. Many reference books have compiled published measurement tools, some of which are specific to instruments used in nursing research.

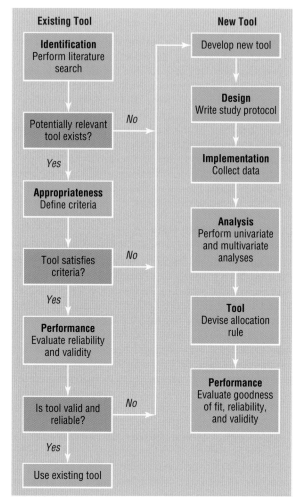

FIGURE 17-13 Flow chart depicting the identification and assessment of an existing tool and development of a new tool.

Dissertations often contain measurement tools that have never been published, so a review of *Dissertation Abstracts* online might be helpful.

Another important source of recently developed measurement tools is word-of-mouth communication among researchers. Information on tools is often presented at research conferences years before publication. There are usually networks of researchers conducting studies on similar nursing phenomena. These researchers are frequently associated with nursing organizations and keep in touch through newsletters, correspondence, telephone, email, computer discussion boards, and Web pages. Researchers are being encouraged to collect data on common elements across studies to advance the research needed for practice. Also the use of common measurement methods is thought to increase understanding of variables (Cohen, Thompson, Yates, Zimmerman, & Pullen, 2015).

Questioning available nurse investigators can lead to a previously unknown tool. These researchers can often be contacted by telephone, letter, or email and are usually willing to share their tools in return for access to the data to facilitate work on developing validity and reliability information. The Sigma Theta Tau *Directory of Nurse Researchers* provides email address and phone information for nurse researchers. In addition, it lists nurse researchers by category according to their area of research (http://www.nihpromis.org/#3). The instruments used in the medical outcome studies are available online at http://www.outcomes-trust.org/instruments.htm.

Waltz et al. (2010) made the following suggestions to facilitate locating existing instruments for studies:

"(1) Search computerized databases by using the name of the instrument or keywords or phrases; (2) generalize the search to the specific area of interest and related topics (research reports are particularly valuable); (3) search for summary articles describing, comparing, contrasting, and evaluating the instruments used to measure a given concept; (4) search journals, such as *Journal of Nursing Measurement,* that are devoted specifically to measurement; (5) after identifying a publication in which relevant instruments are used, use citation indices to locate other publications that used them; (6) examine computer-based and print indices, and compendia of instruments developed by nursing, medicine, and other disciplines; and (7) examine copies of published proceedings and abstracts from relevant scientific meetings." (Waltz et al., 2010, pp. 393–394)

Evaluating Existing Instruments for Appropriateness and Performance

You may need to examine several instruments to find the one most appropriate for your study. When selecting an instrument for research, carefully consider how the instrument was developed, what the instrument measures, and how to administer it. Before you review existing instruments, be sure you have conceptually defined your study variable and are clear on what you desire to measure (see Chapter 6). You then need to address the following questions to determine the best instrument for measuring your study variable:

1. Does this instrument measure what you want to measure?

2. Does the instrument reflect your conceptual definition of the variable?

3. Is the instrument well constructed? The process for constructing a scale is provided later in this chapter.

4. Does your population resemble populations previously studied with the instrument? (Waltz et al., 2010)

5. Is the readability level of the instrument appropriate for your population?

6. How sensitive is the instrument in detecting small differences in the phenomenon you want to measure (what is the effect size)?

7. What is the process for obtaining, administering, and scoring the instrument? Are there costs associated with the instrument?

8. What skills are required to administer the instrument? Do you need training or a particular credential to administer the instrument?

9. How are the scores interpreted?

10. What is the time commitment of the study participants and researcher for administration of the instrument?

11. What evidence is available related to the reliability and validity of the instrument? Have multiple types of validity been examined (content validity; construct validity from factor analysis, convergence and divergence validity; or evidence of criterion-related validity from prediction of concurrent and future events)? Chapter 16 provides a detailed discussion of instrument reliability and validity (also see Table 16-1; Bialocerkowski et al., 2010; DeVon et al., 2007; Streiner et al., 2015; Waltz et al., 2010).

Assessing Readability Levels of Instruments

The readability level of an instrument is a critical factor when selecting an instrument for a study. Regardless of how valid and reliable the instrument is, it cannot be used effectively if study participants do not understand the items. Many word processing programs and computerized grammar checkers report the readability level of written material (see Chapter 16). If the reading level of an instrument is beyond the reading level of the study population, you need to select another instrument for use in your study. Changing the items on an instrument to reduce the reading level can alter the validity and reliability of the instrument.

CONSTRUCTING SCALES

Scale construction is a complex procedure that should not be undertaken lightly. There must be firm evidence of the need for developing another instrument to measure a particular phenomenon important to nursing practice. However, in many cases, measurement methods have not been developed for phenomena of concern to nurse researchers, or measurement tools that have been developed may be poorly constructed and have insufficient evidence of validity to be acceptable for use in studies. It is possible for researchers to carry out instrument development procedures on an existing scale with inadequate evidence of validity before using it in a study. Neophyte nurse researchers could assist experienced researchers in carrying out some of the field studies required to complete the development of scale validity and reliability.

The procedures for developing a scale have been well defined. The following discussion briefly describes this theory-based process and the mathematical logic underlying it. The theories on which scale construction is most frequently based include classic test theory (Cappelleri, Lundy, & Hays, 2014; Nunnally & Bernstein, 1994; Polit & Yang, 2016), item response theory (Streiner et al., 2015), and multidimensional scaling (Borg & Groenen, 2010). Most existing instruments used in nursing research have been developed with classic test theory, which assumes a normal distribution of scores.

Constructing a Scale by Using Classic Test Theory

In classic test theory, the following process is used to construct a scale:

1. *Define the concept.* A scale cannot be constructed to measure a concept until the nature of the concept has been delineated. The more clearly the concept is defined, the easier it is to write items to measure it (Spector, 1992). Concepts are defined through the process of concept analysis, a procedure discussed in Chapter 8.

2. *Design the scale.* Items should be constructed to reflect the concept as fully as possible. The process of construction differs depending on whether the scale is a rating scale, Likert scale, or VAS. Items previously included in other scales can be used if they have been shown empirically to be good indicators of the concept (Cappelleri et al., 2014). A blueprint may ensure that all elements of the concept are covered. Each item must be stated clearly and concisely and express only one idea. The reading level of items must be identified and considered in terms of potential respondents. The number of items constructed must be considerably larger than planned for the completed instrument because items are discarded during the item analysis

step of scale construction. Nunnally and Bernstein (1994) suggested developing an item pool at least twice the size of that desired for the final scale.

3. *Review the items.* As items are constructed, it is advisable to ask qualified individuals to review them. Feedback is needed in relation to accuracy, appropriateness, or relevance to test specifications; technical flaws in item construction; grammar; offensiveness or appearance of bias; and level of readability. The items should be revised according to the critical appraisal. This is part of the development of content validity (see Chapter 16).

4. *Conduct preliminary item tryouts.* While items are still in draft form, it is helpful to test items on a limited number of subjects (15 to 30) who represent the target population. The reactions of respondents should be observed during testing to note behaviors such as long pauses, answer changing, or other indications of confusion about specific items. After testing, a debriefing session needs to be held during which respondents are invited to comment on items and offer suggestions for improvement. Descriptive and exploratory statistical analyses are performed on data from these tryouts while noting means, response distributions, items left blank, and outliers. Items need to be revised based on this analysis and comments from respondents (Streiner et al., 2015).

5. *Perform a field test.* All the items in their final draft form are administered to a large sample of subjects who represent the target population. Spector (1992) recommended a sample size of 100 to 200 subjects. However, the sample size needed for the subsequent statistical analyses depends on the number of items in the instrument. Some experts recommend including 10 subjects for each item being tested. If the final instrument was expected to have 20 items, and 40 items were constructed for the field test, 400 subjects could be required.

6. *Conduct item analyses.* The purpose of item analysis is to identify items that form an internally consistent or reliable scale and to eliminate items that do not meet this criterion. Internal reliability implies that all items are consistently measuring a concept. Before these analyses are conducted, negatively worded items must be reverse-scored or given a score as though the item was stated positively. For example, the item might read "I do not believe exercise is important to health," with the responses of 1 = strongly disagree, 2 = disagree, 3 = uncertain, 4 = agree, and 5 = strongly agree. If the subject marked a 1 for strongly disagree, this item would be reverse-scored and given a 5, indicating the subject

thinks exercise is very important to health. The analyses examine the extent of intercorrelation among the items. The statistical computer programs currently providing the set of statistical procedures needed to perform item analyses (as a package) are SPSS, SPSS/PC, and SYSTAT. These packages perform both item-to-item correlations and item-to-total score correlations. In some cases, the value of the item being examined is subtracted from the total score, and an item-remainder coefficient is calculated. This latter coefficient is most useful in evaluating items for retention in the scale.

7. *Select items to retain.* Depending on the number of items desired in the final scale, items with the highest coefficients are retained. Alternatively, a criterion value for the coefficient (e.g., 0.40) can be set, and all items greater than this value are retained. The greater the number of items retained, the smaller the item-remainder coefficients can be and still have an internally consistent scale. After this selection process, a coefficient alpha is calculated for the scale. This value is a direct function of the number of items and the magnitude of intercorrelations. Thus, one can increase the value of a coefficient alpha by increasing the number of items or raising the intercorrelations through inclusion of more highly intercorrelated items. Values of coefficient alphas range from 0 to 1. The alpha value should be at least 0.70 to indicate sufficient internal consistency in a new tool (Nunnally & Bernstein, 1994). An iterative process of removing or replacing items or both, recalculating item-remainder coefficients, and recalculating the alpha coefficient is repeated until a satisfactory alpha coefficient is obtained. Deleting poorly correlated items raises the alpha coefficient, but decreasing the number of items lowers it (Spector, 1992). The initial attempt at scale development may not achieve a sufficiently high coefficient alpha. In this case, additional items need to be written, more data collected, and the item analysis redone.

8. *Conduct validity studies.* When scale development is judged to be satisfactory, studies must be performed to evaluate the validity of the scale (see Chapter 16 and Table 16-1). These studies require the researcher to collect additional data from large samples. As part of this process, scale scores must be correlated with scores on other variables proposed to be related to the concept being put into operation. Hypotheses must be generated regarding variations in mean values of the scale in different groups. Exploratory and confirmatory factor analysis (discussed in Chapters 16 and 23) is usually performed as part of establishing the validity of the instrument. Collect as many different types of validity evidence as possible (Cappelleri et al., 2014; Streiner et al., 2015; Waltz et al., 2010).

9. *Evaluate the reliability of the scale.* Various statistical procedures are performed to determine the reliability of the scale (see Chapter 16: Polit & Yang, 2016).

10. *Compile norms on the scale.* To determine norms, the scale must be administered to a large sample that is representative of the groups to which the scale is likely to be administered. Norms should be acquired for as many diverse groups as possible. Data acquired during validity and reliability studies can be included for this analysis. To obtain the large samples needed for this purpose, many researchers permit others to use their scale with the condition that data from these studies be provided for compiling norms (Streiner et al., 2015).

11. *Publish the results of scale development.* Scales often are not published for many years after the initial development because of the length of time required to validate the instrument. Some researchers never publish the results of this work. Studies using the scale are published, but the instrument development process may not be available except by writing to the author. This information needs to be added to the body of knowledge, and colleagues should encourage instrument developers to complete the work and submit it for publication (Cappelleri et al., 2014; Lynn, 1989). Klein et al. (2010) provided a detailed discussion of their development of the NPAT that was presented earlier in this chapter. The validity and reliability of the tool were addressed, and a copy of the tool was included in the article (see Figure 17-4).

Constructing a Scale by Using Item Response Theory

Using item response theory to construct a scale proceeds initially in a fashion similar to that of classic test theory. There is an expectation of a well-defined concept to operationalize. Items are initially written in a manner similar to that previously described, and item tryouts and field testing are also similar. However, the process changes with the initiation of item analysis. The statistical procedures used are more sophisticated and complex than the procedures used in classic test theory. Using data from field testing, item characteristic curves are calculated by using logistic regression models (Nunnally & Bernstein, 1994; Polit & Yang, 2016; Streiner et al., 2015). After selecting an appropriate model based on information obtained from the analysis, item parameters are estimated. These parameters are used to select items for the scale. This strategy is used to avoid problems encountered with classic test theory measures.

Scales developed by using classic test theory effectively measure the characteristics of subjects near the mean. The statistical procedures used assume a linear distribution of scale values. Items reflecting responses of respondents closer to the extremes tend to be discarded because of the assumption that scale values should approximate the normal curve. Scales developed in this manner often do not provide a clear understanding of study participants at the high or low end of values.

One purpose of item response theory is to choose items in such a way that estimates of characteristics at each level of the concept being measured are accurate. To accomplish this goal, researchers use maximal likelihood estimates. A curvilinear distribution of scale values is assumed. Rather than choosing items on the basis of the item remainder coefficient, the researcher specifies a test information curve. The scale can be tailored to have the desired measurement accuracy. By comparing a scale developed by classic test theory with one developed from the same items with item response theory, one would find differences in some of the items retained. Biserial correlations among items would be lower in the scale developed from item response theory than in the scale developed from classic test theory. Item bias is lower in scales developed by using item response theory and this is because respondents from different subpopulations having the same amount of an underlying trait have different probabilities of responding to an item positively (Hambleton & Swaminathan, 2010; Streiner et al., 2015).

Constructing a Scale by Using Multidimensional Scaling

Multidimensional scaling is used when the concept being operationalized is actually an abstract construct believed to be represented most accurately by multiple dimensions. The scaling techniques used allow the researcher to uncover the hidden structure in the construct. The analysis techniques use proximities among the measures as input. The outcome of the analysis is a spatial representation, or a geometrical configuration of data points, that reveals the hidden structure. The procedure tends to be used to examine differences in stimuli rather than differences in people. A researcher might use this method to measure differences in perception of pain. Scales developed by using this procedure reveal patterns among items. The procedure is used in the development of rating scales (Borg & Groenen, 2010).

TRANSLATING A SCALE TO ANOTHER LANGUAGE

Contrary to expectations, translating an instrument from the original language to a target language is a complex process. By translating a scale, researchers can compare concepts among respondents of different cultures. The goal of translation is achieving equivalence of the versions of a scale in different languages. Conceptual equivalence, semantic equivalence, and measurement equivalence are important to determine in translating a scale (Streiner et al., 2015). **Conceptual equivalence** is focused on determining whether the people in the two cultures view the construct to be measured in the same way. The comparison requires that they first infer and then validate that the conceptual meaning about which the scale was developed is the same in both cultures. **Semantic equivalence** of the two scales refers to the meaning that is attached to each item on the scale by the different cultures. **Measurement equivalence** is conducted after the translation of a scale to establish the psychometric properties of the translated scale, and to determine its correlation to the original (Streiner et al., 2015).

Four types of translations can be performed: pragmatic translations, aesthetic-poetic translations, ethnographic translations, and linguistic translations. Pragmatic translations communicate the content from the source language accurately in the target language. The primary concern is the information conveyed. An example of this type of translation is the use of translated instructions for assembling a computer. Aesthetic-poetic translations evoke moods, feelings, and affect in the target language that are identical to those evoked by the original material. In ethnographic translations, the purpose is to maintain meaning and cultural content. In this case, translators must be familiar with both languages and cultures. Linguistic translations strive to present grammatical forms with equivalent meanings. Translating a scale is generally done in the ethnographic mode (Hulin, Dasgow, & Parsons, 1983).

One strategy for translating scales is to translate from the original language to the target language and then back-translate from the target language to the original language by using translators not involved in the original translation. Discrepancies are identified, and the procedure is repeated until troublesome problems are resolved. After this procedure, the two versions are administered to bilingual subjects and scored by standard procedures. The resulting sets of scores are examined to determine the extent to which the two versions yield similar information from the subjects. This procedure assumes that the subjects are equally skilled in both languages. One problem with this strategy is that bilingual subjects may interpret meanings of words differently from monolingual subjects. This difference in interpretation is a serious concern because the target subjects for most cross-cultural research are monolingual.

Severinsson (2012) provided a clear description of her process for translating the Manchester Clinical Supervision Scale (MCSS) from English to Norwegian and Swedish versions. The translation process she used is outlined in the following excerpt.

"Translation and Back-Translation Using a Monolingual and Bilingual Test

A number of procedures were employed to achieve cross-cultural validity, including translation and back-translation … The English language version of the MCSS was translated using structured translation and back-translation. First, the scale was translated from English into Norwegian and Swedish by a professional bilingual translator, after which the researcher investigated the semantic and conceptual equivalence between the versions. In the next step, an expert group of academic healthcare professionals checked and commented on the back-translation and reached consensus on one version, which was then submitted to a qualified professional translator for bi-lingual testing, resulting in minor modification of two items. The linguistic differences were compared and discussed until consensus was achieved." (Severinsson, 2012, p. 83)

Severinsson (2012) described her translation process of the MCSS scale, which focused on achieving conceptual and semantic equivalence of the versions of the scale. Measurement equivalence was examined and a detailed discussion of the validity and reliability testing on the new versions of the scale was provided. Severinsson (2012, p. 81) concluded that "Translation of an instrument for cross-cultural nursing research is important; although there are methodological limitations associated with construct validity."

Rather than translating an instrument into each language, Turner, Rogers, Hendershot, Miller, and Thornberry (1996) tested the use of electronic technology involving multilingual audio computer-assisted self-interviewing (Audio-CASI) to enable researchers to include multiple linguistic minorities in nationally representative studies and clinical studies. The Audio-CASI system uses electronic translation from one language to another. In the funded project to develop and test Audio-CASI, a backup phone bank was available to provide multilingual assistance if needed. Whether this strategy will provide equivalent validity of a translated tool is unclear.

▌ KEY POINTS

- Measurement approaches used in nursing research include physiological measures; observations; interviews; questionnaires; scales; and specialized instruments such as Q-sort method, Delphi technique, diaries, and analyses using existing databases.
- Measurements of physiological variables can be either direct or indirect and sometimes require the use of specialized equipment or laboratory analysis.
- The Human Genome Project has increased the opportunities for nurses to be involved in genetic research and to include the measurement of nucleic acids in their studies.
- To measure observations, every variable is observed in a similar manner in each instance, with careful attention given to training data collectors.
- In structured observational studies, category systems must be developed; checklists or rating scales are developed from the category systems and used to guide data collection.
- Interviews involve verbal communication between the researcher and the study participant, during which the researcher acquires information. Interviewers must be trained in the skills of interviewing, and the interview protocol must be pretested.
- A questionnaire is a printed or electronic self-report form designed to elicit information through the responses of a study participant. An item on a questionnaire usually has two parts: a stem or lead-in question and a response set.
- Scales, another form of self-reporting, are more precise in measuring phenomena than are questionnaires and have been developed to measure psychosocial and physiological variables. The types of scales included in this text are rating scale, Likert scale, and VAS.
- A rating scale is a crude form of measurement that includes a list of an ordered series of categories of a variable, which are assumed to be based on an underlying continuum. A numerical value is assigned to each category.
- The Likert scale contains declarative statements with a scale after each statement to determine the opinion or attitude of a study participant.
- The VAS, sometimes referred to as magnitude scaling, is a 100-mm line with right-angle stops at each end with bipolar anchors placed beyond each end of the

line. These end anchors must cover the entire range of sensations possible in the phenomenon being measured.

- Q-sort methodology is a technique of comparative rating that preserves the subjective point of view of the individual. Q-sort methodology might be used in research to determine the importance of selected concepts or variables in a study or to select items for scale development.
- The Delphi technique measures the judgments of a group of experts to assess priorities or make forecasts. It provides a means for researchers to obtain the opinions of a wide variety of experts across the U.S. without the need for the experts to meet.
- A diary, which allows a research participant to record an experience shortly after an event, is more accurate than obtaining the information through recall at an interview. In addition, the reporting level of incidents is higher, and one tends to capture the participant's immediate perception of situations.
- Nurse researchers are expanding their use of data from existing databases to answer their research questions and test their research hypotheses. Health data are usually categorized into secondary data and administrative data.
- The choice of tools for use in a particular study is a critical decision that can have a major impact on the significance of the study. The researcher first must conduct an extensive search for existing tools. Once found, the tools must be carefully evaluated.
- Scale construction is a complex procedure that takes extensive expertise and time to complete. Theories on which scale construction is most frequently based include classic test theory, item response theory, and multidimensional scaling. Most existing instruments used in nursing research have been developed through the use of classic test theory.
- Translating a scale to another language is a complex process that allows concepts among respondents of different cultures to be compared if care is taken to ensure that concepts have the same or similar meanings across cultures.

REFERENCES

Ahn, H., Stechmiller, J., Fillingim, R., Lyon, D., & Garvan, C. (2015). Bodily pain intensity in nursing home residents with pressure ulcers: Analysis of National Minimum Data Set 3.0. *Research in Nursing & Health*, 38(3), 207–212.

Akhtar-Danesh, N., Baumann, A., & Cordingley, L. (2008). Q-methodology in nursing research: A promising method for the study of subjectivity. *Western Journal of Nursing Research*, 30(6), 759–773.

Alaszewski, A. (2006). *Using diaries for social research*. London, UK: Sage.

American Geriatric Society (AGS) Panel on Persistent Pain in Older Persons. (2002). The management of persistent pain in older persons. *Journal of American Geriatrics Society*, 50(Suppl.), S205–S224.

Ancheta, I. B., Carlson, J. M., Battie, C. A., Borja-Hart, N., Cogg, S., & Ancheta, C. V. (2015). One size does not fit all: Cardiovascular health disparities as a function of ethnicity in Asian-American women. *Applied Nursing Research*, 28(2), 99–105.

Aroian, K. J., & Wal, J. S. V. (2007). Measuring elders' symptoms with daily diaries and retrospective reports. *Western Journal of Nursing Research*, 29(3), 322–337.

Bialocerkowski, A., Klupp, N., & Bragge, P. (2010). Research methodology series: How to read and critically appraise a reliability article. *International Journal of Therapy & Rehabilitation*, 17(3), 114–120.

Borg, J., & Groenen, P. J. (2010). *Modern multidimensional scaling: Theory and application* (2nd ed.). New York, NY: Springer.

Brener, N. D., Kann, L., Kinchen, S. A., Grunbaum, J. A., Whalen, L., Eaton, D., et al. (2004). Methodology of the Youth Risk Behavior Surveillance System. *Morbidity & Mortality Weekly Report*, 53(RR–12), 1–13.

Brown, S. J. (2014). *Evidence-based nursing: The research-practice connection* (3rd ed.). Boston, MA: Jones & Bartlett.

Burman, M. E. (1995). Health diaries in nursing research and practice. *Image Journal of Nursing Scholarship*, 27(2), 147–152.

Cappelleri, J. C., Lundy, J. J., & Hays, R. D. (2014). Overview of classical test theory and item response theory for the quantitative assessment of items in developing patient-reported outcomes measures. *Clinical Therapeutics*, 36(5), 648–662.

Cazzell, M. (2010). *College student risk behavior: The implications of religiosity and impulsivity*. Ph.D. dissertation, The University of Texas at Arlington, United States: Texas. Proquest Dissertations & Theses. (Publication No. AAT 3391108).

Clinical and Laboratory Standards Institute. (CLSI, 2015). *Standards: Standards resources*. Retrieved July 15, 2015 from http://clsi.org/standards/about-our-standards/standards-resources/.

Cohen, M. Z., Thompson, C. B., Yates, B., Zimmerman, L., & Pullen, C. H. (2015). Implementing common data elements across studies to advance research. *Nursing Outlook*, 63(2), 181–188.

Couper, M. R. (1984). The Delphi technique: Characteristics and sequence model. *Advances in Nursing Science*, 7(1), 72–77.

Cowan, M. J., Heinrich, J., Lucas, M., Sigmon, H., & Hinshaw, A. S. (1993). Integration of biological and nursing sciences: A 10-year plan to enhance research and training. *Research in Nursing & Health*, 16(1), 3–9.

Coyne, J. C., Brown, G., Datto, C., Bruce, M. L., Schulberg, H. C., & Katz, I. (2001). The benefits of a broader perspective in case-finding for disease management of depression: Early lessons from the PROSPECT Study. *International Journal of Geriatric Psychiatry*, 16(6), 570–576.

Creswell, J. W. (2014). *Research design: Qualitative, quantitative, and mixed methods approaches* (4th ed.). Thousand Oaks, CA: Sage.

Department of Education Genomic Science. (2014). *Human Genome Project information Archive 1990–2003*. Retrieved July 6, 2015 from http://www.ornl.gov/sci/techresources/Human_Genome/home.shtml.

DeVon, H. A., Block, M. E., Moyle-Wright, P., Ernst, D. M., Hayden, S. J., Lazzara, D. J., et al. (2007). A psychometric toolbox for testing validity and reliability. *Journal of Nursing Scholarship*, *39*(2), 155–164.

Dillman, D. A., Smyth, J. D., & Christian, L. M. (2009). *Internet, mail, and mixed-mode surveys: The tailored design method*. Hoboken, NJ: John Wiley & Sons.

Doody, O., & Noonan, M. (2013). Preparing and conducting interviews to collect data. *Nurse Researcher*, *20*(5), 28–32.

Doran, D. M. (2011). *Nursing outcomes: The state of the science* (2nd ed.). Sudbury, MA: Jones & Bartlett.

Edelen, M. O., & Saliba, D. (2010). Correspondence of verbal descriptor and numeric rating scales for pain intensity: An item response theory calibration. *The Journals of Gerontology. Series A, Biological Sciences and Medical Sciences*, *65*(7), 778–785.

Finch, B. K., Kolody, B., & Vega, W. A. (2000). Perceived discrimination and depression among Mexican-origin adults in California. *Journal of Health and Social Behavior*, *41*(3), 295–313.

Froman, R. D. (2014). Editorial: The ins and outs of self-report response options and scales. *Research in Nursing & Health*, *37*(6), 447–451.

Gift, A. G. (1989). Visual analog scales: Measurement of subjective phenomena. *Nursing Research*, *38*(5), 286–288.

Gorden, R. L. (1998). *Basic interviewing skills*. Chicago, IL: Dorsey Press.

Green, A., Gance-Cleveland, B., Smith, A., Toly, V. B., Ely, E., & McDowell, B. M. (2014). Charting the course of pediatric nursing research: The SPN Delphi Study. *Journal of Pediatric Nursing*, *29*(5), 401–409.

Grove, S. K., & Cipher, D. (2017). *Statistics for nursing research: A workbook for evidence-based practice* (2nd ed.). St. Louis, MO: Saunders.

Hambleton, R. K., & Swaminathan, H. (2010). *Item response theory: Principles and applications*. Boston, MA: Kluwer Academic.

Harris, D. F. (2014). *The complete guide to writing questionnaires: How to get better information for better decisions*. Durham, NC: BW&A.

Herr, K. (2011). Pain assessment strategies in older patients. *Journal of Pain*, *12*(3 Suppl. 1), S3–S13.

Holden, A. E. C., Ramirez, A. G., & Gallion, K. (2014). Depressive symptoms in Latina breast cancer survivors: A barrier to cancer screening. *Health Psychology*, *33*(3), 242–248.

Hulin, C. L., Drasgow, F., & Parsons, C. K. (1983). *Item response theory: Application to psychological measurement*. Homewood, IL: Dow Jones-Irwin.

International Organization for Standardization. (ISO, 2015). *Standards development: How does ISO develop standards?* Retrieved July 15, 2015 from <http://www.iso.org/iso/standards_development.htm>.

Johantgen, M. (2010). Using existing administrative and national databases. In C. F. Waltz, O. L. Strickland, & E. R. Lenz (Eds.), *Measurement in nursing and health research* (4th ed., pp. 241–250). New York, NY: Springer.

Jones, J. M. (2004). Nutritional methodology: Development of a nutritional screening or assessment tool using a multivariate technique. *Nutrition (Burbank, Los Angeles County, Calif.)*, *20*(3), 298–306.

Keeney, S., Hasson, F., & McKenna, H. (2011). *The Delphi technique in nursing and health research*. Oxford, UK: Wiley-Blackwell.

Kim, H. G., Harrison, P. A., Godecker, A. L., & Muzyka, C. N. (2014). Posttraumatic stress disorder among women receiving prenatal care at three federally qualified health care centers. *Maternal Child Health Journal*, *18*(5), 1056–1065.

Klein, D. G., Dumpe, M., Katz, E., & Bena, J. (2010). Pain assessment in the intensive care unit: Development and psychometric testing of the nonverbal pain assessment tool. *Heart and Lung: The Journal of Critical Care*, *39*(6), 521–528.

Kubik, M. J., Permenter, T., & Saremian, J. (2015). Specimen age stability for human papilloma virus DNA testing using BD SurePath. *Lab Medicine*, *46*(1), 51–54.

Lee, K. A., & Kieckhefer, G. M. (1989). Measuring human responses using visual analogue scales. *Western Journal of Nursing Research*, *11*(1), 128–132.

Lim, M., Sacks-Davis, R., Aitken, C. K., Hocking, J. S., & Hellard, M. E. (2010). Randomized controlled trial of paper, online, and SMS diaries for collecting sexual behavior information from young people. *Journal of Epidemiology & Community Health*, *64*(10), 885–889.

Liu, H., & Chiu, S. (2015). The effectiveness of vitamin B_{12} for relieving pain in aphthous ulcers: A randomized, double-blind, placebo-controlled trial. *Pain Management Nursing*, *16*(3), 182–187.

Lynn, M. R. (1989). Instrument reliability: How much needs to be published? *Heart and Lung: The Journal of Critical Care*, *18*(4), 421–423.

Marshall, C., & Rossman, G. B. (2016). *Designing qualitative research* (6th ed.). Thousand Oaks, CA: Sage.

McKeown, B., & Thomas, D. (1988). *Q methodology*. Newbury Park, CA: Sage.

McPeake, J., Bateson, M., & O'Neill, A. (2014). Electronic surveys: How to maximize success. *Nurse Research*, *21*(3), 24–26.

Melnyk, B. M., & Fineout-Overholt, E. (2015). *Evidence-based practice in nursing & healthcare: A guide to best practice* (3rd ed.). Philadelphia, PA: Lippincott Williams & Wilkins.

Moon, C., Phelan, C. H., Lauver, D. R., & Bratzke, L. C. (2015). Is sleep quality related to cognition in individuals with heart failure? *Heart and Lung: The Journal of Critical Care*, *44*(3), 212–218.

National Institute of Nursing Research. (NINR, 2011). *About NINR: Mission & strategic plan*. Retrieved July 15, 2015 from http://www.ninr.nih.gov/aboutninr/ninr-mission-and-strategic-plan#.VabFp_lVhBc.

National Institute of Nursing Research. (NINR, 2016). *NINR: Summer Genetics Institute (SGI)*. Retrieved March 14, 2016 from http://www.ninr.nih.gov/training/trainingopportunities intramural/summergeneticsinstitute#.Vumd5OIrKUk.

Ng, K., Wong, S., Lim, S., & Goh, Z. (2010). Evaluation of the Cadi ThermoSENSOR wireless skin-contact thermometer against ear and axillary temperatures in children. *Journal of Pediatric Nursing, 25*(3), 176–186.

Nicholl, H. (2010). Diaries as a method of data collection in research. *Pediatric Nursing, 22*(7), 16–20.

Nunnally, J. C., & Bernstein, I. H. (1994). *Psychometric theory* (3rd ed.). New York, NY: McGraw-Hill.

Polit, D. R., & Yang, F. M. (2016). *Measurement and the measurement of change: A primer for the health professions.* Philadelphia, PA: Wolters Kluwer.

Radloff, L. S. (1977). The CES-D scale: A self-report depression scale for research in the general population. *Applied Psychological Measures, 1*(3), 385–394.

Radloff, L. S. (1991). The use of the Center for Epidemiologic Studies Depression Scale in adolescents and young adults. *Journal of Youth and Adolescence, 20*(2), 149–166.

Raven, E. E., Haverkamp, D., Sierevelt, I. N., Van Montfoort, D. O., Poll, R. G., Blankevoort, L., et al. (2008). Construct validity and reliability of the disability of arm, shoulder, and hand questionnaire for upper extremity complaints in rheumatoid arthritis. *Journal of Rheumatology, 35*(12), 2334–2338.

Rudy, E., & Grady, P. (2005). Biological researchers: Building nursing science. *Nursing Outlook, 53*(2), 88–94.

Ryan-Wenger, N. A. (2010). Evaluation of measurement precision, accuracy, and error in biophysical data for clinical research and practice. In C. F. Waltz, O. L. Strickland, & E. R. Lenz (Eds.), *Measurement in nursing and health research* (4th ed., pp. 371–383). New York, NY: Springer.

Saliba, D., & Buchanan, J. (2008). *Development and validation of a revised nursing home assessment tool: MDS 3.0.* Retrieved January 30, 2015, from http://www.cms.gov/Medicare/Quality-Initiatives-Patient-Assessment-Instruments/.NursingHomeQualityInits/downloads/MDS30FinalReport.pdf.

Saris, W. E., & Gallhofer, I. N. (2007). *Design, evaluation, and analysis of questionnaires for survey research.* Hoboken, NJ: John Wiley & Son.

Sennott-Miller, L., Murdaugh, C., & Hinshaw, A. S. (1988). Magnitude estimation: Issues and practical applications. *Western Journal of Nursing Research, 10*(4), 414–424.

Severinsson, E. (2012). Evaluation of the Manchester Clinical Supervision Scale: Norwegian and Swedish versions. *Journal of Nursing Management, 20*(1), 81–89.

Simpson, S. H. (1989). Use of Q-sort methodology in cross-cultural nutrition and health research. *Nursing Research, 38*(5), 289–290.

Spector, P. E. (1992). *Summated rating scale construction: An introduction.* Newbury Park, CA: Sage.

Stone, K. S., & Frazier, S. K. (2010). Measurement of physiological variables using biomedical instrumentation. In C. F. Waltz, O. L. Strickland, & E. R. Lenz (Eds.), *Measurement in nursing and health research* (4th ed., pp. 335–370). New York, NY: Springer.

Streiner, D. L., Norman, G. R., & Cairney, J. (2015). *Health measurement scales: A practical guide to their development and use* (5th ed.). Oxford, UK: University Press.

Tetting, D. W. (1988). Q-sort update. *Western Journal of Nursing Research, 10*(6), 757–765.

Thomas, S. J. (2004). *Using web and paper questionnaires for data-based decision making: From design to interpretation of the results.* Thousand Oaks, CA: Corwin Press.

Turner, C. F., Rogers, S. M., Hendershot, T. P., Miller, H. G., & Thornberry, J. P. (1996). Improving representation of linguistic minorities in health surveys. *Public Health Reports, 111*(3), 276–279.

U.S. Department of Health and Human Services. (2015). *Health information privacy.* Retrieved July 8, 2015 from http://www.hhs.gov/ocr/privacy/.

U.S. Preventative Task Force. (2002). *Screening for depression: Recommendations and rationale* (Vol. 2006). Rockville, MD: Agency for Healthcare Research and Quality.

Van Hooft, S. M., Dwarswaard, J., Jedeloo, S., Bal, R., & van Staa, A. (2015). Four perspectives on self-management support by nurses for people with chronic conditions: A Q-methodological study. *International Journal of Nursing Studies, 52*(1), 157–166.

Vernon, W. (2009). The Delphi technique: A review. *International Journal of Therapy & Rehabilitation, 16*(2), 69–76.

Waltz, C. F., Strickland, O. L., & Lenz, E. R. (2010). *Measurement in nursing and health research* (4th ed.). New York, NY: Springer.

Wewers, M. E., & Lowe, N. K. (1990). A critical review of visual analogue scales in the measurement of clinical phenomena. *Research in Nursing & Health, 13*(4), 227–236.

Wong-Baker FACES Foundation. (2015). *Wong-Baker FACES® Pain Rating Scale.* Retrieved July 1, 2015 with permission from http://www.wongbakerfaces.org/.

Critical Appraisal of Nursing Studies

Jennifer R. Gray, Susan K. Grove

ⓔ http://evolve.elsevier.com/Gray/practice/

Professional nurses continually strive for evidence-based practice (EBP), which includes critically appraising studies, synthesizing research findings, and applying sound scientific evidence in practice. Nurse researchers also critically appraise studies in a selected area, develop a summary of current knowledge, and identify areas for subsequent study. Thus, all nurses need skills in critically appraising research. The **critical appraisal of research** involves a systematic, unbiased, careful examination of all aspects of studies to judge their strengths, limitations, trustworthiness, meaning, and applicability to practice. This chapter provides a background for critically appraising studies in nursing and other healthcare disciplines. The expanding roles of nurses in conducting critical appraisals of research are addressed. Detailed guidelines are provided to direct you in critically appraising both quantitative and qualitative studies.

EVOLUTION OF CRITICAL APPRAISAL OF RESEARCH IN NURSING

The process for critically appraising research has evolved gradually in nursing from a few to now many nurses who are prepared to conduct comprehensive, scholarly critiques. Public research critiques, written or verbal, were rare before the 1970s, partially because of the harsh critiques that some nurse researchers endured in the 1940s and 1950s (Meleis, 2007). Nurses responding to research presentations in the 1960s and 1970s focused on the strengths of studies, and the weaknesses were minimized. Thus, the effects of the study limitations and other weaknesses on the quality, credibility, and meaning of studies were often lost.

Incomplete critique or the absence of critique may have served to encourage budding nurse researchers as they gained basic research skills. However, now comprehensive critical appraisals of research are essential to evaluate and synthesize knowledge for nursing (Fawcett & Garity, 2009; Knowles & Gray, 2011; Wintersgill & Wheeler, 2012). As a result of advances in the profession over the last 50 years, many nurses have the educational preparation and expertise to conduct critical appraisals of research. Nursing research textbooks, workshops, and conferences provide information on the critical appraisal process.

The critical appraisal of studies is essential for the development and refinement of nursing knowledge. Nurses examine the credibility and meaning of study findings by asking searching questions such as: Was the methodology of a study a valid choice for producing credible findings? Are the study findings trustworthy or an accurate reflection of reality? Do the findings increase our understanding of the nature of phenomena that are important in nursing? Are the findings from the present study consistent with those from previous studies? Are these studies' findings applicable to practice, theory, and/or knowledge development? The answers to these questions require careful examination of the research problem and purpose, the theoretical or philosophical basis of the study, the methodology, findings, and researcher's conclusions. Not only must the mechanics of conducting the study be evaluated, but also the abstract and logical reasoning the researchers used to plan and implement the study (Whiffin & Hasselder, 2013). If the reasoning process used to develop a study contains flaws, there are probably flaws in interpretation of the findings, decreasing the credibility of the study.

All studies have flaws; in fact, science itself is flawed. Science does not completely or perfectly describe, explain, predict, or control reality. However, improved understanding and an increased ability to predict and control phenomena depend on recognizing the weaknesses in studies and in science. In this chapter, **study weaknesses** are the errors or missteps that researchers consciously or unconsciously make in developing, implementing, and/or reporting studies. **Limitations** are specific types of study weaknesses that are reported by researchers, can reduce the quality of study findings; and in quantitative studies, reduce the ability to generalize findings. Study limitations might be identified before, during, or after a study is conducted; are identified in the research report; and are discussed in relationship to the study findings. All studies have limitations and most include weaknesses that are not addressed by the researchers. You must decide whether a study is flawed to the extent that the evidence is not credible and is inappropriate to use in a systematic review of knowledge in an area (Higgins & Green, 2008; Whittemore, Chao, Jang, Minges, & Park, 2014). Although we recognize that knowledge is not absolute, we need to have confidence in the research evidence synthesized for practice.

All studies have strengths as well as weaknesses. Recognition of these strengths is essential to the generation of sound research evidence for practice. If only weaknesses are identified, nurses might discount the value of all studies and refuse to invest time in reading and examining research. The continued work of researchers also depends on recognizing the strengths of their studies. The strong points of a study, added to the strong points from multiple other studies, slowly build solid research evidence for practice (Brown, 2014; Melnyk & Fineout-Overholt, 2015).

WHEN ARE CRITICAL APPRAISALS OF RESEARCH IMPLEMENTED IN NURSING?

In general, research is critically appraised to broaden understanding, summarize knowledge for practice, and provide a knowledge base for future studies. Critical appraisal allows the consumer of research to make an assessment of a study and determine its contribution to nursing. In addition, critical appraisals often are conducted after verbal presentations of studies, after publication of a research report, for an abstract section for a conference, for article selection for publication, and for evaluation of research proposals for implementation and funding. In these instances, they underscore or rebut the research's observations, analyses, syntheses, and conclusions. Nursing students, practicing nurses, nurse educators, and nurse researchers all need to be involved in the critical appraisal of research.

Critical Appraisal of Studies by Students

In nursing education, conducting a critical appraisal of a study is often seen as a first step in learning the research process. Part of learning this process is being able to read and comprehend published research reports. However, conducting a critical appraisal of a study is not a basic skill, and a firm grasp of the content presented in previous chapters is essential for implementing this process. Students usually acquire basic knowledge of the research process and critical appraisal skills early in their baccalaureate nursing education (Grove, Gray, & Burns, 2015). Advanced analysis skills usually are taught at the master's and doctoral levels (Knowles & Gray, 2011; Whiffin & Hasselder, 2013).

By performing critical appraisals, students expand their analysis skills, strengthen their knowledge base, and increase their use of research evidence in practice. The *Essentials of Master's Education in Nursing* (American Association of Colleges of Nursing [AACN], 2011) identifies the competencies that nurses prepared at the master's level should accomplish. One of these competencies is the ability to translate evidence for use in practice in striving for an EBP. The AACN Quality and Safety Education for Nurses (QSEN) Education Consortium (2012) also has a graduate-level competency focused on EBP. EBP requires critical appraisal and synthesis of study findings for practice (Sherwood & Barnsteiner, 2012). Therefore, critical appraisal of studies is an important part of your education and your practice as a nurse.

Critical Appraisal of Research by Practicing Nurses

Practicing nurses must appraise studies critically so that their practice is based on current research evidence and not merely tradition, supplemented by trial and error (Melnyk & Fineout-Overholt, 2015; Spruce, van Wicklin, Hicks, Conner, & Dunn, 2014). Nursing actions must be updated in response to the current evidence, generated through research. Practicing nurses need to formulate strategies for remaining current in their practice areas. Reading research journals, discussing study findings on a social media site, and posting or sharing current studies with peers can increase nurses' awareness of study findings but are insufficient for the purposes of critical appraisal. Nurses need to question the quality of studies and the credibility of findings and share their concerns with other nurses. For example, nurses may form a research journal club in which studies are presented and critically appraised by members of the group (Fothergill & Lipp, 2014; Gloeckner & Robinson, 2010). Skills in critical appraisal of research enable practicing nurses to synthesize the most credible, significant, and appropriate evidence for use in their practice. EBP is essential in healthcare agencies either seeking or maintaining Magnet status. The Magnet Recognition Program® was developed by the American Nurses Credentialing Center (ANCC, 2015) to recognize healthcare organizations that provide nursing excellence with care based on the most current research evidence.

Critical Appraisal of Research by Nurse Educators

Educators critically appraise research to expand their knowledge for practice and to develop and refine the educational process. The careful analysis of current nursing studies provides a basis for updating curriculum content for use in clinical and classroom settings. Educators influence students' perceptions of research and act as role models for their students by examining new studies, evaluating the information obtained from research, and indicating what research evidence to use in practice (Tsai, Cheng, Chang, & Liou, 2014). In addition, educators may conduct or collaborate with others to conduct studies, which require critical appraisal of previous relevant research.

Critical Appraisal of Studies by Nurse Researchers

Nurse researchers critically appraise previous research to plan and implement their next study. Many researchers have programs of research in selected areas, and they update their knowledge base by critiquing new studies in these areas. The outcomes of these appraisals influence the selection of research problems and purposes, the implementation of research methodologies, and the interpretations of study findings.

Critical Appraisal of Research Presentations and Publications

Critical appraisals following research presentations can assist researchers in identifying the strengths and weaknesses of their studies and generating ideas for further research. Experiencing the critical appraisal process can increase the ability of participants to evaluate studies and judge the usefulness of the research evidence for practice. Participants listening to study critiques might also gain insight into the conduct of research.

The nursing research journals *Scholarly Inquiry for Nursing Practice: An International Journal* and *Western Journal of Nursing Research* include commentaries after the research articles. In these journals, other researchers critically appraise the authors' studies, and the authors have a chance to respond to these comments. Published research critical appraisals often increase the reader's understanding of the study and the quality of the study findings (American Psychological Association [APA], 2010; Pyrczak, 2008). Another, more informal critique of a published study might appear in a letter to the editor, in which readers have the opportunity to comment on the strengths and weaknesses of published studies by writing to the journal editor.

Critical Appraisal of Abstracts for Conference Presentations

One of the most difficult types of critical appraisal is examining abstracts. The amount of information available usually is limited because many abstracts are restricted to 100 to 250 words. Nevertheless, reviewers must select the best-designed studies with the most significant outcomes for presentation at professional conferences. This process requires an experienced researcher who needs few cues to determine the quality of a study. Critical appraisal of an abstract usually addresses the following criteria: (1) appropriateness of the study for the program; (2) completeness of the research project; (3) overall quality of the study problem, purpose, methodology, results, and findings; (4) contribution of the study to the knowledge base of nursing; (5) contribution of the study to nursing theory; (6) originality of the work (not previously published); (7) implication of the study findings for practice; and (8) clarity, conciseness, and completeness of the abstract (APA, 2010).

Critical Appraisal of Research Articles for Publication

Nurse researchers who serve as peer reviewers for professional journals evaluate the quality of research articles submitted for publication. The role of these scientists is to ensure that the studies accepted for publication are well designed and contribute to the body of knowledge. Most of these reviews are conducted anonymously so that relationships or reputations do not interfere with the selection process. In most refereed journals, the experts who examine the research report have been selected from an established group of peer reviewers. Their comments or summaries of their comments are sent to the researcher. The editor also uses these comments to make selections for publication. The process for publishing a study is described in Chapter 27.

Critical Appraisal of Research Proposals

Critical appraisals of research proposals are conducted to approve student research projects; to permit data collection in an institution; and to select the best studies for funding by local, state, national, and international organizations and agencies. The process researchers use to seek the approval to conduct a study is presented in Chapter 28. The peer review process in federal funding agencies involves an extremely complex critical appraisal. Nurses are involved in this level of research review through the national funding agencies, such as the National Institute of Nursing Research (NINR, 2015), National Institutes of Health, and the Agency for Healthcare Research and Quality (AHRQ, 2015). Some of the criteria used to evaluate the quality of a proposal for possible funding include the (1) significance of the research problem and purpose for nursing, (2) appropriate use of methodology for the types of questions that the research is designed to answer, (3) appropriate use and interpretation of analysis procedures, (4) evaluation of clinical practice and forecasting of the need for nursing or other appropriate interventions, (5) construction of models to direct the research and interpret the findings, and (6) innovativeness of the study. The NINR (2015) website (http://www.ninr.nih.gov/researchandfunding#.VPNdkvnF-Ck) provides details on grant development and research funding (see Chapter 29 on seeking funding for research).

NURSES' EXPERTISE IN CRITICAL APPRAISAL OF RESEARCH

Conducting a critical appraisal of a study is a complex mental process that is stimulated by raising questions. The three major steps for critical appraisal included in this text are (1) identifying the elements or processes of the study; (2) determining the study strengths and weaknesses; and (3) evaluating the credibility, trustworthiness, and meaning of the study (Box 18-1). The level of critique conducted is influenced by the sophistication of the individual appraising the study (Table 18-1). The initial critical appraisal of research by an undergraduate student often involves the identification of the elements or steps of the research process in a quantitative study.

BOX 18-1 **Critical Appraisal Guidelines for Quantitative and Qualitative Studies**

1. Identifying the elements or processes of the study
2. Determining the study strengths and weaknesses
3. Evaluating the credibility, trustworthiness, and meaning of the study

---

TABLE 18-1 **Educational Level With Associated Expertise in Critical Appraisal of Research**

Educational Level	Expertise in Critical Appraisal of Research
Baccalaureate	Identify the steps of the quantitative research process in a study. Identify the elements of a qualitative study.
Master's	Determine study strengths and weaknesses in quantitative, qualitative, mixed methods, and outcomes studies. Evaluate the credibility, trustworthiness, and meaning of a study and its contribution to nursing knowledge and practice.
Doctorate or postdoctorate	Synthesize multiple studies in systematic reviews, meta-analyses, meta-syntheses, and mixed methods systematic reviews.

Some baccalaureate programs offer more in-depth research courses that also include critical appraisals of the processes of qualitative studies (Grove et al., 2015).

A critical appraisal of research conducted by a student at the master's level usually involves description of study strengths and weaknesses and evaluation of the credibility and meaning of the study findings for nursing knowledge and practice (see Table 18-1). Critical appraisals by master's-level students and practicing nurses focus on a variety of studies, such as quantitative, qualitative, mixed methods, and outcomes studies.

At the doctoral level, students often critically appraise several studies in an area of interest and perform a complex synthesis of the research findings to determine the current empirical knowledge base for the phenomenon (see Table 18-1). These complex syntheses of quantitative, qualitative, mixed methods, and outcomes research include (1) systematic review of research, (2) meta-analysis, (3) meta-synthesis, and (4) mixed methods systematic review (Whittemore et al., 2014). These summaries of current research evidence are essential for providing EBP and directing future research (Craig & Smyth, 2012; Higgins & Green, 2008; Sandelowski & Barroso, 2007). Definitions of these types of complex syntheses are presented in Chapter 2, and Chapter 19 provides guidelines for critically appraising and conducting these research syntheses.

The major focus of this chapter is conducting critical appraisals of quantitative and qualitative studies using the steps previously discussed and outlined in Box 18-1. Critical appraisals of quantitative and qualitative studies involve implementing key principles that are outlined in Box 18-2. These principles stress the importance of examining the expertise of the authors; reviewing the entire study; addressing the strengths and weaknesses of the study; evaluating the credibility, trustworthiness, and meaning of the study findings; determining the usefulness or applicability of the findings for practice; and facilitating the conduct of future research (Creswell, 2013, 2014; Doran, 2011; Fawcett & Garity, 2009; Fothergill & Lipp, 2014; Marshall & Rossman, 2016; Miles, Huberman, & Saldaña, 2014; Morse, 2012; Munhall, 2012; Shadish, Cook, & Campbell, 2002; Tonelli, 2012; Whiffin & Hasselder, 2013). These key principles provide a basis for the critical appraisal process for quantitative research that is discussed in the next section and the critical appraisal process for qualitative research discussed later in this chapter.

CRITICAL APPRAISAL PROCESS FOR QUANTITATIVE RESEARCH

As you critically appraise studies, follow the steps of the **critical appraisal process** presented in Box 18-1. These steps occur in sequence, vary in depth, and presume accomplishment of the preceding steps. However, an individual with critical appraisal experience frequently performs multiple steps of this process simultaneously. This section includes the three steps of the research critical appraisal process applied to quantitative studies and provides relevant questions for each step. These questions are not comprehensive but have been selected as a means for stimulating the logical reasoning and analysis necessary for conducting a study review. Persons experienced in the critical appraisal process formulate additional questions as part of their reasoning processes. We cover the identification of the steps or elements of the research process separately because persons who are

---

BOX 18-2 Key Principles for Critical Appraisal of Research

1. *Examine the research, clinical, and educational background of the authors.* The authors need a scientific and clinical background that is appropriate for the study conducted.
2. *Examine the organization and presentation of the research report.* The title of the research report needs to identify the focus of the study. The report usually includes an abstract, introduction, methods, results, discussion, and references. The abstract of the study needs to present the purpose of the study clearly and to highlight the methodology and major study results and findings. The body of the research report should be complete, concise, logically organized, and clearly presented. The references need to be complete and presented in a consistent format (APA, 2010).
3. *Read and critically appraise the entire study.* A research appraisal involves examining the quality of all aspects of the research report (see Box 18-1 and the critical appraisal guidelines provided throughout this chapter).
4. *Examine the significance of the problem studied for nursing practice and knowledge.* The foci of nursing studies need to be on the generation of quality knowledge to promote evidence-based practice.
5. *As you identify the strengths and weaknesses of the study, provide specific examples of and rationales for the identified strengths and weaknesses of a study.* Address the quality of the problem, purpose, theoretical or philosophical basis, methodology, results, and findings of quantitative and qualitative studies. Include examples and rationales for your critical appraisal and document your ideas with sources from the current literature. This strengthens the quality of your critical appraisal and documents the use of critical thinking skills.
6. *If you determine that the study resulted in valid and trustworthy findings, examine the usefulness or transferability of the findings to practice.* The findings for a study need to be linked with the findings from previous research and examined for use in practice.
7. *Suggest ideas and modifications for future studies.* Identify ideas and modifications for future studies to increase the strengths and decrease the limitations and other weaknesses of the current study.

new to critical appraisal often only conduct this step. The questions for determining the study strengths and weaknesses are covered together because this process occurs simultaneously in the mind of the person conducting the critical appraisal. Evaluation is covered separately because of the increased expertise needed to perform this final step.

Step I: Identifying the Steps of the Quantitative Research Process in Studies

Initial attempts to comprehend research articles are often frustrating because the terminology and stylized manner of the report are unfamiliar. Identification of the steps of the research process in a quantitative study is the first step in critical appraisal. It involves understanding the terms and concepts in the report; identifying study elements; and grasping the nature, significance, and meaning of the study elements. The following guidelines are presented to direct you in the initial critical appraisal of a quantitative study.

Guidelines for Identifying the Steps of the Quantitative Research Process

The first step involves reviewing the study title and abstract and reading the study from beginning to end (review the key principles in Box 18-2). As you read, address the following questions about the research report: Was the writing style of the report clear and concise? Were the different parts of the research report plainly identified (APA, 2010)? Were relevant terms defined? You might underline the terms you do not understand and determine their meaning from the glossary at the end of this textbook. Read the article a second time and highlight or underline each step of the quantitative research process. An overview of these steps is presented in Chapter 3. To write a critical appraisal identifying the study steps, you need to identify each step concisely and respond briefly to the following guidelines and questions:

    I. Introduction
        A. Describe the qualifications of the authors to conduct the study, such as research expertise, clinical experience, and educational preparation. Doctoral education, such as a PhD, and postdoctorate training provide experiences in conducting research. Have the researchers conducted previous studies, especially studies in this area? Are the authors involved in clinical practice or certified in their area of clinical expertise (Fothergill & Lipp, 2014)?
        B. Discuss the clarity of the article title (variables and population identified). Does the

title indicate the general type of study conducted—descriptive, correlational, quasi-experimental, or experimental (Shadish et al., 2002)?
        C. Discuss the quality of the abstract. An abstract should include the study purpose, design, sample, intervention (if applicable), and results; and highlight key findings (APA, 2010).
    II. State the problem (see Chapter 5).
        A. Significance of the problem
        B. Background of the problem
        C. Problem statement
    III. State the purpose (see Chapter 5).
    IV. Examine the literature review (see Chapter 7).
        A. Were relevant previous studies and theories described?
        B. Were the references current? (Number and percentage of sources in the last 10 years and in the last 5 years?)
        C. Were the studies described, critically appraised, and synthesized (Fawcett & Garity, 2009; Hoe & Hoare, 2012)?
        D. Was a summary provided of the current knowledge (what is known and not known) about the research problem (Wakefield, 2014)?
    V. Examine the study framework or theoretical perspective (see Chapter 8).
        A. Was the framework explicitly expressed, or must the reviewer extract the framework from implicit statements in the introduction or literature review?
        B. Is the framework based on tentative, substantive, or scientific theory? Provide a rationale for your answer.
        C. Did the framework identify, define, and describe the relationships among the concepts of interest? Provide examples of this.
        D. Is a model (diagram) of the framework provided for clarity? If a model is not presented, develop one that represents the framework of the study and describe it.
        E. Link the study variables to the relevant concepts in the model.
        F. How was the framework related to the body of knowledge of nursing (Smith & Liehr, 2013)?
    VI. List any research objectives, questions, or hypotheses (see Chapter 6).
    VII. Identify and define (conceptually and operationally) the study variables or concepts that

were identified in the objectives, questions, or hypotheses. If objectives, questions, or hypotheses were not stated, identify and define the variables in the study purpose and the results section of the study. If conceptual definitions were not included, identify possible definitions for each major study variable. Indicate which of the following types of variables were included in the study. A study usually includes independent and dependent variables or research variables but not all three types of variables.

   A. Independent variables: Identify and define conceptually and operationally.

   B. Dependent variables: Identify and define conceptually and operationally.

   C. Research variables or concepts: Identify and define conceptually and operationally.

VIII. Identify demographic variables and other relevant terms.

  IX. Identify the research design.

   A. Identify the specific design of the study. Draw a model of the design by using the sample design models presented in Chapters 10 and 11.

   B. Did the study include a treatment or intervention (see Chapter 11)? If so, is the treatment clearly described with a protocol and consistently implemented, which indicates intervention fidelity (Forbes, 2009; Mittlbock, 2008; Morrison et al., 2009)?

   C. If the study had more than one group, how were subjects assigned to groups (Kerlinger & Lee, 2000; Shadish et al., 2002)?

   D. Were extraneous variables identified and controlled for by the design or methods? Extraneous variables usually are discussed in research reports of quasi-experimental and experimental studies (Shadish et al., 2002).

   E. Were pilot study findings used to design this study? If yes, briefly discuss the pilot and the changes made in the study based on the pilot.

  X. Describe the population, sample, and setting (see Chapter 15).

   A. Identify inclusion or exclusion sample or eligibility criteria that designate the target population.

   B. Identify the specific type of probability or nonprobability sampling method that was used to obtain the sample. Did the researchers identify the sampling frame for the study (Kandola, Banner, Okeefe-McCarthy, & Jassal, 2014; Thompson, 2002)?

   C. Identify the sample size. Discuss the refusal rate and include the rationale for refusal if presented in the article. Discuss the power analysis if this process was used to determine sample size (Aberson, 2010; Cohen, 1988).

   D. Identify the sample attrition (number and percentage). Was a rationale provided for the study attrition?

   E. Identify the characteristics of the sample.

   F. Discuss the institutional review board approval. Describe the informed consent process used in the study (see Chapter 9).

   G. Identify the study setting, and indicate whether it is appropriate for the study purpose.

  XI. Identify and describe each measurement strategy used in the study (see Chapters 16 and 17). The following information should be provided for each measurement method included in a study. Identify each study variable that was measured and link it to a measurement method(s).

   A. Identify the name and author of each measurement strategy.

   B. Identify the type of each measurement strategy (e.g., Likert scale, visual analog scale, and physiological measure).

   C. Identify the level of measurement (nominal, ordinal, interval, or ratio) achieved by each measurement method used in the study (Grove & Cipher, 2017).

   D. Describe the reliability of each scale for previous studies, for this study, and for the pilot study if one was performed. Identify the precision of each physiological measure (Bartlett & Frost, 2008; Bialocerkowski, Klupp, & Bragge, 2010; DeVon et al., 2007; Polit & Yang, 2016).

   E. Identify the validity of each scale and the accuracy of physiological measures (DeVon et al., 2007; Ryan-Wenger, 2010).

   F. If data for the study were obtained from an existing database, did the researchers identify how, where, when, and by whom the original data were collected?

The following table includes the critical information about two measurement methods, the Beck Likert scale to measure depression and the physiological instrument to measure blood pressure. Completing this table allows you to identify essential measurement content for a study (Waltz, Strickland, & Lenz, 2010).

Variable Measured	Name of Measurement Method/ Author	Type of Measurement Method	Level of Measurement	Reliability or Precision	Validity or Accuracy
Depression level	Beck Depression Inventory/ Beck	Likert scale	Interval	Cronbach alpha of 0.82–0.92 from previous studies and 0.84 for this study. Reading level at 6th grade.	Content validity from concept analysis, literature review, and reviews of experts. Construct validity: Convergent validity with Zung Depression Scale. Factor validity from previous research. Successive use validity with previous studies and this study. Criterion-related validity: Predictive validity of patients' future depressive episodes.
Blood pressure (BP)	Omron BP equipment: Healthcare Equipment Company	Physiological measurement method	Ratio	Test-retest values of BP measurements in previous studies. BP equipment new and recalibrated every 50 BP readings in this study. Average three BP readings to determine average BP.	Documented accuracy of systolic and diastolic BPs to 1 mm Hg by company developing Omron BP cuff. Designated protocol for taking BP. Average three BP readings to determine average BP.

XII. Describe the procedures for data collection and management (see Chapter 20).

XIII. Describe the statistical techniques performed to analyze study data (see Chapters 21, 22, 23, 24, and 25).

    A. List the statistical procedures conducted to describe the sample.

    B. Was the level of significance or alpha identified? If so, indicate what it was (0.05, 0.01, or 0.001).

    C. Complete the following table with the analysis techniques conducted in the study: (1) identify the focus (description, relationships, or differences) for each analysis technique; (2) list the statistical analysis technique performed; (3) list the statistic; (4) provide the specific results; and (5) identify the probability (p) of the statistical significance achieved by the result (Gaskin & Happell, 2014; Grove & Cipher, 2017; Hayat, Higgins, Schwartz, & Staggs, 2015; Hoare & Hoe, 2013; Plichta & Kelvin, 2013).

Purpose of Analysis	Analysis Technique	Statistic	Results	Probability (p)
Description of Subjects' Pulse Rate	Mean	M	71.52	NA
	Standard deviation	SD	5.62	NA
	Range	Range	58–97	NA
Difference between men and women in systolic and diastolic blood pressures respectively	t-test t-test	t t	3.75 2.16	0.001 0.042
Differences of diet group, exercise group, and comparison group for pounds lost by adolescents	Analysis of variance	F	4.27	0.04
Relationship of depression and anxiety in elderly adults	Pearson correlation	r	0.46	0.03

XIV. Describe the researcher's interpretation of the study findings (see Chapter 26).
  A. Are the findings related back to the study framework? If so, do the findings support the study framework?
  B. Which findings are consistent with the expected findings?
  C. Which findings were not expected?
  D. Are the findings consistent with previous research findings (Fawcett & Garity, 2009; Tonelli, 2012)?
XV. What study limitations did the researcher identify?
XVI. How did the researcher generalize the findings?
XVII. What were the implications of the findings for nursing?
XVIII. What suggestions for further study were identified?
XIX. Was the researcher's description of the study design and methods sufficiently clear for replication?

Step II: Determining Study Strengths and Weaknesses

The next step in critically appraising a quantitative study requires determining the strengths and weaknesses of the study (see Box 18-1). To do this, you must have knowledge of what each step of the research process should be like from expert sources such as this textbook and other research sources (Aberson, 2010; Bartlett & Frost, 2008; Bialocerkowski et al., 2010; Borglin & Richards, 2010; Creswell, 2014; DeVon et al., 2007; Fawcett & Garity, 2009; Forbes, 2009; Fothergill & Lipp, 2014; Gaskin & Happell, 2014; Grove & Cipher, 2017; Hoe & Hoare, 2012; Hoare & Hoe, 2013; Morrison et al., 2009; Polit & Yang, 2016; Ryan-Wenger, 2010; Shadish et al.,

2002; Tonelli, 2012; Wakefield, 2014; Waltz et al., 2010; Whiffin & Hasselder, 2013). Another source for critical appraisal of research is the Critical Appraisal Skills Programme (CASP) that was developed in the United Kingdom with critical appraisal checklists provided online at http://www.casp-uk.net/#!casp-tools -checklists/c18f8 (CASP, 2013). The ideal ways to conduct the steps of the research process are compared with the actual study steps. During this comparison, you examine the extent to which the researcher followed the rules for an ideal study and identify the study elements that are strengths or weaknesses. Your critical appraisal comments need to be supported with documentation from research sources.

You also need to examine the logical links connecting one study element with another. For example, the problem needs to provide background and direction for the statement of the purpose. In addition, you need to examine the overall flow of logic in the study. The variables identified in the study purpose need to be consistent with the variables identified in the research objectives, questions, or hypotheses. The variables identified in the research objectives, questions, or hypotheses need to be conceptually defined in light of the study framework. The conceptual definitions provide the basis for the development of operational definitions. The study design and analyses need to be appropriate for the investigation of the study purpose and for the specific objectives, questions, or hypotheses (Fawcett & Garity, 2009; Fothergill & Lipp, 2014). Many study weaknesses result from breaks in logical reasoning. For example, biases caused by sampling, measurement methods, and the selected design impair the logical flow from design to interpretation of findings (Borglin & Richards, 2010). The previous level of critical appraisal addressed concrete aspects of the study. During analysis, the process moves to examining abstract dimensions of the study, which requires greater familiarity with the logic behind the research process and increased skill in critical thinking (Whiffin & Hasselder, 2013).

You also need to gain a sense of how clearly the researcher grasped the study situation and expressed it. The clarity of the researchers' explanation of study elements demonstrates their skill in using and expressing ideas that require abstract reasoning. With this examination of the study, you can determine which aspects of the study are strengths and which are weaknesses and provide rationale and documentation for your decisions.

Guidelines for Determining Study Strengths and Weaknesses

The following questions were developed to assist you in examining the different aspects of a study and determining whether they are strengths or weaknesses. The intent is not to answer each of these questions but to read the questions and make judgments about the elements or steps in the study. You need to provide a rationale for your decisions and document from relevant research sources such as those listed in the previous section and in the references at the end of this chapter. For example, you might decide the study purpose is a strength because it addresses the study problem, clarifies the focus of the study, and is feasible to investigate (Fawcett & Garity, 2009; Fothergill & Lipp, 2014).

I. Research problem and purpose
   A. Was the problem sufficiently delimited in scope so that it is researchable but not trivial?
   B. Is the problem significant to nursing (Brown, 2014)?
   C. Does the purpose narrow and clarify the focus of the study? Does the purpose clearly address the gap in the nursing knowledge?
   D. Was this study feasible to conduct in terms of money commitment; the researchers' expertise; availability of subjects, facilities, and equipment; and ethical considerations?

II. Review of literature
   A. Was the literature review organized to show the progressive development of evidence from previous research?
   B. Was a theoretical knowledge base developed for the problem and purpose?
   C. Was a clear, concise summary presented of the current empirical and theoretical knowledge in the area of the study (CASP, 2013; Craig & Smyth, 2012; Fawcett & Garity, 2009; Wakefield, 2014)?

D. Did the literature review summary identify what was known and not known about the research problem, at the beginning of the study process, and provide direction for the formation of the research purpose?

III. Study framework
   A. Is the framework presented with clarity? If a model or conceptual map of the framework is present, is it adequate for explaining the phenomenon of concern?
   B. Is the framework linked to the research purpose? If not, would another framework fit more logically with the study?
   C. Is the framework related to the body of knowledge in nursing and clinical practice at the time the study was conducted?
   D. If a proposition or relationship from a theory is to be tested, is the proposition clearly identified and linked to the study hypotheses (Fawcett & Garity, 2009; Smith & Liehr, 2013)?

IV. Research objectives, questions, or hypotheses
   A. Were the objectives, questions, or hypotheses expressed clearly?
   B. Were the objectives, questions, or hypotheses logically linked to the research purpose (Fothergill & Lipp, 2014)?
   C. Were hypotheses stated to direct the conduct of quasi-experimental and experimental research (Kerlinger & Lee, 2000; Shadish et al., 2002)?
   D. Were the objectives, questions, or hypotheses logically linked to the concepts and relationships (propositions) in the framework (Fawcett & Garity, 2009; Smith & Liehr, 2013)?

V. Variables
   A. Were the variables reflective of the concepts identified in the framework?
   B. Were the variables clearly defined (conceptually and operationally) and based on previous research or theories (Fothergill & Lipp, 2014; Smith & Liehr, 2013)?
   C. Is the conceptual definition of a variable consistent with the operational definition?
   D. Did the operational definitions capture both the concept and the breadth of its manifestations in the population of interest?

VI. Design
   A. Was the design used in the study the most appropriate design to obtain the needed data (Creswell, 2014; Hoe & Hoare, 2012; Shadish et al., 2002)?

B. Did the design provide a means to examine all of the objectives, questions, or hypotheses?

C. Was the treatment clearly described (Forbes, 2009)? Was the treatment appropriate for examining the study purpose and hypotheses? Did the study framework explain the links between the treatment (independent variable) and the proposed outcomes (dependent variables)?

D. Was a protocol developed to promote consistent implementation of the treatment to ensure intervention fidelity? Did the researcher monitor implementation of the treatment to ensure consistency? If the treatment was not consistently implemented, what might be the impact on the findings (Morrison et al., 2009)?

E. Did the researcher identify the threats to design validity (statistical conclusion validity, internal validity, construct validity, and external validity) and minimize them as much as possible? What threats to internal validity were actually controlled for in the design phase, and in what ways? (see Chapters 10 and 11; Shadish et al., 2002)?

F. Was the design logically linked to the sampling method and statistical analyses?

G. If more than one group is included in the study, do the groups appear equivalent?

H. If a treatment was implemented, were subjects randomly assigned to the treatment group, or were the treatment and comparison groups dependent? Were the treatment and comparison group assignments appropriate for the purpose of the study (Borglin & Richards, 2010)?

I. If a quasi-experimental design was implemented instead of an experimental one, was the decision justified by the researcher?

VII. Sample, population, and setting

A. Was the sampling method adequate for producing a sample that was representative of the target population (Kandola et al., 2014)?

B. If random sampling was employed, was the type of sample actually obtained representative of the accessible population?

C. What were the potential biases in the sampling method? Were any subjects excluded from the study because of age, socioeconomic status, or ethnicity without a sound rationale (Borglin & Richards, 2010; Thompson, 2002)?

D. Did the sample include an understudied or vulnerable population, such as young, elderly, pregnant, or minority subjects?

E. Were the sampling criteria (inclusion and exclusion) appropriate for the type of study conducted?

F. Was the sample size sufficient to avoid a Type II error? Was a power analysis conducted to determine sample size? If a power analysis was conducted, were the results of the analysis clearly described and used to determine the final sample size? Was the attrition rate projected in determining the final sample size (Aberson, 2010; Cohen, 1988)?

G. Were the rights of human subjects protected?

H. Was the setting used in the study typical of actual clinical settings (Borglin & Richards, 2010)?

I. What was the refusal rate for the study? If it was greater than 20%, how might this have affected the representativeness of the sample? Did the researchers provide rationale for the refusals?

J. What was the attrition rate for the study? Did the researchers provide a rationale for the attrition of study participants? How did attrition influence the final sample and the study results and findings (Cohen, 1988; Fawcett & Garity, 2009)?

VIII. Measurements

A. Did the measurement methods selected for the study adequately measure the study variables (Polit & Yang, 2016; Waltz et al., 2010)?

B. Were the measurement methods sufficiently sensitive for detection of small differences between subjects? Should additional measurement methods have been used to improve the quality of the study outcomes (Waltz et al., 2010)?

C. Did the measurement methods used in the study have adequate validity and reliability? What additional reliability or validity testing might have improved the quality of the measurement methods (Bartlett & Frost, 2008; Bialocerkowski et al., 2010; DeVon et al., 2007)?

D. Respond to the following questions, which are relevant to the measurement approaches used in the study:

1. Scales and questionnaires
   (a) Were the instruments clearly described?
   (b) Were techniques for completion and scoring of the instruments provided?
   (c) Were validity and reliability of the instruments described (DeVon et al., 2007)?

(d) Did the researcher reexamine the validity and reliability of instruments for the present sample?

(e) If an instrument was developed for the study, was the instrument development process described (Waltz et al., 2010)?

2. Observation

(a) Were the entities that were to be observed clearly identified and defined?

(b) Was interrater reliability described?

(c) Were the techniques for recording observations described (Waltz et al., 2010)?

3. Interviews

(a) Did the interview questions address concerns expressed in the research problem?

(b) Were the interview questions relevant for the research purpose and objectives, questions, or hypotheses?

(c) Did the design of the questions tend to bias subjects' responses?

(d) Did the sequence of questions tend to bias subjects' responses (Waltz et al., 2010)?

4. Physiological measures

(a) Were the physiological measures clearly described (Ryan-Wenger, 2010)? If appropriate, are the brand names, such as Hewlett-Packard, of instruments identified?

(b) Were the accuracy, precision, and error of physiological instruments discussed (Ryan-Wenger, 2010)?

(c) Were the physiological measures appropriate for the research purpose and objectives, questions, or hypotheses?

(d) Were the methods for recording data from physiological measures clearly described? Was the recording of data consistent?

IX. Data collection

A. Was the data collection process clearly described?

B. Were the forms used to collect data organized to facilitate computerizing the data? Did the subjects enter their data into a computer?

C. Was the training of data collectors clearly described and adequate?

D. Was the data collection process conducted in a consistent manner (Borglin & Richards, 2010)?

E. Were the data collection methods ethical?

F. Did the data collected address the research objectives, questions, or hypotheses?

G. Did any adverse events occur during data collection? If adverse events occurred, were these appropriately managed?

X. Data analysis

A. Were data analysis procedures appropriate for the type of data collected (Grove & Cipher, 2017; Hayat et al., 2015; Plichta & Kelvin, 2013)?

B. Were data analysis procedures clearly described? Did the researcher address any problems with missing data and how this problem was managed?

C. Did the data analysis techniques address the study purpose and the research objectives, questions, or hypotheses?

D. Were the results presented in an understandable way by narrative, tables, or figures, or a combination of methods (APA, 2010; Hoare & Hoe, 2013)?

E. Were the statistical analyses logically linked to the design?

F. Is the sample size sufficient to detect significant differences if they are present (Gaskin & Happell, 2014)?

G. Were the results interpreted appropriately?

XI. Interpretation of findings

A. Were findings discussed in relation to each objective, question, or hypothesis?

B. Were various explanations for significant and nonsignificant findings examined?

C. Were the findings clinically significant (Gatchel & Mayer, 2010; Tonelli, 2012)?

D. Were the findings linked to the study framework?

E. Were the study findings an accurate reflection of reality and valid for use in clinical practice?

F. Did the conclusions fit the results from the data analyses? Were the conclusions based on statistically significant and clinically important results?

G. Did the study have weaknesses not identified by the researcher?

H. Did the researcher generalize the findings appropriately?

I. Were the identified implications for practice appropriate, based on the study findings and the findings from previous research (Wintersgill & Wheeler, 2012)?

J. Were quality suggestions made for further research?

Step III: Evaluating a Study

Evaluation involves determining the credibility, trustworthiness, meaning, and usefulness of the study findings. This type of critical appraisal requires more advanced skills and might be performed by master's and doctoral level students in determining current nursing knowledge and its usefulness in practice. Evaluating research involves summarizing the quality of the research process and findings, determining the consistency of the findings with those from previous studies, and determining the usefulness of the findings for practice. The steps of the study are evaluated in light of previous studies, such as an evaluation of present hypotheses based on previous hypotheses, present design based on previous designs, and present methods of measuring variables based on previous methods of measurement. Evaluation builds on conclusions reached during the first two stages of the critical appraisal so that the credibility, meaning, trustworthiness, and usefulness of the study findings can be determined for nursing knowledge, theory, and practice.

Guidelines for Evaluating a Study

You need to reexamine the discussion section of the study focusing on the study findings, conclusions, implications for practice, and suggestions for further study. It is important for you to read previous studies conducted in the area to determine the quality, credibility, and meaning of the study based on previous research. Using the following questions as a guide, summarize your evaluation of the study, and document your responses.

I. Did the study build upon previous research problems, purposes, designs, samples, and measurement methods? Provide examples to support your comments.

II. Could the weaknesses of the study have been corrected? How might that have been accomplished?

III. When the findings are examined in light of previous studies, do the findings build on previous findings?

IV. Do you believe the study findings are credible? How much confidence can be placed in the study findings (Tonelli, 2012)?

V. Based on this study and the findings from previous research, what is now known and not known about the phenomenon under study?

VI. To what populations can the findings be generalized (Cohen, 1988)?

VII. Were the implications of the findings for practice discussed? Based on previous research, are the findings ready for use in practice (Melnyk & Fineout-Overholt, 2015)?

VIII. Were relevant studies suggested for future research?

CRITICAL APPRAISAL PROCESS FOR QUALITATIVE STUDIES

Critical appraisal of qualitative studies requires different detailed guidelines than those used when appraising a quantitative study (Marshall & Rossman, 2016; Sandelowski, 2008), because the different qualitative approaches have different standards of quality than do quantitative approaches. However, appraisals of quantitative and qualitative studies follow the same three major steps in the appraisal process (see Box 18-1) and have a common purpose—determining the credibility and trustworthiness of the findings. The integrity of the design and methods affects the credibility and meaningfulness of qualitative findings and their usefulness in clinical practice (Melnyk & Fineout-Overholt, 2015; Pickler & Butz, 2007). Burns (1989) first described the standards for rigorous qualitative research almost 30 years ago. Since that time, other criteria have been published (Cesario, Morin, & Santa-Donato, 2002; Clissett, 2008; Melnyk & Fineout-Overholt, 2015; Morse, 2012; Pickler & Butz, 2007), including one book on evaluating qualitative research (Roller & Lavrakas, 2015). The standards by which qualitative research should be appraised have been the source of considerable debate (Cohen & Crabtree, 2008; Hannes, 2011; Liamputtong, 2013; Mackey, 2012; Nelson, 2008; Roller & Lavrakas, 2015; Stige, Malterud, & Midtgarden, 2009; Whittemore, Chase, & Mandle, 2001). Nurses critically appraising qualitative studies need three prerequisite characteristics in applying rigorous appraisal standards. Without these prerequisites, nurses may miss potential valuable contributions qualitative studies might make to the knowledge base of nursing. These required prerequisite characteristics are addressed in the following section.

Prerequisites for Critical Appraisal of Qualitative Studies

The first prerequisite for appraising qualitative studies is an appreciation for the philosophical foundation of qualitative research (Melnyk & Fineout-Overholt, 2015) (Box 18-3). Qualitative researchers design their studies to be congruent with one of a wide range of philosophies, such as phenomenology, symbolic interactionism, and hermeneutics, each of which espouses slightly different methods and approaches to gaining new knowledge (Charmaz, 2014; Corbin & Strauss, 2015;

Kaestle, 1992; Marshall & Rossman, 2016; Munhall, 2012; Norlyk & Harder, 2010). Without an appreciation for the philosophical perspective supporting the study being critically appraised, the appraiser may not appropriately apply standards of rigor that are congruent with that perspective (Melnyk & Fineout-Overholt, 2015). Although unique, the qualitative philosophies are similar in their views of the uniqueness of the individual and the value of the individual's perspective. Chapter 4 contains more information on the different philosophies that are foundational to qualitative research.

Guided by an appreciation of qualitative philosophical perspectives, nurses appraising a qualitative study can evaluate the approach used to gather, analyze, and interpret the data (Miles et al., 2014). A basic knowledge of different qualitative approaches is as essential for appraisal of qualitative studies as knowledge of quantitative research designs is for appraising quantitative studies (see Box 18-3; Munhall, 2012). Spending an extended time in the culture, organization, or setting that is the focus of the study is an expectation for ethnography studies but would not be expected for a phenomenological study. A researcher using a grounded theory approach is expected to analyze data to extract social processes and construct connections among emerging concepts (Charmaz, 2014). Phenomenological researchers are expected to produce a rich, detailed description of a lived experience. Knowing these distinctions is a prerequisite to fair and objective critical appraisal of qualitative studies. What one expects to find in a qualitative research report may be the primary determinant of one's appraisal of the quality of that study (Morse, 2012; Sandelowski & Barroso, 2007).

Box 18-3 outlines the prerequisites of philosophical foundation, type of qualitative study, and openness to study participants that direct the implementation of the following guidelines for critically appraising qualitative studies. Appreciating philosophical perspectives and knowing qualitative approaches are superficial, however, without respect for the participant's perspective. Qualitative philosophers are similar in their views of the uniqueness of the individual and the value of the

individuals' perspective. That basic valuing creates an openness to hearing a participant's story and perceiving the person's life, in context. This openness allows qualitative researchers and nurses using the findings to perceive different truths and to acknowledge the depth, richness, and complexity inherent in the lives of all the patients we serve.

Step I: Identifying the Steps of the Qualitative Research Process in Studies

As with quantitative research, you will start by reviewing the title and abstract. Reading the article completely is essential when critically appraising a study, because you need to use all of the information that the researchers provided. If you are unfamiliar with the qualitative approach that was used, this is a good time to look it up in Chapter 4 of this book or in other qualitative research sources listed in the references of this chapter.

Guidelines for Identifying the Steps of the Qualitative Research Process

The following questions are provided to help you identify the key elements of the study.

I. Introduction
   A. Describe the researchers' qualifications. Take note of their employers, professions, levels of educational preparation, clinical expertise, and research experience. Have the researchers conducted previous studies on this topic or with this population? Not all of this information will be available in the article, so you will need to search for additional information about the researchers online (Fothergill & Lipp, 2014).
   B. Does the title give you a clear indication of the concepts studied and the population? Can you determine from the title which qualitative approach was used?
   C. Is the abstract inclusive of the purpose of the study, qualitative approach, and sample (Fothergill & Lipp, 2014)? The abstract should also contain key findings.
II. Research problem
   A. Is the significance of the study established? In other words, why should you care about the problem that inspired the researcher to conduct this study (Liamputtong, 2013)?
   B. Identify the problem statement. Is the research problem explicitly stated?
   C. Does the researcher identify a personal connection or motivation for selecting this topic to study? For example, the researcher may

choose to study the lived experience of men undergoing radiation for prostate cancer after the researcher's father underwent the same treatment. Acknowledging motives and potential biases is an expectation for qualitative researchers, but the researcher may not include this information in the article (Marshall & Rossman, 2016; Munhall, 2012).

III. Purpose and research questions
   A. Identify the purpose of the study. Is the purpose a logical approach to addressing the research problem of the study (Fawcett & Garity, 2009; Munhall, 2012)? Does the purpose have an intuitive fit with the problem?
   B. List research questions that the study was designed to answer.
   C. Are the research questions related to the problem and purpose?
   D. Are qualitative methods appropriate to answer the research questions?

IV. Literature review
   A. Are quantitative and qualitative studies cited that are relevant to the focus of the study? What other types of literature are included?
   B. Were the references current at the time the research was published? For qualitative studies, the author may have included studies older than the 5-year limit typically used for quantitative studies. Findings of older qualitative studies may be relevant to a qualitative study that involves human processes, such as grieving or coping, that transcend time.
   C. Identify the disciplines of the authors of studies cited in the article. Does it appear that the researcher searched databases outside the Cumulative Index to Nursing and Allied Health Literature (CINAHL) for relevant studies? Research publications in other disciplines as well as literary works in the humanities may have relevance for some qualitative studies.
   D. Were the cited studies evaluated and their limitations noted?
   E. Did the literature review include adequate synthesized information to build a logical argument (Marshall & Rossman, 2016; Wakefield, 2014)? Another way to ask the question: Does the author provide enough evidence to support the assertion that the study was needed?

V. Philosophical foundation or theoretical perspective
   The methods used by qualitative researchers are determined by the philosophical foundation of their work. The researcher may or may not state the philosophical stance on which the study is based. Despite this omission, you as a knowledgeable reader can recognize the philosophy through the description of the problem, formulation of the research questions, and selection of the methods to address the research questions.
   A. Was a specific perspective (philosophy or theory) described from which the study was developed? If so, what was that perspective?
   B. If a broad philosophy, such as phenomenology, was identified, was the specific philosopher, such as Husserl or Heidegger, also identified?
   C. Did the researcher cite a primary source for the philosophical foundation or theory (see Chapter 4)?

VI. Qualitative approach
   A. Identify the stated or implied research approach used for the study.
   B. Provide a paraphrased description of the research approach used. In addition to reviewing Chapter 4, refer to Charmaz (2014), Corbin and Strauss (2015), Creswell (2013), and Munhall (2012) for descriptions of the different qualitative research perspectives or traditions.

VII. Sampling and sample
   A. Identify how study participants were selected.
   B. Identify the types of sites where participants were recruited for the study.
   C. Describe the inclusion and exclusion criteria of the sample.
   D. Discuss the sample size. How was the sample size determined (theoretical saturation, no new themes generated, researcher understanding of the essences of the phenomenon, et cetera)?

VIII. Data collection
   A. Describe the data collection method.
   B. Identify the period of time during which data collection occurred, and also the duration of any interviews.
   C. Describe the sequence of data collection events for a participant. For example, were data collected from one interview or a series of interviews? Were focus group participants given an opportunity to provide additional data or review the preliminary conclusions of the researcher?
   D. Describe any changes in the methods in response to the context and early data

collection (Marshall & Rossman, 2016; Miles et al., 2014; Roller & Lavrakas, 2015).

IX. Protection of human study participants
   A. Identify the benefits and risks of participation. Are there benefits or risks the researchers do not identify?
   B. Are recruitment and consent techniques adjusted to accommodate the sensitivity of the subject matter and psychological distress of potential participants?
   C. Describe the data collection and management techniques that acknowledge participant sensitivity and vulnerability. These might include how potential participants are identified or what resources are available if the participant becomes upset (McCosker, Barnard, & Gerber, 2001; Munhall, 2012).

X. Data management and analysis
   A. Describe the data management and analysis methods used in the study, by name if possible (Marshall & Rossman, 2016; Miles et al. 2014; Munhall, 2012).
   B. Is an audit trail mentioned? An audit trail is a record of critical decisions that were made during the development and implementation of the study (see Chapter 4).
   C. Does the researcher describe other strategies used to minimize or allow for the effects of researcher bias (Miles et al., 2014; Patton, 2015)? For example, did two researchers analyze the data independently and compare their analyses?

XI. Findings
   A. What are the findings of the study?
   B. Does the researcher include participants' quotes to support themes or other processes identified as the findings (Corbin & Strauss, 2015; Patton, 2015)?
   C. Do the findings "ring true" to the reader? This resonation, this believing on the part of the reader, in relation to something already experienced in private or professional life, supports the study's veracity.

XII. Discussion
   A. Describe the limitations of the study.
   B. Identify whether the findings are compared to the findings of other studies or other relevant literature (Fawcett & Garity, 2009; Munhall, 2012).
   C. Did the results offer new information about the phenomenon?
   D. What clinical, policy, theoretical, and other types of implications are identified?

Step 2: Determining the Strengths and Weaknesses of the Study

Nurses prepared at the graduate level will compare each component of qualitative studies to the writings of qualitative experts, such as Charmaz (2014), Corbin and Strauss (2015), Creswell (2013), Maxwell (2013), Miles et al. (2014), Morse (2012), Munhall (2012), Roller and Lavrakas (2015), and Sandelowski and Barroso (2007). See also Chapters 4 and 12 in this text to review the processes considered appropriate for qualitative studies. By doing this comparison, you can determine the strengths and weaknesses of the study.

Guidelines for Determining the Strengths and Weaknesses of Qualitative Studies

I. Research report
   A. Are you able to identify easily the elements of the research report?
   B. Are readers able to hear the voice of the participants and gain an understanding of the phenomenon studied?
   C. Does the overall presentation of the study fit its purpose, method, and findings (Fawcett & Garity, 2009; Marshall & Rossman, 2016; Munhall, 2012; Sandelowski & Barroso, 2007)?

II. Research problem, purpose, and questions
   A. Is the purpose a logical approach to addressing the research problem of the study (Fawcett & Garity, 2009; Munhall, 2012)?
   B. Does the purpose have an intuitive fit with the problem?
   C. Are the research questions related to the problem and purpose?

III. Literature review
   A. Is the study based on a broad review of the literature? Does it appear that the author searched databases outside CINAHL for relevant studies?
   B. Is the review of the literature adequately synthesized and presented in a way that builds a logical argument? Another way to ask the question: Do the researchers provide enough evidence to support the conclusion that the study is needed?

IV. Methods
   A. Are the qualitative methods appropriate for the study purpose (Sandelowski & Barroso, 2007)?
   B. Are the methods consistent with the philosophical tradition and qualitative approach that was used? Determining whether there is **methodological congruence** among the elements of the

study is key to the quality of the study (Hannes, 2011).

C. Were the selected participants able to provide data relevant to the study purpose and research questions?

D. Were the methods of data collection effective in obtaining data to address the study purpose?

E. Were resources available to support participants who may have become upset? What resources did the researcher cite? Topics of qualitative studies may be sensitive topics that are difficult to talk about (Cowles, 1988; McCosker et al., 2001). Researchers concerned for their participants ensure that a mental health professional and other resources are available, should the participant become distressed.

F. Was the rationale provided for the selection of the particular data collection method used?

G. Were the data collection procedures proscriptively applied or allowed to emerge with some flexibility? Flexibility within parameters of the method is considered appropriate for qualitative studies (Patton, 2015).

H. Did the data management and analysis methods fit the research purposes and data?

I. Were the data analyzed sufficiently to allow new insights to occur?

J. Were the methods used to ensure rigor adequate for eliciting the reader's confidence in the findings (Miles et al., 2014)? For example, were participants given the opportunity to validate their data after transcription and initial analysis? Did quotes support the themes or descriptions?

V. Findings

A. Do the findings address the purpose of the study (Marshall & Rossman, 2016; Munhall, 2012)?

B. Are the findings of the study consistent with the qualitative approach? For example, findings of a grounded theory study are presented as a description of concepts and social processes and the findings of an ethnography study are a description of a culture.

C. Is there a coherent logic to the presentation of findings (Corbin & Strauss, 2015; Sandelowski & Barroso, 2007?

D. Are the interpretations of data congruent with data collected (Miles et al., 2014)?

E. Did the researcher address variation in the findings by relevant sample characteristics (Corbin & Strauss, 2015)?

VI. Discussion

A. Did the researcher acknowledge the study limitations? Could any of these limitations been corrected before the end of the study?

B. Did the researcher identify implications of the study that are consistent with the data and findings?

C. What new insights or knowledge were gained from the study?

Step 3: Evaluating a Study

"The sense of rightness and feeling of comfort readers experience reading the report of a study constitute the very judgments they make about the validity or trustworthiness of the study itself" (Sandelowski & Barroso, 2007, p. xix). Critical appraisal of research is not complete without making judgments about the validity of the study, or in the case of qualitative studies, making judgments about the trustworthiness. Balancing the strengths against the researcher-identified limitations and other weaknesses of the study, you determine the value or trustworthiness of study findings. Figure 18-1 demonstrates that trustworthiness in qualitative research involves transparency, time, truth, and transformation, leading to transferability. Transparency, time, truth, and transformation are displayed as different aspects or facets of trustworthiness. Each of them plays a key role in whether the findings of a study are trustworthy. The arrow leading from trustworthiness indicates that trustworthy studies can potentially be transferable. Transferability of the findings to other populations is appropriate only if you determine that the findings are trustworthy. These characteristics of high quality qualitative studies were synthesized from sets of criteria that included terms such as credibility, reflexivity, confirmability, and dependability (Hannes, 2011; Lietz & Zayas, 2010;

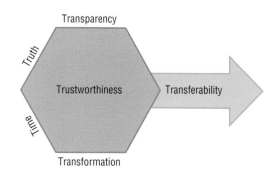

FIGURE 18-1 Criteria for evaluating trustworthiness of qualitative findings.

Marshall & Rossman, 2016: Maxwell, 2013; Miles et al., 2014; Morse, 2012; Munhall, 2012; Roller & Lavrakas, 2015; Stige et al., 2009). By examining transparency, truth, time, and transformation, you can make a judgment about the trustworthiness of the study findings. Although they will be described separately, the four characteristics overlap.

Guidelines for Evaluating a Qualitative Study

I. Transparency

Transparency is the extent to which the researcher provided details about the study processes such as decisions made during data collection and analysis, ethical concerns that were noted, and personal perspectives that may bias the findings (Maxwell, 2013; Roller & Lavrakas, 2015). The researcher may indicate that field notes were written immediately after each interview. For examples, such field notes may include thoughts on what worked or did not work in getting participants to talk freely as well as insights from the researcher's self-reflection of his or her response to the data. The openness of the researcher about how personal bias was managed increases your confidence in the findings. Terms used in assessing qualitative research that have similar meanings as transparency are confirmability, dependability, and rich or thick descriptions (Liamputtong, 2013). The questions are prompts to help you evaluate transparency.

A. Were the researchers' assumptions made explicit about "sample population, data-gathering techniques, and expected outcomes" (Roller & Lavrakas, 2015, p. 93)?

B. Did the researcher describe how personal biases and preconceived ideas were identified and managed (Charmaz, 2014; Lietz & Zayas, 2010; Miles et al., 2014)?

C. Did the researcher indicate the use of journals, field notes, memos, and other forms of documentation written during the study?

D. Were any ethical issues discussed that arose during the study?

E. Were the characteristics of the participants described adequately for you to determine the relevance of the findings?

F. Was the rationale provided for any changes in the study methods?

G. Were the stages of data analysis from raw data to findings described (Miles et al, 2014)?

H. Were quotations or other participant data provided as exemplars of codes, themes, and patterns (Patton, 2015)?

II. Truth

Truth as a characteristic of qualitative studies is not absolute. Your evaluation is influenced by your confidence that the findings can be confirmed by reviewing the audit trail, field notes, or transcripts (note the overlap with transparency). Strategies implemented to increase rigor, such as comparing transcripts to audio recordings, sharing the findings with participants and writing memos, also increase your confidence in the truth of the findings. Truth also includes the conceptual and experiential fit of the findings with your view of the phenomenon. Your view of the phenomenon also may expand as you empathize with the thoughts, feelings, and experiences of the participants. Some describe this as intuition or new insights that emerge as you read the article.

A. What strategies did the researcher use to confirm the accuracy and logic of the findings?

B. How do the findings fit with your previous views related to the phenomenon?

C. Are the findings believable?

III. Time

In qualitative research, the researcher is the instrument (Marshall & Rossman, 2016). Time must be spent in gathering data, developing relationships with participants and key informants, interviewing additional participants based on initial data analysis, and being immersed in the data during analysis and interpretation. These activities take time. Some qualitative experts have described this study characteristic as "prolonged engagement" and "persistent observation" (Roller & Lavrakas, 2015, p. 21). As a researcher, you need time to reflect and analyze your own responses to the data as well as thoroughly analyze the data. One indication of the amount of time spent engaged in the study is the depth and comprehensiveness of the descriptions (note the overlap with transparency).

A. How long did interviews last, how much time was spent in the field, and/or how much time was spent in observation (Sandelowski & Barroso, 2007)?

B. Does the time spent collecting and analyzing data seem adequate based on the size of the sample, complexity of the design, and scope of the phenomenon?

IV. Transformation

Data analysis and interpretation transform the words of participants, the observations of the ethnographer, and the text of a document into findings

(Liamputtong, 2013). Qualitative researchers who analyze the data at a superficial level will report the data as the findings, without evidence of synthesis, comparison across participants, or creation of abstract themes or categories. To transform data, the researcher must organize, interpret, compare, and reorganize phrases and themes until the meaning of the data begins to emerge (Miles et al., 2014). Data analysis is "the heart of qualitative inquiry" (Streubert & Carpenter, 2011, p. 51). As you might expect, for transformation of the data to occur, the researcher must spend time to become focused and immersed in the data. Immersion requires persistent engagement with the data (note overlap with time).

A. Do the findings go beyond reporting facts and words to describing experiences with depth and insight?

B. Are there other possible interpretations of the data?

C. How do the meaning and interpretation of the data match or contrast with previous research findings?

D. What contributions do the findings of the study make to what is known about the phenomenon?

E. Has the researcher taken the time to hone the writing—to transform the stories of the participants to a narrative that exhibits both thoroughness and eloquence?

V. Transferability

Trustworthiness is a necessary, but not sufficient, condition for transferability. Transferability is the applicability of the findings to another population or phenomenon, or stated another way the "ability to do something of value with the outcomes" (Roller & Lavrakas, 2015, p. 23). To be transferable, the findings must have meaning for similar groups or settings. The reader or user of the findings is the one who makes the determination of transferability (Streubert & Carpenter, 2011). If you have answered the previous questions and concluded the study is trustworthy, proceed with answering the following questions to determine the transferability of the findings to your practice.

A. How similar were the study participants to the persons or groups with whom you interact? Are there general truths that emerged from the research that might be used with similar populations, or with people in similar circumstances?

B. What implications may the findings have for your practice?

C. What actions could be taken that are consistent with the findings?

D. How does the study move research, theory, knowledge, education, and practice forward?

KEY POINTS

- Critical appraisal of research involves carefully examining all aspects of a study to judge its strengths, weaknesses, meaning, credibility, and significance in light of previous research experience, knowledge of the topic, and clinical expertise.

- Critical appraisals of research are conducted (1) to summarize evidence for practice, (2) to provide a basis for future research, (3) to evaluate presentations and publications of studies, (4) to select abstracts for a conference, (5) to evaluate whether a manuscript should be published, and (6) to evaluate research proposals for funding and implementation in clinical agencies.

- Nurses' levels of expertise in conducting critical appraisals depend on their educational preparation and experiences; nurses with baccalaureate, masters, doctorate, and postdoctorate preparation all have a role in examining the quality of research.

- The critical appraisal process for research includes the following steps: identifying the steps of the research process in a study; determining the study strengths and weaknesses; and evaluating the credibility, trustworthiness, and meaning of a study to nursing knowledge and practice (see Box 18-1).

- The identification step involves understanding the terms and concepts in the report and identifying the study steps.

- The second step of determining study strengths and weaknesses involves comparing what each step of the research process should be like with how the steps of the study were conducted. The logical development and implementation of the study steps also need to be examined for strengths and weaknesses.

- Study strengths and weaknesses need to be clearly identified, supported with a rationale, and documented with current research sources.

- The evaluation step involves examining the credibility, trustworthiness, and meaning of the study according to set criteria.

- To perform fair critical appraisals of qualitative studies, nurses need the prerequisites of an appreciation for the philosophical foundations of qualitative research, knowledge of different qualitative approaches, and respect for the study participant's perspective (see Box 18-3).

- Each aspect of a qualitative study, such as problem, purpose, research questions, sample, data collection and analysis, and findings, needs to be examined for strengths and weaknesses.
- The trustworthiness of a qualitative study's findings is the extent to which the researcher demonstrated transparency, provided true findings, expended adequate time, and transformed the data into meaningful findings. Transparency, truth, time, and transformation are essential elements or aspects that determine whether a study's findings are trustworthy (see Figure 18-1).
- Trustworthiness of a qualitative study is a necessary, but not sufficient, condition for transferability, the application of the findings to similar groups or settings. A study's findings may be trustworthy, but the sample, setting, or focus of the study may not be similar enough for transferring the findings to your population.

REFERENCES

Aberson, C. L. (2010). *Applied power analysis for the behavioral sciences.* New York, NY: Routledge Taylor & Francis Group.

Agency for Healthcare Research and Quality (AHRQ, 2015). *Funding & grants.* Retrieved February 23, 2015 from http://www.ahrq.gov/funding/index.html.

American Association of Colleges of Nursing (AACN) (2011). *Essentials of master's education in nursing.* Retrieved June 17, 2015 from http://www.aacn.nche.edu/education-resources/MastersEssentials11.pdf.

American Association of Colleges of Nursing (AACN) QSEN Education Consortium. (2012). *Graduate-level QSEN competencies: Knowledge, skills, and attitudes.* Retrieved February 23, 2015 from http://www.aacn.nche.edu/faculty/qsen/competencies.pdf.

American Nurses Credentialing Center (ANCC, 2015). *Magnet program overview.* Retrieved April 25, 2016 from www.nursecredentialing.org/Magnet/ProgramOverview.

American Psychological Association (APA, 2010). *Publication manual of the American Psychological Association* (6th ed.). Washington, DC: Author.

Bartlett, J. W., & Frost, C. (2008). Reliability, repeatability and reproducibility: Analysis of measurement errors in continuous variables. *Ultrasound in Obstetrics and Gynecology, 31*(4), 466–475.

Bialocerkowski, A., Klupp, N., & Bragge, P. (2010). Research methodology series: How to read and critically appraise a reliability article. *International Journal of Therapy and Rehabilitation, 17*(3), 114–120.

Borglin, G., & Richards, D. A. (2010). Bias in experimental nursing research: Strategies to improve the quality and explanatory power of nursing science. *International Journal of Nursing Studies, 47*(1), 123–128.

Brown, S. J. (2014). *Evidence-based nursing: The research-practice connection* (3rd ed.). Sudbury, MA: Jones & Bartlett.

Burns, N. (1989). Standards for qualitative research. *Nursing Science Quarterly, 2*(1), 44–52.

Cesario, S., Morin, K., & Santa-Donato, A. (2002). Evaluating the level of evidence of qualitative research. *Journal of Obstetric, Gynecologic, and Neonatal Nursing, 31*(6), 708–714.

Charmaz, K. (2014). *Constructing grounded theory* (2nd ed.). Los Angeles, CA: Sage.

Clissett, P. (2008). Evaluating qualitative research. *Journal of Orthopedic Nursing, 12*(2), 99–105.

Cohen, D. J., & Crabtree, B. F. (2008). Evaluative criteria for qualitative research in health care: Controversies and recommendations. *Annals of Family Medicine, 6*(4), 331–339.

Cohen, J. (1988). *Statistical power analysis for the behavioral sciences* (2nd ed.). New York, NY: Academic Press.

Corbin, J., & Strauss, A. (2015). *Basics of qualitative research: Techniques and procedures for developing grounded theory* (4th ed.). Los Angeles, CA: Sage.

Cowles, K. V. (1988). Issues in qualitative research on sensitive topics. *Western Journal of Nursing Research, 10*(2), 163–179.

Craig, J. V., & Smyth, R. L. (2012). *The evidence-based practice manual for nurses* (3rd ed.). Edinburgh, UK: Churchill Livingstone.

Creswell, J. W. (2013). *Qualitative inquiry & research design: Chosing among five approaches* (3rd ed.). Thousand Oaks, CA: Sage.

Creswell, J. W. (2014). *Research design: Qualitative, quantitative and mixed methods approaches* (4th ed.). Thousand Oaks, CA: Sage.

Critical Appraisal Skills Programme (CASP, 2013). *CASP checklists.* Retrieved February 23, 2015 from http://www.casp-uk.net/#!casp-tools-checklists/c18f8.

DeVon, H. A., Block, M. E., Moyle-Wright, P., Ernst, D. M., Hayden, S. J., Lazzara, D. J., et al. (2007). A psychometric toolbox for testing validity and reliability. *Journal of Nursing Scholarship, 39*(2), 155–164.

Doran, D. M. (2011). *Nursing-sensitive outcomes: State of the science.* Sudbury, MA: Jones & Bartlett.

Fawcett, J., & Garity, J. (2009). *Evaluating research for evidence-based nursing practice.* Philadelphia, PA: F. A. Davis.

Forbes, A. (2009). Clinical intervention research in nursing. *International Journal of Nursing Studies, 46*(4), 557–568.

Fothergill, A., & Lipp, A. (2014). A guide to critiquing a research paper on clinical supervision: Enhancing skills for practice. *Journal of Psychiatric and Mental Health Nursing, 21*(9), 834–840.

Gaskin, C. J., & Happell, B. (2014). Power, effects, confidence, and significance: An investigation of statistical practices in nursing research. *International Journal of Nursing Studies, 51*(5), 795–806.

Gatchel, R. J., & Mayer, T. G. (2010). Testing minimal clinically important difference: Consensus or conundrum? *The Spine Journal, 35*(19), 1739–1743.

Gloeckner, M. B., & Robinson, C. B. (2010). A nursing journal club thrives through shared governance. *Journal for Nurses in Staff Development, 26*(6), 267–270.

Grove, S. K., & Cipher, D. (2017). *Statistics for nursing research: A workbook for evidence-based practice.* St. Louis, MO: Saunders.

Grove, S. K., Gray, J. R., & Burns, N. (2015). *Understanding nursing research* (6th ed.). Philadelphia, PA: Saunders.

Hannes, K. (2011). Critical appraisal of qualitative research. In J. Noyes, A. Booth, K. Hannes, J. Harris, S. Lewin, & C. Lockwood (Eds.). *Supplementary guidance for inclusion in qualitative research in Cochrane systematic reviews of interventions.* Retrieved February 20, 2016 from http://cqrmg.cochrane.org/supplemental-handbook-guidance.

Hayat, M. J., Higgins, M., Schwartz, T. A., & Staggs, V. S. (2015). Statistical challenges in nursing education and research: An expert panel consensus. *Nursing Educator, 40*(1), 21–25.

Higgins, J. P. T., & Green, S. (2008). *Cochrane handbook for systematic reviews of interventions.* West Sussex, UK: Wiley-Blackwell & The Cochrane Collaboration.

Hoare, Z., & Hoe, J. (2013). Understanding quantitative research: Part 2. *Nursing Standards, 27*(18), 48–55.

Hoe, J., & Hoare, Z. (2012). Understanding quantitative research: Part 1. *Nursing Standards, 27*(15–17), 52–57.

Kaestle, C. (1992). Standards of evidence in historical research: How do we know when we know? *History of Education Society, 32*(3), 361–366.

Kandola, D., Banner, D., Okeefe-McCarthy, S., & Jassal, D. (2014). Sampling methods in cardiovascular nursing research: An overview. *Canadian Journal of Cardiovascular Nursing, 24*(3), 15–18.

Kerlinger, F. N., & Lee, H. B. (2000). *Foundations of behavioral research* (4th ed.). Fort Worth, TX: Harcourt College.

Knowles, J. M., & Gray, M. A. (2011). The experience of critiquing published research: Learning from the student and researcher perspective. *Nurse Education in Practice, 11*(6), 390–394.

Liamputtong, P. (2013). *Qualitative research methods* (4th ed.). South Melbourne, VIC, Australia: Oxford University Press.

Lietz, C., & Zayas, L. (2010). Evaluating qualitative research for social work practitioners. *Advances in Social Work, 11*(2), 188–202.

Mackey, M. C. (2012). Evaluation of qualitative research. In P. L. Munhall (Ed.), *Nursing research: A qualitative perspective* (5th ed., pp. 517–532). Sudbury, MA: Jones & Bartlett.

Marshall, C., & Rossman, G. B. (2016). *Designing qualitative research* (6th ed.). Los Angeles, CA: Sage.

Maxwell, J. (2013). *Qualitative research design: Inductive approach.* Los Angeles, CA: Sage.

McCosker, H., Barnard, A., & Gerber, R. (2001). Undertaking sensitive research: Issues and strategies for meeting the safety needs of all participants. *Qualitative Social Research, 2*(1), Article 22.

Meleis, A. I. (2007). *Theoretical nursing: Development and progress* (4th ed.). Philadelphia, PA: Lippincott.

Melnyk, B. M., & Fineout-Overholt, E. (2015). *Evidence-based practice in nursing & healthcare: A guide to best practice* (3rd ed.). Philadelphia, PA: Lippincott Williams & Wilkins.

Miles, M. B., Huberman, A. M., & Saldaña, J. (2014). *Qualitative data analysis: A methods sourcebook* (3rd ed.). Los Angeles, CA: Sage.

Mittlbock, M. (2008). Critical appraisal of randomized clinical trials: Can we have faith in the conclusions? *Breast Care, 3*(5), 341–346.

Morrison, D. M., Hoppe, M. J., Gillmore, M. R., Kluver, C., Higa, D., & Wells, E. A. (2009). Replicating an intervention: The tension between fidelity and adaptation. *AIDS Education and Prevention, 21*(2), 128–140.

Morse, J. M. (2012). *Qualitative health research: Creating a new discipline.* Walnut Creek, CA: Left Coast Press.

Munhall, P. L. (2012). *Nursing research: A qualitative perspective* (5th ed.). Sudbury, MA: Jones & Bartlett Learning.

National Institute of Nursing Research (NINR, 2015). *Research and funding.* Retrieved April 26, 2016 from http://www.ninr.nih.gov/researchandfunding#.VPNeD_nF-Ck.

Nelson, A. M. (2008). Addressing the threat of evidence-based practice to qualitative inquiry through increasing attention to quality: A discussion paper. *International Journal of Nursing Studies, 45*(2), 316–322.

Norlyk, A., & Harder, I. (2010). What makes a phenomenological study phenomenological? An analysis of peer-reviewed empirical nursing studies. *Qualitative Health Research, 20*(3), 420–431.

Patton, M. (2015). *Qualitative research & evaluation methods* (4th ed.). Los Angeles, CA: Sage.

Pickler, R. H., & Butz, A. (2007). Evaluating qualitative research studies. *Journal of Pediatric Health Care, 21*(3), 195–197.

Plichta, S. B., & Kelvin, E. (2013). *Munro's statistical methods for health care research* (6th ed.). Philadelphia: Lippincott Williams & Wilkins.

Polit, D. F., & Yang, F. M. (2016). *Measurement and the measurement of change.* Philadelphia, PA: Wolters Kluwer.

Pyrczak, F. (2008). *Evaluating research in academic journals: A practical guide to realistic evaluation* (4th ed.). Los Angeles, CA: Pyrczak.

Roller, M., & Lavrakas, P. (2015). *Applied qualitative research design: A total quality framework approach.* New York, NY: Guilford Press.

Ryan-Wenger, N. A. (2010). Evaluation of measurement precision, accuracy, and error in biophysical data for clinical research and practice. In C. F. Waltz, O. L. Strickland, & E. R. Lenz (Eds.), *Measurement in nursing and health research* (4th ed., pp. 371–383). New York, NY: Springer.

Sandelowski, M. (2008). Justifying qualitative research. *Research in Nursing and Health, 31*(3), 193–195.

Sandelowski, M., & Barroso, J. (2007). *Handbook for synthesizing qualitative research.* New York, NY: Springer.

Shadish, W. R., Cook, T. D., & Campbell, D. T. (2002). *Experimental and quasi-experimental designs for generalized causal inference.* Chicago, IL: Rand McNally.

Sherwood, G., & Barnsteiner, J. (2012). *Quality and safety in nursing: A competency approach to improving outcomes.* Ames, IA: Wiley-Blackwell.

Smith, M. J., & Liehr, P. R. (2013). *Middle range theory for nursing* (3rd ed.). New York, NY: Springer.

Spruce, L., van Wicklin, S., Hicks, R., Conner, R., & Dunn, D. (2014). Introducing AORN's new model for evidence rating. *American Association of Operating Nurses Journal, 99*(2), 243–255.

Stige, B., Malterud, K., & Midtgarden, T. (2009). Toward an agenda for evaluation of qualitative research. *Qualitative Health Research, 19*(10), 1504–1516.

Streubert, H., & Carpenter, D. (2011). *Qualitative research in nursing: Advancing the humanistic perspective* (5th ed.). Philadelphia, PA: Lippincott Williams & Wilkins.

Thompson, S. K. (2002). *Sampling* (2nd ed.). New York, NY: John Wiley & Sons.

Tonelli, M. R. (2012). Compellingness: Assessing the practical relevance of clinical research results. *Journal of Evaluation in Clinical Practice*, *18*(5), 962–967.

Tsai, H., Cheng, C., Chang, C., & Liou, S. (2014). Preparing future nurses for nursing research: A creative teaching strategy for RN-to-BSN students. *International Journal of Nursing Practice*, *20*(1), 25–31.

Wakefield, A. (2014). Searching and critiquing the research literature. *Nursing Standard*, *28*(39), 49–57.

Waltz, C. F., Strickland, O. L., & Lenz, E. R. (2010). *Measurement in nursing and health research* (4th ed.). New York, NY: Springer.

Whiffin, C. J., & Hasselder, A. (2013). Making the link between critical appraisal, thinking, and analysis. *British Journal of Nursing*, *22*(14), 831–835.

Whittemore, R., Chao, A., Jang, M., Minges, K. W., & Park, C. (2014). Methods of knowledge synthesis: An overview. *Heart and Lung: The Journal of Critical Care*, *43*(5), 453–461.

Whittemore, R., Chase, S. K., & Mandle, C. L. (2001). Validity in qualitative research. *Qualitative Health Research*, *11*(4), 522–537.

Wintersgill, W., & Wheeler, E. C. (2012). Engaging nurses in research utilization. *Journal for Nurses in Staff Development*, *28*(5), E1–E5.

Evidence Synthesis and Strategies for Implementing Evidence-Based Practice

Susan K. Grove

ⓔ http://evolve.elsevier.com/Gray/practice/

Research evidence has expanded greatly since the 1990s as numerous quality studies in nursing, medicine, and other healthcare disciplines have been conducted and disseminated. These studies are commonly communicated via journal publications, the Internet, books, conferences, and social media. The expectations of society and the goals of healthcare systems are the delivery of high-quality, cost-effective health care to patients, families, and communities. To ensure the delivery of quality health care, the care must be based on the current, best research evidence available. Healthcare agencies are emphasizing the delivery of evidence-based care, and nurses and physicians are focused on developing evidence-based practice (EBP). With the emphasis on EBP over the last two decades, outcomes have improved for patients, healthcare providers, and healthcare agencies (S. Brown, 2014; Doran, 2011; Edward, 2015; Gerrish et al., 2011).

Evidence-based practice (EBP) is an important theme in this textbook and was defined earlier as the conscientious integration of best research evidence with clinical expertise and patient values and needs in the delivery of quality, cost-effective health care (see Chapter 1) (Craig & Smyth, 2012; Sackett, Straus, Richardson, Rosenberg, & Haynes, 2000). **Best research evidence** is produced by the conduct and synthesis of numerous high-quality studies in a selected health-related area. Chapter 2 includes an introduction to the concept best research evidence and the processes for synthesizing research, which in this text include systematic review, meta-analysis, meta-synthesis, and mixed methods

systematic review (Paré, Trudel, Jaana, & Kitsiou, 2015; Whittemore, Chao, Jang, Minges, & Park, 2014).

This chapter builds on previous EBP discussions to provide you with strategies for implementing best research evidence in your practice and moving the profession of nursing toward EBP (Stetler, Ritchie, Rycroft-Malone, & Charns, 2014). Benefits and barriers related to implementing EBP in nursing are discussed. Guidelines are provided for synthesizing research to determine the best research evidence. Two nursing models developed to facilitate EBP in healthcare agencies are introduced. Expert researchers, clinicians, and consumers—through government agencies, professional organizations, and healthcare agencies—have developed an extensive number of evidence-based guidelines. This chapter offers a framework for reviewing the quality of these evidence-based guidelines and for using them in practice. The chapter concludes with a discussion of nationally designated EBP centers and the role of translational research in promoting EBP.

BENEFITS AND BARRIERS RELATED TO EVIDENCE-BASED NURSING PRACTICE

EBP is a goal for the profession of nursing and each practicing nurse. At the present time, some nursing interventions are evidence-based, or supported by the best research knowledge available from research syntheses. However, many nursing interventions require additional research to generate essential knowledge for making changes in practice. Some nurses readily use research-based interventions, and others are slower to make changes in their practice based on research. Some clinical agencies are supportive of EBP and provide resources to facilitate this process, but other agencies provide limited support for the EBP process. This section identifies some of the benefits and barriers related to EBP to assist you in promoting EBP in your agency and delivering evidence-based care to your patients.

Benefits of Evidence-Based Practice in Nursing

The greatest benefits of EBP are improved outcomes for patients, providers, and healthcare agencies (Bridges, 2015; Gillam & Siriwardena, 2014). Organizations and agencies nationally and internationally have promoted the synthesis of the best research evidence in thousands of healthcare areas by teams of expert researchers and clinicians. **Research synthesis** is a summary of relevant studies for a selected healthcare topic that is critical to the advancement of practice, research, and policy (Whittemore et al., 2014). Systematic reviews and meta-analyses are the most common research syntheses conducted to provide support for EBP guidelines. These guidelines identify the best treatment plan or gold standard for patient care in a selected area for promotion of quality healthcare outcomes. Healthcare providers have easy access to numerous evidence-based guidelines to assist them in making the best clinical decisions for their patients. These evidence-based syntheses and guidelines are communicated by presentations and publications and can easily be accessed online through the National Guideline Clearinghouse (NGC, 2015) in the United States, Cochrane Collaboration (2015) in England, and Joanna Briggs Institute and library (2015) in Australia.

Individual studies, research syntheses, and evidence-based guidelines assist students, educators, registered nurses (RNs), and advanced practice nurses (APNs) to provide the best possible care. Expert APNs, such as nurse practitioners (NPs), clinical nurse specialists, nurse anesthetists, and nurse midwives, are resources to other nurses and facilitate access to evidence-based guidelines to ensure that patient care is based on the best research evidence available (Gerrish et al., 2011; Stetler et al., 2014; Wintersgill & Wheeler, 2012). Healthcare agencies are highly supportive of EBP because it promotes quality, cost-effective care for patients and families and meets accreditation requirements. The Joint Commission (2015) revised their accreditation criteria to emphasize patient care quality achieved through EBP.

Many chief nursing officers (CNOs) and healthcare agencies are trying either to obtain or to maintain Magnet status, which documents the excellence of nursing care in an agency. Approval for Magnet status is obtained through the American Nurses Credentialing Center (ANCC, 2015). National and international healthcare agencies that currently have Magnet status can be viewed online at http://www.nursecredentialing .org/FindaMagnetHospital.aspx. The Magnet Recognition Program® recognizes EBP as a way to improve the quality of patient care and to revitalize the nursing environment. Magnet status requires that healthcare agencies promote the following research activities: reading and using research evidence in practice, budgeting for research activities, providing a research infrastructure with the help of consultants, conducting research and mentoring nursing staff in research activities, developing policies for protection of subjects' rights, and documenting internal and external research activities. Important research outcomes documented in a Magnet application include: nursing studies conducted, professional publications, and research presentations. Documentation of a study in a Magnet report must include the study title, principal investigator or investigators, role of nurses in the study, and study status (Horstman & Fanning, 2010).

Barriers of Evidence-Based Practice in Nursing

Barriers to the EBP movement have been both practical and conceptual. One of the most serious barriers is the lack of research evidence available regarding the effectiveness of many nursing interventions (Alzayyat, 2014; Edward, 2015). EBP requires synthesizing research evidence from randomized controlled trials (RCTs) and other types of interventional studies, but these types of studies are still limited in nursing. Mantzoukas (2009) reviewed the research evidence in 10 high-impact nursing journals, including *Nursing Research, Research in Nursing & Health, Western Journal of Nursing Research, Journal of Nursing Scholarship,* and *Advances in Nursing Science,* between 2000 and 2006 and found that the studies were 7% experimental, 6% quasi-experimental, and 39% nonexperimental. In a study of nursing research proposals submitted in 2010–2011 for national funding in France, Dupin, Chami, Petit dit Dariel, Debout, and Rothan-Tondeur (2013) described the designs as 43% RCTs (experimental), 15% interventional non-RCTs (quasi-experimental), and 10% quantitative non-interventional. Identifying the areas in which research evidence is lacking is an important first step in developing the evidence needed for practice. Quality interventional studies such as RCTs, other experimental studies, and quasi-experimental studies are needed to generate sound evidence for practice (see Chapter 11).

Systematic reviews and meta-analyses conducted in nursing have been limited compared with other disciplines. Bolton, Donaldson, Rutledge, Bennett, and Brown (2007, p. 123S) conducted a review of "systematic/integrative reviews and meta-analyses on nursing interventions and patient outcomes in acute care settings." Their literature search covered 1999–2005 and identified 4000 systematic/integrative reviews and 500 meta-analyses covering the following seven topics selected by the authors: staffing, caregivers, incontinence, elder care, symptom management, pressure ulcer prevention and treatment, and developmental care of neonates and infants. The authors found a limited association between nursing interventions and processes and patient outcomes in acute care settings. Their findings included the following.

"The strongest evidence was for the use of patient risk-assessment tools and interventions implemented by nurses to prevent patient harm. We observed significant variation in the methods to measure the effect of independent variables (nursing interventions) on patient outcomes. Results indicate the need for more research measuring the effect of specific nursing interventions that may impact acute care patient outcomes." (Bolton et al., 2007, p. 123S)

Thus, nurses need to be more active in conducting quality syntheses (systematic reviews, meta-analyses, meta-syntheses, and mixed methods systematic reviews) of research evidence in selected areas (Baker & Weeks, 2014; Moore, 2012; Rew, 2011; Whittemore et al., 2014).

Another concern is that the research evidence is generated based on population data and then is applied in practice to individual patients. Sometimes it is difficult to transfer research knowledge to individual patients, who respond in unique ways or have unique needs (Bridges, 2015). More work is needed to promote the use of evidence-based guidelines with individual patients. The National Institutes of Health (NIH, 2015) are supporting translational research to improve the use of research evidence with different patient populations in various settings. Patients who have poor outcomes when managed according to an evidence-based guideline should be reported and, if possible, the particulars of patients' responses published as case studies.

Another concern of the EBP movement is that the development of evidence-based guidelines can lead to a "cookbook" approach to health care, with health professionals thinking they are expected to follow these guidelines in their practice as developed. However, the definition of EBP describes it as the conscientious *integration* of best research evidence with clinical expertise and patient values and needs. Nurse clinicians have a major role in determining how the best research evidence will be implemented to achieve quality care and outcomes. For example, APNs use the national evidence-based guidelines for the diagnosis and management of patients with hypertension (HTN). Two current guidelines exist for the management of HTN: (1) 2014 Evidence-Based Guideline for the Management of High Blood Pressure in Adults by the panel members of the Eighth Joint National Committee (JNC 8; James et al., 2014) and the Clinical Practice guidelines for the Management of Hypertension in the Community by the American Society of Hypertension and the International Society of Hypertension (Weber et al., 2014). These guidelines are discussed in more detail later in this chapter. Evidence-based guidelines provide the gold standard for managing a particular health condition, but the healthcare provider and patient individualize the treatment plan.

Another serious barrier is that some healthcare agencies and administrators do not provide the resources necessary for nurses to implement EBP. Their lack of support might include the following: (1) inadequate access to research journals and other sources of synthesized research findings and evidence-based guidelines, (2) inadequate knowledge on how to implement evidence-based changes in practice, (3) heavy workload with limited time to make research-based changes in practice, (4) limited authority or support to change patient care based on research findings, (5) limited funding to support research projects and research-based changes in practice, and (6) minimal rewards for providing evidence-based care to patients and families (Alzayyat, 2014; Butler, 2011; Edward, 2015; Eizenberg, 2010; Gerrish et al., 2011). The success of EBP is determined by all involved, including healthcare agencies, administrators, nurses, physicians, and other healthcare professionals (Stetler et al., 2014). We all must take an active role in ensuring that the health care provided to patients and families is based on the best research available.

GUIDELINES FOR SYNTHESIZING RESEARCH EVIDENCE

Many nurses lack the expertise and confidence to synthesize research evidence in a selected nursing area

(Edward, 2015). They need additional knowledge and skills in critically appraising and synthesizing studies. Master's and doctoral students often focus on clearly defined interventions when conducting research syntheses. Synthesis of research is best done by more than one individual, including researchers and/or clinicians, and guided by specific guidelines or protocols (Pölkki, Kanste, Kääriäinen, Elo, & Kyngäs, 2013). Novice researchers should seek membership on these teams to increase their understanding of the research synthesis processes.

In this section, guidelines are provided for conducting systematic reviews, meta-analyses, meta-syntheses, and mixed-methods systematic reviews to assist you in synthesizing research evidence for nursing practice. Numerous research syntheses have been conducted in nursing and medicine, so be sure to search for an existing synthesis or review of research in an area before undertaking such a project. Recent data suggest that at least 2500 new systematic reviews are reported in English and indexed in MEDLINE each year (Liberati et al., 2009; Pölkki et al., 2013). Table 19-1 identifies some common databases and EBP organizational websites that nurses can search for syntheses of healthcare research. The Cochrane Collaboration (2015) library of systematic reviews is an excellent resource with more than 11,000 entries relevant to nursing and health care. In 2009, the Cochrane Nursing Care Field was developed to support the conduct and dissemination of research syntheses in nursing. The Joanna Briggs Institute (2015) also provides resources for locating and conducting nursing research syntheses. If you can find no research synthesis for a selected nursing intervention or the review you find is outdated, you might use the following guideline to conduct a systematic review of the relevant research.

Guideline for Implementing and Evaluating Systematic Reviews

A **systematic review** is a structured, comprehensive synthesis of the research literature conducted to determine the best research evidence available for addressing a healthcare question. A systematic review involves identifying, locating, appraising, and synthesizing quality research evidence for expert clinicians to use to promote an EBP (Bettany-Saltikov, 2010a; Craig & Smyth, 2012; Pölkki et al., 2013). Systematic reviews must be conducted with rigorous research methodology to promote the accuracy of the findings and minimize the reviewers' bias. Pölkki et al. (2013) studied the quality of systematic reviews published in high-impact nursing journals and noted that the quality of the reviews varied consid-

erably, and that some reviews were conducted without guidelines or protocols to direct the process.

We recommend using the Preferred Reporting Items for Systematic Reviews and Meta-Analyses (PRISMA) Statement for reporting systematic reviews and meta-analyses (Liberati et al., 2009; Moher, Liberati, Tetzlaff, Altman & PRISMA Group, 2009). The PRISMA Statement was developed by an international group of expert healthcare researchers and clinicians to improve the quality of reporting for systematic reviews and meta-analyses. Table 19-2 provides an adapted checklist of items identified by Moher et al. (2009) to include when reporting the results of systematic reviews or meta-analyses. A systematic review conducted by Catania and colleagues (2015) is presented as an example with the discussion of the steps outlined in Table 19-2. Catania and colleagues (2015, p. 5) used the PRISMA guidelines to conduct a systematic review of quantitative studies to determine the "effectiveness of complex interventions focused on quality-of-life assessment to improve palliative care patients' outcomes."

Step 1: Title of the Literature Synthesis

The title of a literature synthesis needs to clearly reflect the type of synthesis conducted. Thus, the report title needs to identify whether a systematic review, meta-analysis, or both were conducted. Having the type of synthesis in the title makes it easier to identify these sources when conducting a literature search

Step 2: Abstract

The report for a systematic review or meta-analysis should have an abstract that provides a concise summary of the focus, process, and outcomes of the synthesis. The abstract includes the background, objective(s) or question(s) guiding the synthesis, data sources, study eligibility criteria, participants, and interventions for the synthesis. The critical appraisal and synthesis methods should be highlighted as well as key results, limitations, conclusions, and implications of the findings.

Step 3: Introduction of Rationale, Clinical Question, and Protocol to Direct the Review

A systematic review or meta-analysis includes an introduction that provides a background of what is known and not known in a selected area with a rationale for conducting the review. A relevant clinical question is developed to focus the review process. Systematic reviews and meta-analyses need to be conducted using a specified guideline or protocol (see Table 19-2). The PRISMA Statement or guideline is often used because of its international acceptance for promoting

TABLE 19-1 Evidence-Based Practice Resources

Resource	Description
Electronic Databases	
CINAHL (Cumulative Index to Nursing and Allied Health Literature)	CINAHL is an authoritative resource covering the English-language journal literature for nursing and allied health. Database was developed in the U.S. and includes sources published from 1982 forward.
MEDLINE (PubMed—National Library of Medicine)	Database was developed by the National Library of Medicine in the U.S. and provides access to > 11 million MEDLINE citations back to the mid-1960s and additional life science journals.
MEDLINE with MeSH	Database provides authoritative medical information on medicine, nursing, dentistry, veterinary medicine, the healthcare system, preclinical services, and more.
PsycINFO	Database was developed by the American Psychological Association and includes professional and academic literature for psychology and related disciplines from 1887 forward.
CANCERLIT	Database of information on cancer was developed by the U.S. National Cancer Institute.
National Library Sites	
Cochrane Library	Cochrane Library provides high-quality evidence to inform people providing and receiving health care and people responsible for research, teaching, funding, and administration of health care at all levels. Included in the Cochrane Library is the Cochrane Collaboration, which has many systematic reviews of research. Cochrane Reviews are available at http://www.cochrane.org/reviews/.
National Library of Health (NLH)	NLH is located in the United Kingdom. You can search for evidence-based sources at http://www.evidence.nhs.uk/.
Evidence-Based Practice Organizations	
Cochrane Nursing Care Network	Cochrane Collaboration includes 11 different fields, one of which is the Cochrane Nursing Care Field (CNCF), which supports the conduct, dissemination, and use of systematic reviews in nursing; see http://cncf.cochrane.org/.
National Guideline Clearinghouse (NGC)	Agency for Healthcare Research and Quality (AHRQ) developed NGC to house the thousands of evidence-based guidelines that have been developed for use in clinical practice. The guidelines can be accessed online at http://www.guidelines.gov.
National Institute for Health and Clinical Excellence (NICE)	NICE was organized in the United Kingdom to provide access to the evidence-based guidelines that have been developed. These guidelines can be accessed at http://nice.org.uk.
Joanna Briggs Institute	This international evidence-based organization, originating in Australia, has a search website that includes evidence summaries, systematic reviews, systematic review protocols, evidence-based recommendations for practice, best practice information sheets, consumer information sheets, and technical reports; Search the Joanna Briggs Institute at http://joannabriggs.org/.

TABLE 19-2 **Checklist of Items to Include When Reporting a Systematic Review or Meta-Analysis**

Steps	Section/Topic	Checklist Item	Reported on Page No.
Step 1	**Title**	Identify the report as a systematic review, meta-analysis, or both in the study title.	
Step 2	**Abstract**	Provide a structured summary of the systematic review or meta-analysis including: background, objective(s) or question(s) directing the review, eligibility criteria, participants, interventions, study appraisal and synthesis methods, results, limitations, conclusions, and implications of key findings.	
Step 3	**Introduction**		
	Background and rationale	Describe the background and rationale for the review in the context of what is already known and not known.	
	Question(s) or .Objective(s)	Provide an explicit statement of question(s) or objective(s) being addressed with reference to PICOS (participants, interventions, comparisons, outcomes, and study design) format.	
	Guideline or Protocol used	Indicate whether a specific guideline or protocol was used to direct the review. Most of the systematic reviews and meta-analyses are conducted using the Preferred Reporting Items for Systematic Reviews and Meta-Analyses (PRISMA) Statement.	
	Methods		
Step 4	Eligibility criteria	Specify the study eligibility criteria such as type of participants in studies, intervention, measurement methods and report characteristics (e.g., years considered, language, publication status). Provide a rationale for the eligibility criteria selected.	
Step 5	Information sources	Describe all information sources (e.g., databases with dates of coverage, contact with study authors to identify additional studies) in the search and date last searched. List and define all variables for which data were sought (e.g., PICOS, funding sources) and any assumptions and simplifications made.	
Step 6	Literature search	Present full electronic search strategy for at least one database, including any limits used, with enough detail so that it could be repeated by another researcher.	
	Results		
Step 7	Study selection	Describe the study selection process, including the number of studies screened, eligibility criteria assessment, and studies included in review, with reasons for excluding studies. This process is best presented in a flow diagram (see Figure 19-1).	
Step 8	Critical appraisal of studies	Critical appraisal is best accomplished by constructing a table describing the characteristics of the included studies, such as the purpose, population, sampling method, sample size, sample acceptance and attrition rates, design, intervention (independent variable), outcomes (dependent variables), measurement methods for each outcome, and major results.	

TABLE 19-2 Checklist of Items to Include When Reporting a Systematic Review or Meta-Analysis—cont'd

Steps	Section/Topic	Checklist Item	Reported on Page No.
Step 9	Results of the review	Results of the review include descriptions of the studies' participants, settings, interventions, and measurement methods.	
	Population and setting	Describe the methods of handling data and combining results of studies. Describe the participants and settings for the different studies. Critically appraise the quality of the population for the review.	
	Interventions	If appropriate, identify the intervention(s) included in the studies. Critically appraise the similarities and differences of these interventions.	
	Measurement methods	Describe and critically appraise the measurement methods included in the studies for key study variables.	
Step 10	Meta-analysis	If a meta-analysis was included as part of the systematic review, describe the process for selecting the studies to be included in the analysis.	
Step 11	**Discussion** Summary of evidence, limitations, conclusions, implications	Develop a summary of the current best research evidence based on the review. Discuss the limitations or risks of bias in the review. State the conclusions obtained from the systematic review or meta-analysis. Describe the implications of the evidence for practice, policy, and research.	
Step 12	**Publication**	Develop the systematic review or meta-analysis for publication based on the PRISMA guidelines. Identify any sources of funding.	

Adapted from Moher, D., Liberati, A., Tetzlaff, J., Altman, D. G., & PRISMA Group. (2009). Preferred Reporting Items for Systematic Reviews and Meta-Analyses: The PRISMA Statement. Retrieved April 26, 2016 from http://www.prisma -statement.org.

consistency in reporting of systematic reviews and meta-analyses (Moher et al., 2009).

Formulating a question involves identifying a relevant topic, developing a question of interest that is worth investigating, deciding whether the question will generate significant information for practice, and determining whether the question will clearly direct the review process and synthesis of findings. A well-stated question will define the nature and scope of the literature search, identify keywords for the search, determine the best search strategy, provide guidance in selecting articles for the review, and guide the synthesis of results (Bettany-Saltikov, 2010a, 2010b; Higgins & Green, 2008; Liberati et al., 2009; Moher et al., 2009; Rew, 2011).

The question developed might focus on a therapy or intervention, health promotion action, illness prevention strategy, diagnostic process, prognosis, causation, or experience (Bettany-Saltikov, 2010a). One of the most common formats used to develop a relevant clinical question to guide a systematic review is the PICO or PICOS format described in the *Cochrane Handbook for Systematic Reviews of Interventions* (Higgins & Green, 2008). **PICOS format** includes the following elements:

P—Population or participants of interest (see Chapter 15, sampling)

I—Intervention needed for practice (see Chapter 11, discussion of interventions)

C—Comparisons of the intervention with control, placebo, standard care, variations of the same intervention, or different therapies

O—Outcomes needed for practice (see Chapter 13, outcomes research, and Chapter 17, measurement methods)

S—Study design (see Chapters 10 and 11, for study designs)

Catania and colleagues (2015) stated that a large variety of quality of life (QoL) measurements are appropriate for use in palliative care (PC); however, little is known about the effectiveness of interventions focused on QoL assessment in PC settings. Therefore, "The review question was to what extent interventions focused on QoL measurement in clinical practice are effective in improving outcomes in PC patients? This systematic review was conducted according to the recommendations of the ... PRISMA statement" (Catania et al., 2015, p. 7). The authors used the PICO format in developing their research question: *population* was PC patients, *interventions* were focused on QoL assessment, *comparisons* were any in PC settings, and *outcomes* were any PC patient's outcomes.

Step 4: Eligibility Criteria

The methods section of a systematic review includes eligibility criteria for the review, discussion of information sources, and the literature search process (see Table 19-2). Inclusion and exclusion criteria can be used to direct a literature search. The PICOS format might be used to develop the search criteria with more detail being developed for each of the elements. These search criteria might focus on the following: (1) type of research methods, such as quantitative, qualitative, or outcomes research; (2) the population or type of study participants; (3) study designs, such as descriptive, correlational, quasi-experimental, experimental, qualitative, or mixed methods; (4) sampling processes, such as probability or nonprobability sampling methods; (5) intervention and comparison of interventions; and (6) specific outcomes to be measured. The PICOS format is effective in identifying the key terms to be included in the search process. The search criteria also should indicate the years for the review, language, and publication status. The review might be narrowed by limiting the years reviewed, specifying the language as English, and the studies to those in print (Bettany-Saltikov, 2010b; Higgins & Green, 2008; Rew, 2011).

Catania and colleagues (2015) developed exclusion and inclusion criteria to direct their search of the literature. The exclusion criteria included: "Studies on validation aimed at assessing the psychometric properties of a QoL measure. Furthermore, studies focused solely on caregivers' QoL measurement and on the prognostic value of measuring QoL. Editorials, case report, descriptive, and qualitative studies, and dissertations were also excluded" (Catania et al., 2015, p. 7). The inclusion criteria are provided using the following PICOS format:

P—Population: "Any adult patient—aged 18 years or more—with PC needs according to the WHO [World Health Organization] definition and regardless of primary disease in any PC clinical practice setting of care. ..."

I—Intervention: "Any clinical intervention focused on QoL measurement, specifically on QoL measured by either patient's self-report or proxy and including at least two or more QoL dimensions" (Catania et al., 2015, p. 7).

C—Comparison: Any comparisons with QoL assessments.

O—Outcomes: "Any objectively measured patients' outcomes in PC clinical setting" (Catania et al., 2015, p. 7).

S—Types of studies: "This systematic review considered any experimental, quasi-experimental, or observational analytical studies, aimed at describing and/or assessing complex clinical interventions focused on QoL measurement and published in articles written in English (regardless of year of publication)" (Catania et al., 2015, p. 7).

Step 5: Information Sources

Once the eligibility criteria have been identified, relevant information sources are selected. Often searches have been limited to published sources in common databases, which excludes the grey literature from the research synthesis. **Grey literature** refers to studies that have limited distributions, such as theses and dissertations, unpublished research reports, articles in obscure journals, articles in some online journals, conference papers and abstracts, conference proceedings, research reports to funding agencies, and technical reports (Benzies, Premji, Hayden, & Serrett, 2006; Conn, Valentine, Cooper, & Rantz, 2003). Most grey literature is difficult to access through database searches, is often not peer-reviewed, and has limited referencing information. These are some of the main reasons for not including grey literature in searches for systematic reviews and meta-analyses. However, excluding grey literature from these searches might result in misleading, biased results. Studies with significant findings are more likely to be published than studies with nonsignificant findings and are usually published in more high-impact, widely distributed journals that are indexed in computerized databases. Studies with significant findings are more likely to have duplicate publications that need to be excluded when selecting studies to include in a research synthesis. Benzies et al. (2006, p. 60) recommended considering the inclusion of grey literature in a systematic review or meta-analysis in the following situations:

- Interventions and outcomes are complex with multiple components.

- Lack of consensus is present concerning measurement of outcome.
- Context is important to implementing the intervention.
- Availability of research-based evidence is low volume and quality.

Authors of systematic reviews also should identify the search strategies they will use. Often it is best to construct a table that includes the search criteria so that they can be applied consistently throughout the search process (Liberati et al., 2009). Bagnasco and colleagues (2014) developed a protocol to guide them in conducting a systematic review of the factors influencing self-management by patients with type 2 diabetes. This protocol would be very helpful in planning a systematic review. Many sources are identified through searches of electronic databases using the criteria previously discussed. However, publication bias might best be reduced with more rigorous searches of the following areas for grey literature and other unpublished studies:

1. Review the references of identified studies for additional studies. These are **ancestry searches** to use citations in relevant studies to identify additional studies.
2. Hand search certain journals for selected years, especially for older studies that were not identified in the electronic search.
3. Identify expert researchers in an area and search their names in the databases.
4. Contact the expert researchers regarding studies they have conducted that have not yet been published.
5. Search thesis and dissertation databases for relevant studies.
6. Review abstracts and conference reports of relevant professional organizations.
7. Search the websites of funding agencies for relevant research reports.
   (Bagnasco et al., 2014; Bettany-Saltikov, 2010b; Liberati et al., 2009)

Catania and colleagues (2015) designed their literature search strategies and their protocol for conducting the systematic review using sources such as the Cochrane Collaboration handbook (Higgins & Green, 2008) and the PRISMA Statement (Liberati et al., 2009). No date restriction was applied to the search for studies, but only studies reported in English were identified. The databases searched are discussed in Step 6. The researchers did not include grey literature, such as dissertations, but did hand search the references of articles for additional studies.

Step 6: Comprehensive Search of the Research Literature

The next step for conducting a systematic review or meta-analysis requires an extensive search of the literature focused on the inclusion and exclusion criteria and strategies identified in Steps 4 and 5. The different databases searched, date of the search, and search results are recorded for each database (see Chapter 7 for details on conducting and storing searches of databases). Table 19-1 identifies common databases that are searched by nurses in conducting syntheses of research and in searching for evidence-based guidelines. Key search terms usually are identified in the report. Sometimes authors of systematic reviews provide a table that identifies search terms and criteria. The PRISMA Statement recommends presenting the full electronic search strategy used for at least one major database such as CINAHL or MEDLINE (Liberati et al., 2009). Search strategies used to identify grey literature and other unpublished studies should be identified.

Catania and colleagues (2015, p. 7) identified the studies for their review through "searching five databases: CINAHL, EMBASE, MEDLINE, PsycINFO, and the Cochrane Library, and through hand searching from references lists of included articles. One reviewer performed the searches in each database from its inception to June 2012 with no limits of date. … Specific keywords for each database and free text terms were combined with Boolean operators. According to different terms and rules of searching for each database, the effective combination of search terms was designed and set up by one reviewer and discussed with the other three reviewers." The search strategies for the different databases are included in Appendix 1 of their article.

Step 7: Selection of Studies for Review

The results section of a systematic review includes the study selection process, critical appraisal of the selected studies, and results of the review (see Table 19-2). The following sections cover these areas in detail. The selection of studies for inclusion in the systematic review or meta-analysis is a complex process that initially involves review and removal of duplicate sources. Two or more authors and sometimes an external reviewer examine the remaining abstracts to ensure they meet the criteria identified in Step 4. The abstracts might be excluded based on the study participants, interventions, outcomes, or design not meeting the search criteria. Sometimes the abstracts are not in English, are incomplete, or represent studies that are not obtainable. If contacting the authors of the abstracts cannot produce

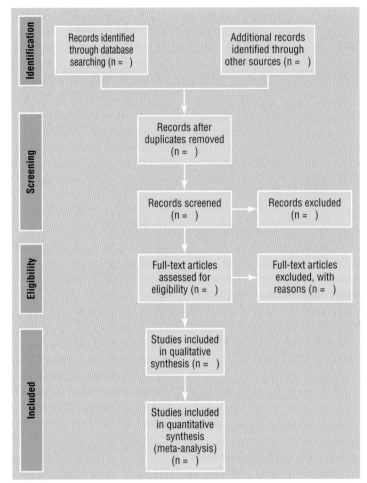

FIGURE 19-1 PRISMA 2009 Flow Diagram. Identification, screening, eligibility, and inclusion of research sources in systematic reviews and meta-analyses. (Adapted from Moher, D., Liberati, A., Tetzlaff, J., Altman, D. G., & PRISMA Group. [2009]. *Preferred Reporting Items for Systematic Reviews and Meta-Analyses: The PRISMA Statement.* Retrieved April 26, 2016 from http://www.prisma-statement.org.)

essential information, often the abstracts are excluded from the review (Bagnasco et al., 2014; Bettany-Saltikov, 2010b; Liberati et al., 2009; Pölkki et al., 2013).

After the abstracts that meet the designated criteria are identified, the next step is to retrieve the full-text citation for each study. It is best to enter these studies into a table and document how each study meets the eligibility criteria. If studies do not meet criteria, they should be removed and a rationale provided. Two or more authors of the review need to examine the studies to ensure that eligibility or inclusion criteria are consistently implemented. Often the study selection process includes all members of the review team. This selection process is best demonstrated by the flow diagram in

Figure 19-1 that was developed by the PRISMA Group (Liberati et al., 2009). This flow diagram includes four phases: (1) identification of the sources, (2) screening of the sources based on set criteria, (3) determining whether the sources meet eligibility requirements, and (4) identifying the studies included in the review.

Catania and colleagues (2015) provided a detailed description of their search results and final selection of sources for their systematic review. Three PC experts and the authors of the review independently searched for eligible studies and assessed the title, abstract and full text against the inclusion criteria. The stages for selection of sources are summarized in Figure 19-2 using the PRISMA flow diagram.

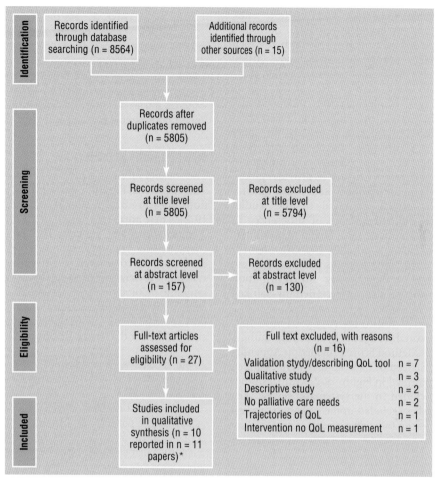

FIGURE 19-2 Study selection flow chart.
QoL, Quality of life.
*Detmar et al. (2002) and Snyder et al. (2011) were pooled because reported different analyses from the same study.
(Adapted from Catania, G., Beccaro, M., Costantini, M., Ugolini, D., De Silvestri, A., Bagnasco, A., et al. [2015]. Effectiveness of complex interventions focused on quality-of-life assessment to improve palliative care patients' outcomes: A systematic review. *Palliative Medicine, 29*[1], 8.)

"The searches of electronic databases and hand searches of reference lists yielded 8579 references, which were included in this review. On the basis of the titles and the abstracts, 27 met the inclusion criteria, and the full-text articles were obtained. After reading the full-text articles, 11 fulfilled the inclusion criteria, and 2 of those were pooled because they reported different analyses from the same study. As a result, 10 studies were submitted to qualitative synthesis." (Catania et al., 2015, p. 8)

Step 8: Critical Appraisal of the Studies Included in the Review

An initial critical appraisal of methodological quality occurs during the selection of studies to be included in the systematic review. Once the studies are selected, a more thorough critical appraisal takes place. This second appraisal is best accomplished by constructing a table describing the characteristics of the included studies, such as the purpose, population, sampling method, sample size, sample acceptance and attrition rates, design, intervention (independent variable), outcomes (dependent variables), measurement methods for each outcome, and major results (Bettany-Saltikov, 2010b; Higgins & Green, 2008; Liberati et al., 2009; Pölkki et al., 2013).

It is best if two or more experts independently review the studies and make judgments about their quality. The authors of the review contact the study investigators if it is necessary to obtain important information about the study design or results not included in the publication. Chapter 18 provides guidelines for critically appraising quantitative and qualitative studies. The critical appraisal of the studies reviewed is often difficult because of differences in types of participants, designs, sampling methods, intervention protocols, outcome variables and measurement methods, and presentation of results. Studies often are rank-ordered, based on their quality and contribution to the development of the review (Bettany-Saltikov 2010b; Liberati et al., 2009).

In the Catania et al. (2015) review, a total of 27 full-text articles were scored for quality by two of the authors using the Edwards Method Score provided in Appendix 2 of their article. Sixteen of these studies were excluded for the reasons identified in Figure 19-2, with 10 studies and 11 papers included in the systematic review. The designs of the studies included in the systematic review are summarized in the following excerpt.

"Study design comprised three randomized controlled trials (RCTs), and one of those was a crossover trial, all designed to evaluate the efficacy of a standardized QoL measurement; one quasi-experimental study designed to compare changes in QoL in two patient groups; and one interrupted time series study and five longitudinal prospective studies designed to identify patient's needs, demonstrate a QoL change over time, and evaluate feasibility of QoL measurement among healthcare professionals (HPs)." (Catania et al., 2015, p. 14)

The authors presented a detailed table of standardized information from each of the 10 studies, which included: authors, year, and country; aims; study design; participants; intervention; outcome measures; results; and Edwards Method Scores. You need to access this systematic review to view their table of studies, the 11 elements of the Edwards Method Score, the final Edwards score for each study, and other critical appraisal strategies implemented.

Catania et al. (2015, p. 14) developed Table 19-3 that identified the studies' designs and concluded that "the quality of the evidence was found to be relatively moderate to low. We identified three RCTs, and the remaining were mostly observational prospective studies with heterogeneity in study designs. One experimental study out of three and six observational studies out of seven did not report how sample size or power was determined."

Step 9: Results of the Review

The results of a systematic review should include a description of the study participants, types of interventions, measurement methods, and outcomes (see Table 19-2). These areas are covered in the following sections.

Populations and settings. The participants, sample characteristics, and settings for each of the studies must be discussed and considered when synthesizing studies for systematic reviews and meta-analyses. The sample size and sampling methods are critically appraised for quality and consistency among the studies. Catania and colleagues (2015) included the following description of participants and settings for the ten studies included in their review.

"Four studies were conducted in the United Kingdom, two studies in the United States, and the remaining were set in Canada, the Netherlands, New Zealand, and Germany. Most of the studies (90%) included advanced-stage cancer patients, at any site, while the remaining study included mostly patients with advanced AIDS. The population across studies was diverse and ranged in size from 30 to 709 participants; the median sample size was 108. Patients formed the study group in six studies, patients and HPs in three studies, and dyads of patients and caregivers in one study. The median proportion of female patients was 53%. The interventions were delivered either in outpatient, inpatient, home care, or combinations of these services." (Catania et al., 2015, p. 14)

Interventions in studies. Creating a table is a very efficient way to organize and summarize the results of different types of interventions. Liberati et al. (2009) recommended inclusion of the following in an intervention table summary: (1) study source; (2) structure of the intervention (stand-alone or multifaceted); (3) specific type of intervention, such as physiological treatment, education, counseling, or behavioral therapy; (4) delivery method such as demonstration and return demonstration, verbal, video, or self-administered; (5) statistical difference between the intervention and the control, standard care, placebo, or alternative intervention groups; and (6) the interventions effect sizes.

TABLE 19-3 **Effect Size of Interventions Focused on QoL Assessment on Patients' Outcomes**			
Outcome	**Study Design**	**Sample (n)**	**Effect Size**
Overall QoL			
Jocham et al., 2009	Longitudinal prospective	121	0.58
Hill, 2002	Quasi-experimental	36	0.40
Mills et al., 2009	Randomized controlled trial	74	−0.38
Symptom			
Bruera et al., 1991	Longitudinal prospective	95	0.53
Hill, 2002	Quasi-experimental	36	0.47
Jocham et al., 2009	Longitudinal prospective		
Pain		121	0.68
Nausea/vomiting		121	0.63
Dyspnea		121	0.51
Fatigue		121	0.47
Lack of appetite		121	0.47
Constipation		121	0.33
Diarrhea		121	0.30
Physical function			
Hill, 2002	Quasi-experimental	36	0.48
Jocham et al., 2009	Longitudinal prospective	121	0.37
Emotional Function			
Jocham et al., 2009	Longitudinal prospective	121	0.60
Chapman et al., 2008	Longitudinal retrospective		
Feeling frustrated		20	0.67
Worry about pain		20	0.53
Social Function			
Jocham et al., 2009	Longitudinal prospective	121	0.55
Role Function			
Jocham et al., 2009	Longitudinal prospective	121	0.30
Cognitive Function			
Jocham et al., 2009	Longitudinal prospective	121	0.27
Satisfaction			
Detmar et al., 2002	Randomized controlled trial	199	0.37
Communication About QoL Topic			
Detmar et al., 2002	Randomized controlled trial	199	0.38

QoL, quality of life
From Catania, G., Beccaro, M., Costantini, M., Ugolini, D., De Silvestri, A., Bagnasco, A., et al. (2015). Effectiveness of complex interventions focused on quality-of-life assessment to improve palliative care patients' outcomes: A systematic review. *Palliative Medicine, 29*(1), 15.

Catania and colleagues (2015) developed a table of the outcomes, study designs, and effect sizes (*ESs*) of the interventions focused on QoL assessment (see Table 19-3). The *ESs* indicate how effective the interventions focused on QoL assessment were in improving the study participants' outcomes. *ESs* are usually expressed with Cohen's *d*. A moderate value is *ES* = 0.3 to 0.5 and a large value is *ES* > 0.5 (see Chapter 15; Cohen, 1988). The following study excerpt describes the effectiveness of the interventions.

"Effectiveness of Interventions Focused on QoL Assessment

Overall, the analysis of the single *ES* could be estimated for 5 out of 10 eligible studies. ... The results of single *ES* for patients' outcomes are presented in Table 19-3. All but one study showed a positive ES ranging from Cohen's *d* = 0.27 (cognitive function) to Cohen's *d* = 0.68 (pain symptom). Only one RCT examining the effect of weekly completion of a patient-held QoL diary on QoL showed a negative *ES* for overall QoL (*d* = −0.38). ... A positive but small *ES* was revealed for the randomized trial ... for satisfaction and communication about QoL topic. The largest magnitude of effect was revealed in pain response (*d* = 0.68)." (Catania et al., 2015, p. 14)

Outcomes of the studies. Specific outcomes, including primary and secondary outcomes, of the studies are effectively summarized in a table. This table might include (1) the study source; (2) outcome variable, with an indication as to whether it was a primary or secondary outcome in the study; (3) measurement method used for each study outcome variable; and (4) the quality of the measurement methods, such as the reliability and validity of a scale or the precision and accuracy of a physiological measure (see Chapter 16). Catania and colleagues (2015) discussed the measurement methods for their review of outcomes in the following excerpt.

"Most of the studies reported using a set of outcome measures for use with PC patients. However, some studies used either validated measures, a non-validated author-developed tool, or a mix of them including checklists and tailor-made multiple-item measures using some items taken from existing questionnaires" (Catania et al., 2015, p. 16).

The outcomes examined in this systematic review are identified in column one of Table 19-3. Most of the outcomes were measured with multi-item Likert type scales in the studies reviewed (see Chapter 17). Many of the scales were valid and reliable but some were newly developed for this study and lacked measures of reliability and validity (see Chapter 16). Thus, Catania et al. (2015) assessed the quality of some of the measurement methods as questionable, limiting both the accuracy of the results and the credibility of conclusions presented in those particular studies.

Step 10: Conduct a Meta-Analysis if Appropriate

Some systematic reviews include published meta-analyses as sources in the review. Because a meta-analysis involves the use of statistics to summarize results of different studies, it usually provides strong, objective information about the effectiveness of an intervention or well-substantiated knowledge about a clinical problem. Some authors conduct meta-analyses in the process of synthesizing sources for their systematic review (Liberati et al., 2009). The authors of the review should provide a rationale for conducting the meta-analysis and detail the process they used. For example, the authors of a review might identify that a meta-analysis was conducted with a small group of similar studies to determine the effect of an intervention. The following section provides more details on the conduct of meta-analyses.

The systematic review conducted by Catania and colleagues (2015) did not include a meta-analysis as a source, and a meta-analysis was not conducted as a part of the review process. A meta-analysis was probably not appropriate because of the limited number and quality of studies that had been conducted to determine the effectiveness of QoL assessment in improving PC patients' outcomes.

Step 11: Discussion Section of the Review

In a systematic review or meta-analysis, discussion of the findings must include an overall evaluation of types of interventions implemented and outcomes measured in the reviewed studies. Methodological issues or limitations of the review also must be addressed. The discussion section requires a theoretical link back to the studies' frameworks to indicate the theoretical implications of the findings. Finally, the authors must present implications for research, practice, education, and policy development (see Table 19-2; Bagnasco et al., 2014; Bettany-Saltikov, 2010b; Higgins & Green, 2008; Liberati et al., 2009). Catania and colleagues (2015) provided the following discussion of their findings, implications for research and practice, limitations, and conclusions.

"As a result of our systematic review, the following evidence can be summarized: interventions focused on QoL assessment can have a moderate practical significance in patients with PC needs on symptoms, psychosocial dimension, and overall QoL" (Catania et al., 2015, p. 16).

Implications for Research and Practice

"Future interventions may benefit from mainly considering that QoL measurement in PC practice is a complex intervention, and as such, research should be conducted (1) including validated QoL tools; (2) scheduling baseline assessment within 3 days from admittance and further assessment 7–10 days after; (3) training staff and educating patients and caregivers; (4) developing a practical way to share and discuss QoL results with patients and their caregiver immediately after performing QoL assessment (e.g., QoL summary profile); (5) using QoL measurement scores to design care plans to address patients' needs involving, whenever possible, patients and their families in any case according to patients' values and preferences; and then (6) identifying a coordinator who could undertake responsibility of the intervention within staff. ..."

Limitations of the Review

Our review has some limitations. First, although three authors according to our eligibility criteria performed the study selection, we cannot be completely sure that we identified all relevant studies. Second, the restriction to the English language could represent a limitation, and it is possible that interventions published in overseas language journals were not identified. Third, the selected studies reported variability in the type of interventions and methodological approaches, thus, it is difficult to compare results between studies, and generalizability could be compromised. ...

Conclusion

Overall, implementing interventions focused on QoL assessment in PC practice does result in improved patients' outcomes. The results of our review should be interpreted with caution because they are based mainly on observational studies with weaknesses in their designs. ... Also, although the level of evidence is limited, results might contribute to a more close professional relationship between HPs, patients, and their families along the disease trajectory through slightly more confidence that the QoL measurement can improve PC patients' outcomes in terms of physical (e.g., pain), psychological, and social dimensions, and overall QoL." (Catania et al., 2015, p. 17)

Step 12: Development of the Final Report for Publication

The final step is the development of the systematic review report for publication. The report should include a title that identifies it as either a systematic review or a meta-analysis for ease of location in database searches. An abstract must be included that provides a concise summary of the review. The body of the report should include the content discussed in the previous steps and outlined in Table 19-2 (see Chapter 27 for details on publishing research reports). If the synthesis process is clearly detailed in the review report, others can replicate the process and verify the findings (Bagnasco et al., 2014; Pölkki et al., 2013). Catania and colleagues (2015) developed a quality systematic review for publication that included the relevant sections and topics identified in Table 19-2.

The PRISMA checklist is an excellent guide for developing a systematic review or meta-analysis for publication and is available at the following website: http://www.prisma-statement.org. Subsequently, the PRISMA group published an additional guideline, with a focus on conducting systematic reviews and meta-analyses of individual participant data (IPD; Stewart et al. 2015). The PRISMA-IPD guideline involves collecting, checking, and reanalyzing individual-level data from studies to address a particular clinical question. The PRISMA-IPD might be considered a gold standard, since the specific participants' data from studies are reanalyzed to determine the results of a research synthesis. However, the difficulty occurs in obtaining the participants' actual data from studies while protecting their rights. For more details on the PRISMA-IPD Statement, read the Stewart et al. (2015) article.

Critical Appraisal of a Published Systematic Review

Your critical appraisal of a systematic review focuses on whether each step of the PRISMA checklist was completed in a quality way, and adhered to the questions presented in Table 19-4. You also will need to provide comments and rationale for the appraised strengths and limitations of the review. Using this list of questions, you could develop a formal critical appraisal paper for a systematic review. In critically appraising systematic reviews and meta-analyses, you might also use methodology articles (Bagnasco et al., 2014; Bettany-Saltikov, 2010a, 2010b; Pölkki et al., 2013), the Cochrane Collaboration handbook (Higgins & Green, 2008), the EBP manual for nurses by Craig and Smyth (2012), and other sources identified by your faculty advisors or experts in this area.

The critical appraisal of a systematic review or meta-analysis also includes an assessment of how current the literature synthesis is. This leads to the following question: How quickly do systematic reviews become outdated? Shojania et al. (2007, p. 224) conducted a survival analysis of 100 quantitative systematic reviews published from 1995–2005 "to estimate the average time to changes in evidence that is sufficiently important to warrant updating systematic reviews." The authors

TABLE 19-4 **Checklist for Critically Appraising Published Systematic Reviews**

Systematic Review Steps	Step Complete (Yes or No)	Comments: Quality and Rationale
1. Were the title and abstract clearly presented?		
2. Was the clinical question clearly expressed and significant? Was the PICOS (participants, intervention, comparative interventions, outcomes, and study design) format used to develop the question and focus the review?		
3. Were the purpose and objectives or questions of the review clearly expressed and used to direct the review?		
4. Were the search criteria clearly identified? Was the PICOS format used to identify the search criteria and were the years covered, language, and publication status of sources identified in the search criteria?		
5. Was a comprehensive, systematic search of the literature conducted using explicit criteria identified in Step 4? Were the search strategies clearly reported with examples? Did the search include published studies, grey literature, and unpublished studies?		
6. Was the process for the selection of studies for the review clearly identified and consistently implemented? Was the selection process expressed in a flow diagram such as Figure 19-1?		
7. Were key elements (population, sampling process, design, intervention, outcomes, and results) of each study clearly identified and presented in a table?		
8. Was a quality critical appraisal of the studies conducted? Were the results related to participants, types of interventions, outcomes, outcome measurement methods, and risks of bias clearly discussed related to each study (i.e., in table and narrative format)?		
9. Were the results of the review clearly described (i.e., in narrative and table)? Were details of the study interventions compared and contrasted in a table? Were the outcome variables clearly identified and the quality of the measurement methods addressed?		
10. Was a meta-analysis conducted as part of the systematic review? Was a rationale provided for conducting the meta-analysis? Were the details of the meta-analysis process and results clearly described?		
11. Did the report conclude with a clear discussion section?		
a. Were the review findings summarized to identify the current best research evidence?		
b. Were the limitations of the review and how they might have affected the findings addressed?		
c. Were the implications for research, practice, education, and policy development addressed?		
12. Did the authors of the review develop a clear, concise, quality report for publication? Was the report inclusive of the items identified in the PRISMA Statement (Liberati et al., 2009)? Were sources of funding identified?		

found that the average time before a systematic review should be updated was 5.5 years. However, 23% of the reviews needed updating within 2 years, and 15% in 1 year. Shojania et al. (2007) stressed that high-quality systematic reviews that were directly relevant to clinical practice require frequent updating to stay current. Numerous nursing and medical research syntheses have been conducted, so knowledge of the elements of systematic reviews and meta-analyses will assist you in critically appraising the quality of these reviews.

Conducting Meta-Analyses to Synthesize Research Evidence

A **meta-analysis** is a research synthesis strategy that involves statistically pooling the samples and results from previous studies with the same research design. Meta-analyses provide one of the highest levels of evidence about the effectiveness of an intervention (Andrel, Keith, & Leiby, 2009; Higgins & Green, 2008; Liberati et al., 2009; Moore, 2012). This approach has objectivity because it includes analysis techniques to determine the effect of an intervention while examining the influences of variations in the studies selected for the meta-analysis. The studies to be included in the analysis must be examined for variations or **heterogeneity** in such areas as sample characteristics, sample size, design, types of interventions, and outcomes variables and measurement methods (Higgins & Green, 2008). Meta-analysis is best conducted using studies that are more homogeneous in these areas. Heterogeneity in the studies to be included in a meta-analysis can lead to different types of biases, which are detailed in the following section.

Statistically combining data from several studies results in a large sample size with increased power to determine the true effect of a specific intervention on a particular outcome (see Chapter 15 for discussion of power). The ultimate goal of a meta-analysis is to determine whether an intervention (1) significantly improves outcomes, (2) has minimal or no effect on outcomes, or (3) increases the risk of adverse events. Meta-analysis is also an effective way to resolve conflicting study findings and controversies that have arisen related to a selected intervention. As mentioned earlier, authors might conduct a meta-analysis as part of a systematic review that includes a group of similar studies to determine the effectiveness of an intervention (Higgins & Green, 2008).

Strong evidence for using an intervention in practice can be generated from a meta-analysis of multiple, quality studies such as RCTs and quasi-experimental studies. However, the conduct of a meta-analysis

---

BOX 19-1 Recommended Reporting in Research Publications to Facilitate Meta-Analysis

Demographic Variables Relevant to Population Studied
 Age
 Gender
 Marital status
 Ethnicity
 Education
 Socioeconomic status

Methodological Characteristics
 Sample size (experimental and control groups)
 Type of sampling method
 Sampling refusal rate and attrition rate
 Sample characteristics
 Research design
 Groups included in study—experimental, control, comparison, placebo groups
 Intervention protocol and fidelity discussion
 Data collection techniques
 Outcome measurements
 Reliability and validity of instruments
 Precision and accuracy of physiological measures

Data Analysis
 Name of statistical tests
 Sample size for each statistical test
 Degrees of freedom for each statistical test
 Exact value of each statistical test
 Exact p value for each test statistic
 One-tailed or two-tailed statistical test
 Measures of central tendency (mean, median, and mode)
 Measures of dispersion (range, standard deviation)
 Post hoc test values for ANOVA (analysis of variance) test of three or more groups

---

depends on the accuracy, clarity, and completeness of information presented in individual study reports. Box 19-1 provides a list of information that should be included in a research report to facilitate the conduct of a meta-analysis.

The steps for conducting a meta-analysis are similar to the steps for conducting a systematic review that were detailed in the previous section. The PRISMA Statement introduced earlier provides clear directions for developing a report for either a systematic review or a meta-analysis (see Table 19-2; Liberati et al., 2009; Moher et al., 2009). The following information is provided to increase your ability to appraise critically meta-analysis studies and to conduct a meta-analysis for a selected intervention. The PRISMA Statement, Cochrane Collaboration guidelines for meta-analysis (Higgins & Green, 2008), and other resources (Andrel et al., 2009; Conn & Rantz, 2003; Moore, 2012; Noordzij, Hooft, Dekker, Zoccali, & Jager, 2009; Turlik, 2010) were used to provide detail for conducting a meta-analysis. Conn's (2010) meta-analysis to examine the effectiveness of physical activity interventions on depressive symptoms in healthy adults is presented as an example.

Clinical Question for Meta-Analysis

The clinical question developed for a meta-analysis is usually clearly focused as: "What is the effectiveness of a selected intervention?" The PICOS (participants, intervention, comparative interventions, outcomes, and study design) format discussed earlier might be used to generate the clinical question (Higgins & Green, 2008; Liberati et al., 2009; Moher et al., 2009). Conn (2010) indicated that only one previous meta-analysis had examined the effect of physical activities (PAs) on depressive symptoms among subjects without clinical depression. Thus, Conn wanted to address the following clinical question: What is the effect of PAs on the outcomes of depressive symptoms in healthy adults?

Purpose and Questions to Direct Meta-Analysis

Researchers must identify clearly the purpose of their meta-analysis and the questions or objectives that guide the analysis. The Cochrane Collaboration identified the following four basic questions to guide a meta-analysis to determine the effect of an intervention:

1. What is the direction of effect?
2. What is the size of effect?
3. Is the effect consistent across studies?
4. What is the strength of evidence for the effect? (Higgins & Green, 2008, p. 244)

Conn clearly identified the following purpose and questions to guide her meta-analysis.

"This meta-analysis synthesized depressive symptom outcomes of supervised and unsupervised PA interventions among healthy adults." (Conn, 2010, p. 128)

"This meta-analysis addressed the following research questions:

(1) What are the overall effects of supervised PA and unsupervised PA interventions on depressive symptoms in healthy adults without clinical depression?

(2) Do interventions' effects on depressive symptom outcomes vary depending on intervention, sample, and research design characteristics?

(3) What are the effects of interventions on depressive symptoms among studies comparing treatment subjects with before versus after interventions?" (Conn, 2010, p. 129)

Search Criteria and Strategies for Meta-Analyses

The methods for identifying search criteria and selecting search strategies are similar for meta-analyses and systematic reviews. Search criteria usually are narrowly focused for meta-analysis, in order to identify selective studies examining the effect of a particular intervention. The search needs to be rigorous and to include published sources identified through varied databases and unpublished studies and other grey literature identified through other types of searches (see previous section). Conn (2010) presented her detailed search strategies in the following excerpt.

Primary Study Search Strategies

Multiple search strategies were used to ensure a comprehensive search and thus limit bias while moving beyond previous reviews. An expert reference librarian searched 11 computerized databases (e.g., MEDLINE, PsycINFO, EMBASE) using broad search terms. … Search terms for depressive symptoms were not used to narrow the search because many PA intervention studies report depressive symptom outcomes but do not consider these the main outcomes of the study and thus papers are not indexed by these terms. Several research registers were examined including Computer Retrieval of Information on Scientific Projects and mRCT, which contains 14 active registers and 16 archived registers. Computerized author searches were completed for project principal investigators located from research registers and for the first three authors on eligible studies. Author searches were completed for dissertation authors to locate published papers. Ancestry searches were conducted on eligible and review papers. Hand searches were completed for 114 journals which frequently report PA intervention research." (Conn, 2010, p. 129)

Possible Biases for Meta-Analyses and Systematic Reviews

Even with rigorous literature searches, authors of meta-analyses and systematic reviews are often limited primarily to published studies. The nature of the sources can lead to biases and flawed or inaccurate conclusions in the research syntheses. The common biases that can occur in conducting and reporting research syntheses include publication bias, such as time lag bias, location bias, duplicate publication bias, citation bias, and language bias; bias from poor study methodology; and outcome reporting bias. **Publication bias** occurs because studies with positive results are more likely to be published than studies with negative or inconclusive results. Higgins and Green (2008) found that the odds were four times greater that positive study results would be published by researchers versus negative results. **Time-lag bias**, a type of publication bias, occurs because studies with negative results are usually published later, sometimes 2 to 3 years later, than studies with positive results. Sometimes studies with negative results are not published at all, whereas studies with positive results might be published more than once (**duplicate publication bias**). **Location bias** can occur if studies are published in lower impact journals and indexed in less-searched databases. A special case of location bias is dissertation research. It is often omitted from systematic reviews and meta-analyses because of the difficulty or cost involved to access it, yet its findings may represent the most current research to date in an area. A **citation bias** occurs when certain studies are cited more often than others and are more likely to be identified in database searchers. **Language bias** can occur if searches focus just on studies in English and important studies exist in other languages.

Biases in studies' methodologies often are related to design and data analysis problems. The strengths and threats to design validity should be examined during critical appraisal of the studies for inclusion in a meta-analysis or systematic review (see Chapters 10 and 11 for discussion of design validity). The analyses conducted in studies need to be appropriate and complete (see Chapters 21 through 25 on data analysis). **Outcome reporting bias** occurs when study results are not reported clearly and with complete accuracy. For example, reporting bias occurs when researchers selectively report positive results and not negative results; or positive results might be addressed in detail with limited discussion of negative results. Higgins and Green (2008) provided a detailed discussion of potential biases in systematic reviews and meta-analyses.

An analysis method called the **funnel plot** can be used to assess for biases in a group of studies. Funnel plots provide graphic representations of possible *ES*s or odds ratios (*OR*s) for interventions in selected studies. To calculate the *ES* or strength of an intervention in a study, determine the difference between the experimen-

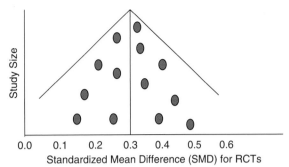

FIGURE 19-3 Funnel plot of standardized mean differences (SMDs) for randomized controlled trials (RCTs) with limited bias.

tal and control groups for the outcome variable. The mean difference between the experimental and control groups for several studies is easily determined if the outcome variable is measured by the same scale or instrument in each study (see Chapter 15 for calculation of *ES*). However, the **standardized mean difference** (SMD) must be calculated in a meta-analysis when the same outcome, such as depression, has been measured by different scales or methods. Figure 19-3 shows an example funnel plot of the SMDs from 13 individual studies. The SMDs from these particular studies are quite symmetrical, and equally divided by the line through the middle of the funnel in the graph. A symmetrical funnel plot indicates little publication bias. Asymmetry of the funnel plot is widely thought to be the result of publication bias, but may also be the result of methodological bias, reporting bias, heterogeneity in individual studies' sample size or in research interventions, or chance (Egger, Smith, Schneider, & Minder, 1997). In Figure 19-3, studies with small sample sizes are toward the bottom of the graph, and studies with larger samples are toward the top.

Figure 19-4 includes two example funnel plots, with the plot in Figure 19-4*A* showing no asymmetry. An unbiased sample of studies should appear basically symmetrical in the funnel with the *OR*s of the studies fairly equally divided on either side of the line (see Chapter 24 for calculating *OR*). The funnel plot shown in Figure 19-4*B* demonstrates asymmetry with possible publication bias in favor of larger studies with positive results when the studies having smaller effect and sample sizes are removed. This collection of studies in a meta-analysis could lead to the conclusion that a treatment was effective when it might not be when looking at a larger collection of studies with negative and positive results as in the plot in Figure 19-4*A*. Conn (2010)

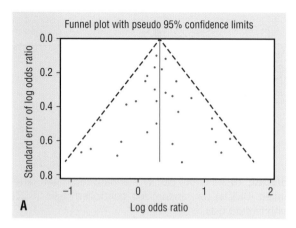

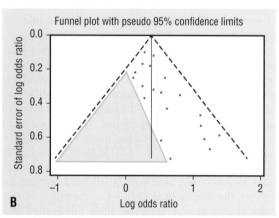

FIGURE 19-4 A and B, Funnel plots examining publication bias. (Adapted from Andrel, J. A., Keith, S. W., & Leiby, B. E. [2009]. Meta-analysis: A brief introduction. *Clinical & Translational Science, 2*[5], 376.)

discussed her search results and risk of publication bias in the following excerpt.

"Comprehensive searchers yielded 70 reports. ... The supervised PA two-group comparison included 1,598 subjects. The unsupervised PA two-group comparison included 1,081 subjects. The treatment single-group comparisons included 1,639 supervised PA and 3,420 unsupervised PA subjects. ... Most primary studies were published articles ($s = 54$), and the remainder were dissertations ($s = 14$), book chapter ($s = 1$), and conference presentation materials ($s = 1$; s indicates the number of reports). Publication bias was evident in the funnel plots for supervised and unsupervised PA two-group outcome comparisons and for treatment group, pre- vs.

post-intervention supervised PA and unsupervised PA comparisons. The control group pre- and post-comparison distributions on the funnel plots suggested less publication bias than plots of treatment groups. Unless otherwise specified, all results are from the treatment vs. control comparisons." (Conn, 2010, p. 131)

Results of Meta-Analysis for Continuous Outcomes

Many nursing studies examine continuous outcomes or outcomes that are measured by methods that produce interval or ratio level data (see Chapter 16). Physiological measures to examine blood pressure (BP) produce ratio level data. Likert scales, such as the Center for Epidemiologic Studies Depression (CES-D) Scale (see Figure 17-8), produce interval level data. Thus, BP and depression are considered continuous outcomes and the data are analyzed with the same statistical tests. Meta-analysis includes a two-step process: Step 1 is the calculation of a summary statistic for each study to describe the intervention effect, and step 2 is the summary (pooled) intervention effect that is the weighted average of the intervention effects, derived from the values of different studies. In step 1, to determine the effect of an intervention on continuous outcomes, the mean difference between two groups is calculated. The **mean difference** is a standard statistic that is calculated to determine the absolute difference between two groups. It is an estimate of the amount of change caused by the intervention (e.g., physical activity) on the outcome (e.g., depressive symptoms) on average compared with the control group. The mean difference can be calculated to determine the effect of an intervention only if the outcome is measured by the same scale in all of the studies (Higgins & Green, 2008).

A **standardized mean difference** (SMD), or *d*, is used in studies as a summary statistic and is calculated in a meta-analysis when the same outcome is measured by different scales or methods across studies. The SMD is also sometimes referred to as the standardized mean effect size. For example, in the meta-analysis by Conn (2010), depression was commonly measured with three different scales: Profile of Mood States, Beck Depression Inventory, and CES-D Scale. Studies that have differences in means in the same proportion to the standard deviations have the same SMD (*d*) regardless of the scales used to measure the outcome variable. The differences in the means and standard deviations in the studies are assumed to be due to the measurement scales and not variability in the outcome (Higgins & Green,

2008). The SMD is calculated by meta-analysis software, and the formula is provided as follows:

$$\text{SMD } (d) = \frac{\text{difference in mean outcome between groups}}{\text{Standard deviation of outcome among participants}}$$

Step 2 of the meta-analysis calculations involves summarizing the effects of an intervention across studies. The pooled intervention effect estimate is "calculated as a weighted average of the intervention effects estimated in the individual studies." A weighted average is defined by Higgins and Green (2008, p. 263) as:

$$\text{Weighted average} = \frac{\text{sum of (estimate} \times \text{weight)}}{\text{sum of weights}}$$

In combining intervention effect estimates across studies, a random-effects meta-analysis model or fixed-effect meta-analysis model can be used. The assumption of using the **random-effects model** is that all of the studies are not estimating the same intervention effect but rather related effects over studies that follow a distribution across studies. When each study is estimating the exact same quality, a **fixed-effects model** is used. Meta-analysis results can be obtained using software from SPSS and SAS statistical packages (see Chapter 21). Cochrane Collaboration Review Manager (RevMan) is software that can be used for conducting meta-analyses. This chapter provides a very basic discussion of key ideas related to conducting meta-analyses, and you are encouraged to review Higgins and Green (2008) and other meta-analysis sources to increase your understanding of this process (Andrel et al., 2009; Fernandez & Tran, 2009; Moore, 2012; Turlik, 2010). We also recommend the assistance of a statistician in conducting these analyses.

Conn's (2010) meta-analysis result identified a standardized mean *ES* of 0.372 between the treatment and the control groups for the 38 supervised PA studies and SMD of 0.522 among the 22 unsupervised PA studies. This meta-analysis documented that supervised and unsupervised PA reduced symptoms of depression in healthy adults or adults without clinical depression. Thus, a decrease in depression is another important reason for encouraging patients to be involved in PA.

Results of Meta-Analysis for Dichotomous Outcomes

If the outcome data to be examined in a meta-analysis are dichotomous, risk ratios, odds ratio, and risk differences usually are calculated to determine the effect of the intervention on the measured outcome. These terms are introduced in this chapter but more information is available in Craig and Smyth (2012), Higgins and Green (2008), and Sackett et al. (2000). With dichotomous data, every participant fits into one of two categories, such as clinical improvement versus no clinical improvement, effective versus ineffective screening device, or alive versus dead. **Risk ratio** (*RR*), also called **relative risk**, is the ratio of the risk of subjects in the intervention group to the risk of subjects in the control group for having a particular health outcome. The intervention group might also be referred to as the exposed group and the control group as the unexposed group in some studies. The health outcome is usually adverse, such as the risk of a disease (e.g., cancer) or the risk of complications or death (Higgins & Green, 2008; Moore, 2012). The calculation for *RR* is:

$$\text{Relative risk } (RR) = \frac{\text{risk of event in experimental group}}{\text{risk of event in control group}}$$

The **odds ratio** (*OR*) is defined as the ratio of the odds of an event occurring in one group, such as the treatment group, to the odds of it occurring in another group, such as the standard care group (Grove & Cipher, 2017). The *OR* is a way of comparing whether two groups have the same odds of a certain event's occurrence (see Chapter 24). An example is the odds of medication adherence or nonadherence for an experimental group receiving an intervention of education and specialized medication packaging intervention versus a group receiving standard care. The calculation for *OR* is:

$$\text{Odds ratio } (OR) = \frac{\text{odds of event in experimental group}}{\text{odds of event in control or comparison group}}$$

The **risk difference** (*RD*), also called the *absolute risk reduction*, is the risk of an event in the experimental group minus the risk of the event in the control or standard care group.

$$\text{Risk difference } (RD) = \text{risk for experimental group} - \text{risk for control group}$$

Meta-analysis results from studies with dichotomous data are often presented using a forest plot. Figure 19-5 provides a format for presenting a forest plot in a

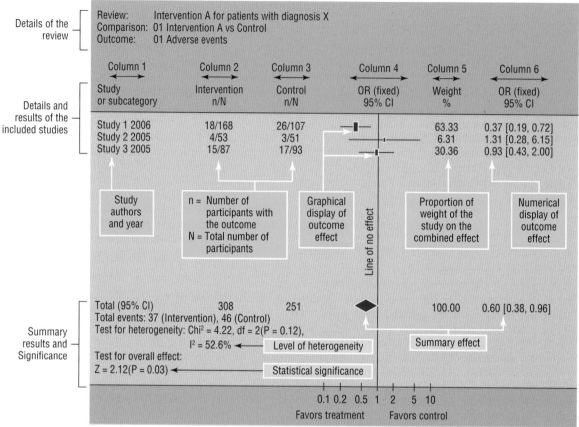

FIGURE 19-5 Meta-analysis graph for dichotomous data. CI, confidence interval; OR, odds ratio. (Adapted from Fernandez, R. S., & Tran, D. T. [2009]. The meta-analysis graph: Clearing the haze. *Clinical Nurse Specialist, 23*[2], 58.)

meta-analysis study (Fernandez & Tran, 2009). A forest plot usually includes the following information: (1) author, year, and name of the study; (2) raw data from the intervention and control groups and total number in each group; (3) point estimate (*OR* or *RR*) and confidence internal (*CI*) for each study shown as a line and block on the graph; (4) numerical values for point estimate (*OR* or *RR*) and *CI* for each study; and (5) percent weights given to each study (Fernandez & Tran, 2009; Higgins & Green, 2008; Moore, 2012). In Figure 19-5, column 1 identifies each of the studies using the clearest format for the studies being analyzed. Column 2 includes the number of participants with the outcome (*n*) and total number of participants in the intervention or experimental group (*N*), expressed as *n/N*. Column 3 includes the number of participants who displayed the outcome and the total number in the control group.

Column 4 graphically presents the *OR* with a block and the 95% *CI* with a line. Column 5 displays the percent weights given to each of the three studies in this example. Column 6 shows the numerical values for the *OR* and 95% *CI*.

The bottom of the forest plot in Figure 19-5 provides a summary of results and significance including total events for intervention and control groups, a test for heterogeneity, and a test for overall effect. The unlabeled line at the very bottom represents the *OR*. The scale of the line is logarithmic, not arithmetic. The large diamond in the plot is the summary of the effect of the studies included in the analysis. If the diamond is situated to the left of the line that is positioned at 1, the results favor the intervention or treatment. The *CI* does not include 1 if the results are statistically significant (Fernandez & Tran, 2009). If the point estimates are consistently more on one side of the vertical line, this shows homogeneity of the studies. If the point estimates are fairly equally distributed on both the left and the right side of the vertical line, this shows heterogeneity of the studies included in the meta-analysis. The term "heterogeneity" was introduced earlier; heterogeneity can exist in the sample size and characteristics, types of an intervention, designs, and outcomes of the studies. Heterogeneity statistics for random-effects meta-analyses include chi-square tests (see Chapter 25), the I^2, and a test for differences across subgroups when it is appropriate (Higgins & Green, 2008).

Magnus, Ping, Shen, Bourgeois, and Magnus (2011) conducted a meta-analysis of the effectiveness of mammography screening in reducing breast cancer mortality in women 39 to 49 years old. Because mammography screening is significant in reducing breast cancer mortality of women older than 50 years and early detection of breast cancer increases survival, annual routine mammography screening has been recommended for all women 40 to 47 years old in the United States. Thus, the "primary aim of the current study was, after a quality assessment of identified randomized controlled trials (RCTs), to conduct a meta-analysis of the effectiveness of mammography screening [*intervention*] in women ages 39–49 years [*population*] in reducing breast cancer mortality [*dichotomous outcome*]. The second aim was to compare and discuss the results of previously published meta-analyses" (Magnus et al., 2011, p. 845). The following excerpts describe the methods, results, and conclusions of this meta-analysis.

Methods: The PubMed/MEDLINE, OVID, Educational Resources Information Center (ERIC) and COCHRANE databases were searched and the extracted studies were assessed. In addition, dissertation abstracts and clinical trials databases were searched to identify unpublished and ongoing research. Two reviewers conducted independent assessments of the studies selected. The meta-analysis conducted by Magnus and colleagues (2011, p. 845) only included RCTs published in English that had "data on women aged 39–49, and reported relative risk (*RR*)/odds ratio (*OR*) or frequency data."

Results: Nine RCTs met eligibility criteria to be included in the meta-analysis. "The individual trials were quality assessed, and the data were extracted using predefined forms. Using the DerSimonian and Laird random effects model, the results from the seven RCTs with the highest quality score were combined, and a significant pooled *RR* estimate of 0.83 (95% confidence interval [CI] 0.72–0.97) was calculated." (Magnus et al., 2011, p. 845)

The results of the study were graphically represented using a forest plot that is presented in Figure 19-6. The plot clearly identifies the names of the seven studies included in the meta-analysis on the left side of the figure. The *RR* and *CI* for each study are identified with a block and horizontal line. The numerical *RR* and 95% *CI* values are identified on the right side of the plot with the percent of weight given to each study. Most of the studies show homogeneity with *ORs* left of the vertical line except for the Stockholm study. The forest plot would have been strengthened by including the results from the test for heterogeneity and the test for overall effect. Magnus et al. (2011, p. 845) concluded, "Mammography screenings were effective and generate a 17% reduction in breast cancer mortality in women 39–49 years of age. The quality of the trials varies, and providers should inform women in this age group about the positive and negative aspects of mammography screenings."

Conducting Meta-Synthesis of Qualitative Research

Qualitative research synthesis is the process and product of systematically reviewing and formally integrating the findings from qualitative studies (Sandelowski & Barroso, 2007). Various synthesis methods for qualitative research have appeared in the literature, such as meta-synthesis, meta-ethnography, meta-study, meta-narrative, qualitative meta-summary, qualitative meta-analysis, and aggregated analysis (Barnett-Page & Thomas, 2009; Kent & Fineout-Overholt, 2008; Korhone, Hakulinen-Viitanen, Jylhä, & Holopainen, 2013; Sandelowski & Barroso, 2007; Walsh & Downe, 2005; Whittemore et al., 2014). Qualitative researchers are not in agreement at the present time about the best method to use for synthesizing qualitative research or whether a single synthesis method would suffice. Although the methodology is not clearly developed for qualitative research synthesis, researchers recognize the importance of summarizing qualitative findings to determine knowledge that might be used in practice and for policy development (Finfgeld-Connett, 2010; Korhonen et al., 2013; Sandelowski & Barroso, 2007; Whittemore et al., 2014). The Cochrane Collaboration recognizes the importance of synthesizing qualitative research, and the Cochrane Qualitative Methods Group was formed as a forum for discussion and development of methodology in this area (Higgins & Green, 2008).

The qualitative research synthesis method that seems to be gaining momentum in the nursing literature is meta-synthesis. Methodological articles have been published to describe meta-synthesis, but this synthesis

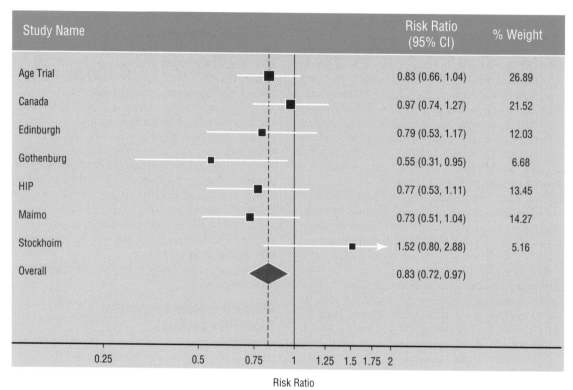

FIGURE 19-6 Forest plot showing the individual randomized controlled trials and the overall pooled estimate from the seven original randomized controlled trials with a high-quality score addressing the impact of mammography screening on breast cancer mortality in women 39 to 49 years old. *CI*, confidence interval. (Redrawn from Magnus, M. C., Ping, M., Shen, M. M., Bourgeois, J., & Magnus, J. H. [2011]. Effectiveness of mammography screening in reducing breast cancer mortality in women aged 39-49 years: A meta-analysis. *Journal of Women's Health*, *20*[6], 848.)

process is still evolving (Finfgeld-Connett, 2010; Kent & Fineout-Overholt, 2008; Korhonen et al., 2013). **Meta-synthesis** is defined as the systematic compiling and integration of qualitative study results to expand understanding and develop a unique interpretation of study findings in a selected area. The focus is on interpretation rather than the combining of study results as with quantitative research synthesis. Meta-synthesis involves the breaking down of findings from different studies to discover essential features and then the combining of these ideas into a unique, transformed whole. Sandelowski and Barroso (2007) identified meta-summary as a step in conducting meta-synthesis. **Meta-summary** is the summarizing of findings across qualitative reports to identify knowledge in a selected area. A process for conducting a meta-synthesis is described in the following section. A meta-synthesis conducted by Denieffe and

Gooney (2011) of the symptom experience of women with breast cancer is presented as an example.

Framing a Meta-Synthesis Exercise

Initially, researchers need to provide a frame for the meta-synthesis to be conducted (Kent & Fineout-Overholt, 2008; Walsh & Downe, 2005). Framing involves identifying the focus and scope of the meta-synthesis to be conducted. The focus of the meta-synthesis is usually an important area of interest for the individuals conducting it and a topic with an adequate body of qualitative studies. The scope of a meta-synthesis is an area of debate, with some qualitative researchers recommending a narrow, precise approach and others recommending a broader, more inclusive approach. However, researchers recognize framing is essential for making the synthesis process manageable and the findings meaningful and potentially transferable to practice. Framing the meta-synthesis is facilitated by the authors' research and clinical expertise, initial review of the relevant qualitative literature, and discussion with expert qualitative researchers. Usually a research question is developed to direct the meta-synthesis process.

Denieffe and Gooney (2011) conducted their meta-synthesis based on the stages developed by Sandelowski and Barroso (2007). These stages included "identifying a research question, collecting relevant data (qualitative studies), appraising the studies, performing a metasummary and meta-synthesis" (Denieffe & Gooney, 2011, p. 425). Denieffe and Gooney developed the following question to direct their meta-synthesis and provided a rationale for their scope and focus.

"In this study the question was set as 'What is the symptom experience of women with breast cancer from time of diagnosis to completion of treatment?' The time frame selected from time of diagnosis to completion of treatment, has been conceptualized ... as the 'acute stage,' encompassing initial diagnosis and treatment in the first of a three-stage process of survivorship." (Denieffe & Gooney, 2011, p. 425)

Searching the Literature and Selecting Sources

Most authors agree that a rigorous search of the literature needs to be conducted. The search should include databases, books and book chapters, and full reports of theses and dissertations. Special search strategies that were identified earlier must be engaged to identify grey literature because qualitative studies might be published in more obscure journals. The search criteria need to identify the years of the search, keywords to be searched, and language of sources. Meta-syntheses usually are limited to qualitative studies only and do not included mixed method studies (Korhonen et al., 2013; Walsh & Downe, 2005). Also, qualitative findings that have not been interpreted but are unanalyzed quotes, field notes, case histories, stories, or poems usually are excluded (Finfgeld-Connett, 2010). The search process is very fluid with the conduct of additional computerized and hand searches to identify more studies. Sandelowski and Barroso (2007) identified a dynamic process of modifying search terms and methods to identify relevant sources. However, it is important for researchers to document systematically the strategies that they used to search the literature and the sources found through these different search strategies.

The final selection of studies to include in the meta-synthesis depends on its focus and scope. Some authors focus on one type of qualitative research, such as ethnography, or one investigator in a particular area. Others include studies with different qualitative methodologies and investigators in a field or related fields. The search criteria should be consistently implemented in determining the studies to be included in or excluded from the synthesis. A flow diagram is useful in identifying the process for selecting studies similar to the one identified for systematic reviews and meta-analyses (see Figure 19-1). Denieffe and Gooney (2011) provided the following description of the literature search, search criteria, and selection of studies for their meta-synthesis.

"Relevant qualitative research studies were located and retrieved using computer searches in CINAHL, PsychLIT, Academic Search Premier, Embase, and MEDLINE. The research reports selected for this synthesis met the following inclusion criteria: (1) the study focused on women with breast cancer; (2) there were explicit references to the use of qualitative research methods; and (3) the study focused on women's perspectives and experiences of symptoms with breast cancer. There were no restrictions related to the date the research was published. Keywords used were *breast cancer, experience, symptom*, and *symptom experience*. ... The search using electronic databases was supplemented by ... footnote chasing using reference lists, citation searching, in addition to hand searching of journals, and consultation with clinical colleagues and researchers in the area. A total of 253 studies were identified as being possibly relevant. ... Only 31 studies were found to be relevant to the research question and included in the meta-synthesis. Reasons for this reduction included papers that provided limited qualitative data, ... did not address the research question, ... addressed post-treatment/survivor concerns, ... or data given may not have related to patients with breast cancer." (Denieffe & Gooney, 2011, pp. 425–426)

Appraisal of Studies and Analysis of Data

The critical appraisal process for qualitative research varies among sources. We recommend the critical appraisal guidelines for qualitative research presented in Chapter 18. These guidelines might be used for examining the quality of individual studies and a group of studies for a meta-synthesis. Usually a table is developed as part of the appraisal process, but this is also an area of debate. The table headings might include (1) author and year of source, (2) aim or goal of the study, (3) philosophical orientation, (4), methodological orientation, (5) type of findings, (6) sampling plan, (7) sample size, and (8) other key content relevant for comparison. This table provides a display of relevant study elements so that a comparative appraisal might be conducted (Sandelowski & Barroso, 2007; Walsh & Downe, 2005). The **comparative analysis** of studies involves examining methodology and findings across studies for similarities and differences. The frequency of similar findings might be recorded. The differences or contradictions in studies should be resolved or explained (or both). Varied analysis techniques often are used by the researchers to translate the findings of the different studies into a new or unique description.

Denieffe and Gooney (2011) developed a detailed comparative analysis table of the 31 studies, which they included in their meta-synthesis. Their table included the headings mentioned in the previous paragraph and the following: time frame from diagnosis, treatment, age range, and ethnic origin. They indicated that the "final stage of data analysis was the qualitative meta-synthesis, interpreting the findings. Constant targeted comparison within and between study findings was undertaken, utilizing external literature to facilitate interpretation of the emerging findings" (Denieffe & Gooney, 2011, p. 426).

Discussion of Meta-Synthesis Findings

A meta-synthesis report might include findings presented in different formats based on the knowledge developed and the perspective of the authors. A synthesis of qualitative studies in an area might result in the discovery of unique or more refined themes explaining the area of synthesis. The findings from a meta-synthesis might be presented in narrative format or graphically presented in a conceptual map or model. The discussion of findings also needs to include identification of the limitations of the meta-synthesis. The report often concludes with recommendations for further research and possibly implications for practice or policy development or both (Korhonen et al., 2013).

The synthesis by Denieffe and Gooney (2011) of 31 qualitative studies in the area of symptoms experienced by women with breast cancer resulted in the identification of four emerging themes: (1) breast cancer and the impact on self, (2) self-image and stigma, (3) self and self-control, and (4) more than just a symptom. The researchers linked each of these themes with the appropriate studies and presented this information clearly in a table. Denieffe and Gooney (2011) also developed a detailed model presented in Figure 19-7 that linked the

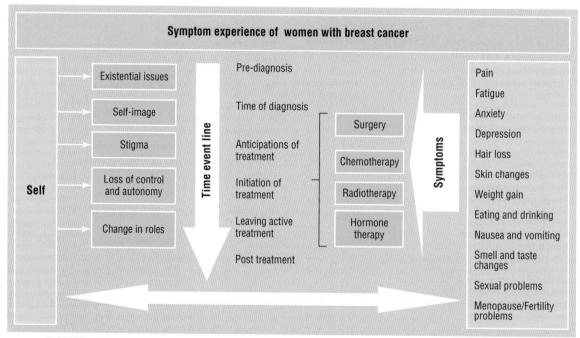

FIGURE 19-7 Overall findings of meta-synthesis. (Adapted from Denieffe, S., & Gooney, M. [2011]. A meta-synthesis of women's symptoms experience and breast cancer. *European Journal of Cancer Care, 20*[4], 430.)

themes about self to the diagnosis and treatment of the women and the symptoms they experienced. The following excerpt provides the conclusions from this meta-synthesis.

"The overarching idea emerging from this meta-synthesis is that the symptoms experience for women with breast cancer has effects on the very 'self' of the individual. Emerging is women's need to consider the existential issues that they face while simultaneously dealing with a multitude of physical and psychological symptoms. This meta-synthesis develops a new, integrated, and more complete interpretation of findings on the symptom experience of women with breast cancer. The results offer the clinician a greater understanding in depth and breadth than the findings from individual studies on symptom experiences." (Denieffe & Gooney, 2011, p. 424)

Mixed-Methods Systematic Reviews

In recent years, nurse researchers have conducted mixed methods studies that include both quantitative and qualitative research methods (Creswell, 2014; see Chapter 14). Researchers recognize the importance of synthesizing the findings of these studies to determine important knowledge for practice and policy development. For some synthesis areas, researchers need to combine the findings from both quantitative and qualitative studies to determine current knowledge in that area. Harden and Thomas (2005) identified this process of combining findings from quantitative and qualitative studies as mixed methods synthesis. Higgins and Green (2008) referred to this synthesis of quantitative, qualitative, and mixed methods studies as a mixed methods systematic review.

The systematic reviews discussed earlier in this chapter included only studies of a quantitative methodology, such as meta-analyses, RCTs, and quasi-experimental studies, to determine the effectiveness of an intervention. Mixed methods systematic reviews might include various study designs, such as qualitative research and quasi-experimental, correlational, and descriptive studies (Bettany-Saltikov, 2010b; Higgins & Green, 2008; Liberati et al., 2009; Whittemore et al., 2014). Reviews that include syntheses of various quantitative and qualitative study designs are referred to as **mixed methods systematic reviews** in this text. Mixed methods systematic reviews have the potential to contribute to Cochrane Interventions reviews for practice and health policy in the following ways:

1. **Informing** reviews by using evidence from qualitative research to help define and refine a question
2. **Enhancing** reviews by synthesizing evidence from qualitative research identified whilst looking for evidence
3. **Extending** reviews by undertaking a search and synthesis specifically of evidence from qualitative studies to address questions directly related to the effectiveness review
4. **Supplementing** reviews by synthesizing qualitative evidence to address questions on aspects other than effectiveness

(Higgins & Green, 2008, p. 574)

Conducting mixed-methods systematic reviews involves implementing a complex synthesis process that includes expertise in synthesizing knowledge from quantitative, qualitative, and mixed methods studies. Higgins and Green (2008) recommended two types of approaches to integrate the findings from quantitative, qualitative, and mixed methods studies: (1) multilevel syntheses and (2) parallel syntheses. **Multilevel synthesis** involves synthesizing the findings from quantitative studies separately from qualitative studies and integrating the findings from these two syntheses in the final report. **Parallel synthesis** involves the separate synthesis of quantitative and qualitative studies, but the findings from the qualitative synthesis are used in interpreting the synthesized quantitative studies.

Further work is needed to develop the methodology for conducting a mixed methods systematic review. The steps overlap with the systematic review and meta-synthesis processes described previously. The process might best be implemented by a team of researchers with expertise in conducting different types of studies and research syntheses. The basic structure for a mixed methods systematic review might include the following: (1) identify purpose and questions or aims of the review; (2) develop the review protocol that includes search strategies for quantitative, qualitative, and mixed methods studies; (3) identify search criteria for quantitative studies; (4) identify search criteria for qualitative and mixed methods studies; (5) conduct a rigorous search of the literature; (6) select relevant quantitative, qualitative, and mixed methods studies for synthesis; (7) construct a table of information of studies to allow comparative appraisal of the studies; (8) conduct critical appraisals of the quality of quantitative and qualitative studies; (9) synthesize study findings; and (10) develop a report that integrates the results of syntheses for quantitative, qualitative, and mixed methods studies. The reader is encouraged to refer to the steps in systematic review and meta-analysis for conducting quantitative research syntheses and to the meta-synthesis discussion for synthesizing qualitative studies.

Purpose and Questions to Focus Review

Shaw, Downe, and Kingdon (2015, p. 1451) conducted a "systematic mixed-methods review of interventions, outcomes, and experiences for pregnant incarcerated women" and their babies. The researchers thought it important to synthesize research in this area because the number of pregnant women imprisoned is increasing and this population is particularly vulnerable. The mixed methods review addressed the following questions:

- How do women who have been incarcerated during pregnancy and/or who give birth while in prison experience maternity care?
- What are the outcomes for incarcerated pregnant and childbearing women and their babies, particularly in the context of new innovations in maternity service delivery?
(Shaw et al., 2015, p. 1453)

Search Methods and Results

Shaw and colleagues detailed their literature search strategies, which included the Cochrane Library, CINAHL, EMBASE, MEDLINE, PsycINFO, and PubMed databases. The results of the search were presented in a PRISMA flow diagram (see Figure 19-1 for the format). A total of 424 citations were identified in the search of the databases and after the application of their inclusion and exclusion criteria, seven papers were selected for inclusion in their mixed-methods systematic review. "Four of the studies were quantitative, two were qualitative; and one used mixed-methods" (Shaw et al., 2015, p. 1451). The seven studies included in the review were assessed and found to have adequate quality. A table of the studies was presented in the article and included the following information: author, year, country, focus, design and methods, sampling strategy, analytic strategies, sample characteristics, quality score, and findings.

Results of the Review

Shaw et al. (2015) found limited published data on the experience and outcomes of incarcerated pregnant women and those giving birth in prison. Their results are summarized in the following excerpt.

"None [of the studies] reported the outcomes of an intervention. Examination of the quantitative data identified a complex picture of potential harms and benefits for babies born in prison. Qualitative data revealed the unique needs of childbearing women in prison, as they continuously negotiate being an inmate, becoming a mother, complex social histories, and the threat of losing their baby, all coalescing with opportunities for transformation offered by pregnancy." (Shaw et al., 2015, p. 1451).

"There is an urgent need for intervention studies. ... Adequate support to facilitate more positive experiences of pregnancy and birth while in prison may also improve long-term health outcomes for mothers and children. ... Continuity of care and support for these families on release should also be a priority." (Shaw et al., 2015, pp. 1460–1461)

MODELS TO PROMOTE EVIDENCE-BASED PRACTICE IN NURSING

Two models commonly used to facilitate EBP in nursing are the Stetler Model of Research Utilization to Facilitate EBP (Stetler, 2001) and the Iowa Model of Evidence-Based Practice to Promote Quality of Care (Titler et al., 2001). This section introduces these two models, which might be used to implement evidence-based protocols, algorithms, and guidelines in clinical agencies.

Stetler Model of Research Utilization to Facilitate Evidence-Based Practice

An initial model for **research utilization** in nursing was developed by Stetler and Marram in 1976 and expanded and refined by Stetler in 1994 and 2001 to promote EBP for nursing. The **Stetler model** (2001), presented in Figure 19-8, provides a comprehensive framework to enhance the use of research evidence by nurses in order to facilitate EBP. The research evidence can be used at the institutional or individual level. At the institutional level, synthesized research knowledge is used to develop or update protocols, algorithms, policies, procedures, or other formal programs implemented in the institution. Individual nurses, including practitioners, educators, and policymakers, summarize research and use the knowledge to influence educational programs, make practice decisions, and impact political decision-making. Stetler's model is included in this text to guide individual nurses and healthcare institutions in using research evidence in practice. The following sections briefly describe the five phases of the Stetler model: (I) preparation, (II) validation, (III) comparative

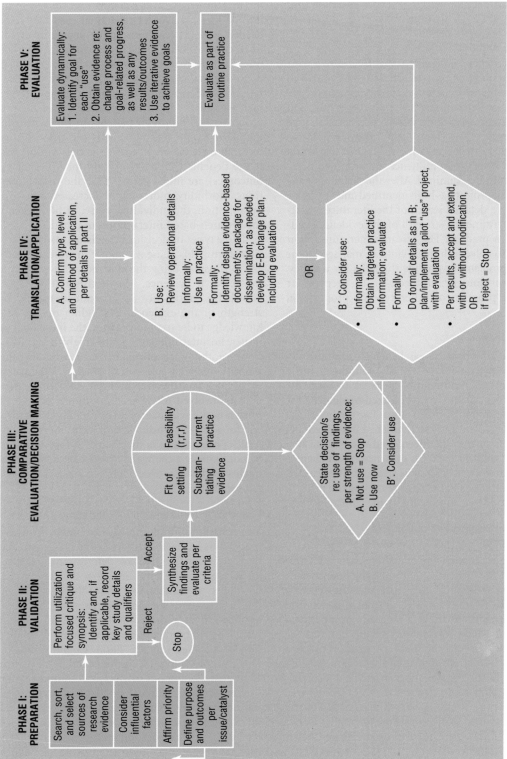

FIGURE 19-8 Stetler Model, part I: Steps of research utilization to facilitate EBP. (Adapted from Stetler, C. B. [2001]. Updating the Stetler Model of Research Utilization to facilitate evidence-based practice. *Nursing Outlook, 42*[6], 276.)

evaluation and decision making, (IV) translation and application, and (V) evaluation.

Phase I: Preparation

The intent of Stetler's model (2001) is to ensure a conscious, critical thinking process is initiated by nurses to use research evidence in practice. The first phase (preparation) involves determining the purpose, focus, and potential outcomes of making an evidence-based change in a clinical agency (see Figure 19-8). The agency's priorities and other external and internal factors that could be influenced by or could influence the proposed practice change must be examined. After the purpose of the evidence-based project has been identified and approved by the agency, a detailed search of the literature is conducted to determine the strength of the evidence available for use in practice. The research literature might be reviewed to solve a difficult clinical, managerial, or educational problem; to provide the basis for a policy, standard, algorithm, or protocol; or to prepare for an in-service program or other type of professional presentation.

Phase II: Validation

In the **validation phase**, research reports are critically appraised to determine their scientific soundness. If the studies are limited in number or are weak or both, the findings and conclusions are considered inadequate for use in practice, and the process stops. The quality of the research evidence is greatly strengthened if a systematic review or meta-analysis has been conducted in the area in which you want to make an evidence-based change. If the research knowledge base is strong in the selected area, a decision needs to be made regarding the priority of using the evidence in practice by the clinical agency.

Phase III: Comparative Evaluation and Decision-Making

Comparative evaluation includes four parts: (1) substantiation of the evidence, (2) fit of the evidence with the healthcare setting, (3) feasibility of using research findings, and (4) concerns with current practice (see Figure 19-8). Substantiating evidence is produced by replication, in which consistent, credible findings are obtained from several studies in similar practice settings. The studies generating the strongest research evidence are RCTs, meta-analyses of RCTs, and quasi-experimental studies. To determine the fit of the evidence in the clinical agency, the characteristics of the setting are examined to determine the forces that would facilitate or inhibit the evidence-based change. Stetler (2001) believed the feasibility of using research evidence

for making changes in practice necessitated examination of the three Rs: (1) potential risks, (2) resources needed, and (3) readiness of the people involved. The final comparison involves determining whether the research information provides credible, empirical evidence for making changes in the current practice. The research evidence must document that an intervention increases quality in current practice by solving practice problems and improving patient outcomes. By conducting phase III, the overall benefits and risks of using the research evidence in a practice setting can be assessed. If the benefits (improved patient, provider, or agency outcomes) are much greater than the risks (complications, morbidity, mortality, or increased costs) for the organization, the individual nurse, or both, then using the research-based intervention in practice is feasible.

Three types of decisions (**decision making**) are possible during this phase: (1) to use the research evidence, (2) to consider using the evidence, and (3) not to use the research evidence. The decision to use research knowledge in practice is determined mainly by the strength of the evidence. Depending on the research knowledge to be used in practice, the individual practitioner, hospital unit, or agency might make this decision. Another decision might be to consider using the available research evidence in practice. When a change is complex and involves multiple disciplines, the individuals involved often need additional time to determine how the evidence might be used and what measures will be taken to coordinate the involvement of different health professionals in the change. A final option might be not to make a change in practice because of the poor quality of the research evidence, costs, and other potential problems.

Phase IV: Translation and Application

The **translation and application phase** involves planning for and using the research evidence in practice. The translation phase involves determining exactly what knowledge will be used and how that knowledge will be applied to practice. The use of the research evidence can be cognitive, instrumental, or symbolic. **Cognitive application** is a more informal use of the research knowledge to modify one's way of thinking or appreciation of an issue (Stetler, 2001). Cognitive application may improve the nurse's understanding of a situation, allow analysis of practice dynamics, or improve problem-solving skills for clinical problems. Instrumental and symbolic applications are formal ways to make changes in practice. **Instrumental application** involves using research evidence to support the need for change in nursing interventions or practice protocols, algorithms, and guidelines. **Symbolic or political use** occurs when information is used to support or change an agency policy. The application phase includes the following steps for planned change: (1) assess the situation to be changed, (2) develop a plan for change, and (3) implement the plan. During the application phase, the protocols, policies, procedures, or algorithms developed with research knowledge are implemented in practice (Stetler, 2001). A pilot project on a single hospital unit might be conducted to implement the change in practice, and the results of this project could be evaluated to determine whether the change should be extended throughout the healthcare agency or corporation.

Phase V: Evaluation

The final stage of Stetler's Model is evaluation of the effect of the evidence-based change on selected agency, personnel, or patient outcomes. The **evaluation** process can include both formal and informal activities that are conducted by administrators, nurse clinicians, and other health professionals (see Figure 19-8). Informal evaluations might include self-monitoring or discussions with patients, families, peers, and other professionals. Formal evaluations can include case studies, audits, quality assurance, and outcomes research projects. The goal of the Stetler model (2001) is to increase the use of research evidence in nursing to facilitate EBP. This model provides detailed steps to encourage nurses to become change agents and make the necessary improvements in practice based on the best current research evidence.

Iowa Model of Evidence-Based Practice

Nurses have a strong commitment to EBP and can benefit from the direction provided by the Iowa model to expand their research-based practice. The **Iowa Model of Evidence-Based Practice** provides direction for the development of EBP in a clinical agency (Figure 19-9). Titler and colleagues initially developed this EBP model in 1994 and revised it in 2001. In a healthcare agency, triggers initiate the need for change, and the focus should always be to make changes based on best research evidence. These triggers can be problem-focused and evolve from risk management data, process improvement data, benchmarking data, financial data, and clinical problems. The triggers can also be knowledge-focused, such as new research findings, changes in national agencies or organizational standards and guidelines, an expanded philosophy of care, or questions from the institutional standards committee (see Figure 19-9). The triggers are evaluated and prioritized based on the needs of the clinical agency. The underlying theme of the Iowa model is that only so many things can be focused upon at once, so

prioritization of triggers is an essential part of the model. If a trigger is considered an agency priority, a group is formed to search for the best evidence to manage the clinical concern (Titler et al., 2001).

In some situations, the research evidence is inadequate to make changes in practice, and additional studies are needed to strengthen the knowledge base. Sometimes the research evidence can be combined with other sources of knowledge (theories, scientific principles, expert opinion, and case reports) to provide fairly strong evidence for developing research-based protocols for practice. The strongest evidence is generated from meta-analyses of several RCTs, systematic reviews that usually include meta-analyses, and individual studies. Systematic reviews provide the best research evidence for developing evidence-based guidelines. Then research-based protocols or evidence-based guidelines are pilot-tested on a particular unit and then evaluated to determine the impact on patient care (see Figure 19-9). If the outcomes of the pilot test are favorable, the change is made in practice and monitored over time to determine its impact on the agency environment, staff, and costs, as well as the patient and family (Titler et al., 2001). An agency can promote EBP by using the Iowa model to identify triggers for change, implement patient care based on the best research evidence, monitor changes in practice to ensure quality care, and then disseminate results of internal evaluations of the change's efficacy. For example, C. Brown (2014) implemented the Iowa Model of EBP to promote quality care in an oncology nursing unit.

IMPLEMENTING EVIDENCE-BASED GUIDELINES IN PRACTICE

Every day, research knowledge is generated and must be critically appraised and synthesized to determine the best evidence for use in practice (S. Brown, 2014; Craig & Smyth, 2012; Melnyk & Fineout-Overholt, 2015; Whittemore et al., 2014). This section focuses on the development of EBP guidelines using the best research evidence and provides a model for using these guidelines in practice. The JNC 8 evidence-based guidelines for the management of high BP in adults is presented as an example (James et al., 2014).

Development of Evidence-Based Guidelines

Once a significant health topic or condition has been selected, guidelines are developed to promote effective assessment, diagnosis, and management of this health condition. Since the 1980s, the Agency for Healthcare Research and Quality (AHRQ) has had a major role in identifying health topics and developing evidence-based

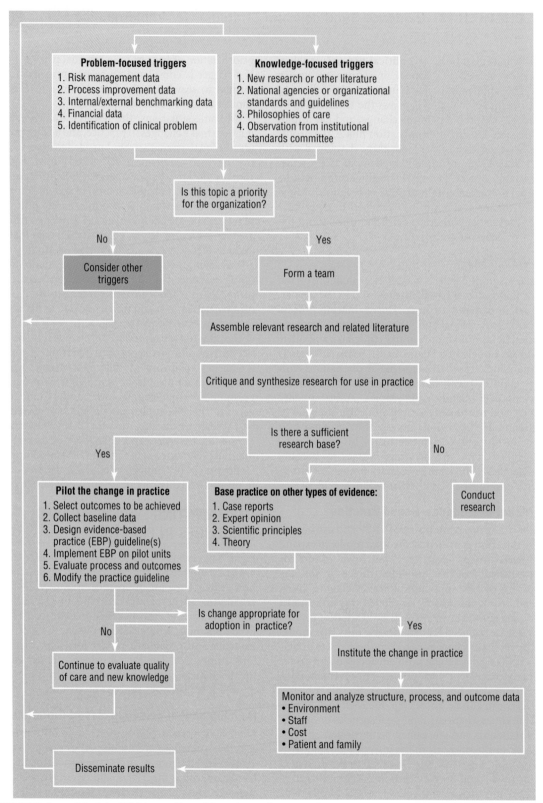

FIGURE 19-9 Iowa Model of Evidence-Based Practice to Promote Quality Care. (Adapted from Titler, M. G., Kleiber, C., Steelman, V. J., Rakel, B. A., Budreau, G., Everett, L. Q., et al. [2001]. The Iowa Model of Evidence-Based Practice to promote quality care. *Critical Care Nursing Clinics of North America, 13*[4], 500.)

guidelines for these topics. In the late 1980s and early 1990s, a panel or team of experts was often charged with developing guidelines. The AHRQ solicited the members of the panel, who usually included nationally recognized researchers in the topic area; expert clinicians, such as physicians, nurses, pharmacists, and social workers; healthcare administrators; policy developers; economists; government representatives; and consumers. The group designated the scope of the guidelines and conducted extensive reviews of the literature including relevant systematic reviews, meta-analyses, qualitative research syntheses, mixed-methods systematic reviews, individual studies, and theories.

The best research evidence available was synthesized to develop recommendations for practice. Most of the evidence-based guidelines included systematic reviews, meta-analyses, and multiple individual studies. The guidelines were examined for their usefulness in clinical practice, their impact on health policy, and their cost-effectiveness. Consultants, other researchers, and additional expert clinicians often were asked to review the guidelines and provide input. Based on the experts' critique, the AHRQ revised and packaged the guidelines for distribution to healthcare professionals. Some of the first guidelines focused on the following healthcare problems: (1) acute pain management in infants, children, and adolescents; (2) prediction and prevention of pressure ulcers in adults; (3) urinary incontinence in adults; (4) management of functional impairments with cataracts; (5) detection, diagnosis, and treatment of depression; (6) screening, diagnosis, management, and counseling about sickle cell disease; (7) management of cancer pain; (8) diagnosis and treatment of heart failure (HF); (9) low back problems; and (10) otitis media diagnosis and management in children.

The AHRQ initiated the NGC (2015) in 1998 to store EBP guidelines. The NGC is a publicly available database of evidence-based clinical practice guidelines and related documents. Free Internet access to guidelines is available at http://www.guideline.gov. The NGC is updated weekly with new content that the AHRQ produces in partnership with the American Medical Association and America's Health Insurance Plans. Some of the critical information on the NGC website includes the following.

- Guidelines by topics are provided with an option to search for a specific guideline you need for practice. Links are provided to full-text guidelines, where available, and/or ordering information for print copies.
- Guideline syntheses are provided, which are systematic comparisons of selected guidelines that address similar topic areas.

- A Guideline Comparison utility is available that gives users the ability to generate side-by-side comparisons for any combination of two or more guidelines.
- An electronic forum, NGC-L, is accessible for exchanging information on clinical practice guidelines, their development, implementation, and use.
- An Annotated Bibliography database exists, where users can search for citations for publications and resources about guidelines, including guideline development and methodology, structure, evaluation, and implementation.
- Guideline resources include complementary websites, mobile device resources, and patient education materials.
- Criteria for submitting EBP guidelines and the application process are provided.
(NGC, 2015, http://www.guideline.gov/).

In addition to evidence-based guidelines, the AHRQ has developed many tools to assess quality of care provided by the evidence-based guidelines. You can search the AHRQ (2015b) website (http://www.qualitymeasures.ahrq.gov/) for an appropriate tool to measure a variable in a research project or to evaluate outcomes of care in a clinical agency.

Numerous government agencies, professional organizations, healthcare agencies, universities, and other groups provide evidence-based guidelines for practice. Websites are as follows:

- Academic Center for Evidence-Based Nursing: http://www.acestar.uthscsa.edu
- Association of Women's Health, Obstetric, and Neonatal Nurses: http://awhonn.org
- Centers for Disease Control Healthcare Providers: http://www.cdc.gov/CDCForYou/healthcare_providers.html
- Centers for Health Evidence: http://www.cche.net
- Guidelines Advisory Committee: http://www.gacguidelines.ca
- Guidelines International Network: http://www.g-i-n.net/
- HerbMed: Evidence-Based Herbal Database, 1998, Alternative Medicine Foundation: http://www.herbmed.org/
- National Association of Neonatal Nurses: http://www.nann.org/
- National Institute for Clinical Excellence (NICE): http://www.nice.org.uk/
- Oncology Nursing Society: http://www.ons.org/

- PIER—the Physicians' Information and Education Resource (authoritative, evidence-based guidance to improve clinical care; ACP-ASIM members only): http://pier.acponline.org/index.html
- Primary Care Clinical Practice Guidelines: http://www.medscape.com/pages/editorial/public/pguidelines/index-primarycare
- U.S. Preventive Services Task Force: http://www.uspreventiveservicestaskforce.org

Implementing the Eighth Joint National Committee Evidence-Based Guidelines for the Management of High Blood Pressure in Adults

Evidence-based guidelines have become the standards for providing care to patients in the United States and other nations. A few nurses have participated on committees that have developed these evidence-based guidelines, and many APNs are using them in their practices. The 2014 evidence-based guideline for the management of high BP in adults is presented as an example. This guideline was developed by the JNC 8 panel members who conducted a systematic review of RCTs to determine the best research evidence for management of HTN. The guideline includes nine revised recommendations for the management of HTN that are available in the James et al. (2014, p. 511) article or through the NGC (2014) Guideline Summary NGC-10397. The JNC 8 guideline also includes the 2014 Hypertension Guideline Management Algorithm. This algorithm provides clinicians with direction for: (1) implementing lifestyle interventions; (2) setting BP goals; and (3) initiating BP lowering medication based on age, diabetes, and chronic kidney disease (CKD; James et al., 2014). Healthcare providers can use this algorithm to select the most appropriate treatment methods for each individual patient diagnosed with HTN.

APNs and RNs need to assess the usefulness and quality of each evidence-based guideline before they implement it in their practice. Figure 19-10 presents the **Grove Model for Implementing Evidence-Based Guidelines in Practice**. In this model, nurses identify a practice problem, search for the best research evidence to manage the problem in their practice, and identify an evidence-based guideline. Assessing the quality and usefulness of the guideline involves examining the following: (1) the authors of the guideline, (2) the significance of the healthcare problem, (3) the strength of the research evidence, (4) the link to national standards, and (5) the cost-effectiveness of using the guideline in

practice. The quality of the JNC 8 guideline is discussed using these five criteria.

Authors of the Guidelines

The panel members of the JNC 8 guideline were specifically selected from more than 400 nominees based on their "expertise in hypertension ($n = 14$), primary care ($n = 6$), … pharmacology ($n = 2$), clinical trials ($n = 6$), evidence-based medicine ($n = 3$), epidemiology ($n = 1$), informatics ($n = 4$), and the development and implementation of clinical guidelines in systems of care ($n = 4$)" (James et al., 2014, p. 508). These panel members were specifically selected based on their strong, varied expertise to develop an evidence-based guideline for HTN.

Significance of Healthcare Problem

James and colleagues (2014) addressed the significance of HTN in the following excerpt:

HTN is the most "common condition seen in primary care and leads to myocardial infarction (MI), stroke, renal failure, and death if not detected early and treated appropriately. Patients want to be assured that BP treatment will reduce their disease burden, while clinicians want guidance on HTN management using the best scientific evidence." (James et al., 2014, p. 507)

Strength of Research Evidence

A modified Delphi technique (see Chapter 17) was used to identify the three highest-ranked questions related to high BP management. The following questions guided the systematic review.

In adults with HTN:
1. "… does initiating antihypertensive pharmacologic therapy at specific BP thresholds improve health outcomes?
2. … does treatment with antihypertensive pharmacologic therapy to a specified BP goal lead to improvements in health outcomes?
3. … do various antihypertensive drugs or drug classes differ in comparative benefits and harms on specific health outcomes?" (James et al., 2014, p. 508)

The evidence review was focused on answering these three questions. The participants in the studies reviewed were adults aged 18 and older with HTN. The studies with less than 100 participants or those with a follow-up period of less than one year were excluded. Only the studies with strong sample sizes and follow-up that was adequate in yielding meaningful health-related

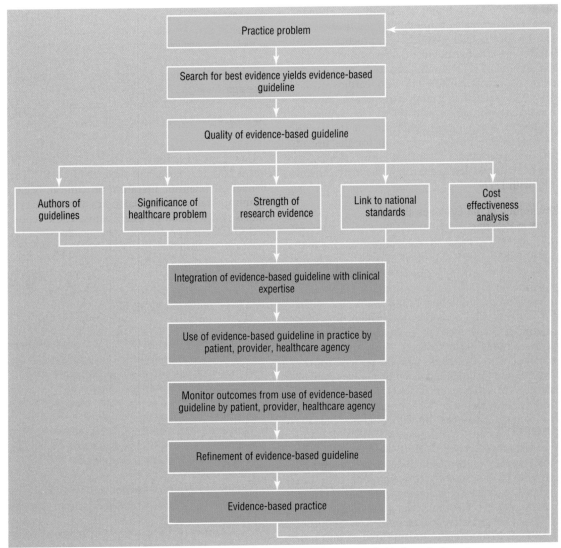

FIGURE 19-10 Grove Model for Implementing Evidence-Based Guidelines in Practice.

outcomes were included in the systematic review. The panel also "limited its evidence review to only randomized controlled trials (RCTs) because they are less subject to bias than other study designs and represent the gold standard for determining efficacy and effectiveness" (James et al., 2014, p. 508).

The JNC 8 panel members had the services of an external methodology team that searched the literature and summarized the data from selected studies into an evidence table (James et al., 2014). From the evidence review, panel members developed evidence statements that provided the basis for a guideline of nine recom-

mendations for the management of HTN. The research evidence for the development of the JNC 8 guideline for management of HTN was extremely strong.

Link to National Standards and Cost-Effectiveness of Evidence-Based Guideline

Quality evidence-based guidelines should link to national standards and be cost-effective (see Figure 19-10). The JNC 8 evidence-based guideline for the management of HTN built upon the JNC 7 national guideline for the assessment, diagnosis, and treatment of HTN. The recommendations from the JNC 7 are supported by the Department of Health and Human Services and disseminated through NIH publication no. 03-5231. Use of the JNC 8 guideline in practice is projected to be cost-effective because the recommendations for management of HTN should lead to decreased incidences of MI, stroke, CKD, HF, and cardiovascular disease (CVD) related mortality and should improve health outcomes for adults with HTN. The Hypertension Guideline Management Algorithm in the James et al. (2014) article provides direction for the use of various antihypertensive drugs or drug classes to improve benefits and decrease harm in the management of adults with HTN.

Implementation of the Evidence-Based Guideline in Practice

The next step is for APNs and physicians to use the JNC 8 evidence-based guideline in their practice (see Figure 19-10). Healthcare providers can assess the adequacy of the guideline for their practice and modify HTN treatments based on the individual health needs and values of their patients. The outcomes for patient, provider, and healthcare agency need to be examined. The outcomes are recorded in the patients' charts and possibly in a database since electronic medical records are the norm and would include the following: (1) BP readings for patients; (2) incidence of diagnosis of HTN based on the JNC 8 guidelines; (3) appropriateness of the pharmacological therapies implemented to manage HTN; and (4) incidence of stroke, MI, HF, CKD, and CVD related mortality over 5, 10, 15, and 20 years. The healthcare agency outcomes include access to care by patients with HTN, patient satisfaction with care, and costs related to diagnosis and management of HTN, in addition to the HTN complications previously mentioned. This EBP guideline will be refined in the future based on clinical outcomes, outcome studies, and new RCTs. The use of this evidence-based guideline and additional guidelines promote an EBP for APNs and RNs (see Figure 19-10).

EVIDENCE-BASED PRACTICE CENTERS

In 1997, the AHRQ launched its initiative to promote EBP by establishing 12 **evidence-based practice centers** (EPCs) in the United States and Canada.

"The EPCs develop evidence reports and technology assessments on topics relevant to clinical, social science/behavioral, economic, and other healthcare organization and delivery issues—specifically those that are common, expensive, and/or significant for the Medicare and Medicaid populations. With this program, AHRQ became a 'science partner' with private and public organizations in their efforts to improve the quality, effectiveness, and appropriateness of health care by synthesizing the evidence and facilitating the translation of evidence-based research findings. Topics are nominated by non-federal partners such as professional societies, health plans, insurers, employers, and patient groups." (AHRQ, 2015a)

Under the EPC Program, the AHRQ awards 5-year contracts to institutions to serve as EPCs. EPCs review all relevant scientific literature on clinical, behavioral, organizational, and financial topics to produce evidence reports and technology assessments. These reports are used to inform and develop coverage decisions, quality measures, educational materials, tools, guidelines, and research agendas. The EPCs also conduct research on methodology of systematic reviews. The AHRQ developed the following criteria as the basis for selecting a topic to be managed by an EPC:

- High incidence or prevalence in the general population and in special populations, including women, racial and ethnic minorities, pediatric and elderly populations, and those of low socioeconomic status.
- Significance for the needs of the Medicare, Medicaid, and other Federal health programs.
- High costs associated with a condition, procedure, treatment, or technology, whether due to the number of people needing care, high unit cost of care, or high indirect costs.
- Controversy or uncertainty about the effectiveness or relative effectiveness of available clinical strategies or technologies.
- Impact potential for informing and improving patient or provider decision making.
- Impact potential for reducing clinically significant variations in the prevention, diagnosis, or management of a disease or condition; in the use of a procedure or technology; or in the health outcomes achieved.
- Availability of scientific data to support the systematic review and analysis of the topic.
- Submission of the nominating organization's plan to incorporate the report into its managerial or policy decision making, as defined above.
- Submission of the nominating organization's plan to disseminate derivative products to its members and plan to measure members' use of these products, and the resultant impact of such use on clinical practice. (AHRQ, 2015a)

The AHRQ (2015a) website (http://www.ahrq.gov/clinic/epc) provides the names of the EPCs and the focus of each center. This site also provides a link to the evidence-based reports produced by these centers. These EPCs have had an important role in the development of evidence-based guidelines since the 1990s and will continue to make significant contributions to EBP in the future.

INTRODUCTION TO TRANSLATIONAL RESEARCH

Some of the barriers to EBP have resulted in the development of a new type of research to improve the translation of research knowledge to practice. This new research strategy is called translational research and is being supported by the NIH (2015). **Translational research** is an evolving concept that is defined by the NIH as the translation of basic scientific discoveries into practical applications. Basic research discoveries from the laboratory setting should be tested in studies with humans before application is considered. In addition, the outcomes from human clinical trials should be adopted and maintained in clinical practice. Translational research is encouraged by both medicine and nursing to increase the implementation of evidence-based interventions in practice and to determine whether these interventions are effective in producing the outcomes desired (Chesla, 2008; NIH, 2015). Translational research was originally part of the National Center for Research Resources. However, in December 2011, the National Center for Advancing Translation Sciences (NCATS) was developed as part of the NIH Institutes and Centers (NIH, 2015).

The NIH wanted to encourage researchers to conduct translational research, so the Clinical and Translational Science Awards (CTSA) Consortium was implemented in October 2006. The consortium started with 12 centers located throughout the United States and expanded to 39 centers in April 2009. The program was fully implemented in 2012 with about 60 institutions involved in clinical and translational science. A website has been developed (http://www.ctsaweb.org/) to enhance communication and encourage sharing of information related to translational research projects.

The CTSA Consortium is primarily focused on expanding the translation of medical research to practice. Titler (2004, p. S1) defined transitional research for the nursing profession as the: "Scientific investigation of methods, interventions, and variables that influence adoption of EBPs by individuals and organizations to improve clinical and operational decision-making in health care. This includes testing the effect of interventions on and promoting and sustaining the adoption of EBPs." Westra and colleagues (2015, p. 600) developed "a national action plan for sharable and comparable nursing data to support practice and translation research." This plan provides direction for the conduct and use of translation research to change nursing practice.

As you search the literature for relevant research syntheses and studies, you will note that translation studies are appearing more frequently. Mello and colleagues (2013) conducted a translation study to promote the use of an alcohol Screening, Brief Intervention, and Referral to Treatment (SBIRT) guideline in pediatric trauma centers. Prior to the study only 11% of the eligible patients were screened and received an intervention. The researchers reported the following results from their translational study.

"After completion of the SBIRT technical assistance activities, all seven participating trauma centers had effectively developed, adopted, and implemented SBIRT policies for injured adolescent inpatients. Furthermore, across all sites, 73% of eligible patients received SBIRT services after both the implementation and maintenance phases." (Mello et al, 2013, p. S301)

Additional translational studies are needed to assist with translating research findings into practice and determining the outcomes of EBP on patients' health. However, national funding is required to expand the conduct of translational research and other relevant outcomes studies in nursing.

▌ KEY POINTS

- EBP is the conscientious integration of best research evidence with clinical expertise and patient values and needs in the delivery of quality, cost-effective health care. Best research evidence is produced by the conduct and synthesis of numerous, high-quality studies in a health-related area.
- There are benefits and barriers associated with EBP. An important benefit is the delivery of care based on the most current research evidence. However, a barrier is the limited amount of interventional research, such as RCTs and quasi-experimental studies, that have been conducted in nursing.
- Guidelines are provided for conducting the research synthesis processes of systematic review, meta-analysis, meta-synthesis, and mixed-methods systematic review.

- A systematic review is a structured, comprehensive synthesis of the research literature to determine the best research evidence available to address a health-care question. A systematic review involves identifying, locating, appraising, and synthesizing quality research evidence for expert clinicians to use to promote EBP.
- Meta-analysis is a synthesis strategy that statistically pools the samples and results from previous studies with the same research design. Meta-analyses provide one of the highest levels of evidence about the effectiveness of an intervention.
- Meta-synthesis is defined as the systematic compiling and integration of qualitative study results to expand understanding and develop a unique interpretation of study findings in a selected area. The focus is on interpretation rather than the combining of study results, as in quantitative research synthesis.
- Reviews that include syntheses of various quantitative, qualitative, and mixed methods studies are referred to as mixed methods systematic reviews in this text.
- Two models have been developed to promote EBP in nursing: the Stetler Model of Research Utilization to Facilitate EBP (Stetler, 2001) and the Iowa Model of Evidence-Based Practice to Promote Quality of Care (Titler et al., 2001).
- The phases of the revised Stetler model are (I) preparation, (II) validation, (III) comparative evaluation and decision making, (IV) translation and application, and (V) evaluation.
- The Iowa model provides guidelines for implementing patient care based on the best research evidence and monitoring changes in practice to ensure quality care. It operates on the basis of responding to clinical triggers.
- The process for developing evidence-based guidelines is introduced, and the national guideline for the management of HTN in adults is provided as an example.
- The Grove Model for Implementing Evidence-Based Guidelines in Practice is provided to assist nurses in determining the quality of evidence-based guidelines and the steps for using these guidelines in practice.
- An excellent source for evidence-based guidelines is the NGC.
- EPCs have an important role in the conduct of research, development of systematic reviews, and formulation of evidence-based guidelines for selected practice areas.
- Translational research is an evolving concept that is defined by the NIH as the translation of basic scientific discoveries into practical applications.

REFERENCES

Agency for Healthcare Research and Quality (AHRQ, 2015a). *Evidence-based practice centers (EPC): Program overview.* Retrieved August 9, 2015 from http://www.ahrq.gov/research/findings/evidence-based-reports/overview/index.html.

Agency for Healthcare Research and Quality (AHRQ, 2015b). *National Quality Measures Clearinghouse (NQMC).* Retrieved August 9, 2015, from http://qualitymeasures.ahrq.gov/.

Alzayyat, A. S. (2014). Barriers to evidence-based practice utilization in psychiatric/mental health nursing. *Issues in Mental Health Nursing, 35*(2), 134–143.

American Nurses Credentialing Center (ANCC, 2015). *Magnet Recognition Program® overview.* Retrieved August 9, 2015 from http://www.nursecredentialing.org/Magnet/ProgramOverview.aspx.

Andrel, J. A., Keith, S. W., & Leiby, B. E. (2009). Meta-analysis: A brief introduction. *Clinical & Translational Science, 2*(5), 374–378.

Bagnasco, A., Di Giacomo, P., Mora, R., Catania, G., Turci, C., Rocco, G., et al. (2014). Factors influencing self-management in patients with type 2 diabetes: A quantitative systematic review protocol. *Journal of Advanced Nursing, 70*(1), 187–199.

Baker, K. A., & Weeks, S. M. (2014). An overview of systematic review. *Journal of Perianesthesia Nursing, 29*(6), 454–458.

Barnett-Page, E., & Thomas, J. (2009). Methods for the synthesis of qualitative research: A critical review. *BMC Medical Research Methodology, 9*, 59. DOI:10.1186/1471-2288-9-59.

Benzies, K. M., Premji, S., Hayden, K. A., & Serrett, K. (2006). State-of-the-evidence reviews: Advantages and challenges of including grey literature. *Worldviews on Evidence-based Nursing, 3*(2), 55–61.

Bettany-Saltikov, J. (2010a). Learning how to undertake a systematic review: Part 1. *Nursing Standard, 24*(50), 47–56.

Bettany-Saltikov, J. (2010b). Learning how to undertake a systematic review: Part 2. *Nursing Standard, 24*(51), 47–58.

Bolton, L. B., Donaldson, N. E., Rutledge, D. N., Bennett, C., & Brown, D. S. (2007). The impact of nursing interventions: Overview of effective interventions, outcomes, measures, and priorities for future research. *Medical Care Research & Review, 64*(Suppl. 2), 123S–143S.

Bridges, E. J. (2015). Research at the bedside: It makes a difference. *American Journal of Critical Care, 24*(4), 283–289.

Brown, C. B. (2014). The Iowa Model of Evidence-Based Practice to promote quality care: An illustrated example in oncology nursing. *Clinical Journal of Oncology Nursing, 18*(2), 157–159.

Brown, S. J. (2014). *Evidence-based nursing: The research-practice connection* (3rd ed.). Sudbury, MA: Jones & Bartlett.

Bruera, E., Kuehn, N., Miller, M. J., Selmser, P., & MacMillan, K. (1991). The Edmonton Symptom Assessment System (ESAS): A simple method for the assessment of palliative care patients. *Journal of Palliative Care, 7*(1), 6–9.

Butler, K. D. (2011). Nurse practitioners and evidence-based nursing practice. *Clinical Scholars Review, 4*(1), 53–57.

Catania, G., Beccaro, M., Costantini, M., Ugolini, D., De Silvestri, A., Bagnasco, A., et al. (2015). Effectiveness of complex interventions focused on quality-of-life assessment to improve palliative care patients' outcomes: A systematic review. *Palliative Medicine, 29*(1), 5–21.

Chapman, E., Whale, J., Landy, A., Hughes, D., Saunders, M., & Palliative & Supportive Care. (2008). Clinical evaluation of the Mood and Symptom Questionnaire (MSQ) in a day therapy unit in a palliative support center in the United Kingdom. *Palliative Support Care, 6*(1), 51–59.

Chesla, C. A. (2008). Translational research: Essential contributions from interpretive nursing science. *Research in Nursing & Health, 31*(4), 381–390.

Cochrane Collaboration. (2015). *Cochrane: Our evidence.* Retrieved August 9, 2015 from http://www.cochrane.org/evidence.

Cohen, J. (1988). *Statistical power analysis for the behavioral sciences* (2nd ed.). New York, NY: Academic Press.

Conn, V. S. (2010). Depressive symptom outcomes of physical activity interventions: Meta-analysis findings. *Annals of Behavioral Medicine, 39*(2), 128–138.

Conn, V. S., & Rantz, M. J. (2003). Research methods: Managing primary study quality in meta-analyses. *Research in Nursing & Health, 26*(4), 322–333.

Conn, V. S., Valentine, J. C., Cooper, H. M., & Rantz, M. J. (2003). Methods: Grey literature in meta-analyses. *Nursing Research, 52*(4), 256–261.

Craig, J. V., & Smyth, R. L. (2012). *The evidence-based practice manual for nurses* (3rd ed.). Edinburgh, UK: Churchill Livingstone.

Creswell, J. W. (2014). *Research design: Qualitative, quantitative and mixed methods approaches* (4th ed.). Thousand Oaks, CA: Sage.

Denieffe, S., & Gooney, M. (2011). A meta-synthesis of women's symptoms experience and breast cancer. *European Journal of Cancer Care, 20*(4), 424–435.

Detmar, S. B., Muller, M. J., Schornagel, J. H., Wever, L. D. V., Aaronson, N. K., & Glass, F. M. (2002). Health-related quality-of-life assessments and patient-physician communication: A randomized controlled trial. *Journal of the American Medical Association, 288*(23), 3027–3034.

Doran, D. (2011). *Nursing-sensitive outcomes: The state of the science* (2nd ed.). Sudbury, MA: Jones & Bartlett Learning.

Dupin, C. M., Chami, K., Petit dit Dariel, O., Debout, C., & Rothan-Tondeur, M. (2013). Trends in nursing research in France: A cross-sectional analysis. *International Nursing Review, 60*(2), 258–266.

Edward, K. L. (2015). A model for increasing appreciation, accessibility, and application of research in nursing. *Journal of Professional Nursing, 31*(2), 119–123.

Egger, M., Smith, G. D., Schneider, M., & Minder, C. (1997). Bias in meta-analysis detected by a simple graphical test. *British Medical Journal, 315*(7109), 629–634.

Eizenberg, M. M. (2010). Implementation of evidence-based nursing practice: Nurses' personal and professional factors? *Journal of Advanced Nursing, 67*(1), 33–42.

Fernandez, R. S., & Tran, D. T. (2009). The meta-analysis graph: Clearing the haze. *Clinical Nurse Specialist, 23*(2), 57–60.

Finfgeld-Connett, D. (2010). Generalizability and transferability of meta-synthesis research findings. *Journal of Advanced Nursing, 66*(2), 246–254.

Gerrish, K., Guillaume, L., Kirshbaum, M., McDonnell, A., Tod, A., & Nolan, M. (2011). Factors influencing the contribution of advanced practice nurses to promoting evidence-based practice among front-line nurses: Findings from a cross-sectional survey. *Journal of Advanced Nursing, 67*(5), 1079–1090.

Gillam, S., & Siriwardena, A. N. (2014). Evidence-based healthcare and quality improvement. *Quality in Primary Care, 22*(3), 125–132.

Grove, S. K., & Cipher, D. (2017). *Statistics for nursing research: A workbook for evidence-based practice* (2nd ed.). St. Louis, MO: Saunders.

Harden, A., & Thomas, J. (2005). Methodological issues in combining diverse study types in systematic reviews. *International Journal of Social Research Methodology, 8*(3), 257–271.

Higgins, J. P. T., & Green, S. (2008). *Cochrane handbook for systematic reviews of interventions.* West Sussex, UK: Wiley-Blackwell & The Cochrane Collaboration.

Hill, N. (2002). Use of quality-of-life scores in care planning in a hospice setting: A comparative study. *International Journal of Palliative Nursing, 8*(11), 540–547.

Horstman, P., & Fanning, M. (2010). Tips for writing magnet evidence. *Journal of Nursing Administration, 40*(1), 4–6.

James, P. A., Oparil, S., Carter, B. L., Crushman, W. C., Denison-Himmelfarb, C., Handler, J., et al. (2014). 2014 evidence-based guideline for the management of high blood pressure in adults: Report from the panel members appointed to the Eighth Joint National Committee (JNC 8). *Journal of American Medical Association, 311*(5), 507–520.

Joanna Briggs Institute. (2015). *Search the Joanna Briggs Institute.* Retrieved August 9, 2015 from http://joannabriggslibrary.org/.

Jocham, H. R., Dassen, T., Widdershoven, G., & Halfens, R. J. G. (2009). Quality-of-life assessment in a palliative care setting in Germany: An outcome evaluation. *International Journal of Palliative Nursing, 15*(7), 338–345.

Kent, B., & Fineout-Overholt, E. (2008). Using meta-synthesis to facilitate evidence-based practice. *Worldviews on Evidence-Based Nursing, 5*(3), 160–162.

Korhonen, A., Hakulinen-Viitanen, T., Jylhä, V., & Holopainen, A. (2013). Meta-synthesis and evidence-based health care—a method for systematic review. *Scandinavian Journal of Caring Sciences, 27*(4), 1027–1034.

Liberati, A., Altman, D. G., Tetzlaff, J., Mulrow, C., Gotzsche, P. C., Ioannidis, J. P., et al. (2009). The PRISMA Statement for reporting systematic reviews and meta-analyses of studies that evaluate healthcare interventions: Explanation and elaboration. *Annals of Internal Medicine, 151*(4), W-65–W-94.

Magnus, M. C., Ping, M., Shen, M. M., Bourgeois, J., & Magnus, J. H. (2011). Effectiveness of mammography screening in reducing breast cancer mortality in women aged 39–49 years: A meta-analysis. *Journal of Women's Health, 20*(6), 845–852.

Mantzoukas, S. (2009). The research evidence published in high impact nursing journals between 2000 and 2006: A quantitative content analysis. *International Journal of Nursing, 46*(4), 479–489.

Mello, M. J., Bromberg, J., Baird, J., Nirenberg, T., Chun, T., Lee, C., et al. (2013). Translation of alcohol screening and brief intervention guidelines to pediatric trauma centers. *Journal of Trauma & Acute Care Surgery, 75*(4), S301–S307.

Melnyk, B. M., & Fineout-Overholt, E. (2015). *Evidence-based practice in nursing & healthcare: A guide to best practice* (3rd ed.). Philadelphia, PA: Lippincott Williams & Wilkins.

Mills, M. E., Murray, L. J., Johnston, B. T., Cardwell, C., & Donnelly, M. (2009). Does a patient-held quality-of-life diary benefit patients with inoperable lung cancer? *Journal of Clinical Oncology, 27*(1), 70–77.

Moher, D., Liberati, A., Tetzlaff, J., Altman, D. G., & PRISMA Group. (2009). *Preferred Reporting Items for Systematic Reviews and Meta-Analyses: The PRISMA Statement.* Retrieved April 26, 2016 from http://www.prisma-statement.org.

Moore, Z. (2012). Meta-analysis in context. *Journal of Clinical Nursing, 21*(19/20), 2798–2807.

National Guideline Clearinghouse (NGC, 2014). *Guideline Summary NGC-10397: 2014 evidence-based guideline for the management of high blood pressure in adults. Report from the panel members appointed by the Eighth Joint National Committee (JNC 8).* Retrieved October 3, 2015, from http://www.guideline.gov/content.aspx?id=48192&search=jnc+8.

National Guideline Clearinghouse (NGC, 2015). *National Guideline Clearinghouse: Guidelines by topics.* Agency for Healthcare Research and Quality. Retrieved August 9, 2015 from http://www.guideline.gov/browse/by-topic.aspx.

National Institutes of Health (NIH, 2015). *NIH: National Center for Advancing Translational Science: Translational science spectrum.* Bethesda, MD: Author. Retrieved August 9, 2015 from http://ncats.nih.gov/translation/spectrum.

Noordzij, M., Hooft, L., Dekker, F. W., Zoccali, C., & Jager, K. J. (2009). Systematic reviews and meta-analyses: When they are useful and when to be careful. *Kidney International, 76*(11), 1130–1136.

Paré, G., Trudel, M., Jaana, M., & Kitsiou, S. (2015). Synthesizing information systems knowledge: A typology of literature reviews. *Information & Management, 52*(1), 183–199.

Pölkki, T., Kanste, O., Kääriäine, M., Elo, S., & Kyngäs, H. (2013). The methodological quality of systematic reviews published in high-impact nursing journals: A review of the literature. *Journal of Clinical Nursing, 23*(3/4), 315–332.

Rew, L. (2011). The systematic review of literature: Synthesizing evidence for practice. *Journal for Specialists in Pediatric Nursing, 16*(1), 64–69.

Sackett, D. L., Straus, S. E., Richardson, W. S., Rosenberg, W., & Haynes, R. B. (2000). *Evidence-based medicine: How to practice & teach EBM* (2nd ed.). London, UK: Churchill Livingstone.

Sandelowski, M., & Barroso, J. (2007). *Handbook for synthesizing qualitative research.* New York, NY: Springer.

Shaw, J., Downe, S., & Kingdon, C. (2015). Systematic mixed-methods review of interventions, outcomes, and experiences for imprisoned pregnant women. *Journal of Advanced Nursing, 7*(7), 1451–1462.

Shojania, K. G., Sampson, M., Ansari, M. T., Ji, J., Doucette, S., & Moher, D. (2007). How quickly do systematic reviews go out of date? Survival analysis. *Annals of Internal Medicine, 147*(4), 224–234.

Snyder, C. F., Blackford, A. L., Aaronson, N. K., Detmar, S. B., Carducci, M. A., & Brundage, M. D. (2011). Can patient-reported outcome measures identify cancer patients' most bothersome issues? *Journal of Clinical Oncology, 29*(9), 1216–1220.

Stetler, C. B. (1994). Refinement of the Stetler/Marram model for application of research findings to practice. *Nursing Outlook, 42*(1), 15–25.

Stetler, C. B. (2001). Updating the Stetler Model of Research Utilization to facilitate evidence-based practice. *Nursing Outlook, 49*(6), 272–279.

Stetler, C. B., & Marram, G. (1976). Evaluating research findings for applicability in practice. *Nursing Outlook, 24*(9), 559–563.

Stetler, C. B., Ritchie, J. A., Rycroft-Malone, J., & Charns, M. P. (2014). Leadership for evidence-based practice: Strategic and functional behaviors for institutionalizing EBP. *Worldviews on Evidence-Based Nursing, 11*(4), 219–226.

Stewart, L. A., Clarke, M., Rovers, M., Riley, R. D., Simmonds, M., Stewart, G., et al. for the PRISMA-IPD Development Group. (2015). Preferred Reporting for a Systematic Review and Meta-analysis of Individual Participant Data: The PRISMA-IPD Statement. *Journal of the American Medical Association, 313*(6), 1657–1665.

The Joint Commission. (2015). *About our standards.* Retrieved August 9, 2015 from http://www.jointcommission.org/standards_information/standards.aspx.

Titler, M. G. (2004). Overview of the U.S. invitational conference "Advancing Quality Care Through Translation Research." *Worldviews on Evidence-based Nursing, 1*(1), S1–S5.

Titler, M. G., Kleiber, C., Steelman, V. J., Rakel, B. A., Budreau, G., Everett, L. Q., et al. (1994). Research-based practice to promote the quality of care. *Nursing Research, 43*(5), 307–313.

Titler, M. G., Kleiber, C., Steelman, V. J., Rakel, B. A., Budreau, G., Everett, L. Q., et al. (2001). The Iowa Model of Evidence-Based Practice to promote quality care. *Critical Care Nursing Clinics of North America, 13*(4), 497–509.

Turlik, M. (2010). *Evaluating the results of a systematic review/meta-analysis.* Podiatry management. Retrieved August 15, 2015 from www.podiatrym.com.

Walsh, D., & Downe, S. (2005). Meta-synthesis method for qualitative research: A literature review. *Journal of Advanced Nursing, 50*(2), 204–211.

Weber, M. A., Schiffrin, E. L., White, W. B., Mann, S., Lindholm, L. H., Kenerson, J. G., et al. (2014). Clinical practice guidelines for the management of hypertension in the community: A statement by the American Society of Hypertension and the International Society of Hypertension. *Journal of Clinical Hypertension, 16*(1), 14–26.

Westra, B. L., Latimer, G. E., Matney, S. A., Park, J. I., Sensmeier, J., Simpson, R. L., et al. (2015). A national action plan for sharable and comparable nursing data to support practice and translation research for transforming health care. *Journal of American Medical Informatics Association, 22*(3), 600–607.

Whittemore, R., Chao, A., Jang, M., Minges, K. E., & Park, C. (2014). Methods for knowledge synthesis: An overview. *Heart and Lung: The Journal of Critical Care, 43*(5), 453–461.

Wintersgill, W., & Wheeler, E. C. (2012). Engaging nurses in research utilization. *Journal for Nurses in Staff Development, 28*(5), E1–E5.

20

Collecting and Managing Data

Jennifer R. Gray

http://evolve.elsevier.com/Gray/practice/

Data collection is one of the most exciting parts of research. After all the planning, writing, and negotiating that precede it, the researcher is eager for this active part of research. However, before beginning, the researcher must spend time carefully preparing for this endeavor and double-checking each step. For quantitative research, preparation begins with clarifying exactly which data will be collected, how they will be collected, and how they will be recorded. The data to be collected are determined by the variables' operational definitions (see Chapter 6). Data collection strategies for qualitative studies are described in Chapter 12.

Data collection is the process of selecting subjects and gathering data from them. The actual steps of collecting data are specific to each study and depend on both research design and measurement methods. Data may be collected from subjects by observing, testing, measuring, questioning, recording, or any combination of these methods, either conducted by the research team or retrieved from data sources. The researcher is actively involved in this process either by collecting data or by supervising data collectors.

This chapter describes practical aspects of quantitative data collection. Consistent with other phases of the research process, decisions made later in the planning process may affect decisions made previously. Although presented in the chapter as a chronological series of steps, preparation for implementing a study, and specifically collecting the data, is actually a circular process that is refined through the planning and pilot study

phases. The first section of the chapter is a brief discussion of the study protocol, which includes recruiting and consenting subjects, assigning subjects to groups if part of the study design, implementing an intervention, and collecting the data. Following that section, the focus of the chapter changes to the specific details of data collection and begins with a description of factors that affect data collection decisions such as cost and time. In the context of these factors, the researcher may need to develop or refine a demographic questionnaire, prepare for data entry, and revise a data collection plan.

Conducting a pilot test with a small group of subjects greatly strengthens the study. After necessary modifications based on the pilot results, the researcher begins data collection, maintaining consistency among data collectors over time. Incoming data are coded and stored in ways that allow easy retrieval to answer the research question. The last sections of the chapter address common problems encountered during data collection and strategies for solving them. The chapter concludes with a discussion of the supports and resources available to the researcher.

STUDY PROTOCOL

By the time you sketch plans for implementation of the study, the bulk of the methods have been decided upon. Refer to previous parts of the study proposal. How did you specify that subjects would be recruited? Were you planning on assigning your subjects randomly to groups? If so, at what point did you plan on making that assignment? It is optimal to assign subjects randomly to an intervention group or control group after baseline data are collected but before introducing the intervention. In this way, all subjects demonstrate the ability to complete questions and measures, but they have the opportunity to decline further participation before group assignment. For an interventional study, the way in which you will enact the research intervention was specified with your definition of the independent variable, but when did you envision that intervention as occurring, relative to baseline measurements?

You as the researcher will develop a flow diagram to illustrate the **study protocol** for implementing the study. A study protocol is the step-by-step plan for recruiting subjects, obtaining consent, collecting data, and implementing an intervention. The Consolidated Standards of Reporting Trials (CONSORT) 2010 Statement was developed from previous CONSORT guidelines for consistency and clarity in reporting randomized trials in publications (Schulz, Altman, & Moher, 2010). The flowchart for screening and enrollment of study participants recommended by the CONSORT 2010 guidelines should be followed. Figure 15-2 in Chapter 15 is the CONSORT figure from Newnam et al.'s (2015) study of extremely low birth weight infants who needed continuous positive airway pressure to support breathing. To create one of these flowcharts, the researcher must keep excellent records of recruitment, enrollment, attrition, and reasons for attrition. Jull and Aye (2015) conducted a systematic review of five high-impact nursing journals and found improvement in the extent to which the CONSORT guidelines were followed, but also identified areas for improvement. Chapters 11 and 15 contain more information on CONSORT guidelines and flowcharts.

FACTORS INFLUENCING DATA COLLECTION

When planning data collection, critical factors to consider are cost, number of researchers, time, availability of data collection tools, and methods of data collection. The researcher balances these with the need to maintain optimal reliability and validity of the study throughout data collection.

Cost Factors

Cost is a major consideration when planning a study. Box 20-1 provides a list of common costs associated with quantitative studies. Measurement tools, such

---

> **BOX 20-1 Common Costs for Data Collection in Quantitative Studies**
>
> - Fee for use of instrument, data collection forms, and manual for scoring and coding
> - Duplication of questionnaires and consent forms
> - Payment of non-volunteer data collectors
> - Equipment purchase or rental, maintenance costs
> - Supplies related to physiological measures, such as glucometer test strips
> - Laboratory analysis or test result analysis
> - Compensation to subjects for time and travel
> - Statistical or other consultation and services

---

as continuous electrocardiogram monitors (Holter monitors), wrist activity monitors (accelerometers), spirometers, pulse oximeters, or glucometers, used in physiological studies, may need to be rented, purchased, or borrowed from the manufacturer, a medical supply company, or a healthcare agency.

Researchers may be required to pay a fee to use instruments or questionnaires. Some of these instruments and questionnaires are available only if a copy is purchased for each participant or if a fee is paid for access of each participant to an electronic instrument. Data collection forms must be formatted or adapted to electronic use. Printing costs for materials such as teaching materials or questionnaires that will be used during the study must be considered. Providing subjects the required copy of the signed consent form doubles the expense of printing consent forms. Small payments to participants in the form of cash or gift cards should be considered as compensation for subjects' time and effort. Sometimes a researcher may choose to provide childcare so that parents and other caregivers who would not otherwise be able to participate in the study can be included. In studies with mailed surveys, postage is a substantial expense. There may be costs involved in coding data for computer entry and for conducting data analysis. Consultation with a statistician early in the development of a research project and during data analysis must also be budgeted. The researcher may need to hire an assistant who can remain blinded for data entry or analysis, or someone who can type the final report, develop graphics or presentations, or type and edit manuscripts for publication.

In addition to these direct costs of a research project, there are costs associated with the researcher's time and travel to and from the study site. The researcher may also include the estimated expense of presenting the research findings at conferences and include those expenses in the budget, if allowable in the budget. To prevent unexpected expenses from delaying the study, estimated costs should be tabulated and totaled in a budget. This can be revised as needed. Seeking funding for at least part of the costs can facilitate the conduct of a study. Some proposals for funding require considerable time to write, so benefit versus cost should be pondered.

Size of Research Team

One researcher can implement a study as the primary investigator, but one-researcher studies require more time to complete. Having a research team of two or more people means having assistance in completing all of the tasks a study requires. The disadvantage of working with a team is that additional time is required for meetings and coordination of the members' activities. The larger, more complex the study, the less likely it is that the study will be implemented by one person. Funded studies are more likely to be implemented by a research team of two or more.

Time Factors

Researchers often underestimate the time required for participants to complete data collection forms and for the research team to recruit and enroll subjects for a study. The first aspect of time—the participant's time commitment—must be determined early in the process because the time needed for participant involvement must be included in the informed consent process and document. While conducting the pilot study, make note of the time required to collect data from a subject. The researcher may need to revise the consent form to reflect the expected time commitment accurately.

The time needed for each individual subject is based on the average time pilot study subjects spent in completing data collection. The number of days, weeks, or months required in order to obtain enough subjects for the research is a more difficult prediction, because unforeseen circumstances may make gaining Institutional Review Board (IRB) approval, securing access to subjects, obtaining consent, and collecting data more extended processes than originally envisioned. For example, a sudden heavy staff workload may make data collection temporarily difficult or impossible, or the number of potential subjects might be reduced for a period. In some situations, researchers must obtain permission from administrators, managers, and even each subject's physician before they are permitted to collect data from the subject. Activities required for these stipulations, such as meeting the person in authority,

explaining the study, and obtaining permission, require extensive time. In some cases, potential subjects are lost before the researcher can obtain permission, extending the time required to obtain the necessary number of subjects.

How long will it take to identify potential subjects, explain the study, and obtain consent? How much time will be needed for activities such as completing questionnaires or obtaining physiological measures? How long will it take to obtain approval of the IRB? Schick-Makaroff and Molzahn (2015) noted that it took a year for them to obtain approval because the IRB was not familiar with electronic data collection tools. The IRB had many questions about security of data and the adequacy of Internet service in study locations.

Novice researchers may have difficulty making reasonable estimates of time and costs related to a study. Validating those estimates with an academic advisor or on-site nurse researcher, after initial pilot study completion, is recommended. If cost and time factors are prohibitive, a "trimmed-down" study measuring fewer variables, using fewer measurement instruments, or consenting fewer subjects is a reasonable solution. The researcher, however, should thoroughly examine the consequences for design validity before making such revisions.

Selection of Instruments

When several instruments or methods are available for measuring a variable, the researcher must select the best one for the specific study. Chapters 16 and 17 provide information to assist researchers in selecting quality measurement methods. Specifically, instruments and other measurements used in a study should fit, or be congruent, with the conceptual definitions for each study concept. In addition, practical considerations for instrument selection include item burden and reading level.

Item burden, which is the number of items a subject is asked to complete, must be considered in selecting an instrument for a study. The researcher balances the scientific quality of each measurement method with its feasibility in terms of cost, availability, and item burden. There is no magical number of items that a researcher can reasonably ask a subject to complete, but the maximum number is influenced by the mental state and physical health of the members of the target population. Asking subjects to complete multiple instruments of 40 or more questions may be unreasonable and result in missing data.

Reading level is another consideration: Does the typical member of the target population have adequate literacy to be able to complete a printed instrument without assistance? If not, the researcher or an assistant should read the questions to each subject. If this is not possible or not feasible, another instrument or measurement method may be more appropriate to use for the study.

Methods of Data Collection

Based on data needed to answer the research question, and on instruments to be used in a study, the researcher must decide whether to present this instrument to subjects as a packet of pencil-paper instruments, a link to a website to access the instruments, or questions on an electronic tablet or other electronic interface. For some studies, the subject is equipped with an electronic sensor to automatically gather pertinent data. What are some of the advantages and disadvantages of different approaches to data collection?

Researcher-Administered and Participant-Completed Instruments

If a subject's accurate BP, height, and weight are demographic variables, a self-report measure may be neither valid nor reliable for the purpose of the study. However, if the purpose of the study can be accomplished with a self-report survey method, you must decide whether the subject will complete the survey or whether the researcher will administer the survey. It may be best for the researcher to administer self-report paper-and-pencil instruments if the potential subjects have minimal language or literacy ability, whereas it may be best to consider electronic data collection or medical record extraction if the subjects are likely to have hearing impairments, transportation problems, or physical difficulties.

If the researcher is administering the survey, will this occur in person or by telephone? If self-administered, will the participant complete a pencil-and-paper copy or an online electronic copy? Internet survey centers specialize in the latter mode of data collection and provide expert help or tutorials for assessing the best mode for the study purpose. For example, in deciding on a telephone survey, how many times will attempts be made to reach a potential subject before stopping, what days of the week or hours of the day will calls be made, how might that bias the sample or their responses, and how will the response rate be determined (Harwood, 2009)? A relatively new factor in using telephones to collect data is that some families no longer have home phone lines, which formerly were the numbers publicly available. If a mailed paper-and-pencil survey will be used, what will be done with undelivered or incomplete

returns? Will the researcher search for correct mailing addresses and undertake a second mailing, to contact subjects with forwarding addresses on record? Will reminders be sent if the survey is not received within a particular time frame, and if so, what time frame will be given respondents, and how many reminders will be sent (Harwood, 2009)?

Scannable Forms

Some target populations may have limited access to technology, requiring use of more conventional types of data collection. Even with paper versions of data collection documents, there are ways to decrease the labor of data entry and improve the accuracy of data entry by preparing special data collection forms that can be scanned. These forms are developed and coded using optical character recognition (OCR). OCR requires exact placement on the page for each potential response. To maintain the precise location of each response on print copies of these instruments, careful attention must be given to printing or copying. The complete form is scanned and responses (data) are automatically recorded in a database. Additional features include data accuracy verification, selective data extraction and analysis, auditing and tracking, and flexible export interfaces. Figure 20-1 shows the first page of a scannable version of the Parents and Newborn Screening Survey developed by Patricia Newcomb, PhD, RN, CPNP, and Barbara True, MSN, CNS. Subjects completing the survey fill in the circle that corresponds to the appropriate option for each question.

Online Data Collection

Computer software packages developed by a variety of companies (e.g., SurveyMonkey and Qualtrics) enable researchers to provide instruments and other data collection forms online to potential subjects. These software programs have unique features that allow the researcher to develop point-and-click automated forms that can be distributed electronically. The following questions should be considered with use of these programs. The first major question is whether computers and online access are available among the target population. For an online survey, is the parent company a secure site for the purposes of confidentiality and anonymity? Is the survey formatted so that it can be completed using other electronic devices such as smartphones and tablets? What strategies can be used to increase the likelihood that only eligible participants complete the survey? Will potential subjects receive a personalized email message with a link to a website? How will email addresses be obtained? Can the researcher

ID | 1 | 0 | 6 | 1

Parents and Newborn Screening Survey
The University of Texas at Arlington College of Nursing
Andrews Women's Hospital

Instructions: Please use a BLACK PEN for completing the survey. Do not use pencil.

Please shade circles like this: ●
Not like this: ✗ ✓

1. My age is:

○ Less than 18   ○ 18-24   ○ 25-30   ○ 31-35   ○ 36+

2. My race/ethnic group is:

○ African-American   ○ Asian   ○ Caucasian   ○ Hispanic   ○ Other

3. My highest level of education is:

○ Less than high school   ○ High school diploma   ○ Some college   ○ Bachelor's degree   ○ Master's degree or more

4. I work in the healthcare field:

○ Yes   ○ No

5. I started pregnancy care:
○ In the first 3 months of my pregnancy
○ In the second 3 months of my pregnancy
○ In the last 3 months of my pregnancy
○ I did not get medical care during my pregnancy

6. My care for this pregnancy and birth was paid for by:
○ Medicaid
○ Private insurance
○ I paid for it by myself
○ I don't know how it will be paid for

7. I learned about newborn screening from (may circle more than one):
○ I never heard of newborn screening before this
○ My doctor or midwife
○ My child's doctor or nurse practitioner
○ A book, video, or brochure
○ My hospital nurse
○ My doctor's nurse
○ Internet
○ Friend or family member
○ Other

109
Parents and Newborn Screening Survey
08/22/2011

0534001092

FIGURE 20-1 Scannable form: Parents and Newborn Screening Survey, Page 1. (Developed by Patricia Newman, PhD, RN, CPN/PN, and Barbara True, MSN, CNS; University of Texas at Arlington College of Nursing and Health Innovation Center for Nursing Research.)

or data collector offer help if subjects have questions about the study?

Online services can be easy to use for both researcher and study participants. Gill, Leslie, Grech, and Latour (2013) chose SurveyMonkey (2011) to conduct a Delphi study electronically. They clearly articulated their reasons for using this particular online tool.

"SurveyMonkey (SM) … was user-friendly, had been used with different web browsers, computer configurations, and Internet services, supported SPSS for data importation and employed high level data protection measures that were consistent with industry standards (Allen & Roberts, 2010; Fan & Yan, 2010; Funke et al., 2011; SurveyMonkey, 2011)." (Gill et al., 2013, p. 1323)

The International Business Machines (IBM) Corporation that owns Statistical Package for Social Sciences (SPSS) data analysis software also markets SPSS Data Collector, a product that, in addition to assisting with survey development, includes the capacity to host online surveys (IBM, n.d.). Because some Internet survey programs are costly and require specific assurances about confidentiality of data and anonymity of subjects, the National Institutes of Health (NIH) funded a project team at Vanderbilt University in 2004 to develop a secure Internet environment for building online data surveys and data management packages (Harris et al., 2009). This free service is called *REDCap* (Research Electronic Data Capture) and is used worldwide by research organizations and universities. For example, a research team of nurse practitioners and physicians used a REDCap database to store data abstracted from medical records about outcomes of treatment for central precocious puberty in their pediatric population (Cafasso et al., 2015). Using this type of database allowed data to be available to multiple users while remaining secure.

Researchers have reported that online or electronically delivered surveys may be more acceptable to subjects when responding to sensitive questions, such as those about sexual behaviors and prejudices (Hunter, 2012). Jones, Hoover, and Lacroix (2013) studied the effect of a soap opera intervention delivered by smartphone on sexual risk behaviors of African American women in urban areas. In their randomized trial, the treatment group ($n = 117$) received a soap opera video about reducing risk behaviors once a week for 12 weeks. The comparison group also received text messages on their smartphones once a week for 12 weeks containing strategies to prevent infection with the human immunodeficiency virus (HIV). The intervention was designed to change the sex scripts of the young women related to unprotected sex. The dependent variable was unprotected sex with high-risk partners, and the incidence of unprotected sex declined in both groups. The decrease was greater in the treatment group but was not statistically significant. The smartphone was identified as a way to deliver the intervention and collect the data in a target population that has a lower proportion of people with access to the Internet (Jones et al., 2013).

An additional advantage of Internet data collection is that all postings are dated and timed. If subjects are instructed to complete a questionnaire before bedtime, time can be verified. If subjects are instructed to complete a daily diary, date of entry is automatically associated with each entry, discouraging subjects from posting all diary entries on the last day, just before returning the diary to the researcher (Fukuoka, Kamitani, Dracup, & Jong, 2011).

Digital Devices for Electronic Data Collection

With the increased sophistication and capacity of laptops, tablet computers, and smartphones, data collectors can code data directly into an electronic file at the data collection site. There is increasing overlap between the functions of mobile phones and computers. Healthcare providers load applications to their smartphones that facilitate accurate assessment, diagnosis, and pharmacological and nonpharmacological management of patients. Some of these applications can be used to collect various data, and new "apps" are being developed for research purposes. When children and adolescents are the study subjects, using an iPad for data collection allows the use of a touchscreen interface on a device familiar to the target audience (Linder et al., 2013). Children and adults with disabilities may be able to use a touchscreen even if unable to manipulate a mouse or type in responses.

Text messaging or short-message services (SMS), mentioned earlier, have been used for decades to remind subjects of return visits and, more recently, to deliver interventions or collect data (Udtha, Nomie, Yu, & Sanner, 2015). Other electronic devices include Medication Event Monitoring Systems (MEMS), which are pill bottle tops that record the times at which the bottle is opened. Because of the expense, in a multiple medication regimen, the cap is placed on the pill bottle containing the most critical medication. Waldrop-Valverde, Dong, and Ownby (2013) used MEMS caps in their study of medication adherence among persons with cocaine addiction and HIV infection and found that adherence declined over time. In addition to researchers using technology at the point of data collection to record data, technology has made it possible to interface physiological monitoring systems with computers for data collection.

Digital devices connected to a computer enable users to collect large amounts of data with few errors, data that can readily be analyzed with a variety of statistical software packages. An advantage of using digital devices for the acquisition and storage of physiological data is the increased accuracy and precision that can be achieved by reducing errors associated with manually recording or transcribing physiological data from a monitor. Chen and Chen (2015) conducted a study to determine the validity of physiological parameters in assessing pain of patients in intensive care units (ICUs). They found support for the discriminant validity of heart rate (HR) and BP for the assessment of pain in this population.

"The physiologic indicators observed in this study were HR [heart rate] and mean arterial pressure (MAP). In ICUs, each bed is equipped with a set of physiologic monitoring devices to track the patient's hemodynamics and vital sign changes. The physiologic monitor used in the ICUs included in this study was the Philips M1205A. One of the monitor's functions is to transmit physiologic signals from the electrodes attached to the patient's chest and display the signals as waves or numbers on the monitor. The displayed physiologic signals are electrocardiogram and respiration. This monitor is also equipped with a non-invasive blood pressure (NIBP) cuff for BP measurement." (Chen & Chen, 2015, p. 107)

Another advantage in electronic monitoring devices is that more data points can be recorded electronically than could be recorded manually. Computers linked to physiological monitoring systems can store multiple data values for multiple indicators, such as BPs, oxygen saturation levels, and sleep stages, storing these as frequently as once per minute. Electronic sensors record signals that transducers translate into data. Because data can be electronically recorded, data collection is less labor intensive, and data are ready for analysis more quickly. The initial cost of equipment may be high, but may be reasonable when compared to the cost of hiring and training human data collectors.

Some of the disadvantages of using electronic devices are the upfront expense, the need to support those unfamiliar with electronic devices, including nurses and subjects, and resistance from healthcare administrators because of concerns about security (Schick-Makaroff & Molzahn, 2015). In addition, using electronic devices does require additional attention to data and device security and availability of wireless Internet or a cellular network (Linder et al., 2013; Schick-Makaroff & Molzahn, 2015). An additional disadvantage of data collection with electronic devices is the potential for technical difficulty, resulting in loss of signal and resultant gaps in the data stream for seconds, minutes, or hours. If the malfunction occurs undetected in a repeated-measures study, some or all of the data for that particular subject may have to be discarded.

Physiological data typically require adequate electronic storage space on a computer or network of computers. Computer-equipment interface machinery may require more space in an already crowded clinical setting; when possible, existing equipment should be used to collect data. Purchasing equipment, setting it up, and installing software can be time-consuming and expensive at the beginning of a project. Thus, initial studies usually require substantial funding. Another concern is that the nurse researcher may focus on the machine and technology, decreasing time spent in observing and interacting with the subject (see Chapter 17 for more detail about physiologic measures).

A serious concern with computerized data collection is the possibility of measurement error that can occur with equipment malfunctions and software errors. This threat can be reduced by regular maintenance and calibrations, reliability checks of the equipment and software, and frequent uploads of the data to **cloud storage**. Cloud storage is an increasingly popular means of storing data across computer servers and the Internet that allows access to the data from anywhere with Internet access. Wilson and Anteneise (2014), researchers at Johns Hopkins University, identified a flaw that threatened the security of cloud-stored data during file sharing. In cloud-based storage, privacy is reportedly protected because even the host company is not able to "see" the data. Encrypted electronic devices and neutral third-party agents are needed to protect the confidentiality of data during transmission. These electronic devices can be misplaced or stolen, threatening confidentiality. Researchers need to protect the data with a security code to ensure that no one but themselves can access data in these formats. However, the use of these devices for research may require considerable preparation, including hiring programmers, purchasing or renting the electronic devices, and setting up security parameters..

Development of a Demographic Questionnaire

A few tested instruments contain demographic questions, but often researchers develop their own demographic questionnaires in order to capture the attributes of the sample as a whole, as well as differences that might be associated with the study variables. Data generated by subjects answering demographic questions are used to describe the sample. As you review the literature on your topic, make note of demographic variables other researchers have used to describe their samples. You may choose to ask other researchers for copies of their demographic questionnaires as a way of exploring options for composition and for different ways to measure demographics. Consider the importance of each piece of data and the subject's time required to collect it. The quantity of information provided should not be redundant. If the data can be obtained from patient records or any other written sources, researchers do not need to ask subjects to provide this information again.

Selecting Demographic Variables

Identifying data includes variables such as patient record number, home address, and date of birth. Avoid collecting these data unless they are essential to answer the research question. For example, collecting a patient's age instead of date of birth is preferred because of the privacy regulations of the Health Insurance Portability and Accountability Act about the participant's health information (see Chapter 9; www.hhs.gov/ocr/hipaa). There are instances in which you do need to obtain contact information from the subjects so that you can contact them in the future for additional data collection.

When the methodology of a study does include contacting subjects later for additional data collection, the researcher needs to obtain the subject's contact information, such as telephone number, email address, and physical address, and protect the information appropriately. Names and contact information of family members or friends may also be useful if subjects are likely to move or may be difficult to contact. This information can be obtained only with subjects' permission as part of their informed consent. To collect data from a patient's records, make sure to include permission to do this in the consent form, and ensure that the IRB has authorized the team to do this.

Common demographic descriptors are gender, race/ethnicity, and age. For gender, the answer responses may be male and female category. The researcher may also want to include an "other" category for participants who are bisexual, transgendered, or transsexual, when this is pertinent for the study focus. Human Rights Campaign (HRC) recommends dividing this question into "gender" and "gender identity," including the latter only if it yields information pertinent to data analysis. HRC recommends use of a self-identification fill-in blank for "gender" as the least-restrictive option (HRC, 2015).

At the writing of this book, federal guidelines regarding determinations of race and ethnicity for federally

> ### BOX 20-2   Race and Ethnicity Questions for Demographic Questionnaires
>
> **Ethnicity**
> (1) Hispanic or Latino
> (2) Non-Hispanic or Latino
>
> **Race**
> (1) American Indian or Alaskan Native
> (2) Asian
> (3) Black or African American
> (4) Native Hawaiian or Other Pacific Islander
> (5) White

supported agencies require two questions, as shown in Box 20-2. How would a subject who is multiple races complete the form? Therefore, researchers may ask for additional demographic information so as to clarify subjects' responses. The researcher may want to word the question to ask the participant's primary race or allow multiple responses. The current questions mandated by federal guidelines are overly simplistic and have resulted in confusing and inaccurate data (Cohn, 2015). The U.S. Census Bureau is conducting pilot testing of different questions for the 2020 Census. One option under consideration is the replacement of the current questions with a single question titled "Categories" that lists all current options plus Middle East and North Africa heritage. The instructions would be for the subject to select all that apply.

Developing Response Options for Demographic Questions

The response options for each single item on a questionnaire that allows only one response to be selected must be mutually exclusive but also exhaustive, which means that any given value for a specific variable fits into only one category. For example, subjects are highly unlikely to recall or want to reveal exact income but would be more willing to indicate that the income is in a particular range. The income ranges would not be mutually exclusive or exhaustive if they were categorized in the following way on a demographic questionnaire:

Income range (please check the range that most accurately reflects your income):
____ (1) $30,000 to $40,000
____ (2) $40,000 to $50,000
____ (3) $50,000 to $59,000
____ (4) $60,000 to $70,000
____ (5) $70,000 or more

These categories are not exclusive because they overlap, and a subject with a $40,000 income could mark category 1 or category 2 or both. Neither are the categories exhaustive because a subject may have an income of either $25,000 or $59,500, yet the questionnaire does not contain categories that include either of these incomes. Box 20-3 lists income ranges that are both exclusive and exhaustive and would be appropriate for collecting demographic data from subjects. The researcher must decide how much detail is actually needed regarding income. Does the researcher seek to discover whether each participant's household income is below poverty level according to U.S. federal poverty guidelines? To determine poverty level, the researcher must collect not only the household income but also how many people live in the household, which allows comparison with federal poverty guidelines (U.S. Department of Health & Human Services, 2015) and classification of each subject as below or above poverty level.

Some researchers have used qualifying for the free or reduced lunch program as a proxy for low socioeconomic status (SES) in studies with children and families (Bohr, Brown, Laurson, Smith, & Bass, 2013). Bohr and colleagues compared the physical fitness of junior high students of higher and lower SES, using free or reduced lunch program as the indicator for lower SES. Boys of higher and lower SES were significantly different for only one type of fitness marker, performing "curl-ups," which was more likely to be a failed item for boys of higher SES than lower; in contrast, lower SES girls were significantly lower on all fitness measures than higher SES girls were. It is interesting that, for boys, differences in body mass index and percentage of body fat were also found to be statistically significant, with lower values found in boys of lower SES. It is not known whether this is a function of anthropometric variation, shortage of adequate calories, or more vigorous activity among boys of lower SES.

BOX 20-3　An Example of Mutually Exclusive, Exhaustive Categories for Income

Income range

Please check the range that most accurately reflects your family's income for a year, before taxes.

_____ (1) Less than $30,000
_____ (2) $30,000 to $49,999
_____ (3) $50,000 to $69,999
_____ (4) $70,000 or greater

Preparation for Data Entry

Preparation for data entry and preparation for data collection often occur simultaneously, as the two aspects of the research process are intertwined. We have chosen to present the preparation for data entry first because it occurs behind the scenes and involves formatting and compiling the instruments that will be used during data collection.

Formatting and Compiling the Instruments

Before collecting data, the researcher must consider carefully the wording of questions on surveys and instruments, as well as the format of response options, to prevent inaccurate subject responses or data entry. Figure 20-2 provides a sample data collection form. It includes four items that could be problematic for coding, data analysis, or both. The blank used to enter "Surgical Procedure Performed" would lead to problems for data entry into a computerized data set. Because multiple surgical procedures could have been performed, developing codes for the various surgical procedures would be difficult and time-consuming. In addition, different words might be used to record the same surgical procedure. It may be necessary to tally the surgical procedures manually. Unless this degree of specification of procedures is important to the study, an alternative would be to develop larger categories of procedures before data collection and place the categories on the data collection form. A category of "Other" might be useful for less frequently performed surgical procedures. This method would require the data collector to make a judgment regarding which category was appropriate for a particular surgical procedure. Another option would be to write in the category code number for a particular surgical procedure after the data collection form is completed but before data entry. If the specific surgical procedure is important to the study, recording the code the facility uses to bill for the procedure may be the best method.

Similar problems occur with the items "Narcotics Ordered after Surgery" and "Narcotic Administration." Unless these data are to be used in statistical analyses, it might be better to categorize this information manually for descriptive purposes. If these items are needed for planned statistical procedures, use care to develop appropriate coding. Detailed information may be needed to know the appropriateness of the narcotic doses given. The researcher might be interested in determining differences in the amount of narcotics administered in a given period in relation to weight and height. For blinded studies, do not record the treatment group assignments on the data collection form. Placing the treatment group code on the data collection form would

---

DATA COLLECTION FORM

Demographics
____Subject Identification Number
____Age
____Gender
   1. Male
   2. Female
____Weight (in pounds)
____Height (in inches)
_____Surgical Procedure Performed
_/_/_Surgery Date (Month/Day/Year)
_/_/_Surgery Time (Hour/Minute/AM or PM)
Narcotics Ordered After Surgery_____

_____

Narcotic Administration

	Date	Time	Narcotic	Dose
1.				
2.				
3.				
4.				
5.				

Instruction on Use of Pain Scale
_/_/_Date (Month/Day/Year)
_/_/_Time (Hour/Minute/AM or PM)
Comments:

__Treatment Group
   1. TENS
   2. Placebo-TENS
   3. No-Treatment Control

Treatment Implemented
_/_/_Date (Month/Day/Year)
_/_/_Time (Hour/Minute/AM or PM)
Comments:

Dressing Change
_/_/_Date (Month/Day/Year)
_/_/_Time (Hour/Minute/AM or PM)
____Hours since surgery
Comments:

Measurement of Pain
____Score on Visual Analogue Pain Scale
_/_/_Date Pain Measured
    (Month/Day/Year)
_/_/_Time Pain Measured
    (Hour/Minute/AM or PM)
____Hours since surgery
Comments:

____Data Collector Code
Comments:

FIGURE 20-2 Data collection form.

---

be a mistake because the information would no longer be blinded and could influence data recorded by data collectors.

Data collection forms offer many response styles. The person completing the form (subject or data collector) might be asked to check a blank space before or after the words "male," "female," or "other" or to circle one of the words. Location of spaces for data on forms is important because careful placement makes it easier for subjects to complete the form without missing an item and for data entry staff to locate responses for computer entry. Locating responses on the left margin seems most efficient for data entry, but this layout may prove problematic for subject completion. The least effective arrangement is that in which data are positioned irregularly on a form, making it more likely that data will be missed during data collection and transcription.

You now have the individual instruments and data collection forms formatted consistently. What is the best order for presenting the instruments? Should you ask subjects to complete the demographic questions first or last? Skilled researchers organize data collection forms and instruments, so that the initial ones begin with less personal types of questions about age and education before asking more sensitive ones. Also, the researchers may choose not to leave the most important items for the last page of the questionnaire because of the risk of missing data if a participant becomes too fatigued or bored to complete all questions. Different types of questions require more or less time to answer, a factor that must be considered. Also, questions may ask for a response related to different time frames. For example, if one questionnaire asks about the past week and two other questionnaires ask about the past month, these should be organized so that the subject is not confused by going back and forth between time frames. If several instruments or forms are being used, putting them together in a booklet may minimize the likelihood that a questionnaire or form will be missed.

Developing a Codebook

All of the decisions the researcher makes about coding variables are documented in a codebook, either physical or virtual. A **codebook** identifies and defines each variable in the study and includes an abbreviated variable name (*income*), a descriptive variable label (*gross household annual income*), and the range of possible numerical values for every variable entered in a computer file (*0 = none; 1 = < \$30,000; ... 6 = > \$100,000*). Prior to electronic files, the codebook was a binder or notebook available for the research team that contained all the information about variables, coding, and categories. Electronic versions of a codebook contain the same information as those in the past and can be shared easily with data collectors and other team members. Some codebooks also identify the source of each datum, linking the codebook with data collection forms and scales. The codebook is a useful repository of information, allowing not only a quick-reference guide for decisions made during planning and analyses processes but a useful reference months or years later when data are analyzed for periodic reports to IRBs and funding agencies, retrieved for publication, reused for secondary analyses, shared anonymously with other researchers, or used for follow-up research on the same sample. Some computer programs, such as SPSS, allow researchers to print out data definitions after setting up a database. Figure 20-3 is an example of data definitions from SPSS for Windows. The standard attributes are labels of characteristics of the variable. For example, the figure indicates that "motivation to migrate because of low pay" was measured at the ordinal level. The valid values are the response options for the item with the corresponding number. Figure 20-4 is another example of codes for two variables. The codebook in Figure 20-4 includes the source of the data for the variable of "mother's feeling on Day 3" as being the diary completed by the mother on Tuesday.

Developing a logical method of abbreviating variable names can be challenging. For example, the researcher might use a quality-of-life (QOL) questionnaire. It will be necessary to develop an abbreviated variable name for each item in the questionnaire. For example, the fourth item on a QOL questionnaire might be given the abbreviated variable name *QOL4*. A question asking the last time a home health nurse visited might be abbreviated *HHNLstvisit,* because variable names cannot have spaces. Although abbreviated variable names usually seem logical at the time the name is created, it is easy to confuse or forget these names unless they are clearly documented with a variable label. Again, the variable name is the abbreviation used to designate the variable and the variable label is the phrase that describes the variable.

Determining the Logistics of Data Entry

If data are being collected on paper forms, the researcher must either scan a specially designed form for data entry or enter each individual datum, as one piece of data is called, into a computer program for analysis. When data are manually entered, the most accurate practice is to have two data collectors enter data separately and then

Q1		Value
Standard Attributes	Position	2
	Label	I was motivated to migrate from my country because my pay was too low.
	Type	Numeric
	Format	F8
	Measurement	Ordinal
	Role	Input
Valid Values	1	Strongly Disagree
	2	Disagree
	3	Neutral
	4	Agree
	5	Strongly Agree
Missing Values	System	

Q 39		Value
Standard Attributes	Position	40
	Label	What is your gender?
	Type	Numeric
	Format	F8
	Measurement	Nominal
	Role	Input
Valid Values	1	Male
	2	Female
Missing Values	System	

Q50		Value
Standard Attributes	Position	54
	Label	Which of the following best describes your current employment situation?
	Type	Numeric
	Format	F8
	Measurement	Nominal
	Role	Input
Valid Values	1	Employed and working full time
	2	Employed and working part time
	3	Employed, currently on leave
	4	Self-Employed
	5	Unemployed
	6	Other
Missing Values	System	

FIGURE 20-3 Example of data definitions from SPSS for Windows. (From the Nurse International Relocation Questionnaire 2 [Gray & Johnson, 2009].)

compare the files for accuracy and to check entered data for out-of-range values (Kupzyk & Cohen, 2015). Kupzyk and Cohen also describe how to format spreadsheets such as those in Microsoft Excel® so that out-of-range values cannot be entered. If data are collected

Variable Name	Variable Label	Source	Value Levels	Valid Range	Missing Data	Comments
A1 to A5	Family Apgar	Q2Family Apgar	1 = never 2 = hardly ever 3 = some of the time 4 = almost always 5 = always	1–5	9	Code as is (CAI)
MF3	Mother's feeling, Day 3	Tuesday diary, mother	1 = poor 2 = average 3 = good	1–3	9	Code 1 to 3 left to right

FIGURE 20-4 Example of coding for hypothetical study.

electronically, data collection and entry are simultaneous. While setting up an online instrument to be completed by subjects, you will indicate the number or variable name and the code for each response for each variable (1 = Strongly disagree, 2 = Disagree, 3 = Neutral, 4 = Agree, 5 = Strongly agree).

Ensure that the question provides data at the level needed for the planned analysis. If you are planning inferential statistical analysis involving age, the question needs to be open-ended to elicit the number of years. However, if you ask the question with a list of options from which the subject selects (18–24 years, 25–32, so forth), the data will be ordinal and not suitable for parametric analyses. Categorical data are assigned a number. For example, for gender, male would be coded as "1," female as "2," and other as "3." The value of the number (lower or higher) does not mean a greater or smaller quantity in this case because measurement is at the nominal level: the number represents a name or category, not a numerical value (see Chapter 16 for more information about levels of measurement). The assigned number allows the data analysis program to count the frequency and percentage of each numbered category. Another common example is an item on a questionnaire about medical diagnoses or surgical procedures. Because multiple responses may need to be marked, each response is treated as a Yes/No question and coded as "1" or "0." If physiological measures are to be included, decisions need to be made about how they will be entered as well. A blood pressure (BP) may need to be entered as separate systolic and diastolic values. The variable name and the variable label, a short abbreviation, are recorded for each variable in the data analysis program.

With the first few pilot study subjects, it is good practice for the researcher to review the values obtained for all variables, in terms of whether the data collected are interpretable and clear as stated. This practice encourages identification of items in questionnaires that might prove to be a problem during data entry because of overlapping or "batched" categories. For instance, the researcher may find that a single question contains not one but five variables: an item that asks whether the subject received support from her or his mother, father, sister, brother, or other relatives, followed by an item that asks the subject to indicate those who provided support, is unnecessarily tangled. It may, at first, seem logical to code mother as "1," father as "2," sister as "3," brother as "4," and other as "5." However, when a questionnaire allows an individual to select more than one source of support, each relative must be coded separately. Thus, mother is one variable and would be a dichotomized value, coded "1" if circled and "0" if not circled. The father would be coded similarly as a second dichotomous variable, and so on. Identifying these items before data collection may allow items on the questionnaire or data collection form to be restructured to simplify computer entry.

Creating Rules for Data Entry

Rules for data entry may be finalized during pilot testing. For example, if a subject selects two responses for a single-response item, two decisions are possible: (1) the variable can be coded as missing, or (2) either the higher or the lower variable can become the default value. In the latter instance, a multiple-choice question indicating how many months have elapsed since a subject visited a dentist might be answered with both "six to eleven months ago" and "twelve to seventeen months ago." The researcher, in this instance, would use "six to eleven months ago" as the default value, because the meaning of the question is not "how long has it been since you saw a dentist?" but, rather, "how long has it been since you *last* saw a dentist?" If feasible, this particular question should then be reworded for the actual study as "When was your last visit to a dentist?"

Even when items and responses are unambiguous, those entering the data will be faced with decisions. Therefore, it is not sufficient to establish general rules for individuals entering data, such as "in this case always do X." This action still requires the person who is entering data to recognize a problem, refer to a general rule, and correct the data before entry. Correcting raw data is a judgment call and should only be undertaken when the person entering data is certain, beyond a doubt, of the actual value.

1. *Missing data.* Provide the data if possible or determine the impact of the missing data. In some cases, the subject must be excluded from at least some of the analyses, so the researcher must determine which data are essential. Leave the variable blank when a datum is missing. Entering a zero (0) will skew data analysis because the analysis program will include the value as a quantity.

2. *Items in which the subject provided two responses when only one was requested.* For example, if the question asked the subject to mark the most important item in a list of ten items and the subject selected two items, a decision must be made by the researcher as to how to resolve this problem, not left to a data entry person to decide. In the codebook and on the form itself, then, the researcher should indicate how that particular datum is to be coded and entered, so that the decision is documented and can be remade in the same manner when other subjects double-select a response.

3. *Items in which the subject has marked a response between two options.* This problem occurs frequently with Likert-type scales, particularly scales using forced-choice options. Given four options, the subject places a mark on the line between response 2 and response 3. In the codebook and on the form, indicate how the datum is to be coded. This is often best coded as a missing value, but coding rules should be consistent. A rationale can be constructed that supports using the highest value, lowest value, or a value halfway between the two. Removing the possibility of not clearly selecting an option is eliminated with electronic data collection, another advantage to that type of data collection.

4. *Items that ask the subject to write in some information such as occupation or diagnosis.* As noted earlier, such items are very time-consuming to code and enter. The researcher should develop a list of codes for entering such data. Rather than leaving it up to the assistant to determine which code matches the subject's written response, the researcher should make decisions concerning coding and make a master list

for any data entry assistants to use, so as to protect data integrity.

For paper instruments, after data have been checked and the necessary codes entered, it is prudent to make a copy of all completed forms rather than turning over the only set to an assistant for data entry. In addition, if someone other than the researcher is to enter the data, that person should receive the following information to facilitate setting up the database in advance:

- Dates for the beginning and ending of data collection
- Estimated number of subjects in the sample and how often batches of data will be entered
- Plan for documenting refusal rate, sample size, and attrition
- Copies of all scales, questionnaires, and data collection forms to be used
- Statistical package to be used for analysis of the data
- Statistical analyses to be conducted to describe the sample and to address the research purpose and the objectives, questions, or hypotheses
- Contact information for the statistician or project director with whom to consult for data entry or data analysis questions
- Computer directory location of the database in which the data will be entered and copied for backup
- Timeline for receiving the data—for example, will the data be delivered in batches, or will all the data be gathered and delivered at the same time

With this information, the assistant can develop the database in preparation for receiving data. The time needed to prepare the database varies depending upon number of variables and complexity of response categories. Approximate dates for completion of data entry, analyses, or both must be negotiated before beginning data collection.

PREPARATION FOR DATA COLLECTION

Creating a Data Collection Plan

Extensive planning increases accuracy of the data collected and validity of the study findings. Validity and strength of the findings from several carefully planned studies increase the quality of the research evidence that is then available for implementation (Melnyk & Fineout-Overholt, 2015). Building on the preparations made for data collection and data entry, a **data collection plan** can now be developed. The data collection plan is a flowchart of interactions with subjects and decisions to be made consistently. The plan for collecting data is specific to the study being conducted, beginning with recruitment. Figure 20-5 is a flowchart of data collection steps that will be followed carefully, to maintain consistency.

A detailed plan ensures consistency of the data collection process. You as a researcher must first envision the overall activities that will occur during data collection. Write each step and develop the forms, training, and equipment needed for that step. Focus on who, what, when, where, why, and how. A data collection plan contains important details to ensure consistency of the data collected across subjects, which is critical to construct validity. Although described related to validity in Chapters 10 and 11, construct validity also is affected by the attention to details in planning and implementing the study. Some of these details include the timing of data collection, training data collectors, and identifying decision points.

Scheduling Data Collection

The specific days and hours of data collection may influence the consistency of the data collected and must be carefully considered. For example, the energy level and state of mind of subjects from whom data are gathered in the morning may differ from that of subjects from whom data are gathered in the evening. With hospitalized study participants, visitors are more likely to be present at certain times of day and may interfere with data collection or influence participant responses. Patient care routines vary with the time of day. Consultation with the nurses and other staff in the areas in which data collection will occur provides insight into the best times for data collection. In some studies, the care recently received or the care currently being provided may alter the data gathered. Subjects approached on Saturday to participate in the study may differ from subjects approached on weekday mornings. Subjects seeking care on Saturday may have full-time jobs, whereas subjects seeking care on weekday mornings may be either unemployed or too ill to work.

Will you collect data from more than one subject at a time, or do you think it would be simpler to focus attention on one subject at a time? How much time will be needed to collect data from each subject? If concurrent data collection is planned for several subjects, the length of time data collection will take per subject is determined by study design, setting, and available space. In addition, if the plan is for three subjects to complete data collection in the morning and three in the afternoon, what are the contingencies for subjects who arrive late or require additional time? Some subjects may be available only during lunch breaks or in the evening, after work hours.

What time of year will data be collected? For example, if the study is conducted during holiday seasons, data about sleeping, eating, or exercising may vary. Pediatric patients with asthma may experience more symptoms during the winter months than during the summer. Planning data collection for a study of symptom management with this population would need to take this possibility into consideration.

Training Data Collectors

A high level of consistency in data collection, across subjects, is the goal. You may decide to collect all the data yourself for that reason. If you decide to use data collectors, they must be trained in responsible conduct of research and issues of informed consent, ethics, and confidentiality and anonymity (see Chapter 9). They must be informed about the research project, become familiar with the instruments to be used, and receive training in the data collection process. In addition to training, data collectors must have written guidelines or protocols that indicate which instruments to use, the order in which to introduce the instruments, how to administer the instruments, and a time frame for the data collection process (Harwood, 2009; Kang, Davis, Habermann, Rice, & Broome, 2005). If nurses and other hospital staff collect the data for the study while performing day-to-day routines of patient care, observing their methods will identify the degree of consistency in both the collection and recording of data.

If more than one person is to collect data, consistency among data collectors (interrater reliability) must be ensured through testing (see Chapter 16). Additional training must continue until interrater reliability estimates are at least 85% to 90% agreement between the expert trainer and the trainees. Waltz, Strickland, and Lenz (2010) suggest that a minimum of 10% of the data should be compared across raters if interrater reliability is to be reported accurately. A newly trained data collector's interrater reliability with the expert trainer should be assessed intermittently throughout data collection to ensure consistency from the first to the last participant in the study. In addition, data collectors must be encouraged to identify and record any problems or variations in the environment that affect the data collection process. The description of the training of data collectors is usually reported in the methods section of an article so that the reader can evaluate the likelihood that consistency resulted (Harwood & Hutchinson, 2009).

ENROLLMENT AND SURVEY ADMINISTRATION PROCEDURES

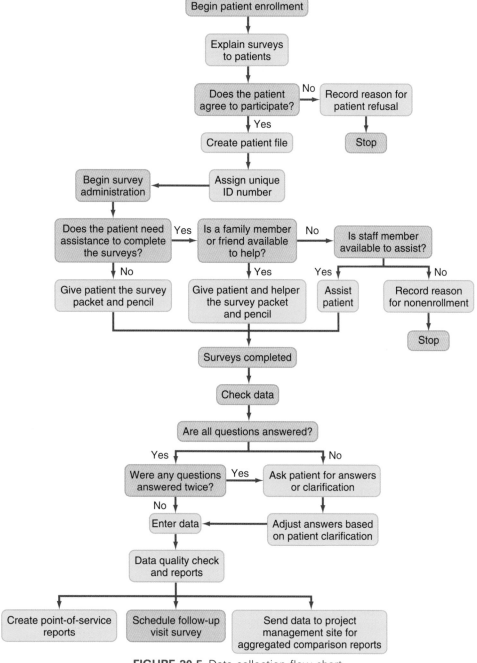

FIGURE 20-5 Data collection flow chart.

Identifying Decision Points

Decision points that occur during data collection must be identified, and all options must be considered. One decision may pertain to whether too few potential subjects are meeting the sampling inclusion criteria. If too few subjects from the potential pool are eligible, at what point will the researcher consider changing exclusion criteria? For example, a study's inclusion criterion is first-time mothers older than 30 years of age, and the plan is to recruit 60 subjects. However, only four subjects have been consented during the first two weeks of the study, and persons younger than 30 who are willing to participate are being turned away, so the research team may reconsider the rationale for the age criterion and perhaps decide either to lower the age range or to seek additional recruitment sites, foreseeing a total data collection period of seven and a half months at this rate of recruitment. In contrast, DeVon, Patmon, Rosenfeld, Fennessey, and Francis (2013) found they were recruiting subjects for a study on acute coronary syndrome (ACS) that were later determined to be ineligible.

> "The initial plan was to have the Symptom Checklist completed by triage nurses, but this plan was modified early in the process because of the challenge of identifying who should be screened. In the first 6 months of data collection, we recruited many more patients who had ACS ruled out than was anticipated. To more accurately identify who was likely to be ruled in, we chose to delay the enrollment process until evidence of ischemia was available." (DeVon et al., 2013, p. 7)

Other decisions include whether the subject understands the information needed to give informed consent, whether the subject comprehends instructions related to providing data, and whether the subject has provided all the data needed. As the researcher reviews the completed data forms, are all responses completed? If the subject skips a page, will the data collector need to return that page to the subject for completion? If the question about income is not completed, how will the missing response be handled? The data collection plan (Figure 20-5) should indicate how much missing data will be allowed per subject. At what point will the subject's responses be excluded due to missing data?

PILOT STUDY

Completing a pilot study is an essential step that saves difficulty later when the final steps of the research process are implemented. A pilot study may be conducted with several different aims. The aims of a pilot test may include identifying problems that may interfere with study validity or challenges in using the instruments. Chapter 3 provides additional reasons to conduct a pilot study, but being clear about the aims will help you determine the appropriate sample size for the pilot study (Hertzog, 2008). If the purpose is to try out the procedures, use the research plan to recruit three to five subjects who meet the eligibility criteria. Use the data collection methods that have been selected and prepared. Pay attention to how long it takes to recruit a subject, obtain informed consent, and collect all data. At the conclusion of data collection, ask the participant to identify questions or aspects of the process that were unclear or confusing. Based on the pilot study and feedback of the first subjects, researchers may choose to modify data collection forms and methods of data collection to ensure the feasibility, validity, and reliability of the study. When the aim of the pilot study is to determine the effect size of an intervention or the internal consistency of an instrument, the necessary sample size to achieve the aim will be larger and can be determined by different statistical analyses (Hertzog, 2008). If no changes are made in the procedures or instruments, pilot subjects are "rolled over" into the study because they meet eligibility criteria.

ROLE OF THE RESEARCHER DURING THE STUDY

The researcher applies ethical principles, people management strategies, and problem-solving skills constantly as data collection tasks are implemented. Even after pilot testing, whether related to the research plan or to situations external to the research, unforeseen events can occur, and support systems occasionally are needed for data collectors. For instance, a data collector in a subject's home may find that family members are neglecting a subject in the study who cannot get out of bed. The data collector will need assistance in reporting this to legal authorities. When multiple data collectors are involved, frequent interactions between data collectors and team leader are essential for assessing any minor or major risks and reporting adverse effects to the IRB. In addition, the researcher's role includes maintaining control and managing the data.

Maintaining Controls and Consistency

Maintaining control and consistency of design and methods during subject selection and data collection protects the integrity or validity of the study. Researchers build controls into the design to minimize the influence of intervening forces on study findings. Maintenance of these controls is essential. For example, a study to describe changes in sleep stages during puberty may require controlling the environment of the bedroom to such an extent that a sleep laboratory is the only setting in which study integrity can be maintained. Control has stringent limitations in natural field settings. In some cases, these tenuous controls can fail without the researcher realizing that anything is amiss.

In addition to maintaining controls identified in the research plan, researchers continually watch for previously unidentified extraneous variables that might have an impact on the data being collected. These variables are often study-specific, becoming apparent during data collection. Extraneous variables identified at this time must be considered during data analysis and interpretation. These variables also must be noted in the research report to allow subsequent researchers to be aware of them. For example, Lee and Gay (2011) studied sleep quality in new mothers and asked about the infant's sleep location, but the location at the beginning of the night was often not the same by morning and could not be controlled for in the home setting.

Data Entry Period

Data must be carefully checked and problems corrected before the data entry phase, which should be essentially automatic and require no decisions regarding the data. Anything that alters the rhythm of data entry increases errors. For example, the subject's entry should be coded as it appears, and any reverse coding that may be needed should be done at a later time by computer manipulation in a consistent manner, rather than trying to have the data entry person recode during data entry. Follow the codebook that you have created very carefully.

If you enter your own data, develop a rhythm to the data entry process. Avoid distractions while entering data, and limit your data entry periods to 2-hour intervals to reduce fatigue and error. Back up the database after each data entry period and store it on an encrypted flash drive, on a secure website, or in a fireproof safe. It is possible for the computer to crash and lose all of your precious data. If an assistant is entering the data, make yourself as available as possible to respond to questions and address problems. After entry, the data should be randomly checked for accuracy. Data checking is discussed in Chapter 21.

Managing Data

Protecting the confidentiality of the data is a primary concern for the researcher. In general, the subject's name should not appear on data collection forms; only the subject's identification number should appear. The researcher may keep a master list of subjects and their code numbers, which is stored in a location separate from other data, and either encrypted in an electronic file or data repository, or locked in a file drawer, to ensure subjects' privacy. Often this master list of subjects and codes is kept with subjects' consent forms in a locked file drawer. This master list is required if contacting subjects again is necessary for additional data collection or if a subject later contacts the researcher to withdraw from the study.

Once data collection begins, the researcher begins to accumulate large quantities of data. To avoid a state of total confusion, careful plans should be in place before data collection begins. Plans are needed to keep all data from a single subject together until analysis is initiated. The researcher must write the subject code number on each page of each form, and check the forms for each subject to ensure that they all are present. Researchers have been known to sort their data by form, such as putting all the scales of one kind together, only to realize afterwards that they have failed to code the forms with subject identification numbers first. They then had no way to link each scale to the individual subject, and valuable data were lost.

Storage and Retrieval of Data

Space must be allotted for storing forms. File folders with a clear method of labeling allow easy access to data. Using different colors for forms is often useful. Large envelopes, approximately $8'' \times 11''$, should be used to hold small pieces of paper or note cards that might fall out of a file folder. Plan to code data and enter them into the computer as soon as possible after data collection to reduce loss or disorganization of data. If data are recorded directly into a computer, data backup and storage in a separate location are imperative.

In this time of electronic storage devices and cloud storage, it is relatively easy to store data. The original data forms and database must be stored for a specified number of years dictated by the IRB, funding source, or journal publisher. There are several reasons to store data. The data can be used for secondary analyses. For example, researchers participating in a project related to a particular research focus may pool data from various studies for access by all members of the group. Data should be available to document the validity of the analyses and the published results of the study. Because of nationally publicized incidents of scientific miscon-duct (see Chapter 9), in which researchers fabricated data and published multiple manuscripts, researchers would be wise to preserve documentation supporting the appropriate and accurate collection of data. Issues that have been raised include how long data should be stored, the need for institutional policy regarding data storage, and access of team members to the data after the study is completed.

Some researchers store their data for five years after publication, whereas others store their data until they retire from a research career. Researchers should check with their funding sponsors and publishers for guide-lines on how long to retain data. Most researchers store data in their offices or laboratories; others archive their data in central locations with storage fees or retrieval fees. Graduate students do have a responsibility to keep and securely store data collected in the course of their studies.

Policies are needed about the access that members of the team have following completion of the initial study (Sarpatwari, Kesselheim, Malin, Gagne, & Schneeweiss, 2014). Will graduate students who assist with a study receive a copy of the raw data or will they have access to it after they leave the institution? The lack of policies related to access to data can have consequences. In the case of the Havasupai tribe vs. Arizona State University (Chapter 9), members of the research team continued to use data and samples after they moved to other uni-versities without permission of the original subjects (McEwen, Boyer, & Sun, 2013).

Problem Solving

Little has been written about the problems encountered by nurse researchers. Research reports often read as though everything went smoothly. Research journals generally do not provide enough space for researchers to describe the problems encountered, and inexperi-enced researchers may receive a rosier impression than is realistic. Some problems are hinted at in a published paper in either the limitations section or in a discussion of areas for subsequent research. A more realistic sense of problems encountered by a researcher can be obtained through personal discussions with the primary author about the process of data collection for a par-ticular sample, or the use of a particular method or instrument.

"If anything can go wrong, it will, and at the worst possible time." This statement is often called **Murphy's Law** and it seems to prevail in research, just as in other dimensions of life. For example, data collection fre-quently requires more time than was anticipated, and

collecting data is often more difficult than expected. A problem can be perceived either as a frustration or as a challenge. The fact that the problem occurred is not as important as successfully resolving it. The final and perhaps most important task during the data collection period may be debriefing with the research team in weekly meetings to resolve problems that arise.

Despite conducting a pilot study, researchers may encounter challenges during the data collection process. Sometimes changes must be made in the way the data are collected, in the specific data collected, or in the timing of data collection. Potential subjects, as well as healthcare workers in a given area, react to a research study in unpredictable ways. Institutional changes may force modifications in the research plan. Unusual or unex-pected events may occur. Data collection processes must be as consistent as possible, but flexibility also is needed in dealing with unforeseen problems. Sometimes stick-ing with the original plan no matter what happens is a mistake. Skills in finding ways to resolve problems that protect the integrity of the study are critical.

In preparation for data collection, possible problems must be anticipated, and solutions for these problems must be explored. The following discussion describes some common problems and concerns and presents possible solutions. Problems that tend to occur with some regularity in studies have been categorized as people problems, researcher problems, institutional problems, and event problems.

People Problems

Nurses cannot place a subject in a laboratory test tube, instill one drop of the independent variable, and then measure the effect. Nursing studies often are conducted by examining subjects as they interact with their envi-ronments. In a laboratory setting, many aspects of the environment can be controlled, but other studies require a natural setting, to generate external validity. When research involves people, nothing is completely predict-able. People, in their complexity and wholeness, have an impact on all aspects of nursing studies. Researchers, potential subjects, family members of subjects, health-care professionals, institutional staff members, and others ("innocent bystanders") interact within the study situation. As a researcher, you must be a keen observer and evaluate these interactions to determine their impact on your study.

Problems recruiting a sample. The first step in initiat-ing data collection, recruiting a sample, may represent the tip of the people problem iceberg. Researchers may find that few people are available who fit the inclusion criteria or that many people refuse to participate in the study even though the request seems reasonable. Appropriate subjects, who were numerous a month earlier, seem to evaporate. Institutional procedures change, making many potential subjects ineligible for participation. At this juncture, inclusion and exclusion criteria may need to be evaluated or additional sites for recruitment identified (see Chapter 15).

In research-rich institutions where studies are plentiful, patients paradoxically may be reluctant to participate in research. This lack of participation might arise because these patients are frequently exposed to studies, or feel manipulated, or misunderstand what participation will involve. Patients may feel that they are being used "as guinea pigs" or fear that they will be harmed in some way that is external to the research. For example, recruiting Spanish-speaking women for a study of stress and acculturation may be met with high refusal rates if these women are worried about revealing their legal status in the U.S. Albrecht and Taylor (2013) conducted a study with a sample of women with advanced ovarian cancer. When accrual of subjects was slow, they reallocated some of their funding to pay for advertisements in local newspapers, which was effective in improving recruitment.

Subject attrition. After the sample is selected, certain problems might cause **subject attrition** (a loss of subjects from the study over time) (see Chapter 15). For example, some subjects may agree to participate but then fail to follow through. Some may not complete needed forms and questionnaires or may fill them out incorrectly, and their data must be discarded.

To reduce these and related problems, a research team member can be available to subjects while they complete essential questions. Some subjects may not return for a second interview or may not be home for a scheduled visit. Although time has been invested to collect data from these subjects, if follow-up reveals that they do not want to continue as research subjects, their data may have to be excluded from analysis because of incompleteness. Generally, the more data collection time points there are in the study's design, the higher the risk for attrition. Attrition can occur because of subject burden accumulating over time, because healthy adults relocate for employment or family reasons, or because of death in a more critically ill population.

Sometimes subjects must be dropped from the study by the research team because of changes in health status. For example, a patient may be transferred out of the ICU in which the study is being conducted. Another possibility might be that the patient's condition may worsen and the patient no longer meets the inclusion criteria. The limits of third-party reimbursement may force the healthcare provider to discontinue the procedures or services being studied. The research team may drop a subject if it appears that participation is unusually burdensome, and that the subject's better interests would be served outside the study, or if a subject initially determined to be mentally competent is re-evaluated as someone with limited ability to consent.

Subject attrition occurs to some extent in all longitudinal studies. One way for you to deal with this problem is to anticipate the attrition rate and increase the planned number of subjects to ensure that a minimally desired number will complete the full study. Review of similar studies can allow you to anticipate your study's attrition rate. For example, Lim, Chiu, Dohrmann, and Tan (2010) reported a 31% attrition rate in their quasi-experimental study of the knowledge of registered nurses employed in long-term care. The investigators collected pretest data from 58 subjects and four weeks later collected posttest data from 40 subjects. If subject attrition is higher than expected, it may be effective to offer a smaller token payment for the time and effort for initial data collection and increase the payment slightly for each data collection. Attrition usually is higher in a placebo or control group, unless equalization of treatment is employed. Sometimes in pretest-posttest or longitudinal studies, the sample size is smaller than expected by the end of the study due to attrition. If so, the effect of a smaller sample on the power of planned statistical analyses must be considered because this smaller sample may be inadequate to test the study's hypotheses. If this is the case, a researcher may apply to the IRB for revision of the estimated size of the sample, resuming recruitment.

Researchers should report information about subjects' acceptance to participate in a study and attrition during the study to determine the degree to which the sample is representative of the study target population. Journal editors often require that manuscripts include a CONSORT flowchart or similar flowchart indicating the number of subjects meeting sample criteria, the numbers refusing to participate, and the reasons for refusal. If data collected over time (repeated measures) or the study intervention is implemented over time, subjects often drop out of a study, and it is important to document when and how much attrition occurred. The flowchart clearly identifies important aspects of the sampling process and reasons for attrition. This information enables researchers and clinicians to evaluate the representativeness of their sample for external validity and for any potential bias in interpreting the results.

Subject as an object. The quality of interactions between the researcher and subjects during the study is a critical dimension for maintaining subject participation. When researchers are under pressure to complete a study, people can be treated as objects rather than as subjects, particularly if electronic data collection is used. In addition to being unethical, such impersonal treatment alters interactions, diminishes subject satisfaction, and increases the likelihood for missing data and subject attrition. Subjects are scarce resources and must be treated with care. Treating the subject as an object can affect another researcher's ability to recruit from this population in the future. Treating the subject as an object can be minimized by building strategies into the consent process, such as offering subjects a personal copy of their results, recognizing their valuable participation with small gifts as tokens of appreciation, or providing monetary reimbursement for their time and effort. Because of their sterling social skills, nurses are valuable members of interdisciplinary research teams: they establish relationships with subjects, aiding in retention.

External influences on subject responses. People external to the research who interact with the subject, the researcher, or both can have an important impact on the data collection process. Family members may not agree to the subject's participation in the study or may not understand the study process. These individuals often influence the subject's decision to participate. Researchers benefit from taking time to explain the study and seeking the cooperation of family members.

Family members or other patients also may influence the subject's responses to scales or interview questions. In some cases, subjects may ask family members, friends, or other patients to complete study forms for them. The subject may discuss questions on the forms with other people who happen to be in the room, and therefore the data recorded may not reflect the subject's perceptions accurately. If interviews are conducted while others are in the room, the subject's responses may depend on his or her need to meet the expectations of the persons present. Sometimes a family member answers questions addressed verbally to the patient by the researcher. The setting in which a questionnaire is completed or an interview is conducted may determine the extent to which answers obtained are a true reflection of a subject's point of view. If the privacy afforded by the setting varies from one subject to another, subjects' responses may also vary and threaten the internal validity of the findings.

Usually, the most desirable setting for questionnaire completion is a private area away from distractions. If it is not possible to arrange for such a setting, the researcher can be present at the time the questionnaire is completed to decrease the influence of others. If the questionnaire is to be completed later or taken home and returned at a later time, the probability of influence by others increases, and return of questionnaire packet becomes less likely, even if the subject is provided with a stamped return envelope. The impact of the influence of others on the integrity of the data depends on the nature of the questionnaire items. For example, a marital relationship questionnaire may have different responses if the subject is allowed to complete it alone and return it immediately to the researcher, versus completing it aloud with the spouse in attendance.

Passive resistance. Healthcare professionals and institutional staff members working with study participants in clinical settings may affect the data collection process. DeVon and colleagues (2013) found that some nurses were initially enthusiastic about the study and later become less so, while another nurse indicated that research was not part of her job. Some professionals may verbalize strong support for the study and yet passively interfere with data collection. For example, nurses providing care may fail to follow guidelines agreed upon for providing specific care activities being studied, or they may forget to include information needed for the study in the patient records. The researcher may not be informed when a potential subject has been admitted, and a physician who has agreed that his or her patients can be participants may decide as each patient is admitted that this one is not quite right for the study. In addition, when the permission of the physician or nurse practitioner is required, the provider might be unavailable to the researcher.

Nonprofessional staff members may not realize the impact of the data collection process on their work patterns until the process begins. The data collection process may violate their beliefs about how care should be provided (or has been provided). If ignored, their resistance can completely undo a carefully designed study. For example, research on skin care may disrupt a bathing routine by nursing assistants so they may continue the normal routine regardless of the study protocol and thus invalidate the study findings. When there is funding to support subject recruitment and data collection, funds can be used to reimburse clinic or hospital staff members for their time, to create a raffle for one substantial gift, to offer a gift certificate to buy something needed for the clinic, or to send a nurse who assisted in data collection to a continuing education course. When funding is limited, staff members' enthusiasm for the study may be enhanced if they are able to participate in the research as authors or presenters in dissemination of the research findings.

Because of the potential impact of these problems, the researcher must maintain open communication and nurture positive relationships with other professionals and staff members during data collection. Early recognition and acknowledgment of problems allow the researcher to resolve issues promptly, ideally with fewer serious consequences to the integrity of the study. However, not all problems can be resolved. Sometimes the researcher may need to seek creative ways to work around an individual or to counteract the harmful consequences of passive resistance.

What is cavalierly referred to as "passive resistance" on the part of staff members is sometimes related to lack of researcher presence. If a researcher, or an assistant, telephones the hospital unit's clerk daily to enquire about new admissions in the past 24 hours and to ask whether those patients are suitable for study inclusion, the unit clerk may wonder why the researcher is not putting in an appearance. The responsible researcher either goes to the research site daily and assesses potential subjects for recruitment, or delegates this daily responsibility to a member of the research team. In addition, being on-site for questions when interventions and documentation of information required by the research team are taking place, and thanking them for their fine work are important ways to build goodwill and an effective quick-check of accuracy and quality.

Researcher Problems

Some problems are a consequence of a researcher's interaction with the study situation or lack of skill in data collection techniques. These problems are often difficult to identify because of the researcher's personal involvement. However, their effect on the study can be serious.

Researcher interactions. Researcher interactions can interfere with data collection in interview situations. To gain the cooperation of the subject, the researcher needs to develop rapport with the subject. One way to do this is to select data collectors who resemble the types of subjects being recruited as much as possible. Rapport may suffer if a young man collects data from female caregivers of elderly adults about their experience with end-of-life care. Similarly, a white middle-aged woman collecting data from young African American men or Hispanic teens is likely to be at more of an initial disadvantage, in terms of establishing immediate rapport, than would be a data collector who shares age or ethnic background with the subjects.

Lack of skill in data collection techniques. The researcher's skill in using a particular quantitative data collection technique can affect the quality of the data collected. A researcher who is unskilled at the beginning of data collection can practice the data collection techniques with the assistance of an experienced researcher. A pilot study to test data collection techniques is always helpful. If data collectors are being used, they also need opportunities to practice data collection techniques before the study is initiated. Sometimes a skill is developed during the course of a study; if this is the case, as one's skill increases, the data being collected may change and confound the study findings and threaten the validity of the study. If more than one data collector is used, the degree to which skills improve may vary across time and data collectors. The consistency of data collectors must be evaluated during the study to detect any changes in their data collection techniques.

Researcher role conflict. As a researcher, one is observing and recording events. Nurses who conduct clinical research often experience a conflict between their researcher role and their clinician role during data collection. In some cases, the researcher's involvement in the event, such as providing physical or emotional care to a patient during data collection, could alter the event and bias the results. It would be difficult to generalize study findings to other situations in which the researcher was not present to intervene. However, the needs of patients must take precedence over the needs of the study.

The dilemma is to determine when the needs of patients are great enough to warrant researcher intervention. Some patient situations are life-threatening, such as respiratory distress and changes in cardiac function, and require immediate action by anyone present, especially when that person is a nurse. Other patient needs are simple, can be addressed by any nurse available, and can be answered if the response is not likely to alter the results of the study. Examples of these interventions include giving the patient a bedpan, informing the nurse of the patient's need for pain medication, or helping the patient open food containers. These situations seldom cause a dilemma.

Solutions to other situations are not as easy. For example, suppose that the study involves examining the emotional responses of family members during and immediately after a patient's surgery. The study includes an experimental group that receives one 30-minute family support session before and during the patient's surgery and a control group that receives no support session. Both sets of families are being monitored for one week after surgery to measure level of anxiety and coping strategies. The researcher is currently collecting data from subjects in the control group. The data consist of demographic information and scales measuring anxiety and coping. After completing demographic information, one of the family members is experiencing great distress and verbally expresses her fears and the lack of support she has received from the nursing staff. Two other subjects from different families hear the expressed distress and concur; they move closer to the conversation and look to the researcher for information and support.

In this situation, a supportive response from the researcher is likely to modify the results of the study because these responses are part of the treatment to be provided to the experimental group only. This interaction is likely to narrow the difference between the two groups and decrease the possibility that the results will show a significant difference between the two groups. How should the researcher respond? Is it obligatory to provide support? To some extent, almost any response would be supportive. One alternative is to provide the needed support and not include these family members in the control group. Another alternative is to recruit the help of a nonprofessional to collect the data from the control group. However, most people would provide some degree of support in the described situation, even though their skills in supportive techniques may vary.

Other dilemmas include witnessing unethical behavior that interferes with patient care or witnessing subjects' unethical or illegal behavior (Humphreys et al., 2012). Consent forms are often required to stipulate that any member of the research team is legally required to report illegal behaviors that pose potential harm to the subject or others, such as neglect or abuse of children and elderly adults. Try to anticipate these dilemmas before data collection whenever possible, and include this information in the consent form (Wong, Tiwari, Fong, Humphreys, & Bullock, 2011).

Pilot studies can help identify dilemmas likely to occur in a study, and allow the research team to build strategies into the design to minimize or avoid them. However, some dilemmas cannot be anticipated and must be responded to spontaneously. There is no prescribed way to handle difficult dilemmas; each case must be dealt with individually. The wise researcher discusses any unethical and illegal behavior with members of the IRB, ethics committee members, or legal advisors. Situations related to potential harm must be reported to the IRB, as well, and experts there can advise on the next step or course of action. After the dilemma is resolved, it is wise to reexamine the situation for its effect on study results and consider options in case the situation arises again.

Another type of conflict arises when a subject makes inaccurate statements or asks a question about health practices or treatment. Rather than offering professional advice or responding to the question, the research nurse should acknowledge that it is a good question, but that the research protocol does not allow for a response during data collection. When data collection is complete, the research nurse can help the subject write down the question for the healthcare provider or provide patient-education materials for more information.

Maintaining perspective. Data collection includes both joys and frustrations. Researchers must be able to maintain some degree of objectivity during the process and yet not take themselves too seriously. A sense of humor is invaluable. You must be able to experience the emotions and then become the rational problem solver. Management skills and mental health are as invaluable to a research career as being obsessive about data collection and data management.

Institutional Problems

Institutions are in a constant state of change. They will not stop changing for the period of a study, and these changes often affect data collection. A nurse who has been most helpful in the study may be promoted or transferred. The unit on which the study is conducted may be reorganized, moved, or closed during data collection. An area used for subject interviews may be transformed into an office or a storeroom. Patient record forms may be revised, omitting data that you and your team are collecting. The medical record personnel may be reorganizing files and temporarily unable to provide needed records. Albrecht and Taylor's (2013) study with women with advanced ovarian cancer involved the pharmacy dispensing the study-related medications. Following IRB approval, it took three months for procedural issues with the pharmacy to be resolved.

These problems are, for the most part, completely outside your control in your role as researcher. Pay attention to the internal communication network of the institution for advanced warning of impending changes. Contacts within the institution's administrative decision makers could warn you about the impact of proposed changes on an ongoing study. In many cases, the IRB in the local hospital will have a nurse representative who can provide needed consultation. However, in many cases, data collection strategies might have to be modified to meet a newly emerging situation. Balancing flexibility with maintaining the integrity of the study may be the key to successful data collection. As a data collection site, the subject's home setting may be more desirable and convenient for a subject than a complex facility or institution, and response rates may improve. The disadvantage is that home visits are time-intensive for the researcher, and the subject may not be home at the agreed-upon appointment time, despite confirmed appointments and reminder calls.

Event Problems

Unpredictable events can be a source of frustration during a study. Research tools ordered from a testing company can be lost in the mail. The printer may stop functioning just before 500 data collection forms are to be printed, or a machine to be used in data collection may break and require several weeks for repair. A computer ordered for data collection may not arrive when promised or may malfunction. Data collection forms can be misplaced, misfiled, or lost.

Local, national, or world events can also influence a subject's response to a questionnaire or the willingness to enroll in a study, as can changes in treatment protocols. Albrecht and Taylor (2013) noted that medical management of advanced ovarian cancer changed between seeking funding and implementing their study and, as a result, many of the women counted in the potential pool of subjects were no longer eligible. If data collection for the entire sample is planned for a single time, a snowstorm or a flood can require the researcher to cancel the session. Weather may decrease attendance far below the number expected at a support group or series of teaching sessions. A bus strike can disrupt transportation systems to such an extent that subjects who depend on public transportation can no longer reach the data collection site. A new health agency may open in the city, which may decrease demand for the care activities being studied. Conversely, an external event can also increase attendance at clinics to such an extent that existing resources are stretched and data collection is no longer possible. These events are also outside the researcher's control and are impossible to anticipate. In most cases, however, restructuring the data collection period can salvage the study. To do so, it is necessary to examine all possible alternatives for collecting the study data. In some cases, data collection can simply be rescheduled; in other situations, changes may need to be more complex. For example, recruiting women to participate in a study that requires an hour or longer of their time may necessitate that the researcher provide childcare. Providing childcare would be more costly and add complexity to the process, but it may be the best alternative for increasing participation.

RESEARCH/RESEARCHER SUPPORT

The researcher must have access to individuals or groups who can provide mentorship, support, and consultation during the data collection period. Support can usually be obtained from academic committees, from IRB staff, and from colleagues on the research team.

Support of Academic Committees

Although thesis and dissertation committees are basically seen as stern keepers of the sanctity of the research process, they also serve as support systems for novice researchers. Committee members must be selected from among faculty who are willing and able to provide the needed expertise and support. Experienced academic researchers are usually more knowledgeable about the types of support needed. Because they are involved directly in research, they tend to be sensitive to the needs of the novice researcher, and more realistic about what can be accomplished within a given period of time.

Institutional Support

A support system within the institution in which the study is conducted is also important. Support might come from people serving on the institutional research committee or from nurses working on the unit in which the study is conducted. These people may have knowledge of how the institution functions, and their closeness to the study can increase their understanding of the problems experienced by the researcher and subjects. Do not overlook their ability to provide useful suggestions and assistance. The ability to resolve some of the problems encountered during data collection may depend on having someone within the power structure of the institution who can intervene.

Colleague Support

In addition to professional support, having at least one peer in your research world with whom to share the joys, frustrations, and current problems of data collection is important. This colleague can often serve as a mirror to allow you to see the situation clearly and perhaps more objectively. With this type of support, the researcher can share and release feelings and gain some distance from the data collection situation. Alternatives for resolving the problem can be discussed dispassionately.

Data Safety and Monitoring Board as Source of Support

If an intervention is being implemented that is deemed to be of low risk to the patient, such as a behavioral intervention to improve sleep quality, a data safety and monitoring plan will suffice. The plan includes monitoring consistent with the intervention's risks and benefits and the complexity of the study (Artinian, Froelicher, & Wall, 2004). In these situations, a plan is deemed adequate when it conforms to the IRB requirements for reporting any adverse event and includes annual progress reports. It requires that the researcher explicitly state the plan to review the data from each set number of subjects or from each 3-month or 6-month batch of recruited subjects, depending on the extent of the study.

If the study involves a vulnerable population (Artinian et al., 2004) or an intervention protocol posing higher than average risk to patient safety, a data safety and monitoring board (DSMB) is required. This board includes members who are not directly involved in the study and who can be objective about the findings. The DSMB will review the results of interim data analyses provided the researcher and compare the results to the criteria for stopping the study, criteria that were determined prior to the beginning of the study. Because of the nature of the work, the DSMB should consist of very experienced researchers and clinical experts.

An example of a study that was terminated by a DSMB was the study conducted by Niemann et al. (2015) to determine whether therapeutic hypothermia resulted in delayed graft function in 500 recipients of deceased-donor kidneys. When the interim data analysis occurred as planned, the DSMB noted the reduced rate of delayed graft function in the hypothermia group as compared to the normothermia group. The DSMB recommended that the study be discontinued early because hypothermia was obviously effective in protecting organ function (Niemann et al., 2015). The DSMB supported the research team's decision to stop the study.

SERENDIPITY

Serendipity is the accidental discovery of something useful or valuable that is not the primary focus of the inquiry. During the data collection phase of studies, researchers often become aware of elements or relationships that they had not identified previously. These aspects may be closely related to the study being conducted or have little connection with it. They come from increased awareness and close observation of the study situation. Serendipitous findings are important for the development of new insights in nursing theory. They can be important for understanding the totality of the phenomenon being examined. Additionally, they lead to areas of research that generate new knowledge. A relatively easy way to capture these insights as they occur is to maintain a research journal or make field notes. These events must be carefully recorded, even if their impact or meaning is not understood at the time, and they should be reported in the study findings.

▮ KEY POINTS

- Careful planning is needed before collecting and managing data.
- A study protocol provides a plan for the implementation of the study.
- Factors such as cost, size of research team, and time affect decisions about data collection.
- The researcher has several decisions to make about measuring the study variables, including cost of the instrument, reading level, and method of data collection.
- Data may be collected with or without the assistance of the researcher. Data may be collected online, on scannable forms, or on printed surveys.
- Demographic questionnaires are developed to include the variables to describe the sample and in a format to promote accuracy of the data.
- To prepare for data entry, the instruments are formatted and compiled prior to creating a codebook to promote consistent data entry.
- The logistics of data entry include who will enter the data and the rules for data entry, such as how missing data will be coded.
- A detailed data collection plan includes the chronology of recruiting and consenting subjects, scheduling data collection, training data collectors, and identifying decision points.
- When a pilot study is conducted, the lessons learned can refine the study protocol and data collection plan.
- During the study, the researcher maintains control and consistency, manages the data collection, and oversees the storage and retrieval of the data.
- Problems that arise during data collection involve recruitment and attrition issues, treatment of the subject as an object, external influences on subject responses, passive resistance from staff members or family, researcher interactions, lack of skill in data collection techniques, and researcher role conflicts.

- A successful study requires support that is often obtained from academic committees, healthcare agencies, work colleagues, and even data safety-monitoring boards.

REFERENCES

Albrecht, T., & Taylor, A. (2013). No stone left unturned: Challenges encountered during recruitment of women with advanced ovarian cancer for a phase I study. *Applied Nursing Research*, *26*(4), 245–250.

Allen, P., & Roberts, L. (2010). The ethics of outsourcing online survey research. *International Journal of Technoethics*, *1*(3), 35–48.

Artinian, N., Froelicher, E., & Wal, J. (2004). Data and safety monitoring during randomized controlled trials of nursing interventions. *Nursing Research*, *53*(6), 414–418.

Bohr, A., Brown, D., Laurson, K., Smith, P., & Bass, R. (2013). Relationship between socioeconomic status and physical fitness in junior high students. *Journal of School Health*, *83*(8), 542–547.

Cafasso, M., Elder, D., Blum, S., Weiss, T., Hornung, L., Khoury, J., et al. (2015). Treatment of central precocious puberty using gonadotropin-releasing hormone agonists. *The Journal of Nurse Practitioners*, *11*(2), 686–694.

Chen, H.-J., & Chen, Y.-M. (2015). Pain assessment: Validity of the physiologic indicators in the ventilated adult patients. *Pain Management Nursing*, *16*(2), 105–111.

Cohn, D. (2015). *Census considers new approach to asking about race-by not using the term at all.* Pew Research Center. Retrieved July 15, 2015, from http://www.pewresearch.org/fact-tank/2015/06/18/census-considers-new-approach-to-asking-about-race-by-not-using-the-term-at-all/.

DeVon, H., Patmon, F., Rosenfeld, A., Fennessy, M., & Francis, D. (2013). Implementing clinical research in the high acuity setting of the emergency department. *Journal of Emergency Nursing*, *39*(1), 6–12.

Fan, W., & Yan, Z. (2010). Factors affecting response rates of the web survey: A systematic review. *Computers in Human Behavior*, *26*(2), 132–139.

Fukuoka, Y., Kamitani, E., Dracup, K., & Jong, S. S. (2011). New insights into compliance with a mobile phone diary and pedometer use in sedentary women. *Journal of Physical Activity & Health*, *8*(3), 398–403.

Funke, G., Reips, U.-D., & Thomas, R. (2011). Sliders for the smart: Type of rating scale on the web interacts with educational level. *Social Science Computer Review*, *29*(2), 221–231.

Gill, F., Leslie, G., Grech, C., & Latour, J. (2013). Using a web-based survey tool to undertake a Delphi study: Application to nursing education research. *Nurse Education Today*, *33*(1), 1322–1328.

Gray, J., & Johnson, L. (2009). *Nurse International Relocation Questionnaire 2.* Unpublished research tool. Retrieved July 20, 2015, from Jennifer.gray@oc.edu.

Harris, P. A., Taylor, R., Thielke, R., Payne, J., Gonzalez, N., & Conde, J. G. (2009). Research electronic data capture (REDCap)—A metadata-driven methodology and workflow process for providing translational research informatics support. *Journal of Biomedical Informatics*, *42*(2), 377–381.

Harwood, E. M. (2009). Data collection methods series: Part 3: Developing protocols for collecting data. *Journal of Wound Ostomy Continence Nursing*, *36*(3), 246–250.

Harwood, E. M., & Hutchinson, E. (2009). Data collection methods series: Part 2: Select the most feasible data collection mode. *Journal of Wound Ostomy Continence Nursing*, *36*(2), 129–135.

Hertzog, M. (2008). Considerations for determining sample size for pilot studies. *Research in Nursing & Health*, *31*(2), 180–191.

Human Rights Campaign. (HRC, 2015). *Resources. Collecting transgender-inclusive gender data in workplace and other surveys.* Retrieved August 1, 2015, from http://www.hrc.org/resources/entry/collecting-transgender-inclusive-gender-data-in-workplace-and-other-surveys.

Humphreys, J., Epel, E. S., Cooper, B. A., Lin, J., Blackburn, E. H., & Lee, K. A. (2012). Telomere shortening in formerly abused and never abused women. *Biological Research for Nursing*, *14*(2), 115–123.

Hunter, L. (2012). Challenging the reported disadvantages of e-questionnaires and addressing methodological issues of online data collection. *Nurse Researcher*, *20*(1), 11–20.

International Business Machines (IBM) Corporation. (n.d.) *IBM SPSS data collection.* Retrieved May 7, 2016, from http://www-01.ibm.com/software/analytics/spss/products/data-collection/.

Jones, R., Hoover, D., & Lacroix, J. (2013). A randomized controlled trial of soap opera videos streamed to smartphones to reduce risk of sexually transmitted human immunodeficiency virus (HIV) in young urban African American women. *Nursing Outlook*, *61*(2), 205–215.

Jull, A., & Aye, P. (2015). Endorsement of the CONSORT guidelines, trial registration, and the quality of reporting randomised controlled trials in leading nursing journals: A cross-sectional analysis. *International Journal of Nursing Studies*, *52*(6), 1071–1079.

Kang, D. H., Davis, L., Habermann, B., Rice, M., & Broome, M. (2005). Hiring the right people and management of research staff. *Western Journal of Nursing Research*, *27*(8), 1059–1066.

Kupzyk, K., & Cohen, M. (2015). Data validation and other strategies for data entry. *Western Journal of Nursing Research*, *37*(4), 546–556.

Lee, K. A., & Gay, C. L. (2011). Can modifications to the bedroom environment improve the sleep of new parents? Two randomized controlled trials. *Research in Nursing & Health*, *34*(1), 7–19.

Lim, L. M., Chiu, L. H., Dohrmann, J., & Tan, K. (2010). Registered nurses' medication management of the elderly in aged care facilities. *International Nursing Review*, *57*(1), 98–106.

Linder, L., Ameringer, S., Erickson, J., Macpherson, C., Stegenga, K., & Linder, W. (2013). Using an iPad in research with children and adolescents. *Journal for Specialists in Pediatric Nursing*, *18*(2), 158–164.

McEwen, J., Boyer, J., & Sun, K. (2013). Evolving approaches to the ethical management of genomic data. *Trends in Genetics*, *29*(6), 375–382.

Melnyk, B. M., & Fineout-Overholt, E. (2015). *Evidence-based practice in nursing and healthcare: A guide to best practice* (3rd ed.). Philadelphia, PA: Wolters-Kluwer.

Newnam, K., McGrath, J., Salyer, J., Estes, T., Jallo, N., & Bass, W. (2015). A comparative effectiveness study of continuous positive airway pressure-related skin breakdown when using different nasal interfaces in the extremely low birth weight neonate. *Applied Nursing Research, 28*(1), 36–41.

Niemann, C., Feiner, J., Swain, S., Bunting, S., Friedman, M., Crutchfield, M., et al. (2015). Therapeutic hypothermia in deceased organ donors and kidney-graft function. *New England Journal of Medicine, 373*(5), 405–414.

Sarpatwari, A., Kesselheim, A., Malin, B., Gagne, J., & Schneeweiss, S. (2014). Ensuring patient privacy in data sharing for postapproval research. *The New England Journal of Medicine, 137*(17), 1644–1649.

Schick-Makaroff, K., & Molzahn, A. (2015). Strategies to use tablet computers for collection of electronic patient-reported outcomes. *Health and Quality of Life Outcomes, 13*, 2. Retrieved May 7, 2016 from http://dx.doi.org/10.1186/s12955-014-0205-1 Article 2.

Schulz, K., Altman, D., & Moher, D. (2010). CONSORT 2010 statement: Updated guidelines for reporting parallel group randomized trials. *Annals of Internal Medicine, 152*(11), 1–8.

SurveyMonkey (2011). *SurveyMonkey user manual.* Retrieved July 15, 2015, from https://www.surveymonkey.com.

Udtha, M., Nomie, K., Yu, E., & Sanner, J. (2015). Novel and emerging strategies for longitudinal data collection. *Journal of Nursing Scholarship, 47*(2), 152–160.

United States Department of Health & Human Services (U.S. DHHS, 2015). *U.S. poverty guidelines.* Retrieved December 14, 2015, from http://aspe.hhs.gov/poverty/15poverty.cfm.

Wadrop-Valverde, D., Dong, C., & Ownby, R. (2013). Medication-taking self-efficacy and medication adherence among HIV-infected cocaine users. *Journal of the Association of Nurses in AIDS Care, 24*(3), 198–206.

Waltz, C. F., Strickland, O. L., & Lenz, E. R. (2010). *Measurement in nursing and health research* (4th ed.). New York, NY: Springer.

Wilson, D., & Anteneise, G. (2014). *"To share or not to share" in client-side encrypted clouds.* Preprinted by ArXiv.org. Retrieved August 1, 2015, from http://arxiv.org/pdf/1404.2697v1.pdf.

Wong, J. Y., Tiwari, A., Fong, D. Y., Humphreys, J., & Bullock, L. (2011). Depression among women experiencing intimate partner violence in a Chinese community. *Nursing Research, 60*(1), 58–65.

21

Introduction to Statistical Analysis

Daisha J. Cipher

http://evolve.elsevier.com/Gray/practice/

Statistical analysis is often considered one of the most exciting steps of the research process. During this phase, you will finally obtain answers to the questions that led to the development of your study. Critical appraisal of the results section of a quantitative study requires you to be able to (1) identify the statistical procedures used; (2) judge whether these statistical procedures were appropriate for the hypotheses, questions, or objectives of the study and for the data available for analysis; (3) comprehend the discussion of statistical analysis results; (4) judge whether the author's interpretation of the results is appropriate; and (5) evaluate the clinical importance of the findings (see Chapter 18 for more details on critical appraisal).

As a neophyte researcher performing a quantitative study, you are confronted with many critical decisions related to statistical analysis that require statistical knowledge. To perform statistical analysis of data from a quantitative study, you need to be able to (1) determine the necessary sample size to power your study adequately; (2) prepare the data for analysis; (3) describe the sample; (4) test the reliability of the measurement methods used in the study; (5) perform exploratory analyses of the data; (6) perform analyses guided by the study objectives, questions, or hypotheses; and (7) interpret the results of statistical procedures. We recommend consulting with a statistician or expert researcher early in the research process to help you develop a plan for accomplishing these seven tasks. A statistician is also invaluable in conducting statistical analysis for a study and interpreting the results (Hayat, Higgins, Schwartz, & Staggs, 2015).

Critical appraisal of the results of studies and statistical analyses both require an understanding of the statistical theory underlying the process of analysis. This chapter and the following four chapters provide you with the information needed for critical appraisal of the results sections of published studies and for performance of statistical procedures to analyze data in studies and in clinical practice. This chapter introduces the concepts of statistical theory and discusses some of the more pragmatic aspects of quantitative statistical analysis: the purposes of statistical analysis, the process of performing statistical analysis, the method for choosing appropriate statistical analysis techniques for a study, and resources for conducting statistical analysis procedures. Chapter 22 explains the use of statistics for descriptive purposes, such as describing the study sample or variables. Chapter 23 focuses on the use of statistics to examine proposed relationships among study variables, such as the relationships among the variables dyspnea, fatigue, anxiety, and quality of life. Chapter 24 explores the use of statistics for prediction, such as using independent variables of age, gender, cholesterol values, and history of hypertension to predict the dependent variable of cardiac risk level. Chapter 25 guides you in using statistics to determine differences between groups, such as determining the difference in muscle strength and falls (dependent variables) between an experimental or intervention group receiving a strength training program (independent variable) and a comparison group receiving standard care.

CONCEPTS OF STATISTICAL THEORY

One reason nurses tend to avoid statistics is that many were taught the mathematical mechanics of calculating statistical formulas and were given little or no explanation of the logic behind the analysis procedure or the meaning of the results (Grove & Cipher, 2017). This mathematical process is usually performed by computer, and information about it offers little assistance to the individuals making statistical decisions or explaining results. We approach statistical analysis from the perspective of enhancing your understanding of the meaning underlying statistical analysis. You can use this understanding either for critical appraisal of studies or for conducting data analyses.

The ensuing discussion explains some of the concepts commonly used in statistical theory. The logic of statistical theory is embedded within the explanations of these concepts. The concepts presented in this chapter include probability theory, classical hypothesis testing, Type I and Type II errors, statistical power, statistical significance versus clinical importance, inference, samples and populations, descriptive and inferential statistical techniques, measures of central tendency, the normal curve, sampling distributions, symmetry, skewness, modality, kurtosis, variation, confidence intervals, and both parametric and nonparametric types of inferential statistical analyses.

Probability Theory

Probability theory addresses statistical analysis as the likelihood of accurately predicting an event or the extent of an effect. Nurse researchers are interested in the probability of a particular nursing outcome in a particular patient care situation. For example, what is the probability of patients older than 75 years of age with cardiac conditions falling when hospitalized? With probability theory, you could determine how much of the variation in your data could be explained by using a particular statistical analysis. In probability theory, the researcher interprets the meaning of statistical results in light of his or her knowledge of the field of study. A finding that would have little meaning in one field of study might be important in another (Good, 1983; Kerlinger & Lee, 2000). Probability is expressed as a lowercase p, with values expressed as a percentage or as a decimal value ranging from 0 to 1. For example, if the exact probability is known to be 0.23, it would be expressed as $p = 0.23$. The p in statistics is defined as the probability of obtaining a statistical value as extreme or greater when the null hypothesis is true (Cohen, 1994). The p should be distinguished from Type I error (α) (discussed later in this chapter), which is the probability of rejecting the null hypothesis when the null is actually true. Nurse researchers typically consider a $p = 0.05$ value or less to indicate a real effect.

Classical Hypothesis Testing

Classical hypothesis testing refers to the process of testing a hypothesis to infer the reality of an effect. This process starts with the statement of a null hypothesis, which assumes no effect (e.g., no difference between groups, or no relationship between variables). The researcher sets the values of two theoretical probabilities: (1) the probability of rejecting the null hypothesis when it is in fact true (alpha [α], **Type I error**) and (2) the probability of retaining the null hypothesis when it is in fact false (beta [β], **Type II error**). In nursing research, alpha is usually set at 0.05, meaning that the researcher will allow a 5% or lower chance of making a Type I error. The beta is frequently set at 0.20, meaning that the researcher will allow for a 20% or lower chance of making a Type II error (Fisher, 1935; 1971).

After conducting the study, the researcher culminates the hypothesis testing process by making a rational decision either to reject or to retain the null hypothesis, based on the statistical results. The following steps outline each of the components of statistical hypothesis testing:

1. State your primary null hypothesis. (Chapter 6 discusses the development of the null hypothesis.)
2. Set your study alpha (Type I error); this is usually $\alpha = 0.05$.
3. Set your study beta (Type II error); this is usually $\beta = 0.20$.
4. Conduct power analyses (Cohen, 1988; Grove & Cipher, 2017).
5. Design and conduct your study.
6. Compute the appropriate statistic on your obtained data.
7. Compare your obtained statistic with its corresponding theoretical distribution in the tables provided in the Appendices at the back of this book. For example, if you analyzed your data with a t-test, you would compare the t value from your study with the critical values of t in the table in Appendix B.
8. If your obtained statistic exceeds the critical value in the distribution table, you can reject your null hypothesis. If not, you must accept your null hypothesis. These ideas are discussed in more depth in Chapters 23 through 25, in which the results of various statistical analyses are presented.

Significance testing addresses whether the data support the conclusion that there is a true effect in the direction of the apparent difference (Cox, 1958). This decision is a judgment and can be in error. The level of statistical significance attained indicates the degree of uncertainty in taking the position that the difference between groups (or the association between variables) is real. Classical hypothesis testing has been widely criticized for such errors in judgments (Cohen, 1994; Loftus 1993). Much emphasis has been placed on researchers providing indicators of effect, rather than just relying on *p* values, specifically, providing the magnitude of the obtained effect (e.g., a difference or relationship) as well as confidence intervals associated with the statistical findings. These additional statistics give consumers of research more information about the phenomenon being studied (Cohen, 1994; Gaskin & Happell, 2014).

Type I and Type II Errors

We choose the probability of making a Type I error when we set alpha, and if we decrease the probability of making a Type I error, we increase the probability of making a Type II error. The relationships between Type I and Type II errors are defined in Table 21-1. Type II error occurs as a result of some degree of overlap between the values of different populations, so in some cases a value with a greater than 5% probability of being within one population may be within the dimensions of another population.

It is impossible to decrease both types of error simultaneously without a corresponding increase in sample size. The researcher must decide which risk poses the greatest threat within a specific study. In nursing research, many studies are conducted with small samples and instruments that lack precision and accuracy in the measurement of study variables (see Chapter 16). Many nursing situations include multiple variables that interact to lead to differences within populations. However, when one is examining only a few of the interacting variables, small differences can be overlooked and could lead to a false conclusion of no differences between the samples. In this case, the risk of a Type II error is a greater concern, and a more lenient level of significance is in order. Nurse researchers usually set the level of significance or $\alpha = 0.05$ for their studies versus a more stringent $\alpha = 0.01$ or 0.001. Setting $\alpha = 0.05$ reduces the

risk of a Type II error of indicating study results are not significant when they are.

Statistical Power

Power is the probability that a statistical test will detect an effect when it actually exists. Power is the inverse of Type II error and is calculated as $1 - \beta$. Type II error is the probability of retaining the null hypothesis when it is in fact false. When the researcher sets Type II error at 0.20 before conducting a study, this means that the power of the planned statistic has been set to 0.80. In other words, the statistic will have an 80% chance of detecting an effect if it actually exists.

Reported studies failing to reject the null hypothesis (in which power is unlikely to have been examined) often have a low power level to detect an effect if one exists. Until more recently, the researcher's primary interest was in preventing a Type I error. Therefore, great emphasis was placed on the selection of a level of significance, but little emphasis was placed on power. However, this point of view is changing as the seriousness of a Type II error is increasingly recognized in nursing studies.

As stated in the steps of classical hypothesis testing previously, step 4 is "conducting a power analysis." Power analysis involves determining the required sample size needed to conduct your study after performing steps 1, 2, and 3. Power analysis can address the number of participants required for a study, or conversely the extent of the power of a statistical test. A power analysis performed prior to the study beginning to determine the required number of participants needed to identify an effect is termed an **a priori power analysis**. A power analysis performed after the study ends to determine the power of the statistical result is termed a **post hoc power analysis**. Optimally, the power analysis is performed prior to the study beginning so that the researcher can plan to include an adequate number of participants. Otherwise, the researcher risks conducting a study with an inadequate number of participants and putting the study at risk for Type II error (Grove & Cipher, 2017).

Cohen (1988) identified four parameters of power: (1) significance level, (2) sample size, (3) effect size, and (4) power (standard of 0.80). If three of the four are known, the fourth can be calculated by using power analysis formulas. Significance level and sample size are straightforward. Chapter 15 provides a detailed discussion of determining sample size in quantitative studies that includes power analysis. **Effect size** is "the degree to which the phenomenon is present in the population or the degree to which the null hypothesis is false" (Cohen, 1988, pp. 9–10). For example, suppose you were

TABLE 21-1	**Type I and Type II Errors**		
		DECISION	
		Reject Null	Accept Null
True Population Status	*Null is True.*	Type I error α	Correct decision $1 - \alpha$
	Null is False.	Correct decision $1 - \beta$	Type II error β

measuring changes in anxiety levels, measured first when the patient is at home and then just before surgery. The effect size would be large if you expected a great change in anxiety. If you expected only a small change in the level of anxiety, the effect size would be small.

Small effect sizes require larger samples to detect these small differences (see Chapter 15 for a detailed discussion of effect size). If the power is too low, it may not be worthwhile to conduct the study unless a large sample can be obtained, because statistical tests are unlikely to detect differences or relationships that exist. Deciding to conduct a study in these circumstances is costly in time and money, frequently does not add to the body of nursing knowledge, and can lead to false conclusions. Power analysis can be conducted with hand calculations, computer software, or online calculators and should be performed to determine the sample size necessary for a particular study (Cohen, 1988). Power analysis can be calculated by using the free power analysis software G*Power (Faul, Erdfelder, Lang, & Buchner, 2007) or statistical software such as NCSS, SAS, and SPSS (Table 21-2). In addition, many free sample size calculators are available online that are easy to use and understand. The workbook by Grove and Cipher (2017) provides step-by-step instructions for six common power analyses using the software G*Power 3.1 (Faul, Erdfelder, Buchner, & Lang, 2009).

The power achieved should be reported with the results of the studies, especially studies that fail to reject the null hypothesis (have nonsignificant results). If power is high, it strengthens the meaning of the findings. If power is low, researchers need to address this issue in the discussion of limitations and implications of the study findings. Modifications in the research methodology that resulted from the use of power analysis also need to be reported.

TABLE 21-2 Software Applications for Statistical Analysis

Software Application	Website
SPSS (Statistical Packages for the Social Sciences)	www.ibm.com/software/analytics/spss/
SAS (Statistical Analysis System)	www.sas.com
NCSS (Number Cruncher Statistical System)	www.ncss.com
Stata	www.stata.com
JMP	www.jmp.com

Statistical Significance Versus Clinical Importance

The findings of a study can be statistically significant but may not be clinically important. For example, one group of patients might have a body temperature 0.1° F higher than that of another group. Statistical analysis might indicate that the temperatures of two groups are significantly different. However, the findings have little or no clinical importance because of the small difference in temperatures between groups. It is often important to know the magnitude of the difference between groups in studies. However, a statistical test that indicates significant differences between groups (e.g., a *t*-test) provides no information on the magnitude of the difference. The extent of the level of significance (0.01 or 0.0001) tells you nothing about the magnitude of the difference between the groups or the relationship between two variables. The magnitude of group differences can best be determined through calculating effect sizes and confidence intervals (see Chapters 22 through 25).

Inference

Statisticians use the terms **inference** and **infer** in a way that is similar to the researcher's use of the term *generalize*. Inference requires the use of inductive reasoning. One infers from a specific case to a general truth, from a part to the whole, from the concrete to the abstract, from the known to the unknown. When using inferential reasoning, you can never prove things; you can never be certain. However, one of the reasons for the rules that have been established with regard to statistical procedures is to increase the probability that inferences are accurate. Inferences are made cautiously and with great care. Researchers use inferences to infer from the sample in their study to the larger population.

Samples and Populations

Use of the terms *statistic* and *parameter* can be confusing because of the various populations referred to in statistical theory. A **statistic**, such as a mean ($\overline{X}$), is a numerical value obtained from a sample. A **parameter** is a true (but unknown) numerical characteristic of a population. For example, μ is the population mean or arithmetic average. The mean of the sampling distribution (mean of samples' means) can also be shown to be equal to μ. A numerical value that is the mean ($\overline{X}$) of the sample is a statistic; a numerical value that is the mean of the population (μ) is a parameter (Barnett, 1982).

Relating a statistic to a parameter requires an inference as one moves from the sample to the sampling distribution and then from the sampling distribution to the population. The population referred to is in one sense real (concrete) and in another sense abstract. These ideas are illustrated as follows:

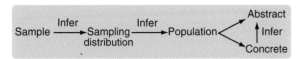

For example, perhaps you are interested in the cholesterol levels of women in the United States (U.S.). Your population is women in the U.S. You cannot measure the cholesterol level of every woman in the U.S.; therefore, you select a sample of women from this population. Because you wish your sample to be as representative of the population as possible, you obtain your sample by using random sampling techniques (see Chapter 15). To determine whether the cholesterol levels in your sample are similar to those in the population, you must compare the sample with the population. One strategy would be to compare the mean of your sample with the mean of the entire population. However, it is highly unlikely that you *know* the mean of the entire population; you must make an estimate of the mean of that population. You need to know how good your sample statistics are as estimators of the parameters of the population. First, you make some assumptions. You assume that the mean scores of cholesterol levels from multiple, randomly selected samples of this population would be normally distributed. This assumption implies another assumption: that the cholesterol levels of the population will be distributed according to the theoretical normal curve—that difference scores and standard deviations can be equated to those in the normal curve. The normal curve is discussed in Chapter 22.

If you assume that the population in your study is normally distributed, you can also assume that this population can be represented by a normal sampling distribution. You infer from your sample to the sampling distribution, the mathematically developed theoretical population made up of parameters such as the mean of means and the standard error. The parameters of this theoretical population are the measures of the dimensions identified in the sampling distribution. You can infer from the sampling distribution to the population. You have both a concrete population and an abstract population. The concrete population consists of all the individuals who meet your study sample criteria, whereas the abstract population consists of individuals who will meet your sample criteria in the future or the groups addressed theoretically by your framework (see Chapter 8).

TYPES OF STATISTICS

There are two major classes of statistics: descriptive statistics and inferential statistics. **Descriptive statistics** are computed to reveal characteristics of the sample and to describe study variables. **Inferential statistics** are computed to draw conclusions and make inferences about the population, based on the sample data set (Plichta & Kelvin, 2013). The following sections define the concepts and rationale associated with descriptive and inferential statistics.

Descriptive Statistics

A basic yet important way to begin describing a sample is to create a frequency distribution of the variable or variables being studied. A frequency distribution is a plot of one variable, whereby the x-axis consists of the possible values of that variable, and the y-axis is the tally of each value. For example, if you assessed a sample for a variable such as pain using a visual analog scale, and your subjects reported particular values for pain, you could create a frequency distribution as illustrated in Figure 21-1.

Measures of Central Tendency

The measures of central tendency are descriptive statistics. The statistics that represent **measures of central tendency** are the mean, median, and mode. All of these statistics are representations or descriptions of the center or middle of a frequency distribution. The **mean** is the arithmetic average of all of the values of a variable. The **median** is the exact middle value (or the average of the middle two values if there is an even number of observations). The **mode** is the most commonly occurring value in a data set (Grove & Cipher, 2017; Zar, 2010). It is possible to have more than one mode in a sample, which is discussed in Chapter 22. In a normal curve, the mean, median, and mode are equal or approximately equal (see Figure 21-2).

Normal Curve

The theoretical **normal curve** is an expression of statistical theory. It is a theoretical frequency distribution of all *possible* scores (see Figure 21-2). However, no real distribution fits the normal curve exactly. The idea of the normal curve was developed by an 18-year-old mathematician, Gauss, in 1795, who found that data measured repeatedly in many samples from the same population by using scales based on an underlying continuum can be combined into one large sample (Gauss, 1809). From this large sample, one can develop a more accurate representation of the pattern of the curve in

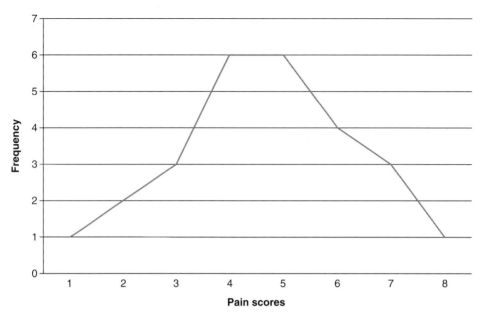

FIGURE 21-1 Frequency distribution of visual analog scale pain scores.

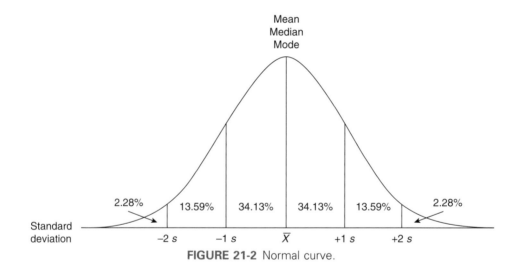

FIGURE 21-2 Normal curve.

that population than is possible with only one sample. In most cases, the curve is similar, regardless of the specific data that have been examined or the population being studied. This theoretical normal curve is symmetrical and unimodal and has continuous values. The mean, median, and mode are equal. The distribution is completely defined by the mean and standard deviation, which are calculated and discussed further in Chapter 22.

Sampling Distributions

The shape of the distribution provides important information about the data. The outline of the distribution shape is obtained by using a histogram. Within this outline, the mean, median, mode, and standard deviation can be graphically illustrated (see Figure 21-2). This visual presentation of combined summary statistics provides insight into the nature of the distribution. As the sample size becomes larger, the shape of the distribution more accurately reflects the shape of the population from which the sample was taken. Even when statistics, such as means, come from a population with a skewed (asymmetrical) distribution, the sampling distribution developed from multiple means obtained from that skewed population tends to fit the pattern of the normal curve. This phenomenon is referred to as the **central limit theorem**.

Symmetry

Several terms are used to describe the shape of the curve (and the nature of a particular distribution). The shape of a curve is usually discussed in terms of symmetry, skewness, modality, and kurtosis. A **symmetrical curve** is one in which the left side is a mirror image of the right side (Figure 21-3). In these curves, the mean, median, and mode are equal and are the dividing point between the left and right sides of the curve.

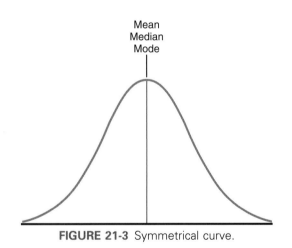

FIGURE 21-3 Symmetrical curve.

Skewness

Any curve that is not symmetrical is referred to as **skewed** or **asymmetrical**. Skewness may be exhibited in the curve in various ways. A curve may be **positively skewed**, which means that the largest portion of data is below the mean. For example, data on length of enrollment in hospice are positively skewed. Most people die within the first 3 weeks of enrollment, whereas increasingly smaller numbers survive as time increases. A curve can also be **negatively skewed**, which means that the largest portion of data is above the mean. For example, data on the occurrence of chronic illness by age in a population are negatively skewed, with most chronic illnesses occurring in older age groups. Figure 21-4 includes both a positively skewed distribution and a negatively skewed distribution.

In a **skewed distribution,** the mean, median, and mode are not equal. Skewness interferes with the validity of many statistical analyses; therefore, statistical procedures have been developed to measure the skewness of the distribution of the sample being studied. Few samples are perfectly symmetrical; however, as the deviation from symmetry increases, the seriousness of the impact on statistical analysis increases (Plichta & Kelvin, 2013). In a positively skewed distribution, the mean is greater than the median, which is greater than the mode. In a negatively skewed distribution, the mean is less than the median, which is less than the mode (see Figure 21-4).

Modality

Another characteristic of distributions is their modality. Most curves found in practice are **unimodal**, which means that they have one mode, and frequencies progressively decline as they move away from the mode. Symmetrical distributions are usually unimodal.

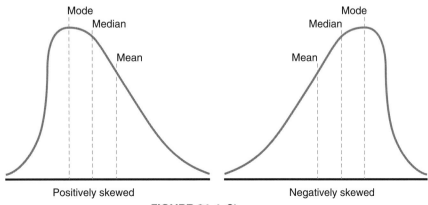

Positively skewed   Negatively skewed

FIGURE 21-4 Skewness.

However, curves can also be **bimodal** (Figure 21-5) or multimodal. When you find a bimodal sample, it may mean that you have not defined your population adequately.

Kurtosis

Another term used to describe the shape of the distribution curve is kurtosis. **Kurtosis** explains the degree of peakedness of the curve, which is related to the spread or variance of scores. An extremely peaked curve is referred to as **leptokurtic**, an intermediate degree of kurtosis is referred to as **mesokurtic**, and a relatively flat curve is referred to as **platykurtic** (Figure 21-6). Extreme kurtosis can affect the validity of statistical analysis because the scores have little variation in a leptokurtic curve. Many computer programs analyze kurtosis before conducting statistical analyses. A kurtosis of zero indicates that the curve is mesokurtic. Kurtosis values above zero indicate that the curve is leptokurtic, and values below zero that are negative indicate a platykurtic curve (Box, Hunter, & Hunter, 1978).

Tests of Normality

Statistics are computed to obtain an indication of the skewness and kurtosis of a given frequency distribution. The **Shapiro-Wilk W test** is a formal test of normality that assesses whether the distribution of a variable is skewed, kurtotic, or both. This test has the ability to calculate both skewness and kurtosis for a study variable such as pain measured with a visual analog scale. For large samples ($n > 2000$), the **Kolmogorov-Smirnov D test** is an alternative test of normality for large samples (Grove & Cipher, 2017).

Variation

The range, standard deviation, and variance are statistics that describe the extent to which the values in the sample vary from one another. The most common of these statistics to be reported in the literature is the standard deviation because of its direct association with the normal curve. If the frequency distribution of any given variable is approximately normal, knowing the standard deviation of that variable allows us to know what percentages of subjects' values on that variable fall between +1 and −1 standard deviation. Referring back to the hypothetical frequency distribution of pain in Figure 21-1, when we calculate a standard deviation, we know that 34.13% of the subjects' pain scores were between the mean pain score and 1 standard deviation above the mean pain score. We also know that 34.13% of the subjects' pain scores were between the mean pain score and 1 standard deviation below the mean. The middle 95.44% of the subjects' scores were between −2 standard deviations and +2 standard deviations.

Confidence Intervals

When the probability of including the value of the parameter within the interval estimate is known, this is referred to as a **confidence interval**. Calculating a confidence interval involves the use of two formulas to identify the upper and lower ends of the interval (see Chapter 22 for calculations). Confidence intervals are usually expressed as "(38.6, 41.4)," with 38.6 being the lower end and 41.4 being the upper end of the interval. Theoretically, we can produce a confidence interval for any parameter of a distribution. It is a generic statistical

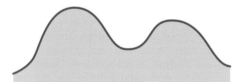

FIGURE 21-5 Bimodal distribution.

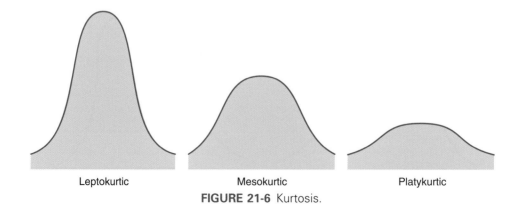

Leptokurtic   Mesokurtic   Platykurtic

FIGURE 21-6 Kurtosis.

procedure. Confidence intervals can also be developed around correlation coefficients (Glass & Stanley, 1970). Estimation can be used for a single population or for multiple populations. In **estimation**, we are inferring the value of a parameter from sample data and have no preconceived notion of the value of the parameter. In contrast, in **hypothesis testing**, we have an a priori theory about the value of the parameter or parameters or some combination of parameters. A formula is provided for calculating confidence intervals and example confidence intervals are provided for different analysis results in Chapters 22 through 25.

Inferential Statistics

Inferential statistics are computed to draw conclusions and make inferences about the greater population, based on the sample data set. There are two classes of inferential statistics: parametric and nonparametric statistics.

Parametric Statistics

The most commonly used type of statistical analysis is parametric statistics. The analysis is referred to as **parametric statistical analysis** because the findings are inferred to the parameters of a normally distributed population. These approaches to analysis emerged from the work of Fisher (1935) and require meeting the following three assumptions before they can justifiably be used:

1. The sample was drawn from a population for which the variance can be calculated. The distribution is usually expected to be normal or approximately normal (Conover, 1971; Zar, 2010).
2. Because most parametric techniques deal with continuous variables rather than discrete variables, the level of measurement should be at least interval level data or ordinal data with an approximately normal distribution.
3. The data can be treated as random samples (Box et al., 1978).

Nonparametric Statistics

Nonparametric statistical analyses, or distribution-free techniques, can be used in studies that do not meet the first two assumptions of normal distribution and at least interval-level data. Nonparametric analyses are conducted to analyze nominal and ordinal levels of data and interval-level data that are skewed. Most nonparametric techniques are not as powerful as their parametric counterparts (Tanizaki, 1997). In other words, nonparametric techniques are less able to detect differences and have a greater risk of a Type II error if the data meet the assumptions of parametric procedures;

this is generally because nonparametric statistics are actually performed on ranks of the original data. When data have been converted into ranks, they inevitably lose accuracy. Because nonparametric statistics have lower statistical power, many researchers choose to submit ordinal data to parametric statistical procedures. If the instrument or measurement procedure yielding ordinal data has been rigorously evaluated, parametric statistics are justified (de Winter & Dodou, 2010). For example, researchers often analyze data from a Likert scale with strong reliability and validity as though they are interval-level data (see Chapter 17 for a description of Likert scales).

PRACTICAL ASPECTS OF STATISTICAL ANALYSIS

Statistics can be conducted for a variety of purposes, such as to (1) summarize, (2) explore the meaning of deviations in the data, (3) compare or contrast descriptively, (4) test the proposed relationships in a theoretical model, (5) infer that the findings from the sample are indicative of the entire population, (6) examine causality, (7) predict, or (8) infer from the sample to a theoretical model. These different purposes for statistical analysis are addressed in Chapters 22 through 25.

The process of quantitative statistical analysis consists of several stages: (1) preparation of the data for analysis; (2) description of the sample; (3) testing the reliability of measurement; (4) exploratory analysis of the data; (5) confirmatory analysis guided by the hypotheses, questions, or objectives; and (6) post hoc analysis. Statisticians such as Tukey (1977) divided the role of statistics into two parts: exploratory statistical analysis and confirmatory statistical analysis. You can perform **exploratory statistical analysis** to obtain a preliminary indication of the nature of the data and to search the data for hidden structure or models. **Confirmatory statistical analysis** involves traditional inferential statistics, which you can use to make an inference about a population or a process based on evidence from the study sample.

Although not all of these six stages are reflected in the final published report of the study, they all contribute to the insight you can gain from analyzing the data. Many novice researchers do not plan the details of statistical analysis until the data are collected and they are confronted with the analysis task. This research technique is poor and often leads to the collection of unusable data or the failure to collect the data needed to answer the research questions. Plans for statistical analysis need to be made during development of the study methodology. The following section covers the six stages of quantitative statistical analysis.

Preparing the Data for Analysis

Except in very small studies, computers are almost universally used for statistical analysis. When computers are used for analysis, the first step of the process is entering the data into a software package designed for data and/or statistical analyses. Table 21-2 lists examples of common statistical packages used for nursing research.

Before entering data, a codebook should be created that describes the measurement, coding, and scoring information for each variable as described in Chapter 20. Each variable must be labeled in the statistical software so that the variables involved in a particular analysis are clearly designated in the output. Develop a systematic plan for data entry that is designed to reduce errors during the entry phase, and enter data during periods when you have few interruptions. In some studies, the data are already in a database and no data entry is needed. Examples of existing databases are electronic medical records and online surveys for which the responses are collected electronically.

In some cases, data must be reverse-scored before initiating statistical analysis. Items in scales are often arranged so that sometimes a higher numbered response indicates more of the construct being studied. For example, on a scale of 1 to 5, five designates higher levels of coping. Sometimes a higher numbered response indicates less of the construct being studied. In the example of the coping scale, resilience might be measured 1 to 5, with 1 representing higher levels of resilience and 5 representing lower levels of resilience. This arrangement prevents the subject from giving a global response to all items in the scale. To reduce errors, the values on these items need to be entered into the statistical software exactly as they appear on the data collection form. Values on the items are reversed by software commands.

Cleaning the Data

To examine the data carefully for errors, begin by printing a paper copy of the data file. When the size of the data file allows, you need to cross-check every datum on the printout with the original datum for accuracy. Otherwise, randomly check the accuracy of data points. Correct all errors found in the computer file. Perform an analysis of the frequencies of each value of every variable as a second check of the accuracy of the data. Search for values outside the appropriate range of values for that variable. Data that have been scanned into a computer program are less likely to have errors but should still be checked.

Identifying Missing Data

Identify all missing data points. Determine whether the information can be obtained and entered into the data file. If a large number of subjects have missing data on specific variables, you need to make a judgment regarding the availability of sufficient data to perform analysis with those variables. In some cases, subjects must be excluded from the analysis because of missing essential data. Missing data can also be imputed (estimated) via missing data statistical procedures. The rules involving the appropriateness of missing data imputations are complex, and there are many choices of statistical applications. The seminal publication on the subject of missing data imputation was written by Rubin (1976).

Data Transformations

Skewed or non-normally distributed data that do not meet the assumptions of parametric analysis can sometimes be transformed in such a way that the values are distributed closer to the normal curve. Various mathematical operations are used for this purpose. Examples of these operations include squaring each value, calculating the square root of each value, or calculating the logarithm of each value. These operations can allow the researcher to yield a frequency distribution that more closely approximates normality, freeing the researcher to compute parametric statistics.

Data Calculations and Scoring

Sometimes a variable used in the analysis is not collected but calculated from other variables and is referred to as a **calculated variable**. For example, if data are collected on the number of patients on a nursing unit and on the number of nurses on a shift, one might calculate a ratio of nurse to patient for a particular shift. The data are more accurate if this calculation is performed with statistical software rather than manually. The results can be stored in the data file as a variable rather than being recalculated each time the variable is used in an analysis (Shortliffe & Cimino, 2006).

Data Storage and Documentation

When the data-cleaning process is complete, backups need to be made again; labeled as the complete, cleaned data set; and carefully stored. Data cleaning is a time-consuming process that you will not wish to repeat unnecessarily. Be sure to back up the information each time you enter more data. It is wise to keep a second copy of the data filed at a separate, carefully protected site. If your data are being stored on a network, ensure that the network drive is being backed up at least once a day. After data entry, you need to store the original data in secure files for safekeeping. The data files need to be secured as designated by institutional review board policies. This usually includes password-protecting data files or storing data on encrypted flash drives to which only the research team has access.

Rather than keep paper printouts of statistical output, it is recommended that you make portable document format (pdf) files of each output file and store these files in the same folder as your data sets and reports. There are many free pdf converters available on the Internet for download. A pdf converter allows you to convert any file into a pdf file, which can be read by most computer operating systems. Converting output files into pdf files allows the researcher to transport those files and read them on any computer, even a computer that does not house the statistical software that created the original output file.

All files, including data sets and output files, need to be systematically named to allow easy access later when theses or dissertations are being written or research papers are being prepared for publication. We recommend naming files by time sequence. Name the file by its contents, and at the end of the file name, identify the date (month, day, and year) that the file was created or the analysis was performed. For example, the files named *Rehab Outcomes Data 020318* and *Means and Standard Deviations of Pain Subscales 062318* represent a data file saved on February 3, 2018 and a statistical output file containing means and standard deviations of subscale scores saved on June 23, 2018, respectively.

Description of the Sample

After the data have been successfully entered into the software, saved, and stored, researchers start conducting the essential analysis techniques for their studies. The first step is to obtain as complete a picture as possible of the sample. The demographic variables such as age, gender, race, and ethnicity are analyzed with the appropriate analysis techniques and used to develop the characteristics of the sample. The analysis techniques used in describing the sample are covered in Chapter 22.

Testing the Reliability of Measurement Methods

Examine the reliability of the methods of measurement used in the study. The reliability of observational measures or physiological measures may have been obtained during the data collection phase, but it needs to be noted at this point. Additional examination of the reliability of measurement methods, such as a Likert scale, is possible at this point. If you used an instrument that contained self-report items, such as true-false or Likert scale responses, internal consistency coefficients need to be calculated (see Chapter 16; Waltz, Strickland, & Lenz, 2010). The value of the coefficient needs to be compared with values obtained for the instrument in previous studies. If the coefficient is unacceptably low (< 0.6), you need to determine whether you are justified in performing analysis on data from the instrument (see Chapter 16).

Exploratory Analysis of the Data

Examine all the data descriptively, with the intent of becoming as familiar as possible with the nature of the data. You might explore the data by conducting measures of central tendency and dispersion and examining outliers of the data. Neophyte researchers often omit this step and jump immediately into the analyses that were designed to test their hypotheses, questions, or objectives. However, they omit this step at the risk of missing important information in the data and performing analyses that are inappropriate for the data. The researcher needs to examine data on each variable by using measures of central tendency and dispersion. Are the data skewed or normally distributed? What is the nature of the variation in the data? Are there **outliers** with extreme values that appear different from the rest of the sample that cause the distribution to be skewed? The most valuable insights from a study sometimes come from careful examination of outliers (Tukey, 1977).

In many cases, as a part of exploratory analysis, inferential statistical procedures are used to examine differences and associations within the sample. From an exploratory perspective, these analyses are relevant only to the sample under study. There should be no intent to infer to a population. If group comparisons are made, effect sizes need to be determined for the variables involved in the analyses.

In some nursing studies, the purpose of the study is exploratory. In such studies, it is often found that sample sizes are small, power is low, measurement methods have limited reliability and validity, and the field of study is relatively new. If treatments are tested, the procedure might be approached as a pilot study. The most immediate need is tentative exploration of the phenomena under study. Confirming the findings of these studies requires more rigorously designed studies with much larger samples. Many of these exploratory studies are reported in the literature as confirmatory studies, and attempts are made to infer to larger populations. Because of the unacceptably high risk of a Type II error in these studies, negative findings should be viewed with caution.

Using Tables and Graphs for Exploratory Analysis

Although tables and graphs are commonly thought of as a way of presenting the findings of a study, these tools may be even more useful in helping the researcher to become familiar with the data (see Figure 21-1 of the frequency distribution of visual analog scale pain scores). Tables and graphs need to illustrate the descriptive analyses being performed, even though they will probably not be included in a research report. These tables and figures are prepared for the sole purpose of helping researchers to identify patterns in their data and interpret exploratory findings, but they are sometimes useful in reporting study results to selected groups (Tukey, 1977). Visualizing the data in various ways can greatly increase insight regarding the nature of the data (see Chapter 22).

Confirmatory Analysis

As the name implies, **confirmatory analysis** is performed to confirm expectations regarding the data that are expressed as hypotheses, questions, or objectives. The findings are inferred from the sample to the population. Thus, inferential statistical procedures are used. The design of the study, the methods of measurement, and the sample size must be sufficient for this confirmatory process to be justified. A written analysis plan needs to describe clearly the confirmatory analyses that will be performed to examine each hypothesis, question, or objective.

1. Identify the level of measurement of the data available for analysis with regard to the research objective, question, or hypothesis (see Chapter 16).
2. Select a statistical procedure or procedures appropriate for the level of measurement that will respond to the objective, answer the question, or test the hypothesis (Grove & Cipher, 2017; Plichta & Kelvin, 2013).
3. Select the level of significance that you will use to interpret the results, which is usually $\alpha = 0.05$.
4. Choose a one-tailed or two-tailed test if appropriate to your analysis. The extremes of the normal curve are referred to as **tails**. In a **one-tailed test of significance**, the hypothesis is directional, and the extreme statistical values that occur in a single tail of the curve are of interest. In a **two-tailed test of significance**, the hypothesis is nondirectional or null, and the extreme statistical values in both ends of the curve are of interest. Tailedness is discussed in more detail in Chapter 25.
5. Determine the risk of a Type II error in the analysis by performing a power analysis.

6. Determine the sample size available for the analysis. If several groups will be used in the analysis, identify the size of each group (Cohen, 1988; Grove & Cipher, 2017).
7. Evaluate the representativeness of the sample (see Chapter 15).
8. Develop dummy tables and graphics to illustrate the methods that you will use to display your results in relation to your hypotheses, questions, or objectives.
9. Perform the statistical analyses.
10. Most analyses are conducted by statistical software, and the output includes the statistical value obtained by analyzing the data, p value, and degrees of freedom (*df*) for each inferential analysis technique.
11. Reexamine the analysis to ensure that the procedure was performed with the appropriate variables and that the statistical procedure was correctly specified in the software program.
12. Interpret the results of the analysis in terms of the hypothesis, question, or objective.
13. Interpret the results in terms of the framework.

Post Hoc Analysis

Post hoc analyses are commonly performed in studies with more than two groups when the analysis indicates that the groups are significantly different, but does not indicate which groups are different. For example, an analysis of variance is conducted to examine the differences among three groups—experimental group, control group, and placebo group—and the groups are found to be significantly different. A post hoc analysis must be performed to determine which of the three groups are significantly different. Post hoc analysis is discussed in more detail in Chapter 25. In other studies, the insights obtained through the planned analyses generate further questions that can be examined with the available data.

CHOOSING APPROPRIATE STATISTICAL PROCEDURES FOR A STUDY

Multiple factors are involved in determining the suitability of a statistical procedure for a particular study. These factors can be related to the nature of the study, the nature of the researcher, and the nature of statistical theory. Specific factors include (1) the purpose of the study; (2) hypotheses, questions, or objectives; (3) research design; (4) level of measurement; (5) previous experience in statistical analysis; (6) statistical knowledge level; (7) availability of statistical consultation; (8) financial resources; and (9) access to statistical software. Use items 1 to 4 to identify statistical procedures that meet the requirements of the study, and narrow your options further through the process of elimination based on items 5 through 9.

The most important factor to examine when choosing a statistical procedure is the study hypothesis. The hypothesis that is clearly stated indicates the statistics needed to test it. An example of a clearly developed hypothesis is, "There is a difference in employment rates between veterans who receive vocational rehabilitation and veterans who are on a wait-list control." This statement tells the researcher that a statistic to determine differences between two groups is appropriate for addressing this hypothesis.

One approach to selecting an appropriate statistical procedure or judging the appropriateness of an analysis technique is to use a decision tree. A decision tree directs your choices by gradually narrowing your options through the decisions you make. A decision tree that can been helpful in selecting statistical procedures is presented in Figure 21-7.

One disadvantage of decision trees is that if you make an incorrect or uninformed decision (guess), you can be led down a path where you might select an inappropriate statistical procedure for your study. Decision trees are often constrained by space and do not include all of the information needed to make an appropriate selection. Detailed explanations and examples of how to use a statistical decision tree can be found in *Statistics for Nursing Research: A Workbook for Evidence-Based Practice* by Grove and Cipher (2017). The following examples of questions designed to guide the selection or evaluation of statistical procedures were extracted from this book (Andrews et al., 1981):

1. How many variables does the problem involve?
2. How do you want to treat the variables with respect to the scale of measurement?
3. What do you want to know about the distribution of the variable?
4. Do you want to treat outlying cases differently from others?
5. How will you handle missing data?
6. What is the form of the distribution?
7. Is a distinction made between a dependent and an independent variable?
8. Do you want to test whether the means of the two variables are equal?
9. Do you want to treat the relationship between variables as linear?
10. How many of the variables are dichotomous?
11. Do you want to treat the ranks of ordered categories as interval scales?
12. Do the variables have the same distribution?
13. Do you want to treat the ordinal variable as though it were based on an underlying normally distributed interval variable?
14. Is the dependent variable at least at the interval level of measurement?
15. Do you want a measure of the strength of the relationship between the variables or a test of the statistical significance of differences between groups?
16. Are you willing to assume that an interval-scaled variable is normally distributed in the population?
17. Is there more than one dependent variable?
18. Do you want to statistically remove the linear effects of one or more covariates from the dependent variable?
19. Do you want to treat the relationships among the variables as additive?
20. Do you want to analyze patterns existing among variables or among individual cases?
21. Do you want to find clusters of variables that are more strongly related to one another than to the remaining variables? (Andrews et al, 1981; Grove & Cipher, 2017)

Each question confronts you with a decision. The decision you make narrows the field of available statistical procedures (see Figure 21-7). Decisions must be made regarding the following:

1. Research design
2. Number of variables (one, two, or more than two)
3. Level of measurement (nominal, ordinal, or interval)
4. Type of variable (independent, dependent, or research)
5. Distribution of variable (normal or non-normal)
6. Type of relationship (linear or nonlinear)
7. What you want to measure (strength of relationship or difference between groups)
8. Nature of the groups (equal or unequal in size, matched or unmatched, dependent [paired] or independent)
9. Type of analysis (descriptive, classification, methodological, relational, comparison, predicting outcomes, intervention testing, causal modeling, examining changes across time)

Examples

The following are some examples of using the questions listed previously, along with Figure 21-7, to select the appropriate statistic:

1. A researcher has an associational study design and a research question that involves the linear association between two normally distributed variables that are

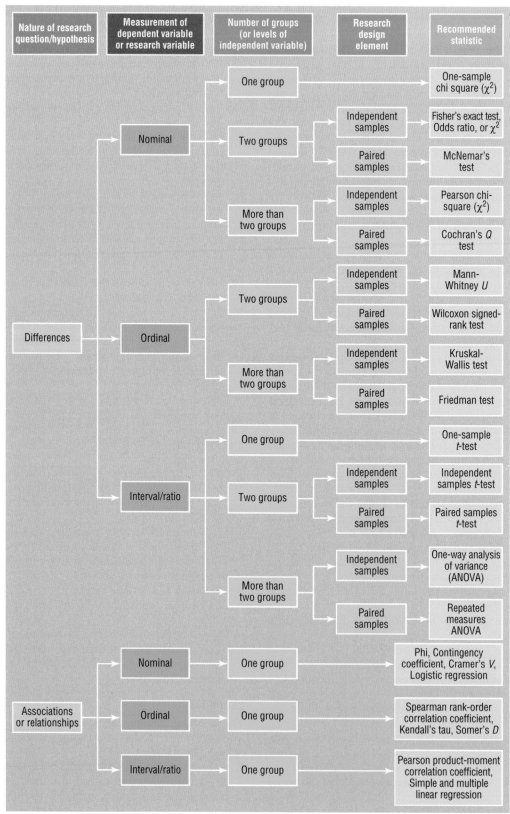

FIGURE 21-7 Statistical decision tree for selecting an appropriate analysis technique.

both measured on an interval scale. The appropriate statistic would be the Pearson r correlation.

2. A researcher has an experimental study design with a comparative research question involving the difference between two groups on a dichotomous dependent variable. The Pearson chi-square test would be the appropriate statistic to test the difference between two groups on a dichotomous variable.

3. A researcher has an experimental study design with a comparative research question involving the difference between three independent groups on a normally distributed dependent variable measured on an interval scale. The appropriate statistic would be a one-way analysis of variance (ANOVA).

4. A researcher has an associational study design and a predictive research question that involves the linear association between a set of predictors and one normally distributed dependent variable that is measured on an interval scale. Multiple linear regression is the appropriate statistical procedure that tests the extent to which a set of variables predicts a normally distributed dependent variable.

In summary, selecting and evaluating statistical procedures requires that you make many judgments regarding the nature of the data and what you want to know. Knowledge of the statistical procedures and their assumptions is necessary for selecting appropriate procedures. You must weigh the advantages and disadvantages of various statistical options. Access to a statistician can be invaluable in selecting the appropriate procedures.

KEY POINTS

- This chapter introduces you to the concepts of statistical theory and discusses some of the more pragmatic aspects of quantitative statistical analysis, including the purposes of statistical analysis, the process of performing statistical analysis, the choice of the appropriate statistical procedures for a study, and resources for statistical analysis.
- Two types of errors can occur when making decisions about the meaning of a value obtained from a statistical test: Type I errors and Type II errors.
- A Type I error occurs when the researcher concludes a significant effect when no significant effect actually exists.
- A Type II error occurs when the researcher concludes no significant effect when an effect actually exists.
- The formal definition of the level of significance, or alpha (α), is the probability of making a Type I error when the null hypothesis is true.

- The p value is the exact value that can be calculated during a statistical computation to indicate the probability of obtaining a statistical value as extreme or greater when the null hypothesis is true.
- Power is the probability that a statistical test will detect a significant effect when it actually exists.
- Statistics can be used for various purposes, such as to (1) summarize, (2) explore the meaning of deviations in the data, (3) compare or contrast descriptively, (4) test the proposed relationships in a theoretical model, (5) infer that the findings from the sample are indicative of the entire population, (6) examine causality, (7) predict, or (8) infer from the sample to a theoretical model.
- The quantitative statistical analysis process consists of several stages: (1) preparation of the data for analysis; (2) description of the sample; (3) testing the reliability of measurement; (4) exploratory analysis of the data; (5) confirmatory analysis guided by hypotheses, questions, or objectives; and (6) post hoc analysis.
- A decision tree is provided to assist you in selecting appropriate analysis techniques to use in analyzing study or clinical data.

REFERENCES

Andrews, F. M., Klem, L., Davidson, T. N., O'Malley, P. M., & Rodgers, W. L. (1981). *A guide for selecting statistical techniques for analyzing social science data* (2nd ed.). Ann Arbor, MI: Survey Research Center, Institute for Social Research, University of Michigan.

Barnett, V. (1982). *Comparative statistical inference.* New York, NY: Wiley.

Box, G. E. P., Hunter, W. G., & Hunter, J. S. (1978). *Statistics for experimenters.* New York, NY: Wiley.

Cohen, J. (1988). *Statistical power analysis for the behavioral sciences* (2nd ed.). New York, NY: Academic Press.

Cohen, J. (1994). The earth is round ($p < .05$). *American Psychologist, 49*(12), 997–1003.

Conover, W. J. (1971). *Practical nonparametric statistics.* New York, NY: Wiley.

Cox, D. R. (1958). *Planning of experiments.* New York, NY: Wiley.

de Winter, J. C. F., & Dodou, D. (2010). Five-point Likert items: t test versus Mann-Whitney-Wilcoxon. *Practical Assessment, Research, and Evaluation, 15*(11), 1–16.

Faul, F., Erdfelder, E., Buchner, A., & Lang, A. (2009). Statistical power analyses using G*Power 3.1: Tests for correlation and regression analyses. *Behavior Research Methods, 41*(4), 1149–1160.

Faul, F., Erdfelder, E., Lang, A.-G., & Buchner, A. (2007). G*Power 3: A flexible statistical power analysis program for the social, behavioral, and biomedical sciences. *Behavior Research Methods, 39*(2), 175–191.

Fisher, R. A. (1935). *The design of experiments*. New York, NY: Hafner.

Fisher, R. A. (1971). *The design of experiments* (9th ed.). New York, NY: MacMillan.

Gaskin, C. J., & Happell, B. (2014). Power, effects, confidence, and significance: An investigation of statistical practices in nursing research. *International Journal of Nursing Studies, 51*(5), 795–806.

Gauss, C. F. (1809). *Theoria motus corporum coelestium in sectionibus conicis solem ambientium*. Hamburg: Friedrich Perthes and I.H. Besser.

Glass, G. V., & Stanley, J. C. (1970). *Statistical methods in education and psychology*. Englewood Cliffs, NJ: Prentice-Hall.

Good, I. J. (1983). *Good thinking: The foundations of probability and its applications*. Minneapolis, MN: University of Minnesota Press.

Grove, S. K., & Cipher, D. J. (2017). *Statistics for nursing research: A workbook for evidence-based practice* (2nd ed.). St. Louis, MO: Saunders.

Hayat, M. J., Higgins, M., Schwartz, T. A., & Staggs, V. S. (2015). Statistical challenges in nursing education and research: An expert panel consensus. *Nurse Educator, 40*(1), 21–25.

Kerlinger, F. N., & Lee, H. B. (2000). *Foundations of behavioral research* (4th ed.). New York, NY: Harcourt Brace.

Loftus, G. R. (1993). A picture is worth a thousand *p* values: On the irrelevance of hypothesis testing in the microcomputer age. *Behavior Research Methods, Instrumentation, & Computers, 25*(2), 250–256.

Plichta, S. B., & Kelvin, E. A. (2013). *Munro's statistical methods for health care research*. Philadelphia, PA: Wolters Kluwer/Lippincott Williams & Wilkins.

Rubin, D. B. (1976). Inference and missing data. *Biometrika, 63*(3), 581–592.

Shortliffe, E. H., & Cimino, J. J. (2006). *Biomedical informatics: Computer applications in health care and biomedicine*. New York, NY: Springer Science.

Tanizaki, H. (1997). Power comparison of non-parametric tests: Small-sample properties from Monte Carlo experiments. *Journal of Applied Statistics, 24*(5), 603–632.

Tukey, J. W. (1977). *Exploratory data analysis*. Reading, MA: Addison-Wesley.

Waltz, C. F., Strickland, O. L., & Lenz, E. R. (2010). *Measurement in nursing and health research* (4th ed.). New York, NY: Springer.

Zar, J. H. (2010). *Biostatistical analysis* (5th ed.). Upper Saddle River, NJ: Pearson Prentice-Hall.

22

Using Statistics to Describe Variables

Daisha J. Cipher

There are two major classes of statistics: descriptive statistics and inferential statistics. Descriptive statistics are computed to reveal characteristics of the sample data set. Inferential statistics are computed to gain information about effects in the population being studied. For some types of studies, descriptive statistics are the only approach to analysis of the data. For other studies, descriptive statistics are the first step in the statistical analysis process, to be followed by inferential statistics. For all studies that involve numerical data, descriptive statistics are crucial to understanding the fundamental properties of the variables being studied. This chapter focuses on descriptive statistics and includes the most common descriptive statistics conducted in nursing research with examples from clinical studies.

USING STATISTICS TO SUMMARIZE DATA

Frequency Distributions

A basic yet important way to begin describing a sample is to create a **frequency distribution** of the variable or variables being studied. A frequency distribution can be displayed in a table or figure. A line graph figure can be used to plot one variable, whereby the x-axis consists of the possible values of that variable, and the y-axis is the tally of each value. The frequency distributions presented in this chapter include values of continuous variables. With a **continuous variable**, the higher numbers represent more of that variable, and the lower numbers represent less of that variable. Continuous variables may be ordinal, interval, or ratio scales of measurement. Common examples of continuous variables are age, income, blood pressure, weight, height, pain levels, and perception of quality of life.

The frequency distribution of a variable can be presented in a **frequency table**, which is a way of organizing the data by listing every possible value in the first column of numbers and the frequency (tally) of each value in the second column of numbers. For example, consider the following hypothetical age data for patients from a primary care clinic. The ages of 20 patients were:

45, 26, 59, 51, 42, 28, 26, 32, 31, 55,
43, 47, 67, 39, 52, 48, 36, 42, 61, 57

First, we must sort the patients' ages from lowest to highest values:

26
26
28
31
32
36
39
42
42
43
45
47
48
51
52
55
57
59
61
67

Next, each age value is tallied to create the frequency. This is an example of an ungrouped frequency distribution. In an **ungrouped frequency distribution**, researchers list all categories of the variable for which they have data and tally each observation (Grove & Cipher, 2017). In this example, all the different ages of the 20 patients are listed and then tallied for each age.

Age	Frequency
26	2
28	1
31	1
32	1
36	1
39	1
42	2
43	1
45	1
47	1
48	1
51	1
52	1
55	1
57	1
59	1
61	1
67	1

Because most of the ages in this data set have frequencies of "1," it is better to group the ages into ranges of values. These ranges must be mutually exclusive. A patient's age can be classified into only one of the ranges. In addition, the ranges must be exhaustive, meaning that each patient's age fits into at least one of the categories. For example, one may choose to have ranges of 10, so that the age ranges are 20 to 29, 30 to 39, 40 to 49, 50 to 59, and 60 to 69. A researcher may choose to have ranges of 5, so that the age ranges are 20 to 24, 25 to 29, 30 to 34, and so on. The grouping should be devised to provide the greatest possible meaning to the purpose of the study. If the data are to be compared with data in other studies, groupings should be similar to groupings of other studies in this field of research. Classifying data into groups results in the development of a **grouped frequency distribution** (Grove & Cipher, 2017). Table 22-1 presents a grouped frequency distribution of patient ages classified by ranges of 10 years. The range starts at "20" because there are no patient ages lower than 20; also, there are no ages higher than 69.

Table 22-1 also includes percentages of patients with an age in each range and the cumulative percentages for the sample, which should add to 100%. This table pro-

TABLE 22-1   Grouped Frequency Distribution of Patient Ages With Percentages

Adult Age Range	Frequency (*f*)	Percentage	Cumulative Percentage
20-29	3	15%	15%
30-39	4	20%	35%
40-49	6	30%	65%
50-59	5	25%	90%
60-69	2	10%	100%
Total	**20**	**100%**	

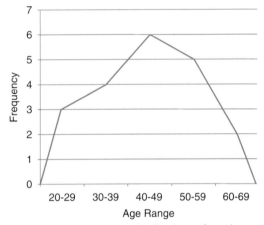

FIGURE 22-1 Frequency distribution of patient age ranges.

vides an example of a **percentage distribution** that indicates the percentage of the sample with scores falling in a specific group or range (Grove & Cipher, 2017). Percentage distributions are particularly useful in comparing the data of the present study with results from other studies.

As discussed earlier, frequency distributions can be presented in figures. Frequencies are commonly presented in graphs, charts, histograms, and frequency polygons. Figure 22-1 is the frequency distribution for age ranges, where the x-axis (horizontal line) represents the different age ranges, and the y-axis (vertical line) represents the frequencies of patients with ages in each of the ranges.

A frequency table is also an important method to represent nominal data (Grove & Cipher, 2017; Tukey, 1977). For example, a common nominal variable is

TABLE 22-2 Frequency Table of Smoking Status		
Smoking Status	Frequency	Percentage (%)
Current smoker	142	34.0%
Former smoker	174	41.6%
Never smoked	102	24.4%
Total	**418**	**100%**

TABLE 22-3 Body Mass Index (BMI) Values in 10 Veterans With Inflammatory Bowel Disease	
BMI	BMI
20.0	31.0
24.4	31.7
28.1	34.2
28.1	36.8
28.7	36.9

FIGURE 22-2 Histogram of smoking status.

smoking history. Many researchers assess subjects' history of smoking using nominal categories such as "never smoked," "former smoker," and "current smoker." Table 22-2 presents frequency and percentage distributions for data extracted from a sample of veterans with rheumatoid arthritis (Tran, Hooker, Cipher, & Reimold, 2009).

As shown in Table 22-2, the frequencies indicate that of 418 veterans, 142 (34.0%) were current smokers, 174 (41.6%) were former smokers, and 102 (24.4%) never smoked. For nominal variables such as smoking status, tables are a helpful method to inform researchers and others about the variable being studied. Graphically representing the values in a frequency table can yield visually important trends. Figure 22-2 is a histogram that was developed to represent the smoking status data visually.

Measures of Central Tendency

A **measure of central tendency** is a statistic that represents the center or middle of a frequency distribution (Zar, 2010). The three measures of central tendency commonly reported in nursing studies include mode,

median (MD), and mean ($\bar{X}$). The mode, median, and mean are defined and calculated in this section using a simulated subset of data collected from veterans with inflammatory bowel disease (Flores, Burstein, Cipher, & Feagins, 2015). Table 22-3 contains the body mass index (BMI) data collected from a subset of 10 veterans with inflammatory bowel disease. The BMI, a measure of body fat based on height and weight that applies to adult men and women, is considered an indicator of obesity when 30 or greater (National Heart, Lung, and Blood Institute, 2013). Because the number of study subjects represented is 10, the correct statistical notation to reflect that number is:

$$n = 10$$

The letter "n" is lowercase because it refers to a sample of veterans and italicized because it represents a statistic. If the data being presented represented the entire population of veterans, the correct notation would be uppercase "N" (Zar, 2010). Because most nursing research is conducted using samples, not populations, all formulas in Chapters 22 to 25 incorporate the sample notation, n.

Mode

The **mode** is the numerical value or score that occurs with the greatest frequency in a data set. It does not indicate the center of the data set. The data in Table 22-3 contain one mode: 28.1. The BMI value of 28.1 occurred twice in the data set. When two modes exist, the data set is referred to as **bimodal** (see Chapter 21). A data set that contains more than two modes is referred to as **multimodal** (Zar, 2010).

Median

The **median** (MD) is the score at the exact center of the ungrouped frequency distribution. It is the 50th percentile. To obtain the MD, sort the values from lowest to highest. If the number of values is an uneven number, the *MD* is the exact middle number in the data set. If the number of values is an even number, the *MD* is the average of the two middle values; thus, the *MD* may not be an actual value in the data set (Zar, 2010). For example, the data in Table 22-3 consist of 10 observations, and the *MD* is calculated as the average of the two middle values.

$$MD = \frac{(28.7 + 31)}{2} = 29.85$$

Mean

The **mean** is the arithmetic average of all the values of a variable in a study and is the most commonly reported measure of central tendency. The mean is the sum of the scores divided by the number of scores being summed. Similar to the *MD,* the mean may not be a member of the data set. The formula for calculating the mean is as follows:

$$\bar{X} = \frac{\Sigma X}{n}$$

where
$\bar{X}$ = mean
Σ = sigma, the statistical symbol for summation
X = a single value in the sample
n = total number of values in the sample
The mean BMI for the veterans with inflammatory bowel disease is calculated as follows:

$$\bar{X} = \frac{(20.1 + 24.4 + 28.1 + 28.1 + 28.7 + 31.0 + 31.7 + 34.2 + 36.8 + 36.9)}{10}$$

$$\bar{X} = \frac{300}{10} = 30.0$$

The mean is an appropriate measure of central tendency to calculate for approximately normally distributed populations with variables measured at the interval or ratio levels. It is also appropriate for ordinal-level data such as Likert scale or rating scale values (as described in Chapter 17), where higher numbers represent more of the construct being measured and lower numbers represent less of the construct, such as a 5-point rating scale, on which 1 represents excellent perceived health and 5 represents poor perceived health (Hooker, Cipher, & Sekscenski, 2005).

The mean is sensitive to extreme scores such as outliers. An **outlier** is a value in a sample data set that is unusually low or unusually high in the context of the rest of the sample data (Zar, 2010). An example of an outlier in the data presented in Table 22-3 might be a value such as a BMI of 55. The existing values range from 20.1 to 36.9, indicating that no veteran had a BMI value greater than 36.9. If an additional veteran was added to the sample, and that person had a BMI of 55, the mean would be larger: 32.27 (mean = 355 ÷ 11 = 32.27). The outlier would also change the frequency distribution. Without the outlier, the frequency distribution is approximately normal, as shown in Figure 22-3. The inclusion of the outlier changes the shape

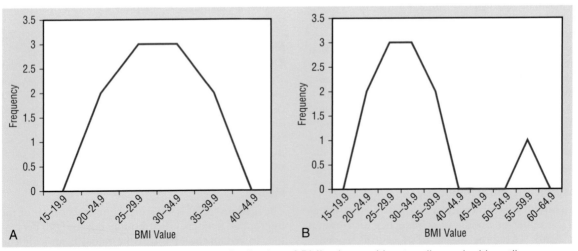

FIGURE 22-3 **A** and **B,** Frequency distribution of BMI values, without outlier and with outlier.

from an approximately normal distribution to a positively skewed distribution (see Figure 22-3) (Zar, 2010). The median is a better measure of central tendency than the mean for data that are positively skewed by an outlier (see Chapter 21 for discussion of skewness).

USING STATISTICS TO EXPLORE DEVIATIONS IN THE DATA

Although the use of summary statistics has been the traditional approach to describing data or describing the characteristics of the sample before inferential statistical analysis, the ability of summary statistics to clarify the nature of data is limited. For example, using measures of central tendency, particularly the mean, to describe the nature of the data obscures the impact of extreme values or deviations in the data. Significant features in the data may be concealed or misrepresented. Measures of dispersion, such as the range, difference scores, variance, and standard deviation, provide important insight into the nature of the data.

Measures of Dispersion

Measures of dispersion or variability are measures of individual differences of the members of the population and sample (Zar, 2010). They indicate how values in a sample are dispersed around the mean. These measures provide information about the data that is not available from measures of central tendency. They indicate how different the scores are—the extent to which individual values deviate from one another. If the individual values are similar, measures of variability are small, and the sample is relatively **homogeneous** in terms of those values. When there are wide variations or differences in the scores, the sample is considered **heterogeneous**. The **heterogeneity** of sample scores or values is determined by measures of dispersion or variability (Grove & Cipher, 2017). The measures of dispersion most commonly reported in nursing research are range, difference scores, variance, and standard deviation.

Range

The simplest measure of dispersion is the **range**. In published studies, range is presented in two ways: (1) the range is the lowest and highest scores, or (2) the range is calculated by subtracting the lowest score from the highest score. The range for the scores in Table 22-3 is 20.1 to 36.9 or can be calculated as follows: 36.9 − 20.1 = 16.8. In this form, the range is a difference score that uses only the two extreme scores for the comparison. The range is generally reported in published studies but is not used in further analyses.

Difference Scores

Difference scores are obtained by subtracting the mean from each score. Sometimes a difference score is referred to as a **deviation score** because it indicates the extent to which a score deviates from the mean. Most variables in nursing research are not "scores"; however, the term *difference score* is used to represent the deviation of a value from the mean. The difference score is positive when the score is above the mean, and it is negative when the score is below the mean. The difference scores (both positive and negative) add to zero or approximately zero based on rounding. Difference scores are the basis for many statistical analyses and can be found within many statistical equations. The formula for difference scores is:

$$X - \bar{X}$$

The **mean deviation** is the average difference score, using the absolute values. The formula for the mean deviation is:

$$\bar{X}_{deviation} = \frac{\sum |X - \bar{X}|}{n}$$

$$\bar{X}_{deviation} = \frac{9.9 + 5.6 + 1.9 + 1.9 + 1.3 + 1 + 1.7 + 4.2 + 6.8 + 6.9}{10}$$

$$\bar{X}_{deviation} = \frac{41.2}{10}$$

$$\bar{X}_{deviation} = 4.12$$

In this example using the data from Table 22-4, the mean deviation is 4.12. The result indicates that, on average, veterans' BMI values deviated from the mean by 4.12.

TABLE 22-4 Difference Scores of Body Mass Index			
X	**−$\bar{X}$**	**X − $\bar{X}$**	**|X − $\bar{X}$|**
20.1	−30	−9.9	9.9
24.4	−30	−5.6	5.6
28.1	−30	−1.9	1.9
28.1	−30	−1.9	1.9
28.7	−30	−1.3	1.3
31.0	−30	1.0	1.0
31.7	−30	1.7	1.7
34.2	−30	4.2	4.2
36.8	−30	6.8	6.8
36.9	−30	6.9	6.9
		Σ of absolute values = 41.2	

Variance

Variance is another measure of dispersion commonly used in statistical analysis. The equation for a sample variance (s^2) is provided. The lowercase letter "s^2" is used to represent a sample variance. The lowercase Greek sigma "σ^2" is used to represent a population variance, in which the denominator is "N" instead of "$n-1$." Because most nursing research is conducted using samples, not populations, all formulas in the next several chapters that contain a variance or standard deviation incorporate the sample notation and use "$n-1$" as the denominator. Statistical software packages compute the variance and standard deviation using the sample formulas, not the population formulas.

$$s^2 = \frac{\sum (X - \bar{X})^2}{n-1}$$

The variance is always a positive value and has no upper limit. In general, the larger the calculated variance for a study variable is, the larger the dispersion or spread of scores is for the variable. Table 22-4 displays how you might compute a variance by hand, using the BMI data. Table 22-5 shows calculation of variance for BMI.

$$s^2 = \frac{253.66}{9}$$

$$s^2 = 28.18$$

Standard Deviation

Standard deviation (s) is a measure of dispersion that is the square root of the variance. The equation for obtaining a standard deviation is:

$$s = \sqrt{\frac{\sum (X - \bar{X})^2}{n-1}}$$

Table 22-5 displays the computations for the variance. To compute the standard deviation, simply take the square root of the variance. You know that the variance of BMI values is $s^2 = 28.18$. Therefore, the standard deviation of BMI values is $s = 5.31$. In published studies, sometimes the statistic reported by researchers for standard deviation is *SD*. Either *SD* or *s* might be used in a research report to indicate the standard deviation for a study variable.

The standard deviation is an important statistic, both for understanding dispersion within a distribution and for interpreting the relationship of a particular value to the distribution. The statistical workbook by Grove and Cipher (2017) provides you with a resource for calculating and interpreting the measures of central tendency and measures of dispersion in published studies, as well as computing those measures with statistical software. The following section summarizes the properties of the standard deviation as it relates to a normal distribution.

Normal Curve

The standard deviation of a variable tells researchers much about the entire sample of values. A frequency distribution of a variable that is *perfectly normally distributed* is shown in Figure 22-4, otherwise known as the **normal curve**.

The normal curve is a perfectly symmetrical frequency distribution. The value at the exact center of a normal curve is the mean of the values. Note the vertical lines to the left and to the right of the mean. Those lines are drawn at +1 standard deviation (which indicates 1 *s* above the mean) and −1 standard deviation (which indicates 1 *s* below the mean), +2 standard deviations above the mean, −2 standard deviations below the mean, and so forth. When a frequency distribution is shaped like the normal curve, we know that 34.13% of the subjects scored between the mean and 1 standard deviation above the mean, and 34.13% of the subjects scored between the mean and 1 standard deviation below the mean. Because the normal curve is perfectly symmetrical, we also know that 50% of the subjects scored above the mean, and 50% of the subjects scored below the mean.

We can also say that 68.26% of the subjects scored between −1 and +1 standard deviation. This number is obtained by adding 34.13% and 34.13%. Furthermore, we can say that 95.44% of the subjects scored between −2

TABLE 22-5 **Calculation of Variance for Body Mass Index**			
X	$-\bar{X}$	$X - \bar{X}$	$(X - \bar{X})^2$
20.1	−30	−9.9	98.01
24.4	−30	−5.6	31.36
28.1	−30	−1.9	3.61
28.1	−30	−1.9	3.61
28.7	−30	−1.3	1.69
31.0	−30	1.0	1
31.7	−30	1.7	2.89
34.2	−30	4.2	17.64
36.8	−30	6.8	46.24
36.9	−30	6.9	47.61
		Σ	253.66

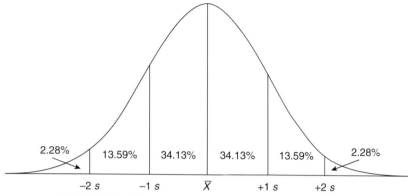

FIGURE 22-4 Normal curve. s = Standard deviation (SD)

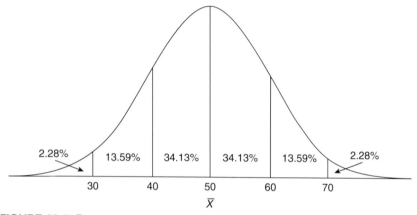

FIGURE 22-5 Frequency distribution of SF-36 Physical Functioning Scale values.

and +2 standard deviations. If we are given a mean and a standard deviation value for any variable that is normally distributed, we know certain facts about those data. For example, consider a score obtained on a subscale of the Short Form (36) Health survey (SF-36). The SF-36 is a widely used health survey that yields eight subscales that each represent a domain of subjective health status (Ware & Sherbourne, 1992). The subscales have been normed on populations of respondents as having a mean of 50 and standard deviation of 10. The frequency distribution of responses for the subscale "Physical Functioning" can be drawn as seen in Figure 22-5.

The mean is marked as "50" in the middle, and the standard deviations are marked at the lines. Therefore, you know that 34.13% of the population scores fall between a 50 and a 60 on the Physical Functioning subscale. You also know that 95.44% of the population scores fall between 30 and 70 on the Physical Functioning subscale. Figure 22-5 shows that only 2.28% of the

population scores fall above the value of 70 (this is computed by subtracting 34.13% and 13.59% from 50%). Likewise, only 2.28% of the population scores fall below the value of 30.

When using examples such as these, researchers often use the statistic "z" instead of the term "standard deviation." A z value is synonymous with a standard deviation unit. A z value of 1.0 represents 1 standard deviation unit above the mean. A z value of −1.0 represents 1 standard deviation unit below the mean (Appendix A: z Values Table). Although a standard deviation value cannot have a negative value, a z value can be negative or positive. A z of 0 represents exactly the mean value. Any value in a data set can be converted to a z by using the following formula:

$$z = \frac{(X - \bar{X})}{s}$$

For example, a person scoring a 61 on the SF-36 Physical Functioning scale would have a z value of 1.1:

$$z = \frac{(61-50)}{10}$$

$$z = 1.1$$

It is important to note how z values represent standard deviations on the normal curve because this knowledge becomes necessary when performing significance testing in inferential statistics. For example, observe how a z value of 1.0 or −1.0 is much more common than a z value of 3.0 or −3.0. The farther the z value is from the mean, the more uncommon, unusual, and unlikely that value is to occur. This principle is revisited in Chapters 23 through 25.

The distribution of the normal curve is drawn once more in Figure 22-6 but this time with the z statistic, where z represents 1 standard deviation unit. Common values of z are smaller values and closer to the mean. Uncommon and unusual z values are farther away from the mean (either lower than the mean or higher than the mean). When a variable is normally distributed, 95% of z values for that variable fall somewhere between a z of −1.96 and 1.96; 99% of z values for that variable fall somewhere between a z of −2.58 and 2.58 (see Figure 22-6). A table of z values can be found in Appendix A.

Sampling Error

A standard error describes the extent of **sampling error**. A **standard error of the mean** is calculated to determine the magnitude of the variability associated with the mean. A small standard error is an indication that the sample mean is close to the population mean. A large standard error yields less certainty that the sample mean approximates the population mean. The formula for the standard error of the mean ($s_{\bar{x}}$) is:

$$s_{\bar{x}} = \frac{s}{\sqrt{n}}$$

where
$s_{\bar{x}}$ = standard error of the mean
s = standard deviation
n = sample size

Using the BMI data for the veterans with inflammatory bowel disease, we know that the standard deviation of BMI values is $s = 5.31$. Therefore, the standard error of the mean for BMI values is computed as follows:

$$s_{\bar{x}} = \frac{5.31}{\sqrt{10}}$$

$$s_{\bar{x}} = 1.68$$

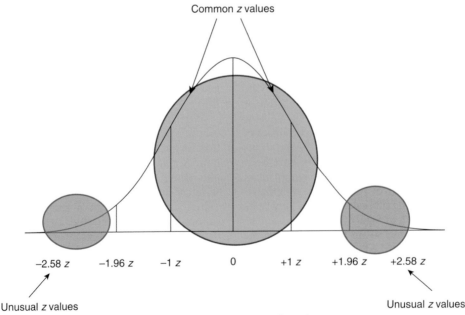

FIGURE 22-6 Distribution of z values.

The standard error of the mean for BMI data in this sample of veterans is 1.68.

A **standard error of the proportion** is calculated to determine the magnitude of the variability associated with a proportion, also expressed as a percentage. A small standard error of proportion is an indication that the sample proportion is close to the population proportion. The formula for the standard error of the proportion (s_p) is:

$$s_p = \sqrt{\frac{p(1-p)}{n}}$$

where
s_p = standard error of the proportion
p = proportion observed
n = sample size

Using the smoking example from Table 22-2, we know that the percentage of veterans with rheumatoid arthritis who never smoked is 24.4% (Tran et al., 2009). Therefore, "p" would be 0.244. Therefore, the standard error of the proportion for veterans who never smoked is computed as follows:

$$s_p = \sqrt{\frac{0.244(1-0.244)}{418}}$$

$$s_p = \sqrt{\frac{0.184}{418}}$$

$$s_p = 0.021$$

The standard error of the proportion for veterans with rheumatoid arthritis who never smoked is 0.021, or 2.1%.

Confidence Intervals

To determine how closely the sample mean approximates the population mean, or the sample proportion approximates the population proportion, the standard error is used to build a **confidence interval**. A confidence interval can be created for many statistics, such as a mean, proportion, odds ratio, and correlation. To build a confidence interval around a statistic, you must have the standard error value and the t value to adjust the standard error. The t is a statistic for the t-test that is calculated to determine group differences and is discussed in more detail in Chapter 25. The degrees of freedom (df) calculation for a confidence interval is as follows:

$$df = n - 1$$

To compute the confidence interval for a mean, the lower and upper limits of that interval are created by multiplying the standard error by the t statistic, where $df = n - 1$. For a 95% confidence interval, the t value should be selected at alpha $(\alpha) = 0.05$. For a 99% confidence interval, the t value should be selected at $\alpha = 0.01$.

Using the BMI data, we know that the standard error of the mean for BMI values is $s_{\bar{x}} = 1.68$. The mean BMI is 30.0. The 95% confidence interval for the mean BMI is computed as follows:

$$\bar{X} \pm s_{\bar{x}}t$$
$$30.0 \pm (1.68)(2.26)$$
$$30.0 \pm 3.80$$

As referenced in Appendix B, the t value required for the 95% confidence interval with $df = 9$ for a two-tailed test is 2.26. The previous computation results in a lower limit of 26.2 and an upper limit of 33.8.

This means that our confidence interval of 26.2–33.8 estimates the population mean BMI among veterans with inflammatory bowel disease with 95% confidence (Kline, 2004). Technically and mathematically, it means that if we computed the mean BMI on an infinite number of groups of veterans, and a confidence interval for each of those means, exactly 95% of the confidence intervals would contain the true population mean, and 5% would not contain the population mean (Gliner, Morgan, & Leech, 2009).

If we were to compute a 99% confidence interval, we would require the t value that is referenced at $\alpha = 0.01$ for a two-tailed test. The 99% confidence interval for BMI is computed as follows:

$$30.0 \pm (1.68)(3.25)$$
$$30.0 \pm 5.46$$

As referenced in Appendix B, the t value required for the 99% confidence interval with $df = 9$ for a two-tailed test is 3.25. The previous computation results in a lower limit of 24.54 and an upper limit of 35.46. Thus, our confidence interval of 24.54–35.46 estimates the population mean BMI among veterans with inflammatory bowel disease with 99% confidence.

Using the smoking data, we know that the percentage of veterans who never smoked is 24.4%, and the standard error of the proportion is $(s_p) = 2.1\%$. The 95% confidence interval for the percentage of veterans who never smoked is computed as follows:

$$p \pm s_p t$$
$$24.4\% \pm (2.1\%)(1.96)$$
$$24.4\% \pm 4.12\%$$

As referenced in Appendix B, the t value required for the 95% confidence interval with $df = 417$ for a two-tailed test is 1.96. As can be observed from the table, any df larger than $df = 300$ would require a t of 1.96 for a 95% confidence interval. The previous computation results in a lower limit of 20.28% and an upper limit of 28.52%. This means that our confidence interval of 20.28%–28.52% estimates the population percentage of veterans with rheumatoid arthritis who never smoked with 95% confidence.

Degrees of Freedom

The concept of degrees of freedom was used in reference to computing a confidence interval. For any statistical computation, **degrees of freedom (*df*)** is the number of independent pieces of information that are free to vary to estimate another piece of information (Zar, 2010). In the case of the confidence interval, the df is $n - 1$. This means that there are $n - 1$ independent observations in the sample that are free to vary (to be any value) to estimate the lower and upper limits of the confidence interval.

▮ KEY POINTS

- Data analysis begins with descriptive statistics in any study in which the data are numerical, including demographic variables for samples in quantitative and qualitative studies.
- Descriptive statistics allow the researcher to organize the data in ways that facilitate meaning and insight.
- Three measures of central tendency are the mode, median, and mean.
- The measures of dispersion most commonly reported in nursing studies are range, difference scores, variance, and standard deviation.
- The standard deviation and z represent certain properties of the normal curve that are used in significance testing.
- Standard error indicates the extent of sampling error.
- To determine how closely the sample mean approximates the population mean, the standard error of the mean is used to build a confidence interval.
- For any statistical computation, degrees of freedom are the number of independent pieces of information that are free to vary to estimate another piece of information.

REFERENCES

Flores, A., Burstein, E., Cipher, D. J., & Feagins, L. A. (2015). Obesity in inflammatory bowel disease: A marker of less severe disease. *Digestive Diseases and Sciences, 60*(8), 2436–2445.

Gliner, J. A., Morgan, G. A., & Leech, N. L. (2009). *Research methods in applied settings* (2nd ed.). New York, NY: Routledge.

Grove, S. K., & Cipher, D. J. (2017). *Statistics for nursing research: A workbook for evidence-based practice* (2nd ed.). St. Louis, MO: Elsevier.

Hooker, R. S., Cipher, D. J., & Sekscenski, E. (2005). Patient satisfaction with physician assistant, nurse practitioner, and physician care: A national survey of Medicare recipients. *Journal of Clinical Outcomes Management, 12*(2), 88–92.

Kline, R. B. (2004). *Beyond significance testing.* Washington, DC: American Psychological Association.

National Heart, Lung, and Blood Institute. (2013). *Managing overweight and obesity in adults: Systematic evidence review from the obesity expert panel.* Retrieved from http://www.nhlbi.nih .gov/sites/www.nhlbi.nih.gov/files/obesity-evidence-review.pdf.

Tran, S., Hooker, R. S., Cipher, D. J., & Reimold, A. (2009). Patterns of biologic use in inflammatory diseases: An institution-focused, observational post-marketing study. *Drugs and Aging, 26*(7), 607–615.

Tukey, J. W. (1977). *Exploratory data analysis.* Reading, MA: Addison-Wesley.

Ware, J. E., & Sherbourne, C. D. (1992). The MOS 36-Item Short-Form Health Survey (SF-36[r]): Conceptual framework and item selection. *Medical Care, 30*(6), 473–483.

Zar, J. H. (2010). *Biostatistical analysis* (5th ed.). Upper Saddle River, NJ: Prentice-Hall.

23

Using Statistics to Examine Relationships

Daisha J. Cipher

ⓔ http://evolve.elsevier.com/Gray/practice/

Correlational analyses identify relationships or associations among variables. There are many different kinds of statistics that yield a measure of correlation. All of these statistics address a research question or hypothesis that involves an association or a relationship. Examples of research questions that are answered with correlation statistics are as follows: "Is there an association between weight loss and depression?" "Is there a relationship between patient satisfaction and health status?" A hypothesis is developed to identify the nature (positive or negative) of the relationship between the variables being studied. For example, a researcher may hypothesize that higher levels of depression are associated with lower levels of glycemic control among persons with diabetes (Mancuso, 2010).

This chapter presents the common analysis techniques used to examine relationships in studies. The analysis techniques discussed include the use of scatter diagrams before correlational analysis, bivariate correlational analysis, testing the significance of a correlational coefficient, spurious correlations, correlations between two raters or measurements, the role of correlation in understanding causality, and the multivariate correlational procedure of factor analysis.

SCATTER DIAGRAMS

Scatter plots or **scatter diagrams** provide useful preliminary information about the nature of the relationship between variables (Plichta & Kelvin, 2013). The researcher should develop and examine scatter diagrams before performing a correlational analysis. Scatter plots may be useful for selecting appropriate correlational procedures, but most correlational procedures are useful for examining linear relationships only. A scatter plot can be used to identify nonlinear relationships; if the data are nonlinear, the researcher should select statistical alternatives such as nonlinear regression analysis (Zar, 2010). A scatter plot is created by plotting the values of two variables on an *x*-axis and *y*-axis. As shown in Figure 23-1, the ages at which veterans received a diagnosis of ulcerative colitis were plotted against their body mass indices (BMIs) (Flores, Burstein, Cipher, & Feagins, 2015). Specifically, each veteran's pair of values (age at diagnosis, BMI) was plotted on the diagram. The resulting scatter plot reveals a linear trend whereby older diagnostic ages tend to correspond with higher BMI values. The line drawn in Figure 23-1 is a regression line that represents the concept of **least-squares**. A **least-squares regression line** is a line drawn through a scatter plot that represents the smallest distance between each value and the regression line (Cohen & Cohen, 1983). Regression analysis is discussed in detail in Chapter 24.

BIVARIATE CORRELATIONAL ANALYSIS

Bivariate correlational analysis measures the magnitude of a **linear relationship** between two variables and is performed on data collected from a single sample (Zar, 2010). The particular correlation statistic that is computed depends on the scale of measurement of each variable. Correlational techniques are available for all levels of data: nominal (phi, contingency coefficient, Cramer's *V*, and lambda), ordinal (Spearman rank order correlation coefficient, gamma, Kendall's tau, and Somers' *D*), or interval and ratio (Pearson product-moment correlation coefficient). Figure 21-7 in Chapter 21 illustrates the level of measurement for which each of these statistics is appropriate. Many of the correlational techniques (Kendall's tau, contingency coefficient, phi, and Cramer's *V*) are used in conjunction with contingency tables, which illustrate how values of one variable vary with values for a second variable. Contingency tables are explained further in Chapter 25.

Correlational analysis provides two pieces of information about the data: the nature or direction of the linear relationship (positive or negative) between the two variables, and the magnitude (or strength) of the linear relationship. *Correlation statistics are not an indication of causality,* no matter how strong the statistical result.

In a **positive linear relationship**, the values being correlated vary together (in the same direction). When one value is high, the other value tends to be high; when one value is low, the other value tends to be low. The relationship between weight and blood pressure is considered positive because the more a patient weighs, usually the higher his or her blood pressure. In a **negative linear relationship**, when one value is high, the other value tends to be low. There is a negative linear relationship between level of pain and functional capacity because the more pain a person is experiencing, the lower the person's ability to function. A negative linear relationship is sometimes referred to as an **inverse linear relationship**—the terms *negative* and *inverse* are synonymous in correlation statistics.

Sometimes the relationship between two variables is **curvilinear**, which reflects a relationship between the variables that changes over the range of both variables. For example, one of the most famous curvilinear relationships is that of stress and test performance. Test performance tends to be better as test-takers have more stress but only up to a point. When students experience very high stress levels, test performance deteriorates (Lupien, Maheu, Tu, Fiocco, & Schramek, 2007; Yerkes & Dodson, 1908). Analyses designed to test for linear relationships or associations between two variables, such as Pearson correlation, cannot detect a curvilinear relationship.

Pearson Product-Moment Correlation Coefficient

The Pearson product-moment correlation was one of the first of the correlation measures developed and is the most commonly used (Plichta & Kelvin, 2013; Zar, 2010). This coefficient (statistic) is represented by the letter *r*, and the value of *r* is always between −1.00 and +1.00. A value of zero indicates no relationship between the two variables. A positive correlation indicates that higher values of *x* are associated with higher values of *y*, and lower values of *x* are associated with lower values of *y*. A negative or inverse correlation indicates that higher values of *x* are associated with lower values of *y*. The *r* value is indicative of the slope of the line (called a regression line) that can be drawn through a standard scatter plot of the values of two paired variables. The strengths of different associations are identified in Table 23-1 (Cohen, 1988; Grove & Cipher, 2017). Figure 23-2 represents an *r* value approximately equal to zero, indicating no relationship or association between the two variables. An *r* value is rarely, if ever, exactly equal to zero. Figure 23-3 shows an *r* value equal to 0.50, which is a moderate positive relationship. Figure 23-4 shows an *r* value equal to −0.50, which is a moderate negative or inverse relationship.

As discussed earlier, the **Pearson product-moment correlation coefficient** is used to determine the relationship between two variables measured at least at the interval level of measurement. The formula for the Pearson correlation coefficient is based on the following assumptions:

1. Interval or ratio measurement of both variables (e.g., age, income, blood pressure, cholesterol levels). However, if the variables are measured with a Likert

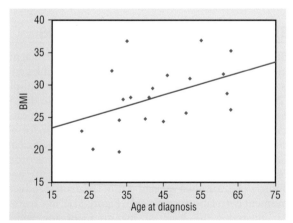

FIGURE 23-1 Scatter plot of BMI and age at diagnosis among veterans with ulcerative colitis.

TABLE 23-1	**Strength of Association for Pearson *r***	
Strength of Association	**Positive Association**	**Negative Association**
Weak	0.00 to 0.29	0.00 to −0.29
Moderate	0.30 to 0.49	−0.49 to −0.30
Strong	0.50 to 1.00	−1.00 to −0.50

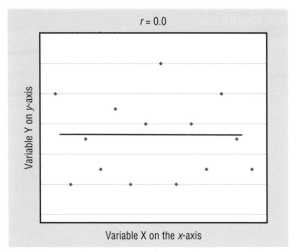

FIGURE 23-2 Scatter plot of *r* equal to approximately 0.00, representing no relationship between two variables.

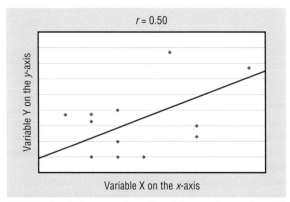

FIGURE 23-3 Scatter plot of variables where *r* is 0.50, representing a moderate positive correlation.

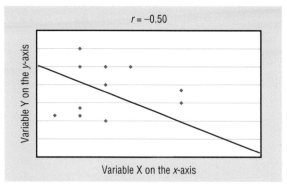

FIGURE 23-4 Scatter plot of variables where *r* is -0.50, representing a moderate inverse correlation.

scale, and the frequency distribution is approximately normally distributed, these data are usually considered interval level measurement and are appropriate for the Pearson *r* (de Winter & Dodou, 2010; Rasmussen, 1989).

2. Normal distribution of at least one variable.
3. Independence of observational pairs.
4. Homoscedasticity.

Data that are **homoscedastic** are evenly dispersed both above and below the regression line, which indicates a linear relationship on a scatterplot (see Chapter 24 for more information on heteroscedasticity). Homoscedasticity reflects equal variance of both vari-

ables. In other words, for every value of *x*, the distribution of *y* values should have equal variability with respect to the regression line. If the data for the two variables being correlated are not homoscedastic, inferences made during significance testing could be invalid (Cohen & Cohen, 1983).

Calculation

The Pearson product-moment correlation coefficient is computed using one of several formulas; the following formula is considered the "computational formula" because it makes computation by hand easier (Zar, 2010).

$$r = \frac{n\sum xy - \sum x \sum y}{\sqrt{[n\sum x^2 - (\sum x)^2][n\sum y^2 - (\sum y)^2]}}$$

where
r = Pearson correlation coefficient
n = total number of subjects
x = value of the first variable
y = value of the second variable
xy = *x* multiplied by *y*
Table 23-2 displays how one would set up data to compute a Pearson correlation coefficient. The data are composed of a simulated subset of data from veterans with a type of inflammatory bowel disease called ulcerative colitis (Flores et al., 2015). The two variables are BMIs and the patient's age at the initial diagnosis of ulcerative colitis. The BMI, a measure of body fat based on height and weight that applies to adult men and women, is considered an indicator of obesity when 30 or greater (National Heart, Lung, and Blood Institute [NHLBI], 2016). The null hypothesis is: *There is no*

TABLE 23-2 Computation of Pearson _r_ Correlation Coefficient

Participant Number	x (Age at Diagnosis)	y (BMI)	x^2	y^2	xy
1	33	19.7	1089	388.09	650.1
2	26	20.1	676	404.01	522.6
3	23	22.9	529	524.41	526.7
4	45	24.4	2025	595.36	1098
5	33	24.6	1089	605.16	811.8
6	40	24.8	1600	615.04	992
7	51	25.7	2601	660.49	1310.7
8	63	26.2	3969	686.44	1650.6
9	34	27.8	1156	772.84	945.2
10	41	28.1	1681	789.61	1152.1
11	36	28.1	1296	789.61	1011.6
12	62	28.7	3844	823.69	1779.4
13	42	29.5	1764	870.25	1239
14	46	31.5	2116	992.25	1449
15	52	31	2704	961	1612
16	61	31.7	3721	1004.89	1933.7
17	31	32.2	961	1036.84	998.2
18	63	35.3	3969	1246.09	2223.9
19	35	36.8	1225	1354.24	1288
20	55	36.9	3025	1361.61	2029.5
sum Σ	872	566	41040	16481.92	25224.10

correlation between age at diagnosis and BMI among veterans with ulcerative colitis.

A simulated subset of 20 veterans was randomly selected for this example so that the computations would be small and manageable. In actuality, studies involving Pearson correlations need to be adequately powered (Cohen, 1988). Observe that the data in Table 23-2 are arranged in columns, which correspond to the elements of the formula. The summed values in the last row of Table 23-2 are inserted into the appropriate place in the Pearson _r_ formula.

$$r = \frac{20(25224.1) - (872)(566)}{\sqrt{[(20)(41040) - 872^2][(20)(16481.92) - 566^2]}}$$

$$r = \frac{20(25224.1) - (872)(566)}{\sqrt{[60416][9282.4]}}$$

$$r = \frac{504482 - 493552}{\sqrt{[60416][9282.4]}}$$

$$r = \frac{10930}{23681.3} = 0.46$$

Interpretation of Results

The _r_ is 0.46, indicating a moderate positive correlation between BMI and age at diagnosis among veterans with ulcerative colitis. To determine whether this relationship is improbable to have been caused by chance alone, we consult the _r_ probability distribution table in Appendix C. The formula for **degrees of freedom** (_df_) for a Pearson _r_ is _n_ − 2. Recall from Chapter 22 that every inferential statistic has its own formula for degrees of freedom (numbers of values that are free to vary). In our analysis, the _df_ is 20 − 2 = 18. With _r_ of 0.46 and _df_ = 18, you need to consult the table in Appendix C to identify the critical value of _r_ for a two-tailed test. The critical _r_ value at alpha = 0.05, _df_ = 18 is 0.4438 that was rounded to 0.444 for this discussion. Our obtained _r_ was 0.46, which exceeds the critical value in the table. Therefore, we can conclude that: _There was a significant correlation between BMI and age at diagnosis among veterans with ulcerative colitis, r(18) = 0.46, p < 0.05. Higher BMI values were associated with older ages at which the diagnosis occurred._ The null hypothesis is rejected.

Every inferential statistic can be reflected by a **probability distribution** of that statistic. The table to which we referred in Appendix C to determine the significance of our obtained r was actually drawn from the probability distribution of r values. Chapter 22 illustrated the probability distribution of z, which appears identical to the normal curve. The Pearson r can be reflected by a theoretical distribution of r values. The shape of this distribution changes, depending on the size of the sample. When a Pearson correlation is computed using a large number of values ($n > 120$), the corresponding distribution of r values appears similar to the normal curve. The smaller the sample size, the flatter the r distribution, and the larger the sample size, the more the r distribution approximates the normal curve, reflecting the range of paired values obtained. Sample size matters because the shape of the probability distribution determines whether our obtained statistic is statistically significant (Plichta & Kelvin, 2013; Zar, 2010).

For example, consider our obtained r of 0.46, previously calculated. At 18 df, the r probability distribution looks like that of Figure 23-5. With a sample size of 20 (and 18 df), the middle 95% of the r probability distribution is delimited by −0.444 and 0.444. The mean r, theoretically, is $r = 0$. That is, most correlation coefficients computed between two variables equal zero, reflecting no relationships between the two variables.

Therefore, an r value of 0 is the most common and probable r value. It is much more improbable to obtain a high r value. At 18 df, r values within the limits of −0.444 and 0.444 are considered common and likely, and values outside these limits are uncommon, unlikely, and improbable to have occurred by chance. The values outside these limits constitute 5% of the r distribution, which is where the concept of alpha (Type I error) originates. We obtained an r of 0.46 and rejected the null hypothesis that there was no association between age at diagnosis and BMI. Thus, there is an association between age at diagnosis and BMI among veterans with ulcerative colitis. In rejecting the null hypothesis, there is less than a 5% chance that we are making a Type I error.

Compare Figure 23-5 with Figure 23-6, in which the probability distribution of r at $df = 100$ is displayed. Appendix C indicates that the critical r value at alpha (α) = 0.05, $df = 100$ (and a sample size of 102) for a two-tailed test is $r = 0.1946$, rounded to 0.19. This means that the middle 95% of the r probability distribution at $df = 100$ is delimited by −0.19 and 0.19. Furthermore, r values within the limits of −0.19 and 0.19 are considered common and likely, and values outside these limits are uncommon, unlikely, and improbable to have occurred by chance. Observe the difference that the larger sample

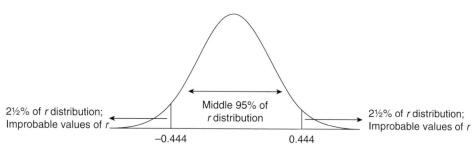

FIGURE 23-5 Probability distribution of r at $df = 18$.

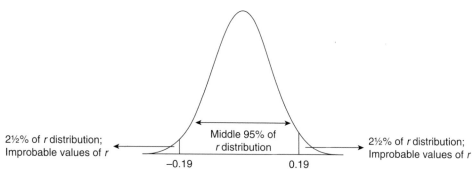

FIGURE 23-6 Probability distribution of r at $df = 100$.

size makes in the critical r value needed to achieve significance. The larger the sample size, the smaller the r value needed to demonstrate statistical significance.

Effect Size

After establishing the statistical significance of r, the relationship subsequently must be examined for clinical importance. There are ranges for strength of association suggested by Cohen (1988), as displayed in Table 23-1. One can also assess the magnitude of association by obtaining the **coefficient of determination** for the Pearson correlation. Computing the coefficient of determination simply involves squaring the r value. The r^2 (multiplied by 100%) represents the percentage of variance shared between the two variables (Cohen & Cohen, 1983). In our example, the r was 0.46, and therefore the r^2 was 0.21116, rounded to 0.211. This indicates that age at diagnosis and BMI shared 21.1% (0.211 × 100%) of the same variance. More specifically, 21.1% of the variance in age at diagnosis can be explained by knowing the veteran's BMI, and vice versa—21.1% of the variance in BMI can be explained by knowing the veteran's age at diagnosis. Statistical textbooks and online resources provide more direction in interpreting the Pearson correlation coefficient (r) and explaining its calculations (Grove & Cipher, 2017).

Nonparametric Alternatives

If one or both of your variables do not meet the assumptions for a Pearson correlation, both **Spearman rank-order correlation coefficient** and **Kendall's tau** are more appropriate statistics. The Spearman rank-order correlation coefficient and Kendall's tau calculations involve converting the data to ranks, discarding any variance or normality issues associated with the original values.

If your data meet the assumptions for the Pearson correlation coefficient, it is the preferred analysis procedure. You would calculate a nonparametric alternative only if your data violate those assumptions. Because Spearman correlation and Kendall's tau are based on ranks of the data, the properties of the original data are lost when they are converted to ranks. Because of this fact, most nonparametric statistics of association yield lower statistical power (Daniel, 2000). The statistical workbook by Grove and Cipher (2017) provides examples of Spearman rank-order correlation coefficient from published studies and provides guidance in the interpretation of these results.

If both of your variables are dichotomous, the phi coefficient is the appropriate statistic for determining an association. If both of your variables are nominal and one or both has more than two categories, Cramer's V statistic is the appropriate statistic. Spearman rank-order correlation coefficient, Kendall's tau, phi, and Cramer's V are addressed in detail by Daniel (2000).

Role of Correlation in Understanding Causality

In any situation involving causality, a relationship exists between the factors involved in the causal process. Therefore, the first clue to the possibility of a causal link is the existence of a relationship. However, *a relationship does not mean causality*. For example, blood glucose level may be related to or correlated with body temperature; however, this does not mean that one *causes* the other. Two variables can be highly correlated but have no causal relationship. However, as the strength of a relationship increases, the possibility of a causal link increases. The absence of a relationship precludes the possibility of a causal connection between the two variables being examined, given adequate measurement of the variables and absence of other variables that might mask the relationship (Cohen & Cohen, 1983). A correlational study can be the first step in determining the connections among variables important to nursing practice within a particular population. Determining these dynamics can allow us to increase our ability to predict and control the situation studied. However, correlation cannot be used to show causality.

Spurious Correlations

Spurious correlations are relationships between variables that are not true. In some cases, these significant relationships are a consequence of chance and have no meaning. When you choose a level of significance of $\alpha = 0.05$, 1 in 20 correlations that you compute will be statistically significant by chance alone. There is really no true relationship between the two variables under study in the population; you just happened to draw a sample that showed a relationship where there typically is none. Other pairs of variables may be correlated because of the influence of other unrelated or confounding variables. For example, you might find a positive correlation between the number of deaths on a nursing unit and the number of nurses working on the unit. The number of deaths cannot be explained as occurring because of increases in the number of nurses. It is more likely that a third variable (units having patients with more critical conditions) explains both the increased number of nurses and the increased number of deaths. In many cases, the "other" variable remains unknown, although the researcher can use reasoning to identify and exclude most of these spurious correlations.

BLAND AND ALTMAN PLOTS

Bland and Altman plots are used to examine the extent of agreement between two measurement techniques (Bland & Altman, 1986, 2010). In nursing research, Bland and Altman plots are used to display visually the extent of interrater agreement and test-retest agreement (see Chapter 16 for discussion of reliability). For both instances, pairs of data are collected from each subject (from rater 1 and rater 2, or administration 1 and administration 2), and each subject's two values are subtracted from one another. The differences are plotted on a graph, displaying a scatter diagram of the differences plotted against the averages. Limits of agreement are defined as twice the standard deviation above and below the mean. Bland and Altman plots are primarily used to see how many of the values are outside these limits. Acceptable interrater or test-retest agreement is considered to be reflected when at least 95% of the values are within the limits of agreement on the plot (Altman, 1991).

Example

Table 23-3 displays a simulated subset of test-retest data from veterans with inflammatory bowel disease. These values are BMIs collected from 20 veterans, one month apart. Each veteran's BMI value at Assessment 1 and Assessment 2 is displayed in Table 23-3, along with the difference between each pair of scores.

A Bland and Altman plot of these data is illustrated in Figure 23-7. The line of perfect agreement is drawn as a red line in the exact horizontal middle of the graph. The mean difference of the sample data is represented by the dotted middle line, and the limits of agreement are the two outside dotted lines. Observe that there are no values outside of the limits of agreement. Therefore, all 20 pairs of data were within the limits of agreement. Incidentally, the r between the first and second assessments of the BMI was 0.97. However, the Bland and Altman plot does not always corroborate a Pearson correlation coefficient, and vice versa, because they are distinctly different methods (Bland & Altman, 1986).

Bland and Altman (1986) created the coefficient of repeatability as an indication of the repeatability of a single method of measurement. Because the same method is being measured repeatedly, the mean difference should be zero. Use the following formula to calculate a coefficient of repeatability (CR), where $s_{x_1 - x_2}$ is the standard deviation of the difference scores.

$$CR = 1.96\,(s_{x_1 - x_2})$$

Table 23-3 displays each difference score, of which the mean is −0.315. The standard deviation of the difference scores is $s_{x_1 - x_2} = 1.17$. Therefore, the CR is calculated as:

$$CR = 1.96\,(1.17)$$

$$CR = 2.29$$

TABLE 23-3 Test-Retest Data for Body Mass Index Values Among Veterans With Inflammatory Bowel Disease

Assessment 1	Assessment 2	Difference
19.7	20.9	−1.2
20.1	20.7	−0.6
22.9	22.2	0.7
24.4	26.6	−2.2
24.6	24.4	0.2
24.8	25.3	−0.5
25.7	27.5	−1.8
26.2	25.2	1
27.8	29.2	−1.4
28.1	30.1	−2
28.1	27.3	0.8
28.7	28.4	0.3
29.5	31.3	−1.8
31.5	32.4	−0.9
31	29.8	1.2
31.7	30.7	1
32.2	32.5	−0.3
35.3	36.0	−0.7
36.8	35.3	1.5
36.9	36.5	0.4
		$\bar{X}$: −0.315

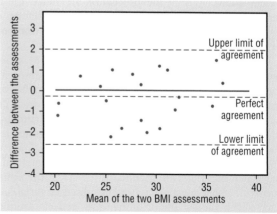

FIGURE 23-7 Bland and Altman plot of test-retest data for body mass index (BMI) values for veterans with inflammatory bowel disease.

Interpretation of Results

The mean difference between the two assessments of BMI was −0.315 (Table 23-3). In other words, the average difference between the first and second assessments of BMI values was −0.315. A perfect average agreement would be 0, meaning that, on average, the two sets of values were exactly the same. The *CR* value, 2.29, is added to and subtracted from the mean difference to create lower and upper limits of acceptable agreement: −0.315 ± 2.29. Differences within −0.315 ± 2.29 (−2.61, 1.98) would not be deemed clinically important, according to Bland and Altman (2010). Differences between the two administrations that are less than −2.61 and greater than 1.98 are "unacceptable for clinical purposes" (Bland & Altman, 2010). The *CR* is not an inferential statistic, and values of lower and upper limits of agreement are not interpreted the way one would interpret a confidence interval. Rather, they are formulas invented by Bland and Altman for heuristic purposes to make decisions on the extent of agreement between two measurements.

FACTOR ANALYSIS

Factor analysis refers to a collection of statistical techniques designed to examine interrelationships among large numbers of variables to reduce them to a smaller set of variables and to identify clusters of variables that are most closely linked together (**factors**). Factors are hypothetical constructs created from the original variables. The term "factor analysis" may apply to the statistical applications of exploratory factor analysis (EFA) (sometimes called "principal components analysis") and confirmatory factor analysis (Tabachnick & Fidell, 2006). EFA is the procedure of choice for a researcher who is primarily interested in reducing a large number of variables down to a smaller number of components.

A common reason for performing EFA is to assist with validity investigations of a new measurement method or scale, particularly subjective assessments or instruments that pertain to attitudes, beliefs, values, or opinions. When researchers develop a new instrument, EFA can serve to assist the researcher in investigating its content and construct validity, as described in Chapter 16. The results of EFA assist researchers in understanding which questions are redundant (or assess the same concept), which questions represent subsets of variables, and which items stand alone and reflect unique concepts.

Mathematically, EFA extracts maximum variance (explanatory "power" to predict one variable's value from another's value) from the data set with each "factor." The first factor is the linear combination of the variables (or instrument items) that maximizes the variance of their factor scores. The second component is formed from residual correlations. Subsequent factors are formed from the residual correlations that have not yet been created.

Once the factors have been identified mathematically, the researcher attempts to explain why the variables are grouped as they are. Factor analysis aids in the identification of theoretical constructs and is also used to confirm the accuracy of a theoretically developed construct.

Example

The following example describes how EFA was used to investigate content and construct validity for the Maslach Burnout Inventory (MBI; Poghosyan, Aiken, & Sloane, 2009). The MBI was developed in 1981 to assess burnout experienced by nurses (Maslach & Jackson, 1981). The MBI has been reported in many factor analytic studies since its original publication (Worley, Vassar, Wheeler, & Barnes, 2008). Poghosyan and colleagues (2009) investigated the factor structure of the MBI in 54,738 nurses living in one of eight countries. The 22 items were answered on a 7-point Likert scale, ranging from never having those feelings to having those feelings a few times a week. Of the 22 items, all loaded on at least one of the subscales (with a factor loading of > 0.30). Using EFA, three factors were identified, confirming prior factor analytic reports. The factor loadings from the United States nurses (the other countries were excluded for this example) are listed in Table 23-4.

The first factor, Emotional Exhaustion, accounted for the majority of the variance extracted from the EFA solution, followed by smaller percentages of variance explained by the second and third factors. Table 23-4 lists the factor loadings of each item. **Factor loadings** are the correlations between the item and the new factor. The MBI items that were not highly correlated with a factor (the factor loadings that were < 0.30) are not listed with that factor in Table 23-4. The first factor, named Emotional Exhaustion by the researchers, represented feelings of being exhausted and overextended by work. This factor was correlated with nine of the MBI items, and the factor loadings ranged from 0.58 to 0.94. The second factor, Personal Accomplishment, was correlated with eight of the MBI items, all of which pertained to feelings of successful achievement and competence in the workplace. The factor loadings ranged from 0.40 to 0.73. The third factor, named

TABLE 23-4 Item Factor Loadings on Three MBI Subscales

Factor Loading*	MBI Item
EMOTIONAL EXHAUSTION SUBSCALE	
0.93	Feel emotionally drained from work
0.94	Feel used up at the end of the workday
0.86	Feel fatigued when getting up in the morning
0.58	Feel like at the end of the rope
0.77	Feel burned out from work
0.75	Feel frustrated by job
0.72	Feel working too hard on the job
0.59	Working with people puts too much stress
0.60	Working with patients is a strain
PERSONAL ACCOMPLISHMENT SUBSCALE	
0.40	Can easily understand patients' feelings
0.50	Deal effectively with the patients' problems
0.64	Feel positively influencing people's lives
0.46	Feel very energetic
0.62	Can easily create a relaxed atmosphere
0.63	Feel exhilarated after working with patients
0.73	Have accomplished worthwhile things in job
0.52	Deal with emotional problems calmly
DEPERSONALIZATION SUBSCALE	
0.61	Treat patients as impersonal "objects"
0.79	Become more callous toward people
0.71	Worry that job is hardening emotionally
0.64	Don't really care what happens to patients
0.41	Feel patients are to blame for their problems

*From United States sample.
MBI, Maslach Burnout Inventory.
Adapted from Poghosyan, L., Aiken, L.H., & Sloane, D.M. (2009). Factor structure of the Maslach Burnout Inventory: An analysis of data from large scale cross-sectional surveys of nurses from eight countries. *International Journal of Nursing Studies, 46*(7), 894–902.

Depersonalization, was correlated with five of the MBI items, all of which pertained to the respondent feeling impersonal and/or emotionless when delivering care to the patient. The factor loadings ranged from 0.41 to 0.79.

"Naming" the Factor

The three factors generated from the EFA were named according to the nature of the items that loaded on those factors. When naming the factor, the researcher must examine the items that cluster together in a factor and seem to explain that clustering. Variables with high loadings on the factor must be included, even if they do not fit the researcher's preconceived theoretical notions of which items *fit* together because they reflect a similar concept. The purpose is to identify the broad construct of meaning that has caused these particular variables to be so strongly intercorrelated. Naming this construct is an important part of the procedure because naming of the factor provides theoretical meaning.

Factor Scores

After the initial factor analysis, additional studies are conducted to examine changes in the phenomenon in various situations and to determine the relationships of the factors with other concepts. **Factor scores** are used during statistical analysis in these additional studies. To obtain factor scores, the variables included in the factor are identified, and the scores on these variables are summed for each study participant. Thus, each participant has a score for each factor in the instrument. There are several methods of computing factor scores. One of the most common methods involves simply adding the participant's scores on the items that load on a factor. Using the MBI results as an example, to obtain a factor score for Depersonalization, a respondent's score on the items that loaded on the Depersonalizations subscale would be summed. For example, if a participant scored a 4 on "Treat patients as impersonal objects," 2 on "Become more callous toward people," 5 on "Worry that job is hardening emotionally," 2 on "Don't really care what happens to patients," and 3 on "Feel patients are to blame for their problems," that individual's factor score for Depersonalization would be:

$$4 + 2 + 5 + 2 + 3 = 16$$

Another common method of computing a factor score is using the factor loadings to weight each study participant's score. Applying the same hypothetical scores as before, the factor loadings are multiplied by the item scores to create the factor score:

$$(0.61)4 + (0.79)2 + (0.71)5 + (0.64)2 + (0.41)3$$
$$= 2.44 + 1.58 + 3.55 + 1.28 + 1.23 = 10.08$$

In the first method, each item is weighted equally in the equation because the weight is essentially "1." In the second method, each item is adjusted for the extent to which that item loads on that factor. The advantages and disadvantages of these factor score methods, in addition to descriptions of other methods for obtaining factor scores, are reviewed by DiStefano, Zhu, and Mîndrilă (2009).

KEY POINTS

- Correlational analyses identify relationships or associations between or among variables.
- The purpose of correlational analysis is also to clarify relationships among theoretical concepts or help identify potentially causal relationships, which can be tested by inferential analysis.
- All data for the analysis should have been obtained from a single population from which values are available for all variables to be examined.
- Correlational analysis provides two pieces of information about the data: the nature of a linear relationship (positive or negative) between the two variables and the magnitude (or strength) of the linear relationship.
- The Pearson product-moment correlation coefficient is the preferred computation when investigating the association among two variables measured at the interval or ratio level and when the variables meet the other required statistical assumptions.
- Spearman rank-order correlation coefficient and Kendall's tau are both nonparametric statistics that are calculated when the assumptions of a Pearson correlation cannot be met, such as variables that are non-normally distributed.
- The first clue to the possibility of a causal link is the existence of a relationship, but a relationship does not mean causality.
- Bland and Altman plots are a graphical display of agreement between two administrations of an instrument or assessment, or two raters of a clinician-rated instrument.
- The coefficient of repeatability (*CR*) is a value that is used to determine acceptable lower and upper limits of interrater agreement and test-retest agreement.

- Exploratory factor analysis is a procedure that reduces a large number of variables down to a smaller number of components and is most often used during the construction of a new measurement method or scale.
- The results of exploratory factor analysis assist the researcher in understanding which questions assess the same concept and are redundant, which questions represent subsets of variables, and which items stand alone.

REFERENCES

Altman, D. G. (1991). *Practical statistics for medical research* (1st ed.). London, UK: Chapman & Hall.

Bland, J. M., & Altman, D. M. (1986). Statistical methods for assessing agreement between two methods of clinical measurement. *Lancet*, *1*(8476), 307–310.

Bland, J. M., & Altman, D. M. (2010). Statistical methods for assessing agreement between two methods of clinical measurement. *International Journal of Nursing Studies*, *47*(8), 931–936.

Cohen, J. (1988). *Statistical power analysis for the behavioral sciences* (2nd ed.). Hillsdale, NJ: Lawrence Erlbaum Associates.

Cohen, J., & Cohen, P. (1983). *Applied multiple regression/correlation analysis for the behavioral sciences* (2nd ed.). Hillsdale, NJ: Erlbaum.

Daniel, W. W. (2000). *Applied nonparametric statistics* (2nd ed.). Pacific Grove, CA: Duxbury Press.

de Winter, J. C. F., & Dodou, D. (2010). Five-point Likert items: *t* test versus Mann-Whitney-Wilcoxon. *Practical Assessment, Research, and Evaluation*, *15*(11), 1–16.

DiStefano, C., Zhu, M., & Mîndrilă, D. (2009). Understanding and using factor scores: Considerations for the applied researcher. *Practical Assessment, Research Evaluation*, *14*(20), 1–9.

Flores, A., Burstein, E., Cipher, D. J., & Feagins, L. A. (2015). Obesity in inflammatory bowel disease: A marker of less severe disease. *Digestive Diseases and Sciences*, *60*(8), 2436–2445.

Grove, S. K., & Cipher, D. J. (2017). *Statistics for nursing research: A workbook for evidence-based practice* (2nd ed.). St. Louis, MO: Saunders.

Lupien, S. J., Maheu, F., Tu, M., Fiocco, A., & Schramek, T. E. (2007). The effects of stress and stress hormones on human cognition: Implications for the field of brain and cognition. *Brain & Cognition*, *65*(3), 209–237.

Mancuso, J. M. (2010). Impact of health literacy and patient trust on glycemic control in an urban USA populations. *Nursing & Health Sciences*, *12*(1), 94–104.

Maslach, C., & Jackson, S. E. (1981). The measurement of experienced burnout. *Journal of Occupational Behaviour*, *2*(2), 99–113.

National Heart, Lung, and Blood Institute (NHLBI). Managing overweight and obesity in adults: Systematic evidence review from the obesity expert panel. (2016). Retrieved June 21, 2016 from http://www.nhlbi.nih.gov/sites/www.nhlbi.nih.gov/files/obesity-evidence-review.pdf.

Plichta, S. B., & Kelvin, E. (2013). *Munro's statistical methods for health care research* (6th ed.). Philadelphia, PA: Wolters Kluwer/ Lippincott Williams & Wilkins.

Poghosyan, L., Aiken, L. H., & Sloane, D. M. (2009). Factor structure of the Maslach Burnout Inventory: An analysis of data from large scale cross-sectional surveys of nurses from eight countries. *International Journal of Nursing Studies*, 46(7), 894–902.

Rasmussen, J. L. (1989). Analysis of Likert-scale data: A reinterpretation of Gregoire and Driver. *Psychological Bulletin*, 105(1), 167–170.

Tabachnick, B. G., & Fidell, L. S. (2006). *Using multivariate statistics* (5th ed.). Needham Heights, MA: Allyn & Bacon.

Worley, J. A., Vassar, M., Wheeler, D. L., & Barnes, L. B. (2008). Factor structure of scores from the Maslach Burnout Inventory: A review and meta-analysis of 45 exploratory and confirmatory factor-analytic studies. *Educational and Psychological Measurement*, 68(5), 797–823.

Yerkes, R. M., & Dodson, J. D. (1908). The relation of strength of stimulus to rapidity of habit-formation. *Journal of Comparative Neurology & Psychology*, 18(5), 459–482.

Zar, J. H. (2010). *Biostatistical analysis* (5th ed.). Upper Saddle River, NJ: Prentice-Hall.

24

Using Statistics to Predict

Daisha J. Cipher

http://evolve.elsevier.com/Gray/practice/

In nursing practice, the ability to predict future events is crucial. Clinical researchers might investigate whether hospital length of stay can be predicted by severity of illness. Health outcome researchers want to know what factors play an important role in responses of patients to health promotion, illness prevention, and rehabilitation interventions. Educators are interested in knowing which variables are most effective in predicting scores of undergraduate nurses on the National Council Licensure Examination (NCLEX). Advanced practice nurses are interested in what variables predict their success in passing their national certification examinations.

The statistical procedure most commonly used for prediction is regression analysis. The purpose of a regression analysis is to identify which factor or factors predict or explain the value of a dependent (outcome) variable. In some cases, the analysis is exploratory, and the focus is prediction. In others, selection of variables is based on a theoretical proposition, and the purpose is to develop an explanation that confirms the theoretical proposition (Cohen & Cohen, 1983).

In **regression analysis**, the independent (predictor) variable or variables influence variation or change in the value of the dependent variable. The goal is to determine how accurately one can predict the value of an outcome (or dependent) variable based on the value or values of one or more predictor (or independent) variables. This chapter describes some common statistical procedures used for prediction. These procedures include simple linear regression, multiple regression, logistic regression, and Cox proportional hazards regression.

SIMPLE LINEAR REGRESSION

Simple linear regression is a procedure that estimates the value of a dependent variable based on the value of an independent variable. Simple linear regression is an effort to explain the dynamics within a scatter plot by drawing a straight line (the **line of best fit**) through the plotted scores. This line is drawn to best explain the **linear relationship** or association between two variables. Knowing that linear relationship, we can, with some degree of accuracy, use regression analysis to predict the value of one variable if we know the value of the other variable (Cohen & Cohen, 1983). Figure 24-1 illustrates the linear relationship between gestational age and birth weight. As shown in the scatter plot, there is a strong positive association in preterm births between the two variables. In premature infants, more advanced gestational ages predict higher birth weights.

Use of simple linear regression involves the following assumptions (Zar, 2010):
1. Normal distribution of the dependent (y) variable
2. Linear relationship between x and y
3. Independent observations
4. No (or little) multicollinearity
5. Homoscedasticity

Data that are **homoscedastic** are symmetrically dispersed both above and below the regression line throughout the range of values, which indicates a linear relationship on a scatterplot. Homoscedasticity reflects equal variance of both variables. In other words, for all values of x, the distribution of y values should have equal variability. If the data for the predictor and dependent variables are not homoscedastic, inferences made

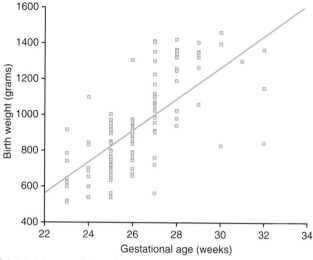

FIGURE 24-1 Linear relationship between gestational age and birth weight.

during significance testing could be invalid (Cohen & Cohen, 1983; Grove & Cipher, 2017).

The homoscedasticity assumption can be checked by visual examination of a plot of the standardized residuals (the errors) by the regression standardized predicted value. Ideally, residuals are randomly scattered around 0 (the horizontal line) providing a relatively even distribution. **Heteroscedasticity** is indicated when the residuals are not evenly scattered around the line. Heteroscedasticity manifests itself in all kinds of uneven shapes. When the plot of residuals appears to deviate substantially from normal, more formal tests for heteroscedasticity should be performed. Formal tests for heteroscedasticity include the Breusch-Pagan test (Breusch & Pagan, 1979) and White test (White, 1980).

Formulas

In simple linear regression, the dependent variable is continuous, and the predictor can be any scale of measurement. However, if the predictor is nominal, it must be correctly coded prior to analysis with statistical software. Examples of coding nominal variables are presented later in this chapter. Once the data are ready, the parameters a and b are computed to obtain a regression equation. To understand the mathematical process, recall the algebraic equation for a straight line:

$$y = bx + a$$

where
y = dependent variable (outcome)
x = independent variable (predictor)

b = **slope of the line** (beta, or what the increase in value is along the x-axis for every unit of increase in the y value)

a = **y-intercept** (the point where the regression line intersects the y-axis)

A regression equation can be generated with a data set containing participants' x and y values. When this equation is generated, it can be used to predict y values of other participants, given only their x values. In simple or bivariate regression, predictions are made in cases with two variables. The score on variable y (dependent variable) is predicted from the same individual's known score on variable x (independent variable).

No single regression line can be used to predict with complete accuracy every y value from every x value. You could draw an infinite number of lines through the scattered paired values. However, the purpose of the regression equation is to develop the line that allows the highest degree of prediction possible—the **line of best fit**. The procedure for developing the line of best fit is the **method of least squares**. The formulas for the beta (b) and y-intercept (a) of the regression equation are computed as follows. Note that when the b is calculated, that value is inserted into the formula for a.

$$b = \frac{n\sum xy - \sum x \sum y}{n\sum x^2 - \left(\sum x\right)^2} \qquad a = \frac{\sum y - b\sum x}{n}$$

where
b = beta
a = y-intercept

n = total number of subjects
x = value of the predictor
y = value of the dependent variable
xy = x multiplied by y

Calculation of Simple Linear Regression

Table 24-1 displays how one would arrange data to perform linear regression by hand. Regression analysis is conducted with a computer for most studies, but this calculation is provided to increase your understanding of the aspects of regression analysis and how to interpret the results. This example uses data collected from a study of students enrolled in a registered nurse (RN) to bachelor's of science in nursing (BSN) program (Mancini, Ashwill, & Cipher, 2015). The predictor in this example is number of academic degrees obtained by the student prior to enrollment, and the dependent variable was number of months it took for the student to complete the RN to BSN program. The null hypothesis is "Number of degrees does not predict the number of months until completion of an RN to BSN program."

The data are presented in Table 24-1. A simulated subset of 20 students was selected for this example so that the computations would be small and manageable. In actuality, studies involving linear regression must be adequately powered (Cohen, 1988; Grove & Cipher, 2017). Observe that the data in Table 24-1 are arranged in columns, which correspond to the elements of the formula. The summed values in the last row of the table are inserted into the appropriate place in the formula for b.

Calculation Steps

Step 1: Calculate b

From the values in Table 24-1, we know that $n = 20$, $\Sigma x = 20$, $\Sigma y = 267$, $\Sigma x^2 = 30$, and $\Sigma xy = 238$. These values are inserted into the formula for b, as follows:

$$b = \frac{20(238) - (20)(267)}{20(30) - 20^2}$$

$$b = \frac{-580}{200}$$

$$b = -2.9$$

Step 2: Calculate a

From Step 1, we now know that $b = -2.9$, and we insert this value into the formula for a.

$$a = \frac{267 - (-2.9)(20)}{20}$$

$$a = \frac{325}{20}$$

$$a = 16.25$$

Step 3: Write the new regression equation:

$$y = -2.9x + 16.25$$

Step 4: Calculate R

We can use our new regression equation from Step 3 to compute predicted program completion for each student, using their number of degrees. The extent to which predicted program completion is the same as actual program completion is determined by the multiple R. The **multiple R** is defined as the correlation between the actual y values and the predicted y values using the new regression equation. The predicted y value using the new equation is represented by the symbol $\hat{y}$ to differentiate from y, which represents the

TABLE 24-1	Computation of Linear Regression Equation			
Student ID	x (Number of Degrees)	y (Months to Completion)	x^2	xy
1	1	17	1	17
2	2	9	4	18
3	0	17	0	0
4	1	9	1	9
5	0	16	0	0
6	1	11	1	11
7	0	15	0	0
8	0	12	0	0
9	1	15	1	15
10	1	12	1	12
11	1	14	1	14
12	1	10	1	10
13	1	17	1	17
14	0	20	0	0
15	2	9	4	18
16	2	12	4	24
17	1	14	1	14
18	2	10	4	20
19	1	17	1	17
20	2	11	4	22
sum Σ	20	267	30	238

actual y values in the data set. For example, Student #1 had earned 1 academic degree prior to enrollment, and the predicted months to completion for Student 1 is calculated as:

$$\hat{y} = -2.9(1) + 16.25$$

$$\hat{y} = 13.35$$

Thus, the predicted $\hat{y}$ for Student #1 is 13.35 months for RN to BSN program completion. This procedure would be continued for the rest of the students, and the Pearson correlation between the actual months to completion (y) and the predicted months to completion ($\hat{y}$) would yield the multiple R value. In this example, the R = 0.638. The higher the R, the more likely that the new regression equation accurately predicts y because the higher the correlation, the closer the actual y values are to the predicted $\hat{y}$ values. Figure 24-2 displays the regression line for which the x axis represents possible numbers of degrees, and the y axis represents the predicted months to program completion ($\hat{y}$ values).

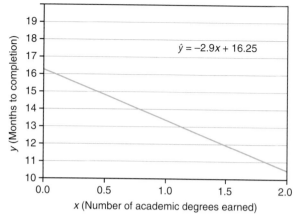

FIGURE 24-2 Regression line represented by regression equation of months of program completion predicted by number of academic degrees earned. (From Grove, S. K., & Cipher, D. J. [2017]. *Statistics for nursing research: A workbook for evidence-based practice* [2nd ed.]. St. Louis, MO: Elsevier.)

Step 5: Determine whether the predictor significantly predicts y

To know whether the predictor significantly predicts y, the beta must be tested against zero. In simple regression, this is most easily accomplished by using the R value from Step 4:

$$t = R\sqrt{\frac{n-2}{1-R^2}}$$

$$t = 0.638\sqrt{\frac{20-2}{1-0.407}}$$

$$t = 3.52$$

The t value is then compared to the t probability distribution table (see Appendix B). The df for this t statistic is $n - 2$. The critical t value for a two-tailed test at alpha (α) = 0.05, df = 18 is 2.101, rounded to 2.10. Our obtained t was 3.52, which exceeds the critical value in the table, thereby indicating a significant association between the predictor x and y (outcome).

Step 6: Calculate R^2

After establishing the statistical significance of the R value, it must subsequently be examined for actual importance. This is accomplished by obtaining **the coefficient of determination** for regression—which simply involves squaring the R value. The R^2 represents the percentage of variance explained in y by the predictor. Cohen describes R^2 values of 0.02 as small, 0.15 as moderate, and 0.26 or higher as large effect sizes (Cohen, 1988). In our example, the R was 0.638, and therefore, the R^2 was 0.407. Multiplying 0.407 × 100% indicates that 40.7% of the variance in months to program completion can be explained by knowing the student's number of earned academic degrees at admission (Cohen & Cohen, 1983).

The R^2 can be very helpful in testing more than one predictor in a regression model. Unlike R, the R^2 for one regression model can be compared with another regression model that contains additional predictors (Cohen & Cohen, 1983). For example, a researcher could add another predictor, such as student's admission grade-point average (GPA), to the regression model of months to completion. The R^2 values of both models would be compared, the first with number of academic degrees as the sole predictor and the second with number of academic degrees and enrollment GPA as predictors. The R^2 values of the two models would be statistically compared to indicate whether the proportion of variance in $\hat{y}$ was significantly increased by including the second predictor, enrollment GPA, in the model.

The standardized beta (β) is another statistic that represents the magnitude of the association between x and y. β has the same limits as a Pearson r, meaning that the standardized β cannot be lower than -1.00 or higher than 1.00. This value can be calculated by hand, but is best computed with statistical software. The standardized beta (β) is calculated by converting the x and y values to z scores, and then correlating the x and y values using the

Pearson r formula. The standardized beta (β) is often reported in literature instead of the unstandardized b, because b does not have lower or upper limits and therefore, the magnitude of b cannot be judged. β, on the other hand, is interpreted as a Pearson r and the descriptions of the magnitude of β (as recommended by Cohen, 1988) can be applied to β. In this example, the standardized beta (β) is -0.638. Thus, the magnitude of the association between x and y in this example is considered a large predictive association (Cohen, 1988).

Interpretation of Results

The following summative statements are written in APA (American Psychological Association, 2010) format, as one might read the results in an article. *Simple linear regression was performed with number of earned academic degrees prior to enrollment as the predictor and months to program completion as the dependent variable. The student's number of degrees significantly predicted months to completion among students in an RN to BSN program, $\beta = -0.638$, $p < 0.05$, $R^2 = 40.7\%$. Higher numbers of earned academic degrees significantly predicted shorter program completion time.*

MULTIPLE REGRESSION

Multiple linear regression analysis is an extension of simple linear regression in which more than one independent variable is entered into the analysis (Grove & Cipher, 2017; Stevens, 2009). Because the relationships between multiple predictors and y are tested simultaneously, the calculations involved in multiple regression analysis are very complex. Multiple regression is best conducted using a statistical software package such as those presented in Table 21-2. However, full explanations and examples of the matrix algebraic computations of

multiple regression are presented by Stevens (2009) and Tabachnick and Fidell (2006).

Interpretations of multiple regression findings are the same as with simple regression. The beta (b) values of each predictor are tested for significance, and a multiple R and R^2 are computed. The only difference is that in multiple regression, when all predictors are tested simultaneously, each b has been adjusted for every other predictor in the regression model. The b represents the independent relationship between that predictor and y, even after controlling for (or accounting for) the presence of every other predictor in the model.

Mancuso (2010) conducted a study of 102 subjects with diabetes to develop a predictive model of glycemic control, as measured by glycosylated hemoglobin (HbA_{1c}). The five predictors for HbA_{1c} were health literacy, patient trust, knowledge of diabetes, performance of self-care activities, and depression. The five predictors of glycemic control were tested with multiple regression analysis. The analysis yielded five b and β values, each with a corresponding p value. As shown in Table 24-2, patient trust and depression were significant predictors of glycemic control (HbA_{1c}), even after adjusting for the presence or contribution of every other predictor in the model. The p values for these two predictors were less than 0.05. Health literacy, diabetes knowledge, and performance of self-care activities did not significantly predict HbA_{1c} levels ($p > 0.05$). R^2 was 0.285, indicating that patient trust and depression accounted for 28.5% of the variance in HbA_{1c} (the measure of glycemic control).

The findings from this study have potential implications for the management of patients with diabetes. Because lower levels of patient trust were associated with higher HbA_{1c} values, fostering communication and trusting collaboration between the patient and the healthcare

TABLE 24-2	Predictors of Glycosylated Hemoglobin (HbA₁c) in Patients With Diabetes				
	UNSTANDARDIZED COEFFICIENTS		**STANDARDIZED COEFFICIENT**		
Independent Variable	**B**	**SE**	**β**	**t**	**Significance (p)**
Health literacy	−0.063	0.080	−0.070	−0.782	0.436
Patient trust	−0.873	0.165	−0.459	−5.288	0.000*
Diabetes knowledge	0.012	0.011	0.100	1.116	0.267
Performance of self-care activities	0.005	0.135	0.003	0.040	0.968
Depression	0.036	0.014	0.226	2.589	0.011*

*$p < 0.05$, significant.
Data from Mancuso, J. M. (2010). Impact of health literacy and patient trust on glycemic control in an urban USA populations. *Nursing & Health Sciences, 12*(1), 94–104.

provider could directly or indirectly improve glycemic control. Higher levels of depression were also associated with higher HbA_{1c} values, and early interventions or referrals aimed at addressing depressive symptoms could be important in improving glycemic control. However, it is important to note that regression analysis is not an indication of cause and effect. Rather, these results can serve as a basis for further research aimed at investigating the influence of patient factors such as trust and depression on glycemic control.

Multicollinearity

Multicollinearity occurs when the independent variables in a multiple regression equation are strongly correlated with one another. The presence of multicollinearity does not affect predictive power (the capacity of the independent variables to predict values of the dependent variable in a specific sample); rather, it causes problems related to generalizability and to the stability of the findings. If multicollinearity is present, the equation lacks **predictive validity**, and the amount of variance explained by each variable in the equation is inflated. Additionally, when cross-validation is performed, the *b* values do not remain consistent across samples (Cohen & Cohen, 1983). Multicollinearity is minimized by carefully selecting the independent variables and thoroughly determining their correlation before the regression analysis. If highly correlated independent variables are found, the correlated predictors might be combined into one score or value yielding one predictor, or only one of the measures (scores) might be included in the regression equation.

The first step in identifying multicollinearity is to examine the correlations among the independent variables. Therefore, you would perform multiple correlation analyses before conducting the regression analyses. The correlation matrix is carefully examined for evidence of multicollinearity. Many statistical software packages, such as SPSS, provide two statistics—tolerance and variance inflation factor (VIF)—that describe the extent to which your model has a multicollinearity problem. A tolerance of less than 0.20 and/or a VIF of 10 and above indicates a multicollinearity problem (Allison, 1999).

Types of Predictor Variables Used in Regression Analyses

Variables in a regression equation can take many forms. Traditionally, as with most multivariate analyses, variables are measured at the interval or ratio level. However, researchers also use nominal variables (referred to as **dummy variables**), multiplicative terms,

and transformed terms. A mixture of types of variables may be used in a single regression equation. The following discussion describes the treatment of dummy variables in regression equations.

Dummy Variables

To use categorical variables in regression analysis, a coding system is developed to represent group membership. Categorical variables of interest in nursing that might be used in regression analysis include gender, income, ethnicity, social status, level of education, and diagnosis. If the variable is dichotomous, such as gender, members of one category are assigned the number 1, and all others are assigned the number 0. In this case, for gender the coding could be the following:

1 = female
0 = male

If the categorical variable has three values, two dummy variables are used; for example, social class could be classified as lower class, middle class, or upper class. The first dummy variable (X_1) would be classified as:

1 = lower class
0 = not lower class

The second dummy variable (X_2) would be classified as the following:

1 = middle class
0 = not middle class

The three social classes would be represented in the data set in the following manner:

Lower class $X_1 = 1$, $X_2 = 0$
Middle class $X_1 = 0$, $X_2 = 1$
Upper class $X_1 = 0$, $X_2 = 0$

The variables lower class and middle class would be entered as predictors in the regression equation, in which both are tested against the reference category, upper class. Specifically, the *b* values for these two variables would represent whether *y* differs by lower class versus upper class and middle class versus upper class. When more than three categories define the values of the variable, increased numbers of dummy variables are used. The number of dummy variables is always one less than the number of categories (Aiken & West, 1991). An example of how one might analyze dichotomous dummy variables is presented in the next section.

ODDS RATIO

When both the predictor and the dependent variable are dichotomous (having only two values), the **odds ratio** (*OR*) is a statistic commonly used to obtain an indication of association and is defined as the ratio of the odds of an event occurring in one group to the odds of it occurring in another group (Gordis, 2014). Put simply, the *OR* is a way of comparing whether the odds of a certain event is the same for two groups. For example, the use of angiotensin-converting enzyme (ACE) inhibitors in a sample of veterans was examined in relation to having advanced adenomatous colon polyps (Kedika et al.,2011). The *OR* was 0.63, indicating that ACE inhibitor use was associated with a lower likelihood of developing adenomatous colon polyps in veterans.

Statistical Formula and Assumptions

Use of the OR involves the following assumptions (Gordis, 2014):

1. Only one datum entry is made for each subject in the sample. Therefore, if repeated measures from the same subject are being used for analysis, such as pretests and posttests, the odds ratio is not an appropriate test.
2. The variables must be dichotomous, either inherently or transformed to nominal values from quantitative values (ordinal, interval, or ratio). The formula for the odds ratio is:

$$OR = \frac{ad}{bc}$$

The formula for the *OR* designates the odds of occurrence in the numerator when the predictor is present, and the odds of occurrence in the denominator when the predictor is absent. Note that the values must be coded accordingly. Table 24-3 displays the following notation to assist you in calculating the *OR*, by noting which cells represent *a*, *b*, *c*, and *d*. For example, "*a*" represents the number of homeless veterans who had had one or more ED visits.

Calculation of Odds Ratio

A retrospective associational study examined the medical utilization by homeless veterans receiving treatment in a Veterans Affairs Healthcare System (LePage, Bradshaw, Cipher, Crawford, & Hooshyar, 2014). A sample of veterans seen in the Veterans Affairs North

Texas Health Care System in 2010 (*N* = 102,034) was evaluated for homelessness at any point during the year, as well as chronic medical and psychiatric diseases, and medical utilization. The two variables in this example are dichotomous: homelessness in 2010 (yes/no), and having made at least one visit to the emergency department (ED) in 2010 (yes/no). The data are presented in Table 24-4. The null hypothesis is "There is no association between homelessness and emergency department visits among veterans."

Calculation Steps

The computations for the odds ratio are as follows:

Step 1: Fit the cell values into the *OR* formula:

$$OR = \frac{ad}{bc} = \frac{(807)(84631)}{(1398)(15198)} = \frac{68297217}{21246804} = 3.21$$

$$OR = 3.21$$

Step 2: Compute the 95% confidence interval for the odds ratio. *OR* values are often accompanied by a confidence interval, which consists of a lower and upper limit value. An *OR* of 1.0 is an indication of no association between the variables (null hypothesis). In this example, the calculated OR of 3.21 will possibly allow rejection of that null hypothesis if the confidence interval around 3.21 does not include the value 1.00. As demonstrated in Chapter 22, the confidence interval for any statistic is composed of three components: [computed statistic]± *SE(t)*. To compute a 95% confidence interval for the *OR*, you must first convert the *OR* into the natural logarithm (*ln*) of the *OR*. The natural logarithm of a number *X* is the power to which *e* would have to be raised to equal *X* (where *e* is approximately 2.718288, a mathematical constant). For example, the natural logarithm of *e* itself would be 1, because $e^1 = 2.718288$.

Convert the *OR* to the *ln*(OR)

$$ln(3.21) = 1.17$$

TABLE 24-3 Notation in Cells of the Odds Ratio Table		
	≥1 ED Visit	No ED Visits
Homeless	a	b
Not Homeless	c	d

ED, Emergency department.

TABLE 24-4 Homelessness and Emergency Department Visits		
	≥1 ED Visit	No ED Visits
Homeless	807	1,398
Not Homeless	15,198	84,631

ED, Emergency department.

Step 3: Compute the standard error of $ln(OR)$:

$$SE_{ln(OR)} = \sqrt{\frac{1}{a} + \frac{1}{b} + \frac{1}{c} + \frac{1}{d}}$$

$$SE_{ln(OR)} = \sqrt{\frac{1}{807} + \frac{1}{1398} + \frac{1}{15198} + \frac{1}{84631}}$$

$$SE_{ln(OR)} = \sqrt{\frac{.001239 + .000715}{+ .0000658 + .0000118}}$$

$$SE_{ln(OR)} = 0.045$$

Step 4: Create the confidence interval (*CI*) still using the $ln(OR)$, with a *t* of 1.96

$$95\% \; CI = ln(OR) \pm SE(t)$$

$$95\% \; CI = 1.17 \pm 0.045(1.96)$$

$$[1.082, 1.258]$$

Step 5: Convert the lower and upper limits of the *CI* back to the original *OR* unit:
Place the lower limit, 1.082, as the exponent of *e*:
$e^{1.082} = \mathbf{2.95}$
Place the upper limit, 1.258, as the exponent of *e*:
$e^{1.258} = \mathbf{3.52}$

This means that the interval of 2.95 to 3.52 estimates the population *OR* with 95% confidence (Kline, 2004). Moreover, because the *CI* does not include the number 1.0, the odds ratio indicates a significant association between homelessness and ED visits.

Step 6: Interpret the directionality of the odds ratio
An *OR* of $\cong$ 1.0 indicates that exposure (to homelessness) does not affect the odds of the outcome (ED visit).
An *OR* of > 1.0 indicates that exposure (to homelessness) is associated with a higher odds of the outcome (ED visit).
An *OR* of < 1.0 indicates that exposure (to homelessness) is associated with a lower odds of the outcome (ED visit).

The *OR* for the study was 3.21, indicating that the odds of having made an ED visit among veterans who were homeless was higher than those who were not homeless. We can further note that homeless veterans were *over three times more likely, or 221% more likely to have made an emergency department visit* (LePage et al., 2014). This value was computed by subtracting 1.00

from the *OR* (3.21 − 1.00) = 2.21 × 100% = 221%. The difference between the obtained *OR* and 1.00 represents the extent of the lesser or greater likelihood of the event occurring.

The following summative statements are written in APA (2010) format, as one might read the results in an article. *An odds ratio was computed to assess the association between homelessness and emergency department visits. Homeless veterans were significantly more likely to have made an emergency department visit in 2010 than the non-homeless veterans (36.6% versus 15.2%, respectively; OR = 3.21, 95% CI [2.94, 3.51]).*

LOGISTIC REGRESSION

Logistic regression replaces linear regression when the researcher wants to test a predictor or predictors of a dichotomous dependent variable. The output yields an adjusted *OR* for each predictor, meaning that each predictor's *OR* represents the relationship between that predictor and *Y*, after adjusting for the presence of the other predictors in the model (Tabachnick & Fidell, 2006). As is the case with multiple linear regression, each predictor serves as a covariate to every other predictor in the model. In other words, when all predictors are tested simultaneously, each *b* has been adjusted for every other predictor in the regression model. Logistic regression is best conducted using a statistical software package. Full explanations and examples of the mathematical computations of logistic regression are presented in Tabachnick and Fidell (2006). A brief overview is provided in this chapter, with an example of simple logistic regression using actual clinical data.

Some common examples of dependent variables that are analyzed with logistic regression are: patient lived or died, responded or did not respond to treatment, and employed or unemployed. The logistic regression model can be considered more flexible than linear regression in the following ways:

1. Logistic regression can have continuous predictors, nominal predictors, or a combination of the two, with no assumptions regarding normality of the distribution.
2. Logistic regression can test predictors with a non-linear relationship between the predictor (independent) variable and the outcome (dependent) variable.
3. With a logistic regression model, you can compute the odds of a person's outcome. Each predictor is associated with an *OR* that represents the independent association between that predictor and the outcome (*y*) (Tabachnick & Fidell, 2006).

Because the dependent variable is either 1 or 0, logistic regression analysis produces a regression equation that yields probabilities of the outcome occurring for each person. If the predictor is continuous, we can determine the probability of the outcome occurring with a predictor score of some value x. If the predictor is dichotomous, we can determine the probability of the outcome occurring with a predictor value of "1" and a predictor value of "0."

Calculation of Logistic Regression

Because the dependent variable in logistic regression is dichotomous, the predicted $\hat{y}$ is always in the range of 0 to 1, which is interpreted as a probability. Similar to linear regression, the predicted $\hat{y}$ values are calculated from a b (or more than one b in the case of multiple predictors) and a y-intercept. In contrast to linear regression, the b and y-intercept are the exponents of the number e (2.718). An exponent of e is commonly referred to as the natural logarithm. In other words, the natural logarithm of a given number is the power to which e would have to be raised to equal that number. When the b and y-intercept serve as natural logarithms, it allows the result to yield a probability (a value between 0 and 1).

Recall the example from the homelessness and ED visits data (LePage et al., 2014). If a veteran was homeless, the probability of that veteran making at least one ED visit is calculated:

Given: For these data, $b = 1.17$, and the y-intercept (a) is -1.72.

$$\hat{Y} = \frac{e^{1.17(1)+-1.72}}{1+e^{1.17(1)+-1.72}}$$

$$\hat{Y} = \frac{e^{-0.55}}{1+e^{-0.55}} \quad \text{SO} \quad \hat{Y} = \frac{0.577}{1.577} = 0.37$$

The probability of making an ED visit if the veteran was homeless was $0.37 \times 100\%$, or 37%. The probability of making an ED visit if the veteran was *not* homeless is 15%, as shown in the next calculation. The risk of making an ED visit was greater if the veteran was homeless.

$$\hat{y} = \frac{e^{1.17(0)+-1.72}}{1+e^{1.17(0)+-1.72}}$$

$$\hat{y} = \frac{e^{-1.72}}{1+e^{-1.72}} \quad \text{SO} \quad \hat{y} = \frac{0.18}{1.18} = 0.15$$

Odds Ratio (*OR*) in Logistic Regression

Each predictor is associated with an *OR* in a logistic regression model. If the predictor is dichotomous, the

OR is interpreted as: with an x value of "yes," the odds of the outcome occurring is [*OR* value] times as likely. The homelessness and ED visits example yielded an *OR* of 3.21. As was stated previously, this *OR* indicates that homeless veterans were 3.21 times as likely to make an ED visit.

If the predictor is continuous, the *OR* is interpreted as: for every 1-unit increase in x, the odds of the outcome occurring are [*OR* value] times as likely. For example, the association between years of education and obtaining employment among persons with a spinal cord injury was investigated (Ottomanelli, Sippel, Cipher, & Goetz, 2011). The predictor was age, and the dependent variable was employment (yes/no). The *OR* was 1.10, indicating that for every year older in age, the patient was 1.10 times as likely (or 10% more likely) to have obtained employment.

In the same study, the association between being male and obtaining employment among persons with spinal cord injury was investigated (Ottomanelli et al., 2011). The predictor was being male (yes/no), and the dependent variable was employment (yes/no). The *OR* was 1.00, indicating that patients who were male were 1.00 times as likely (or just as likely) as females to have obtained employment. In other words, the likelihood of employment was equal among males and females.

COX PROPORTIONAL HAZARDS REGRESSION

When testing predictors of a dependent variable that is time-related, the appropriate statistical procedure is Cox proportional hazards regression (or Cox regression) (Hosmer, Lemeshow, & May, 2008). The dependent variable in Cox regression is called the **hazard**, a neutral word intended to describe the risk of event occurrence (e.g., risk of obtaining an illness, risk of complications from medications, or risk of relapse). The primary output in a Cox regression analysis represents the relationship between each predictor variable and the *hazard*, or rate of event occurrence.

Cox regression is a type of survival analysis that can answer questions pertaining to the amount of time that elapses until an event occurs. Examples of the types of questions that can be answered using Cox regression follow. A group of nurse practitioners begins a doctoral program. What variables predict how long it will take the students to graduate? A group of depressed adults completes a cognitive therapy program. What variables predict the time elapsed from the end of treatment until a patient's first relapse?

The major difference between using Cox regression as opposed to linear regression is the ability of survival

TABLE 24-5 Cox Proportional Hazards Regression Results of Major Adverse Cardiovascular Events in Veterans With Rheumatoid Arthritis

Predictor	Hazard Ratio (Unadjusted)	p Value	Hazard Ratio (Adjusted)*	p Value
DAS score	1.29	0.02	1.31	0.01
Age	1.01	0.62	0.99	0.83
Hypertension	2.55	0.03	2.43	0.08
Tobacco use	1.37	0.33	1.12	0.78
Diabetes	1.3	0.33	0.99	0.99
Hyperlipidemia	2.63	< 0.01	2.45	0.01
History of vascular disease	2.36	< 0.01	2.54	< 0.01
DMARD use	0.63	0.06	0.52	< 0.01
aTNF-α use	0.65	0.23	0.81	0.02
DMARD + aTNF-α use	0.68	0.34	0.82	0.83

Note: Full explanations and examples of the computations of Cox regression are presented in Hosmer, Lemeshow, & May (2008).

aTNF- , Anti–tumor necrosis factor-α medication; *DAS,* disease activity score; *DMARD,* disease-modifying antirheumatic drug.
*Adjusted for all other model predictors.
Data from Banerjee, S., Compton, A. P., Hooker, R. S., Cipher, D. J., Reimold, A., Brilakis, E. S., et al. (2008). Cardiovascular outcomes in male veterans with rheumatoid arthritis. *American Journal of Cardiology, 101*(8), 1204; and Hosmer, D. W., Lemeshow, S., & May, S. (2008). *Applied survival analysis: Regression modeling of time to event data* (2nd ed.). Hoboken, NJ: John Wiley & Sons.

analysis to handle cases where survival time is unknown. For example, in the study of treatment for streptococcal pharyngitis (strep throat), perhaps only 20% of cases relapse. The other 80% do not relapse by the end of the researcher's study. Thus, it is unknown how long it will be until the patients relapse. Survival times that are known only to exceed a certain value are called **censored data**. Censored data can also occur when a participant drops out of the study. Cox regression calculations take into account censored data when estimating the relationships between predictors and y—in contrast to linear regression analyses, which would delete or exclude those cases from analysis (Hosmer et al., 2008).

Logistic regression yields an odds ratio for each predictor that represents the association between each predictor and y, whereas Cox regression yields a **hazard ratio** (HR). An HR is interpreted almost identically to an OR with the exception that the HR represents the risk of the event occurring *sooner*.

An example of Cox regression used in clinical research is presented in Table 24-5. Predictors of major adverse cardiovascular events (MACE) in a sample of 312 veterans with rheumatoid arthritis were tested with Cox regression (Banerjee et al., 2008). There were 10 predictors of cardiovascular events tested, and the analysis yielded 10 HRs, each with a corresponding p value. As shown in Table 24-5, the disease activity score (DAS)

for extent of rheumatoid arthritis, hypertension, hyperlipidemia, and history of vascular disease were significant predictors of a cardiovascular event when each predictor was tested separately. However, when all 10 predictors were tested simultaneously, the HRs were called **adjusted hazard ratios**, which means that each HR has been adjusted for every other predictor in the regression model. The results of the adjusted HR values indicated that DAS, hyperlipidemia, history of vascular disease, disease-modifying antirheumatic drug (DMARD) use, and anti–tumor necrosis factor (anti-TNF) medication use all were significant predictors of a MACE, even after controlling for the presence of every other predictor in the model. Full explanations and examples of the computations of Cox regression are presented by Hosmer and colleagues (2008).

The findings from this study could have indications for the treatment of rheumatoid arthritis in clinical practice. Because higher levels of rheumatoid arthritis disease activity were associated with a greater likelihood of MACE, it could be that the successful control of rheumatoid arthritis symptoms might directly or indirectly reduce the risk of MACE. DMARD and anti-TNF use were associated with a lower risk of MACE, and so proper medication management of these patients might be an important factor in reducing the risk of MACE. Traditional cardiovascular risk factors studied in other populations (e.g., age, diabetes, smoking history) did not predict MACE in this sample (D'Agostino et al., 2000; Kannel, McGee, & Gordon, 1976). Therefore, male veterans with rheumatoid arthritis seem to be unique with regard to the experience of MACE and may require tailored treatment specific to their demographics to minimize cardiovascular events.

◼ KEY POINTS

- The purpose of a regression analysis is to predict or explain as much of the variance in the value of the dependent variable as possible.
- The independent (predictor) variable or variables cause variation in the value of the dependent (outcome) variable.
- Simple linear regression provides a means to estimate the value of a dependent variable based on the value of an independent variable.
- Multiple regression analysis is an extension of simple linear regression in which more than one independent variable is entered into the analysis to predict a dependent variable.
- Multicollinearity occurs when the predictors in a multiple regression equation are strongly intercorrelated and result in unstable findings.
- The odds ratio is a way of comparing whether the odds of a certain event are the same for two groups.
- Logistic regression replaces linear regression when the intent is to test a predictor or predictors of a dichotomous dependent variable.
- When testing predictors of a dependent variable that is time-related, the appropriate statistical procedure is Cox proportional hazards regression (or Cox regression).
- The hazard ratio represents the risk of the event occurring sooner than the end-time specified in the study.

REFERENCES

Aiken, L. S., & West, S. G. (1991). *Multiple regression: Testing and interpreting interactions.* Newbury Park, UK: Sage.

Allison, P. D. (1999). *Multiple regression: A primer.* Thousand Oaks, CA: Pine Forge Press.

American Psychological Association (2010). *Publication manual of the American Psychological Association* (6th ed.). Washington, DC: American Psychological Association.

Banerjee, S., Compton, A. P., Hooker, R. S., Cipher, D. J., Reimold, A., Brilakis, E. S., et al. (2008). Cardiovascular outcomes in male veterans with rheumatoid arthritis. *American Journal of Cardiology, 101*(8), 1201–1205.

Breusch, T. S., & Pagan, A. R. (1979). A simple test for heteroscedasticity and random coefficient variation. *Econometrica: Journal of the Econometric Society, 47*(5), 1287–1294.

Cohen, J. (1988). *Statistical power analysis for the behavioral sciences* (2nd ed.). New York, NY: Academic Press.

Cohen, J., & Cohen, P. (1983). *Applied multiple regression/correlation analysis for the behavioral sciences* (2nd ed.). Hillsdale, NJ: Erlbaum.

D'Agostino, R. B., Russell, M. W., Huse, D. M., Ellison, R. C., Silbershatz, H., Wilson, P. W., et al. (2000). Primary and subsequent coronary risk appraisal: New results from the Framingham Study. *American Heart Journal, 139*(2 Pt. 1), 272–281.

Gordis, L. (2014). *Epidemiology* (5th ed.). Philadelphia, PA: Saunders.

Grove, S. K., & Cipher, D. J. (2017). *Statistics for nursing research: A workbook for evidence-based practice* (2nd ed.). St. Louis, MO: Saunders.

Hosmer, D. W., Lemeshow, S., & May, S. (2008). *Applied survival analysis: Regression modeling of time to event data* (2nd ed.). Hoboken, NJ: John Wiley & Sons.

Kannel, W. B., McGee, D., & Gordon, T. (1976). A general cardiovascular risk profile: The Framingham Study. *American Journal of Cardiology, 38*(1), 46–51.

Kedika, R., Patel, M., Pena Sahdala, H. N., Mahgoub, A., Cipher, D. J., & Siddiqui, A. A. (2011). Long-term use of angiotensin converting enzyme inhibitors is associated with decreased incidence of advanced adenomatous colon polyps. *Journal of Clinical Gastroenterology, 45*(2), e12–e16.

Kline, R. B. (2004). *Beyond significance testing: Reforming data analysis methods in behavioural research.* Washington, DC: American Psychological Association.

LePage, J. P., Bradshaw, L. D., Cipher, D. J., Crawford, A. M., & Hooshyar, D. (2014). The effects of homelessness on veterans' healthcare service use: An evaluation of independence from comorbidities. *Public Health, 128*(11), 985–992.

Mancini, M. E., Ashwill, J., & Cipher, D. J. (2015). A comparative analysis of demographic and academic success characteristics of on-line and on-campus RN-to-BSN students. *Journal of Professional Nursing, 31*(1), 71–76.

Mancuso, J. M. (2010). Impact of health literacy and patient trust on glycemic control in an urban USA populations. *Nursing & Health Sciences, 12*(1), 94–104.

Ottomanelli, L., Sippel, J., Cipher, D. J., & Goetz, L. (2011). Factors associated with employment among veterans with spinal cord injury. *Journal of Vocational Rehabilitation, 34*(1), 141–150.

Stevens, J. P. (2009). *Applied multivariate statistics for the social sciences* (5th ed.). London, UK: Psychology Press.

Tabachnick, B. G., & Fidell, L. S. (2006). *Using multivariate statistics* (5th ed.). Needham Heights, MA: Allyn & Bacon.

White, H. (1980). A heteroskedasticity-consistent covariance matrix estimator and a direct test for heteroskedasticity. *Econometrica: Journal of the Econometric Society, 48*(4), 817–838.

Zar, J. H. (2010). *Biostatistical analysis* (5th ed.). Upper Saddle River, NJ: Prentice Hall.

25

Using Statistics to Determine Differences

Daisha J. Cipher

http://evolve.elsevier.com/Gray/practice/

The statistical procedures in this chapter examine differences between or among groups. Statistical procedures are available for examining difference with nominal, ordinal, and interval/ratio level data. The procedures vary considerably in their power to detect differences and in their complexity. How one interprets the results of these statistics depends on the design of the study. If the design is quasi-experimental or experimental and the study is well designed and has no major issues in regard to threats to internal and external validity, causality can be considered, and the results can be inferred or generalized to the target population. If the design is comparative descriptive, differences identified are associated only with the sample under study. The parametric statistics used to determine differences that are discussed in this chapter are the independent samples *t*-test, paired or dependent samples *t*-test, and analysis of variance (ANOVA). If the assumptions for parametric analyses are not achieved or if study data are at the ordinal level, the nonparametric analyses of Mann-Whitney *U*, Wilcoxon signed-rank test, and Kruskal-Wallis *H* are appropriate techniques to use to test the researcher's hypotheses. This chapter concludes with a discussion of the Pearson chi-square test, which is a nonparametric technique for analyzing nominal level data.

CHOOSING PARAMETRIC VERSUS NONPARAMETRIC STATISTICS TO DETERMINE DIFFERENCES

Parametric statistics are always associated with a certain set of assumptions that the data must meet; this is because the formulas of parametric statistics yield valid results only when the properties of the data are within the confines of these assumptions (Grove & Cipher, 2017; Zar, 2010). If the data do not meet the parametric assumptions, there are nonparametric alternatives that do not require those assumptions to be met, usually because nonparametric statistical procedures convert the original data to rank-ordered data.

Many statistical tests can assist the researcher in determining whether his or her data meet the assumptions for a given parametric test. The most common assumption (that accompanies all parametric tests) is that the data are normally distributed. The K^2 test and the Shapiro-Wilk test are formal tests of normality that assess whether distribution of a variable is non-normal—that is, skewed or kurtotic (see Chapter 21; D'Agostino, Belanger, & D'Agostino, 1990). The Shapiro-Wilk test is used with samples with less than 1000 subjects. When the sample is larger, the Kolmogorov-Smirnov D test is more appropriate. All of these statistics are found in mainstream statistical software packages and are accompanied by a *p* value. Significant normality tests with $p \leq 0.05$ indicate that the distribution being tested is significantly different from the normal curve, violating the normality assumption. The nonparametric statistical alternative is listed in each section in the event that the data do not meet the assumptions of each parametric test illustrated in this chapter.

t-TESTS

One of the most common parametric analyses used to test for significant differences between group means of two samples is the ***t*-test**. The **independent samples *t*-test** was developed to examine differences between two independent groups; the **paired or dependent *t*-test** was developed to examine differences between two matched or paired groups, or a comparison of two measurements in the same group. The details of the independent and paired t-tests are described in this section.

t-Test for Independent Samples

The most common parametric analysis technique used in nursing studies to test for significant differences between two independent samples is the **independent samples t-test**. The samples are independent if the study participants in one group are unrelated to or different from the participants in the second group. Use of the t-test for independent samples involves the following assumptions (Zar, 2010):

1. Sample means from the population are normally distributed.
2. The dependent or outcome variable is measured at the interval/ratio level.
3. The two samples have equal variance.
4. All observations within each sample are independent.

The t-test is robust to moderate violation of its assumptions. **Robustness** means that the results of analysis can still be relied on to be accurate when an assumption has been violated. If the dependent variable is measured with a Likert scale, and the frequency distribution is approximately normally distributed, these data are usually considered interval-level measurement and are appropriate for an independent samples t-test (de Winter & Dodou, 2010; Rasmussen, 1989). The t-test is not robust with respect to the between-samples or within-samples independence assumptions, and it is not robust with respect to an extreme violation of the normality assumption unless the sample sizes are extremely large. Sample groups do not have to be equal for this analysis—instead, the concern is for equal variance. A variety of t-tests have been developed for various types of samples. The formula and calculation of the independent samples t-test is presented next.

Calculation

The formula for the t-test is:

$$t = \frac{\bar{X}_1 - \bar{X}_2}{s_{\bar{X}_1 - \bar{X}_2}}$$

where

$\bar{X}_1$ = mean of group 1
$\bar{X}_2$ = mean of group 2
$s_{\bar{X}_1 - \bar{X}_2}$ = the standard error of the difference between the two groups.

To compute the t-test, one must compute the denominator in the formula, which is the standard error of the difference between the means. If the two groups have different sample sizes, one must use this formula:

$$s_{\bar{X}_1 - \bar{X}_2} = \sqrt{\frac{(n_1 - 1)s_1^2 + (n_2 - 1)s_2^2}{n_1 + n_2 - 2}\left(\frac{1}{n_1} + \frac{1}{n_2}\right)}$$

where

n_1 = group 1 sample size
n_2 = group 2 sample size
s_1 = group 1 variance
s_2 = group 2 variance

If the two groups have the same number of subjects in each group, one can use this simplified formula:

$$s_{\bar{X}_1 - \bar{X}_2} = \sqrt{\frac{s_1^2 + s_2^2}{n}}$$

where

n = sample size in *each* group, because this "short" formula is based on equal n per group.

A retrospective associational or correlational study was conducted to examine the medical utilization of homeless veterans receiving treatment in a Veterans Affairs healthcare system (LePage, Bradshaw, Cipher, Crawford, & Hooshyar, 2014). A sample of veterans seen in the Veterans Affairs healthcare system in 2010 ($N = 102,034$) was evaluated for homelessness at any point during the year, as well as chronic medical and psychiatric diseases, and medical utilization.

A simulated subset of data for these patients was selected for this example so that the computation would be small and manageable (Table 25-1). In actuality, studies involving t-tests need to be adequately powered to identify significant differences between groups accurately (Aberson, 2010; Cohen, 1988; Grove & Cipher, 2017). The independent variable in this example is homelessness in 2010 (yes/no), and the dependent variable is the total number of outpatient visits in 2010 (ratio scale of measurement). The null hypothesis is: *There is no difference between homeless and non-homeless veterans for the number of outpatient visits.*

The computations for the t-test are as follows:

Step 1: Compute means for both groups, which involves the sum of scores for each group divided by the number in the group.

The mean for Group 1, Homeless: $\bar{X}_1 = 24.7$
The mean for Group 2, Not Homeless: $\bar{X}_2 = 15.4$

Step 2: Compute the numerator of the t-test:

$$24.7 - 15.4 = 9.3$$

It does not matter which group is designated as "Group 1" or "Group 2." Another possible correct method for Step 2 is to subtract Group 1's mean from Group 2's mean, such as: $\overline{X}_2 - \overline{X}_1 = 15.4 - 24.7 = -9.3$ This will result in the exact same *t*-test results and interpretation for a two-tailed test, although the *t*-test value will be negative instead of positive. The sign of the *t*-test does not matter in the interpretation of the results— only the *magnitude* of the *t*-test.

Step 3: Compute the standard error of the difference

a. Compute the variances for each group
   s^2 for Group 1 = 100.68
   s^2 for Group 2 = 89.82

TABLE 25-1 Outpatient Visits by Veteran Homelessness Status

Patient Number	Homeless Veterans' Number of Outpatient Visits	Patient Number	Non-Homeless Veterans' Number of Outpatient Visits
1	36	11	28
2	18	12	33
3	23	13	3
4	15	14	9
5	28	15	13
6	40	16	16
7	18	17	22
8	38	18	10
9	15	19	12
10	16	20	8
Σ	247		154

b. Insert into the standard error of the difference formula

$$s_{\overline{X}_1 - \overline{X}_2} = \sqrt{\frac{s_1^2 + s_2^2}{n}}$$

$$s_{\overline{X}_1 - \overline{X}_2} = \sqrt{\frac{100.68 + 89.82}{10}}$$

$$s_{\overline{X}_1 - \overline{X}_2} = \sqrt{19.05}$$

$$s_{\overline{X}_1 - \overline{X}_2} = 4.36$$

Step 4: Compute *t* value:

$$t = \frac{\overline{X}_1 - \overline{X}_2}{s_{\overline{X}_1 - \overline{X}_2}}$$

$$t = \frac{9.3}{4.36}$$

$$t = 2.13$$

Step 5: Compute the degrees of freedom:

$$df = n_1 + n_2 - 2$$
$$df = 10 + 10 - 2$$
$$df = 18$$

Step 6: Locate the critical *t* value in the *t* distribution table (Appendix B) and compare it to the obtained *t* value.

The critical *t* value for a two-tailed test with 18 degrees of freedom at alpha (α) = 0.05 is 2.101, which was rounded to 2.10. This means that if we viewed the *t* distribution for $df = 18$, the middle 95% of the distribution would be delimited by −2.10 and 2.10, as shown in Figure 25-1.

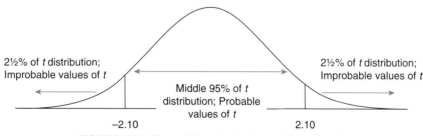

FIGURE 25-1 Probability distribution of *t* at $df = 18$.

Interpretation of Results

Our obtained t is 2.13, exceeding the critical value, which means that the t-test is *significant* and represents a real difference between the two groups. The following summative statement is written in the American Psychological Association (APA, 2010) format, as one might read the results in an article. *An independent samples t-test computed on number of outpatient visits revealed that homeless veterans had significantly higher numbers of outpatient visits in 2010 than non-homeless veterans, t (18) = 2.13, p < 0.05; $\overline{X}$ = 24.7 versus 15.4.* With additional research in this area, knowledge of housing status might assist healthcare professionals to improve the healthcare needs of homeless veterans. This knowledge could lead to the more frequent implementation of preventive and health maintenance programs for the homeless veteran population (LePage et al., 2014).

Nonparametric Alternative

If the data do not meet the assumptions involving normality or equal variances for an independent samples t-test, the nonparametric alternative is the **Mann-Whitney U test**. Mann-Whitney U calculations involve converting the data to ranks, discarding any variance or normality issues associated with the original values. In some studies, the data collected are ordinal level, and the Mann-Whitney U test is appropriate for analysis of the data. The Mann-Whitney U test is 95% as powerful as the t-test in determining differences between two groups. For a more detailed description of the Mann-Whitney U test, see the statistical textbooks by Daniel (2000) and Plichta and Kelvin (2013). The statistical workbook by Grove and Cipher (2017) has exercises for expanding your understanding of t-tests and Mann-Whitney U results from published studies.

t-Tests for Paired Samples

When samples are related, the formula used to calculate the t statistic is different from the formula previously described for independent groups. One type of **paired samples** refers to a research design that assesses the same group of people two or more times, a design commonly referred to as a **repeated measures design**. Another research design for which a paired samples t-test is appropriate is the case-control research design. **Case-control designs** involve a matching procedure whereby a control subject is matched to each case, in which the cases and controls are different people but matched demographically (Gordis, 2014). Paired or dependent samples t-tests can also be applied to a **crossover** study design, in which subjects receive one kind of treatment and subsequently receive a comparison treatment (Gliner, Morgan, & Leech, 2009; Gordis, 2014). However, similar to the independent samples t-test, this t-test requires that differences between the paired scores be independent and normally or approximately normally distributed.

Calculation

The formula for the paired samples t-test is:

$$t = \frac{\overline{D}}{s_{\overline{D}}}$$

where
$\overline{D}$ = mean difference of the paired data
$s_{\overline{D}}$ = standard error of the difference
To compute the t-test, one must compute the denominator in the formula, the standard error of the difference:

$$s_{\overline{D}} = \frac{s_D}{\sqrt{n}}$$

where
s_D = standard deviation of the differences between the paired data
n = number of subjects in the sample
Using an example from a study examining the level of functional impairment among 10 adults receiving rehabilitation for a painful injury, changes over time were investigated (Cipher, Kurian, Fulda, Snider, & Van Beest, 2007). These data are presented in Table 25-2. A

Patient Number	Baseline Functional Impairment Scores	Posttreatment Functional Impairment Scores	Difference
1	2.9	1.7	1.2
2	5.7	2.9	2.8
3	2.3	2.9	−0.6
4	3.9	3	0.9
5	3.8	3.1	0.7
6	3.3	3.2	0.1
7	2.9	3.2	−0.3
8	4.7	3.2	1.5
9	3.2	2.1	1.1
10	4.9	3.4	1.5
Σ	37.6	28.7	8.9

TABLE 25-2 Functional Impairment Levels at Baseline and After Treatment

simulated subset was selected for this example so that the computations would be small and manageable. In actuality, studies involving both independent and dependent samples *t*-tests need to be adequately powered (Aberson 2010; Cohen, 1988; Grove & Cipher, 2017).

The independent variable in this example was treatment over time, meaning that the whole sample received rehabilitation for their injury for three weeks. The dependent variable was functional impairment, which was represented by patients' scores on the Interference subscale of the Multidimensional Pain Inventory (MPI; Kerns, Turk, & Rudy, 1985), with higher scores representing more functional impairment. The null hypothesis is: *There is no reduction in functional impairment from baseline to post-treatment for patients in a rehabilitation program.*

The computations for the *t*-test are as follows:

Step 1: Compute the difference between each subject's pair of data (see last column of Table 25-2).

Step 2: Compute the mean of the difference scores, which becomes the numerator of the *t*-test:

$$\bar{D} = 0.89$$

Step 3: Compute the standard error of the difference.

a. Compute the standard deviation of the difference scores:

$$s_D = 0.99$$

b. Insert into the standard error of the difference formula:

$$s_{\bar{D}} = \frac{s_D}{\sqrt{N}}$$

$$s_{\bar{D}} = \frac{0.99}{\sqrt{10}}$$

$$s_{\bar{D}} = \frac{0.99}{3.16}$$

$$s_{\bar{D}} = 0.313$$

Step 4: Compute *t* value:

$$t = \frac{\bar{D}}{s_{\bar{D}}}$$

$$t = \frac{0.89}{0.313}$$

$$t = 2.84$$

Step 5: Compute degrees of freedom:

$$df = n - 1$$

$$df = 10 - 1$$

$$df = 9$$

Step 6: Locate the critical *t* value on the *t* distribution table in Appendix B and compare it with the obtained *t* value.

The critical *t* value for 9 degrees of freedom for a two-tailed test at alpha (α) = 0.05 is 2.262 rounded to 2.26. Our obtained *t* is 2.84, exceeding the critical value (see *t* Table in Appendix B). This means that if we viewed the *t* distribution for *df* = 9, the middle 95% of the distribution would be delimited by −2.26 and 2.26.

Interpretation of Results

Our obtained *t* = 2.84 exceeds the critical *t* value in the table, which means that the *t*-test is statistically significant and represents a real difference between participants' pre-intervention and post-intervention functional impairment scores. The following summative statement is written in APA (2010) format, as one might read the results in an article. *A paired samples t-test computed on MPI functional impairment scores revealed that the patients undergoing rehabilitation had significantly lower functional impairment levels from baseline to post-treatment, t(9) = 2.84, p < 0.05; $\bar{X}$ = 3.8 versus 2.9.* During the 3-week rehabilitation program, patients successfully reduced their functional impairment levels. After additional research in this area, this knowledge might be used to facilitate evidence-based practice interventions in rehabilitation facilities to improve patients' functional status (Melnyk & Fineout-Overholt, 2015).

Nonparametric Alternative

If the interval/ratio level data do not meet the normality assumptions for a paired samples *t*-test, the nonparametric alternative is the **Wilcoxon signed-rank test**. The Wilcoxon signed-rank test calculations involve converting the data to ranks, discarding any variance or normality issues associated with the original values. This analysis technique is also appropriate when the study data are ordinal level, such as self-care abilities identified as low, moderate, and high based on the Orem Self-Care Model (Orem, 2001). This test is thoroughly addressed by Daniel (2000) and Plichta and Kelvin (2013) in their statistical textbooks. The statistical workbook for nursing research by Grove and Cipher (2017) has an exercise for expanding your understanding of the Wilcoxon signed-rank results from published studies.

ONE-WAY ANALYSIS OF VARIANCE

Analysis of variance (**ANOVA**) is a statistical procedure that compares data between two or more groups or conditions to investigate the presence of differences between those groups on some continuous dependent variable. In this chapter, we will focus on the *one-way ANOVA*, which involves testing one independent variable and one dependent variable (as opposed to other types of ANOVAs such as factorial ANOVAs that incorporate multiple independent variables).

Why ANOVA and not a *t*-test? Remember that a *t*-test is formulated to compare two sets of data or two groups at one time. Thus, data generated from a clinical trial that involves four experimental groups, Treatment 1, Treatment 2, Treatment 1 & 2 combined, and a Control, would require six *t*-tests. Consequently, the chance of making a Type I error (alpha error) increases substantially (or is inflated) because so many computations are being performed. Specifically, the chance of making a Type I error is the number of comparisons multiplied by the alpha level. Thus, ANOVA is the recommended statistical technique for examining differences between more than two groups (Zar, 2010).

ANOVA is a procedure that culminates in a statistic called the **F statistic**. This value is compared against an F distribution (see Appendix D) to determine whether the groups significantly differ from one another on the dependent variable studied. The basic formula for the F is:

$$F = \frac{\text{Mean square between groups}}{\text{Mean square within groups}}$$

The term *mean square* (MS) is used interchangeably with the word "variance." The formulas for ANOVA compute two estimates of variance: the between-groups variance and the within-groups variance. The **between-groups variance** represents differences between the groups or conditions being compared, and the **within-groups variance** represents differences among (within) each group's data.

Calculation

A randomized experimental study examined the impact of a special type of vocational rehabilitation on employment variables among spinal cord–injured veterans, in which posttreatment hours worked were examined (Ottomanelli et al., 2012). Participants were randomized to receive supported employment or standard care. A third group, also a standard care group, consisted of a non-randomized observational group of participants. Supported employment (SE) refers to a type of specialized interdisciplinary vocational rehabilitation designed to help people with disabilities obtain and maintain community-based competitive employment in their chosen occupation (Bond, 2004). Standard care (named "treatment as usual" in the study, or TAU) consisted of referral to a vocation rehabilitation provider outside Veterans Affairs, which the veteran may or may not have pursued.

The independent variable in this example is treatment group (SE, TAU randomized, and TAU observational/not randomized), and the dependent variable is the number of hours worked posttreatment. The null hypothesis is: *There is no difference between the treatment groups and the control group in posttreatment number of hours worked among veterans with spinal cord injuries.* A simulated subset was selected for this example so that the computations would be small and manageable (Table 25-3). In actuality, studies involving ANOVA must be adequately powered to detect differences accurately among study groups (Aberson 2010; Cohen, 1988; Grove & Cipher, 2017).

TABLE 25-3 Posttreatment Employment Hours Worked by Treatment Group

Participant Number	TAU Observational	Participant Number	TAU Randomized	Participant Number	Supported Employment
1	8	6	15	11	25
2	9	7	18	12	28
3	15	8	9	13	35
4	17	9	18	14	30
5	24	10	16	15	15
Σ	73		76		133
Grand total (G)					282

TAU, treatment as usual.

The steps to perform an ANOVA are as follows:

Step 1: Compute correction term, C.

$$C = \frac{G^2}{N}$$

Square the grand sum (G), and divide by total N:

$$C = \frac{282^2}{15} = 5301.60$$

Step 2: Compute total sum of squares.

$$\left(\Sigma X^2\right) - C$$

Square every value in data set, sum, and subtract C:

$$(8^2 + 9^2 + 15^2 + 17^2 + 24^2 + 15^2 + 18^2 \ldots + 15^2)$$
$$- 5301.6 = 6204 - 5301.6 = 902.4$$

Step 3: Compute between groups sum of squares.

$$\Sigma \frac{\left(\Sigma X_{group}\right)^2}{n} - C$$

Square the sum of each column and divide by N. Add each, and then subtract C.

$$\frac{73^2}{5} + \frac{76^2}{5} + \frac{133^2}{5} - 5301.6$$

$$(1065.8 + 1155.2 + 3537.8) - 5301.6 = 457.2$$

Step 4: Compute within groups sum of squares.

$$SS_{within} = SS_{total} - SS_{between}$$

Subtract the between groups sum of squares (Step 3) from total sum of squares (Step 2).

$$902.4 - 457.2 = 445.2$$

Step 5: Create an ANOVA summary table similar to Table 25-4.

a. Insert the sum of squares values in the first column.

b. The degrees of freedom are in the second column. Because the F is a ratio of two separate statistics (mean square between groups and mean square

TABLE 25-4 Analysis of Variance Summary Table

Source of Variation	SS	df	MS	F
Between groups	457.2	2	228.6	6.16
Within groups	445.2	12	37.1	
Total	902.4	14		

within groups) both have different df formulas—one for the "numerator" and one for the "denominator":
Mean square between groups df = number of groups − 1
Mean square within groups $df = N$ − number of groups
For this example, the df for the numerator is 3 − 1 = 2. The df for the denominator is 15 − 3 = 12.

c. The mean square between groups and mean square within groups are in the third column in Table 25-4. These values are computed by dividing the SS by the df. Therefore, the MS between = 457.2 ÷ 2 = 228.6. The MS within = 445.2 ÷ 12 = 37.1.

d. The F is the final column and is computed by dividing the MS between by the MS within. Therefore, $F = 228.6 ÷ 37.1 = 6.16$.

Step 6: Locate the critical F value on the F distribution table (see Appendix D) and compare the obtained F value with it. The critical F value for 2 and 12 df at alpha (α) = 0.05 is 3.89. Our obtained F is 6.16, which exceeds the critical value.

Interpretation of Results

The obtained $F = 6.16$ exceeds the critical value in the table, which means that the F is statistically significant and that the population means are not equal. We can reject our null hypothesis that the three groups have the same number of hours worked posttreatment. However, the F does not tell us which treatment groups differ from one another. Further testing, termed *multiple comparison tests* or *post hoc tests*, are required to complete the ANOVA process and determine all of the significant differences among the study groups.

Post hoc tests have been developed specifically to determine the location of group differences after ANOVA is performed on data from more than two groups. For example, is the significant difference between SE and TAU randomized, between SE and TAU observational, or between TAU randomized and TAU observational? These tests were developed to reduce the incidence of a Type I error. Frequently used post hoc tests are the Tukey Honestly Significant Difference (HSD) test, the Newman-Keuls test, the Scheffé test, and the Dunnett test (Plichta & Kelvin, 2013). When these tests are calculated, the alpha level is reduced in proportion to the number of additional tests required to locate statistically significant differences. For example, for several of the aforementioned post hoc tests, if many groups' mean values are being compared, the magnitude of the difference is set higher than if only two groups are being compared. Post hoc tests are tedious to perform by hand and are best handled with statistical computer software programs. The statistical workbook for nursing research by Grove and Cipher (2017) has exercises for expanding your interpretation and understanding of ANOVA and post hoc procedure results from published studies.

The following summative statements are written in APA (2010) format, as one might read the results in an article. The Tukey Honestly Significant post hoc test is reported here as an example of how to write the results of a post hoc test. *Analysis of variance performed on employment hours revealed significant differences between the three treatment groups, F (2, 12) = 6.16, p < 0.05. Post hoc comparisons using the Tukey HSD comparison test indicated that the veterans in the SE group worked significantly more hours than the veterans in both the TAU observational group and the TAU randomized group ($\overline{X}$ = 26.26 versus 14.6 and 15.2, respectively). There were no significant differences in the hours worked between the TAU observational group and the TAU randomized group.* Thus, the particular type of vocational rehabilitation approach implemented to increase the work activity of spinal cord injured veterans appeared to have been more effective than standard practice.

Nonparametric Alternative

If the data do not meet the normality assumptions for an ANOVA, the nonparametric alternative is the Kruskal-Wallis test. Calculations for the Kruskal-Wallis test involve converting the data to ranks, discarding any variance or normality issues associated with the original values. Similar to the ANOVA, the **Kruskal-Wallis test** is a nonparametric analysis technique that can accommodate the comparisons of more than two groups. This test is thoroughly addressed in textbooks by Daniel (2000) and Plichta and Kelvin (2013).

Other ANOVA Procedures

There are other kinds of ANOVA that accommodate other research designs involving various numbers of

independent and dependent variables, such as factorial ANOVA, repeated measures ANOVA, and mixed factorial ANOVA. These ANOVA procedures are presented and explained in comprehensive statistics textbooks such as Zar's text (2010).

PEARSON CHI-SQUARE TEST

The chi-square (χ^2) test compares differences in proportions of nominal level variables. When a study requires that researchers compare proportions (percentages) in one category versus another category, the χ^2 is a statistic that reveals whether the difference in proportion is statistically improbable. The χ^2 has its own theoretical distribution and associated χ^2 table (see Appendix E).

A **one-way chi-square** is a statistic that compares different levels of one variable only. For example, a researcher may collect information on gender and compare the proportions of males to females. If the one-way chi-square is statistically significant, it would indicate that the difference in gender proportions was significantly greater than what would be expected by chance (Daniel, 2000).

A **two-way chi-square** is a statistic that tests whether proportions in levels of one variable are significantly different from proportions of the second variable. For example, the presence of advanced colon polyps was studied in three groups of patients: patients having a normal body mass index (BMI), patients who were overweight, and patients who were obese (Siddiqui et al., 2009). The research question tested was: *Is there a significant difference between the three groups (normal, overweight, and obese) in the presence of advanced colon polyps?* The results of the chi-square analysis indicated that a larger proportion of obese patients fell into the category of having advanced colon polyps compared with normal-weight and overweight patients, suggesting that obesity may be a risk factor for developing advanced colon polyps.

Assumptions

The use of the Pearson chi-square involves the following assumptions (Daniel, 2000):

1. Only one datum entry is made for each subject in the sample. Therefore, if repeated measures from the same subject are being used for analysis, such as pretests and posttests, a chi-square is not an appropriate test (the **McNemar test** is the appropriate test; Daniel, 2000).
2. The variables must be categorical (nominal), either inherently or transformed to categorical from ordinal, interval, or ratio values. For example,

body mass index values might be categorized into normal and overweight.

3. For each variable, the categories are mutually exclusive and exhaustive. No cells may have an *expected* frequency of zero. In the actual data, the *observed* cell frequency may be zero. However, the Pearson chi-square test is not sensitive to small sample sizes, and other tests such as the Fisher's exact test are more appropriate when testing very small samples (Daniel, 2000; Yates, 1934).

The test is distribution-free, or nonparametric, which means that no assumption has been made for a normal distribution of values in the population from which the sample was taken (Daniel, 2000).

The formula for a two-way chi-square is:

$$\chi^2 = \frac{n[(A)(D) - (B)(C)]^2}{(A+B)(C+D)(A+C)(B+D)}$$

A **contingency table** is a table that displays the relationship between two or more categorical variables (Daniel, 2000). The contingency table is labeled as follows:

A	B
C	D

With any chi-square analysis, the degrees of freedom (*df*) must be calculated to determine the significance of the value of the statistic. The following formula is used for this calculation:

$$df = (R-1)(C-1)$$

where
R = Number of rows
C = Number of columns

Calculation

A retrospective comparative study examined whether longer antibiotic treatment courses were associated with increased antimicrobial resistance in patients with spinal cord injury (Lee et al., 2014). Using urine cultures from a sample of spinal cord injured veterans, two groups were created: those with evidence of antibiotic resistance, and those with no evidence of antibiotic resistance. All veterans were divided into two groups based on having had a history of recent (in the last six months) antibiotic use for more than two weeks, or no history of recent antibiotic use for more than two weeks.

The data are presented in Table 25-5. The null hypothesis is: *There is no difference between antibiotic*

TABLE 25-5 Antibiotic Use and Antibiotic Resistance in Veterans With Spinal Cord Injuries

	Antibiotic Use	No Recent Antibiotic Use	Total
Antibiotic Resistance	8	7	15
No Antibiotic Resistance	6	21	27
Total	14	28	Grand Total = 42

users and non-users on the presence of antibiotic resistance.

The computations for the Pearson chi-square test are as follows:

Step 1: Create contingency table of the two nominal variables (see Table 25-5).

Step 2: Fit the cells into the formula:

$$\chi^2 = \frac{n[(A)(D) - (B)(C)]^2}{(A+B)(C+D)(A+C)(B+D)}$$

$$\chi^2 = \frac{42[(8)(21) - (7)(6)]^2}{(8+7)(6+21)(8+6)(7+21)}$$

$$\chi^2 = \frac{42[126]^2}{(15)(27)(14)(28)}$$

$$\chi^2 = \frac{666792}{158760}$$

$$\chi^2 = 4.20$$

Step 3: Compute the degrees of freedom:

$$df = (2-1)(2-1) = 1$$

Step 4: Locate the critical χ^2 value in the χ^2 distribution table in Appendix E and compare it to the obtained χ^2 value.

The chi-square table in Appendix E includes the critical values of chi-square for specific degrees of freedom at selected levels of significance. The obtained χ^2 value is compared with the table's χ^2 values. If the value of the statistic is equal to or greater than the value identified in the chi-square table, the difference between the two variables is statistically significant. The critical χ^2 for *df*

= 1 is 3.8415 rounded to 3.84, and our obtained χ^2 is 4.20, thereby exceeding the critical value and indicating a significant difference between antibiotic users and non-users on the presence of antibiotic resistance.

Furthermore, we can compute the rates of antibiotic resistance among antibiotic users and non-users by using the numbers in the contingency Table 25-5 from Step 1. The antibiotic resistance rate among the antibiotic users can be calculated as: $8 \div 14 = 0.571 \times 100\% = 57.1\%$. The antibiotic resistance rate among the non-antibiotic users can be calculated as: $7 \div 28 = 0.25 \times 100\% = 25\%$.

Interpretation of Results

The following summative statement is written in APA (2010) format, as one might read the results in an article. *A Pearson chi-square analysis indicated that two-week antibiotic users had significantly higher rates of antibiotic resistance than those who had not recently used antibiotics, $\chi^2(1) = 4.20$, $p < 0.05$ (57.1% versus 25%, respectively).* This finding suggests that extended antibiotic use may be a risk factor for developing resistance in spinal cord injured patients, and further research is needed to investigate resistance as a direct effect of antibiotics.

▌ KEY POINTS

- Parametric statistics used to determine differences are accompanied by certain assumptions, and the data must be tested for whether they meet those assumptions before computing the statistic.
- Many tests of normality can assist the researcher in determining the suitability of the data for the use of parametric statistics.
- In the event that the data do not meet the assumptions of the parametric statistic, there are nonparametric alternatives that do not adhere to the assumptions of the parametric test.
- The *t*-test is one of the most commonly used parametric analyses to test for significant differences between statistical measures of two samples or groups.
- The independent samples *t*-test indicates a difference between two groups of subjects, whereas the paired samples *t*-test indicates a difference in two assessments of the same subjects or two groups matched on selected variables.
- The Mann-Whitney *U* test is the nonparametric alternative to the independent samples *t*-test when the study data violate one or more of the independent samples *t*-test assumptions.

- The Wilcoxon signed-rank test is the nonparametric alternative to the paired or dependent samples *t*-test when the study data violate one or more of the paired samples *t*-test assumptions.
- A one-way ANOVA can be used to examine data from two or more groups and compares the variance within each group with the variance between groups.
- A one-way ANOVA conducted on three or more groups that yields a significant result requires the use of post hoc analysis procedures for determining the location of group differences.
- The Kruskal-Wallis test is the nonparametric alternative to the ANOVA when the study data violate one or more of the ANOVA assumptions.
- The chi-square test compares proportions (percentages) in one category of a variable of interest with proportions in another category.
- The McNemar test is the appropriate statistical test to use when analyzing nominal level data obtained from repeated measures from the same subject, such as pretests and posttests.

REFERENCES

Aberson, C. L. (2010). *Applied power analysis for the behavioral sciences*. New York, NY: Routledge.

American Psychological Association (APA). (2010). *Publication Manual of the American Psychological Association* (6th ed.). Washington, DC: American Psychological Association.

Bond, G. R. (2004). Supported employment: Evidence for an evidence based practice. *Psychiatric Rehabilitation Journal, 27*(4), 345–359.

Cipher, D. J., Kurian, A. K., Fulda, K. G., Snider, R., & Van Beest, J. (2007). Using the MBMD to delineate treatment outcomes in rehabilitation. *Journal of Clinical Psychology in Medical Settings, 14*(2), 102–112.

Cohen, J. (1988). *Statistical power analysis for the behavioral sciences* (2nd ed.). New York: Academic Press.

D'Agostino, R. B., Belanger, A., & D'Agostino, R. B., Jr. (1990). A suggestion for using powerful and informative tests of normality. *The American Statistician, 44*(4), 316–321.

Daniel, W. W. (2000). *Applied nonparametric statistics* (2nd ed.). Pacific Grove, CA: Duxbury Press.

de Winter, J. C. F., & Dodou, D. (2010). Five-point Likert items: *t*-test versus Mann-Whitney-Wilcoxon. *Practical Assessment, Research, and Evaluation, 15*(11), 1–16.

Gliner, J. A., Morgan, G. A., & Leech, N. L. (2009). *Research methods in applied settings* (2nd ed.). New York, NY: Routledge.

Gordis, L. (2014). *Epidemiology* (5th ed.). Philadelphia, PA: Saunders.

Grove, S. K., & Cipher, D. J. (2017). *Statistics for nursing research: A workbook for evidence-based practice* (2nd ed.). St. Louis, MO: Saunders.

Kerns, R. D., Turk, D. C., & Rudy, T. E. (1985). The West-Haven Yale Multidimensional Pain Inventory (WHYMPI). *Pain, 23*(4), 345–356.

Lee, Y. R., Tashjian, C. A., Brouse, S. D., Bedimo, R. J., Goetz, L. L., Cipher, D. J., et al. (2014). Antibiotic therapy and bacterial resistance in patients with spinal cord injury. *Federal Practitioner, 31*(3), 13–17.

LePage, J. P., Bradshaw, L. D., Cipher, D. J., Crawford, A. M., & Hooshyar, D. (2014). The effects of homelessness on veterans' healthcare service use: An evaluation of independence from comorbidities. *Public Health, 128*(11), 985–992.

Melnyk, B. M., & Fineout-Overholt, E. (2015). *Evidence-based practice in nursing & healthcare: A guide to best practice* (3rd ed.). Philadelphia, PA: Lippincott Williams & Wilkins.

Orem, D. E. (2001). *Nursing: concepts of practice* (6th ed.). St. Louis, MO: Mosby.

Ottomanelli, L., Goetz, L. L., Suris, A., McGeough, C., Sinnott, P. L., Toscano, R., et al. (2012). The effectiveness of supported employment for veterans with spinal cord injuries: Results from a randomized multi-site study. *Archives of Physical Medicine and Rehabilitation, 93*(5), 740–747.

Plichta, S. B., & Kelvin, E. (2013). *Munro's statistical methods for health care research* (6th ed.). Philadelphia, PA: Wolters Kluwer/Lippincott Williams & Wilkins.

Rasmussen, J. L. (1989). Analysis of Likert-scale data: A reinterpretation of Gregoire and Driver. *Psychological Bulletin, 105*(1), 167–170.

Siddiqui, A. A., Nazario, H., Mahgoub, A., Pandove, S., Cipher, D. J., & Spechler, S. J. (2009). Obesity is associated with an increased prevalence of advanced adenomatous colon polyps in a male veteran population. *Digestive Disease & Sciences, 54*(7), 1560–1564.

Yates, F. (1934). Contingency tables involving small numbers and the χ^2 test. *Journal of Royal Statistical Society, 1*(2), 217–235.

Zar, J. H. (2010). *Biostatistical analysis* (5th ed.). Upper Saddle River, NJ: Prentice-Hall.

Interpreting Research Outcomes

Jennifer R. Gray

http://evolve.elsevier.com/Gray/practice/

When data analysis is complete, there is a feeling that the answers are known and the study is finished. However, there remains the need to finish the process by interpreting results of statistical and qualitative analyses. Even a first-time researcher amasses considerable knowledge of the problem area, related literature, potential applications, and needs of the discipline, and may have a beginning understanding of what the study signifies and the extent to which the findings can be generalized. Because of all the preparation that went into the study, the researcher is very knowledgeable in this particular area of inquiry. For masters and doctoral students, aside from the thesis or dissertation committee members, hardly anyone understands all that the researcher understands. Healthcare professionals, in general, represent the primary audience for the results of the research, either through presentation or publication. So before dissemination, the results must be explained, so that others will understand their significance. This detailed explanation is called **interpretation of research outcomes.**

Interpretation of research outcomes requires reflection upon three general aspects of the research and their interactions: the primary findings, validity issues, and the resultant body of knowledge in the area of investigation. These issues will determine how the researcher writes the Discussion section of the research report, presenting the findings, limitations, conclusions, generalizations, usefulness of the research, and recommendations for subsequent inquiry in the area. There is a tendency to rush the interpretation of the findings, but it is not a step to be minimized or hurried. The process takes time for reflection. The researchers may need to step back from the details of the study and reexamine the big picture. The researcher must consider these

dispassionately, as if another person had conducted the study: possessive ownership does not assist the process. Discussion with others in the field such as fellow healthcare workers, and with peers and other academically based persons and mentors, is helpful as well. How do they view the study, in relation to the area of inquiry? What do they envision for application potential, either now or with subsequent research that builds upon this and other studies?

This chapter focuses on the interpretation of outcomes from quantitative and outcomes research. Interpretations of results for qualitative research are presented in Chapter 12. The process of interpreting quantitative research findings includes several steps (Box 26-1). Incorporated into the explanation of each of these steps are examples from a quantitative correlational study conducted by Lambert et al. (2015).

EXAMPLE STUDY

Lambert and colleagues (2015) determined there was a need for their study by comparing HIV-infected women with the general population. When compared to the general population, HIV-infected women are five times more likely to develop cervical cancer in their lifetimes, usually caused by a secondary infection with human papillomavirus (HPV) due to their immunosuppression.

The purpose of this study was to "evaluate the relationships between Pap test adherence during the previous year and the following variables: HPV and cervical cancer knowledge, and perceived susceptibility, perceived seriousness, perceived barriers, perceived benefits, and perceived self-efficacy." (Lambert et al., 2015, p. 272)

Previous research had focused on perceived susceptibility and perceived seriousness in other female populations, but not women with HIV infection. To address this knowledge gap, Lambert et al. (2015) placed their study within the framework of the Health Belief Model (HBM) (Rosenstock, Stretcher, & Becker, 1988). Among the instruments they selected were two they used, Champion's Health Belief Model (CHBM) and the Self-Efficacy Scale (CSE), to measure five concepts of the HBM (Table 26-1). Example quotes from the Lambert et al. (2015) study are presented in the following sections, focusing on identification of study findings, limitations, conclusions, generalizations, implications for nursing, and recommendations for further study.

IDENTIFICATION OF STUDY FINDINGS

The first step the researcher makes in interpretation is examination of the results of the study, and then phrasing those results as language instead of statistical test printouts. Evaluating evidence, translating the study results, and interpreting them provide the basis for developing the **findings**. Although much of the process of developing findings from results occurs in the mind of the researcher, evidence of such thinking can be found in published research reports (Pyrczak & Bruce, 2005). As noted earlier, it is important during this process to talk with colleagues or mentors to clarify meanings or expand implications of the research findings. The study results and findings are presented for the study conducted by Lambert and colleagues (2015). As is common practice, the researchers began the results section by describing the participants of the study.

BOX 26-1 The Process of Interpreting Quantitative Research Outcomes

1. Examine the evidence and identify study findings.
2. Identify limitations through examination of design validity.
3. Generalize the findings in light of the limitations.
4. Consider implications for practice, theory, and knowledge.
5. Suggest further research.
6. Form final conclusions.

TABLE 26-1 Summary of Study Measures and Scoring

Variable	Measure
Pap testing	Self-report of when last Pap test occurred.
Perceived susceptibility	Perceived susceptibility subscale of Champion's Health Belief Model Scale, comprised of four questions. Response set from "strongly agree" to "strongly disagree" (5-point Likert scale). Range is 4 to 20.
Perceived seriousness (severity)	Perceived seriousness subscale of Champion's Health Belief Model Scale, comprised of seven questions. Response set from "strongly agree" to "strongly disagree" (5-point Likert scale). Range is 7 to 35.
Perceived benefits	Perceived benefits subscale of Champion's Health Belief Model Scale, comprised of four questions. Response set from "strongly agree" to "strongly disagree" (5-point Likert scale). Range is 4 to 20.
Perceived barriers	Perceived barriers subscale of Champion's Health Belief Model Scale, comprised of 14 items. Response set from "strongly agree" to "strongly disagree" (5-point Likert scale). Range is 14 to 70.
Self-efficacy	Champion's Self-Efficacy (CSE) Scale consisting of 10 questions. Response set from "strongly agree" to "strongly disagree" (5-point Likert scale). Higher score is interpreted as higher confidence (Champion, Skinner, & Menon, 2005).
Knowledge of HPV and cervical cancer	Selected questions from Ingledue, Cottrell, and Benard's (2004) questionnaire with 40 questions; 15 multiple-choice questions selected specific to HPV and cervical cancer knowledge. One correct answer per question. Each correct question counted as 1 point. Scores range from 0 to 15. Higher scores = greater knowledge.

Data from Lambert, C., Chandler, R., McMillan, S., Kromrey, J., Johnson-Mallard, V., & Kurtyka, D. (2015). Pap test adherence, cervical cancer perceptions, and HPV knowledge among HIV-infected women in a community health setting. *Journal of the Association of Nurses in AIDS Care, 26*(3), 271-280.

"Descriptive

The sample consisted of 300 participants who were recruited from two (one rural and the other metropolitan) ambulatory HIV care clinics in Florida. Participants reported their race as Black/African American (68%), Hispanic-Latina (14%), Caucasian (16.3%), or other (1.7%). The women reported their levels of education as high school or vocational education (50.3%), less than a high school education (33%), or college educated (16.7%). The participants' ages ranged from 18 to 70 years, with a mean age of 45.4 (SD = 11).... Seventy-five percent of the women reported having a Pap test during the previous year; however, according to the medical record, approximately 44% of the women had had a Pap test at the clinic during the previous year. One reason for the reported and observed differences in Pap test utilization could be that some of the participants had received Pap testing from an outside health care provider." (Lambert et al., 2015, p. 275)

TABLE 26-2   **Means and Standard Deviation for Subscales and Age**

Variables	Range	Mean	Standard Deviation
Age	18-70	45.40	11.00
Perceived susceptibility	4-20	9.59	4.06
Perceived benefits	4-20	15.93	3.20
Perceived seriousness	7-35	20.88	6.12
Perceived self-efficacy	10-50	40.22	6.98
Perceived barriers	14-56	29.16	9.09
Knowledge	0-14	6.02	3.59

Note: n = 300.
From Lambert, C., Chandler, R., McMillan, S., Kromrey, J., Johnson-Mallard, V., & Kurtyka, D. (2015). Pap test adherence, cervical cancer perceptions, and HPV knowledge among HIV-infected women in a community health setting. *Journal of the Association of Nurses in AIDS Care, 26*(3), 271-280.

In the results section, Lambert et al. (2015) also provided the results of the descriptive statistics for the primary variables. Table 26-2 contains these results. The researchers also provided some interpretation of whether the scores were low or high and possible reasons.

"The constructs of HBM were evaluated using several subscales.... Perceived susceptibility scores were low, indicating that, on average, the women did not perceive that they were susceptible to cervical cancer ... women in this study did not perceive that cervical cancer was serious.... Perceived benefits scores were high, indicating that women in our study perceived Pap testing as beneficial.... Perceived barriers scores were low, indicating that the women did not perceive barriers to obtaining Pap testing.... Knowledge scores were low, indicating that the women were not aware of risk factors for HPV and cervical cancer...." (Lambert et al., 2015, p. 275)

After describing the sample and the primary variables, the researcher considers the statistical output relative to the hypotheses.

Data Analysis Results for Hypotheses

Interpretation of results for each research hypothesis yields five possible results: (1) significant results that are in keeping with the results predicted by the researcher; (2) nonsignificant results; (3) significant results that oppose the results predicted by the researcher, some-

times referred to as "unexpected" results; (4) mixed results; and (5) serendipitous results (Shadish, Cook, & Campbell, 2002). Table 26-3 provides a listing of possible results with a published example of each.

Significant and Predicted Results

Significant results that coincide with the researcher's predictions validate the proposed logical links among the elements of a study. These results support the logical links developed by the researcher among the purpose, framework, questions, variables, and measurement methods (Shadish et al., 2002). Although this outcome is very gratifying, the researcher needs to consider alternative explanations for the positive findings. What other elements could possibly have led to the significant results? Are the statistically significant results meaningful? Sometimes with very large sample sizes, a result will be statistically significant but the effect size may be very small, or the result may lack clinical significance (O'Halloran, 2013).

Nonsignificant Results

Unpredicted **nonsignificant** or inconclusive **results** are often referred to as **negative results**. The negative results could be a true reflection of reality (Teixeira da Silva, 2015). In this case, the reasoning of the researcher or the theory used by the researcher to develop the hypothesis is in error, but the study was scientifically sound. If so, the negative findings are an important addition to the body of knowledge. Negative results could help refine the hypotheses for a subsequent study.

TABLE 26-3 Interpretation of Results for Hypothesis Testing

Result	Example
Significant, predicted results	Perceived barriers to having a Pap test were lower in women who reported a Pap test in the past year when compared to women who did not report having had a Pap test in the past year (Lambert et al., 2015).
Nonsignificant results	"No significant differences were found between participants on the subscale variables of knowledge, perceived susceptibility, perceived seriousness, and perceived benefits" (Lambert et al., 2015, p. 276).
Significant results but opposite of predictions (unexpected)	Because cervical cancer mortality was higher among African American women in Tuscaloosa County, AL, Morrison, Moody, and Shelton (2010) hypothesized that they had lower rates of screening for cervical cancer than did white women. They instead found that African American women had significantly higher rates of screening than white women.
Mixed results	The age of internationally educated nurses was consistently correlated with interpersonal skills, but other demographic characteristics produced mixed results (Shen, Xu, Staples, & Bolstad, 2014). "Explanations for these observed differences are unclear" (Shen et al., 2014, p. 177).
Serendipitous results	Keough, Schlomer, and Bollenberg (2003) surveyed emergency department nurses about their educational needs. The researchers added an open-ended question to explore the issues and challenges experienced by the nurses in the ED. Their reasoning was that understanding these challenges would allow them to better meet the nurses' educational needs. The researchers identified their serendipitous findings to be that nurses were extremely frustrated and overburdened. The nurses identified their "greatest concerns: (1) insufficient, inexperienced staff; (2) increased responsibilities; (3) lack of administrative support; (4) lack of rewards or incentives to stay; (5) low morale among staff; (6) difficulty balancing work and family; and (7) increasing violence in the emergency department" (Keough et al., 2003, p. 17).

With nonsignificant results, it is important to determine whether adequate power of 0.8 or higher was achieved for the data analysis. The researcher needs to conduct a power analysis to determine whether the sample size was adequate to prevent the risk of a Type II error (Aberson, 2010; O'Halloran, 2013; Shadish et al., 2002). A Type II error means that in reality the findings were significant, but because sample size was inadequate, statistical tests failed to show significance.

Negative results could also be due to poor operationalization of variables, a confounding variable, a sample that was inexplicably nonrepresentative, uncontrolled-for and unmeasured extraneous variables, use of inappropriate statistical techniques, or faulty analysis. Unless these weak links are detected, the reported results could lead to faulty information in the body of knowledge (Teixeira da Silva, 2015). Negative results, to reiterate, do not mean that there are no relationships among the variables or differences between groups; they indicate that the study failed to find any relationships or differences.

Significant and Not Predicted Results

Significant results that are the opposite of those predicted, if the results are valid, are an important addition to the body of knowledge. These are sometimes referred to as "unexpected results." An example would be a study in which the researchers proposed that social support and ego strength were positively related. If the study showed that high social support was related to low ego strength, the result would be the opposite of that predicted. Such results, when verified by other studies, indicate that the theory being tested needs modification and refinement. Because these types of studies can affect nursing practice, this information is important.

Mixed Results

Mixed results are probably the most common outcome of studies that examine more than one relationship. In this case, one variable may uphold the characteristics predicted, whereas another does not, or two dependent measures of the same variable may show opposite results. Each result should be considered individually for interpretation.

Serendipitous Results

Serendipitous results are discoveries or researcher observations that were not the focus of the study. Most researchers examine as many elements of data as possible in addition to the elements directed by the research objectives, questions, or hypotheses. In doing so, they sometimes discover a relationship or variable distribution heretofore unearthed. Serendipitous results should be reported because they are legitimate discoveries of the study.

Lambert et al. (2015) presented their results in the usual order, with description of the sample and primary variables followed by results of analyses relative to the research questions or hypotheses. The discussion for a descriptive study includes only descriptive results, but with other designs, both descriptive and inferential results are discussed, both statistically significant and not. Lambert et al. (2015) reported results of correlational testing, statistically significant and nonsignificant. One of the purposes of the study was to evaluate the relationships among the HBM variables, knowledge, and whether the woman had had a Pap test within the stipulated time. They included results of the analysis using Pearson correlation coefficients in the narrative, indicating those that were significant and what the relationship meant. The presentation of these results would have been clearer in a correlation table, but the journal may have limited the number of tables per article. Because of multiple analyses, the researchers used tables to present other results.

"Statistically significant correlations existed between knowledge and perceived self-efficacy, r (300) = .30, $p < .01$; knowledge and perceived barriers, r (300) = −.18, $p < .01$; and knowledge and perceived benefits, r (300) = .16, $p < .01$. As perceived seriousness increased, perceived susceptibility, perceived benefits, and perceived barriers increased, r (300) = .37, $p < .01$; r (300) = .13, $p < .05$; and r (300) = .30, $p < .01$, respectively. A strong correlation existed between perceived self-efficacy and perceived benefits, r (300) = .53, $p < .01$. Perceived susceptibility and perceived barriers were weakly correlated, r (300) = .28, $p < .01$." (Lambert et al., 2015, p. 276)

The outcome variable of Pap testing was a self-reported measure. However, the researchers attempted to validate the information in the medical record and found a discrepancy (75% self-report; 44% medical record). The researchers described the Pap testing as being self-reported throughout the remainder of the article, but provided only one reason for the discrepancy, which was that the women might have had a Pap test when seeing an out-of-network provider. Another possible explanation may have been the influence of social desirability. Social desirability occurs when subjects recognize what the "correct" answer is and subconsciously overestimate their compliance. In this study, women may have recognized the researcher's belief that the Pap test was needed. Social desirability means women in the study may have, therefore, reported they had the test within the stipulated time period. Also, the women may have truly believed they had had a test in the past year but did not accurately remember the length of time since the test. (See additional discussion of the effects of this result on the study validity in the section on construct validity.)

"A one-way ANOVA examined differences in subscale variables by participants who reported having and participants who reported not having a Pap test during the previous year. No significant differences were found between participants on the subscale variables of knowledge, perceived susceptibility, perceived seriousness, and perceived benefits. Women who reported having had a Pap test during the previous year perceived fewer barriers ($p < .001$) and higher self-efficacy ($p = .029$) than women who reported having had a Pap test more than 1 year ago." (Lambert et al., 2015, p. 276)

The final analysis of the study variables was a logistic regression, the appropriate analysis when the dependent variable is dichotomous. In the study, the dichotomous variable was a Pap test in the last year (Yes or No).

"Perceived barriers and perceived susceptibility were significant predictors of self-reported Pap test adherence. The overall predictive model was statistically significant (likelihood $\chi^2 = 24.58$, $df = 8$, $p < .01$). The probability of adhering to Pap testing during the previous year was contingent upon the perceived barriers level. Women with higher barriers scores were less likely to adhere to annual Pap testing. Women who felt more susceptible to cervical cancer were more likely to adhere to annual Pap testing. Overall, perceived susceptibility and perceived barriers accounted for 11% of the variance (Nagelkerke $R^2 = .116$). The overall predictive accuracy of the model was 76%." (Lambert et al., 2015, p. 276-277)

Lambert and colleagues (2015) continued their discussion of what the statistical results meant. Their descriptive findings were useful in helping the reader interpret the correlational results.

"The HPV and cervical cancer knowledge scores of the women in our study were low, and the mean score was lower than mean scores in other studies with a similar sample size.... The data suggest that these women may be confused about the purpose of Pap testing and their risks for HPV and cervical cancer. The women were either not receiving information about cervical cancer, Pap test, or HPV during their health care visits or they did not retain and act on the information.... Although not all concepts were statistically related to Pap test adherence, perceived barriers and self-efficacy were significantly related, indicating that differences in Pap test adherence existed for the women who perceived fewer barriers and higher perceived self-efficacy.... The relationship between knowledge and Pap test adherence was not significant in our study, however. The ability of the HBM to explain Pap test adherence varies in different populations ..." (Lambert et al., 2015, p. 277–278)

Comparison With the Literature

The results of a study should be examined in light of previous findings. In the Discussion portion of a research report, selected individual results are discussed, both those related to demographics and those examining study variables. The results are not presented again in their entirety because that would be redundant with the Results section. Here the results are discussed in relation to whether the major results were expected or unexpected and whether they were consistent or inconsistent with similar findings in the literature. Consistency in findings across studies is important for developing theories and

refining scientific knowledge for the nursing profession. Therefore, any inconsistencies must be explored to determine reasons for the differences. Replication of studies and synthesis of findings from existing studies using meta-analyses and systematic reviews are critical for the development of empirical knowledge for an evidence-based practice (Brown, 2014; Craig & Smyth, 2012; Melnyk & Fineout-Overholt, 2015).

IDENTIFICATION OF LIMITATIONS THROUGH EXAMINATION OF DESIGN VALIDITY

Limitations of a study may include the scope and its methodology but are essentially validity-based limitations to generalizations of the findings. It is critical for the development of science and evidence-based practice that limitations are acknowledged (Ioannidis, 2007). The suggested language in reports and critiques is "limitation," not "weakness" or "shortcoming," because limitations address usefulness instead of impaired worth. There are four elements of design validity: **construct validity**, **internal validity**, **external validity**, and **statistical conclusion validity** (see Chapters 3, 10, and 11). Each type of validity should be examined before writing the Discussion portion of a research report. Each type of design validity will be reviewed and applied to the Lambert et al. (2015) study.

Construct Validity Limitations

Construct validity issues involve whether or not a central study concept was operationalized, or made measurable, in the way that best represented the concept's presence or range of values (Creswell, 2014). Construct validity is

Element of Design Validity	General Underlying Flaw	Relationship to Limitations
Construct validity	Inaccurate operationalization; measurement irregularities	Results and findings related to the poorly operationalized or poorly measured construct are flawed and may be invalid.
Internal validity	Failure to measure the effect of, or control for, extraneous variables' effects	Hypothesis-testing results may be inapplicable to the concepts studied. Descriptive tests may be valid.
External validity	Population not well represented by the sample	Results pertain to a subset of the population similar in geographical location, language, gender, age, race, underlying health system, and sometimes all of these.
Statistical conclusion validity	Inappropriate statistical test (rarely identified); inadequate sample size	Sample size, because if statistically significant results were not achieved, the research generates no empirical evidence.

TABLE 26-4 The Four Elements of Design Validity—Their Impact on Limitations

examined using theoretical substruction (Dulock & Holzemer, 1991), as discussed in earlier chapters. Construct validity may be due to faulty reasoning that occurs when the researcher selects measurements for study variables (Table 26-4). However, measurement options for some concepts and constructs are limited, and the researcher must make trade-offs and select the most feasible instrument or method to measure the construct from the available options.

For purposes of writing the Discussion section, instrument validity is considered a subtype of construct validity, because it reflects operationalization of variables. If the validity of an instrument is poor, this is a construct validity issue: the instrument did not measure what it was intended to measure (see Chapter 16 for a detailed discussion of construct validity). If the reliability of an instrument is poor, a different problem is present: the instrument's exact values cannot be trusted. However, when the range of error of an instrument with poor reliability can be determined, meaningful statistical analysis based on broad categories of value instead of exact values is still possible.

Lambert et al. (2015) provided a detailed description of their instruments and how they were scored (see Table 26-1). The principal investigator developed the demographic questionnaire based on a literature review. Validity and reliability were addressed in the following study excerpt:

"**Champion's Health Belief Model**
Perceived susceptibility, perceived seriousness (severity), perceived benefits, and perceived barriers were measured using an adapted version of the CHBM scale for cervical cancer and Pap test.... Reported internal consistency for perceived susceptibility, seriousness, and barriers was at least .70 in three studies (Champion, 1984; Guvenc et al., 2011; Medina-Shepherd & Kleier, 2010). Internal consistency for perceived benefits varied, ranging from .62 to .80. Test-retest reliability coefficients for perceived benefits, barriers, seriousness, and susceptibility ranged from .65 to .88. Construct validity for perceived benefits, barriers, seriousness, and susceptibility was examined by factor analysis, and most of the items loaded on their perspective factors at .35 and higher (Champion, 1984, 1999; Guvenc et al., 2011; Medina-Shepherd & Kleier, 2010). In our study, internal consistency as measured by Cronbach's alpha was .92 for perceived susceptibility scale, .85 for perceived seriousness, .72 for perceived benefits, and .89 for perceived barriers. All of the scales had high reliability except the perceived benefits scale, which was acceptable... (George & Mallery, 2006).

Self-efficacy
Self-efficacy (confidence) was measured using Champion's Self-Efficacy (CSE) scale.... The CSE scale has not been widely used in research. The scale has a Cronbach's alpha of .87 and a Pearson's coefficient of .52 for test-retest reliability. For our study, the Cronbach's alpha for perceived self-efficacy was .92, indicating high reliability.

Knowledge
HPV and cervical cancer knowledge was measured by 15 multiple-choice questions.... Content validity for the knowledge portion of the test was determined by a panel consisting of two gynecologists, two professors of health education, and a medical professional from the Breast and Cervical Program (Ingledue et al., 2004). Test-retest reliability for knowledge was .90 (Ingledue et al., 2004). For our study, Kuder-Richardson-20 (KR20) was used to determine internal consistency of the HPV and cervical cancer knowledge scale; the KR20 was .81, indicating high reliability." (Lambert et al., 2015, p. 274)

The researchers described evidence for the validity of the scales from previous studies. In this study, the instruments had acceptable internal consistency as measured by Cronbach's alpha and KR20. The lowest result related to reliability was .72 for the perceived benefits scale. The discussion of measurement methods would have been strengthened by an expanded explanation of the process for selecting the 15 items from the original 40-item Knowledge Scale. There was also a discrepancy between the total number of items on the four subscales (29 items) and the researchers' description of the scale as having 28 items. However, this is a small issue and probably has no impact upon the validity of the researchers' conclusions.

One of the primary study variables, however, having had a Pap test within the past year (Lambert et al., 2015), was measured by self-report and poses a threat to construct validity. Verification of that measurement was called into question by the authors themselves, with their observation that instead of 75% adherence, as subjects reported, clinic records showed that only 44% of the subjects had had Pap tests there within the previous year.

"Phase one consisted of a self-administered survey completed by the participant. The survey could be completed in 45 minutes or less. Phase two consisted of a review of the participant's chart by the researcher.... Seventy-five percent of the women reported having a Pap test during the previous year; however, according to the medical record, approximately 44% of the women had had a Pap test at the clinic during the previous year.... One reason for the reported and observed differences in Pap test utilization could be that some of the participants had received Pap testing from an outside health care provider." (Lambert et al., 2015, p. 274–275)

The researchers' explanation is an appropriate inclusion in the discussion, but they could not definitely state that this possibility accounted for the entire difference between the two values. The use of the self-report measure to divide the sample into two groups—women who had and had not had a Pap test in the past year according to self-report—undermines the construct validity of the study. Possibly, a better way to ask the question about the last Pap test could have been a request to provide the month, year, and location of the last Pap test. For the women who answered the question with information about a Pap test at another clinic, the researchers could have obtained permission to verify the Pap test date with the other clinic. Another approach would have been to divide the group by the more conservative indicator—a Pap test or no Pap test in the past year documented by clinical records. Lambert and colleagues (2015) did not identify the discrepancy between self-report and clinical records as a limitation of their research. They did mention it in their descriptive results, but did not address this limitation in either the limitations section or in the recommendations of their report.

Problems With Study Implementation

In studies with an intervention, problems with implementation can cause validity issues. Intervention fidelity is one of these. Did the research team implement the intervention the same way every time, thereby achieving intervention fidelity (Melnyk, Morrison-Beedy, & Cole, 2015; Stein, Sargent, & Rafaels, 2007)? If not, construct validity may be flawed. The intervention, which is the independent variable, is defined in a certain way at the beginning of the study and establishes the way the independent variable should be enacted throughout the study.

Sometimes data collection does not proceed as planned and unforeseen situations alter the collection of data. This is a problem of construct validity when the variables are not measured as planned for all study subjects. What is the effect if one subject completes the instruments at home and another completes them at the community center before a support group? What is the effect if one day during the study, the blood pressure

is measured using a different machine than is used the other days of the study? In the Lambert et al. (2015) study, the subjects were recruited from the waiting room of two clinics but it is not clear where the subjects were when they completed the instruments and whether it was before, after, or interrupted by the visit with the healthcare provider. Not all of these factors that alter results can be avoided, or even detected, so the researcher must be alert for subject factors that could compromise data integrity. If the researcher is aware of discrepancies in the measurement procedures, they should be noted in the Discussion section. Reporting of this information depends on the integrity of the researcher (Creswell, 2014; Fawcett & Garity, 2009; Kerlinger & Lee, 2000; Pyrczak & Bruce, 2005; Stein et al., 2007).

Internal Validity Limitations

Internal validity is the extent to which the researcher controls for the effect of extraneous variables in the design or methods of a study. Extraneous variables are those that might affect the value of dependent and outcome variables and are neither controlled for nor measured in the study design. Internal validity determines the confidence the researcher can have that the intervention caused the difference in the outcome variable, as opposed to some other factor (Creswell, 2014). Sample selection, method of subject assignment to group if applicable, and timing of measurements, among other decisions, can also introduce extraneous variables in both interventional and noninterventional studies. Depending on design, the researcher may control for the most powerful of the apparent extraneous variables before the study begins. However, there are dozens of potentially extraneous variables, and the researcher can control only for a small number of them in the design phase (Shadish et al., 2002). Lambert et al.'s (2015) study did not present internal validity issues. These types of issues are more likely to occur in interventional research.

External Validity Limitations

External validity is the extent to which study results are generalizable to the target population. The way a sample is selected is the largest determinant of the research's eventual external validity (Shadish et al., 2002). External validity is strongest for studies with large, randomly selected samples, and it is still stronger when that sample is drawn from many different sites. Is the sample representative of the target population for the variable of interest? When a researcher reports the results of a study conducted with a nonrandomly obtained sample, it strengthens the external validity of the results when the researcher can provide population demographics and demonstrate that the sample demographics are markedly similar to those of the entire population. Lambert and colleagues (2015) identified limitations of their study related to external validity in the following excerpt:

"Limitations

Particular limitations should influence the interpretation of our study findings. First, the majority of participants lived in a metropolitan area and all participants received care at a Ryan White Program-Funded facility. In addition, we did not capture HIV-infected women not in care who were also at increased risk for acquiring HPV and developing cervical cancer. Finally, our convenience sampling method limits generalizability to other women infected with HIV." (Lambert et al., 2015, p. 278)

Stated in other words, all limitations identified in Lambert et al.'s (2015) study were external validity limitations. One limitation was geographical due to data collection in only one city. Other limitations were that the participants comprised a convenience sample and received care at a federally funded facility, with the study not being generalizable to HIV-infected women in privately funded care or to those not in care.

Lambert et al. (2015) provided limited detail on recruitment and sample selection. Did the study have a high refusal rate for subject participation? The authors conducted a power analysis based on an odds ratio value of "at least 2" (p. 273), which indicated that a sample of at least 276 should be used. The authors obtained several statistically significant values using a sample of 300, indicating that the sample size was sufficient to identify significant results. The analysis would have been strengthened by a post-hoc power analysis for the non-significant results. If the power of the study was .80 or greater, the reader could have increased confidence that the non-significant results are accurate. Attrition is non-applicable because the study included only a one-time data collection. Note in the excerpt that Lambert et al. (2015) received a waiver for documentation of informed consent to protect the confidentiality of the women.

"Data collection began after the Florida Department of Health's Institutional Review Board approved the study. Participants were recruited from the waiting rooms of two local ambulatory HIV care clinics. To reduce the risk to participant anonymity, the researcher requested a waiver of documentation of consent because the consent form would be the only document to identify participants by name. Each participant was given an informed consent cover letter, a survey, and an envelope. The informed consent cover letter informed participants that their involvement was voluntary and would not influence the care they received. Participants implied consent to the study by completing the survey. Each survey was assigned a unique identifier, which was written on the top of both surveys. The unique identifier allowed the researcher to match the participant's completed survey to the chart review questionnaire." (Lambert et al., 2015, p. 274)

Statistical Conclusion Validity Limitations

Error intrudes in all measurement (Waltz, Strickland, & Lenz, 2010) and, subsequently, additional errors occur during the processes of data management and analysis. Choosing the correct statistical test is critical during the planning of the study, and consultation with a biostatistician is recommended. Continuing consultation with the biostatistician during data analysis is also recommended to ensure that the data meet the assumptions of the selected tests and missing data are handled appropriately. The Grove and Cipher (2017) text provides an algorithm with detailed explanations and examples to assist you in selecting appropriate statistical techniques when conducting data analyses. Lambert and colleagues (2015) did not provide information about how missing data were handled, but their process of having a researcher review the self-assessment questionnaire in real time, while subjects remained on-site, implied that few, if any, data were missing.

Before submitting a study for publication, each analysis reported in the paper should be double-checked, and the interpretations of the statistical analyses checked. Documentation for each statistical value or analysis statement reported in the paper is filed with a copy of the article. The documentation includes the date of the analyses, the page number of the computer printout showing the results or the electronic file containing the output of the statistical analyses, the sample size for each analysis, and the number of missing values (Fawcett & Garity, 2009; Grove & Cipher, 2017). The following excerpt from Lambert et al. (2015) describes their data analyses:

"Data Analysis

The data were analyzed using SPSS statistical software (Version 21; IBM, Armonk, NY). Descriptive statistics were used to describe sample characteristics and Pap test adherence.... Pearson's correlation coefficients were calculated to assess the relationship within the HBM variables. Analysis of variance (ANOVA) was used to determine whether mean differences existed for perceived susceptibility, perceived seriousness, perceived barriers, perceived benefits, perceived self-efficacy, and HPV and cervical cancer knowledge between women who reported having had a Pap test during the past year and women reporting not having had a Pap test during the past year and to obtain η^2. Multiple logistic regression was used to determine whether perceived susceptibility, perceived seriousness, perceived barriers, perceived benefits, perceived self-efficacy, and HPV and cervical cancer knowledge predicted cervical cancer screening adherence." (Lambert et al., 2015, p. 275)

The data analysis section clearly addressed the sample size of the study, analysis software package used, and types of analyses conducted. The researchers included the effect size (η^2) for the analysis of variance (ANOVA), which provides additional information about whether differences are clinically meaningful. The section could have been strengthened by including the significance level (p) for the analyses and any correction of the significance level due to multiple comparisons.

An insufficient sample size can be a threat to statistical conclusion validity. When negative results are obtained, the researcher may conduct a post hoc power analysis to determine whether the study had sufficient power to detect relationships or differences that were present. For example, the *a priori* power analysis may have been calculated using an overestimate of the effect size (strength of the relationships or differences or the effect of the intervention). Such overestimation would cause the projected sample size to be too small. Lambert et al. (2015) noted that a power analysis was conducted to estimate sample size, but did not mention calculation of power for non-significant analyses. An insufficient sample size is often the cause of a Type II error. A Type II error is a serious study limitation. Very little can be salvaged from an interventional study that exhibits this flaw in statistical conclusion. The results could be reported for descriptive purposes but the original research question cannot be answered.

GENERALIZING THE FINDINGS

Generalization extends the implications of the findings from the sample studied to a larger population or from the situation studied to similar situations, within the limitations imposed by design validity issues (see Chapters 10 and 11). It is important to note that some generalization may be possible in the presence of limitations to both internal and external validity. However, in the presence of multiple limitations, generalizability is limited to the sample and accessible population.

Table 26-5 summarizes the effect of threats to validity on the generalization of study findings. When the measurement of a construct is flawed, the study findings related to the construct also are flawed. As a result, no generalizations of findings related to the flawed construct or constructs should be made (Shadish et al., 2002). An internal validity limitation must be considered in terms of both variables and study outcome. The design selected or the implementation of the study did not control for extraneous factors adequately. For example, members of a control group are inadvertently

TABLE 26-5 **The Four Elements of Design Validity—Generalization**		
Element of Design Validity	**General Underlying Flaw**	**Relationship to Generalization**
Construct validity	Inaccurate operationalization; measurement irregularities	No generalizations using the poorly operationalized or poorly measured construct or constructs can be made.
Internal validity	Failure to measure the effect of, or control for, extraneous variables' effects	Generalization must be made conditionally, so as to include possible effects of the extraneous variable.
External validity	Population not well represented by the sample	Cautious generalization to other samples or groups who have similar demographic characteristics.
Statistical conclusion validity	Inappropriate statistical test (rarely identified); inadequate sample size	No empirical evidence was generated, but if the results show "trends," they can inform the reader.

provided the study intervention, or the setting for the study undergoes a change in ownership during a study of nurse satisfaction. These threats to internal validity should be noted in the limitations section of the research report, and they directly affect the extent to which the findings can be generalized. When external validity is limited, generalization can always be made back to the sample itself and possibly to other groups at the same or similar sites, with similar demographic characteristics. For limitations to statistical conclusion validity that involve inadequate sample size, no generalizations related to the research question can be made at all.

Generalizations apply to the current study findings, in conjunction with previous studies in the same area. For instance, an interventional study comparing toothbrushing and plaque-removal-focused toothbrushing in intubated patients in the intensive care unit would build upon recent literature comparing various styles of oral hygiene for their effectiveness in reducing bacterial overgrowth. Because there is extensive evidence already in this problem area, cautious generalization of findings could be made based on the study results and the evidence provided by other studies. Generalizations like these, based on accumulated evidence from many studies, are called **empirical generalizations**. These generalizations are important for verifying hypotheses and theoretical statements, and can contribute to development of new theories. Empirical generalizations are foundational to scientific discovery and, within nursing, provide a basis for generating evidence-based guidelines to manage specific practice problems (Brown, 2014; Craig & Smyth, 2012; Melnyk & Fineout-Overholt, 2015). Chapter 19 provides a detailed discussion of research synthesis processes and strategies for promoting evidence-based nursing practice.

How far can generalizations be made? The answer to this question is debatable. From a narrow perspective, one cannot really generalize from the sample with which the study was conducted because samples differ from the population. The conservative position, represented by Kerlinger and Lee (2000), recommends caution in considering the extent of generalization. Conservatives consider generalization particularly risky if the sample was small, homogeneous, and not randomly selected (Kandola, Banner, O'Keefe-McCarthy, & Jassal, 2014).

The less conservative view allows generalization from the sample to the accessible population (the population from which the sample was drawn) if the population demographics are essentially the same as those of the sample. If an intervention is effective in an outpatient clinic that sees only three or four subjects with a certain disorder each week, it will most likely continue to be effective in the same clinic with subsequent outpatients. In practice, this is exactly what occurs. If an intervention seems to work, it is continued at the same site. If the researchers publish their findings, by the time the study is published, other outpatients will have been treated as well, producing more results that may contradict or strengthen the findings.

The least conservative view also considers what will be generalized and the implications of false generalization. For example, single-site small-sample research is conducted to test the intervention of having a one-minute strategic planning session with the patient early in the shift, so that the patient is aware of the nurse's plans for tasks to be completed and the nurse is aware of the patient's planned activities for the shift. The dependent variables are complaints, amount of sleep, and morning glucose values. If the research demonstrates that, for this sample, the intervention resulted in fewer complaints, more sleep, and more in-range morning glucose values, what would be the generalization potential of the research?

This intervention is benign, cost-free, and takes very little of the nurse's time. The intervention is also consistent with nursing theories and can be classified as a socially appropriate step toward involving the patient in care. If a Type I error occurred in the research and the intervention was in actuality ineffective, what would be the implications of false generalization? The least conservative view might recommend this intervention in a research report based on related literature on patient involvement in care and on the low risk of making a false generalization relate to the intervention.

Lambert et al. (2015) seemed to take the conservative approach to generalizability in this excerpt.

"... our convenience sampling method limits generalizability to other women infected with HIV. The study does, however, provide suggestions for future studies and extends the existing body of literature." (Lambert et al., 2015, p. 278)

Unfortunately, the primary limitation to generalizability of the findings from the Lambert et al. (2015) study is related to construct validity, which the researchers did not identify as a limitation. Therefore, the conservative approach to generalization is appropriate.

CONSIDERING IMPLICATIONS FOR PRACTICE, THEORY, AND KNOWLEDGE

Implications of research findings for nursing are the meanings of the results for the body of nursing practice and knowledge. As with generalizations, implications for practice can be summative, including both the current study and related literature in the same area of evidence. Implications for practices are often based, in part, on whether treatment decisions or outcomes would be different in view of the study findings.

In terms of practice, implications can be drawn from any part of the study findings, descriptive or inferential, but they must arise from those findings, not merely from general principles of nursing practice. The researcher must be cautious and base the implications on the findings. This legitimate identification of implications includes generalizations for teaching or early intervention when description of subjects includes knowledge deficits or potential for harm. Such is the case for Lambert et al.'s (2015) identified implications for practice, which addressed knowledge deficit, which was not a study focus.

> **"Implications for Practice**
> In practice, the rationale for procedures and results must be explained … the provider should provide information in a way that patients can understand, and the provider should ask the patient to repeat the information to assess the patient's level of comprehension. The results of our study suggest that many women lack information regarding HPV and cervical cancer. There are many possible reasons for low HPV and cervical cancer knowledge, including missed opportunities to teach due to the complexity of ambulatory HIV care visits. It is essential for providers to remain abreast of current health care guidelines to improve patient outcomes, educate patients, and decrease health care costs." (Lambert et al., 2015, p. 278–279)

Implications for knowledge development exist in practically all research that generates valid findings. Each study, even if its findings are all negative ones, contributes to the body of knowledge in the discipline.

SUGGESTING FURTHER RESEARCH

Examining a study's implications and making generalizations should culminate in **recommendations for further research** that emerge from the present study and from previous studies in the same area of interest. In every study, the researcher gains knowledge and experience that can be used to design "a better study next time." Formulating recommendations for future studies will stimulate you to define more clearly how your study might have been improved.

These recommendations must also take into consideration the design validity-related limitations identified in the current study. For instance, if construct validity was seriously flawed, further research recommendations might include redesigning the research and conducting it again, not replicating it, because a replication would include the same flawed operational definition(s). If negative findings and low power indicate the possibility of a Type II error, recommending repeating the study with a larger sample may be appropriate. However, if other factors contributed to statistical conclusion validity, the study should be redesigned and these flaws corrected prior to repeating the study.

Recommendations for further research related to internal validity limitations might include a different type of design that eliminates subjects with the extraneous variable of concern, matches subjects in intervention and control groups with respect to the variable, or measures the extraneous variable's effects. The researcher is in the best position to make suggestions as to how an important extraneous variable might be controlled for in the design process.

Recommendations for further research related to external validity limitations are specific to sample selection, sample size, and number of sites used in the research. Recommendations for future studies should reverse those limitations, making the study stronger, larger, more representative. When nonrandom sampling has been used, subsequent research with random sampling allows improved external validity. When a small, single-site sample has been used, further research with a larger sample, using two or more sites, improves external validity.

Lambert and colleagues (2015) provided the following suggestions for future research:

> **"Implications for Research**
> Our findings suggest that similar studies should be repeated (a) in rural areas and private clinics, (b) with HIV-infected women who are not in care, and (c) on the cultural components of care for African American women. Future studies should also address the utility of mobile Pap screenings in underserved areas and the use of telemedicine with the option to perform self-sampling or self-administered Pap tests.
> Future research is essential to better understand HIV-infected women's attitudes, perceptions, and knowledge regarding HPV, cervical cancer, and Pap testing. Future studies assessing the relationships between factors such as perceived barriers, perceived susceptibility, perceived self-efficacy, and HPV and cervical cancer knowledge are

essential prior to intervention development. Our study highlighted the finding that chronic diseases such as HIV can impact health behaviors in ways that are currently not well understood ... future interventions with the goal of increasing awareness and adherence, and improving health care outcomes for HIV-infected women are essential." (Lambert et al., 2015, p. 279)

FORMING FINAL CONCLUSIONS

Conclusions are derived from the study findings and are a synthesis of what the researcher deems the most important findings. Preliminary conclusions are formed when the output of data analyses is reviewed, but they are refined during the process of interpretation. Most researchers provide a summary of their conclusions at the end of the research report. As the researcher's last word on the topic, it is the most likely aspect of the paper to be remembered by the reader.

One of the risks in developing conclusions in research is going beyond the data—specifically, forming conclusions that the data do not warrant, as noted related to causality. Going beyond the data may be due to faulty logic or preconceived ideas and allowing personal biases to influence the conclusions. When forming conclusions, it is important to remember that research never proves anything; rather, research offers support for a position when the study design and statistical analyses were appropriate. A common flaw in logic occurs when the researcher finds statistically significant relationships between A and B by correlational analysis and then concludes that A causes B. This conclusion is inaccurate because a correlational study does not examine causality. Another example of a flawed conclusion occurs when the researcher tests the causal statement that A *causes* B and finds statistical support for the statement under the study's conditions. It is inappropriate to state that, absolutely, in all situations, a causal relationship exists between A and B. This conclusion cannot be scientifically proven. A more credible conclusion is to state the conditional probabilities of a causal relationship. For example, stating that if A occurs, then B occurs under conditions x, y, and z is more appropriate (Kerlinger & Lee, 2000; Shadish et al., 2002). Another way to appropriately state the conclusion is that if A occurs, then B has an 80% probability of occurring. In the Results section, Lambert and colleagues (2015) tentatively described their conclusions related to the HIV-positive women's low levels of knowledge about Pap testing.

"The data suggest that these women may be confused about the purpose of Pap testing and their risks for HPV and cervical cancer. The women were either not receiving information about cervical cancer, Pap test, or HPV during their health care visits or they did not retain and act on the information." (Lambert et al., 2015, p. 277)

"The relationship between knowledge and Pap test adherence was not significant in our study, however ... our study provides evidence that there are relationships between perceived barriers, perceived self-efficacy, and Pap test adherence in HIV-infected women, which suggests that reducing barriers and increasing women's perceived self-efficacy has the potential to increase the likelihood that HIV-infected women will adhere to Pap testing. The data suggest a directional relationship not implying causality." (Lambert et al., 2015, p. 278)

Going beyond the data occurs more frequently in published studies than one would like to believe. Be sure to check the validity of your logic related to the conclusions before disseminating your findings. After noting the implications for practice and research, Lambert and colleagues (2015) provided a conclusion section with additional thoughts on their study findings.

"Conclusion
Despite the inability of CHBM, in its entirety, to explain Pap test adherence in HIV-infected women, many of the concepts have important implications for health care and future research. The increased risk of the population coupled with low HPV and cervical cancer knowledge indicates a need for more HPV education. In addition, it suggests the need to assess the HPV and cervical cancer knowledge of health care providers because patients may be unaware because their providers are unaware. Health care providers must remain competent, build strong relationships with their patients, reduce barriers, and increase health awareness to promote patient self-care management with the purpose of improving health outcomes and cost effectiveness." (Lambert et al., 2015, p. 279)

▌ KEY POINTS

- Interpretation of research outcomes requires reflection upon three general aspects of the research and their interactions: the primary findings, validity issues, and the resultant body of knowledge in the area of investigation.
- Interpretation includes several intellectual activitie, such as examining evidence, forming conclusions,

identifying study limitations, generalizing the findings, considering implications, and suggesting further research.
- The first step in interpretation is examining all of the evidence available that supports or contradicts the validity of the results. Evidence is obtained from various sources, including the research plan, measurement reliability and validity (or precision and accuracy), data collection process, data analysis process, data analysis results, and previous studies.
- The outcomes of data analysis are the most direct evidence available of the results related to the research purpose and the objectives, questions, or hypotheses.
- Five possible results are (1) significant results that are in keeping with those predicted by the researcher, (2) nonsignificant results, (3) significant results that are opposite those predicted by the researcher, (4) mixed results, and (5) serendipitous results.
- Findings are a consequence of evaluating evidence, which includes the findings from previous studies.
- Conclusions are derived from the findings and are a synthesis of the findings.
- The limitations of a study decrease the generlizability of the findings. Limitations may be related to threats to construct validity, internal validity, external validity, and statistical conclusion validity. Each aspect of validity should be clearly identified and discussed in relation to the conclusions of the study.
- Generalization extends the implications of the findings from the sample studied to a larger target population.
- Implications of the study for nursing are the meanings of study conclusions for the body of nursing knowledge, theory, and practice.
- Completion of a study and examination of implications should culminate in recommending future studies that emerge from the present study and previous studies.
- The conclusions are a summary of your most important study findings. Use caution to not go beyond what you found however, emphasize one or two main findings you want the reader to remember.

REFERENCES

Aberson, C. L. (2010). *Applied power analysis for the behavioral sciences.* New York, NY: Routledge.

Brown, S. J. (2014). *Evidence-based nursing: The research-practice connection* (3rd ed.). Sudbury, MA: Jones & Bartlett.

Champion, V. L. (1984). Instrument development for health belief model constructs. *Advances in Nursing Science, 6*(3), 73–85.

Champion, V. L. (1999). Revised susceptibility, benefits, and barriers scale for mammography screening. *Research in Nursing and Health, 22*(4), 341–348.

Champion, V., Skinner, C. S., & Menon, U. (2005). Development of a self-efficacy scale for mammography. *Research in Nursing and Health, 28*(4), 329–336.

Craig, J. V., & Smyth, R. L. (2012). *The evidence-based practice manual for nurses* (3rd ed.). Edinburgh, UK: Churchill Livingstone.

Creswell, J. (2014). *Research design: Qualitative, quantitative, and mixed methods approaches* (4th ed.). Los Angeles, CA: Sage.

Dulock, H., & Holzemer, W. (1991). Substruction: Improving the linkage from theory to method. *Nursing Science Quarterly, 4*(2), 83–87.

Fawcett, J., & Garity, J. (2009). *Evaluating research for evidence-based nursing practice.* Philadelphia, PA: F. A. Davis.

George, D., & Mallery, P. (2006). *SPSS for Windows step by step: A simple guide and reference.* Boston, MA: Pearson Education.

Grove, S. K., & Cipher, D. J. (2017). *Statistics for nursing research: A workbook for evidence-based practice* (2nd ed.). St. Louis, MO: Saunders.

Guvenc, G., Akyuz, A., & Acikel, C. H. (2011). Health Belief Model Scale for cervical cancer and Pap smear test: Psychometric testing. *Journal of Advanced Nursing, 67*(2), 428–437.

Ingledue, K. C., Cottrell, R., & Benard, A. (2004). College women's knowledge, perceptions, and preventative behaviors regarding human papillomavirus infection and cervical cancer. *American Journal of Health Studies, 19*(1), 28–34.

Ioannidis, J. (2007). Limitations are not properly acknowledged in the scientific literature. *Journal of Clinical Epidemiology, 60*(4), 324–329.

Kandola, D., Banner, D., O'Keefe-McCarthy, S., & Jassal, D. (2014). Sampling methods in cardiovascular nursing research: An overview. *Canadian Journal of Cardiovascular Nursing, 24*(3), 15–18.

Keough, V., Schlomer, R., & Bollenberg, B. (2003). Serendipitous findings from an Illinois ED nursing educational survey reflect a crisis in emergency nursing. *Journal of Emergency Nursing, 29*(1), 17–22.

Kerlinger, F. N., & Lee, H. P. (2000). *Foundations of behavioral research* (4th ed.). Fort Worth, TX: Harcourt College.

Lambert, C., Chandler, R., McMillan, S., Kromrey, J., Johnson-Mallard, V., & Kurtyka, D. (2015). Pap test adherence, cervical cancer perceptions, and HPV knowledge among HIV-infected women in a community health setting. *Journal of the Association of Nurses in AIDS Care, 26*(3), 271–280.

Medina-Shepherd, R., & Kleier, J. A. (2010). Spanish translation and adaptation of Victoria Champion's Health Belief Model scales for breast cancer screening-mammography. *Cancer Nursing, 33*(2), 93–101.

Melnyk, B. M., & Fineout-Overholt, E. (2015). *Evidence-based practice in nursing & healthcare: A guide to best practice* (3rd ed.). Philadelphia, PA: Lippincott Williams & Wilkins.

Melnyk, B., Morrison-Beedy, D., & Cole, R. (2015). Generating evidence through quantitative research. In B. Melnyk & E. Fineout-Overholt (Eds.), *Evidence-based practice in nursing & healthcare* (3rd ed.). Philadelphia, PA: Wolters Kluwer.

Morrison, R., Moody, P., & Shelton, M. (2010). Pap smear rates: Predictor of cervical cancer mortality disparity? *Online Journal of Rural Nursing and Health Care, 10*(2), 21–27.

O'Halloran, P. (2013). How to read and make sense of statistical data. In P. Liamputtong (Ed.), *Research methods in health: Foundations for evidence-based practice* (2nd ed., pp. 41–424). Sydney, NSW: Oxford University Press.

Pyrczak, F., & Bruce, R. R. (2005). *Writing empirical research reports* (5th ed.). Glendale, CA: Pyrczak.

Rosenstock, I. M., Strecher, V. J., & Becker, M. H. (1988). Social learning theory and the Health Belief Model. *Health Education Quarterly, 15*(2), 175–183.

Shadish, W. R., Cook, T. D., & Campbell, D. T. (2002). *Experimental and quasi-experimental designs for generalization causal inference.* Chicago, IL: Rand McNally.

Shen, J., Xu, Y., Staples, S., & Bolstad, A. (2014). Using the Interpersonal Skills tool to assess interpersonal skills of internationally educated nurses. *Japan Journal of Nursing Science, 11*(3), 171–179.

Stein, K. F., Sargent, J. T., & Rafaels, N. (2007). Intervention research: Establishing fidelity of the independent variable in nursing clinical trials. *Nursing Research, 56*(1), 54–62.

Teixeira da Silva, J. (2015). Negative results: Negative perceptions limit their potential for increasing reproducibility. *Journal of Negative Results in Biomedicine, 14*, Article 12. Retrieved on August 1, 2015, from http://jnrbm.biomedcentral.com/articles/10.1186/s12952-015-0033-9.

Waltz, C. F., Strickland, O. L., & Lenz, E. R. (2010). *Measurement in nursing and health research* (4th ed.). New York, NY: Springer.

27

Disseminating Research Findings

Jennifer R. Gray

The study is completed and the researcher breathes a sigh of relief. Maybe the researcher feels unskilled in presenting the information and overwhelmed by the idea of publishing. Maybe the researcher is so exhausted by the labor-intensive process of completing the thesis or dissertation that dissemination of the findings beyond the academic requirements is delayed. The study documents are placed in a drawer with the intent to communicate the findings *someday*. Time passes, and disseminating the findings becomes less and less of a priority.

Whether caused by lack of knowledge, feelings of inadequacy, fatigue, or competing priorities, the findings of valuable nursing studies are not communicated and the benefit of the knowledge gained is lost. Failure to communicate research findings may be considered a failure to fulfill the promise to subjects that their input would be used to increase knowledge and benefit others with the same condition. After involving members of an institutional review board (IRB) committee to approve your study and after subjects consented and participated in your study, you have an ethical obligation to complete the process. When researchers do not disseminate, the valuable resources of time, funding, and data are wasted.

Communicating research findings, the final step in the research process, involves developing a research report and disseminating the study findings through presentations and publications to audiences of nurses, healthcare professionals, policymakers, and healthcare consumers. Disseminating study findings provides many advantages for the researcher, the nursing profession, and the consumer of nursing services. By presenting and publishing findings, researchers advance the knowledge of a discipline, which is essential for providing evidence-based practice. For individual researchers, communicating study findings often leads to professional advancement and recognition as a researcher in one's field of specialization. By communicating research findings, the researcher also promotes critical analysis of previous studies, encourages research replication, and identifies additional research problems. Over time, findings from many studies are synthesized with the ultimate goal of providing evidence-based health care to patients, families, and communities (Craig & Smyth, 2012; Melnyk & Fineout-Overholt, 2015).

To facilitate communication of research findings for nurse clinicians and researchers, this chapter describes the basic content of a research report common to quantitative and qualitative studies. Then differences in the report content related to the type of study will be shared. Other types of dissemination will be described as well, such as presentations.

COMPONENTS OF A RESEARCH REPORT

A **research report** is the written description of a completed study designed to communicate study findings efficiently and effectively to nurses and other healthcare professionals. The information included in the report depends on the study, the intended audience, and the mechanisms chosen for dissemination. Usually research reports include four major sections or content areas: (1) introduction, (2) methods, (3) results, and (4) discussion of the findings (Pyrczak & Bruce, 2007). Box 27-1 contains a general outline for the content in each section. Specific journals may require other sections, or your university might include other sections in the final thesis or dissertation report. Some journals limit the

BOX 27-1   Outline for a Research Report

Introduction
- Background and significance of the problem
- Purpose of study
- Brief review of relevant literature (may include theoretical framework and conceptual definitions)
- Gap in knowledge the study will address
- Research objectives, questions, or hypotheses

Methods
- Research design
  Quantitative study: include intervention if applicable
  Qualitative study: approach to the study such as phenomenology or ethnography
- Setting
- Sampling method, consent process
- Human subject protections, including IRB approval
- Data collection methods
  Quantitative studies: measurement with instrument descriptions and scoring
  Qualitative studies: interviews, observation, document analysis, focus groups
- Data collection process
- Data analysis

Results
- Description of sample (may use tables or figures)
- Presentation of results of data analysis
  Quantitative studies results: organized by objectives, questions, or hypotheses
  Qualitative studies results: may be organized by themes or cultural characteristics
- Use narrative, tables, and figures to present results

Discussion
- Major findings compared with previous research
- Limitations of study
- Conclusions
- Implications
- Future studies that are needed

References
- Include references cited in paper, using format specified by journal

Introduction section to two or three brief paragraphs that include a statement about the theoretical framework for the study, a sufficient review of the literature to identify the gap in knowledge, and the clear purpose of the study. Other journals may require a Background section that includes the significance of the study and a review of literature. The Methods section describes how the study was implemented including sampling, data collection, and data analysis. When preparing to publish the results of your thesis or dissertation, recognize the need to drastically reduce the content and revise the paper to fit the format and tone of the journal. The Results sections of reports for qualitative studies are usually longer than those of quantitative studies because of the inclusion of quotes from participants, but may include fewer tables than quantitative studies do. The Discussion section briefly acknowledges the limitations of the study, presents the findings in relation to other literature, and discusses the implications of the findings for the intended journal audience.

Title

The title of your research report must indicate what you have studied so as to attract the attention of interested readers. The title should be concise and consistent with the study purpose and the research objectives, questions, or hypotheses. A title may include the major study variables and population and the type of study conducted, but should not include the results or conclusions of a study (Pyrczak & Bruce, 2007). Some journals limit the length of manuscript titles; others discourage use of colons. The Public Library of Science ([PLOS], n.d.) publishes several open-accessed, online scientific journals. Their submission guidelines request that authors submit a long title of 250 characters or less and a short title of 50 characters or less. The *International Journal of Nursing Studies* website (Elsevier, 2015) provides a specific format for manuscript titles. The title begins with the topic or question of the study. Following a colon, the subtitle includes the study design or type of paper and the population. If more consistent with the study question, the population can be replaced by the care setting in the subtitle.

An example of a title for a mixed methods study is *Change in sexual activity after a cardiac event: The role of medications, comorbidity, and psychosocial factors* (Steinke, Mosack, & Hill, 2015). This title would have been stronger if it had indicated that the researchers used mixed methods with a focus on gender differences in sexual activity by class of medication. Shin, Habermann, and Pretzer-Aboff (2015) provided a descriptive title for their research report, *Challenges and strategies of medication adherence in Parkinson's disease: A qualitative study.* The title states the design of the study (qualitative), the key concept (medication adherence), and the population (persons with Parkinson's disease [PD]).

Abstract

The abstract of a study summarizes the key aspects of the study in 100 to 300 words and is the first component of a research report. In addition, an abstract may be written for submission to seek the opportunity for a poster or oral presentation at a conference. More information about preparing an abstract for that purpose is included later in this chapter.

Structured abstracts have specific headings such as problem, purpose, framework, methods, sample size, key results, and conclusions (Pyrczak & Bruce, 2007). Mallah, Nassar, and Kurdahi Badr (2015) provided a structured abstract for their comparison of hospital acquired pressure ulcer prevalence before and after implementation of a bundle of interventions.

"*Background:* Pressure ulcers (PUs) are associated with high mortality, morbidity, and health care costs. In addition to being costly, PUs cause pain, suffering, infection, a lower quality of life, extended hospital stay and even death. Although several nursing interventions have been advocated in the literature, there is a paucity of research on what constitutes the most effective nursing intervention.

Objectives: To determine the efficacy of multidisciplinary intervention and to assess which component of the intervention was most predictive of decreasing the prevalence of Hospital acquired pressure ulcers (HAPU) in a tertiary setting in Lebanon.

Design: An evaluation prospective research design was utilized with data before and after the intervention. The sample consisted of 468 patients admitted to the hospital from January 2012 to April 2013.

Results: The prevalence of HAPU was significantly reduced from 6.63% in 2012 to 2.47. Sensitivity of the Braden scale in predicting a HAPU was 92.30% and specificity was 60.04%. A logistic multiple regression equation found that two factors significantly predicted the development of a HAPU; skin care and Braden scores.

Conclusion: The multidisciplinary approach was effective in decreasing the prevalence of HAPUs. Skin care management which was a significant predictor of PUs should alert nurses to the cost effectiveness of this intervention. Lower Braden scores also were predictive of HAPUs" (Mallah et al., 2015, p. 106).

Unstructured abstracts include the same elements but are written in narrative format. Shin and colleagues (2015) provided an unstructured abstract in their study's report.

"Little is known about strategies used by people with Parkinson's disease (PD) to facilitate medication adherence in the U.S. The purpose of this study was to describe challenges in adherence to medication regimens and to identify strategies used to facilitate adherence to medication regimens. A qualitative research design was used to interview sixteen community-dwelling people with PD and five caregivers. Data analysis was performed using content analysis. The majority of the participants (81.3%) reported decreased adherence to medication regimens. Seven themes emerged from the data. The main challenges of medication adherence included medication responses, cost of medications, and forgetfulness. Strategies used to facilitate adherence to medication regimens included seeking knowledge about antiparkinsonian medications, seeking advice from family and friends, use of devices, and use of reminders. These findings may be important in formulating interventions to improve adherence to medication regimens for people living with PD." (Shin et al., 2015, p. 192)

Following the abstract are the four major sections of a research report: Introduction, Methods, Results, and Discussion.

Introduction

The Introduction section of a research report discusses the background and significance of the problem, so as to inform the reader of the reason the study was conducted (see Box 27-1). Statements are supported with citations from the literature. The introduction may also describe the study framework or philosophical perspective, and identify the research purpose (aims, objectives, questions, or hypotheses if applicable). The study aim or purpose and specific research questions flow from the phenomenon or research problem, clarify the study focus, and identify expected outcomes of the investigation (see Chapters 5 and 6). You developed this content for the research proposal; now, you summarize it in the final report. Depending on the type of research report, the review of literature and framework might be separate sections or separate chapters, as in a thesis or dissertation.

Review of Literature

The review of literature section of a research report documents the current knowledge of the problem investigated. The sources included in the literature review are the sources that you used to develop your study and interpret the findings. A review of literature can be two or three paragraphs or several pages long. In journal articles, the review of literature is concise and usually includes a maximum of 15 to 20 sources. Theses and dissertations frequently include an extensive literature review to document the student's knowledge of the research problem. The summary of the literature review clearly identifies what is known, what is not known or the gap in knowledge, and the contribution of this study to the current knowledge base. The objectives, questions, or hypotheses that were used to direct the study often are stated at the end of the literature review. See Chapter 7 for more information on writing a review of the literature.

Framework

A research report includes the study framework. In this section, you identify and define the major concepts in the framework and describe the relationships among the concepts (see Chapter 8). You can develop a schematic map or model to clarify the logic within the framework. If a particular proposition or relationship is being tested in a quantitative study, that proposition should be stated clearly. Developing a framework and identifying the proposition or propositions examined in a study serve to connect the framework and research purpose to the objectives, questions, or hypotheses. The concepts in the framework must be linked to the study variables and are used to define the variables conceptually (see Chapters 6 and 8 for examples). A framework for a qualitative study may provide theoretical context for the concepts and possibly structure for the data collection, such as interview questions.

Methods

The Methods section of a research report describes how the study was conducted. This section needs to be concise, yet provide sufficient detail for nurses to appraise critically or replicate the study procedures. In this section, you will describe the study design, sample, setting, data collection tools and process, and plan for data analysis. If the research project included a pilot study, the researcher describes the reason for the pilot, its implementation, and its results succinctly. You will also describe any changes made in the research project based on the pilot study (Pyrczak & Bruce, 2007), and mention whether pilot data were or were not included in the analysis of results.

Design

The study design should be explicitly stated. Review Chapters 10 and 11 for information on quantitative study designs and Chapter 12 for qualitative study

methods. Ma, Zhou, Huang, and Huang (2015) were explicit by stating the following:

> "A cross-sectional design was adopted to facilitate the survey about SRH [self-rated health] status, BP [blood pressure] control levels and determinants of SRH." (Ma et al., 2015, p. 347)

Because a cross-sectional design may be descriptive or correlational, it would be better to state here, "a cross-sectional predictive correlational design." The researchers matched their design to the study's purpose and used appropriate analyses to investigate the determinants of SRH.

Sample and Setting

This section of the research report should describe the sampling method, criteria for selecting the sample, sample size, and sample characteristics (see Chapter 15). Details about subject recruitment, including refusal or acceptance rates, should be reported. Ma et al. (2015) described subject recruitment and the inclusion/exclusion criteria in the methods section and included the refusal and acceptance rates in the description of the sample.

Researchers can present the demographic characteristics of their sample in narrative format; however, most quantitative researchers present the characteristics of their sample in a table. Guidelines for preparing tables will be discussed later in the chapter.

> "The study adopted a convenient sampling method to enlist the subjects. The subjects were recruited from the cardiovascular outpatient department of two community health centers. Inclusion criteria: (1) Subjects older than 18 years of age, agreed to attend the study; (2) Subjects diagnosed as essential hypertension by cardiovascular physician (Wang, 2011). Exclusion criteria: (1) secondary hypertensive patients; (2) women with pregnancy. . . . Nine hundred forty-two subjects were invited for the study, of which 93 refused to participate, 42 did not meet inclusion criteria, and 807 completed the survey." (Ma et al., 2015, pp. 348–349)

In the section about the sample and subjects, researchers are expected to include information about how subjects' rights were protected and informed consent was obtained. In a published study, the setting is often described in one or two sentences, and agencies are not identified by name unless permission has been obtained.

Data Collection Process and Procedures

This section of the report describes the methods used to collect data. The description of the data collection process in the research report includes details such as who collected the data, the types of data collected and whether collected through measurement or a qualitative method, and the procedure for collecting data including frequency and timing. In the Methods section of a quantitative study, instruments and their reliability and validity are described. For qualitative studies, how and where interviews, focus groups, or observations occurred are included. Because of different approaches to research problems, data collection is an area of the report that varies greatly depending on the type of study.

Analysis Plan

Data must be transformed into results through analysis. For quantitative reports, the analysis plan consists of statistical analyses for each research aim, question, or hypothesis. For qualitative study reports, this section highlights the name of the method of analysis and documentation of decisions about the analysis such as use of an audit trail. For mixed methods studies, the analysis plan includes analyses for both quantitative and qualitative data but more important, the processes the researcher used to combine the two types of data into a comprehensive whole.

Results

The Results section usually begins with a description of the sample and subgroups, if applicable, followed by what was learned through implementation of the study methods. For each research objective, question, or hypothesis, the results are provided. Statistical results are reported in narrative description accompanied by tables (Grove & Cipher, 2017; see Chapters 21–25). Themes from qualitative analysis are supported by quotes from the participants. A grounded theory study is reported by describing the emergent theory often accompanied by a model or diagram of the concepts identified (see Chapter 12).

Discussion

The Discussion section ties the other sections of your research report together by connecting parts of the report with one another. For instance, the introduction plus the methods are logically connected to the conclusions. The review of the literature plus the results should have produced the conclusions. It includes your major findings, limitations of the study, conclusions drawn from the findings, implications of the findings for nursing, and recommendations for further research. Your major findings are actually an interpretation of the results and should be discussed in relation to the overriding theoretical framework as well as the research problem, purpose, and questions or hypotheses. Researchers should compare their findings with those from previous research and describe how what you found extends existing knowledge. Discussion of the findings also includes the limitations that were identified while conducting the study. The limitations are threats to validity and should be noted as such. For example, limitations related to measurement such as self-report for unhealthy behaviors are threats to construct validity. A study might have other limitations related to the sample (e.g., size, response rate, attrition) that threaten external validity and the design (e.g., convenience sample, only one clinical site, lack of randomization) that threaten internal validity. These limitations influence the generalizability of the findings (Pyrczak & Bruce, 2007). Refer to Chapter 26 for more information on how to interpret study findings.

The research report includes the conclusions or the knowledge generated from the findings. Conclusions are frequently stated in tentative or speculative terms, because one study by itself does not produce conclusive findings that can be generalized to the larger population. If your study is valid and the findings are consistent with previous studies, you will make a statement related to generalization. You might provide a brief rationale for accepting certain conclusions and rejecting others. The conclusions should be discussed in light of their implications for knowledge, theory, and practice. If there is enough evidence for application, you will describe how the findings and conclusions might be implemented in specific practice areas.

Conclude your research report with recommendations for further research. Based on the limitations, identify how revising the methods for future studies on the same topic may produce findings with greater validity. For example, are the findings sufficient for application? If not, what designs may result in a more rigorous study? If several descriptive studies have been reported, should a correlational study be the next step? If correlational evidence has been reported, is it time to develop a model or test for causation with a quasi-experimental study? The Discussion section of the report demonstrates the value of conducting the study by describing its contribution to knowledge. By the time the study is published, career researchers are conducting that next study to address their own recommendations for future research.

Reference Citations

The final section of the research report is the reference list, which includes all sources that were cited in the report. Most of the sources in the reference list are relevant studies that provided a knowledge base for conducting the study or reference books supporting the methods. The editors of many nursing and psychology journals require the format in the *Publication Manual of the American Psychological Association* (American Psychological Association [APA], 2010). Sources must be cited in the text of the report using a consistent format. It is very important to follow the format guidelines for the journal to which you plan to submit your manuscript for publication. Some journals request that the references include only citations published in the past 5 years, except for landmark studies. Other journals may limit the number of references to less than 50. (*Nursing Research* limits the number of references to 40 at this time.).

TYPES OF RESEARCH REPORTS

Quantitative Research Reports

In reports of quantitative studies, you would expect to see numerical information that you would not find in qualitative research reports. For example, when a clinical trial or experiment is involved, the report must also address the statistical power analysis used to determine how many subjects per group would be needed to find a statistically significant difference if significance is set at $\alpha \le 0.05$ or another alpha level. If fewer subjects enroll or complete the study than what was indicated in the original power analysis, statistically significant findings may be absent, even if the group difference appears to be clinically relevant. Lack of statistically significant findings due to a too-small sample is known as a Type II statistical error (see Chapter 15).

The number of subjects completing the study should be identified in the report. If your subjects were divided into groups (experimental, comparison, or control groups), identify the method for assigning subjects to groups and the number of subjects in each group. For randomized clinical trials (RCTs), the expectation is that you will follow the Consolidated Standards for Reporting Trials (CONSORT, 2010). The guidelines recommend a flow diagram of the enrollment, recruitment, response rate, size of groups, and attrition rate (Schulz, Altman, & Moher, 2010). Jull and Aye (2015) searched top nursing journals for reports of RCTs published in 2012 and examined the reports for compliance with the CONSORT Statement. Of these top journals, half had endorsed CONSORT, but actual reports appearing in the journals did not immediately reflect the newly endorsed CONSORT format. Following the guidelines

facilitates systematic reviews by providing the information reviewers need to determine the quality of a study. Wilson, Roll, Corbett, and Barbosa-Leiker (2015) provided a patient flowchart according to CONSORT guidelines (Figure 27-1) for their randomized controlled trial of a pain management intervention.

Details about the measures or instruments used in the data collection process are crucial if nurses are to critically appraise and replicate a study. The details include each measure's scaling and range of scores, and the frequency with which the instrument was used. These details about scaling, subscales, range of scores, and scoring can be provided most concisely in a table. Table 27-1 is an example. Reliability and validity information previously published for the instrument should also be provided. In addition, the report includes the instrument's reliability in the current study and any further support of validity obtained from the current study. If you have used physiological measures, be sure to address their accuracy, precision, selectivity, sensitivity, and sources of error (Pyrczak & Bruce, 2007; see Chapter 16).

The presentation of results depends on the end product of the data analysis, your own preference, and any journal instructions. Generally, what is presented in a table is not restated in the text of the narrative. When reporting results in a narrative format, the value of the calculated statistic (t, F, r, or χ^2), the degrees of freedom (df), and probability (p value) should be included (Grove & Cipher, 2017). Word-processing programs include the Greek-letter statistics in the collection of symbols that the user can insert into a manuscript. When reporting any nonsignificant results, it is important to include the effect size and power level for that analysis so that readers would be able to evaluate the risk of Type II error (see Chapter 21).

Students often have difficulty putting all these Greek-letter statistical findings back into words for the text of the Results section. The APA *Publication Manual* (APA, 2010) provides direction for how to present various statistical results in a research report. Statistical values should be reported with two decimal digits of accuracy. Although computer output of data may include results reported to several decimal places, this is unnecessary for the report. For example, reporting the χ^2 value as 11.14 is sufficient, even if the computed value is 11.13965 (APA, 2010). The *p*-value, on the other hand, should be reported as the exact value. The exception is that if the computer output reads $p = 0.0000$, it should be reported as $p < 0.001$ because the computer rounds the value to zero, whereas p cannot actually assume that value (Grove & Cipher, 2017).

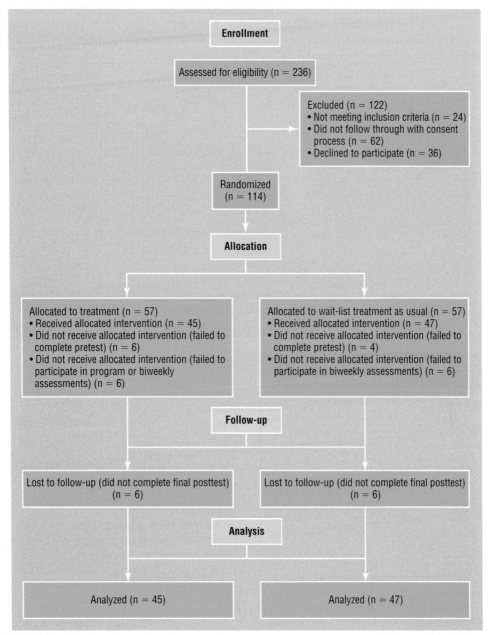

FIGURE 27-1 Patient flow chart for test of a pain management program. (Adapted from Wilson, M., Roll, J., & Barbosa-Leiker, C. [2015]. Empowering patients with persistent pain using an Internet-based self management program. *Pain Management Nursing, 16*[4], 506.)

Presentation of Results in Figures and Tables

Figures and tables are used to present a large amount of detailed information concisely and clearly. Researchers use figures and tables to demonstrate relationship and to document change over time, so as to reduce the number of words in the text of the report (APA, 2010; Saver, 2006). However, figures and tables are useful only if they are appropriate for the results you have generated and if they are well constructed (Saver, 2006). Box 27-2 provides guidelines for developing accurate and clear

TABLE 27-1   Variables, Instruments, and Scoring Used by Wilson et al. (2015) to Test a Pain Management Program

Variable	Instrument Description	Instrument Scoring
Pain intensity	Pain severity subscale of Brief Pain Inventory (Cleeland, 2009), four items with 11-point numerical rating scale (0 = no pain; 10 = pain as bad as you can imagine)	Mean score on the four items; the higher the score, the greater the pain intensity
Functional interference	Pain interference subscale of Brief Pain Inventory (Cleeland, 2009), seven items with 11-point numerical rating scale (0 = no pain; 10 = pain as bad as you can imagine)	Mean score on the seven items; the higher the score, the greater the functional interference
Depression	Short version Personal Health Questionnaire Depression Scale (PHQ-8) (Kroenke, Spitzer, Williams, & Löwe, 2010), eight items with 4-point rating scale (0 = not at all to 3 = nearly every day)	Sum score on the eight items; the higher the score, the greater the depression
Pain self-efficacy	Pain Self-Efficacy Questionnaire (PSEQ) (Tonkin, 2008); 10 items with 7-point Likert scale (0 = not at all confident to 6 = completely confident)	Sum score on the 10 items; the higher the score, the greater the self-efficacy
Opioid misuse	Current Opioid Misuse Measure (COMM) (Inflexxion, 2010); 17-item self assessment of pain-related symptoms and behaviors with 5-point Likert scale (0 = never to 4 = very often)	Sum score on the 17 items; the higher the score, the greater the opioid misuse

---

BOX 27-2   Guidelines for Developing Tables and Figures in Research Reports

- Select the results to include in the report.
- Identify a few key tables and figures that explain or support the major points.
- Develop simple tables and figures.
- Consider a table or figure for each research question or objective.
- Ensure that tables and figures are complete and clear without reference to the narrative.
- Give each table or figure a brief title.
- Number tables and figures separately in the report (e.g., Table 1, 2; Figure 1, 2).
- Review figures and tables in the journal to which you plan to submit your manuscript for formats acceptable to the journal.
- Use descriptive headings, labels, and symbols—may need to provide a key for abbreviations or symbols used in the the tables or figures.
- Include actual probability values or indicate whether statistically significant by asterisks.
- Refer to each table and figure in the narrative (e.g., Table 1 presents . . .).
- Use the narrative to summarize main ideas, without repeating the specifics of figures and tables.

Compiled from APA, 2010; Pallant, 2007; Pyrczak & Bruce, 2007.

---

figures and tables for a research report. More extensive guidelines and examples for developing tables and figures for research reports can be found in the APA *Publication Manual* (APA, 2010). For meta-analysis reports that synthesize the results of many studies, particular figures, called forest plots, are very important in the presentation of results (Floyd, Galvin, Roop, Oermann, & Nordstom, 2010). Refer to Chapter 19 for more information on forest plots and their appearance (Figure 19-6), and other figures used to report meta-analyses.

Figures. Figures are diagrams or pictures that illustrate either a conceptual framework or the study results. Researchers often use computer programs to generate sophisticated black-and-white or color figures. Conceptual frameworks are described both in the text and graphically. See examples in Chapter 8. Other common figures included in nursing research reports are bar graphs and line graphs. Journals often require high-resolution images for reproduction. The APA manual (APA, 2010, p. 167) has a figure checklist for you to review when deciding whether or not to include a figure. Generally, figures require specific formatting and may have less detail than readers want, so potential authors should carefully check with journal guidelines (Saver, 2006).

Bar graphs typically have horizontal or vertical bars that represent the size or amount of the group or variable studied. The bar graph is also a means of comparing one group with another. Henderson, Ossenberg, and Tyler (2015) conducted a mixed methods study of novice nurses' perceptions of the learning environment in a structured program to facilitate the assimilation of new graduates. The quantitative data they collected included the nurses' responses to a survey that measured recognition, affiliation, accomplishment, influence, and dissatisfaction. They added items to the influence subscale to address influence up and influence down and included an engagement subscale from another instrument. Henderson et al. (2015) reported the means on the subscales using a bar graph (Figure 27-2), on which the higher bar displayed a higher mean. The researchers placed the mean for each subscale in a table below the bar. Providing the numerical results effectively supplemented the graph, but it could have been improved by including the standard deviation as well. The researchers included a second bar graph in which 100% of each bar of the graph was divided into sections that represented the percentage of participants selecting that response (Figure 27-3).

A **line graph** is developed by joining a series of points with a line. It displays the values of a variable in comparison with a second variable, usually time. In this type of graph, the vertical scale (y-axis) is used to display the values of the first variable, and the horizontal scale (x-axis) is used to display the values of the second variable. A line graph figure requires at least three data points on the horizontal axis to show a trend or pattern. However, complexity does not enhance the ability to convey the data in a meaningful way, so it is recommended that no more than 10 time points should be included on a single line graph, and there should be no more than four lines or groups per graph, except when physiological data for intervals of seconds or minutes are presented. Figure 27-4 is a simpler line graph developed by Mallah et al. (2015) to depict the change in the prevalence of hospital-acquired pressure ulcers (HAPU) after interventions in a clinical facility. Figure 27-4 is easy to interpret because it includes five data points along the x-axis (quarters of the year) and the y-axis represents percentage prevalence. The figure clearly shows the effect of a group of interventions that were implemented in the third quarter

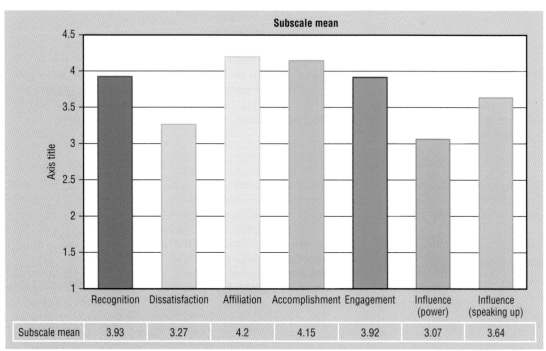

Subscale mean	Recognition	Dissatisfaction	Affiliation	Accomplishment	Engagement	Influence (power)	Influence (speaking up)
Subscale mean	3.93	3.27	4.2	4.15	3.92	3.07	3.64

FIGURE 27-2 Novice nurses' ($n = 78$) perceptions of the clinical learning organizational culture: Bar graph of subscale means. (Adapted from Henderson, A., Ossenberg, C., & Tyler, S. [2015]. "What matters to graduates": An evaluation of a structured clinical support program for newly graduated nurses. *Nurse Education in Practice, 15*[3], 228.)

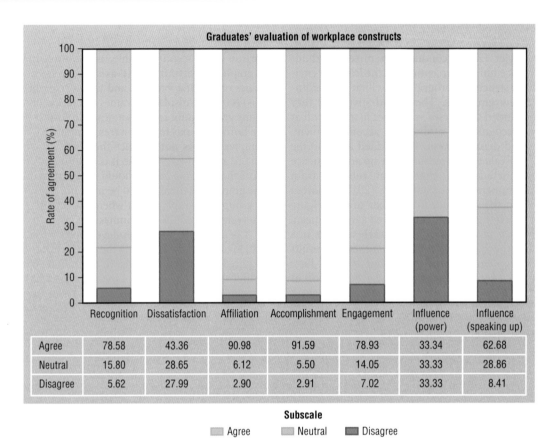

FIGURE 27-3 Novice nurses' (*n* = 78) evaluation of the characteristics of the clinical learning organizational culture: Bar graph with percentage of participants selecting a response. (Adapted from Henderson, A., Ossenberg, C., & Tyler, S. [2015]. "What matters to graduates": An evaluation of a structured clinical support program for newly graduated nurses. *Nurse Education in Practice, 15*[3], 225-231.)

of 2012. The researchers found that there was a statistically significant difference in prevalence rates from the first quarter of 2012 to the first quarter of 2013 (χ^2 = 7.64, $p < 0.01$).

Researchers may use other types of figures to display sample characteristics. A pie chart is an example of a figure that is seen less frequently in publications but fairly often in slides accompanying an oral conference presentation. Remember when preparing figures to provide sufficient and clear information so that the figure is meaningful even without accompanying narrative. For example, the caption and explanation for a figure should include information about the study, such as key concepts, type and size of the sample, and abbreviation used in the figure.

Tables. **Tables** are used more frequently in research reports than figures and can be developed to present

results from numerous statistical analyses in a small amount of space. Tabular results are presented in columns and rows so that the reader can review them easily. Table 27-2 is an example that presents descriptive statistics for the sample and variables, using means (*Ms*), ranges, and standard deviations (*SDs*). *Ms* and *SDs* of the study variables should be included in the published study because they allow other researchers to compare across studies, calculate the effect sizes to estimate sample size for new studies, and conduct meta-analyses (Conn & Rantz, 2003; Craig & Smyth 2012; Sandelowski, 2008). The sample size for each column should be included if the *n* varies from the total sample, reflecting missing values. Newnam et al. (2015, p. 37) conducted a "three group prospective randomized experimental study" with extremely low birth weight neonates who required continuous positive airway pressure (CPAP) due to neonatal respiratory distress syndrome. In these vulnerable neonates, nasal injury and skin breakdown are not uncommon. Newnam and colleagues compared the effects of mask interfaces and prong nasal interfaces with a third group, rotated between mask and prong interfaces every four hours.

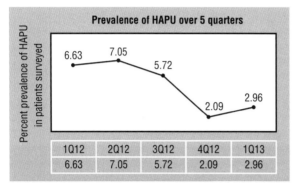

FIGURE 27-4 Prevalence of hospital-acquired pressure ulcers (HAPU) over time: Before and after intervention. (Adapted from Mallah, Z., Nassar, N., & Badr, L. [2015]. The effectiveness of a pressure ulcer intervention program on the prevalence of hospital acquired pressure ulcers: Controlled before and after study. *Applied Nursing Research, 28*[2], 110.) Note: 1st quarter of 2012 (1Q12), 2nd quarter of 2012 (2Q12), 3rd quarter of 2012 (3Q12), 4th quarter of 2012 (4Q15), 1st quarter of 2013 (1Q13).

Table 27-2 was descriptive of the key variables for the total sample but would have been stronger if birth weight and gestational age had been displayed separately by group. Newnam et al. (2015) did carefully note that two of the n's were for the number of participants ($n = 78$) and the remaining n's reflected the number of data collection episodes ($n = 730$). In the same study, the researchers conducted a regression analysis. Table 27-3 is an example of the results of the regression analysis. Newnam et al. (2015) provided a summary of the table in the text of the article as well.

"To best evaluate the effect of additional risk factors and their influence on the incidence and frequency of skin breakdown, a regression model was developed, guided by factors identified in the literature. Factors included in the model were BW [birth weight], length of therapy, PMA [post menstrual age] at the time of CPAP, environmental temperature, amount of CPAP flow administered and nursing interventions that include positioning techniques, nasal suctioning type (oral/nasal), suctioning interval and the use of nasal saline during suctioning (see Table 27-3). The mean PMA made the largest unique contribution (16% variance explained; $\beta = 0.46$; $p < 0.001$) although the number of CPAP days also made a statistically significant contribution (25% variance explained; $\beta = 0.31$; $p = 0.006$). The model accounted for 22% of total variance of skin breakdown ($R^2 = 0.22$; $F = 11.51$, $p = 0.006$)." (Newnam et al., 2015, p. 39)

TABLE 27-2 Sample Description

Demographic Variables for Total Sample

Variable	N	Mean	Minimum	Maximum	SD
Birth weight (g)	78*	873.36	500.00	1460.00	220.70
Birth gestational age (weeks)	78*	26.77	23.00	32.00	1.90
Current weight (g)	730**	1065.24	720.00	3170.00	373.99
Current age (weeks)	730**	3.87	0.14	14.43	3.23
Time to CPAP initiation (weeks)	730**	3.87	0.14	14.43	3.23
Number of CPAP days	730**	4.32	1.00	16.00	3.22
CPAP flow rate (lpm)	730**	5.35	4.00	7.00	0.66
Oxygen supplementation (%)	730**	0.25	0.21	0.60	0.60
Amount of humidity provided (C)	730**	25.59	0.00	86.00	34.26

CPAP, Continuous positive airway pressure; *lpm*, liter per minute; *C*, Celsius.
* Total number of participants in the study.
** Number of data collection episodes.
From Newnam, K., McGrath, J., Salyer, J., Estes, J., Jallo, N., & Bass, W. (2015). A comparative effectiveness study of continuous positive airway pressure-related skin breakdown when using different nasal interfaces in the extremely low birth weight neonate. *Applied Nursing Research, 28*(1), 39.

TABLE 27-3 Regression Model: Identified Predictors of Skin Breakdown Risk Factors During Nasal CPAP Use in the Neonate < 1500 g

Model	R	R^2	Standard Error	Df1	Df2	F	p-value
Model 1: mean post menstrual age at time of nasal CPAP (constant)	0.309	0.159	0.48	1	73	13.82	< 0.001
Model 2: mean post menstrual age at time of nasal CPAP; number of CPAP days (constant)	0.492	0.221	0.46	1	72	11.51	0.006

Note: Dependent variable: mean NSCS sum score.
CPAP, Continuous positive airway pressure.
From Newnam, K., McGrath, J., Salyer, J., Estes, J., Jallo, N., & Bass, W. (2015). A comparative effectiveness study of continuous positive airway pressure-related skin breakdown when using different nasal interfaces in the extremely low birth weight neonate. *Applied Nursing Research, 28*(1), 40.

Tables also are used to identify correlations among variables, and often the table presents a correlation matrix generated from the data analysis. The correlation matrix indicates the correlation values (coefficients) obtained when examining relationships between pairs of variables (bivariate correlations). The table identifies the correlation coefficients (Pearson *r* value) between pairs of variables, and the significance of each of these coefficients. The reader must carefully interpret the significance (*p* value) of each correlation coefficient because significance is sample-size dependent. The asterisks (***) indicate that this correlation is significant at $p \leq 0.001$ (some journals would require the exact *p* value). Smith, Theeke, Culp, Clark, and Pinto (2014) conducted a study of psychosocial factors in female university students who were obese. A body mass index (BMI) of 30 or greater was the criterion for obesity. Table 27-4 displays their correlation table of the relationships among sleep quality, perceived stress, loneliness, and self-esteem. Smith et al. (2014) found statistically significant correlations among all the variables. The three correlations between self-esteem and each of the other three variables indicated negative moderate to strong relationships, while the correlations between other paired variables indicated positive moderate relationships.

In addition to the other elements of the Discussion section that are common to all research reports, reports of quantitative studies usually address the generalizability of the findings to other samples and populations. Demographic and health characteristics of the sample are compared to the same characteristics of the population to examine the extent to which the sample is representative of the target population. Convenience

TABLE 27-4 Correlation Coefficients for Major Study Variables: Relationships Among Psychosocial Variables and Self-Rated Health in Adult Obese Women (*n* = 68)

Variable	Perceived Stress	Sleep Quality	Loneliness
Sleep quality	0.414**		
Loneliness	0.560**	0.414**	
Self-esteem	−0.600**	−0.365*	−0.688**

*p < 0.01.
**p < 0.001.
From Smith, M., Theeke, L., Culp, S., Clark, K., & Pinto, S. (2014). Psychosocial variables and self-rated health in young adult obese women. *Applied Nursing Research, 27*(1), 69.

samples are less representative of the target population than are randomly selected samples.

Qualitative Research Report

Reports for qualitative research are as diverse as the different types of qualitative studies. The types of qualitative research are presented in Chapter 4, and methods from specific qualitative studies are presented in Chapter 12. The intent of a qualitative research report is to describe the dynamic implementation of the research project and the unique, creative findings obtained (Marshall & Rossman, 2016). Similar to a quantitative report, a qualitative research report needs a clear, concise title that identifies the focus of the study.

The abstract for a qualitative research report briefly summarizes the key parts of the study and usually includes the following: (1) aim of the study; (2) qualitative approach (e.g., phenomenology, grounded theory, ethnography, exploratory-descriptive, or historical); (3) methods including sample, setting, and methods of data collection; (4) brief synopsis of findings; and (5) implications of the findings (Munhall, 2012). The example of an unstructured abstract provided earlier in the chapter was developed for a qualitative study (Shin et al., 2015) and contains all five of these elements.

The Methods section for a qualitative study includes the specific qualitative design (e.g., phenomenology, grounded theory, or ethnography); a detailed description of the data collection method such as interview or observation; and the data management and analysis plan. In the presentation of the qualitative approach, the researcher provides the philosophical basis for and the assumptions of the qualitative method with citations from the primary sources. In addition, a rationale for selecting this type of qualitative study should be specified (Marshall & Rossman, 2016).

Unique to qualitative research, the researchers may be expected to describe their relevant educational and clinical background for conducting the study. This documentation helps the reader evaluate the worth of the study because the researcher serves as a primary data-gathering instrument and analyses occur within the reasoning processes of the researcher (Munhall, 2012). The researcher provides detail about all data collection processes, including training of project staff, entry into the setting, selection of participants, and ethical considerations extended to the participants throughout the study. When data collection tools are used, such as observation guides, initial questions for open-ended interviews, or forms to record extracted facts from historical documents, they are described and a copy provided in the report as an inset or as an appendix. The flexible, dynamic way in which the researcher collects data is described, including time spent collecting interview or observational data, how data were recorded, and amount of data collected. For example, if your data collection involved participant observation, you should describe the number, length, structure, and focus of the observation and participation periods. In addition, you should identify the tools (e.g., digital devices) for recording the data from these periods of observation and participation. What processes were used to transcribe audio recordings for analysis? How was the accuracy of the transcription confirmed? The plan described in the methods section for analyzing the data includes the person or persons who coded the data, how they were trained, and the software product used, if any.

Data analysis procedures are performed during or after the data collection process, depending on method, and this timing should be specified (Marshall & Rossman, 2016; Munhall, 2012). Present your results in a manner that clarifies for the reader the phenomenon under investigation. These results include descriptions, themes, social processes, and theories that emerged from the study of life experiences, cultures, or historical events. Sometimes, these theoretical ideas are organized into conceptual maps, models, or tables. Researchers often gather additional data or reexamine existing data to verify their theoretical conclusions, and this process is described in the report (Marshall & Rossman, 2016). Some qualitative study findings lack clarity and quality, which makes it difficult for practitioners to understand and apply them. Some of the problems with qualitative study results are misuse of quotes and theory, lack of clarity in identifying patterns and themes in the data, and misrepresentation of data and data analysis procedures in the report (Sandelowski, 2010). Researchers must clearly and accurately develop their findings and present them in a way that a diverse audience of practitioners and researchers can understand. Sandelowski and Leeman (2012) recommended writing sentences that reflect the identified themes. Clearly writing themes will take practice, because you want to preserve "the complexity of the phenomena these ideas were meant to represent" and yet summarize key ideas (Sandelowski & Leeman, 2012, p. 1407).

The Discussion section includes conclusions, study limitations, implications for nursing, and recommendations for further research in the same manner that quantitative research reports do. The conclusions are a synthesis of the study findings and the relevant theoretical and empirical literature. Limitations are identified and their influence on the formulation of the conclusions is addressed. Small sample size in qualitative research is not a limitation: failure to explain the phenomenon of interest fully due to inadequate data collection and analysis is.

In Australia, Tong, Sainsbury, and Craig (2007) developed a checklist that included three domains to be included in qualitative research reports: "(i) research team and reflexivity, (ii) study design, and (iii) data analysis and reporting" (p. 349). The Consolidated Criteria for Reporting Qualitative Research (COREQ) is their 32-item checklist for studies in which the data are collected through interviews and focus groups. COREQ has not had the widespread acceptance of the CONSORT Statement, but provides a standard by which qualitative researchers can evaluate the thoroughness of their research report.

Theses and Dissertations

Theses and **dissertations** are research reports that students develop in depth as part of the requirements for a degree. The university, nursing school or college, and members of the student's research committee provide specific requirements for the final thesis or dissertation. Traditionally, theses and dissertations are organized by chapters, the content of which are specified by the college or university. The content included in a thesis follows the general outline of reports (see Box 27-1). Chapter 28 also provides guidelines for the content of thesis and dissertation proposals. Baggs (2011) discussed the option of publishable papers as chapters for a dissertation and issues to consider regarding copyright and intellectual property. Morse (2005) raised additional issues in qualitative dissertations that are comprised of publishable articles, and considered these a move away from the richness and depth of qualitative inquiry when an article of limited pages (15 or fewer) is the goal. The advantages for graduates are the experience of writing for publication and the presence of publications on their curriculum vitae (resumé) when they apply for academic positions.

AUDIENCES FOR COMMUNICATION OF RESEARCH FINDINGS

Before developing a research report, you need to determine who will benefit from knowing the findings. The greatest impact on nursing practice can be achieved by communicating nursing research findings to a variety of audiences, including nurses, other health professionals, healthcare consumers, and policymakers.

Nurses and Other Healthcare Professionals

Nurses, including administrators, educators, practitioners, and researchers, must be aware of research findings for use in practice and as a basis for conducting additional studies. Other health professionals need to be aware of the knowledge generated by nurse researchers and facilitate the use of that knowledge in the healthcare system as part of the delivery of evidence-based practice (Craig & Smyth, 2012). Nurse researchers communicate their research more broadly by presenting at conferences sponsored by specialty organizations such as the American Heart Association, American Public Health Association, American Cancer Society, American Lung Association, National Hospice Organization, and National Rural Health Association, at which attendees have an active interest in application of findings. Nurse researchers and other health professionals conducting research on the same problem might collaborate to publish an article, a series of articles, a book chapter, or a book. This type of interdisciplinary collaboration increases communication of research findings and facilitates synthesis of research knowledge to promote evidence-based practice.

Policymakers

Policymakers at the local, state, and federal levels use research findings to generate health policy that has an impact on consumers, individual practitioners, and the healthcare system. Rather than the more common research with individuals as the source of data, Chapman, Wides, and Spetz (2010) provided an excellent example of communicating policy-related research findings using the *Medicare Claims Processing Manual,* reports from the National Council of State Boards of Nursing, and congressional reports as their sources of data. They tabulated their data and concluded that more data are needed in these documents about the type of care provided. They also concluded from their analysis that the payment system for advanced practice nurses needs to be remodeled (Chapman et al., 2010).

Consumers

Nurse researchers frequently neglect healthcare consumers as an audience for research reports. Consumers are interested in research findings about illnesses that they or family members currently face. There is a need to provide consumers with evidence-based guidelines and educational materials to assist them in making quality healthcare decisions.

The findings from nursing studies can be communicated rapidly to the public through a variety of means. Some universities may prepare and disseminate press releases about research findings. The researcher may write a summary of the study for a local newspaper. Even local articles have the potential of being picked up by a national wire service and published in other papers across the U.S. Findings can also be communicated to consumers by being published in news magazines, such as *Time* and *Newsweek,* or popular health magazines, such as *American Baby* and *Health.* Health articles published for consumer magazines and online distribution reach millions of readers at a time (e.g., webmd.com or *WebMD, the Magazine*). Television and radio are other valuable media for communicating research findings to consumers and other healthcare providers. Freelance journalists often contact authors of scientific articles, and these writers have the skills to translate research findings into language for consumers. Lee and Gay (2011) conducted a study entitled, "Can Modifications to the Bedroom Environment Improve the Sleep of New

Parents? Two Randomized Controlled Trials." A skilled journalist writing for *Parenting Magazine* subsequently was able to catch consumers' attention with the title, "Desperately Seeking Sleep," to disseminate the same data contained in the research publication but for a targeted public audience (Bernstein, 2011). (Paraphrased results reported in lay publications are not considered duplicate publications, so they do not represent scientific misconduct.) In addition to print media, the increase of digital media allows the nurse researcher wide dissemination of study findings. One caution of digital media is that the report must be clear about study limitations and additional confirmatory studies that must be conducted before generalization is appropriate.

STRATEGIES FOR PRESENTATION AND PUBLICATION OF RESEARCH FINDINGS

The formal research report must be edited for dissemination. The specifics of conference presentation and manuscript preparation require judicious selection of the most relevant parts of the total study.

Conferences

Nurses communicate research findings to their peers through **presentations** at conferences and meetings. Presentations are structured, formal reports of a completed research study that are communicated orally or through a poster. Sigma Theta Tau, the international honor society for nursing, sponsors international, national, regional, and local research conferences. Specialty organizations, such as the American Association of Critical Care Nurses, Oncology Nurses' Society, and Association of Women's Health, Obstetrics, and Neonatal Nursing, sponsor research conferences. Many universities and some healthcare agencies provide financial support (sponsorship) for research conferences. For various reasons, nurses are not always able to attend these research conferences. To increase the communication of research findings and disseminate the new knowledge more widely, conference sponsors often provide websites with electronic posters and recordings of the research presentations. Some sponsors publish abstracts of studies with the conference proceedings, publish the abstracts in a research journal supplement, or provide materials electronically on their websites. To be selected to present at a conference, the researcher must submit an abstract describing the study.

The Abstract Submission Process

The sponsors of a research conference circulate a call for abstracts months, sometimes as much as a year, before the conference. Many research journals and newsletters publish these requests for abstracts, and they are available electronically. In addition, conference sponsors email requests for abstracts to universities, major healthcare agencies, and nurse researcher listservs.

Acceptance as a presenter is based on the quality of the submitted abstract. The abstract should be based on the theme of the conference and the organizers' criteria for reviewing the abstract. As noted earlier, an **abstract** is a clear, concise summary of a study that has a word limit. The abstract submitted for a verbal presentation is usually based on results from a completed study that is not yet published.

Before submitting an abstract for a conference, pay attention to the description of the conference, which includes its overview, goal, and expected attendees. How well does your study fit with the goals of the conference? Will attendees be interested in your study? The call for abstracts stipulates the format for the abstract. Frequently, abstracts are limited to one page, single-spaced, and include the content outlined in Box 27-3. Use the abstract guidelines for the specific conference to ensure that all required elements are included. When abstracts are submitted online, you may be limited to a specific number of characters instead of words. For electronic submissions, write and revise the abstract in a separate document. Depending on the instructions, you may

---

BOX 27-3 Outline for an Abstract Submitted for a Conference

I. Title of the Study

II. Introduction
Statement of the problem and purpose
Identification of the framework

III. Methodology
Design
Sample size
Identification of data analysis methods

IV. Results
Major findings
Conclusions
Implications for nursing
Recommendations for further research

Note: The title and authors with affiliations, a conflict-of-interest statement, a brief reference list of one or two key citations, and the acknowledgment of funding source are not usually considered in the word limitations for the abstract.

copy and paste the text in a box on the webpage or attach the file.

The title of your abstract must create interest, and the body of your abstract "sells" the study to the reviewers. Names and affiliations are removed for review. Writing an abstract requires practice; frequently, a researcher rewrites an abstract many times until it meets all the criteria, including the word limit, outlined by the conference sponsors. Careful attention to the criteria of the sponsoring agency should assist you in developing and refining your abstract and increase your chances of having the abstract accepted for either a podium or a poster presentation. The Western Institute of Nursing (WIN) has an excellent online tutorial called, "Writing a WINning abstract" by Lentz (2011).

Some conference organizers ask that you specify whether you want to be considered for an oral podium presentation or a poster presentation, whereas others decide on a poster versus oral podium presentation based on their own criteria or scoring system. Generally, abstracts that describe smaller sample sizes and describe preliminary findings or pilot studies are less likely to be accepted for an oral podium presentation. Some conference planning committees require that you submit two versions of your abstract: one with names and affiliations that would be in their program or published abstracts, and another that removes all names and affiliations so that the abstract is anonymous and reviewers are blinded. Read the instructions carefully because they sometimes require that the content of the abstract has not been published or presented elsewhere. Instructions also indicate whether or not accepted abstracts are published, usually as a supplemental issue of the sponsor's affiliated professional journal.

Podium Presentation Research Findings

Through podium presentations, researchers have an opportunity to share their findings with many persons at one time, answer a limited number of questions about their studies, interact formally with other interested professionals, and receive a small amount of immediate feedback on their study, concisely provided. Research project findings frequently are presented at conferences as preliminary findings of completed studies. The researchers may not have completely finalized the implications and conclusions, but the interaction with other researchers may facilitate that process and expand their thinking. When research findings are published, the data must not be published elsewhere, and any presentation of these data at a conference should be acknowledged. In addition to having your abstract accepted, presenting findings at a conference verbally also involves develop-ing a research report, delivering the report, and responding to questions.

Developing an oral research presentation. The presentation developed depends on the audience and the time designated for each presentation. The interests and size of the audience will vary depending on whether you were accepted for a concurrent session with an audience that selects your presentation to attend based on the title and their interest, or for a general session with the entire audience of conference participants. If you are unsure of the composition of your conference audience, ask others who have attended the conference or ask the contact person for the conference.

Time is probably the most important factor in developing a presentation because many presenters are limited to 10 or 15 minutes, with an additional 5 minutes for questions. As a guideline, you want to aim for one slide per minute. Your title slide, acknowledgment slide, and final slide of references or slide calling for questions from the audience should be included in the timing because other factors may encroach on your time. For example, the moderator will introduce you and may give other instructions to the attendees, tasks that may last a few minutes. Your presentation should be designed to fit your allocated time. Your audience is there to hear what is new in your area of research, not to hear the entire background and review of literature that brought you to this current research. Although it is important to address the major sections of a research report (Introduction, Methods, Results, and Discussion) in your presentation, most attendees are more interested in the study results and findings than a review of the literature or history of a tool's development. For guidance, in a 10-minute presentation you should spend 20% (two minutes or two slides) of your total time on the title and introduction, 20% on the methodology, 40% on the results, and 20% on the discussion and implications for practice and research. In planning your allotted time for the presentation, it also is helpful to know whether questions from the audience will be allowed during your presentation, allowed at the end of your presentation, or held until the end of the entire session, at which time participants direct their questions to any one of the presenters in the session.

Your title slide should provide the audience with the gap in knowledge that you addressed in your study. Your introduction should acknowledge funding sources and collaborators, if applicable, as well as any conflict of interest. A very brief review of key background literature and a simple diagram of the conceptual framework should lead directly into the research questions or hypotheses that address the knowledge gap. The methodology content includes a brief identification of the design, sampling method, measurement techniques, and analysis plan. The content covered in the results section should start with a simple table of the sample characteristics followed by a slide of results for each question or hypothesis. The presentation should conclude with a brief discussion of findings, implications of your findings for clinical practice, and recommendations for future research. Most presenters find that the shorter the presentation time, the greater the preparation time needed. If you are limited to 10 minutes, you must be very selective about which one or two research questions or hypotheses will be your focus. If you have 15 or 20 minutes, you may still choose to limit your presentation to three research questions or hypothesis but allow more time to discuss the details regarding the contributions and limitations of your research. Start the development of your presentation early, because some conferences require that you submit your slides up to six weeks prior to the conference. The conference organizers download the presentations to be given in a specific room at a particular time on a laptop computer or tablet to save time on the day of the presentation.

For longer presentations, consider using figures, pictures, or possibly some animation, to emphasize key points and maintain the audience's attention. The information presented on each slide should be limited to eight lines or fewer, with six or fewer words per line. A single slide should contain information that can be easily read and examined in 30 seconds to 1 minute. All words in both title and body of a slide should be bolded, so that they will be visible throughout the audience. Only major points are presented on visuals, so use single words, short phrases, or bulleted points to convey ideas, not complete sentences. Figures such as bar graphs and line graphs may convey ideas more clearly than do tables. Tables and figures that are included should contain only the most important information and be in a font that can be seen clearly by the audience. If a large table is needed, provide it to attendees as a handout and focus on the key points from the table on your slide. Pictures of the research setting and equipment and photographs of the research team help the audience visualize the research project. A laser pointer may be useful to guide the audience to your key point on the slide, but the deliberate and careful use of color is more appealing to the audience, can increase the clarity of the information presented, and can call attention to a particular important statistical test and p value without the need for a laser pointer. However, avoid using particular shades of red color for bulleted points or highlighted wording, particularly if you have a dark background; red

may display correctly on a computer monitor, but it becomes difficult to see when projected to a large audience.

Preparing the script and visuals for a presentation is difficult, so enlist the assistance of an experienced researcher and audiovisual expert. *Rehearse* your presentation in a large room with experienced researchers, so as to confirm readability, and use their comments to refine your script, slides, and presentation style. If your presentation is too long, synthesize parts of your script into handouts for important content. You may want to prepare handouts for the participants, even if your presentation is shorter. Be sure that the handouts include your name, contact information, name of your employer, and acknowledgment of any funding you received to conduct the study.

PowerPoint slides provide an excellent format for presenting an oral research report; they include easy-to-read fonts, color, creative backgrounds, visuals or pictures to clarify points, and animation options. Although you can construct your own PowerPoint presentation, consulting an audiovisual expert will ensure that your materials are clear and properly constructed, with the print large enough and dark enough for the audience to read. When the PowerPoint slides have been developed, view them from the same vantage point as the audience to ensure that each slide is clear and can be visualized without totally darkening the room. Remember to **bold** anything on-screen to ensure that the text is readable from the audience.

Delivering a research report and responding to questions. A novice researcher may benefit from attending conferences and examining the presentation styles of other researchers before preparing an oral report. Even though each researcher needs to develop his or her own presentation style, observing others can promote an effective style. An effective presentation requires practice. You need to rehearse your presentation several times, with the script, until you are comfortable with the timing, the content, and your presentation style. When practicing, use the visuals so that you are comfortable with the equipment.

The first thing the audience hears from you should not be, "(tap-tap) Is this thing on?" Rehearse with special attention to verbal mannerisms such as, "Umm," "you know," "like," and tongue clicks, and to visual mannerisms and body language. Stand up straight. Enunciate. SLOW DOWN. Take a deep breath and slow down even more. If the audience cannot understand what you say, your presentation is wasted. The rules, "Never alibi, never complain" are good to remember. It is always advantageous to check out the room in which you will be presenting to see how chairs are arranged and how the podium and screen are situated. Before your turn to present, check to make sure that your slides are available on the computer, practice opening the file, and ensure that you know how to advance from one slide to the next.

Most conferences organize their oral presentations by topic into a session moderated by an expert in the field. The session usually includes a presentation by the researcher, a comment by the session's moderator, and a question period before moving to the next speaker. If your presentation is too long for the allotted time, the moderator may stop your presentation to proceed to the next speaker or there will be no opportunity for questions from the audience. When preparing for a presentation, try to anticipate the questions that members of the audience might ask and rehearse your answers. As you practice your presentation with colleagues, ask them to raise questions. Frequently, the questions they pose will be the same ones the audience will raise. If you practice making clear, concise responses to specific questions, you will be less anxious during your presentation. When giving a presentation, have someone make notes of the audience's questions, suggestions, or comments, because this input is often useful when preparing a manuscript for publication or developing the next study.

Poster Presentation of Research Findings

Your research abstract may be accepted at a conference as a poster presentation rather than a podium presentation. A **poster session** is a collection of all the posters being displayed in one central location at a conference. A poster is a visual presentation of your study, all on one surface. Through poster presentation, researchers have an opportunity to share their findings with a handful of persons at one time, answer unlimited questions, interact informally with other interested professionals, and receive thoughtful feedback, gently offered. Having the opportunity to present a poster should not be minimized. In nursing, poster presentations are a legitimate means of communicating findings, in fact as legitimate as podium presentations.

Before developing a poster, read the directions. Follow the conference sponsor's specifications for (1) the size limitations or format restrictions for the poster, (2) the size of the poster display area, and (3) the background and potential number of conference participants. Your institution may have a template with the logo that you are required to use for the audience to identify your affiliation more easily. A poster usually includes the following content: the title of the study; investigator and institution names; purpose; research

---

BOX 27-4 **Principles for Developing a Poster**
1. Start planning early with a clear focus.
2. Follow conference guidelines carefully.
a. Poster size
b. Hanging or free-standing
3. Use bullet points or abbreviated wording.
4. Include pictures and graphics that add to the content.
5. Balance text and pictures with white space.
6. Use a large font size for viewing from a distance.

From Forsyth, D., Wright, T., Scherb, C., & Gaspar, P. (2010). Disseminating evidence-based projects: Poster design and evaluation. *Clinical Scholars Review, 3*(1), 14-21.

---

objectives, questions, or hypotheses (if applicable); framework; design; sample; instruments; essential data collection procedures; results; conclusions; implications for nursing; recommendations for further research; a few key references; and acknowledgments. Box 27-4 provides suggestions for developing a poster.

A quality poster presents a study completely, yet can be comprehended in five minutes or less. For clarity and visual appeal, a poster often uses pictures, tables, or figures to communicate the study. High-quality posters have a polished, professional look and present the key aspects of the study using a balance of text, figures, and color. Bold headings are used for the different parts of the research report, followed by concise narratives or bulleted phrases. Summary and implications sections are placed prominently and at eye level, given the limited time for viewing many posters during a session and your desire to make the findings known. Because rich narrative text is so meaningful in qualitative studies, authors are advised to bold and enlarge the font for a few particularly meaningful quotes, and use artwork or photos that conceptualize the quote in a visual way. The size of the text on a poster needs to be large enough to be read at 3 feet (approximately 20 font size), but the title or banner should be readable at 20 feet (Shelledy, 2004). Matte finish is preferable to glossy finish because in less favorable lighting, glossy finishes predispose to glare. Lamination protects the poster from damage and lends to the finished product a slight shine that does not produce glare.

Posters usually take 10 to 20 hours to develop, depending on the complexity of the study and the experience of the researcher. Novice researchers usually need more than 20 hours to develop a poster. Important points in poster development include planning ahead, seeking the assistance of others, and limiting the information on the poster (Shelledy, 2004). Many universities provide detailed online information about poster presentation (New York University Libraries, 2015). There are several modalities for creation of a visually engaging and well-organized poster, including PowerPoint, with which most new researchers are familiar. Many universities have digital laboratories and personnel available to assist in poster development for a study that was completed to meet academic requirements.

Conference organizers often provide boards for displaying posters. The poster can be rolled to prevent creases and easily transported to the conference in a protective tube. Office supply stores and shipping companies provide online services such as designing, printing, and shipping the poster to the conference venue. Posters can also be printed on fabric and easily packed in a suitcase, which is especially nice for an international conference. Because accidents can occur, it is wise to email oneself the poster: if the actual poster is lost or damaged in transit, it can be reprinted onsite.

Poster sessions usually last one to two hours; you should remain by your poster during this time and offer to answer any questions when a viewer is present. Most researchers provide conference participants with a copy of the accepted abstract. You may choose to prepare a single-page handout of the poster with your contact information, particularly if you cannot stand by the poster for the entire allotted time. Some conferences require posters to be displayed for the entire run of the conference. Leaving contact information on or near the poster can help interested attendees who want to communicate with you.

One major advantage of a poster session is the opportunity for one-to-one interaction between the researcher and the viewer. Frequently, at the end of the poster session individuals interested in a study stay to speak with the researcher. Have a notepad on hand to record comments and contact information for individuals conducting similar research. Exchanging business cards and writing key information on the back of the card is a useful practice. Poster sessions provide an excellent opportunity to begin networking with other researchers involved in the same area of research. Conference participants occasionally request your study instruments or other items, so it is essential that you keep a record of their contact information and specific requests.

Publishing Research Findings

Podium and poster presentations are valuable means of rapidly communicating findings, but their impact is limited, and findings should not have been published previously. Even if the accepted abstract is published in a supplemental volume of a journal associated with the conference sponsors, you should be planning publication of the full findings for a research journal as you prepare for the oral podium or poster presentation. **Published research** findings are permanently recorded in a journal or book and usually reach a larger audience than do presentations. Because journals are the most common venue used by nurses to disseminate findings in print, we will focus on that type of publication.

When study findings have been presented prior to publication, there should be an acknowledgment in the published report that the contents of the paper were presented at a particular research conference. The presentation and comments from the audience can provide a basis for finalizing your article for publication. Many journal editors are conference attendees and may request your paper for an article when they hear your oral presentation or see your poster. Many researchers present their findings at a conference or two and never submit the paper for publication.

Studies with negative findings (no significant difference or relationship) are frequently not submitted for publication (Teixeira da Silva, 2015), which can contribute to scientific bias. When statistical power is sufficient and measures are reliable, negative findings may be an accurate reflection of reality. Negative findings can be as important to the development of knowledge as positive findings are because they inform other researchers of what did not work. By eliminating rival hypotheses, science can be advanced (Teixeira da Silva, 2015). Many authors strategize placing these nonsignificant findings within a journal that has previously published an article describing positive findings on the same topic.

While you are developing your study and writing the proposal, outline your plans for dissemination of the findings. Now, at the outset of the endeavor, you and other members of your research team should discuss and determine authorship credit. This discussion can become a complex issue when the research is a collaborative project among individuals from different disciplines with varied degrees of research education and experience.

There are several terms related to authorship credit that are important to understand. Honorary authorship refers to listing a senior researcher's name on an article with that person making *no* contribution to the manuscript (Shamoo & Resnik, 2015). Ghost authorship is the situation in which an individual or company was involved in a study and the manuscript but is not listed

---

BOX 27-5   Authorship Criteria of the International Committee of Medical Journal Editors: Requirements to Be an Author

- Substantial contributions to the conception or design of the work; or the acquisition, analysis, or interpretation of data for the work; AND
- Drafting the work or revising it critically for important intellectual content; AND
- Final approval of the version to be published; AND
- Agreement to be accountable for all aspects of the work in ensuring that questions related to the accuracy or integrity of any part of the work are appropriately investigated and resolved.

From International Committee of Medical Journal Editors [ICMJE]. (2016). *Defining the role of authors and contributors.* Retrieved May 11, 2016, from http://www.icmje.org/recommendations/browse/roles-and-responsibilities/defining-the-role-of-authors-and-contributors.html The ICMJE periodically updates "Recommendations for the Conduct, Reporting, Editing, and Publication of Scholarly Work in Medical Journals." The most recent version is available at www.icmje.org.

---

as an author to avoid the appearance of a conflict of interest (i.e., the manufacturer of a medication used in a study) (Shamoo & Resnik, 2015). Both types of authorship are unethical. To avoid such situations, the International Committee of Medical Journal Editors (ICMJE) developed authorship guidelines that have become the standard for most professional journals. Journal editors require authors to specify their contributions to a study and to the manuscript, including signing a form that documents the contributions. Box 27-5 lists the four criteria on which authorship should be based (ICMJE, 2016). Shamoo and Resnik (2015) provide additional discussion related to authorship that may be helpful for specific situations such as non-research manuscripts and faculty-student relationships.

Journals

Developing a manuscript for publication includes the following steps: (1) selecting a journal, (2) developing a query letter, (3) preparing a manuscript, (4) submitting the manuscript for review, and (5) revising the manuscript.

Selecting a journal. Selecting a journal for publication of your study requires knowledge of the basic requirements of the journal, the journal's review process, and recent articles published in the journal. A **refereed**

journal is peer-reviewed and uses referees or expert reviewers to determine whether a manuscript is acceptable for publication. In nonrefereed journals, the editor makes the decision to accept or reject a manuscript, but this decision is usually made after consultation with a nursing expert. In recent years, there has been an increase in what are termed predatory journals. For these open-access electronic publications, editors solicit manuscripts but require authors to pay an "article-processing charge" of hundreds or thousands of dollars to have a manuscript published. In funded studies, the charge may be paid with grant funds. A faculty author may have the fee paid by the university. Occasionally, the fees may be waived. Some of these journals require peer-review of submitted manuscripts, similar to non-predatory journals. Ensure that the journal you select is a reputable journal that is indexed in databases such as the Cumulative Index to Nursing and Allied Health Literature (CINAHL).

Most refereed journals require manuscripts to be reviewed anonymously, or blinded, by two or three reviewers. Expertise and objectivity are characteristics of ideal reviewers (Shamoo & Resnik, 2015), who can evaluate the quality of a manuscript and its potential contribution to knowledge. In some cases, there are two reviewers for the scientific content and one reviewer for particular attention to the statistical content (Henly, Bennett, & Dougherty, 2010). Reviewers are asked to determine the strengths and weaknesses of a manuscript, and their comments are sent anonymously from the journal editor to the contact author. Most academic institutions support the refereed system and may recognize only publications that appear in peer-reviewed journals for faculty members seeking tenure and promotion.

Opportunities to publish research have grown as research journals have become more plentiful. Publishing opportunities in nursing continue to increase. The *Journal Citation Reports* (Thomson Reuters, 2015) includes at least 88 journals with "nursing" or "nurse" in their titles. The Nursing and Allied Health Resources Section (NAHRS) of the Medical Library Association created a report of the over 200 nursing journals in 2012. The report incorporates the type of review that manuscripts receive, the percentage of submitted manuscripts accepted for publication, and the types of articles published (NAHRS, 2012). When deciding on a potential journal for a study, the NAHRS report, the *Journal Citations Report,* and other similar reports can provide invaluable information about four criteria to consider when selecting a journal: (1) the intended readers that would benefit from reading the findings, (2) the fit of the study's topic to the journal's focus, (3) the journal's reported elapsed time between acceptance of a manuscript and its publication, and (4) the impact factor for the journal. The content for a study may be most suitable for a small specialty group audience, or perhaps a broader spectrum of nurses would think the research interesting and pertinent to their practice. Nurse researchers should not limit their options to nursing journals if a wider audience of health professionals is the proper target for findings of the study. Additional clues about possible audiences can be found in the references cited in the research report. For example, if your reference list includes several articles from genomics journals, one of those journals may be appropriate choice for your article. If it is important for the findings to be reported as soon as possible, consider an online journal or a journal that has monthly issues rather than quarterly issues.

Having a manuscript accepted for publication depends not only on the quality of the manuscript but also on how closely the manuscript matches the goals of the journal and its subscribers or audience (Dougherty, Freda, Kearney, Baggs & Broome, 2011). Reviewing articles recently published in the journal being considered can be helpful in assessing this match. A detailed review of this sort lets you know whether a research topic has recently been addressed and whether the research findings would be of interest to that journal's readers. This process enables you to identify and prioritize a few journals that would be appropriate for publishing your findings. Reviewing the journal's impact factor, the timeline for their review process, and the waiting period from acceptance to publication date can also impact your decision on submission targets for your manuscript.

Journal impact factor. *Journal Citation Report* (Thomson Reuter, 2015) provides quantitative measures for evaluating scientific journals, including data on journal impact factors. The **impact factor** is a measure of the frequency with which the "average article" in a journal has been cited in a given period of time (Garfield, 2006). The impact factor for a journal is calculated based on a 3-year period and can be considered to be the average number of times published papers are cited up to 2 years after publication. The impact factor cannot be calculated until the publication of a year's worth of issues; for that reason, the most current impact factor available may reflect data from 1 to 2 years earlier. The impact factor for a journal can usually be found at the journal's website. The higher the number, the better. Generally, specialty journals in nursing have lower impact factors than broad-based journals such as *Journal*

of the American Medical Association or *New England Journal of Medicine.*

Developing a query letter. A **query letter** is a letter an author sends to an editor, to ask about the editor's interest in reviewing a manuscript. This letter should be no more than one page in length and usually includes the abstract and the researcher's qualifications for writing the article. The length of the manuscript and the numbers of tables or figures may be useful information to include, and the editor may be interested to know when, if ever, something on this topic was last published in their journal. Some editors appreciate a list of potential reviewers that you might suggest. Address your query letter in an email to the current editor of a journal. Indicate in the letter the title of the manuscript you would like to submit, why publishing the manuscript is important, and why the readers of the journal would be interested in reading the manuscript. Even if a letter is not required by a journal, some researchers send a query letter because the response (positive or negative) enables them to make the final selection for submitting their manuscript to a journal. Often an editor responds that the journal is planning a special issue on a particular topic and provides the due dates so that you can prepare well in advance. Other journals, such as *Advances in Nursing Science,* publish only special topic issues. You can select an appropriate issue for your submission by reviewing their websites with due dates by topic.

Preparing a manuscript. A manuscript is written according to the format outlined by each different journal. Guidelines for developing a manuscript usually are published in the individual issues of the journal or on journal websites. Follow these author guidelines explicitly to increase the probability of your manuscript being accepted for publication. Author guidelines are comprised of directions for manuscript preparation, a discussion of copyright and conflict of interest, and guidelines for submission of the manuscript. Most journals accept only online submissions of electronic files.

Writing research reports for publication requires skills in technical writing that are not used in other types of publications. Technical writing condenses information and is stylistic. The *Publication Manual of the American Psychological Association* (APA, 2010); *A Manual for Writers of Research Papers, Theses, Dissertations* (Turabian, Booth, Colomb, & Williams, 2013); and the *Chicago Manual of Style* (University of Chicago Press Staff, 2010) are considered useful sources for quality technical writing. Most journals stipulate the format style required for their journal. In a review of 65 nursing journals, Northam, Yarbough, Haas, and Duke (2010) noted that 36 (55%) required APA format. If a journal requires a format different from that of your original manuscript, there are format "translators" available through most universities that will convert one format to another. Computer programs are available with bibliography systems that enable you to compile a consistent reference list formatted in any commonly accepted journal style. With these programs, researchers can maintain a permanent file of reference citations. When a reference list is needed for a manuscript, the researchers can select the appropriate references from the collection and use the program to format for the requirements of a particular journal.

A quality research report has no errors in punctuation, spelling, or sentence structure. It is also important to avoid confusing words, clichés, jargon, and excessive wordiness and abbreviations. Word processing programs have "tools" that have the capacity to proofread manuscripts for errors. However, as the author, you still need to respond to the software's prompts and correct the sentences that the program has identified as problematic. These program tools also perform a word count, to ensure that your manuscript adheres to the limitations specified in the journal guidelines.

Knowledge about the author guidelines provided by the journal and a background in technical writing will help you develop an outline for a proposed manuscript. You can use the outline to develop a rough draft of your article, which you will revise numerous times. Present the content of your article logically and concisely under clear headings, and select a title that creates interest and reflects the content. The APA manual (APA, 2010) provides detailed directions regarding appropriate terms to use in describing study results and manuscript preparation. Consider using an article from the journal as a guide or template; this can help inform you as to the general length of the Introduction and Discussion sections, the presentation format for tables, the reference citation format, and the wording of acknowledgments.

Developing a well-written manuscript is difficult. Often universities and other agencies offer writing seminars to assist students and faculty members in preparing a publication. Graduate students might consider working with a faculty member to publish a manuscript. Some faculty members who chair thesis and dissertation committees assist their students in developing an article for publication in exchange for second authorship. The APA manual (APA, 2010) has a section on how to reduce the content of a thesis or dissertation so as to create a manuscript of suitable size for publication.

When you are satisfied with your manuscript, ask one or two colleagues to review it for accuracy, organization, completeness of content, and writing style. If you are writing the article with a research team, your coauthors are the colleagues whom you would ask to review the manuscript. Ask a friend or family member who is not a health professional to read the article as well. Although friends and family members may not understand the topic or statistical results, they should be able to read the paper and understand the primary messages being communicated. If the journal has an international focus, it would be important to specify that your sample is from a particular geographic area such as the U.S. For example, if the journal is British, appropriate spelling is important (e.g., "hospitalization" would be spelled "hospitalisation"); software spell check tools have options for American English, British English, and other languages. The reference list for the manuscript must be complete and in the correct format. Double-check all references to ensure that they are accurate.

Submitting a manuscript for review. Guidelines in each journal indicate the name of the editor and the address for manuscript submission. Submit your manuscript to only one journal at a time; only when you confirm that your manuscript is not accepted should you submit to a different journal. Most journals now accept only manuscripts submitted electronically, and the editor provides a portable document format (PDF) version to reviewers when they accept the offer to review the manuscript. When submitting the manuscript, include your complete mailing address, phone number, fax number, and e-mail address. The corresponding author who submits the manuscript usually receives notification of receipt of the manuscript within 24 to 48 hours if submitted electronically, and in many cases the notification is sent to all authors listed on the title page of the manuscript.

Peer review. Scholarly journals use a peer review process to evaluate the quality of manuscripts submitted for publication. As noted previously in the chapter, peer reviewers who do not know the identity of the authors evaluate the quality and acceptability of the manuscript. For reviewers to remain blinded, journal instructions will indicate that any materials in the manuscript that identify the authors or institutions should be omitted and replaced with brackets to indicate that something was intentionally removed from the text—"[removed for blind review]."

For research papers, reviewers are asked to evaluate the validity of the study. Reviewers consider whether the methodology was adequate to address the research question or hypotheses and whether the findings are trustworthy and correctly interpreted. For example, if results were not statistically significant, was a power analysis performed? Reviewers also evaluate whether the discussion was appropriate, given the findings, and whether the author adequately discussed clinical implications of the findings without going beyond the actual data. Reviewers are also asked to comment on the relevance of the reference citations, the usefulness of any tables or figures, and the consistency among title, abstract, and text. Reviewers also look for the strengths and limitations of the study, which the authors should convey in their discussion. Every study has its limitations, and a limitation is not a reason for rejecting the manuscript. However, reviewers want to see that the authors have accurately identified and addressed limitations for the readers.

Responding to requests to revise a manuscript. After reviewing a manuscript, the journal editor gathers the evaluations of all reviewers and reaches one of four possible decisions: (1) acceptance of the manuscript as submitted; (2) acceptance of the manuscript, pending minor revisions; (3) tentative acceptance of the manuscript pending major revisions; or (4) rejection of the manuscript. Acceptance of a manuscript as submitted is extremely rare. When this occurs, the editor sends a letter that indicates acceptance and the likely date of publication.

Most manuscripts are accepted pending revisions or accepted tentatively and returned to the author for minor or major revisions, before publication. Unfortunately, too many of these returned manuscripts are never revised. If you perceive the review to be negative, you may need to set aside the review for a few days to allow the emotional response to subside. An author may also incorrectly interpret the request for revision as a rejection and assume that a revised manuscript would also be rejected. This assumption is not usually true because revising a manuscript based on reviewers' comments improves the quality of the manuscript. When editors return a manuscript for revision, they include reviewers' actual comments or a summary of the comments to direct the revision. These reviewers and the editor have devoted time to reviewing your manuscript, and you should make the necessary revisions or respond with your rationale for not making a specific change requested by a reviewer and return the revised manuscript to the same journal for reconsideration.

On a practical note, create a two-column table in a new document, number all the reviewers' comments, and list them in separate rows in the first column. Review each comment carefully and decide whether the recommendation or modification will improve the quality of the research report without making inaccurate statements about the study. When appropriate, revise accordingly and note the page number where the changes can be found in the second column on the row corresponding to the comment. In some cases, you may disagree with a reviewer's recommendation. If so, provide a rationale for your disagreement with literature support in the second column, but do not ignore any comment or recommendation. If two reviewers provided conflicting comments, consult the journal editor who will provide guidance about how to respond to the suggestions. When you have revised your manuscript based on the reviewers' comments, it should be resubmitted with a cover letter and the table with comments and responses. Sometimes the revised manuscript and your cover letter are returned to the reviewers, and still further modification is requested in the paper before it is published. Some published manuscripts have been revised three times before being accepted by the first journal to which they were submitted. Although these experiences are frustrating, they provide the opportunity to improve your writing skills and logical development of ideas.

In the case that the manuscript is rejected, realize that manuscripts are rejected for various reasons. The editor or reviewers may determine that the topic is not relevant to the journal's audience. A group of nursing journal editors surveyed manuscript reviewers and asked them to identify the most important indicators for a manuscript's contribution to nursing, a major consideration in whether a manuscript is published (Dougherty et al., 2011). Of the list provided, the manuscript reviewers selected five characteristics most frequently. The first was the knowledge or research evidence in the manuscript and the second was the timeliness or current interest in the topic. Closely related to timeliness was the novelty or newness of the emerging ideas. Generalizability across populations or international boundaries and contributions to theory completed the top five. Although these characteristics were determined during the development and implementation of the study, when preparing the article an author may be able to link the topic to a current issue in nursing or health care. When a manuscript is rejected, make changes as appropriate, correct any writing concerns the reviewers identified, and send the manuscript to another journal.

Online Journals

Many print journals have converted to online formats. These journals continue to provide their traditional print version but also maintain a website with access to some or all of the articles in the printed journal. The number of nursing journals being published only online also is growing.

Not all online journals are refereed or provide peer review, however. The author should investigate potential online journals by determining whether submissions are peer reviewed and whether the journal has an editorial board (see earlier comments about predatory journals). Peer review is essential to scholars in the university tenure track system and to the development of nursing science. Because online journals do not have advertisers to offset their operating costs, some journals require a processing fee for submitting and publishing an article in the journal. Carefully review the information provided on the journal's website for specific information on fees and other charges. A way to establish the legitimacy of an online journal is to determine whether the journal, and subsequently each article, has a Digital Object Identifier (DOI). The International DOI Foundation assigns permanent DOIs to all types of digital work. The DOI will never change, even if the location for that work does change. The use of DOIs is expected to increase and become accepted as the permanent identifier for scientific and scholarly publications (International DOI Foundation, 2016).

Online publication has several advantages, including "continuous publication." There is no wait for approved articles to be published because the editor does not have to wait until the next issue is scheduled for publication. The notion of an "issue" is becoming antiquated as a result of electronic publishing. Approved articles are placed online almost immediately. Rapid availability of research findings can facilitate the development of science and promote evidence-based practice. The constraint on length of the manuscript, imposed because of the cost of print publishing, usually does not exist. Multiple tables, figures, graphics, and even streaming audio and video are possibilities with online journals. Animations can be created to assist the reader to visualize ideas. Links may be established with full-text versions of citations from other online sources. It is possible to track the number of times the article has been accessed to assess its impact on the scientific community. Electronic listservs and chat rooms may be available to discuss the paper. All of these capabilities are not currently available with every online journal. The technology to provide them exists, but online journals with some of these advanced technologies cover their costs by charging subscription fees.

Books

Research findings may be disseminated in printed reports and books. Foundations and federal agencies that sponsor a research project may provide paper-based reports of studies that have been conducted or are in progress. Due to the costs of printing, many of these organizations are publishing their reports online. Some qualitative studies and large, complex quantitative studies are published as chapters within books, as monographs, or as free-standing books. Publishing a book requires extensive commitment on the part of the researcher. In addition, the researcher must select a publisher and convince the publisher to support the book project. A prospectus must be developed that identifies the proposed content of the book, describes the market readership for the book, and includes a rationale for publishing the book. The publisher and researcher must negotiate a contract that is mutually acceptable regarding (1) the content and length of the book, (2) the time required to complete the book, (3) the percentage of royalties that the author will receive, (4) any financial coverage to be offered in advance, and (5) how the book will be marketed. The researcher must fulfill the obligations of the contract by producing the proposed book within the agreed time frame. Publishing a book is a significant accomplishment and an effective, but sometimes slow, means of communicating research findings.

Errors to Avoid

Plagiarism is intentionally or inadvertently failing to cite a reference or properly attribute a quotation from another author. When this occurs, the author is implying that the words and ideas are one's own (Shamoo & Resnik, 2015). Many journal editors screen a manuscript for plagiarism using software programs. Plagiarism is unethical behavior (Gennaro, 2012). If portions of the material have been presented at a scientific meeting in the form of an oral podium or poster presentation, this should be acknowledged along with funding sources and any potential conflict of interest.

Journals require the submission of an original manuscript, not previously published. Submitting a manuscript that has been previously published without referencing the duplicate work or notifying the editor of the previous publication is unethical and a form of scientific misconduct (Poster, Pearson, & Pierson, 2012). **Duplicate publication** is the practice of publishing the same article or major portions of the article in two or more print or electronic media without notifying the editors and copyright holders or referencing the other publication in the reference list (Broome, Dougherty, Freda, Kearney, & Baggs, 2010). It is not uncommon, however, to publish more than one article from a single study. Previous publications related to the study must be disclosed and cited in the text of the manuscript and the reference list (Hicks & Berg, 2014). Editors have the responsibility of developing a policy on duplicate publications and informing all authors, reviewers, and readers of this policy (Committee on Publication Ethics, n.d.). In addition, editors must ensure that readers are informed of duplicate materials by adequate citation of the materials in the article's text and reference list. A duplicate publication can result in retractions and refusal to accept other manuscripts for review from the author (ICMJE, 2011). In keeping with the standards of nursing as a profession, dissemination of research findings must occur according to the highest standards for ethical behavior.

■ KEY POINTS

- Communicating research findings, the final step in the research process, involves developing a research report and disseminating it. Disseminating study findings is part of your obligation to your research subjects and to the nursing profession.
- The greatest impact on nursing practice can be achieved by communicating nursing research findings to nurses, other health professionals, policymakers, and healthcare consumers.
- Both quantitative and qualitative research reports include four basic sections: (1) Introduction, (2) Methods, (3) Results, and (4) Discussion.
- The Introduction section provides background for the research topic and the significance of the study.
- The Methods section describes how the study was conducted, including any instruments, equipment, and other means of data collection such as interviews and observation.
- The Results sections of quantitative and qualitative research reports are similar in that each begins with a description of the sample, but they vary greatly for the rest of the report because of the type of data and methods of analysis.
- Quantitative research reports contain the presentation of statistical results in text, tables, or figures.
- Qualitative research reports contain the presentation of themes, sometimes supported by quotations from the participants, within context.
- The Discussion section includes validity-based limitations, conclusions that support or refute other published work, implications for nursing practice, and recommendations for further research.
- Research findings are presented at conferences and meetings through oral podium and poster presentations of selected portions of the study; the content of

the report depends on the focus of the conference, the audience, and the time designated for each presentation.
- A poster presentation is a visual display of a study, presented at the "poster session" of a conference. Conference sponsors provide information concerning (1) size limitations or format restrictions for the poster and (2) the size of the poster display area. The home institution should provide (1) the institution's logo to place with your title and affiliations and (2) any requirements for the poster's color scheme.
- Developing a manuscript for publication includes the following steps: (1) selecting a journal, (2) writing a query letter, (3) preparing an original manuscript, (4) submitting the manuscript for review, and (5) responding to requests for revision of the manuscript.
- Selecting a journal for publication of a study requires knowledge of the basic requirements of the journal, the journal's refereed status, its impact factor, and recent articles published in the journal.
- Researchers must exercise care to avoid plagiarism, self-plagiarism, and duplicate publications by using plagiarism detection systems, receiving permission to use content previously published, and referencing their own and others' publications in the reference list.

REFERENCES

American Psychological Association (APA). (2010). *Publication manual of the American Psychological Association* (6th ed.). Washington, DC: Author.

Baggs, J. G. (2011). The dissertation manuscript option, Internet posting, and publication [Editorial]. *Research in Nursing & Health, 34*(2), 89–90.

Bernstein, N. (2011). *Desperately seeking sleep.* Parenting Magazine. Retrieved May 11, 2016, from http://www.parenting.com/article/desperately-seeking-sleep-21354392?page=0,2.

Broome, M., Dougherty, M., Freda, M., Kearney, M., & Baggs, J. (2010). Ethical concerns of nursing reviewers: An international study. *Nursing Ethics, 17*(6), 741–748.

Chapman, S. A., Wides, C. D., & Spetz, J. (2010). Payment regulations for advanced practice nurses: Implications for primary care. *Policy, Politics, & Nursing Practice, 11*(2), 89–98.

Cleeland, C. (2009). *The Brief Pain Inventory user guide.* Retrieved May 11, 2016, from http://www.mdanderson.org/education-and-research/departments-programs-and-labs/departments-and-divisions/symptom-research/symptom-assessment-tools/BPI_UserGuide.pdf.

Committee on Publication Ethics (COPE). (n.d.). *COPE guide.* Retrieved May 11, 2016, from http://publicationethics.org/about/guide.

Conn, V. S., & Rantz, M. J. (2003). Research methods: Managing primary study quality in meta-analyses. *Research in Nursing & Health*, 26(4), 322–333.

Consolidated Standards of Reporting (CONSORT). (2010). *CONSORT statement*. Retrieved May 11, 2016, from http://www.consort-statement.org/consort-2010.

Craig, J. V., & Smyth, R. L. (2012). *The evidence-based practice manual for nurses* (3rd ed.). Edinburgh, UK: Churchill Livingstone.

Dougherty, M. C., Freda, M. C., Kearney, M. H., Baggs, J. G., & Broome, M. (2011). Online survey of nursing journal peer reviewers: Indicators of quality in manuscripts. *Western Journal of Nursing Research*, 33(4), 506–521.

Elsevier Publisher. (2015). *Guide for authors*. Retrieved May 11, 2016, from https://www.elsevier.com/journals/learning-and-instruction/0959-4752/guide-for-authors.

Floyd, J. A., Galvin, E. A., Roop, J. C., Oermann, M. H., & Nordstrom, C. K. (2010). Graphics for dissemination of meta-analyses to staff nurses. *Nursing Research*, 18(1), 72–86.

Forsyth, D., Wright, T., Scherb, C., & Gaspar, P. (2010). Disseminating evidence-based projects: Poster design and evaluation. *Clinical Scholars Review*, 3(1), 14–21.

Garfield, E. (2006). The history and meaning of the journal impact factor. *Journal of the American Medical Association*, 295(1), 90–93.

Gennaro, S. (2012). Ideas and words: The ethics of scholarship [Editorial]. *Journal of Nursing Scholarship*, 44(2), 109–110.

Grove, S. K., & Cipher, D. J. (2017). *Statistics for nursing research: A workbook for evidence-based practice* (2nd ed.). St. Louis, MO: Saunders.

Henderson, A., Ossenberg, C., & Tyler, S. (2015). "What matters to graduates": An evaluation of a structured clinical support program for newly graduated nurses. *Nurse Education in Practice*, 15(3), 225–231.

Henly, S. J., Bennett, J. A., & Dougherty, M. C. (2010). Scientific and statistical reviews of manuscripts submitted to *Nursing Research*: Comparison of completeness, quality, and usefulness. *Nursing Outlook*, 58(4), 188–199.

Hicks, R., & Berg, J. (2014). Multiple publications from a single study: Ethical dilemmas. *Journal of the American Association of Nurse Practitioners*, 26(5), 233–235.

Inflexxion. (2010). *Current Opioid Misuse Measure (COMM)*. Retrieved May 11, 2016, from http://nationalpaincentre.mcmaster.ca/documents/comm_sample_watermarked.pdf.

International Committee of Medical Journal Editors [ICMJE]. (2016). *Defining the roles of authors and contributors*. Retrieved on June 12, 2016, from http://www.icmje.org/recommendations/browse/roles-and-responsibilities/defining-the-role-of-authors-and-contributors.html.

International Committee of Medical Journal Editors [ICMJE]. (2011). *Uniform requirements for manuscripts submitted to biomedical journals: Writing and editing for biomedical publication*. Retrieved May 11, 2016, from http://www.icmje.org/index.html.

International DOI Foundation. (2016). *DOI® handbook*. Retrieved May 11, 2016, from http://www.doi.org/hb.html.

Jull, A., & Aye, P. (2015). Endorsement of the CONSORT guidelines, trial registration, and the quality of reporting randomized controlled trials in leading nursing journals: A cross-sectional analysis. *International Journal of Nursing Studies*, 54(6), 1071–1079.

Kroenke, K., Spitzer, R., Williams, J., & Löwe, B. (2010). The Patient Health Questionnaire somatic, anxiety, and social depressive symptoms scales: A systematic review. *General Hospital Psychiatry*, 32(4), 345–359.

Lee, K. A., & Gay, C. L. (2011). Can modifications to the bedroom environment improve the sleep of new parents? Two randomized controlled trials. *Research in Nursing & Health*, 34(1), 7–19.

Lentz, M. (2011). *Writing a WINning abstract*. Retrieved May 11, 2016, from https://view.officeapps.live.com/op/view.aspx?src=http%3A%2F%2Fwinursing.org%2F~mcneilp%2Fdocuments%2Fwinningabstract.ppt.

Ma, C., Zhou, W., Huang, C., & Huang, S. (2015). A cross-sectional survey of self-rated health and its determinants in patients with hypertension. *Applied Nursing Research*, 28(4), 347–351.

Mallah, Z., Nassar, N., & Kurdahi Badr, L. (2015). The effectiveness of a pressure ulcer intervention program on the prevalence of hospital acquired pressure ulcers: Controlled before and after study. *Applied Nursing Research*, 28(2), 106–113.

Marshall, C., & Rossman, G. B. (2016). *Designing qualitative research* (6th ed.). Thousand Oaks, CA: Sage.

Melnyk, B. M., & Fineout-Overholt, E. (2015). *Evidence-based practice in nursing & healthcare: A guide to best practice* (3rd ed.). Philadelphia, PA: Lippincott Williams & Wilkins.

Morse, J. (2005). Feigning independence: The article dissertation [Editorial]. *Qualitative Health Research*, 15(9), 1147–1148.

Munhall, P. (2012). *Nursing research: A qualitative perspective* (5th ed.). Sudbury, MA: Jones & Bartlett Learning.

Newnam, K., McGrath, J., Salyer, J., Estes, J., Jallo, N., & Bass, W. (2015). A comparative effectiveness study of continuous positive airway pressure-related skin breakdown when using different nasal interfaces in the extremely low birth weight neonate. *Applied Nursing Research*, 28(1), 36–41.

New York University Libraries (NYU Libraries). (2015). *New York University Libraries. How to create a research poster: Poster basics*. Retrieved May 11, 2016, from http://guides.nyu.edu/posters.

Northam, S., Yarbough, S., Haas, B., & Duke, G. (2010). Journal editor survey: Information to help authors publish. *Nurse Educator*, 35(1), 29–36.

Nursing and Allied Health Resources Section (NAHRS). (2012). *Selected list of nursing journals*. Retrieved May 11, 2016, from http://nahrs.mlanet.org/home/.

Pallant, J. (2007). *SPSS survival manual*. New York, NY: Open University Press, McGraw-Hill.

Poster, E., Pearson, G., & Pierson, C. (2012). Publication ethics: Its importance to readers, authors, and the profession. *Journal of Child and Adolescent Psychiatric Nursing*, 25(1), 1–2.

Public Library of Science (PLOS). (n.d.). *Submission guidelines*. Retrieved May 11, 2016, from http://journals.plos.org/plosone/s/submission-guidelines.

Pyrczak, F., & Bruce, R. (2007). *Writing empirical research reports: A basic guide for students of the social and behavioral sciences* (6th ed.). Los Angeles, CA: Pyrczak.

Sandelowski, M. (2008). Reading, writing and systematic review. *Journal of Advanced Nursing*, 64(1), 104–110.

Sandelowski, M. J. (2010). Getting it right [Editorial]. *Research in Nursing & Health*, 33(1), 1–3.

Sandeloswki, M., & Leeman, J. (2012). Writing usable qualitative research findings. *Qualitative Health Research*, 22(10), 1404–1413.

Saver, C. (2006). Tables and figures: Adding vitality to your article. *AORN Journal*, 84(6), 945–950.

Schulz, K., Altman, D., Moher, D., & for the CONSORT Group. (2010). CONSORT statement: Updated guidelines for reporting parallel group trials. *BMJ (Clinical Research Ed.)*, 340. Retrieved May 11, 2016, from http://dx.doi.org/10.1136/bmj.c332.

Shamoo, A., & Resnik, D. (2015). *Responsible conduct of research* (3rd ed.). Oxford, England: Oxford University Press.

Shelledy, D. C. (2004). How to make an effective poster. *Respiratory Care*, 49(10), 1213–1216.

Shin, J., Habermann, B., & Pretzer-Aboff, I. (2015). Challenges and strategies of medication adherence in Parkinson's disease: A qualitative study. *Geriatric Nursing*, 36(3), 192–196.

Smith, M., Theeke, L., Culp, S., Clark, K., & Pinto, S. (2014). Psychosocial variables and self-rated health in young adult obese women. *Applied Nursing Research*, 27(1), 67–71.

Steinke, E., Mosack, V., & Hill, T. (2015). Change in sexual activity after a cardiac event: The role of medications, comorbidity, and psychosocial factors. *Applied Nursing Research*, 28(3), 244–250.

Teixeira da Silva, J. (2015). Negative results: Negative perceptions limit their potential for increasing reproducibility. *Journal of Negative Results in Biomedicine*, 14, Article 12.

Thomson Reuters. (2015). *Journal citation report 2015*. Retrieved May 11, 2016, from http://about.jcr.incites.thomsonreuters.com/full-titles-2015.pdf.

Tong, A., Sainsbury, P., & Craig, J. (2007). Consolidated criteria for reporting qualitative research (COREQ): A 32-item checklist for interviews and focus groups. *International Journal for Quality in Health Care: Journal of the International Society for Quality in Health Care/ISQua*, 19(6), 349–357.

Tonkin, L. (2008). The pain self-efficacy questionnaire. *The Australian Journal of Physiotherapy*, 54(1), 77.

Turabian, K. L., Booth, W. C., Colomb, G. G., & Williams, J. M. (2013). *A manual for writers of research papers, theses, dissertations: Chicago style for students & researchers* (8th ed.). Chicago, IL: University of Chicago Press.

University of Chicago Press Staff. (2010). *The Chicago manual of style* (16th ed.). Chicago, IL: University of Chicago Press.

Wang, J. Y. (2011). *Medicine*. Peking: People's Medical Publishing House.

Wilson, M., Roll, J., & Barbosa-Leiker, C. (2015). Empowering patients with persistent pain using an Internet-based self management program. *Pain Management Nursing*, 16(4), 503–514.

28

Writing Research Proposals

Susan K. Grove, Jennifer R. Gray, Kathryn Daniel

http://evolve.elsevier.com/Gray/practice/

With a background in quantitative, qualitative, mixed methods, and outcomes research methodologies, you are ready to propose a study. A **research proposal** is a written plan that identifies the major elements of a study, such as the research problem, purpose, literature review, and framework, and outlines the methods and procedures for conducting the proposed study. A proposal is a formal way of communicating a plan for a study and seeking approval and funding to conduct it. Researchers who seek approval to conduct a study submit a proposal to a select group for review and, in many situations, verbally defend the proposal. Receiving approval to conduct research has become more complicated because of the increasing complexity of nursing studies, the difficulty involved in recruiting study participants, and increasing concerns over legal and ethical issues. In many large hospitals and healthcare corporations, both the institution's legal representatives and the institutional review boards (IRBs) evaluate research proposals. The expanded number of healthcare studies being conducted has led to competition for potential subjects in some settings, as well as increased competition for funding. Researchers must develop a quality study proposal to facilitate university and clinical agency IRB approval, obtain funding, and conduct the study successfully. This chapter provides students with guidelines for writing a research proposal and seeking approval to conduct a study. Chapter 29 presents the process of seeking funding for research.

WRITING A RESEARCH PROPOSAL

A well-written proposal communicates a significant, carefully planned research project; shows the qualifications of the researchers; and generates support for the project. Conducting research requires precision and rigorous attention to detail. Reviewers often judge a researcher's ability to conduct a study by the quality of the proposal. A quality study proposal is clear, concise, and complete. Writing a quality proposal involves (1) developing ideas logically, (2) determining the depth or detail of the content of the proposal, (3) identifying critical points in the proposal, and (4) developing an esthetically appealing copy (Bradbury-Jones & Taylor, 2014; Martin & Fleming, 2010; Merrill, 2011; Offredy & Vickers, 2010).

Developing Ideas Logically

The ideas in a research proposal must logically build on each other to justify or defend a study, just as a lawyer would logically organize information in the defense of a client. The researcher builds a case to justify why a problem should be studied and proposes the appropriate methodology for conducting the study. Each step in the research proposal builds on the problem and purpose statements to provide a clear picture of the study and its merit (Merrill, 2011). Universities, medical centers, federal funding agencies, and grant writing consultants have developed websites to help researchers write successful proposals for quantitative, qualitative, mixed methods, and outcomes research. For example, the

University of Michigan Medical School (2015) provides an online guide for proposal development with examples of strong proposals and links to other resources. The National Institute of Nursing Research (NINR, 2015) provides online training on their website for developing nurse scientists. You can use a search engine of your choice, such as Google, and search for research proposal development training, proposal-writing tips, courses on proposal development, and proposal guidelines. In addition, various publications have been developed to help individuals improve their scientific writing skills (American Psychological Association [APA], 2010; Booth, Colomb, Williams, & The University of Chicago Press Editorial Staff, 2013; Munhall & Chenail, 2008; Offredy & Vickers, 2010; The University of Chicago Press Staff, 2010).

Determining the Depth of a Proposal

The depth or detail of the content of a proposal is determined by guidelines developed by colleges or schools of nursing, funding agencies, and institutions where research is conducted. Guidelines provide specific directions for the development of a proposal and should be followed *explicitly*. Omission or misinterpretation of a guideline is frequently the basis for proposal rejection, or request for resubmission with revisions. In addition to following the guidelines, you need to determine the amount of information necessary to describe each step of your study clearly. Often the reviewers of your proposal have varied expertise in the area of your study. The content in a proposal needs to be detailed and clear enough to inform different types of readers, yet concise enough to be interesting and easily reviewed (Martin & Fleming, 2010). The guidelines often stipulate a page limit, which determines the depth of the proposal.

Identifying Critical Points

The key or critical points in a proposal must be evident, even to a hasty reader. You might highlight your critical points with bold or italicized type. Sometimes researchers create headings to emphasize critical content, or they may organize the content into tables or graphs. A research proposal needs to include the background and significance of the research problem and purpose, study methodology, and research implementation plans (data collection and analysis plan, personnel, schedule, and budget) (APA, 2010; Booth et al., 2013; Offredy & Vickers, 2010).

Developing an Aesthetically Appealing Copy

An esthetically appealing copy is typed without spelling, punctuation, or grammatical errors. A proposal with excellent content that is poorly typed or formatted is not likely to receive the full attention or respect of the reviewers. The format used in typing the proposal should follow *exactly* the guidelines developed by the reviewers or organization, with attention to the correct font size, line spacing, and reference style. If no particular format is requested, nursing students and researchers commonly follow APA (2010) format. An appealing copy is legible and uses appropriate tables and figures to communicate essential information. You need to submit the proposal by the means requested as a mailed hard copy, an email attachment, or an uploaded file.

TYPES OF RESEARCH PROPOSALS

This section introduces the common proposals developed in nursing: (1) student proposals, (2) condensed research proposals, and (3) letters of intent or preproposals. The content of a proposal is written with the interest and expertise of the reviewers in mind. Proposals are typically reviewed by faculty, clinical agency IRB members, and representatives of funding institutions. The content and type of a proposal varies in accordance with the expected reviewers, the guidelines developed for the review, and the methodology of the proposed study (quantitative or qualitative).

Student Proposals

Student researchers develop proposals to communicate their research projects to the faculty and members of university and agency IRBs (see Chapter 9 for details on IRB membership and the approval process). Student proposals are written to satisfy requirements for a degree and are developed according to guidelines outlined by the university, the graduate division, and/or the school's or college's faculty. The faculty member who will be assisting with the research project (the chair of the student's thesis or dissertation committee) generally reviews these guidelines with the student. Each faculty member has a unique way of interpreting and emphasizing aspects of the guidelines. In addition, a student needs to evaluate the faculty member's background regarding a research topic of interest and determine whether a productive working relationship can be developed. Faculty members who are actively involved in their own research have extensive knowledge and expertise that can be helpful to a novice researcher. Both the student and the faculty member may benefit when a student becomes involved in an aspect of a faculty member's research. This collaborative relationship can lead to the development of essential knowledge for providing evidenced-based nursing practice (Brown, 2014; Craig

& Smyth, 2012; Johnson, Lizama, Harrison, Bayly, & Bowyer, 2014; Melnyk & Fineout-Overholt, 2015). The major content areas of quantitative and qualitative student research proposals are discussed later in this chapter.

Condensed Proposals

Condensed proposals often are developed for review by clinical agencies and funding institutions. However, even though these proposals are condensed, the logical links among components of the study need to be clearly shown. A condensed proposal often includes the problem and purpose, a short summary of previous research that has been conducted in an area (usually limited to three to five studies), the framework, variables, design, sample, ethical considerations, and plans for data collection and analysis and dissemination of findings.

A proposal submitted to a clinical agency needs to identify the setting clearly, such as the intensive care unit or primary care clinic, and the projected time span for the study. Members of clinical agencies are particularly interested in the data collection process, especially if the data include protected health information and involve institutional personnel in the study. The researcher needs to identify any expected disruptions in institutional functioning, with plans for preventing these disruptions when possible. The researcher must recognize that anything that slows down or disrupts employee functioning costs the agency money and can interfere with the quality of patient care. Showing that you are aware of these concerns and proposing ways to minimize their effects increases the probability of obtaining approval to conduct your study.

Various companies, corporations, and organizations provide funding for research projects. A proposal developed for these types of funding sources frequently includes a brief description of the study, the significance of the study to the institution, a timetable, and a budget. Most of these proposals are brief and might contain a one-page summary sheet or abstract at the beginning of the proposal that summarizes the steps of the study. The salient points of the study are included on this page in easy-to-read, nontechnical terminology. Some proposal reviewers for funding institutions are laypersons with no background in research or nursing. Write the proposal as if the reviewer does not know anything about the topic. An inability to understand the terminology might put the reviewer on the defensive or create a negative reaction, which could lead to disapproval of the study. When an institution is evaluating multiple studies for possible funding, the summary sheet is often the

basis for final decisions. The summary should be concise, informative, and designed to facilitate the funding of the study.

In proposals for both clinical and funding agencies, the investigator needs to document his or her research background by supplying a resume, known in academic circles as a **curriculum vitae**. The research review committee for approval of funding will be interested in previous research, research publications, and clinical expertise, especially if a clinical study is proposed. If you are a graduate student, the committee may request the name of the chair or faculty sponsor for your study, and verification that your proposal has been approved by your school or college committee and by the university IRB.

Letters of Intent or Preproposals

Sometimes a researcher sends a preproposal or letter of intent, rather than a proposal, to a funding institution. For instance, the National Institutes of Health (2015) indicated that a letter of intent was requested for some of the Funding Opportunity Announcements. For sources requesting the letter of intent, it should include the following: descriptive title of the proposed research; name, address, and telephone number of the principal investigators; names of other key personnel; participating institutions; brief description of the proposed study; and number and title of the funding opportunity. Malasanos (1976) identified a **preproposal** as a short document that explores the funding possibilities for a research project by businesses and corporations. The parts of the preproposal usually include (1) the letter of transmittal, (2) the brief proposal of a study, (3) a listing of members of the research team and personnel, (4) an identification of facility or facilities to be used as research sites, and (5) the study budget. The preproposal provides a brief overview of the proposed project, including the research problem, purpose, and methodology (brief description), and, most important, a statement of the significance of the work for knowledge in general and to the funding institution, in particular. By developing a letter of intent or a preproposal, researchers are able to determine the agencies interested in funding their study and limit submission of their proposals to institutions that indicate an interest.

CONTENTS OF STUDENT PROPOSALS

The content of a student proposal usually requires greater detail than a proposal developed for an agency or funding organization. This proposal is often the first three or four chapters of the student's thesis or dissertation. The proposed study is discussed in the future tense—that is, what the student *will do* in conducting the research. A student research proposal usually includes a title page with the title of the proposal, the name and credentials of the investigator, the university name, and the date. You need to devote time to developing the title so that it accurately reflects the scope and content of the proposed study (Martin & Fleming, 2010). This section covers the contents of both quantitative and qualitative student research proposals.

Content of a Quantitative Research Proposal

A **quantitative research proposal** usually includes a table of contents that reflects the following chapters or sections: (1) introduction, (2) review of relevant literature, (3) framework, and (4) methods and procedures. Some graduate schools require in-depth development of these sections, whereas others require a condensed version of the same content. Another approach is that proposals for theses and dissertations may be required to be written in a format that can be transformed readily into a publication or publications. Table 28-1 outlines the content often covered in the chapters of a student quantitative research proposal.

Chapter 1: Introduction

The introductory chapter of a proposal identifies the research topic and problem and discusses their significance and background. The significance of the problem addresses its importance in nursing practice, the social impact of the research, and the expected usefulness of the findings (Bradbury-Jones & Taylor, 2014). The importance of a problem is partly determined by the interest of nurses, other healthcare professionals, policymakers, and healthcare consumers at the local, state, national, or international level. You can document this interest with citations from the literature. The social impact of a study addressing a clinical problem may be supported by the number of people affected, the expected morbidity and mortality of the health problem, and the cost of the problem in money and in human suffering. The background describes how the problem was identified and historically links the problem to nursing practice. Your background information might also include one or two major studies conducted to resolve the problem, some key theoretical ideas related to the problem, and possible solutions to the problem. The background and significance form the basis for your problem statement, which identifies what is not known and establishes the need for further research. Follow your problem statement with a succinct

statement of the research purpose or the goal of the study (see Chapter 5; Martin & Fleming, 2010; Merrill, 2011).

Chapter 2: Review of Relevant Literature

The review of relevant literature provides an overview of essential information that will guide you as you develop your study and usually includes relevant theoretical and empirical literature (see Table 28-1). Theoretical literature provides a background for defining and interrelating relevant study concepts, whereas empirical literature includes a summary and critical appraisal of previous studies. Here you will discuss the recommendations made by other researchers, such as replicating, changing or expanding a study, in relation to your proposed study. The depth of the literature review varies; it might include only recent studies and theorists' works, or it might be extensive and include a description and critical appraisal of many past and current studies and an in-depth discussion of theorists' works. The literature review might be presented in a narrative format or in a table that summarizes relevant studies (see Chapter 7). The literature review demonstrates to the reader that you have a command of the current empirical and theoretical knowledge regarding the proposed problem (Merrill, 2011; Offredy & Vickers, 2010; Wakefield, 2014).

Chapter 2 concludes with a summary. The summary includes a synthesis of the theoretical literature and findings from previous research that describe the current knowledge of a problem (Merrill, 2011). Gaps in the knowledge base are also identified, with a description of how the proposed study is expected to contribute to nursing knowledge.

Chapter 3: Framework

A framework provides the basis for generating and refining the research problem and purpose and linking them to the relevant theoretical knowledge in nursing or related fields. The framework includes concepts and relationships among concepts or propositions, which are sometimes represented in a model or a map (see Chapter 8). Middle-range theories from nursing and other disciplines frequently are used as frameworks for quantitative studies, and the proposition(s) to be tested from the theory need to be identified (Smith & Liehr, 2013). The framework needs to include the concepts to be examined in the study, their definitions, and their links to the study variables (see Table 28-1). If you use another theorist's or researcher's model from a journal article or book, letters documenting permission to use this model from the publisher and the theorist or

TABLE 28-1	**Quantitative Research Proposal Guidelines for Students**
Chapter 1	**Introduction** A. Background and significance of the problem B. Statement of the problem C. Statement of the purpose
Chapter 2	**Review of Relevant Literature** A. Review of theoretical literature B. Review of relevant research C. Summary
Chapter 3	**Framework** A. Development of a framework (Develop a map of the study framework, define concepts in the map, describe relationships or propositions in the map, indicate the focus of the study, and link concepts to study variables) B. Formulation of objectives, questions, or hypotheses C. Definitions (conceptual and operational) of study variables D. Definition of relevant terms
Chapter 4	**Methods and Procedures** A. Description of the research design (Model of the design, strengths, and limitations of the design validity) (Describe if a pilot study is to be conducted and how the findings will be incorporated) B. Identification of the population and sample (Sampling criteria, sample size, use of power analysis, and sampling method including strengths and limitations) C. Selection of a setting (Strengths and limitations of the setting) D. Presentation of ethical considerations (Protection of subjects' rights and university and healthcare agency review processes) E. Description of the intervention if appropriate for the type of study (Provide a protocol for the intervention, identify who will implement the intervention, and describe how intervention fidelity is ensured) F. Selection of measurement methods (Reliability, validity, scoring, and level of measurement of the instruments as well as plans for examining reliability and validity of the instruments in the present study; precision and accuracy of physiological measures) G. Plan for data collection (Data collection process, training of data collectors if appropriate, schedule, data collection forms, and management of data) H. Plan for data analysis (Analysis of demographic data; analyses for research objectives, questions, or hypotheses; level of significance; and other analysis techniques) I. Identification of limitations J. Discussion of communication of findings
References	Include references cited in the proposal and follow APA (2010) format
Appendices	Presentation of a study budget, timetable, and tables or figures for results

researcher need to be included in your proposal appendices.

In some studies, research objectives, questions, or hypotheses are developed to direct the study (see Chapter 6). The objectives, questions, or hypotheses evolve from the research purpose and study framework, in particular, the proposition to be tested, and identify the study variables. The variables are conceptually defined to show the link to the framework, and they are operationally defined to describe the procedures for manipulating or measuring the study variables. You also will need to define any relevant terms and to identify assumptions that provide a basis for your study.

Chapter 4: Methods and Procedures

The researcher describes the design or general strategy for conducting the study, sometimes including a diagram of the design (see Chapters 10 and 11). Designs for descriptive and correlational studies are flexible and can be made unique for the study being conducted (Creswell, 2014; Kerlinger & Lee, 2000). Because of this uniqueness, the descriptions need to include the design's strengths and limitations (see Chapters 10 and 11). Presenting designs for quasi-experimental and experimental studies involves (1) describing how the research situation will be structured; (2) detailing the treatment to be implemented (Chlan, Guttormson, & Savik, 2011); (3) explaining how the effect of the treatment will be measured; (4) specifying the variables to be controlled and the methods for controlling them; (5) identifying uncontrolled extraneous variables and determining their impact on the findings; (6) describing the methods for assigning subjects to the treatment group, comparison or control group, and/or placebo group; and (7) exploring the strengths and limitations of the design (Shadish, Cook, & Campbell, 2002). The design needs to account for all the objectives, questions, or hypotheses identified in the proposal. If a pilot study is planned, the design should include the procedure for conducting the pilot and for incorporating the results into the proposed study (see Table 28-1).

Your proposal should identify the target population to which the study findings will be generalized and the accessible population from which the sample will be selected. You need to outline the inclusion and exclusion criteria you will use to select study participants and to present the rationale for these sampling criteria (Kandola, Banner, Okeefe-McCarthy, & Jassal, 2014). For example, a participant might be selected according to the following sampling criteria: female, ages 18 to 60 years, hospitalized, and first day following abdominal surgery. The rationale for these criteria might be that

the researcher wants to examine the effects of a selected pain management intervention for women who have recently undergone hospitalization and abdominal surgery. The sampling method and the approximate sample size are discussed in terms of their adequacy and limitations in investigating the research purpose (Thompson, 2002). A power analysis should be conducted to determine an adequate sample size to identify significant relationships and differences in studies (see Chapter 15; Aberson, 2010).

A proposal includes a description of the proposed study setting, which frequently includes the name of the agency and the structure of the units or sites in which the study is to be conducted. The specific setting often is identified in the proposal but not in the final research report. The agency you select should have the potential to generate the type and size of sample required for the study. Your proposal might include the number of individuals who meet the sample criteria and are cared for by the agency in a given time period. In addition, the structure and activities in the agency need to be able to accommodate the proposed design of the study. If you are not affiliated with this agency, it is important for you to have a letter of support for your study from the agency.

Ethical considerations in a proposal include the rights of the subjects and the rights of the agency where the study is to be conducted. Describe how you plan to protect subjects' rights as well as the risks and potential benefits of your study. Also, address the steps you will take to reduce any risks that the study might present. Healthcare agencies require a written consent form, and that form often is included in the appendices of the proposal (see Chapter 9). With the implementation of the Health Insurance Portability and Accountability Act (HIPAA), healthcare agencies and providers must have a signed authorization form from patients to release their health information for research. You must also address the risks and potential benefits of the study for the institution (Martin & Fleming, 2010; Offredy & Vickers, 2010). If your study places the agency at risk, outline the steps you will take to reduce or eliminate these risks. You need to state that the proposal will be reviewed by the thesis or dissertation committee, university IRB, and agency IRB.

Some quantitative studies are focused on testing the effectiveness of an intervention, such as quasi-experimental studies or randomized controlled trials. In these types of studies, the elements of the intervention and the process for implementing the intervention must be detailed (Bulecheck, Butcher, & Dochterman, 2008). You need to develop a protocol that details the elements of the intervention and the process for implementing them (see Chapter 11 and the example quasi-experimental study proposal at the end of this chapter). Intervention fidelity needs to be ensured during a study so that the intervention is consistently implemented to designated study participants (Chlan et al., 2011).

When proposing a quantitative study, describe the methods you will use to measure study variables, including each instrument's reliability, validity, methods of scoring, and level of measurement (see Chapter 16). A plan for examining the reliability and validity of the instruments in the present study must be addressed. If an instrument has no reported reliability and validity, conducting a pilot study to examine these qualities is indicated. If the intent of the proposed study is to develop an instrument, describe the process of instrument development (Waltz, Strickland, & Lenz, 2010). If physiological measures are used, address the accuracy, precision, and error rate of the measures (Ryan-Wenger, 2010). A copy of the interview questions, questionnaires, scales, physiological measures, or other tools to be used in the study is usually included in the proposal appendices (see Chapter 17). You must obtain permission from the authors to use copyrighted instruments. Letters documenting that permission has been obtained must be included in the proposal appendices.

The data collection plan clarifies what data are to be collected and the process for collecting the data. In this plan you will identify the data collectors, describe the data collection procedures, and present a schedule for data collection activities. If more than one person will be involved in data collection, it is important to describe methods used to train your data collectors and to document the interrater reliability achieved (see Chapter 16). The method of recording data often is described, and sample data recording sheets are placed in the proposal appendices. Also, discuss any special equipment you will use or develop to collect data for the study, and address data security, including the methods of data storage (see Chapter 20).

The plan for data analysis identifies the analysis techniques that will be used to summarize the demographic data and answer the research objectives, questions, or hypotheses. The analysis section is best organized by the study objectives, questions, or hypotheses. The analysis techniques identified need to be appropriate for the type of data collected (Grove & Cipher, 2017; Plichta & Kelvin, 2013). For example, if an associative hypothesis is developed, correlational analysis is planned. If a researcher plans to determine differences among groups, the analysis techniques might include a t-test or analysis of variance (ANOVA). A level of significance or alpha ($\alpha = 0.05$, 0.01, or 0.001) is also identified, which is usually set at $\alpha = 0.05$ in nursing studies (Gaskin & Happell, 2014). Often, a researcher projects the type of results that will be generated from data analysis (see Chapters 21 through 25). Dummy tables, graphs, and charts can be developed to present these results and are included in the proposal appendices if required by the guidelines. The researcher might project possible findings for a study and indicate what support of a proposed hypothesis would mean in light of the study framework and previous research findings (Gatchel & Mayer, 2010).

The methods and procedures chapter of a proposal usually concludes with a discussion of the study's limitations and a plan for communication of the findings. Limitations related to the study methodology might include weaknesses in the design, sampling method, sample size, measurement tools, data collection procedures, or data analysis techniques. The accuracy with which the conceptual definitions and relational statements in a theory reflect reality has a direct impact on the generalization of study findings. Theory that has withstood frequent testing through research provides a strong framework for the interpretation and generalization of findings. A plan is included for communicating the research through presentations to audiences of nurses, other health professionals, policymakers, and healthcare consumers, as well as publication of the research report (see Chapter 27).

A budget and timetable frequently are included in the proposal appendices. The budget projects the expenses for the study, which might include the cost for data collection tools and procedures; special equipment; consultants for data analysis; computer time; travel related to data collection and analysis; typing; copying; and developing, presenting, and publishing the final report. Study budgets requesting external funding for researchers' time include investigators' salaries and secretarial costs. You need a timetable to direct the steps of your research project and increase the chance that you will complete the project on schedule. A timetable identifies the tasks to be done, who will accomplish these tasks, and when these tasks will be completed. An example proposal for a quasi-experimental study is presented at the end of this chapter to guide you in developing your study proposal.

Content of a Qualitative Research Proposal

Qualitative research proposals are unique because the methods for the planned study are described, with the caveat that the methods may be revised as data are analyzed and new questions emerge. For example, during a phenomenological study, the researcher may learn that the lived experience of adaptation following a myocardial infarction is perceived by some participants to be overwhelming due to the number of lifestyle changes that they are encouraged to make. The researcher, in subsequent interviews, may ask participants about lifestyle changes, a question that was not planned as part of the initial study. A qualitative proposal usually includes the following sections: (1) introduction and background, (2) review of the literature, (3) philosophical foundation for the selected method, and (4) method of inquiry (Marshall & Rossman, 2016; Munhall, 2012; Munhall & Chenail, 2008). Guidelines are presented in Table 28-2 to assist you in developing a qualitative research proposal.

Chapter 1: Introduction and Background

The introduction usually provides a general background for the proposed study by identifying the phenomenon, clinical problem, issue, or situation to be investigated and linking it to nursing knowledge. The general aim or purpose of the study is identified and provides the focus for the qualitative study to be conducted. The study purpose might be followed by research questions that direct the investigation (Munhall, 2012; Munhall & Chenail, 2008; Offredy & Vickers, 2010). For example, a possible aim or purpose for a phenomenological study might be to "describe the experience of losing an adult child to suicide." The corresponding research question may be a rephrasing of the purpose as a question: What is the lived experience of losing an adult child to suicide? In other phenomenological studies, the researcher will identify specific aspects of the experience to address, such as the following: "What life events preceded the suicide?" "Would you tell me about learning of the suicide? "How has your life changed since the suicide?"

The background is incorporated into the introduction and includes the study's potential significance to nursing practice, patients, the healthcare system, and health policy (Bradbury-Jones & Taylor, 2014; Liamputtong, 2013). Pertinent to this discussion are the personal and professional motivations for conducting the study, also called the experiential context. Depending on the topic, how the problem developed, may also need to be described and documented from the literature (Munhall, 2012). The significance of a study may include the number of people affected, how this phenomenon affects health and quality of life, and the consequences of not understanding this phenomenon. Marshall and Rossman (2016) identified the following questions to assess the significance of a study: (1) Who has an interest in this domain of inquiry? (2) What do we already know about the topic? (3) What has not been answered

adequately in previous research and practice? and (4) How will this research add to knowledge, practice, and policy in this area? The introduction and background section concludes with an overview of the remaining sections that are covered in the proposal.

Chapter 2: Review of Relevant Literature

The role of the review of relevant literature depends on the qualitative approach being proposed (see Chapters 4 and 12). As a result, the breadth and depth of the initial literature review will vary between methods. A very limited review of literature will be done prior to the study when conducting phenomenological and grounded theory studies. With both approaches, the researcher may conduct a preliminary review of the literature to document the need for the study, but will otherwise limit the review until after data analysis is complete. At that point, the researcher compares the emerging themes and theory to published theories and research. In grounded theory research, the literature is used to explain, support, and extend the theory generated in the study (Glaser & Strauss, 1965). The primary method of data collection in historical studies is an extensive review and analysis of documents and older literature. In ethnography and exploratory-descriptive studies, the review of the literature may be organized and presented very similarly to the review of the literature for quantitative studies. The reports of completed qualitative studies, no matter what the qualitative approach, will include an examination of the findings in light of the existing literature (see Chapter 12).

Chapter 3: Philosophical Foundation for the Selected Method

This section introduces the philosophical and conceptual foundation for the qualitative research method (phenomenological research, ethnographic research, grounded theory research, exploratory-descriptive qualitative research, or historical research) selected for the proposed study. The researcher introduces the philosophy, the essential elements of the philosophy, and the assumptions for the specific type of qualitative research to be conducted (see Table 28-2).

The philosophy varies for the different types of qualitative research and guides the conduct of the study. For example, a proposal for a grounded theory study might indicate the purpose of the study is to "seek to understand parents' perspectives about the impact of having a child with severe food allergies and adjustments required to effectively manage the condition" (Broome, Lutz, & Cook, 2015, p. 533). The researchers indicated that the study would provide data that could become

TABLE 28-2	**Qualitative Research Proposal Guidelines for Students**

Chapter 1	**Introduction and Background**
	A. Identify the phenomenon to be studied.
	B. Describe the knowledge gap that the study will address.
	C. Identify the study purpose or aim and the qualitative approach to be used.
	D. State the study questions or objectives.
	E. Describe the background of the study.
	   1. Provide a rationale for conducting the study.
	   2. Discuss the significance of the study to nursing.

Chapter 2	**Review of Relevant Literature (the Depth and Breadth of the Initial Literature Review Will Vary, Depending on the Qualitative Method.)** A. Review theoretical literature pertinent to the topic. B. Review relevant research. C. Summarize.
Chapter 3	**Philosophical Foundation for the Selected Method** A. Identify the type of qualitative research to be conducted (phenomenological research, grounded theory research, ethnographic research, exploratory-descriptive qualitative research, and historical research). B. Describe the philosophical basis for the research method. C. Explain the guiding theory, if one is being used. D. Provide preliminary definitions of concepts or terms.

Chapter 4	**Method of Inquiry**
	A. Provide an overview of the qualitative approach.
	B. Select a site and population.
	C. Describe the plan for the following:
	   1. Entry into the site and approval to collect data
	   2. Selection of study participants
	   3. Ethical considerations
	D. Describe the plan for data collection.
	   1. Data to be collected
	   2. Procedures for data collection
	   3. Procedures for recording data during data collection
	   4. Procedures for preparing transcripts and field notes for analysis
	E. Describe the plan for data analysis that begins during data collection.
	   1. Steps for coding information if appropriate to the type of inquiry
	   2. Use of specific data analysis procedures consistent with the specific research method (Miles, Huberman, & Saldaña, 2014)
	   3. Discuss procedures to remain open to unexpected information
	   4. Steps to be taken to increase rigor and credibility, including support from more experienced researchers
	   5. Discuss limitations of the study
	   6. Identify plans for communication of findings (Marshall & Rossman, 2016; Munhall, 2012)

References	Include references cited in the proposal and follow APA (2010) format, other method required by chair or university
Appendices	Present the study budget and timetable

the basis for a family-centered intervention to address the needs of all involved. Consistent with the grounded theory approach to research, symbolic interactionism was the underlying philosophy (Broome et al., 2015). Assumptions about the nature of the knowledge and the reality that underlie the type of qualitative research to be conducted are also identified. The assumptions and philosophy provide a theoretical perspective for the study that influences the focus of the study, data collection and analysis, and articulation of the findings. For exploratory-descriptive studies, and even some phenomenological studies, the researcher may be approaching the study from a specific theoretical perspective. If a theoretical perspective is identified, it is evident in the research questions being asked. As a doctoral student, you might propose an exploratory-descriptive study on the coping strategies of Hispanic first-time mothers. The theoretical perspective may be a theory of stress, appraisal, and coping (Lazarus & Folkman, 1984) or Roy's Adaptation Model (Roy & Andrews, 2008). Having a theoretical framework may help graduate students propose relevant interview questions or identify an appropriate sample.

Chapter 4: Method of Inquiry

Developing and implementing the methodology of qualitative research require an expertise that some believe can be obtained only through a mentorship relationship with an experienced qualitative researcher. Through a one-to-one relationship, an experienced researcher can provide insights to the intricacies of data collection and be available for debriefing and exploring alternative meanings of the data. Planning the methods of a qualitative study requires knowledge of relevant sources that describe the different qualitative research techniques and procedures (Creswell, 2014; Marshall & Rossman, 2016; Miles, Huberman, & Saldaña, 2014; Munhall, 2012; Roller & Lavrakas, 2015). Chapter 12 provides details on qualitative research methods.

Identifying the methods for conducting a qualitative study is a difficult task because sometimes the specifics of the design emerge during the conduct of the study. In contrast to quantitative research, in which the design is a fixed blueprint for a study, the design in qualitative research emerges or evolves as the study is conducted. You must document the logic and appropriateness of the qualitative method and develop a tentative plan for conducting your study. Because this plan is tentative, researchers reserve the right to modify or change the plan as needed during the conduct of the study (Miles et al., 2014). However, the well-conceived design or plan will be consistent with the philosophical approach, study purpose, and specific research aims or questions (Fawcett & Garity, 2009; Munhall, 2012). The tentative plan describes the process for selecting a site and population and the initial steps taken to gain access to the site. Having access to the site includes establishing relationships that facilitate recruitment of the participants necessary to address the research purpose and answer the research questions. For the study of parents whose children have food allergies, participants were recruited electronically through a nonprofit organization providing information and resources related to food allergies (Broome et al., 2015). The organization published an electronic newsletter in which the study was advertised and data collection was done online through an iterative process. Parents who agreed to participate were asked to provide two or three written narratives about their experiences. The research team completed the initial data analysis and followed up individually with each participant by asking specific questions related to the narratives.

The researcher must gain entry into the setting, develop a rapport with the participants that will facilitate the detailed data collection process, and protect the rights of the participants (Jessiman, 2013; Marshall & Rossman, 2016). You need to address the following questions in describing the researcher's role: (1) What is the best setting for the study? (2) What will ease my entry into the research site? (3) How will I gain access to the participants? (4) What actions will I take to encourage the participants to cooperate? and (5) What precautions will I take to protect the rights of the participants and to prevent the setting and the participants from being harmed? You need to describe the process you will follow to obtain informed consent and the actions you will take to decrease study risks (see Chapter 9). The sensitive nature of some qualitative studies increases the risk for participants, which makes ethical concerns and decisions a major focus of the proposal (Jessiman, 2013; Munhall, 2012). For studies on sensitive topics, the researcher needs a plan in place for participants to receive follow-up care with a counselor if they become distressed in telling their story. The researcher might need to be debriefed with an experienced researcher when studying sensitive topics.

In qualitative research, the primary data collection techniques are observation, in-depth interviewing, focus groups, and document analysis. Observations can range from highly detailed, structured notations of behaviors to ambiguous descriptions of behaviors or events. The interview can range from structured, closed-ended questions to unstructured, open-ended questions (Marshall & Rossman, 2016; Munhall, 2012). Focus groups may be conducted with each group in a study, including persons with different perspectives on a topic, such as studying nurse burnout with one focus group of administrators, another with nurses who have worked for 10 years or more, and another with nurses who have worked less than 10 years. The researcher proposing a historical study ought to specify the type, location, and availability of relevant documents.

You need to address several questions when describing the proposed data collection process. What data will be collected? For example, will the data be field notes from memory, audio recordings of interviews, transcripts of conversations, video recordings of events, or examination of existing documents? What techniques or procedures will the research team use to collect the data? For example, if interviews are to be conducted, will a list of the proposed questions be included in the appendix? Another key question is deciding who will collect data and provide any training required for the data collectors. In historical research, the proposal will identify where the sources of data are located. As data collection transpires, how will the data be recorded and stored? (See Chapter 12 for information about source documents for historical research.)

The methods section also needs to address how you will develop an audit trail during data collection and analysis (see Chapter 12). For example, you might keep a research journal or diary during the course of the study. These notes can document day-to-day activities, methodological decisions, data analysis processes, and personal notes about the informants. This information becomes part of the audit trail that you will provide to ensure the quality of the study (Marshall & Rossman, 2016; Miles et al., 2014; Munhall, 2012).

The methods section of the proposal also includes the analysis techniques and the steps for conducting these techniques. In some types of qualitative research, data collection and analysis occur simultaneously. The data are usually in the form of notes, digital files, audio recordings, video recordings, and other material obtained from observation, interviews, and questionnaires. Through qualitative analysis, these data are organized to allow the researcher to "see" the data differently with the goals of promoting insight and determining meaning (see Chapter 12; Liamputtong, 2013). Researchers who use data analysis software to assist in the coding and aggregation of data will need to describe the software and the plan for its use.

Rigor, transferability, and credibility do not happen by accident. Specific actions that will be taken to demonstrate the quality of the study methods must be included in the proposal (Marshall & Rossman, 2016).

Conclude your proposal by describing how you plan to communicate your findings to various audiences through presentations and publications. Often, a realistic budget and timetable are provided in the appendix. A qualitative study budget is similar to a quantitative study budget and includes costs for data collection tools, software, and recording devices; consultants for data analysis; travel related to data collection and analysis; transcription of recordings; copying related to data collection and analysis; and developing, presenting, and publishing the final report. However, one of the greatest expenditures in qualitative research is the researcher's time. Develop a timetable to project how long the study will take; often a period of several months is designated for data collection and analysis (Marshall & Rossman, 2016; Munhall, 2012; Roller & Lavrakas, 2015). You can use your budget and timetable to make decisions regarding the need for funding.

Excellent websites have been developed to assist novice researchers in identifying an idea and developing a proposal for qualitative study. You can use these websites and other publications, such as those cited in this chapter, to promote the quality of your qualitative research proposal. The quality of a proposal may be evaluated according to the potential scientific contribution of the research to nursing knowledge; the congruence of the philosophical foundation and the research methods; and the knowledge, skills, and resources available to the investigators (Marshall & Rossman, 2016; Miles et al., 2014; Munhall, 2012; Roller & Lavrakas, 2015).

SEEKING APPROVAL FOR A STUDY

Seeking approval to conduct a study is an action that should be based on knowledge and guided by purpose. Obtaining approval for a study from a research review committee or IRB requires understanding the approval process, writing a research proposal for review that addresses critical ethical concerns, and, in many cases, verbally defending the proposal. Little has been written to guide the researcher who is going through the labyrinth of approval mechanisms for the first time (Johnson et al., 2014). This section provides a background for obtaining approval to conduct a study.

Clinical agencies and healthcare corporations review studies to evaluate the quality of the study and to ensure that adequate measures are being taken to protect human subjects. The administrators of an institution in which the study is planned also evaluate the impact of the study on the reviewing institution (Bradbury-Jones & Taylor, 2014; Merrill, 2011; Offredy & Vickers, 2010).

Researchers hope to receive approval to collect data at the reviewing institution and to obtain support for the proposed study. IRB reviews sometimes identify potential risks or problems related to studies that must be resolved before the studies are approved.

Approval Process

An initial step in seeking approval is to determine exactly what committees in which agencies must grant approval before the study can be conducted. You need to take the initiative to determine the formal approval process rather than assume that you will be told whether a formal review system exists. Information on the formal research review system might be obtained from administrative personnel, an online website, special projects or grant officers, chairs of IRBs in clinical agencies, clinicians who have previously conducted research, university IRB chairs, and university faculty who are involved in research.

Graduate students usually require approval from their thesis or dissertation committee, the university IRB, and the agency IRB in which the data are to be collected. University faculty members conducting research seek approval for their studies from the university IRB and the agency IRB. Nurses conducting research in an agency in which they are employed must seek approval at that agency only. If researchers seek outside funding, additional review committees are involved. Not all studies require full review by the IRB (see Chapter 9 for the types of studies that qualify for exempt or expedited review). *However, the IRB, not the researcher, determines the type of review that the study requires for conduct in that agency.*

When several committees must review a study, sometimes they agree mutually that one of them shall initiate the review for the protection of human subjects, with those findings receiving general acceptance by the other committees. For example, if the university IRB examines and approves a proposal for the protection of human subjects, funding agencies usually recognize that review as sufficient. Reviews in other committees then focus on approval to conduct the study within the institution or decisions to provide study funding.

As part of the approval process, the researcher must determine the agency's policy regarding the (1) use of the name of the clinical facility in reporting findings, (2) presentation and publication of the research report, and (3) authorship of publications. The facility's name is used only with prior written administrative approval when presenting or publishing a study. The researcher may feel freer to report findings that could be interpreted negatively in terms of the institution if the agency is not identified. Some institutions have rules that limit what is presented or published in a study, where it is presented or published, and who is the presenter or author. Before conducting a study, researchers, especially employees of healthcare agencies, must clarify the rules and regulations of the agency regarding authorship, presentations, and publications. In some cases, recognition of these rules must be included in the proposal if it is to be approved.

Preparing Proposals for Review Committees

The initial proposals for theses and dissertations may be developed as part of a formal class. In this case, the faculty members teaching the class provide students with specific proposal guidelines approved by the graduate faculty and assist them in developing their initial proposals. If students elect to conduct a thesis or dissertation, they ask an appropriate faculty member to serve as chair. With the assistance of the chair, the student identifies committee members with expertise in the focus of the proposed study or in conducting research who can work effectively together to refine the final proposal. The number of committee members varies across universities, but usually will include at least the chair and two additional faculty members. The thesis or dissertation committee members must approve the proposal before the student can seek IRB approval from the university. The student's chairperson usually provides direction and support in obtaining university IRB approval. The IRB review within universities usually requires the completion of a form related to the protection of study participants. These forms are similar but vary based on the requirements of the university. Once university IRB approval is obtained, students can seek approval for their studies from agency IRBs.

Conducting research in a clinical agency requires approval by the agency IRB. The department that supports the IRB committee of the agency can provide researchers with copies of institutional policies and requirements and assist the researcher with the IRB process. The staff in these departments can provide essential insight into studies that will be acceptable to the committee. Frequently, staff persons screen proposals for conducting research in the agency. The approval process policy and proposal guidelines usually are available from the chair of the IRB, and the guidelines should be followed carefully, particularly page limitations. Some committees refuse to review proposals that exceed these limitations. Reviewers on these committees usually evaluate proposals in addition to other full-time responsibilities, and their time is limited.

Investigators also should familiarize themselves with the IRB's process for screening proposals. In addition to scientific merit and human subjects protection, most agency IRBs evaluate proposals for the congruence of the study with the agency's research agenda and the impact of the study on patient care (Bradbury-Jones & Taylor, 2014; Merrill, 2011). Researchers should develop their proposals with these ideas in mind. They also must determine whether the committee requires specific forms to be completed and submitted with the research proposal. Other important information can be gathered by addressing the following questions: (1) How often does the committee meet? (2) When are the committee's regularly scheduled meetings? (3) What materials should be submitted before the meeting? (4) When should these materials be submitted? (5) How many copies of the proposal are required? and (6) What period of time is usually involved in committee review?

Social and Political Factors

Social and political factors play an important role in obtaining approval to conduct a study. You need to treat the review process with as much care as development of the study. The dynamics of the relationships among committee members is important to assess. Seek guidance from your chair on navigating any areas that may be sensitive to one or more committee members. This detail is especially important in the selection of a thesis or dissertation committee to ensure that the members are willing to work together productively. Thorough assessment of the social and political situation in which the study will be reviewed and implemented may be crucial to the success of a study (Bradbury-Jones & Taylor, 2014).

Clinical agency IRBs may include nurse clinicians who have never conducted research, nurse researchers, and researchers in other disciplines (see Chapter 9). The reactions of each of these groups to a study could be very different. Sometimes IRB committees are made up primarily of physicians, which is frequently the case in health science centers. Physicians often are not oriented to nursing research methods, especially qualitative methods, and might need additional explanations related to the research methodology. However, many physicians are strong supporters of nursing research, helpful in suggesting changes in design to strengthen the study, and eager to facilitate access to study participants.

The researcher needs to anticipate potential responses of committee members and to prepare the proposal to elicit a favorable response. It is wise to meet with the chair of the agency IRB or a designee early in the development of a proposal. This meeting could facilitate proposal development, rapport between the researcher and agency personnel, and approval of the research proposal.

In addition to the formal committee approval mechanisms, you will need the tacit approval of the administrative personnel and staff who are affected by the conduct of your study. Obtaining informal approval and support often depends on the way in which a person is approached. Demonstrate interest in the institution and the personnel as well as interest in the research project. The relationships formed with agency personnel should be equal, sharing ones, because these people often can provide ideas and strategies for conducting the study that you may not have considered. The support of agency personnel during data collection can also make the difference between a successful and an unsuccessful study (Merrill, 2011).

Conducting nursing research can benefit the institution as well as the researcher. Clinicians have an opportunity to see nursing research in action, which can influence their thinking and clinical practice if the relationship with the researcher is positive. Conceivably, this is the first close contact some of these clinicians may have had with a researcher, and interpretation of the researcher's role and the aspects of the study may be necessary (Johnson et al., 2014). In addition, clinicians tend to be more oriented in the present than researchers are, and they need to see the immediate impact that the study findings can have on nursing practice in their institution. Interactions with researchers might help clinicians see the importance of research in providing evidence-based practice and encourage them to become involved in study activities in the future (Offredy & Vickers, 2010). Conducting research and providing evidence-based practice are essential if a hospital is to achieve and maintain Magnet status. The award of Magnet status from the American Nurses Credentialing Center (ANCC, 2015) is prestigious to an institution and validates the excellence in evidence-based care that nurses provide in the facility.

Verbal Presentation of a Proposal

Graduate students writing theses or dissertations frequently are required to present their proposals verbally to university committee members in meetings that are called thesis or dissertation proposal defenses. Most clinical agencies require researchers to meet with the IRB to discuss their proposals. In a verbal presentation of a proposal, reviewers can evaluate the researcher as a person, the researcher's knowledge and understanding of the content of the proposal, and his or her ability to reason and provide logical explanations related to the study. These face-to-face meetings give the researcher the opportunity to encourage committee members to approve his or her study.

Appearance is important in a personal presentation because it can give an impression of competence or incompetence. These presentations are business-like, with logical and rational interactions, so one should dress in a business-like manner. The committee might perceive individuals who are casually dressed as not valuing the review process or being careless about research procedures.

Nonverbal behaviors are important during the meeting as well; appearing calm, in control, and confident projects a positive image. Plan and rehearse your presentation to reduce anxiety. Obtain information on the personalities of committee members, their relationships with one another, the vested interests of each member, and their areas of expertise because this can increase your confidence and provide a sense of control. It is important to arrive at the meeting early to assess the environment for the meeting and consider where you could sit so that all members of the committee will be able to see you. However, selecting a seat on one side of a table with all of the committee members on the other side could make you feel uncomfortable and simulate an interrogation rather than a scholarly interaction. Sitting at the side of a table rather than at the head might be a strategic move to elicit support. As a guest in the meeting, you may be invited into the meeting after the committee members are seated. In this case, the chair of the IRB will probably identify where you are to sit.

The verbal presentation of the proposal usually begins with a brief overview of the study. Your presentation needs to be carefully planned, timed, and rehearsed. Salient points should be highlighted, which you can accomplish with the use of audiovisuals. Anticipate questions from the committee members. Be prepared to defend or justify the methods and procedures used in your study. With your committee chair or mentor, practice answers to questions that you are likely to receive. This rehearsal will help you determine the best way to defend your ideas without appearing defensive. When the meeting ends, thank the members of the committee for their time and their input. If the committee did not make a decision regarding the study during the meeting, ask when the decision will be made and how you will be notified of the decision.

Revising a Proposal

Reviewers sometimes suggest changes in a proposal that improve the study methodology; however, some of the changes requested may benefit the institution but not the study. Remain receptive to the suggestions, explore with the committee the impact of the changes on the proposed study, and try to resolve any conflicts. Usually reviewers make valuable suggestions that might improve the quality of a study or facilitate the data collection process. Revision of the proposal is often based on these suggestions before the study is implemented.

Sometimes a study requires revision while it is being conducted because of problems with data collection tools or subjects' participation. However, if clinical agency personnel or representatives of funding institutions have approved a proposal, the researcher needs to consult with those who have approved and/or funded the study before making major changes in the study. Before revising a proposal, address three questions: (1) What needs to be changed? (2) Why is the change necessary? and (3) How will the change affect implementation of the study and the study findings? Students must seek advice from the faculty committee members before revising their studies. Sometimes it is beneficial for seasoned researchers to discuss their proposed study changes with other researchers or agency personnel for suggestions and additional viewpoints.

If a revision is necessary, revise your proposal and discuss the change with members of the IRB in the agency in which the study is being conducted. Most IRB committees have a form to complete requesting a study modification. The IRB members might indicate that the investigators can proceed with the study or that the revised proposal might need additional review. If a study is funded, the study changes must be discussed with the representatives of the funding agency. The funding agency has the power to approve or disapprove the changes. However, realistic changes that are clearly described and backed with a rationale will probably be approved.

EXAMPLE QUANTITATIVE RESEARCH PROPOSAL

An example proposal of a quasi-experimental study is included to guide you in developing a research proposal for a thesis, dissertation, or research project in your clinical agency. The content of this proposal is brief and does not include the detail normally presented in a thesis or dissertation proposal. However, the example provides you with ideas regarding the content areas that would be covered in developing a proposal for a quantitative study. Dr. Kathy Daniel (2015), an associate professor at The University of Texas at Arlington College of Nursing and Health Innovation, developed the proposal that is provided as the example.

"The Effect of Nurse Practitioner Directed Transitional Care on Medication Adherence and Readmission Outcomes of Elderly Congestive Heart Failure Patients"

Kathryn Daniel, PhD, RN, ANP-BC, GNP-BC

Chapter 1

Introduction

Hospitalized patients with chronic health diagnoses such as congestive heart failure (CHF), pneumonia, and stroke are often readmitted to acute care hospitals within a 30-day interval for potentially preventable etiologies. These unnecessary readmissions carry a significant cost to Medicare and have been targeted for non-reimbursement. Hospitals and healthcare systems are eager to implement programs that can safely and effectively reduce unnecessary readmissions. Their interests are also tempered by the realization that either way, whether by administrative non-reimbursement policy or actual prevention of unnecessary readmissions, such admissions will no longer be the source of revenue, but rather a cost to the organization. Even though some readmissions will not be preventable, the burden will likely be on the hospital organization to justify payment (Stauffer et al., 2011).

Estimates of the prevalence of heart failure vary. However, older adults, defined as those 65 years of age and older, have documented higher rates of CHF, 6%–10%. The trends over the past decade are an older age at first hospital admission for adults with CHF and an older age at death. This is probably secondary to technological advances and evidence-based guidelines for the care of individuals with heart failure. Despite these trends, the cost for management of CHF in the United States (U.S.) accounts for nearly 2% of the total cost of health care in the country (Mosterd & Hoes, 2007; Solomon et al., 2005).

CHF patients have one of the highest readmission rates to the hospital within 30 days of any diagnosis. Nationally 25% of patients discharged from the hospital after an acute care stay for heart failure, are readmitted to the hospital within 30 days (Jencks, Williams, & Coleman, 2009). Reports are as high as 50% of those readmitted from the community had no follow-up with their primary care provider prior to readmission. When patients are readmitted to the hospital within the 30-day period, hospitals may not be reimbursed for subsequent hospitalizations. In 2004, premature CHF readmissions cost the Medicare system an estimated 17.4 billion dollars (Jencks et al., 2009).

Prognosis remains poor once CHF is diagnosed. From the date of index hospitalization, the 30-day mortality rate is between 10% and 20%. Mortality at one year, and five years is estimated between 30% to 40% and 60% to 70% respectively. Most individuals will die with progressively worsening symptoms while others will succumb to fatal arrhythmias (Mosterd & Hoes, 2007; Solomon et al., 2005). With these high morbidity and mortality rates, individuals with CHF need additional health care in the community to manage their disease and decrease their rates of premature hospital readmission.

Chapter 2

Review of Relevant Literature

Care for this population is fragmented and uncoordinated. Systems of care today often are connected to sites of care, so when patients are discharged from acute care settings to home or to other settings and back again, there are many opportunities for gaps in care. Vulnerable complex frail patients with new problems or questions about management of existing problems have few knowledgeable resources to help them navigate the new landscape of their health. More and more hospital care is rendered by hospitalist providers who do not follow patients after discharge from the acute care setting, but refer patients back to their outpatient providers for care after discharge. Communication between inpatient and outpatient silos of care may be absent and is frequently delayed. Studies designed to use predictive modeling to identify patients at risk for re-admission have had low predictive sensitivity (Billings et al., 2012).

Medically complex patients who have multiple chronic diseases and few socioeconomic resources are the most vulnerable within this group and most likely to be readmitted. Silverstein, Qin, Mercer, Fong, and Haydar (2008) found that male African American patients over age 75 with multiple medical comorbidities, admitted to a medicine service (not surgical) and who had Medicare only as a payer source have the highest risk of readmission. CHF was the highest single predictor of readmission, but other co-morbidities such as cancer, chronic obstructive pulmonary disease (COPD), or chronic renal failure were also contributing factors. The period of greatest vulnerability for readmission is the first month after hospitalization, before patients have been seen by their primary care provider (PCP).

Adverse drug events are a leading cause of readmission (Morrissey, McElnay, Scott, & McConnell, 2003). Medication reconciliation and adherence are important in the post discharge situation. Patients and families do the best they can to relay their drug information to inpatient providers, but they may forget things or assume the provider knows what they are taking. Because patients have had an acute change in their health, their medication regimens are often modified during their hospital stay. In addition, inpatient medication choices are influenced by hospital formularies. Even when diligent providers discharge patients with prescriptions for their new or modified medications, these choices may not be available on the patients' drug formulary plan. So when they present these prescriptions to their local pharmacy after discharge from the hospital, the new medication may not be available to them or is too costly for them to afford. Inpatient providers may also be unaware of all the medications that the patient already has at home and duplicate drugs or drug classes that the patient has on hand (Corbett, Setter, Daratha, Neumiller, & Wood, 2010).

Early physician follow-up (within seven days) has been identified as a possible target for reducing re-admissions (Hernandez et al., 2010), but in most cases requires that the patient be capable of navigating and transferring within an ambulatory care practice rapidly after hospital discharge. Home visits by nurse practitioners (NPs) are an efficient and logical method of delivering a similar quality service.

NPs are educated to manage chronic diseases and understand systems of care. Thus, they are in a unique position within the healthcare system to have significant positive effects on patient outcomes, thereby decreasing readmissions, improving patient physical and mental health outcomes, and decreasing the costs of care (Naylor, 2004). Trials using the transitional care model have been very favorable, both in controlled research settings and in real world settings. Patients followed by a transitional care NP have had substantial reduction in 30-day readmissions (Naylor, 2004; Neff, Madigan, & Narsavage, 2003; Stauffer et al., 2011; Zhao & Wong, 2009). Yet in spite of success in prevention of unnecessary readmissions, balancing the cost of such programs must be weighed against decreasing revenue streams before hospitals will support them (Stauffer et al., 2011).

Within the past 10 years, multiple interventions regarding medication reconciliation (Young, Barnason, Hays, & Do, 2015), discrepancies (Kostas et al., 2013), and management (Crotty, Rowett, Spurling, Giles, & Phillips, 2004; Davis, 2015), have been implemented to address management of medications across care transitions. Although NPs were among the treating providers within these study samples, they were not identified or controlled for in the studies. Medication discrepancies,

reconciliation, and adherence all continue to be targets in the quest to reduce re-admissions (Coleman, Smith, Raha, & Min, 2005).

We know that transitional care programs utilizing advanced practice nurses have consistently reduced readmissions of vulnerable patients. Medication management is an important part of the transitional care NP role. What is not known is the effect of a transitional care NP program focused on medication management on readmission rates and medication adherence of elderly individuals with CHF. Thus, the purpose of this study is to examine the effects of an NP directed transitional care program on the hospital readmission rate and medication adherence of elderly CHF patients.

Chapter 3
Framework

The Transitional Care Model provides comprehensive in-hospital planning and home follow-up for chronically ill, high-risk older adults hospitalized for common medical and surgical conditions (Figure 28-1). This model was initially developed by Dorothy Brooten in the 1980s with a population of high risk pregnant women and low birth weight infants (Brooten et al., 1987; Brooten et al., 1994). Later Naylor and colleagues developed it further in high risk elderly populations focusing on patients with CHF (Brooten et al., 2002; Naylor, 2004). Multiple randomized controlled trials (RCTs) support its effectiveness in reducing unnecessary readmissions (Naylor, 2004; Neff et al., 2003; Ornstein, Smith, Foer, Lopez-Cantor, & Soriano, 2011; Williams, Akroyd, & Burke, 2010; Zhao & Wong, 2009).

The goals of care provided by the transitional care model focus on empowering the patient and family through coordination of care and medical management of disease and co-morbidities as needed with the ability to make changes immediately based on set protocols, health literacy, self-care management, and collaboration with other providers and families to prevent unnecessary hospital readmissions. Figure 28-1 illustrates the inter-relationship of concepts in this model (Transitional care model—when you or a loved one requires care). Patients who are more vulnerable, either socially or physically, or complex, would utilize more aspects of the transitional care model, whereas patients with more resources (social and physical) need less support during transitions of care. According to this model's conceptual relationships, when advanced practice nurses educate patients about self-management skills, they are more adherent to the overall

Continued

"The Effect of Nurse Practitioner Directed Transitional Care on Medication Adherence and Readmission Outcomes of Elderly Congestive Heart Failure Patients"—cont'd

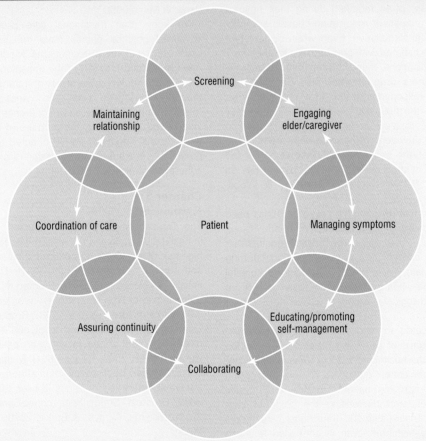

FIGURE 28-1 Transitional Care Model. (Adapted from Transitional Care Model. Retrieved February 1, 2015 from http://www.transitionalcare.info/.)

plan of care. Thus, these chronically ill individuals have fewer unnecessary readmissions and greater medication adherence (Brooten, Youngblut, Kutcher, & Bobo, 2004).

The purpose of this study is to determine the effect of an NP directed transitional care program on medication adherence and hospital readmission rate of discharged elderly adults with CHF. The independent variable (IV) is the NP directed transitional care program and the dependent variables (DVs) are medication adherence and hospital readmission rates. This study will compare the medication adherence and readmission rate of medically complex elderly CHF patients who receive NP directed transitional care with medication management, and those who receive standard home health nursing services. The following table summarizes the conceptual and operational definitions for the independent variable (IV) and dependent variables (DV) in this study.

Variables	Conceptual Definitions	Operational Definitions
IV: Nurse practitioner (NP) directed transitional care program	Time-limited services delivered by specially trained NPs to at risk populations designed to ensure continuity and avoid preventable poor outcomes as they move across sites of care and among multiple providers (Brooten et al., 1987; Coleman & Boult, 2003).	Enrolment and participation in a NP directed transitional care program including medication management after an acute care hospital stay for CHF (see protocol in Appendix A).

Variables	Conceptual Definitions	Operational Definitions
DV: Hospital readmission rate	Outcome which reflects inadequate training and preparation of patients/family to manage new/chronic health conditions or breakdown in communication between patient/family and provider (Coleman & Boult, 2003).	Any unplanned readmission to an acute care hospital reported to study investigators within 30 days of hospital discharge. Number of days from hospital discharge to readmission will be measured.
DV: Medication adherence	Adherence to the medical plan of care which reflects shared values, goals, and decision-making between patients, families, and providers (Rich, Gray, Beckham, Wittenberg, & Luther, 1996).	Score on the Morisky Medication Adherence Scale measured on intake and 30 days from index hospitalization discharge (Morisky, Ang, Krousel-Wood, & Ward, 2008).

Hypotheses

1. CHF patients receiving an NP directed transitional care program with medication management have greater medication adherence than CHF patients who receive standard home health nursing services after discharge from an acute care hospitalization for CHF.
2. CHF patients receiving an NP directed transitional care program with medication management have fewer readmissions within 30 days of discharge from index hospitalization and number of days to readmission are greater than CHF patients who receive standard home health nursing services after discharge from an acute care hospitalization for CHF.

Chapter 4
Methods and Procedures
Design

The design for this study will be a quasi-experimental pretest posttest design comparing readmission outcomes of patients who received NP led transitional care with similar patients who did not receive transitional care at 30 days after index hospitalization discharge (Grove,

Burns, & Gray, 2013). Figure 28-2 provides a model of the study design identifying the implementation of the IV (see Appendix A) and the measurement of the DVs. The study will also compare pretest posttest medication adherence scores between the experimental and standard care groups at 30 days. The protocol for conducting the study is presented in Appendix B. The proposal will be submitted to the Institutional Review Boards (IRBs) of The University of Texas at Arlington (UTA) and a selected healthcare system for approval. After approvals are obtained, patients admitted to one of the participating hospitals in the system who have an admitting diagnosis of CHF will be screened for eligibility. Eligible patients will be approached by study personnel who will explain the opportunity to participate in the study after discharge from the hospital. Patients who consent to participate will be randomized into either the experimental (intervention) group or the comparison (standard care) group. Demographic information, medical status, and pretest medication adherence will be collected from all patients who consent to be in the study before discharge from the hospital. Outcome measures (hospital readmission rate and posttest medication adherence) will be recorded at 30 days after discharge using the data collection form in Appendix C. The pretest and posttest design with a comparison group has uncontrolled threats to validity due to selection, maturation, instrumentation, and the possible interaction between selection and history (Grove et al., 2013; Shadish, Cook, & Campbell, 2002). Randomization of subjects to the treatment, controlled implementation of the study treatment, and quality measurement methods strengthen the study design.

Ethical Considerations

University and Clinical Agency IRB approvals will be obtained. All study personnel who have access to the data or to participants will complete human subject protection training before beginning to participate in study delivery. All participants will have the study explained to them in detail and have all of their questions answered before signing consent forms to participate in the study. The consent form for this study is presented in Appendix D. The participants will receive a copy of their signed consent form.

Time frame: This entire study is projected to take one year. Subject recruitment will begin after IRB approval and informational in-services are presented to the nursing and social work staff in the participating hospitals. Data

Continued

"The Effect of Nurse Practitioner Directed Transitional Care on Medication Adherence and Readmission Outcomes of Elderly Congestive Heart Failure Patients"—cont'd

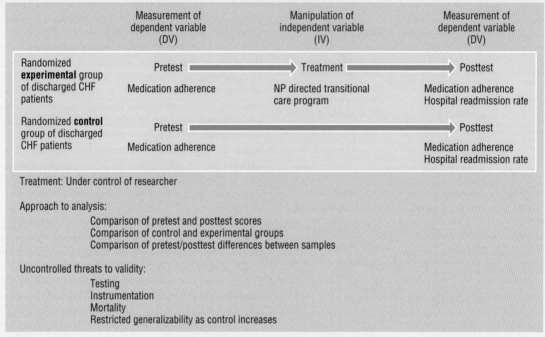

FIGURE 28-2 Classic experimental design.

collection and analysis of readmission outcomes and mortality will begin with the recruitment of participants and will end 30 days after the last participant is recruited (see the Study Protocol in Appendix B).

Intervention and Procedures

Patients who consent to participate in the study will be visited by the transitional care NP who will be following them after discharge for an intake visit before they are discharged from the hospital. The same NP will visit the patient in their home within 24 hours of discharge from the hospital to monitor the patient's condition, review the goals and plans for care, provide patient education as needed, and manage any new issues as they emerge. The NP will also manage all aspects of the patients' medications. The NP will make at least weekly home visits for the entire study period, carefully inquiring about any interval emergency department visits or hospital admissions. Patients who are readmitted to the hospital may be retained in the study for the full study period (30 days) even though they have already reached the endpoint of readmission so that medication adherence can be measured. At the end of the 30 days, all patients in the study will be contacted and/or visited at home by study staff to capture outcome measures. The intervention and study protocols were developed to ensure

intervention fidelity (see Appendices A and B) (Dumas, Lynch, Laughlin, Smith, & Prinz, 2001; Erlen & Sereika, 2006; Moncher & Prinz, 1991).

NPs who will be delivering transitional care to study patients will receive study related training that explicitly reviews the 2009 Focused Update incorporated into the American College of Cardiology Foundation/American Heart Associated (ACCF/AHA) 2005 Guidelines for the Diagnosis and Management of Heart Failure in Adults (Jessup et al., 2009) as well as training in study protocols (weekly visits) and study related measures. Because only 40 patients will be in the intervention group, one NP is expected to be able to manage 40 patients over a one year period. To ensure study continuity and coverage for holidays and scheduled absences, a second NP employed in the agency will also be trained. Study recruitment and outcome measures will be accomplished via a study registered nurse (RN) who will be trained on study information and procedures (see Appendix B and the patient consent process.

Subjects and Setting

Sample criteria: An electronic search of the inpatient database each night at midnight will reveal all patients in the participating hospitals with qualifying diagnosis of CHF who are age 75 or older. Other inclusion criteria are the patient must have a minimum of three chronic disease states, male gender, and have Medicare, Medicaid, and or charity status as a payer source. These criteria are selected based on information from Billings and Silverstein (Billings et al., 2012; Silverstein et al., 2008), which revealed these characteristics specifically increased risk of readmission in a similar population. Study personnel will eliminate any patients who have already been offered participation. Patients who are on ventilator support or vasoactive drips will be deferred until they are stable enough to begin discharge planning. Patients who are being discharged on hospice or who have already participated are not eligible to participate. Patients who are on dialysis will be excluded due to their unique needs and resources.

A power analysis was conducted to determine the desired sample size. Because this intervention is known to be effective in preventing readmission with a moderate effect size, the effect size of 0.45 was chosen with $\alpha = 0.05$ and power of 0.80, indicating a sample size of 70 was required for the study with 35 participants in both the intervention and comparison groups (Aberson, 2010). Ten percent will be added to each group to accommodate for attrition. This leaves a final required sample size of 40 for each group. When the required sample size of 80 has been secured, recruitment will stop. Due to the large population of elderly CHF patients in these hospitals, the sample is hoped to be obtained in 4–6 months.

Demographic variables of interest will be collected to describe the study sample and compare the sample with the population for representativeness. Race, gender, age, chronic illnesses, marital status, educational level, and healthcare insurance will be collected using the data collection form in Appendix C. Socioeconomic status and literacy are known predictors of health status and utilization (Silverstein et al., 2008). Describing relationships between these factors and patient outcomes may be important in explaining study outcomes. The study participants' addresses will be obtained also for contact by NPs following hospital discharge.

Instruments

The Morisky Medication Adherence Scale will be administered to all subjects who agree to participate in the study during intake and at 30 days post initial hospital discharge (Morisky et al., 2008). This tool has established sensitivity of 93% and specificity of 53% when used with a similar population of older adults taking anti-hypertensive medications. It consists of eight questions, seven asking for yes/no answers about the patient's self-reported adherence over the preceding two weeks and a final question with a five point Likert style question. High adherence is associated with a score greater than six on the scale (see Appendix E). Low/medium adherence was significantly associated with poor blood pressure control, while high adhering patients (80.3%) were more likely to have blood pressure controlled (Morisky et al., 2008). Test-retest procedures were utilized to produce consistency of performance measures from one group of subjects on two separate occasions, which were then correlated with the norm reference of actual blood pressure measurements (Waltz, Strickland, & Lenz, 2010). Item-total correlations were > 0.30 for each of the eight items in the scale with Cronbach's alpha of 0.83. Confirmatory factor analysis revealed a unidimensional scale with all items loading to a single factor.

The Morisky Medication Adherence Scale is appropriate for the proposed study because it was validated on a similar population of older outpatients who were mostly minority (76.5% black). The questions specifically ask about "blood pressure medicines," which are the primary medications used in CHF management. This eight question instrument is derived from a previously validated four question version (Morisky, Green, & Levine, 1986).

Procedure

Eligible participants will have the study explained to them by the study recruiter who will obtain consent from those who are willing to participate. The recruiter, a RN who is part of the study team, will also capture demographic and medical data, and administer the Morisky Medication Adherence Scale to all participants (see Appendix E). Patients assigned to the transitional care intervention will be visited by a transitional care NP before being discharged home (see Appendix B for Study Protocol).

On the day after discharge, the transitional care NP will visit the patients in their home to evaluate their home situation and resources as well as review the plan of care. For the next 30 days, the transitional care NP will visit the patient on at least a weekly basis. The visit will conform to the transitional care visit guideline in Appendix A so that intervention fidelity will be maintained. At all times a transitional care NP will be available by telephone. Outcome measures (hospital readmissions and medication adherence) will be measured at 30 days after discharge using the data collection form in Appendix C and the Morisky Medication Adherence Scale in Appendix E. The study recruiter will also do these measures to decrease potential for bias.

Continued

"The Effect of Nurse Practitioner Directed Transitional Care on Medication Adherence and Readmission Outcomes of Elderly Congestive Heart Failure Patients"—cont'd

Plan for Data Management and Analysis

Demographic data will be analyzed and NP actions and their frequency of use will be examined using descriptive statistics. All encounter content with patients will be recorded in the electronic health record, which all transitional care staff will have access to at all times. The documentation of weekly scheduled visits from the transitional care NP will follow a template so that all areas are consistently addressed with all study participants and intervention fidelity is assured (Erlen & Sereika, 2006). Differences in the interval level data produced by the Morisky Medication Adherence Scale will be examined with a t-test at pre-test between the intervention and comparison groups to ensure the groups were similar at the start of the study. Differences will also be examined between pretest and posttest, and at posttest between the intervention and comparison groups. Differences in readmission rates will be examined at 30 days between the intervention and comparison groups. IBM Statistical Package for Social Sciences Statistics 21 will be used to analyze the data. Alpha will be set at 0.05 to conclude statistical difference. The statistical tests will be an independent t-test between two groups and a dependent t-test comparing pre- and posttests. Bonferroni correction for multiple t-tests will be done to reduce the risk of a Type I error (Grove & Cipher, 2017; Plitchta & Kelvin, 2013).

References

Aberson, C. L. (2010). *Applied power analysis for the behavioral sciences.* New York, NY: Routledge.

Billings, J., Blunt, I., Steventon, A., Georghiou, T., Lewis, G., & Bardsley, M. (2012). Development of a predictive model to identify inpatients at risk of re-admission within 30 days of discharge (PARR-30). *BMJ Open, 2*(4), 10.1136/bmjopen-2012-001667. Print 2012. doi:10.1136/bmjopen-2012-001667 [doi].

Brooten, D., Kumar, S., Brown, L. P., Butts, P., Finkler, S. A., Bakewell-Sachs, S., et al. (1987). A randomized clinical trial of early hospital discharge and home follow-up of very-low-birth-weight infants. In L. T. Rinke (Ed.), *Outcome measures in home care: Research* (pp. 95–106). New York, NY: National League for Nursing.

Brooten, D., Naylor, M. D., York, R., Brown, L. P., Munro, B. H., Hollingsworth, A. O., et al. (2002). Lessons learned from testing the quality cost model of advanced practice nursing (APN) transitional care. *Journal of Nursing Scholarship, 34*(4), 369–375.

Brooten, D., Roncoli, M., Finkler, S., Arnold, L., Cohen, A., & Mennuti, M. (1994). A randomized trial of early hospital discharge and home follow-up of women having cesarean birth. *Obstetrics and Gynecology, 84*(5), 832–838.

Brooten, D., Youngblut, J. M., Kutcher, J., & Bobo, C. (2004). Quality and the nursing workforce: APNs, patient outcomes and health care costs. *Nursing Outlook, 52*(1), 45–52.

Coleman, E. A., & Boult, C. (2003). Improving the quality of transitional care for persons with complex care needs. *Journal of the American Geriatrics Society, 51*(4), 556–557.

Coleman, E. A., Smith, J. D., Raha, D., & Min, S. (2005). Posthospital medication discrepancies: Prevalence and contributing factors. *Archives of Internal Medicine, 165*(16), 1842–1847.

Corbett, C. F., Setter, S. M., Daratha, K. B., Neumiller, J. J., & Wood, L. D. (2010). Nurse identified hospital to home medication discrepancies: Implications for improving transitional care. *Geriatric Nursing, 31*(3), 188–196.

Crotty, M., Rowett, D., Spurling, L., Giles, L. C., & Phillips, P. A. (2004). Does the addition of a pharmacist transition coordinator improve evidence-based medication management and health outcomes in older adults moving from the hospital to a long-term care facility? Results of a randomized, controlled trial. *The American Journal of Geriatric Pharmacotherapy, 2*(4), 257–264.

Davis, D. (2015). *A medication management intervention across care transitions.* University of Massachusetts Amherst, Amherst, MA: Capstone DNP Project.

Dumas, J. E., Lynch, A. M., Laughlin, J. E., Smith, E. P., & Prinz, R. J. (2001). Promoting intervention fidelity: Conceptual issues, methods, and preliminary results from the EARLY ALLIANCE prevention trial. *American Journal of Preventive Medicine, 20*(1), 38–47.

Erlen, J. A., & Sereika, S. M. (2006). Fidelity to a 12-week structured medication adherence intervention in patients with HIV. *Nursing Research, 55*(2), S17–S22.

Grove, S. K., Burns, N., & Gray, J. (2013). *The practice of nursing research: Appraisal, synthesis, and generation of evidence* (7th ed.). St. Louis, MO: Elsevier/Saunders.

Grove, S. K., & Cipher, D. (2017). *Statistics for nursing research: A workbook for evidence-based practice* (2nd ed.). St. Louis, MO: Saunders.

Hernandez, A. F., Greiner, M. A., Fonarow, G. C., Hammill, B. G., Heidenreich, P. A., Yancy, C. W., et al. (2010). Relationship between early physician follow-up and 30-day readmission among Medicare beneficiaries hospitalized for heart failure. *JAMA, 303*(17), 1716–1722.

Jencks, S. F., Williams, M. V., & Coleman, E. A. (2009). Rehospitalizations among patients in the Medicare fee-for-service program. *The New England Journal of Medicine, 360*(14), 1418–1428.

Jessup, M., Abraham, W. T., Casey, D. E., Feldman, A. M., Francis, G. S., Ganiats, T. G., et al. (2009). 2009 Focused update: ACCF/AHA guidelines for the diagnosis and management of heart failure in adults: A report of the American College of Cardiology Foundation/American Heart Association task force on practice guidelines: Developed in collaboration with the International Society for Heart and Lung Transplantation. *Circulation, 119*(4), 1977–2016.

Kostas, T., Paquin, A. M., Zimmerman, K., Simone, M., Skarf, L. M., & Rudolph, J. L. (2013). Characterizing medication discrepancies among older adults during transitions of care: A systematic review focusing on discrepancy synonyms, data sources and classification terms. *Aging Health, 9*, 497–508.

Moncher, F. J., & Prinz, R. J. (1991). Treatment fidelity in outcome studies. *Clinical Psychology Review*, *11*(3), 247–266.

Morisky, D. E., Ang, A., Krousel-Wood, M., & Ward, H. J. (2008). Predictive validity of a medication adherence measure in an outpatient setting. *Journal of Clinical Hypertension*, *10*(5), 348–354.

Morisky, D. E., Green, L. W., & Levine, D. M. (1986). Concurrent and predictive validity of a self-reported measure of medication adherence. *Medical Care*, *24*(1), 67–74.

Morrissey, E. F. R., McElnay, J. C., Scott, M., & McConnell, B. J. (2003). Influence of drugs, demographics and medical history on hospital readmission of elderly patients: A predictive model. *Clinical Drug Investigation*, *23*(2), 119–128.

Mosterd, A., & Hoes, A. W. (2007). Clinical epidemiology of heart failure. *Heart (British Cardiac Society)*, *93*(9), 1137–1146.

Naylor, M. (2004). Transitional care for older adults: A cost-effective model. *LDI Issue Brief*, *9*(6), 1–4.

Neff, D. F., Madigan, E., & Narsavage, G. (2003). APN-directed transitional home care model: Achieving positive outcomes for patients with COPD. *Home Healthcare Nurse*, *21*(8), 543–550.

Ornstein, K., Smith, K. L., Foer, D. H., Lopez-Cantor, M., & Soriano, T. (2011). To the hospital and back home again: A nurse practitioner-based transitional care program for hospitalized homebound people. *Journal of the American Geriatrics Society*, *59*(3), 544–551.

Plichta, S. B., & Kelvin, E. (2013). *Munro's statistical methods for health care research* (6th ed.). Philadelphia, PA: Lippincott Williams & Wilkins.

Rich, M. W., Gray, D. B., Beckham, V., Wittenberg, C., & Luther, P. (1996). Effect of a multidisciplinary intervention on medication compliance in elderly patients with congestive heart failure. *The American Journal of Medicine*, *101*(3), 270–276.

Shadish, W. R., Cook, T. D., & Campbell, D. T. (2002). *Experimental and quasi-experimental designs for generalized causal inference*. Boston, MA: Houghton Mifflin.

Silverstein, M. D., Qin, H., Mercer, S. Q., Fong, J., & Haydar, Z. (2008). Risk factors for 30-day hospital readmission in patients <GT> or = 65 years of age. *Baylor University Medical Center Proceedings*, *21*(4), 363–372.

Solomon, S. D., Zelenkofske, S., McMurray, J. J. V., Finn, P. V., Velazquez, E., Ertl, G., et al. (2005). Sudden death in patients with myocardial infarction and left ventricular dysfunction, heart failure, or both. *The New England Journal of Medicine*, *352*(25), 2581–2588.

Stauffer, B., Fullerton, C., Fleming, N., Ogola, G., Herrin, J., Stafford, P., et al. (2011). Effectiveness and cost of a transitional care program for heart failure: A prospective study with concurrent controls. *Archives of Internal Medicine*, *14*(14), 1238–1243.

Waltz, C. F., Strickland, O. L., & Lenz, E. R. (2010). *Measurement in nursing and health research* (4th ed.). New York, NY: Springer.

Williams, G., Akroyd, K., & Burke, L. (2010). Evaluation of the transitional care model in chronic heart failure. *British journal of nursing : BJN*, *19*(22), 1402–1407.

Young, L., Barnason, S., Hays, K., & Do, V. (2015). Nurse practitioner–led medication reconciliation in critical access hospitals. *The Journal for Nurse Practitioners*, *11*(5), 511–518.

Zhao. Y., & Wong, F. K. Y. (2009). Effects of a postdischarge transitional care programme for patients with coronary heart disease in China: A randomised controlled trial. *Journal of Clinical Nursing*, *18*(17), 2444–2455.

APPENDIX A Intervention Protocol for Transitional Care Nurse Practitioner (TCNP) Visit Protocol

1. Patients are initially visited within 24–48 hours of discharge from the hospital.
2. Only NPs who have been trained on CHF protocols and transitional care protocols and are included on the study IRB protocol may visit/interact with study patients.
3. On the first visit the TCNP will review the hospital discharge plan of care with the patient. A family caregiver is identified on the hospital visit or first home visit. This person should be present and included in all visits and supervise the patient's needs in the home. On every visit the following will be addressed by the TCNP.
   a. Review the plan of care given to the patient on discharge from the hospital.
   b. On all visits after the initial visit, inquire about any unplanned visits to any hospital.
   c. Ask about any new problems, issues, or symptoms that have arisen since hospital discharge.
   d. Conduct a brief review of systems, looking specifically for any changes since discharge from the hospital.
   e. Review log of daily weights/teach if needed to do daily weights before breakfast and after voiding each morning.
   f. Conduct a focused physical exam with careful attention to cardiovascular and respiratory exam on every visit; other systems as indicated by any patient complaints.
   g. Review all recommended medications with the patient and caregiver by physically viewing the supply. On the first visit to the home, if the patient does not have a "medminder," the TCNP will provide one to the patient/family at no cost and set

Continued

APPENDIX A Intervention Protocol for Transitional Care Nurse Practitioner (TCNP) Visit Protocol—cont'd

up the medications for the first week. The available quantities and dosages on hand will be monitored on all medications, not just CHF medications. (Anticipate unexpected problems to arise here with possible duplication of drug classes, unavailable meds, etc.)

h. Review indication, rationale, schedule, and possible side effects of every medication.

i. Provide patient/family education as needed on dietary choices, exercise, as needed medications, and so forth.

j. When possible and needed the TCNP will adjust medications as required to accommodate individual patient plan formulary.

k. Adjust/titrate meds as indicated to achieve goals of care.

l. Order lab tests necessary to monitor patient response to medication changes.

m. Order any other medications/tests/referrals indicated by patient exam and complaints.

n. Consult immediately with primary care provider (PCP)/cardiologist for any unexpected deterioration in patient condition.

o. Communicate any changes in medication regimen in writing for patient/caregiver.

p. Record visit in electronic health record (EHR); forward copy to patient's PCP for review. Visit template in EHR will include fields to capture the previous items c–p.

q. On final home visit at the end of 4th week, collect Morisky Medication Adherence Scale for study.

r. After final visit at the end of the 4th week, compose discharge summary and send to PCP.

Study RN Protocol for Comparison Group

a. The study RN will recruit, consent, and randomize patients. After consent is obtained, she will also obtain demographic information and the pre-test Morisky Medication Adherence Scale on all participants.

b. The study RN will contact all usual care patients by telephone at the end of each week during the study period of four weeks to inquire about any interval hospital admissions.

c. On the final telephone call to the usual care participant at the end of week four, the study RN will also collect the posttest Morisky Medication Adherence Scale.

d. The study RN will also contact all transitional care participants at the end of week four to collect posttest Morisky Medication Adherence Scale.

APPENDIX B Study Protocol

Recruiting/Intake—Study RN

1. Generate CHF list from hospital IT.
2. Compare list to track daily discharges of patients already recruited.
3. Screening for eligibility: Inclusion sample criteria
   a. Service area is 30 miles from the hospital: Use Internet directions program if you are unsure about how far the patient lives from the facility.
   b. Must have heart failure diagnosis
   c. 75 and + in age
   d. African American
   e. Male gender
   f. Medicare, non-funded or Medicaid
   g. Patient resides in a private residence, assisted living facility, or residential care home.
4. Exclusion sample criteria:
   a. Patients discharged home on hospice
   b. Patients on dialysis
   c. Patients on ventilators or vasoactive drips should not be approached until they are in the discharge planning stage.

5. If patient meets all of the previous inclusion and exclusion sample criteria, they will be approached for study participation.
6. Introduce yourself to the patient and family.
7. Explain the opportunity to participate in the study after discharge from the hospital and what is involved. If patients agree to participate, give them consent to read or read to them if desired.
8. Ask them to sign consent if they wish to participate.
9. If they decline to participate, thank them for giving you their time. Make a note in the chart that they were offered study participation and have refused, that they are not in the study.
10. For those patients who consent to participate in the study:
    a. Collect patients' demographic, medical, and educational information.
    b. Administer the Morisky medication adherence scale.
    c. Confirm their address and phone number.
    d. Give them your card and phone number.

e. Randomize participant to either the intervention or comparison group. Let them know which group they will be in and when to expect contact again.

f. Intervention group will be visited by NP in hospital and within 24 hours of discharge from hospital in their residence, then weekly throughout study period. Place a transitional care "sticker" on the chart to alert inpatient staff that we are following the patient who was assigned to the intervention group.

g. Usual care group will receive weekly phone call from study RN to determine any hospital readmissions, plus one end of study data collection of Morisky medication adherence scale.

Intervention Group

A transitional care nurse practitioner is preferably certified as an Adult/Gerontology Primary Care NP, although other NPs with significant geriatric expertise will be considered. Other types of advanced practice nurses will not be included in this trial although they were included in much of the original studies by Brooten et al. (2004) and Naylor (2004). All transitional care NPs will complete a standardized orientation and training program focusing on a review of national heart failure guidelines as well as principles of geriatric care, patient and caregiver goal setting, and educational and behavioral strategies focused on patient and caregiver needs.

Scripting for Transitional Care Program Introduction During Inpatient Visit

1. Introduce yourself to the patient/family.
2. You were randomly chosen to be in the Transitional Care group. The goal of the program is to help people (and their families) with heart problems learn how to best manage their illness at home.
   a. Heart failure has more hospital readmissions than any other problem in the United States.
   b. 20% of all people discharged with this problem return to the hospital within 30 days.
   c. Patients followed in transitional care programs have had lower readmission rates.
3. This is how the program works:
   a. I meet you here in the hospital (probably one time only).
   b. I come to see you very soon after you go home; I will be there within 24–48 hours.
   c. I will see you every week for one month at a minimum; we can add more visits to this if needed for you and your family.

4. I work with your doctors and keep them informed of how things are going at home. I am an NP; I am not a home healthcare nurse, although I will work with your home healthcare nurse as needed. Go into more explanation re: differences etc. as needed, give them brochure on "What is an NP."
   a. Why NPs can do more.
   b. NP can prescribe and make medication changes if necessary and keep your physician informed.
   c. NP can address new problems that might come up.
   d. Your Medicare benefit and supplemental insurance will pay for my visits; you will not be billed for any uncovered co-pays.
5. The goal of the program is not to slow you down, we do not want to interfere with your other activities, and we want you to continue to be able to do as much as you can do.
   a. We will review your medications at every visit.
   b. I will ask you each week about any readmissions to any hospital since the previous visit.
   c. Each week we will review your plan of care, how you are doing, and about any new problems or issues that arise.
   d. The study RN who recruited you to the study will contact you at the end of the study and ask you the same questions that she asked after you initially consented to participate (Morisky Medication Adherence Scale).
6. There will be different levels of coordination involved with each patient.
   a. I may discuss your case with your hospital nurse and hospitalist/cardiologist if needed.
   b. I may discuss your case with your primary care provider if needed during intervention period; he/she will receive a copy of the record for every visit.
   c. I will provide a comprehensive discharge summary to your PCP when discharged from transitional care service after one month.

Study RN—Data Collection on Comparison Group Patients

1. Call all usual care patients at 7, 14, 21, and 30 days after discharge. On each occasion, he/she will update the database on any hospitalizations that have occurred since the last interval data collection (specifically how many days since discharge to readmission). On the final call, the Morisky Medication Adherence Scale will also be collected.

Continued

APPENDIX C   Data Collection Form

Study ID	Age	Gender	Race	Years of Education	Pretest Morisky Medication Adherence Score	Heart Failure Diagnosis (ICD-9 Code)	All Other Diagnoses (One Line/ ICD-9 Code)	Days Since Discharge Without Readmission				Posttest Morisky Medication Adherence Score
								End of Week 1	End of Week 2	End of Week 3	End of Week 4	

Data Collection Form

APPENDIX D   Informed Consent

Principal Investigator Name
Kathryn Daniel, PhD, RN, ANP-BC, GNP-BC

Title of Project
The Effect of Nurse Practitioner Directed Transitional Care on Medication Adherence and Readmission Outcomes of Elderly Congestive Heart Failure Patients

Introduction
You are being asked to participate in a research study. Your participation is voluntary. Please ask questions if there is anything you do not understand.

Purpose
This study is designed to examine the effects of nurse practitioner directed transitional care program on medication adherence and hospital readmission of elderly patients who have congestive heart failure. Nationally, 20% or more of patients who are hospitalized with congestive heart failure are readmitted to the hospital within 30 days, often for reasons that are preventable. Transitional care using nurse practitioners has been shown to have positive benefits for

many people like you after they are discharged from the hospital. This study is designed to determine whether medication adherence is also related to decreased hospital readmissions.

Duration
This study will last for 4 weeks after you are discharged from the hospital.

Procedures
After you have read this form and agreed to participate, the intake nurse will gather some basic information from you. Then you will be randomly assigned to receive usual care or transitional care after you are discharged from the hospital.

  If you are assigned to the **usual care group**, you will be given the care your physician orders for you to receive upon discharge from the hospital. In addition, you will be telephoned at your home once per week for 4 weeks by a study nurse who will ask you whether you have been back to the hospital. On the 4th and final week's call, she or he will also ask you some additional questions about how you take your medications.

  "If you are assigned to the **transitional care nurse practitioner group**, your assigned transitional care nurse practitioner will come to your room and introduce herself or himself to you before you are discharged from the hospital. You will also receive the care ordered by your doctor after you are discharged from the hospital including at least weekly visits and telephone support from the transitional care nurse practitioner. The transitional care nurse practitioner will work with you and your doctors to bridge the gap between hospital discharge and your return to your usual primary healthcare provider as you learn to manage the changes in your health.

Possible Benefits
There are no direct benefits to you for participating in this research; however, your participation will help us determine whether nurse practitioner led transitional care can decrease unnecessary hospital readmissions and improve medication adherence. It is possible that having direct access to the transitional care nurse practitioner may provide you with more timely evaluation and management of problems that occur during the 4 weeks after discharge from the hospital.

Compensation
You will not receive any compensation for your participation in this study.

Possible Risks/Discomforts
You may return to your usual state of health and activities rapidly and thus not feel the need for a visit from the nurse practitioner or a phone call from the study nurse every week for 4 weeks.

Alternative Procedures/Treatments
There are no alternatives to participation, except not participating. You will always receive the care ordered by your physician.

Withdrawal From the Study
You may discontinue your participation in this study at any time without any penalty or loss of benefits.

Number of Participants
We expect 80 participants to enroll in this study.

Confidentiality
If in the unlikely event it becomes necessary for the Institutional Review Board to review your research records, then The University of Texas (UT) at Arlington will protect the confidentiality of those records to the extent permitted by law. Your research records will not be released without your consent unless required by law or a court order. The data resulting from your participation may be made available to other researchers in the future for research purposes not detailed within this consent form. In these cases, the data will contain no identifying information that could associate you with it, or with your participation in any study.

  If the results of this research are published or presented at scientific meetings, your identity will not be disclosed.

Continued

APPENDIX D   Informed Consent—cont'd

Contact for Questions

Questions about this research or your rights as a research subject may be directed to Kathryn Daniel at (xxx)-xxx-xxxx. You may contact the chairperson of the UT Arlington Institutional Review Board at (xxx)-xxx-xxxx in the event of a research-related injury to the subject.

Consent Signatures

As a representative of this study, I have explained the purpose, the procedures, the benefits, and the risks that are involved in this research study:

_____

Signature   Date
(Signature and printed name of principal investigator or person obtaining consent / Date)

By signing below, you confirm that you have read or had this document read to you.

You have been informed about this study's purpose, procedures, possible benefits and risks, and you have received a copy of this form. You have been given the opportunity to ask questions before you sign, and you have been told that you can ask other questions at any time. You voluntarily agree to participate in this study. By signing this form, you are not waiving any of your legal rights. Refusal to participate will involve no penalty or loss of benefits to which you are otherwise entitled, and you may discontinue participation at any time without penalty or loss of benefits, to which you are otherwise entitled.

_____

Signature   Date
(Signature of volunteer / Date)

APPENDIX E   Morisky Medication Adherence Scale

Please complete the following scale by circling the best response that fits you:

1. Do you sometimes forget to take your medications? Yes/No
2. Over the past 2 weeks, were there any days when you did not take your medication? Yes/No
3. Have you ever cut back or stopped taking your medication without telling your doctor because you felt worse when you took it? Yes/No
4. When you travel or leave home, do you sometimes forget to bring along your medications? Yes/No
5. Did you take your medicine yesterday? Yes/No
6. When you feel like your blood pressure is under control, do you sometimes stop taking your medication? Yes/No

7. Taking medication every day is a real inconvenience for some people. Do you ever feel hassled about sticking to your blood pressure treatment plan? Yes/No
8. How often do you have difficulty remembering to take all of your medications? (Select one.)

Never
Occasionally, but less than half of the time
About half of the time
More than half of the time
Almost all of the time

Morisky, D. E., Ang, A., Krousel-Wood, M., & Ward, H. J. (2008). Predictive validity of a medication adherence measure in an outpatient setting. *Journal of Clinical Hypertension, 10*(5), 348-354.

▌KEY POINTS

- This chapter focuses on writing a research proposal and seeking approval to conduct a study.
- A research proposal is a written plan that identifies the major elements of a study, such as the problem, purpose, review of literature, and framework, and outlines the methods and procedures to conduct a study.
- Writing a quality proposal involves (1) developing the ideas logically, (2) determining the depth or detail of the proposal content, (3) identifying the critical points in the proposal, and (4) developing an aesthetically appealing copy.

- Most clinical agencies and funding institutions require a condensed proposal, which usually includes a problem and purpose, previous research conducted in the area, a framework, variables, design, sample, ethical considerations, a plan for data collection and analysis, and a plan for dissemination of findings.
- Sometimes a researcher will send a preproposal or letter of intent to funding organizations, rather than a proposal. The parts of the preproposal are logically ordered as follows: (1) a letter of transmittal, (2) proposal for a study, (3) personnel, (4) facilities, and (5) budget.
- A quantitative research proposal usually has four chapters or sections: (1) introduction, (2) review of relevant literature, (3) framework, and (4) methods and procedures.
- A qualitative research proposal generally includes the following chapters or sections: (1) introduction and background, (2) review of relevant literature, (3) philosophical foundation of the selected method, and (4) method of inquiry.
- Seeking approval for the conduct or funding of a study is a process that involves submission of a proposal to a selected group for review and, in many situations, verbally defending that proposal.
- Research proposals are reviewed to (1) evaluate the quality of the study, (2) ensure that adequate measures are being taken to protect human subjects, and (3) evaluate the impact of conducting the study on the reviewing institution.
- Proposals sometimes require revision before or during the implementation of a study; if a change is necessary, the researcher should discuss the change with the members of the university and clinical agency IRBs and the funding institution.
- An example of a brief quantitative research proposal of a quasi-experimental study is provided.

REFERENCES

Aberson, C. L. (2010). *Applied power analysis for the behavioral sciences.* New York, NY: Routledge.

American Nurses Credentialing Center. (ANCC, 2015). *Magnet Recognition Program® overview.* Retrieved July 19, 2015 from http://www.nursecredentialing.org/Magnet/ProgramOverview.aspx.

American Psychological Association (APA, 2010). *Publication manual of the American Psychological Association* (6th ed.). Washington, DC: Author.

Booth, W. C., Colomb, G. G., Williams, J. M., & The University of Chicago Press Editorial Staff. (2013). *Kate L. Turabian: A manual for writers of research papers, theses, and dissertations: Chicago style for students and researchers* (8th ed.). Chicago, IL: University of Chicago Press.

Bradbury-Jones, C., & Taylor, J. (2014). Applying social impact assessment in nursing research. *Nursing Standard, 28*(48), 45–49.

Broome, S., Lutz, B., & Cook, C. (2015). Becoming the parent of a child with life-threatening food allergies. *Journal of Pediatric Nursing, 30*(4), 532–542.

Brown, S. J. (2014). *Evidence-based nursing: The research-practice connection* (3rd ed.). Sudbury, MA: Jones & Bartlett.

Bulecheck, G., Butcher, H., & Dochterman, J. (Eds.), (2008). *Nursing interventions classification (NIC)* (5th ed.). St. Louis, MO: Elsevier.

Chlan, L. L., Guttormson, J. L., & Savik, K. (2011). Methods: Tailoring a treatment fidelity framework for an intensive care unit clinical trial. *Nursing Research, 60*(5), 348–353.

Craig, J. V., & Smyth, R. L. (2012). *The evidence-based practice manual for nurses* (3rd ed.). Edinburgh, UK: Churchill Livingstone.

Creswell, J. W. (2014). *Research design: Qualitative, quantitative and mixed methods approaches* (4th ed.). Thousand Oaks, CA: Sage.

Daniel, K. (2015). *The effect of nurse practitioner directed transitional care on medication adherence and readmission outcomes of elderly congestive heart failure patients.* Unpublished proposal.

Fawcett, J., & Garity, J. (2009). *Evaluating research for evidence-based nursing practice.* Philadelphia, PA: F. A. Davis.

Gaskin, C. J., & Happell, B. (2014). Power, effects, confidence, and significance: An investigation of statistical practices in nursing research. *International Journal of Nursing Studies, 51*(5), 795–806.

Gatchel, R. J., & Mayer, T. G. (2010). Testing minimal clinically important difference: Consensus or conundrum? *The Spine Journal, 35*(19), 1739–1743.

Glaser, B., & Strauss, A. L. (1965). Discovery of substantive theory: A basic strategy underlying qualitative research. *American Behavioral Scientist, 8*(1), 5–12.

Grove, S. K., & Cipher, D. J. (2017). *Statistics for nursing research: A workbook for evidence-based practice* (2nd ed.). St. Louis, MO: Saunders.

Jessiman, W. (2013). 'To be honest, I haven't even thought about it' – recruitment in small-scale, qualitative research in primary care. *Nurse Researcher, 21*(2), 18–23.

Johnson, C., Lizama, C., Harrison, M., Bayly, E., & Bowyer, J. (2014). Cancer health professionals needing funding, time, research knowledge and skills to be involved in health services research. *Journal of Cancer Education, 29*(2), 389–394.

Kandola, D., Banner, D., Okeefe-McCarthy, S., & Jassal, D. (2014). Sampling methods in cardiovascular nursing research: An overview. *Canadian Journal of Cardiovascular Nursing, 24*(3), 15–18.

Kerlinger, F. N., & Lee, H. B. (2000). *Foundations of behavioral research* (4th ed.). Fort Worth, TX: Harcourt College.

Lazarus, R., & Folkman, S. (1984). *Stress, appraisal, and coping.* New York, NY: Springer.

Liamputtong, P. (2013). *Qualitative research methods* (4th ed.). South Melbourne, AU: Oxford University Press.

Malasanos, L. J. (1976). What is the preproposal? What are its component parts? Is it an effective instrument in assessing funding potential of research ideas? *Nursing Research, 25*(3), 223–224.

Marshall, C., & Rossman, G. B. (2016). *Designing qualitative research* (6th ed.). Los Angeles, CA: Sage.

Martin, C. J. H., & Fleming, V. (2010). A 15-step model for writing a research proposal. *British Journal of Midwifery, 15*(12), 791–798.

Melnyk, B. M., & Fineout-Overholt, E. (2015). *Evidence-based practice in nursing & healthcare: A guide to best practice* (3rd ed.). Philadelphia, PA: Lippincott Williams & Wilkins.

Merrill, K. C. (2011). Developing an effective quantitative research proposal. *Journal of Infusion Nursing: The Official Publication of the Infusion Nurses Society, 34*(3), 181–186.

Miles, M. B., Huberman, A. M., & Saldaña, J. (2014). *Qualitative data analysis: A methods sourcebook* (3rd ed.). Beverly Hills, CA: Sage.

Munhall, P. L. (2012). *Nursing research: A qualitative perspective* (5th ed.). Sudbury, MA: Jones & Bartlett.

Munhall, P. L., & Chenail, R. (2008). *Qualitative research proposals and reports: A guide* (3rd ed.). Boston, MA: Jones and Bartlett.

National Institutes of Health. (NIH, 2015). *Letter of intent.* Retrieved August 11, 2015 from http://www.nimh.nih.gov/funding/grant-writing-and-application-process/letter-of-intent.shtml.

National Institute of Nursing Research. (NINR, 2015). *Online: Developing nurse scientists.* Retrieved July 19, 2015 from http://www.ninr.nih.gov/training/online-developing-nurse-scientists#.Vav4aPlVhBc.

Offredy, M., & Vickers, P. (2010). *Developing a healthcare research proposal: An interactive student guide.* Oxford, UK: Wiley-Blackwell.

Plichta, S. B., & Kelvin, E. (2013). *Munro's statistical methods for health care research* (6th ed.). Philadelphia, PA: Lippincott Williams & Wilkins.

Roller, M., & Lavrakas, P. (2015). *Applied qualitative research design: A total quality framework approach.* New York, NY: Guilford Press.

Roy, C., & Andrews, H. A. (2008). *Roy's Adaptation Model for Nursing* (3rd ed.). Stamford, CT: Appleton & Lange.

Ryan-Wenger, N. A. (2010). Evaluation of measurement precision, accuracy, and error in biophysical data for clinical research and practice. In C. F. Waltz, O. L. Strickland, & E. R. Lenz (Eds.), *Measurement in nursing and health research* (4th ed., pp. 371–383). New York, NY: Springer.

Shadish, W. R., Cook, T. D., & Campbell, D. T. (2002). *Experimental and quasi-experimental designs for generalized causal inference.* Chicago, IL: Rand McNally.

Smith, M. J., & Liehr, P. R. (2013). *Middle range theory for nursing* (3rd ed.). New York, NY: Springer.

Thompson, S. K. (2002). *Sampling* (2nd ed.). New York, NY: John Wiley & Sons.

The University of Chicago Press Staff. (2010). *The Chicago manual of style* (16th ed.). Chicago, IL: University of Chicago Press.

University of Michigan Medical School. (2015). *Proposal preparation.* Retrieved August 11, 2015 from http://medicine.umich.edu/medschool/research/office-research/research-development-support/proposal-preparation.

Wakefield, A. (2014). Searching and critiquing the research literature. *Nursing Standard, 28*(39), 49–57.

Waltz, C. F., Strickland, O. L., & Lenz, E. R. (2010). *Measurement in nursing and health research* (4th ed.). New York, NY: Springer.

29

Seeking Funding for Research

Jennifer R. Gray

http://evolve.elsevier.com/Gray/practice/

Research funding is necessary for implementation of complex, well-designed studies. Simpler studies may be completed with fewer resources, but even mailing a survey to an adequate-sized sample can be expensive. As the rigor and complexity of a study's design increase, cost tends to increase proportionately. In addition to paying for expenses, funding adds credibility to a study because it indicates that others have reviewed the proposal and recognized its scientific and social merit. The scientific credibility of the profession is related to the quality of studies conducted by its researchers. Thus, scientific credibility and funding for research are interrelated.

The nursing profession has invested a great deal of energy in increasing the sources of funding and amount of money available for nursing research. Receiving funding enhances the professional status of the recipient and increases the possibilities of greater funding for later studies. In an academic setting, funding is advantageous for faculty members, because a grant may reimburse part or all of their salary and release them from other institutional responsibilities, allowing the research team to devote time to conducting the study. Funding may provide resources to hire assistants and study coordinators to assist with conducting the study, thus enhancing the research team's productivity. Skills in seeking funding for research are essential to developing knowledge in your specialty. This chapter describes building a program of research, different sources of funding, and strategies to increase your success in receiving funding.

BUILDING A PROGRAM OF RESEARCH

As a novice researcher, you may have the goal of writing a grant proposal to the federal government or a national foundation for your first study and receiving a large grant that covers your salary, equipment, computers, payments to subjects for their time and effort, and salaries of research assistants and secretarial support. In reality, this scenario seldom occurs for an inexperienced researcher. Even experienced researchers with previous federal funding are not always funded when they submit grant proposals. A new researcher is usually caught in the difficult position of needing experience to get funded and needing funding to get time away from normal duties to conduct research and gain the needed experience. One way of resolving this dilemma is to design initial studies that can realistically be completed without release time and with little or no funding. This approach requires a commitment to put in extra hours of work, which is often unrewarded monetarily or socially. However, when well conducted, and the findings published, small unfunded studies provide the credibility one needs to begin the process toward major grant funding. Guidelines for proposals for federal funding usually include a section of the proposal in which researchers are expected to describe their own prior research, either completed or in progress, especially studies that are precursors to the one proposed. Grant reviewers want evidence of the ability to conceptualize, implement a study, and disseminate findings. Funders seek assurance that if they fund a proposal, their money will not be wasted and that the findings of the study will be published.

An aspiring career researcher should plan to initiate a program of research in a specific area of study and seek funding in this area. A program of research consists of the studies that a researcher conducts, starting with small, simple ones and moving to larger, complex endeavors over time, usually focusing on closely related problem areas. It sounds simplistic, but if your research interest is promotion of health in rural areas, you need to plan a series of studies that focus on promoting rural health. Early studies may be small, with each successive effort building on the findings of the previous one. Successive findings suggest new solutions or provide evidence that a hoped-for solution is ineffective, a learning program is promising, a trend analysis reveals unforeseen patterns in health and illness, or an old strategy has a new application.

Dr. Jean McSweeney, PhD, RN, FAHA, FAAN, is an example of a nurse researcher who has built a program of research. She is a professor and Director of the PhD Program at the College of Nursing, University of Arkansas of Medical Sciences. When she first worked as a nurse, Dr. McSweeney's area of clinical practice was critical care. In critical care, she became very interested in cardiac patients (American Nurses Association [ANA], 2008). To complete her PhD degree, she conducted a qualitative study with patients and their significant others to explore behavior changes after a myocardial infarction (MI). Her first post-dissertation study was a qualitative study of women's motivations to change their behavior after an MI. She continued by conducting a series of quantitative studies that built on her own qualitative findings. She was the first researcher to document the ways in which women's symptoms of a MI were different from men's typical symptoms, such as crushing chest pain. One symptom that may be an indicator of an impending MI in women is severe fatigue. Her research findings provided the impetus for recognition of these gender differences in the assessment of women (ANA, 2008). While she pursued publication in peer-reviewed journals, Dr. McSweeney capitalized on opportunities to share her findings in the mass media by agreeing to be interviewed by reporters for newspapers and national news programs. Box 29-1 provides some of the publications written by Dr. McSweeney. She has written other articles, as she has

---

BOX 29-1   Publications Reflecting a Program of Research: Exemplar of McSweeney's Research in Cardiovascular Health of Women

Citations From Oldest to Most Recent

McSweeney, J. C. (1993). Explanatory models of a myocardial event: Linkages between perceived causes and modifiable health behaviors. *Rehabilitation Nursing Research, 2*(1), 39–49.

McSweeney, J. C., & Crane, P. B. (2001). An act of courage: Women's decision-making processes regarding outpatient cardiac rehabilitation attendance. *Rehabilitation Nursing, 26*(4), 132–140.

Crane, P. B., & McSweeney, J. C. (2003). Exploring older women's lifestyle changes after myocardial infarction. *Medsurg Nursing, 12*(3), 170–176.

McSweeney, J. C., Cody, M., O'Sullivan, P., Elberson, D., Moser, D. K., & Gavin, B. J. (2003). Women's early warning symptoms of acute myocardial infarction. *Circulation, 108*(21), 2619–2623.

McSweeney, J. C., O'Sullivan, P., Cody, M., & Crane, P. B. (2004). Development of the McSweeney Acute and Prodromal Myocardial Infarction Symptom Survey. *Journal of Cardiovascular Nursing, 19*(1), 58–67.

McSweeney, J. C., & Coon, S. (2004). Women's inhibitors and facilitators associated with making behavioral changes after myocardial infarction. *Medsurg Nursing, 13*(1), 49–56.

McSweeney, J. C., Lefler, L. L., & Crowder, B. F. (2005). What's wrong with me? Women's coronary heart disease diagnostic experiences. *Progress in Cardiovascular Nursing, 20*(2), 48–57.

McSweeney, J. C., Lefler, L. L., Fischer, E. P., Naylor, A. J., & Evans, L. K. (2007). Women's prehospital delay associated with myocardial infarction: Does race really matter? *The Journal of Cardiovascular Nursing, 22*(4), 279–285.

McSweeney, J. C., Pettey, C. M., Fischer, E. P., & Spellman (2009). Going the distance. *Research in Gerontological Nursing, 2*(4), 256–264.

McSweeney, J. C., Cleves, J. A., Zhao, W., Lefler, L. L., & Yang, S. (2010). Cluster analysis of women's prodromal and acute myocardial infarction by race and other characteristics. *The Journal of Cardiovascular Nursing, 25*(4), 104–110.

McSweeney, J. C., O'Sullivan, P., Cleves, M. A., Lefler, L. L., Cody, M., Dunn, K. et al. (2010). Racial differences in women's prodromal and acute symptoms of myocardial infarction. *American Journal of Critical Care, 19*(1), 63–73.

Beck, C., McSweeney, J. C., Richards, K. C., Roberson, P. K., Tsai, P. F., & Souder, E. (2010). Challenges in tailored intervention research. *Nursing Outlook, 58*(2), 104–110.

McSweeney, J. C., Pettey, C. M., Souder, E., & Rhoads, S. (2011). Disparities in women's cardiovascular health. *Journal of Obstetric, Gynecologic, and Neonatal Nursing, 40*(3), 362–371.

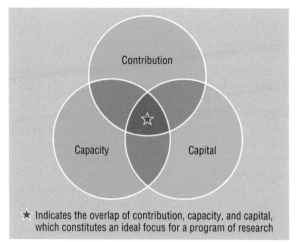

★ Indicates the overlap of contribution, capacity, and capital, which constitutes an ideal focus for a program of research

FIGURE 29-1 Ideal focus for a program of research: The intersection of contribution, capital, and capacity.

also published articles on related topics with clinical partners and PhD students, but perusal of the titles of the articles reveals a common thread of cardiac disease in women. Publication of funded studies increased her credibility and provided the foundation for future funding.

How do you decide on the focus of your program of research? The ideal focus of a program of research is the intersection of a potential contribution to science, your capacity, and the capital that you can assemble. Figure 29-1 shows the ideal program of research with overlapping circles of contribution, capacity, and capital—the three Cs.

Contribution

Contribution refers to the gap in knowledge that your research will address. Is there a contribution to be made in this area? Reviewing the literature and finding a significant gap in knowledge is where you start. Dr. McSweeney identified that little was known about patients' perceptions of cardiac illness. The research focus is broader than a single study. There is no need to develop a program of research in an area that has been extensively studied unless you identify a major gap or perspective that is missing.

Capacity

Once you identify an area in which there is a research gap, assess your capacity to address the gap. Capacity is the second "C." Capacity may be divided into two parts: your connection to the topic and your relevant expertise. Which areas of nursing and health stimulate your curiosity and sustain your interest? Think about the topics or areas of nursing practice in which you are the most interested. Which patients or clinical areas stimulate your curiosity? Maybe you have a personal connection to a particular area, such as a nurse researcher who is interested in autism because of a son with autism. Maybe you work in the newborn nursery and notice the challenges of helping mothers with a history of substance abuse bond with their babies. Your research focus may evolve over time and ideally, your passion for a specific topic or group of patients would provide the basis for a long research career. Research is hard work and a personal connection can lend perseverance for sustained work in an area.

Capacity includes internal resources you possess, such as experience, emotional maturity, intellect, knowledge, skills, and tenacity. Your expertise may arise from educational programs, personal study, and clinical experience. If you are interested in genomics research, what is your knowledge of genes and the interactions between them and the environment? Have you completed a course in genetics or mastered the laboratory skills to gather and analyze cellular-level data? If you are interested in the effects of positioning on the hemodynamics of unstable, acute patients, have you ever worked in a critical care unit? One aspect of building a research career is to continue to expand your capacity in a focus area but, in the beginning, selecting an area in which you have baseline knowledge is helpful.

Capital

Capital refers to resources, specifically available funding, institutional support, and people. The primary purpose of this chapter is to describe how to increase your monetary capital. Review the websites of organizations, foundations, and agencies, including the National Institutes of Health, to learn their research priorities and the types of grants they fund. Although you may have a passion for understanding nurses' experiences in caring for terminally ill patients, you may be unable to find a funder with that priority. If your goal is a lifelong career as a full-time researcher, you must select a topic that is fundable.

Evaluate the institution in which you work. Is the environment supportive of research? Administrators of a non-Magnet hospital may be less supportive of research than those of a hospital designated by the American Nurses Credentialing Center as a Magnet® Hospital through the Magnet Recognition Program®. A teaching hospital or a clinic in a health sciences center may be more supportive of research then a community hospital or private physician's office. If you are a nurse faculty member, a research-intensive university with graduate programs is more likely to demonstrate support of research than is a liberal arts university focused on undergraduate education. In an institution with a research focus, you are more likely to find a reference group.

Peers who share common values, ways of thinking, and activities can be a **reference group** for a novice researcher. Generally speaking, a reference group is the group with which a person identifies, and from which a person assimilates standards and attitudes. You tend to evaluate your own values and behavior in relation to those of the group. A new researcher may need to switch from a reference group that views research and grant writing to be too difficult or irrelevant to a group that values this activity. From this group, you may receive support and feedback necessary to develop grant-writing skills and enact a program of research. In addition, you will have the opportunity to provide similar support and feedback to your peers. There are additional people who can support your program of research, including mentors and experienced researchers with whom you can apprentice. These support persons will be discussed later in the chapter.

When a potential contribution to science, your capacity, and available capital overlap, you have found an ideal focus for your research career (see Figure 29-1). Your focus may shift over time based on findings of your early studies, changes in the healthcare environment, and the availability of funding, but a focus that considers possible contribution, capital, and capacity is a place to start.

BUILDING CAPITAL

Your personal capital may need to be enhanced. How can you build your capital? What type and level of commitment do you have? Who are your support persons and mentors? Do you have a reference group to provide feedback and encouragement?

Level of Commitment

Writing proposals for funding is hard work. Before beginning, reflect on whether your motivation is external or internal. If your motivation is external, you are committed to seeking funding because of the potential to receive rewards from your employer, to earn the high regard of your peers, or to be eligible for a promotion or for a different position. If your motivation is internal, you are convinced that more knowledge is needed to benefit your patients. Both external and internal motivation are valid reasons to be committed to a program

of research; however, an internally motivated researcher may be more likely to conduct studies with limited funding and continue to seek additional funding even in the absence of external funding. As an element of capacity, your level of commitment will determine your ability to persevere and develop a program of research.

Support of Other People

Even the most internally motivated person may experience times of discouragement and need the support of peers. Rarely, if ever, is an investigator funded to conduct a study alone. Funded research projects usually require a team of people with varied skills. As a novice researcher, it is important to work with others who have more experience in seeking and receiving funding (Villalba & Young, 2012).

Networking is a process of developing channels of communication among people with common interests who may not work for the same employer and may be geographically scattered. Contacts may be made through social media, computer networks, mail, telephone, or arrangements to meet at a conference (Adegbola, 2011). Strong networks are based on reciprocal relationships. A professional network can provide opportunities for brainstorming, sharing ideas and problems, and discussing grant-writing opportunities. In some cases, networking may lead to the members of a professional network writing a grant that will be a multisite study with data collected in each member's home institution. When a proposal is being developed, the network, which might also become your reference group, can provide feedback at various stages of proposal development. Adegbola (2011) provides practical tips on how to develop and maintain a professional network such as sitting by people you do not know at a conference and sending a follow-up email to researchers you meet at a conference. Adegbola (2013) further developed the idea of networking to be "scholarly tailgating," the idea of taking charge of your research development and reaching out to leaders in your topic area.

Through networking, nurses interested in a particular area of study can find peers, content experts, and mentors. A **content expert** may be a clinician or researcher who is known for his or her work in the area in which you are interested. Through your review of the literature, you identify a researcher who has developed an instrument to measure a variable that you have decided to include in your proposed study. For example, you want to measure a biological marker of stress and you have read several studies in which an experienced researcher measured the variable using a specific piece of equipment. Contact the researcher through email and make a telephone appointment to discuss the strengths and weaknesses of this particular measurement. You may also arrange to meet at an upcoming conference.

A **mentor** is a person who is more experienced professionally and willing to work with a less experienced professional to achieve his or her goals. Because funded nursing researchers are few, the need for mentoring is greater than the number of available mentors (Maas, Conn, Buckwalter, Herr, & Tripp-Reimer, 2009). Finding a mentor may take time and require significant effort. Grant-writing activities are best learned in a mentor relationship that includes actual participation, because so much of the essential information is transmitted verbally. This type of relationship requires a willingness by both professionals to invest time and energy. A mentor relationship at this level has characteristics of both a teacher-learner relationship and a close friendship. Each individual must have an affinity for the other, from which a close working relationship can be developed. The relationship usually continues for a long period of time.

Grantsmanship

Grantsmanship, the ability to write proposals that are funded, is not an innate skill: it must be learned. Learning grant-related skills requires a commitment of both time and energy. However, the rewards can be great. Strategies used to learn grantsmanship are described in the following sections and are listed in order of increasing time commitment, involvement, and level of expertise needed. These strategies are attending grantsmanship courses, working with experienced researchers, joining research organizations, and participating on research committees or review panels.

Attending Courses and Workshops

Some universities offer elective courses on grantsmanship. Continuing education programs or professional conferences sometimes offer topics related to grantsmanship. The content of these sessions may include the process of grant writing, techniques for obtaining grant funds, and sources of grant funds. In some cases, representatives of funding agencies are invited to explain funding procedures. This information is useful for understanding agency priorities and developing skill in writing proposals. Not all courses or educational opportunities for learning grantsmanship require attendance at a conference because some seminars are offered as webinars or online courses.

Experienced Researchers

Volunteering to assist with the activities of an experienced researcher is an excellent way to learn research and grantsmanship. As graduate students, you can be paid and can gain this experience by becoming graduate research assistants. Through directly working with a funded researcher, you can gain experience in writing grants and reading proposals that have been funded. Examining proposals that have been rejected and the comments of the review committee can be useful as well. The criticisms of the review committee point out the weaknesses of the study and clarify the reasons why the proposal was rejected. Examining these comments on the proposal can increase your insight as a new grant writer and prepare you for similar experiences. Some researchers are sensitive about these criticisms and may be reluctant to share them. If an experienced researcher is willing, however, it is enlightening to hear his or her perceptions and opinions about the criticisms. Ideally, by working closely with an experienced researcher, you will have the opportunity to demonstrate your commitment, and the researcher may invite you to become a permanent member of a research team.

Regional Nursing Research Organizations

In the United States (U.S.), nurse researchers in each region have formed regional research organizations. Table 29-1 lists these organizations and their websites. Each of these regional organizations holds an annual conference and provides opportunities for nursing students to display a poster or present findings of a pilot study or initial phases of a study. These conferences are an excellent opportunity to network and meet more experienced researchers (Adegbola, 2011). These regional research organizations may also fund small grants for which members can apply.

Serving on Research Committees

Research committees and institutional review boards exist in many healthcare and professional organizations.

TABLE 29-1	**Regional Nursing Research Organizations**
Region	**Website**
Eastern Nursing Research Society	http://www.enrs-go.org
Southern Nursing Research Society	http://www.snrs.org
Midwest Nursing Research Society	http://www.mnrs.org
Western Institute of Nursing	http://www.winursing.org

Hospitals, healthcare systems, foundations, and professional nursing organizations have research committees. Through membership on these committees, contacts with researchers can be made. Also, many research committees are involved in reviewing proposals for the funding of small grants or granting approval to collect data in an institution. Often reading proposals for approval for research involving human subjects or for funding can give the novice researcher insight into the importance of clarity and organization in the research proposal. Reviewing proposals and making decisions about funding are experiences that may help researchers become better able to critique and revise their own proposals before submitting them for review.

IDENTIFYING FUNDING SOURCES

Funding sources seek proposals of different types, because the types of studies they fund vary. The next section provides an overview of a few types of grants and donors.

Types of Grants

Two main types of grants are sought in nursing: project grants and research grants. **Project grant proposals** are written to obtain funding for the development of new educational programs in nursing, such as a program designed to teach nurses to provide a new type of nursing care or as a project to support nursing students seeking advanced degrees. These grants may fund a project manager to achieve the goals of the grant. Although these programs may involve evaluation, they seldom involve research. For example, the effectiveness of a new approach to patient care may be evaluated, but the findings can seldom be generalized beyond the unit or institution in which the patient care was provided. The emphasis is on implementing the project, not on conducting research.

Research grants provide funding to conduct a study. Although the two types of grant proposals have similarities, they have important differences in writing techniques, flow of ideas, and content. This chapter focuses on seeking funding for research. Within research grants, proposals vary depending on the source of funding. Proposals for federal funding are the most complex and include a significant amount of information about your institution's resources and capacity to support the study. The section on Government Funding provides additional information on types of federal proposals.

Private or Local Funding

The first step is to determine potential sources for small amounts of research money. In some cases, management in the employing institution can supply limited funding for research activities if a logical, compelling argument is presented for the usefulness of the study to the institution. Healthcare institutions are very interested in saving money and decreasing risks for patients. A funding proposal is stronger when it enumerates benefits to the institution. In many universities, funds are available for intramural grants, which you can obtain competitively by submitting a brief proposal to a university committee. Local chapters of nursing organizations have money available for research activities. Sigma Theta Tau International, the honor society for nurses, provides small grants for nursing research that can be obtained through submission to local, regional, national, or international review committees. Organizations are sources of funding, for instance the local chapters of the American Cancer Society and the American Heart Association. Although grants from the national offices of these organizations require sophisticated research, local or state levels of the organization may have small amounts of funds available for studies in the organization's area of interest, and the studies need not be complex.

Private individuals who are locally active in philanthropy may be willing to provide financial assistance for a small study in an area appealing to them. You need to know of the person whom you might approach and how and when to make that approach to increase the probability of successful funding. Sometimes this approach requires knowing someone who knows someone who might be willing to provide financial support. Acquiring funds from private individuals requires more assertiveness than do other approaches to funding.

Requests for funding need not be limited to a single source. If you anticipate requiring a larger amount of money than one source can supply, seek funds from one source for a specific research need and from another source for another research need, within that line of inquiry. For example, one funder may support the preliminary phase of the research while another funder supports the next phase of the study. Another strategy is to approach different funders about different budget items, such as asking one for mailing costs and another for the salary of a research assistant.

Seeking funding from local sources is less demanding in terms of formality and length of the proposal than is the case with other types of grants. Often, the process is informal and may require only a two- or three-page description of the study. Provide a clear, straightforward description of the study and the way in which the findings will contribute to practice or further study. The important thing is to know what funds are available and how to apply for them. Some of these funds go unused each year because nurses are unaware of their existence, or think that they are unlikely to be successful in obtaining the money. This unused money leads granting agencies or potential donors to conclude that nurses do not need more money for research.

Small grants do more than merely provide the funds necessary to conduct the research. They are the first step you take toward being recognized as a credible researcher and in being considered for more substantial grants for later studies. When you receive a grant, no matter how small, include this information on your curriculum vitae or resumé. Also, list your participation in funded studies, even if you were not the principal investigator (PI). These entries are evidence of first-level recognition as a researcher.

National Nursing Organizations

Many nursing specialty organizations provide support for studies relevant to that specialty, including nurse practitioner groups. These organizations often provide guidance to new, less experienced researchers who need assistance in beginning the process of planning and seeking funding for research. To determine the resources provided by a particular nursing organization, search the organization's website or contact the organization by email, letter, or phone. Table 29-2 provides information about a select group of large nursing specialty organizations that provide grant funding.

Two national nursing organizations that provide small grants not linked to a specialty are the American Nurses Foundation and Sigma Theta Tau International. These grants are usually for less than $7500 each year, are very competitive, and are awarded to new investigators with promising ideas. Receiving funding from these organizations is held in high regard. Information regarding these grants is available from the American Nurses Foundation (2015) and Sigma Theta Tau International (2015).

Industry

Industry may be a good source of funding for nursing studies, particularly if one of the company's products is involved in the study. For example, if a particular type of equipment is being used during an experimental treatment, the company that developed the equipment may be willing to provide equipment for the study without charge, or may be willing to fund the study. If a comparison study examining outcomes of one type of dressing versus another is to be conducted, the company that produces one of the products might provide the product or fund the study. Industry-supported research

TABLE 29-2 National Specialty Nursing Organizations That Fund Research

Organization or Association	Website
Academy of Medical-Surgical Nurses	http://www.amsn.org
American Association of Critical-Care Nurses	http://www.aacn.org
Association of Nurses in AIDS Care	http://www.nursesinaidscare.org
Association of Women's Health, Obstetric and Neonatal Nurses	http://www.awhonn.org
Emergency Nurses Association	http://www.ena.org
Hospice and Palliative Nurses Association	http://www.hpna.org
National Association of Orthopaedic Nurses	http://www.orthonurse.org
National Gerontological Nursing Association	http://www.ngna.org
Oncology Nursing Society	http://www.ons.org
Society of Pediatric Nurses	http://www.pedsnurses.org
Wound Ostomy and Continence Nurses Society	http://www.wocn.org

has been heavily scrutinized because of publicized incidents in which possible conflicts of interest resulted in harm to a subject or may have prevented the publication of unfavorable findings (Fry-Revere & Malmstrom, 2009). The ethics of seeking such funding should be carefully considered because there is sometimes a risk that the researcher might not be unbiased in interpreting study results. A written agreement must be signed among the researcher, employing institution, and company prior to the conduct of the study, describing in detail what will be provided and the rights of the researcher to publish all findings, regardless of the nature of the results.

Foundations

Many foundations in the U.S. provide funding for research, but the problem is to determine which foundations have interests in a particular field of study. The board of a foundation may evaluate the foundation's priorities annually, resulting in different priorities each year. You must learn the characteristics of the foundation, such as what it will fund. A foundation may fund studies only by female researchers, or it may be interested only in studies of low-income groups. A foundation may fund only studies being conducted in a specific geographical region. The average amount of money awarded for a single grant and the ranges of awards are determined by each foundation. If the average award of a particular foundation is $2,500 but $30,000 is needed, that foundation is not the most desirable source of funds. Identify foundations that match your research topic, geographical location, and funding needs. Review carefully the foundation's guidelines for submitting funding requests. Making a personal visit to the foundation or contacting the staff person responsible for funding is desirable in some cases. You can increase your likelihood of funding by revising your proposal to align with the foundation's priorities.

Several publications list foundations and their interests. If you work in a hospital or university, the development department or other department responsible for fundraising for the institution can be very helpful because it has access to information about foundations. That department is likely to have access to a computerized information system, the Sponsored Programs Information Network. This system allows searches for information on specific foundations or on specific health conditions that are funded. You can then locate the most appropriate funding sources to support your research interests. The database contains approximately 2000 programs that provide information on federal agencies, private foundations, and corporate foundations. Check with your development office or administrators to find out whether you have access to this resource.

Other Funders

Despite federal agencies distributing billions of dollars for health research, gaps continue to exist regarding understanding the benefits and processes of selecting one treatment over another. Studies that focus on "decision making by physicians and patients" (Sox & Greenfield, 2009, p. 203) are categorized as being **comparative effectiveness research** (CER). Studies that are classified as being CER are those in which different treatments are evaluated for their outcomes within a select group of people, such as adults with hypertension and hypercholesteremia. In 2006, the Institute of Medicine convened a committee of distinguished researchers, healthcare professionals, and policymakers to set priorities for CER and patient-focused research (Frank et al., 2015). Their report was published by the Institute of Medicine ([IOM], 2008) as *Knowing What Works in Health Care*.

Based on the IOM report, the Patient Protection and Affordable Care Act of Recovery and Revitalization (U.S. Congress, 2010) contained a section (§§ 6301) that authorized the Patient-Centered Outcomes Research Institute (PCORI) to fund CER. PCORI is a nongovernmental, nonprofit corporation run by a board of governors. Patients, healthcare professionals, and insurance companies are involved in studies from conceptualization to dissemination of the findings to the end users (PCORI, 2014).

Another source of funding may be condition-specific organizations in which patients and families are involved, such as the Multiple Sclerosis Association or the National Organization for Rare Disorders. These organizations are similar to foundations in that they have specific funding priorities. A proposal seeking funding must target one of the organization's priorities and the patients with this condition to be successful.

Government Funding

The largest source of grant monies in the US is the federal government—so much so that the federal government influences what is studied and what is not. Information on funding agencies can be obtained from a government entity called the Catalog of Federal Domestic Assistance (n.d.) that allows someone seeking a grant to search for all types of government funding, including funding for healthcare research. The National Institutes of Health (NIH), particularly the National Institute for Nursing Research and the Agency for Healthcare Research and Quality, solicit nursing proposals. Each agency has areas of focus and priorities for funding that change over time.

Federal agencies seek researchers through two paths (Figure 29-2). As the researcher, you can identify a significant problem, develop a study to examine it, and submit a proposal for the study to the appropriate federal funding agency. This type of proposal is called an **investigator-initiated research proposal**. An agency or group of agencies may release periodically a **program announcement** (PA) to remind researchers of priority areas and generate interest in these priority areas. Proposals submitted in response to a PA are considered investigator-initiated proposals. Alternatively, an agency within the federal government can identify a significant problem, develop a plan by which the problem can be studied, and publish a **request for proposals (RFP)** or a **request for applications (RFA)** from researchers (see Figure 29-2).

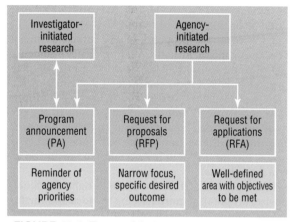

FIGURE 29-2 Types of federal research proposals.

When preparing an investigator-initiated proposal, refine your ideas and contact an official within the government agency early in the planning process to inform the agency of your intent to submit a proposal. Each agency has established dates, usually three times a year, when proposals are reviewed. You will need to start preparing your proposal months ahead of this deadline, and some agencies are willing to provide assistance and feedback to the researcher during development of the proposal. This assistance may occur through email or telephone conversations. NIH program officers, and NIH staff members responsible for specific areas of research, frequently attend regional and national research conferences and make themselves available for appointments to discuss research ideas.

The NIH issues an RFP when scientists advising the institutes have identified a specific need to move an area of knowledge forward. An RFA may be broader than an RFP but still has a focus and a list of objectives that an institute or center within the NIH has identified. An RFA has a single application deadline. The amount that has been budgeted for the successful applications is indicated, and the RFA remains open for several funding cycles.

SUBMITTING A PROPOSAL FOR A FEDERAL GRANT

Federal funding for research is very competitive. To be successful in obtaining funding, you need a strong institutional support and propose an innovative study. The review process has multiple layers at the federal level. You need to allocate extensive time to writing the study plan as well as completing all the required application components. If a proposal is not funded, be prepared to revise and resubmit by the next funding deadline.

Ensuring a Unique Proposal

During your review of the literature, you may have read the findings of funded studies, but the literature does not include recently completed or ongoing funded studies. Early in the process of planning a study for which you intend to seek federal funding, it is wise to determine the studies on your topic of interest that have been funded previously and the funded studies currently in process. This information is available at the website, NIH Research Portfolio Online Reporting Tools—Expenditures and Results (RePORTER), which is maintained by the NIH Office of Extramural Research (NIH, 2015a). The institutes and agencies that fund studies and projects, and are included in the RePORTER, are listed in Table 29-3. You can search the database by state, subject, type of grant, funding agency, or investigator.

Reviewing proposals that are funded by a particular agency can be helpful. Although the agency cannot provide access to these proposals, researchers can sometimes obtain copies of them by contacting the PI of the study personally. In some cases, a researcher writing a proposal may choose to travel to Washington to meet with an agency representative. Project officers, the agency personnel who manage studies on a specified topic, may also travel to regional and national research conferences to be available to meet with potential researchers. This type of contact allows the researcher to modify the proposal to fit more closely within agency guidelines, increasing the probability of funding. In many cases, proposals will fit within the interests of more than one government agency at the time of submission. It is permissible and perhaps desirable to request that the proposal be assigned to two agencies for review and potential funding.

Verifying Institutional Support

Grant awards are most commonly made to institutions rather than to individuals. It is important to determine the willingness of the institution to receive the grant and support the study. This willingness needs to be documented in the proposal. Supporting the study involves agreeing with the appropriateness of the study topic; ensuring the adequacy of facilities and services; providing space needed for the study; contributing to the study in non-monetary ways, such as staff time, equipment, or data processing; and overseeing the rights of human subjects. The study's budget will include a category called **indirect costs** to pay the

TABLE 29-3   **Federal Agencies That Fund Grants and Are Included in the National Institutes of Health Research Portfolio Online Reporting Tools—Expenditures and Results (RePORTER)**

Agency	Types of Projects Funded
Agency for Health Care Research and Quality (AHRQ)	Projects to produce evidence to improve the quality, safety, and accessibility of health care
Centers for Disease Control and Prevention (CDC)	Research studies and projects to improve public health
Food and Drug Administration (FDA)	Grants and cooperative agreements to protect food and drug safety
Health Resources and Services Administration (HRSA)	Program grants to prepare and develop health professionals to care for diverse populations and improve access to care
National Institutes of Health (NIH)	Studies and research training programs on wide range of topics, through its centers and institutes
Substance Abuse and Mental Health Services Administration (SAMHSA)	Research studies and projects to prevent and treat substance abuse and mental illness
U.S. Department of Veterans Affairs	Projects and studies to benefit military veterans

institution's expenses, as compared to **direct costs,** the funds necessary to conduct the study. Direct costs are used to pay a portion of the researcher's salary, and the salaries of data collectors or other research assistants, obtain equipment for the study, and provide a small payment to study participants to acknowledge their time and effort. For federal grants, indirect costs may by equal to direct costs, meaning that 50% of the requested amount will be for direct costs and the other half for indirect costs.

Making Time to Write

Recognize that writing a proposal requires a significant amount of time (see Chapter 28 for how to write a proposal). In a survey of astronomy and psychology researchers ($n = 195$), von Hippel and von Hippel (2015) found even experienced researchers spent over 115 hours writing the proposal. Allow sufficient time to write the proposal. Read the funding agency's guidelines carefully and completely before starting to write. Keep the guidelines nearby as you write so that you can easily refer back to them. Strictly adhere to the page limitations and required font sizes. The sections of the proposal are uploaded separately into an online system. Be sure that all the sections agree with one another on details, such as names of instruments and inclusion criteria for subjects.

Writing your first proposal on a tight deadline is unwise. Proposals require refining the idea and method and rewriting the text several times. Allow 6 to 12 months for proposal development, beginning from the point of early development of your research ideas. As soon as you have a complete draft, ask a peer or mentor to read the proposal to check for errors in logic. As people review your proposal informally, recognize their questions as indications that an idea was not clearly presented and may need to be rewritten: their questions and comments are very valuable. Before submission, it is highly recommended that you have a content expert or other researcher who is not at your institution critique the proposal.

Understanding the Review Process

The Center for Scientific Review has the administrative responsibility for ensuring a fair, equitable review of all proposals submitted to NIH or other Public Health Services agencies. After submission, the staff person assigned to your grant will determine which integrated review group will review your proposal for its technical and scientific merit. Within the integrated review group, each grant is assigned to a study section for scientific evaluation. The study section is comprised of active funded researchers. Peer review of research funding proposals is what gives research its scientific credibility (Barnett et al., 2015). The study sections have no alignment with the funding agency. Thus, staff persons in the agencies have no influence on the committee's work of judging the scientific merit of the proposal. The proposal is given to two or more reviewers who are considered qualified to evaluate the proposal and have no conflicts of interest. The reviewers rate the proposal on the core criteria and overall impact and submit a written critique of the study. Box 29-2 lists the core criteria on which proposals are evaluated. Each member may have 50 to 100 proposals to read in a 1- to 2-month period. A meeting of the full study section is then held. The persons who critiqued the proposal discuss each

BOX 29-2   **Review Criteria for NIH Research Grant Proposals**

- Overall impact
- Significance
- Investigator(s)
- Innovation
- Approach
- Environment

Extracted from http://grants.nih.gov/grants/peer/guidelines_general/Review_Criteria_at_a_glance.pdf.

application, and other members comment or ask questions before recording their scores.

Proposals are assigned a numerical score used to develop a priority rating for funding. A study that is scored is not necessarily funded. The PI may review the progress of the proposal through the stages of review by accessing an online system, called the Electronic Research Administration (eRA) Commons. Funding begins with the proposal that has the highest rank order and continues until available funds are depleted. This process can take 6 months or longer. Because of this process, researchers may not receive grant money for up to a year after submitting the proposal.

Many proposals are rejected (or scored but not funded) with the first submission. The critique of the scientific committee, called a **summary statement**, is available to the researcher via his or her eRA Commons account. Frequently, the agency staff encourages the researcher to rewrite the proposal with guidance from the comments and resubmit it to the same agency. The probability of funding is greater the second time if the researcher has followed the suggestions.

Responding to Rejected Grant Proposals

If your proposal is unfunded, you are not alone. In 2014, only 21% of all proposals submitted to NIH were funded (NIH, 2015b). For NINR, the rate was 16.7% to 26.7% depending on the mechanism (NIH, 2015b). The researcher's reaction to a rejected proposal is usually anger and then depression. The frustrated researcher may want to abandon the proposal. There seems to be no way to avoid the subjective reaction to a rejection because of the significant emotion and time invested in writing the proposal. However, after a few weeks, it is advisable to examine the rejection letter and summary statement again. The comments can be useful in revising the proposal for resubmission. The learning experience of rewriting the proposal and evaluating the comments will provide a background for seeking funding for

another study. Considering the low rate of acceptance, the researcher must be committed to submitting proposals repeatedly to achieve grant funding (Roebber & Schultz, 2011).

GRANT MANAGEMENT

Receiving notice that a grant proposal is funded is one of the highlights in a researcher's career and warrants a celebration. However, work on the study must begin as soon as possible. You included a detailed plan of activities in the proposal that is ready to be implemented. To avoid problems, you need to consider the practicalities of managing the budget, hiring and training research personnel, maintaining the promised timetable, and coordinating activities of the study.

Managing the Budget

Although the supporting institution is ultimately responsible for dispensing and controlling grant monies, the PI is responsible for monitoring budget expenditures and making decisions about how the money is to be spent (Devine, 2009). If this grant is the first one received, a PI who has no previous administrative experience may need guidance in how to keep records and make reasonable budget decisions. If funding is through a federal agency, the PI will be required to provide interim reports as well as updates on the progress of the study.

Training Research Personnel

When a new grant is initiated, set aside time to interview, hire, and train grant personnel (Martin & Fleming, 2010). The personnel who will be involved in data collection need to learn the process, and then data collection needs to be refined to ensure that each data collector is consistent with the other data collectors. This process helps evaluate interrater reliability. The PI needs to set aside time to oversee the work of personnel hired for the grant.

Maintaining the Study Schedule

The timetable submitted with the proposal needs to be adhered to whenever possible, which requires careful planning. Otherwise, work activities and other responsibilities are likely to take precedence and delay the grant work. Unexpected events do happen. However, careful planning can minimize their impact. The PI needs to refer back to the timetable constantly to evaluate progress. If the project falls behind schedule, action needs to be taken to return to the original schedule or to readjust the timetable.

Coordinating Activities

During a large study with several investigators and other grant personnel, coordinating activities can be a problem. Arrange meetings of all grant workers at intervals to share ideas and solve problems. Keep records of the discussions at these meetings. These actions can lead to a more smoothly functioning team.

Submitting Reports

As mentioned, federal grants require the submission of interim reports according to preset deadlines. The notice of a grant award sent as a PDF (Portable Document Format) document via email will include guidelines for the content of the reports, which will consist of a description of grant activities. Set aside time to prepare the report, which usually requires uploading data and other information about the study into the federal electronic record system. In addition to the electronic reports, it is often useful to maintain contact with the appropriate staff at the federal agency.

PLANNING YOUR NEXT GRANT

The researcher should not wait until funding from the first grant has ended to begin seeking funds for a second study because of the length of time required to obtain funding. It may be wise to have several ongoing studies in various stages of implementation. For example, you could be planning one study, collecting data on a second study, analyzing data on a third, and writing papers for publication on a fourth. A full-time researcher could have completed one funded study, be in the last year of funding for a second, be in the first year of funding for a third study, and be seeking funding for a fourth. This scenario may sound unrealistic, but with planning, it is not. This strategy not only provides continuous funding for research activities but also facilitates a rhythm of research that prevents time pressures and makes use of lulls in activity in a particular study. To increase the ease of obtaining funding, all studies should be within the same area of research, each building on the last.

▮ KEY POINTS

- Building a program of research requires conducting a series of studies on a topic, with each study building on the findings of the previous one.
- The ideal topic around which to build a research program can be identified by considering topics for which the researcher has or can gain the expertise to conduct studies (capacity), funding is available (capital), and the potential exists for the researcher

to make a difference (contribution). Capacity can be expanded by working with others with different types of skills and knowledge.

- Writing a grant proposal for funding requires a commitment to working extra hours.
- To receive funding, researchers need to learn grantsmanship skills.
- The first studies a researcher completes usually are conducted with personal funding or small grants.
- Nongovernmental sources of funding include private donors, local organizations, nursing organizations, and foundations.
- Before submitting a proposal to seek federal funding, the researcher should successfully complete two or more small studies and disseminate the findings.
- The researcher identifies a significant problem, develops a study to examine it, and submits a proposal for the study to an appropriate federal funding agency.
- The PI is responsible for keeping within the budget, training research personnel, maintaining the schedule, and coordinating activities.
- Grants require the submission of interim and final reports of expenditures, activities, and achievements.
- A researcher should not wait until funding from one grant ends before seeking funds for the next grant.

REFERENCES

Adegbola, M. (2011). Soar like geese: Building developmental network relationships for scholarship. *Nursing Education Perspectives, 32*(1), 51–53.

Adegbola, M. (2013). Scholarly tailgating defined: A diverse, giant network. *The ABNF Journal: Official Journal of the Association of Black Nursing Faculty in Higher Education, Inc, 24*(1), 17–20.

American Nurses Association. (2008). Leading the way in research on women and heart disease. *The American Nurse, 40*(1), 12.

American Nurses Foundation. (2015). *Nursing research grant.* Retrieved May 12, 2016, from http://www.anfonline.org/MainCategory/NursingResearchGrant.aspx.

Barnett, A., Herbert, D., Campbell, M., Daly, N., Roberts, J., Mudge, A., et al. (2015). *BMC Health Services Research, 15*, Article 55. doi:10.1186/s12913-015-0721-7.

Catalog of Federal Domestic Assistance (CFDA). (n.d.). *CDFA overview.* Retrieved May 12, 2016, from https://www.cfda.gov/?s=generalinfo&mode=list&tab=list&tabmode=list.

Devine, E. B. (2009). The art of obtaining grants. *American Journal of Health-System Pharmacy, 66*(6), 580–587.

Frank, L., Forsythe, L., Ellis, L., Schrandt, S., Sheridan, S., Gerson, J., et al. (2015). Conceptual and practical foundations of patient engagement in research at the Patient-Centered Outcomes Research Institute. *Quality of Life Research: An International*

Journal of Quality of Life Aspects of Treatment, Care and Rehabilitation, 24(5), 1033–1041.

Fry-Revere, S., & Malmstrom, D. B. (2009). More regulation of industry-supported biomedical research: Are we asking the right questions? *The Journal of Law, Medicine & Ethics: A Journal of the American Society of Law, Medicine & Ethics, 29*(3), 420–430.

Institute of Medicine (IOM). (2008). *Knowing what works in health care: A roadmap for the nation.* Washington, DC: National Academies Press.

Martin, C. J. H., & Fleming, V. (2010). A 15-step model for writing a research proposal. *British Journal of Midwifery, 18*(12), 791–798.

Maas, M. L., Conn, V., Buckwalter, K. C., Herr, K., & Tripp-Reimer, T. (2009). Increasing nurse faculty research: The Iowa Gerontological Nurse Research and Regional Research Consortium Strategies. *Journal of Nursing Scholarship, 41*(4), 411–419.

National Institutes of Health. (NIH). (2015a). *Research Portfolio Online Reporting Tools (RePORT).* Retrieved May 12, 2016, from https://projectreporter.nih.gov/reporter.cfm.

National Institutes of Health (NIH). (2015b). *Table #205A: Research project grants and other mechanisms: Competing applications, awards, success rates, and total funding: Fiscal year 2014.* Retrieved October 28, 2015, from http://report.nih.gov/success_rates/index.aspx.

Patient-Centered Outcomes Research Institute. (PCORI). (2014). *About us.* Retrieved October 20, 2015, from http://www.pcori.org/about-us.

Roebber, P., & Schultz, D. (2011). Peer review, program officers and science funding. *PLoS ONE, 6*(4), e18680.

Sigma Theta Tau International. (2015). *Nursing research grants.* Retrieved October 15, 2015, from http://www.nursingsociety.org/advance-elevate/research/research-grants.

Sox, H., & Greenfield, S. (2009). Comparative effectiveness research: A report from the Institute of Medicine. *Annals of Internal Medicine, 151*(3), 203–205.

United States (U.S.) Congress. (2010). *Patient Protection and Affordable Care Act, Subtitle D of Title VI, §§ 6301 Patient-Centered Outcomes Research.* Retrieved October 20, 2015, from http://www.pcori.org/sites/default/files/PCORI_Authorizing_Legislation.pdf.

Villalba, J., & Young, J. (2012). Externally funded research in counselor education: An overview of the process. *Counselor Education & Supervision, 51*(2), 141–155.

von Hippel, T., & von Hippel, C. (2015). To apply or not to apply: A survey analysis of grant writing costs and benefits. *PLoS ONE, 10*(3), e0118494.

A | APPENDIX

z Values Table

z Score	From Mean to z (%)	z Score	From Mean to z (%)	z Score	From Mean to z (%)
.00	.00	.36	14.06	.72	26.42
.01	.40	.37	14.43	.73	26.73
.02	.80	.38	14.80	.74	27.04
.03	1.20	.39	15.17	.75	27.34
.04	1.60	.40	15.54	.76	27.64
.05	1.99	.41	15.91	.77	27.94
.06	2.39	.42	16.28	.78	28.23
.07	2.79	.43	16.64	.79	28.52
.08	3.19	.44	17.00	.80	28.81
.09	3.59	.45	17.36	.81	29.10
.10	3.98	.46	17.72	.82	29.39
.11	4.38	.47	18.08	.83	29.67
.12	4.78	.48	18.44	.84	29.95
.13	5.17	.49	18.79	.85	30.23
.14	5.57	.50	19.15	.86	30.51
.15	5.96	.51	19.50	.87	30.78
.16	6.36	.52	19.85	.88	31.06
.17	6.75	.53	20.19	.89	31.33
.18	7.14	.54	20.54	.90	31.59
.19	7.53	.55	20.88	.91	31.86
.20	7.93	.56	21.23	.92	32.12
.21	8.32	.57	21.57	.93	32.38
.22	8.71	.58	21.90	.94	32.64
.23	9.10	.59	22.24	.95	32.89
.24	9.48	.60	22.57	.96	33.15
.25	9.87	.61	22.91	.97	33.40
.26	10.26	.62	23.24	.98	33.65
.27	10.64	.63	23.57	.99	33.89
.28	11.03	.64	23.89	1.00	34.13
.29	11.41	.65	24.22	1.01	34.38
.30	11.79	.66	24.54	1.02	34.61
.31	12.17	.67	24.86	1.03	34.85
.32	12.55	.68	25.17	1.04	35.08
.33	12.93	.69	25.49	1.05	35.31
.34	13.31	.70	25.80	1.06	35.54
.35	13.68	.71	26.11	1.07	35.77

z Score	From Mean to z (%)	z Score	From Mean to z (%)	z Score	From Mean to z (%)
1.08	35.99	1.58	44.29	2.08	48.12
1.09	36.21	1.59	44.41	2.09	48.17
1.10	36.43	1.60	44.52	2.10	48.21
1.11	36.65	1.61	44.63	2.11	48.26
1.12	36.86	1.62	44.74	2.12	48.30
1.13	37.08	1.63	44.84	2.13	48.34
1.14	37.29	1.64	44.95	2.14	48.38
1.15	37.49	1.65	45.05	2.15	48.42
1.16	37.70	1.66	45.15	2.16	48.46
1.17	37.90	1.67	45.25	2.17	48.50
1.18	38.10	1.68	45.35	2.18	48.54
1.19	38.30	1.69	45.45	2.19	48.57
1.20	38.49	1.70	45.54	2.20	48.61
1.21	38.69	1.71	45.64	2.21	48.64
1.22	38.88	1.72	45.73	2.22	48.68
1.23	39.07	1.73	45.82	2.23	48.71
1.24	39.25	1.74	45.91	2.24	48.75
1.25	39.44	1.75	45.99	2.25	48.78
1.26	39.62	1.76	46.08	2.26	48.81
1.27	39.80	1.77	46.16	2.27	48.84
1.28	39.97	1.78	46.25	2.28	48.87
1.29	40.15	1.79	46.33	2.29	48.90
1.30	40.32	1.80	46.41	2.30	48.93
1.31	40.49	1.81	46.49	2.31	48.96
1.32	40.66	1.82	46.56	2.32	48.98
1.33	40.82	1.83	46.64	2.33	49.01
1.34	40.99	1.84	46.71	2.34	49.04
1.35	41.15	1.85	46.78	2.35	49.06
1.36	41.31	1.86	46.86	2.36	49.09
1.37	41.47	1.87	46.93	2.37	49.11
1.38	41.62	1.88	46.99	2.38	49.13
1.39	41.77	1.89	47.06	2.39	49.16
1.40	41.92	1.90	47.13	2.40	49.18
1.41	42.07	1.91	47.19	2.41	49.20
1.42	42.22	1.92	47.26	2.42	49.22
1.43	42.36	1.93	47.32	2.43	49.25
1.44	42.51	1.94	47.38	2.44	49.27
1.45	42.65	1.95	47.44	2.45	49.29
1.46	42.79	1.96	47.50	2.46	49.31
1.47	42.92	1.97	47.56	2.47	49.32
1.48	43.06	1.98	47.61	2.48	49.34
1.49	43.19	1.99	47.67	2.49	49.36
1.50	43.32	2.00	47.72	2.50	49.38
1.51	43.45	2.01	47.78	2.51	49.40
1.52	43.57	2.02	47.83	2.52	49.41
1.53	43.70	2.03	47.88	2.53	49.43
1.54	43.82	2.04	47.93	2.54	49.45
1.55	43.94	2.05	47.98	2.55	49.46
1.56	44.06	2.06	48.03	2.56	49.48
1.57	44.18	2.07	48.08	2.57	49.49

Continued

z Score	From Mean to *z* (%)	*z* Score	From Mean to *z* (%)	*z* Score	From Mean to *z* (%)
2.58	49.51	2.73	49.68	2.88	49.801
2.59	49.52	2.74	49.69	2.89	49.807
2.60	49.53	2.75	49.702	2.90	49.813
2.61	49.55	2.76	49.711	2.91	49.819
2.62	49.56	2.77	49.720	2.92	49.825
2.63	49.57	2.78	49.728	2.93	49.831
2.64	49.59	2.79	49.736	2.94	49.836
2.65	49.60	2.80	49.744	2.95	49.841
2.66	49.61	2.81	49.752	2.96	49.846
2.67	49.62	2.82	49.760	2.97	49.851
2.68	49.63	2.83	49.767	2.98	49.856
2.69	49.64	2.84	49.774	2.99	49.861
2.70	49.65	2.85	49.781	3.00	49.865
2.71	49.66	2.86	49.788		
2.72	49.67	2.87	49.795		

Critical Values for Student's *t* Distribution

Level of Significance (α), One-Tailed Test					
0.001	0.005	0.01	0.025	0.05	0.10

Level of Significance (α), Two-Tailed Test					
df	0.002	0.01	0.02	0.05	0.10	0.20
2	22.327	9.925	6.965	4.303	2.920	1.886
3	10.215	5.841	4.541	3.182	2.353	1.638
4	7.173	4.604	3.747	2.776	2.132	1.533
5	5.893	4.032	3.365	2.571	2.015	1.476
6	5.208	3.707	3.143	2.447	1.943	1.440
7	4.785	3.499	2.998	2.365	1.895	1.415
8	4.501	3.355	2.896	2.306	1.860	1.397
9	4.297	3.250	2.821	2.262	1.833	1.383
10	4.144	3.169	2.764	2.228	1.812	1.372
11	4.025	3.106	2.718	2.201	1.796	1.363
12	3.930	3.055	2.681	2.179	1.782	1.356
13	3.852	3.012	2.650	2.160	1.771	1.350
14	3.787	2.977	2.624	2.145	1.761	1.345
15	3.733	2.947	2.602	2.131	1.753	1.341
16	3.686	2.921	2.583	2.120	1.746	1.337
17	3.646	2.898	2.567	2.110	1.740	1.333
18	3.610	2.878	2.552	2.101	1.734	1.330
19	3.579	2.861	2.539	2.093	1.729	1.328
20	3.552	2.845	2.528	2.086	1.725	1.325
21	3.527	2.831	2.518	2.080	1.721	1.323
22	3.505	2.819	2.508	2.074	1.717	1.321
23	3.485	2.807	2.500	2.069	1.714	1.319
24	3.467	2.797	2.492	2.064	1.711	1.318
25	3.450	2.787	2.485	2.060	1.708	1.316
26	3.435	2.779	2.479	2.056	1.706	1.315
27	3.421	2.771	2.473	2.052	1.703	1.314
28	3.408	2.763	2.467	2.048	1.701	1.313
29	3.396	2.756	2.462	2.045	1.699	1.311
30	3.385	2.750	2.457	2.042	1.697	1.310
31	3.375	2.744	2.453	2.040	1.696	1.309
32	3.365	2.738	2.449	2.037	1.694	1.309
33	3.356	2.733	2.445	2.035	1.692	1.308
34	3.348	2.728	2.441	2.032	1.691	1.307

df, Degrees of Freedom.

Continued

Level of Significance (α), One-Tailed Test					
0.001	0.005	0.01	0.025	0.05	0.10

Level of Significance (α), Two-Tailed Test—cont'd

df	0.002	0.01	0.02	0.05	0.10	0.20
35	3.340	2.724	2.438	2.030	1.690	1.306
36	3.333	2.719	2.434	2.028	1.688	1.306
37	3.326	2.715	2.431	2.026	1.687	1.305
38	3.319	2.712	2.429	2.024	1.686	1.304
39	3.313	2.708	2.426	2.023	1.685	1.304
40	3.307	2.704	2.423	2.021	1.684	1.303
45	3.281	2.690	2.412	2.014	1.679	1.301
50	3.261	2.678	2.403	2.009	1.676	1.299
55	3.245	2.668	2.396	2.004	1.673	1.297
60	3.232	2.660	2.390	2.000	1.671	1.296
65	3.220	2.654	2.385	1.997	1.669	1.295
70	3.211	2.648	2.381	1.994	1.667	1.294
75	3.202	2.643	2.377	1.992	1.665	1.293
80	3.195	2.639	2.374	1.990	1.664	1.292
85	3.189	2.635	2.371	1.988	1.663	1.292
90	3.183	2.632	2.368	1.987	1.662	1.291
95	3.178	2.629	2.366	1.985	1.661	1.291
100	3.174	2.626	2.364	1.984	1.660	1.290
200	3.131	2.601	2.345	1.972	1.653	1.286
300	3.118	2.592	2.339	1.968	1.650	1.284
∞	3.1	2.58	2.33	1.96	1.65	1.28

df, Degrees of Freedom.

Critical Values of *r* for Pearson Product Moment Correlation Coefficient

Level of Significance (α), One-Tailed Test								
0.05	0.025	0.01	0.005		0.05	0.025	0.01	0.005

Level of Significance (α), Two-Tailed Test								
df = N − 2	0.10	0.05	0.02	0.01	*df* = N − 2	0.10	0.05	0.02	0.01
1	0.9877	0.9969	0.9995	0.9999	39	0.2605	0.3081	0.3621	0.3978
2	0.9000	0.9500	0.9800	0.9900	40	0.2573	0.3044	0.3578	0.3932
3	0.8054	0.8783	0.9343	0.9587	41	0.2542	0.3008	0.3536	0.3887
4	0.7293	0.8114	0.8822	0.9172	42	0.2512	0.2973	0.3496	0.3843
5	0.6694	0.7545	0.8329	0.8745	43	0.2483	0.2940	0.3458	0.3801
6	0.6215	0.7067	0.7887	0.8343	44	0.2455	0.2907	0.3420	0.3761
7	0.5822	0.6664	0.7498	0.7977	45	0.2429	0.2876	0.3384	0.3721
8	0.5493	0.6319	0.7155	0.7646	46	0.2403	0.2845	0.3348	0.3683
9	0.5214	0.6021	0.6851	0.7348	47	0.2377	0.2816	0.3314	0.3646
10	0.4973	0.5760	0.6581	0.7079	48	0.2353	0.2787	0.3281	0.3610
11	0.4762	0.5529	0.6339	0.6835	49	0.2329	0.2759	0.3249	0.3575
12	0.4575	0.5324	0.6120	0.6614	50	0.2306	0.2732	0.3218	0.3542
13	0.4409	0.5140	0.5923	0.6411	55	0.2201	0.2609	0.3074	0.3385
14	0.4259	0.4973	0.5742	0.6226	60	0.2108	0.2500	0.2948	0.3248
15	0.4124	0.4821	0.5577	0.6055	65	0.2027	0.2404	0.2837	0.3126
16	0.4000	0.4683	0.5426	0.5897	70	0.1954	0.2319	0.2737	0.3017
17	0.3887	0.4555	0.5285	0.5751	75	0.1888	0.2242	0.2647	0.2919
18	0.3783	0.4438	0.5155	0.5614	80	0.1829	0.2172	0.2565	0.2830
19	0.3687	0.4329	0.5034	0.5487	85	0.1775	0.2108	0.2491	0.2748
20	0.3598	0.4227	0.4921	0.5368	90	0.1726	0.2050	0.2422	0.2673
21	0.3515	0.4132	0.4815	0.5256	95	0.1680	0.1996	0.2359	0.2604
22	0.3438	0.4044	0.4716	0.5151	100	0.1638	0.1946	0.2301	0.2540
23	0.3365	0.3961	0.4622	0.5052	120	0.1496	0.1779	0.2104	0.2324
24	0.3297	0.3882	0.4534	0.4958	140	0.1386	0.1648	0.1951	0.2155
25	0.3233	0.3809	0.4451	0.4869	160	0.1297	0.1543	0.1827	0.2019
26	0.3172	0.3739	0.4372	0.4785	180	0.1223	0.1455	0.1723	0.1905
27	0.3115	0.3673	0.4297	0.4705	200	0.1161	0.1381	0.1636	0.1809
28	0.3061	0.3610	0.4226	0.4629	250	0.1039	0.1236	0.1465	0.1620
29	0.3009	0.3550	0.4158	0.4556	300	0.0948	0.1129	0.1338	0.1480
30	0.2960	0.3494	0.4093	0.4487	350	0.0878	0.1046	0.1240	0.1371
31	0.2913	0.3440	0.4031	0.4421	400	0.0822	0.0978	0.1160	0.1283
32	0.2869	0.3388	0.3973	0.4357	450	0.0775	0.0922	0.1094	0.1210
33	0.2826	0.3338	0.3916	0.4297	500	0.0735	0.0875	0.1038	0.1149
34	0.2785	0.3291	0.3862	0.4238	600	0.0671	0.0799	0.0948	0.1049
35	0.2746	0.3246	0.3810	0.4182	700	0.0621	0.0740	0.0878	0.0972
36	0.2709	0.3202	0.3760	0.4128	800	0.0581	0.0692	0.0821	0.0909
37	0.2673	0.3160	0.3712	0.4076	900	0.0548	0.0653	0.0774	0.0857
38	0.2638	0.3120	0.3665	0.4026	1000	0.0520	0.0619	0.0735	0.0813

df, Degrees of Freedom.

D APPENDIX

Critical Values of F for α = 0.05 and α = 0.01

Critical Values of F for α = 0.05

df Denominator	\multicolumn{19}{c}{DEGREES OF FREEDOM (df) NUMERATOR}
	1	2	3	4	5	6	7	8	9	10	12	15	20	24	30	40	60	120	∞
1	161.4	199.5	215.7	224.6	230.2	234.0	236.8	238.9	240.5	241.9	243.9	245.9	248.0	249.1	250.1	251.1	252.2	253.3	254.3
2	18.51	19.00	19.16	19.25	19.30	19.33	19.35	19.37	19.38	19.40	19.41	19.43	19.45	19.45	19.46	19.47	19.48	19.49	19.50
3	10.13	9.55	9.28	9.12	9.01	8.94	8.89	8.85	8.81	8.79	8.74	8.70	8.66	8.64	8.62	8.59	8.57	8.55	8.53
4	7.71	6.94	6.59	6.39	6.26	6.16	6.09	6.04	6.00	5.96	5.91	5.86	5.80	5.77	5.75	5.72	5.69	5.66	5.63
5	6.61	5.79	5.41	5.19	5.05	4.95	4.88	4.82	4.77	4.74	4.68	4.62	4.56	4.53	4.50	4.46	4.43	4.40	4.36
6	5.99	5.14	4.76	4.53	4.39	4.28	4.21	4.15	4.10	4.06	4.00	3.94	3.87	3.84	3.81	3.77	3.74	3.70	3.67
7	5.59	4.74	4.35	4.12	3.97	3.87	3.79	3.73	3.68	3.64	3.57	3.51	3.44	3.41	3.38	3.34	3.30	3.27	3.23
8	5.32	4.46	4.07	3.84	3.69	3.58	3.50	3.44	3.39	3.35	3.28	3.22	3.15	3.12	3.08	3.04	3.01	2.97	2.93
9	5.12	4.26	3.86	3.63	3.48	3.37	3.29	3.23	3.18	3.14	3.07	3.01	2.94	2.90	2.86	2.83	2.79	2.75	2.71
10	4.96	4.10	3.71	3.48	3.33	3.22	3.14	3.07	3.02	2.98	2.91	2.85	2.77	2.74	2.70	2.66	2.62	2.58	2.54
11	4.84	3.98	3.59	3.36	3.20	3.09	3.01	2.95	2.90	2.85	2.79	2.72	2.65	2.61	2.57	2.53	2.49	2.45	2.40
12	4.75	3.89	3.49	3.26	3.11	3.00	2.91	2.85	2.80	2.75	2.69	2.62	2.54	2.51	2.47	2.43	2.38	2.34	2.30
13	4.67	3.81	3.41	3.18	3.03	2.92	2.83	2.77	2.71	2.67	2.60	2.53	2.46	2.42	2.38	2.34	2.30	2.25	2.21
14	4.60	3.74	3.34	3.11	2.96	2.85	2.76	2.70	2.65	2.60	2.53	2.46	2.39	2.35	2.31	2.27	2.22	2.18	2.13
15	4.54	3.68	3.29	3.06	2.90	2.79	2.71	2.64	2.59	2.54	2.48	2.40	2.33	2.29	2.25	2.20	2.16	2.11	2.07
16	4.49	3.63	3.24	3.01	2.85	2.74	2.66	2.59	2.54	2.49	2.42	2.35	2.28	2.24	2.19	2.15	2.11	2.06	2.01
17	4.45	3.59	3.20	2.96	2.81	2.70	2.61	2.55	2.49	2.45	2.38	2.31	2.23	2.19	2.15	2.10	2.06	2.01	1.96
18	4.41	3.55	3.16	2.93	2.77	2.66	2.58	2.51	2.46	2.41	2.34	2.27	2.19	2.15	2.11	2.06	2.02	1.97	1.92
19	4.38	3.52	3.13	2.90	2.74	2.63	2.54	2.48	2.42	2.38	2.31	2.23	2.16	2.11	2.07	2.03	1.98	1.93	1.88
20	4.35	3.49	3.10	2.87	2.71	2.60	2.51	2.45	2.39	2.35	2.28	2.20	2.12	2.08	2.04	1.99	1.95	1.90	1.84
21	4.32	3.47	3.07	2.84	2.68	2.57	2.49	2.42	2.37	2.32	2.25	2.18	2.10	2.05	2.01	1.96	1.92	1.87	1.81
22	4.30	3.44	3.05	2.82	2.66	2.55	2.46	2.40	2.34	2.30	2.23	2.15	2.07	2.03	1.98	1.94	1.89	1.84	1.78
23	4.28	3.42	3.03	2.80	2.64	2.53	2.44	2.37	2.32	2.27	2.20	2.13	2.05	2.01	1.96	1.91	1.86	1.81	1.76
24	4.26	3.40	3.01	2.78	2.62	2.51	2.42	2.36	2.30	2.25	2.18	2.11	2.03	1.98	1.94	1.89	1.84	1.79	1.73
25	4.24	3.39	2.99	2.76	2.60	2.49	2.40	2.34	2.28	2.24	2.16	2.09	2.01	1.96	1.92	1.87	1.82	1.77	1.71
26	4.23	3.37	2.98	2.74	2.59	2.47	2.39	2.32	2.27	2.22	2.15	2.07	1.99	1.95	1.90	1.85	1.80	1.75	1.69
27	4.21	3.35	2.96	2.73	2.57	2.46	2.37	2.31	2.25	2.20	2.13	2.06	1.97	1.93	1.88	1.84	1.79	1.73	1.67
28	4.20	3.34	2.95	2.71	2.56	2.45	2.36	2.29	2.24	2.19	2.12	2.04	1.96	1.91	1.87	1.82	1.77	1.71	1.65
29	4.18	3.33	2.93	2.70	2.55	2.43	2.35	2.28	2.22	2.18	2.10	2.03	1.94	1.90	1.85	1.81	1.75	1.70	1.64
30	4.17	3.32	2.92	2.69	2.53	2.42	2.33	2.27	2.21	2.16	2.09	2.01	1.93	1.89	1.84	1.79	1.74	1.68	1.62
40	4.08	3.23	2.84	2.61	2.45	2.34	2.25	2.18	2.12	2.08	2.00	1.92	1.84	1.79	1.74	1.69	1.64	1.58	1.51
60	4.00	3.15	2.76	2.53	2.37	2.25	2.17	2.10	2.04	1.99	1.92	1.84	1.75	1.70	1.65	1.59	1.53	1.47	1.39
120	3.92	3.07	2.68	2.45	2.29	2.17	2.09	2.02	1.96	1.91	1.83	1.75	1.66	1.61	1.55	1.50	1.43	1.35	1.25
∞	3.84	3.00	2.60	2.37	2.21	2.10	2.01	1.94	1.88	1.83	1.75	1.67	1.57	1.52	1.46	1.39	1.32	1.22	1.00

From Merrington, M., & Thompson, C.M. (1943). Tables of percentage points of the inverted beta (F) distribution. *Biometrika, 33*(1), 80-81.

Critical Values of F for $\alpha = 0.01$

df Denominator	df NUMERATOR																		
	1	2	3	4	5	6	7	8	9	10	12	15	20	24	30	40	60	120	∞
1	4052	4999.5	5403	5625	5764	5859	5928	5982	6022	6056	6106	6157	6209	6235	6261	6287	6313	6339	6366
2	98.50	99.00	99.17	99.25	99.30	99.33	99.36	99.37	99.39	99.40	99.42	99.43	99.45	99.46	99.47	99.47	99.48	99.49	99.50
3	34.12	30.82	29.46	28.71	28.24	27.91	27.67	27.49	27.35	27.23	27.05	26.87	26.69	26.60	26.50	26.41	26.32	26.22	26.13
4	21.20	18.00	16.69	15.98	15.52	15.21	14.98	14.80	14.66	14.55	14.37	14.20	14.02	13.93	13.84	13.75	13.65	13.56	13.46
5	16.26	13.27	12.06	11.39	10.97	10.67	10.46	10.29	10.16	10.05	9.89	9.72	9.55	9.47	9.38	9.29	9.20	9.11	9.02
6	13.75	10.92	9.78	9.15	8.75	8.47	8.26	8.10	7.98	7.87	7.72	7.56	7.40	7.31	7.23	7.14	7.06	6.97	6.88
7	12.25	9.55	8.45	7.85	7.46	7.19	6.99	6.84	6.72	6.62	6.47	6.31	6.16	6.07	5.99	5.91	5.82	5.74	5.65
8	11.26	8.65	7.59	7.01	6.63	6.37	6.18	6.03	5.91	5.81	5.67	5.52	5.36	5.28	5.20	5.12	5.03	4.95	4.86
9	10.56	8.02	6.99	6.42	6.06	5.80	5.61	5.47	5.35	5.26	5.11	4.96	4.81	4.73	4.65	4.57	4.48	4.40	4.31
10	10.04	7.56	6.55	5.99	5.64	5.39	5.20	5.06	4.94	4.85	4.71	4.56	4.41	4.33	4.25	4.17	4.08	4.00	3.91
11	9.65	7.21	6.22	5.67	5.32	5.07	4.89	4.74	4.63	4.54	4.40	4.25	4.10	4.02	3.94	3.86	3.78	3.69	3.60
12	9.33	6.93	5.95	5.41	5.06	4.82	4.64	4.50	4.39	4.30	4.16	4.01	3.86	3.78	3.70	3.62	3.54	3.45	3.36
13	9.07	6.70	5.74	5.21	4.86	4.62	4.44	4.30	4.19	4.10	3.96	3.82	3.66	3.59	3.51	3.43	3.34	3.25	3.17
14	8.86	6.51	5.56	5.04	4.69	4.46	4.28	4.14	4.03	3.94	3.80	3.66	3.51	3.43	3.35	3.27	3.18	3.09	3.00
15	8.68	6.36	5.42	4.89	4.56	4.32	4.14	4.00	3.89	3.80	3.67	3.52	3.37	3.29	3.21	3.13	3.05	2.96	2.87
16	8.53	6.23	5.29	4.77	4.44	4.20	4.03	3.89	3.78	3.69	3.55	3.41	3.26	3.18	3.10	3.02	2.93	2.84	2.75
17	8.40	6.11	5.18	4.67	4.34	4.10	3.93	3.79	3.68	3.59	3.46	3.31	3.16	3.08	3.00	2.92	2.83	2.75	2.65
18	8.29	6.01	5.09	4.58	4.25	4.01	3.84	3.71	3.60	3.51	3.37	3.23	3.08	3.00	2.92	2.84	2.75	2.66	2.57
19	8.18	5.93	5.01	4.50	4.17	3.94	3.77	3.63	3.52	3.43	3.30	3.15	3.00	2.92	2.84	2.76	2.67	2.58	2.49
20	8.10	5.85	4.94	4.43	4.10	3.87	3.70	3.56	3.46	3.37	3.23	3.09	2.94	2.86	2.78	2.69	2.61	2.52	2.42
21	8.02	5.78	4.87	4.37	4.04	3.81	3.64	3.51	3.40	3.31	3.17	3.03	2.88	2.80	2.72	2.64	2.55	2.46	2.36
22	7.95	5.72	4.82	4.31	3.99	3.76	3.59	3.45	3.35	3.26	3.12	2.98	2.83	2.75	2.67	2.58	2.50	2.40	2.31
23	7.88	5.66	4.76	4.26	3.94	3.71	3.54	3.41	3.30	3.21	3.07	2.93	2.78	2.70	2.62	2.54	2.45	2.35	2.26
24	7.82	5.61	4.72	4.22	3.90	3.67	3.50	3.36	3.26	3.17	3.03	2.89	2.74	2.66	2.58	2.49	2.40	2.31	2.21
25	7.77	5.57	4.68	4.18	3.85	3.63	3.46	3.32	3.22	3.13	2.99	2.85	2.70	2.62	2.54	2.45	2.36	2.27	2.17
26	7.72	5.53	4.64	4.14	3.82	3.59	3.42	3.29	3.18	3.09	2.96	2.81	2.66	2.58	2.50	2.42	2.33	2.23	2.13
27	7.68	5.49	4.60	4.11	3.78	3.56	3.39	3.26	3.15	3.06	2.93	2.78	2.63	2.55	2.47	2.38	2.29	2.20	2.10
28	7.64	5.45	4.57	4.07	3.75	3.53	3.36	3.23	3.12	3.03	2.90	2.75	2.60	2.52	2.44	2.35	2.26	2.17	2.06
29	7.60	5.42	4.54	4.04	3.73	3.50	3.33	3.20	3.09	3.00	2.87	2.73	2.57	2.49	2.41	2.33	2.23	2.14	2.03
30	7.56	5.39	4.51	4.02	3.70	3.47	3.30	3.17	3.07	2.98	2.84	2.70	2.55	2.47	2.39	2.30	2.21	2.11	2.01
40	7.31	5.18	4.31	3.83	3.51	3.29	3.12	2.99	2.89	2.80	2.66	2.52	2.37	2.29	2.20	2.11	2.02	1.92	1.80
60	7.08	4.98	4.13	3.65	3.34	3.12	2.95	2.82	2.72	2.63	2.50	2.35	2.20	2.12	2.03	1.94	1.84	1.73	1.60
120	6.85	4.79	3.95	3.48	3.17	2.96	2.79	2.66	2.56	2.47	2.34	2.19	2.03	1.95	1.86	1.76	1.66	1.53	1.38
∞	6.63	4.61	3.78	3.32	3.02	2.80	2.64	2.51	2.41	2.32	2.18	2.04	1.88	1.79	1.70	1.59	1.47	1.32	1.00

From Merrington, M., & Thompson, C.M. (1943). Tables of percentage points of the inverted beta (F) distribution. *Biometrika, 33*(1), 84-85.

APPENDIX E

Critical Values of the χ^2 Distribution

Degrees of Freedom (df)	ALPHA (α) LEVEL			Degrees of Freedom (df)	ALPHA (α) LEVEL		
	0.05	0.01	0.001		0.05	0.01	0.001
1	3.842	6.635	10.828	24	36.415	42.980	51.179
2	5.992	9.210	13.816	25	37.653	44.314	52.620
3	7.815	11.345	16.266	26	38.885	45.642	54.052
4	9.488	13.277	18.467	27	40.113	46.963	55.476
5	11.071	15.086	20.515	28	41.337	48.278	56.892
6	12.592	16.812	22.458	29	42.557	49.588	58.301
7	14.067	18.475	24.322	30	43.773	50.892	59.703
8	15.507	20.090	26.125	31	44.985	52.191	61.098
9	16.919	21.666	27.877	32	46.194	53.486	62.487
10	18.307	23.209	29.588	33	47.400	54.776	63.870
11	19.675	24.725	31.264	34	48.602	56.061	65.247
12	21.026	26.217	32.910	35	49.802	57.342	66.619
13	22.362	27.688	34.528	36	50.999	58.619	67.985
14	23.685	29.141	36.123	37	52.192	59.893	69.347
15	24.996	30.578	37.697	38	53.384	61.162	70.703
16	26.296	32.000	39.252	39	54.572	62.428	72.055
17	27.587	33.409	40.790	40	55.759	63.691	73.402
18	28.869	34.805	42.312	41	56.942	64.950	74.745
19	30.144	36.191	43.820	42	58.124	66.206	76.084
20	31.410	37.566	45.315	43	59.304	67.459	77.419
21	32.671	38.932	46.797	44	60.481	68.710	78.750
22	33.924	40.289	48.268	45	61.656	69.957	80.077
23	35.173	41.638	49.728				

A

absolute zero point Point at which a value of zero indicates the absence of the property being measured. Ratio-level measurements, such as weight scales, vital signs, and laboratory values, have an absolute zero point.

abstract Clear, concise summary of a study, usually limited to 100 to 250 words.

abstract thinking Thinking that is oriented toward the development of an idea without application to or association with a particular instance, and independent of time and space. Abstract thinkers tend to look for meaning, patterns, relationships, and philosophical implications.

acceptance rate Number or percentage of the subjects who agree to participate in a study. The percentage is calculated by dividing the number of subjects agreeing to participate by the number of subjects approached. For example, if 100 subjects are approached and 90 agree to participate, the acceptance rate is 90% ([90 ÷ 100] × 100% = 90%).

accessible population Portion of a target population to which the researcher has reasonable access.

accidental or convenience sampling Nonprobability sampling technique in which subjects are included in the study because they happened to be in the right place at the right time. Available subjects who meet inclusion criteria are entered into the study until the desired sample size is reached.

accuracy The closeness of the agreement between the measured value and the true value of the quantity being measured.

accuracy in physiological measures Comparable to validity, the extent to which the instrument measures the concept that is defined in the study.

accuracy of a screening test The ability of a screening test to assess correctly the true presence or absence of a disease or condition.

adjusted hazard ratio The likelihood of an event occurring that has been modified to account for every other predictor in the regression model.

administrative databases Databases with standardized sets of data for enormous numbers of patients and providers that are created by insurance companies, government agencies, and others not directly involved in providing patient care.

Agency for Healthcare Research and Quality (AHRQ) Federal government agency originally created in 1989 as Agency for Health Care Policy and Research. The mission of the AHRQ is to carry out research; establish policy; and develop evidence-based guidelines, training, and research dissemination activities, with respect to healthcare services and systems. The focus of this agency is to promote evidence-based health care.

allocative efficiency The degree to which resources go to the area in which they will do the most good, in terms of delivery of services: effectiveness, usefulness to persons served, number of persons actually reached, and adherence rates.

alpha (α) Level of significance or cut-off point used to determine whether the samples being tested are members of the same population (nonsignificant) or different populations (significant); alpha is commonly set at 0.05, 0.01, or 0.001. Alpha is also the probability of making a Type I error.

alternate-forms reliability Also referred to as *parallel forms reliability*, and involves comparing the scores for two versions of the same paper-and-pencil instrument, as a test of equivalence.

analysis of sources Process of determining the true value of a published reference or other source for a particular study. The source is critically appraised and then compared with that of other sources to determine degree of accuracy or consistency.

analysis of variance (ANOVA) A statistical test that enables the researcher to determine whether there is a difference between or among groups on some continuous dependent or outcome variable.

ancestry search Examination of references for relevant studies to identify previous studies that are pertinent to the search; used when conducting research syntheses or an exhaustive literature search for a study.

anonymity Meaning literally "without a name"; in research, the removal of all names and identifiers from data.

applied research Scientific investigation conducted to generate knowledge, the results of which have potential for direct application to practice.

assent The affirmative agreement to participate in research provided by a person not legally able to provide consent, most usually a child or a person with permanently or temporarily diminished capacity.

associative hypothesis Statement of a proposed noncausative relationship between or among variables. None of the variables in the hypothesis are posited to cause any of the other variables: two or more of them merely may vary in unison.

associative relationship A noncausative relationship between or among variables.

assumption A belief that is accepted as true, without proof. In statistical testing, a belief related to a data set that, if untrue, may invalidate the test's results for that particular set.

asymmetrical relationship A relationship between variables A and B in which a change in the value of A is always accompanied by a change in the value of B; however, the reverse is not always true.

attrition A threat to internal validity that results from subjects withdrawing from a study before its completion. Attrition makes the originally assigned groups less similar to one another.

attrition rate The number or percentage of subjects or study participants who withdraw from a study before its completion. For example, if the sample size is 100 subjects and 20 subjects drop our of the study, the attrition rate is 20% ([20 division sign 100] × 100% = 20%).

authority Person with expertise and power who is able to influence opinion and behavior.

B

background for a research problem Part of the research problem that indicates what is known or identifies key research publications in the problem area.

bar graph Figure or illustration that uses a series of rectangular bars to provide a representation of the results of statistical analysis of a data set. These graphs consist of horizontal or vertical bars that represent the size or amount of the group or variable studied.

basic research Scientific investigation directed toward better understanding of physical or psychological processes, without any emphasis on application.

being A term in phenomenological research indicating a person's subjective awareness of experiencing life in relation to self and others.

beneficence, principle of The ethical position that compels the researcher to actively strive to do good and confer benefit, in respect to the study subjects or participants. Its ethical counterpart is nonmaleficence, which compels the researcher to actively strive to do no harm to research participants.

benefit-risk ratio Means by which researchers and reviewers of research judge the potential gains posed to a subject as a result of research participation, in comparison with the potential harm posed. The benefit-to-risk ratio is one determinant of the ethics of a study.

best interest standard In determining whether an individual should participate in a study, the researcher needs to do what is best for the individual subjects on the basis of balancing risks and benefits in a study.

best research evidence The strongest empirical knowledge available that is generated from the synthesis of quality study findings to address a practice problem.

between-groups variance Variance of the group means around the grand mean (the mean of the total sample) that is examined in analysis of variance (ANOVA).

bias Any influence or action in a study that distorts the findings or slants them away from the true or expected. A distortion. Also used to refer to a point of view that differs from the objective truth.

bibliographical database Database that either consists of citations relevant to a specific discipline or is a broad collection of citations from a variety of disciplines.

bimodal Distribution of scores that has two modes (most frequently occurring scores).

bivariate analysis Statistical procedures that involve comparison of the same variable measured in two different groups, or measurement of two distinct variables within a single group.

bivariate correlation analysis Analysis techniques that measure the extent of the linear relationship between two variables.

Bland and Altman chart or plot A graphical method of displaying agreement between measurement techniques, which may be used to compare repeated measurements of a single method of measurement or to compare a new technique with an established one. Accompanied by a Bland and Altman analysis, which determines extent of agreement.

blinding Strategy in interventional research by which the patient's status as an experimental subject versus a control subject is hidden from the patient, from those providing care to the patient, or from both.

block In research design, refers to stratum or level of a variable. Blocking is the strategy of assigning subjects to groups in two or more stages, so as to assure equal distribution of a potentially extraneous variable between or among groups.

body of knowledge Information, principles, theories, and empirical evidence that are organized by the beliefs accepted in a discipline at a given time.

Bonferroni procedure Post hoc analysis to determine differences among three or more groups without inflating Type I error. When a design involves multiple comparisons, the procedure may be done during the planning phase of a study to adjust the significance level so as not to inflate Type I error.

borrowing Appropriation and use of knowledge from other disciplines to guide nursing practice.

bracketing Practice used in some forms of Husserlian phenomenology, in which the researcher identifies personal preconceptions and beliefs and consciously sets them aside, for the duration of the study.

breach of confidentiality Accidental or direct action that allows an unauthorized person to have access to a subject's identity information and study data.

C

calculated variable A variable used in data analysis that is not collected but is calculated from other variables.

care maps Flow diagrams that display usual care for treatment of an injury or illness, depicting anticipated patient progress. Synonymous with care pathways, clinical pathways, and critical pathways.

carryover effect Effects from a previous intervention that may continue to affect the dependent variable in subsequent interventions.

case-control design An epidemiological design in which subjects or "cases" are members of a certain group, and "controls" are not members of that group. The case group is most commonly comprised of individuals with a certain condition or disease, and the control group lacks the disease. Selection of controls is made on the basis of demographic similarity, yielding a control group that is demographically almost identical to that of the "cases."

case study design A qualitative design that guides the intensive exploration of a single unit of study, such as a person, family, group, community, or institution. It is similar to historical research, in that it tells the story of the unit of study.

causal connection The link between the independent variable (cause) and the dependent variable (outcome or effect) that is examined in quasi-experimental and experimental research.

causal hypothesis or relationship Relationship between two variables in which one variable (independent variable) is thought to cause the presence of the other variable (dependent variable). Some causal hypotheses include more than one independent or dependent variable.

causality A relationship in which one variable causes a change in another. Causality has three conditions: (1) there must be a strong relationship between the proposed cause and effect, (2) the proposed cause must precede the effect in time, and (3) the cause must be present whenever the effect occurs.

cell Intersection between the row and column in a table or matrix, into which a specific value is inserted.

censored data A data point that is known to exceed the limits of measurement parameters but whose exact value is unknown. Examples of this are "relapsed before three months," "beyond retirement age," "survived more than five years," and "too young to attend kindergarten."

central limit theorem The statistical axiom that applies when statistics, such as means, come from a population with a skewed (asymmetrical) distribution. The sampling distribution developed from multiple means obtained from that skewed population will tend to fit the pattern of the normal curve.

chain sampling See *network sampling*.

chi-square test Compares differences in proportions of nominal-level (categorical) variables.

citation The act of quoting a source, using it as an example, or presenting it as support for a position taken. A citation should be accompanied by the appropriate reference to its source.

citation bias The situation that occurs when certain studies are cited more often than others and are more likely to be identified in database searches.

classical hypothesis testing Refers to the process of testing a hypothesis so that the researcher can infer that a relationship exists.

cleaning data Checking raw data to determine errors in data recording, coding, or entry, and to eliminate impossible data points.

clinical databases Databases of patient, provider, and healthcare agency information that are developed by healthcare agencies and sometimes providers to document care delivery and outcomes.

clinical expertise In healthcare, the cumulative effect of a practitioner's knowledge, skills, and past experience in accurately assessing, diagnosing, and managing an individual's health needs. Presumably, expertise increases with experience and may not be translatable from one practice area to another.

clinical guidelines Standardized, current guidelines for the assessment, diagnosis, and management of patient conditions, developed by clinical guideline panels or

professional groups to improve the outcomes of care and promote evidence-based health care.

clinical importance The impact a positive statistical finding would have, if applied to clinical practice. The sensible question associated with this is, "Will this make a meaningful difference to the patient experience or outcomes?"

clinical judgment The quality of reasoned decision making in healthcare practice.

clinical pathways Flow diagrams that display usual care for treatment of an injury or illness, depicting anticipated patient progress. Synonymous with care maps, care pathways and critical pathways.

clinical trial Any study that prospectively assigns human participants or groups of humans to one or more health-related interventions to evaluate the effects on health outcomes, as defined in 2014 by the National Institutes of Health.

cloud storage Multiple-server storage of electronic data, for the purpose of convenient retrieval and assurance against loss.

cluster sampling A sampling method in which locations, institutions, or organizations are chosen from among all possible options, instead of individual subjects, because individual subjects' identities are not yet known. It is used most often when the accessible population is widespread, and the research is multi-site in nature.

code A symbol or abbreviation used to label words or phrases in qualitative data sets during the data-analysis phase the data-analysis phase.

codebook Identifies and defines each variable in a study and includes an abbreviated variable name, a descriptive variable label, and the range of possible numerical values of every variable entered into a computer file.

coding In qualitative studies, the process of labeling phrases and quotations so as to identify themes and patterns. In quantitative research, the process of transforming quantitative or qualitative data into numerical symbols that can be analyzed statistically.

coefficient of determination (r^2) The square of the correlation value, which represents the percentage of variance two variables share.

coefficient of multiple determination (R^2) The percentage of the total variation that can be explained by all the variables the researcher includes in the final predictive equation.

coefficient of stability Result of a correlational analysis of the scores of an educational test or scale administered at two different measurement times.

coercion Overt threat of harm or excessive reward intentionally presented by one person to another to obtain compliance.

cohorts Usually synonymous with groups. Used in medical and epidemiologic studies to refer to a group that shares at least one characteristic that is the focus of the research.

communicating research findings Sharing the findings of a study, either verbally or in print, informally or formally.

comparative analysis Examination of methodology and findings across studies for similarities and differences.

comparative descriptive design A design used to describe differences in a variable's value in two or more different groups.

comparative effectiveness research Descriptive or correlational research that compares different treatment options, for their risks and benefits.

comparative evaluation The part of the Stetler's Model in which research findings are assessed for accuracy, fit in a given healthcare setting, feasibility, and the likelihood that the intervention will produce change in current practice.

comparison group A group of subjects that is not selected through random sampling and, because of design structure, does not control for the effects of extraneous variables.

compensatory equalization of treatment Extra attention or advantages provided to control group subjects by staff or family members, in compensation for what experimental subjects receive.

complete IRB review One of the three types of designations made by the institutional review board (IRB) committee. In complete review, because the study poses greater than minimal risk, the entire IRB reads and makes a judgment about whether the research will be permitted.

complete observation Data collection strategy in which the researcher is passive and has no direct social interaction in the setting.

complete participation Qualitative data collection strategy in which the researcher becomes a member of the group and conceals the researcher role.

complex hypothesis Predicts the relationship (associative or causal) among three or more variables.

comprehending a source Reading an entire source carefully and focusing on understanding the major concepts and the logical flow of ideas within the source.

concept An abstract idea. A concept's definition applies to the entire group of ideas, processes, or objects that fit that definition.

concept analysis Strategy through which a set of characteristics essential to the connotative meaning or conceptual definition of a concept are identified.

concept derivation Process of extracting and defining concepts from theories in other disciplines. The derived concepts describe or define an aspect of nursing in an innovative way that is meaningful.

concept synthesis Process of describing and naming a previously unidentified concept, using sources in which the concept is used in order to establish common elements.

conceptual definition Provides a variable or concept with connotative (abstract, comprehensive, theoretical) meaning and is established through concept analysis, concept derivation, or concept synthesis. The conceptual definition of a variable in a study is often developed from the study framework and is the link between the study framework and the operational definition of the variable.

conceptual map The visual representation of a research framework. It depicts the study's concepts and relational statements by use of a diagram.

conceptual model Set of highly abstract, related constructs that broadly explains phenomena of interest, expresses assumptions, and usually reflects a philosophical stance.

conclusions Syntheses and clarifications of the meanings of study findings. They provide a basis for identifying nursing implications and suggesting further studies.

concrete thinking Thinking that is oriented toward and limited by tangible things or events observed and experienced in reality.

concurrent relationship Relationship in which two concepts occur at the same time or are measured at the same time.

concurrent validity The extent to which a subject's individual score on an instrument or scale can be used to estimate concurrent performance for a different instrument, scale, quality, criterion, or other variable.

condensed proposal A brief or shortened proposal developed for review by clinical agencies and funding institutions.

confidence interval The probability of including the value of a parameter within an interval estimate.

confidentiality Management of data provided by a subject so that the information will not be shared with others without the subject's authorization. This implies that access to data will be guarded carefully, to prevent breaches of confidentiality.

confirmatory data analysis Use of inferential statistics to confirm expectations regarding the data that are expressed as hypotheses.

confirmatory studies Conducted only after a large body of knowledge has been generated with exploratory studies. Confirmatory studies are expected to have large samples and to use random sampling techniques. The results are intended for wide generalization.

confounding variables A special subtype of extraneous variable, unique in that it is embedded in the study design because it is intertwined with the independent variable. It is the result of poor initial operationalization of the independent variable.

connotative definition Refers to something suggested by a word, external to its literal meaning.

consent form Printed form containing the requisite information about a study to ensure a potential subject has been adequately informed about a study and can make a decision about whether to participate. The subjects sign consent forms to indicate agreement and willingness to participate in a study.

construct validity The degree to which a study measures all aspects of the concept it purports to measure. This depends on the skill with which the researcher has conceptually defined and then operationally defined a study variable.

constructs Concepts at very high levels of abstraction that have general meanings.

content analysis Qualitative analysis technique whereby the words in a text are classified into categories, according to repeated ideas or patterns of thought.

content expert A clinician or researcher who is known for broad and deep knowledge in a specific content area.

content validity Examines the extent to which the measurement method includes all the major elements relevant to the construct being measured. Evidence for this type of validity is obtained from the literature, representatives of the relevant populations, and relevant experts.

content validity ratio A calculation by researchers of each item on a scale, made by rating it a 0 (not necessary), 1 (useful), or 3 (essential).

content validity index A ratio score of the proportion of the number of experts who agree the items of an instrument measure the desired concept to the total number of experts performing the review. The score is calculated for a complete instrument.

contingent relationship A statistical relationship between two variables that exists only if a third variable or concept is present. The third variable is called either an *intervening* or a *mediating* variable.

continuous variable Variable with an unlimited number of potential values, including decimals and fractions. Values in the "gaps" between whole numbers are possible. If a variable is not continuous, it is termed a *discrete variable*.

control Design decisions made by the researcher to decrease the intrusion of the effects of extraneous variables that could alter research findings and consequently force an incorrect conclusion.

control group Group of elements or subjects not exposed to the experimental treatment. The term *control group* is always used in studies with random assignment to group, and sometimes used for research without random assignment, if the presence of the group allows control of the effects of extraneous variables.

convenience sampling See *accidental sampling.*

convergent concurrent strategy A mixed methods strategy selected when a researcher wishes to use quantitative and qualitative methods in an attempt to confirm, cross-validate, or corroborate findings within a single study. Quantitative and qualitative data collection processes are conducted concurrently.

convergent validity Type of measurement validity obtained by using two instruments to measure the same variable, such as depression, and correlating the results from these instruments. Evidence of validity from examining convergence is achieved if the data from the two instruments have a moderate to strong positive correlation.

correlational analysis Statistical procedure conducted to determine the direction (positive or negative) and magnitude (or strength) of the relationship between two variables.

correlational coefficient Indicates the degree of relationship between two variables; coefficients range in value from +1.00 (perfect positive relationship) to 0.00 (no relationship) to −1.00 (perfect negative or inverse relationship).

correlation matrix A table of the bivariate correlations of every pair of variables in a data set. Along the diagonal through the matrix the variables are correlated with themselves, with the left and right sides of the table being mirror images of each other.

correlational research Systematic investigation of relationships between two or more variables to explain the direction (positive or negative) and strength of the relationship, but never cause and effect.

correlational study designs Variety of study designs developed to examine relationships among variables.

costs of care In outcomes research, costs to the patient or family. Costs of care can be direct or indirect.

counterbalancing Administration of various treatments in random order rather than consistently in the same sequence.

covert data collection Data collection that occurs when subjects are unaware that research data are being collected.

criterion-referenced testing Comparison of a subject's score with a criterion of achievement that includes the definition of target behaviors. When the subject has mastered the behaviors, he or she is considered proficient in these behaviors, such as being proficient in the behaviors of a nurse practitioner.

criterion sampling Recruiting participants for a qualitative study who do or do not have specific characteristics relevant to the phenomenon. Criterion sampling may be used to create homogenous samples or focus groups.

critical appraisal of research Systematic, unbiased, careful examination of all aspects of a study to judge the merits, weaknesses, meaning, and significance based on previous research experience and knowledge of the topic. The following three steps are used in the process: (1) identifying the steps of the research process, (2) determining the study's strengths and weaknesses, and (3) evaluating the credibility, trustworthiness, and meaning of a study to nursing knowledge and practice.

critical appraisal process for qualitative research Evaluating the quality of a qualitative study using standards appropriate for qualitative research, such as congruence of the methods to the philosophical basis of the research approach and transferability of the findings.

critical appraisal process for quantitative research Examination of the quality of a quantitative study using standards appropriate for quantitative research, such as threats to internal and external validity.

critical cases Cases that make a point clearly, or are extremely important in understanding the purpose of the study, and are identified through purposive sampling.

critical pathways See *clinical pathways.*

critical value In quantitative data analysis, the value at which statistical significance is achieved in a study.

crossover or counterbalanced design Two-phase design in which half of the sample is administered an intervention, with the other half acting as control group; then, in a second phase, assignments are reversed, so that the initial control group receives the intervention while the initial experimental group does not. This type of research sometimes is conducted using more than two groups or more than two phases.

cross-sectional designs Research strategies used to simultaneously examine groups of subjects in various stages of a process, with the intent of inferring trends over time.

cultural immersion The spending of extended periods of time in the culture one is studying using ethnographic methods to gain increased familiarity with such things as language, sociocultural norms, and traditions in a culture.

curvilinear relationship A relationship between two variables, in which the strength of the relationship varies over the range of values so that the graph of the relationship is a curved line rather than a straight one.

cutoff point The value at which a decision is made.

D

data (plural) Pieces of information that are collected during a study (singular: datum).

data analysis In quantitative studies, statistical testing of prevalence, relationship, and cause. In qualitative research, reduction and organization of data, and revelation of meaning.

data collection Precise, systematic gathering of information relevant to the research purpose and the specific objectives, questions, or hypotheses of a study.

data collection forms Forms researchers develop or adapt, and use for collecting or recording demographic data, information excerpted from patient records, observations, or values from physiological measures.

data collection plan A detailed flowchart of the chronology of interactions with subjects and responses at different points in the data collection.

data saturation The point in the qualitative research process at which new data begin to be redundant with what already has been found, and no new themes can be identified.

data use agreement Pre-existent document that limits how the data set for a study may be used and how it will be protected to meet Health Insurance Portability and Accountability Act (HIPAA) requirements. This usually stipulates that data accessed must not contain names or personal identifiers.

datum (singular) One piece of information collected for research.

debriefing Meeting at the end of a process, intended for exchange of factual information. In research, may refer to conferences among the researchers, or between a researcher and a subject. When data collection has been clandestine, or deception of subjects has occurred, debriefing is used to disclose hidden information to subjects, including the true purpose of the study and its results.

deception Deliberate deceit. In research, refers to misinforming subjects for research purposes.

decision making Cognitive process of assessing a situation and deciding on a course of action, which is important for conducting research and providing health care. Phase III in the Stetler Model of Research Utilization to Facilitate Evidence-Based Practice.

Declaration of Helsinki Ethical code based on the Nuremberg Code (1964) that described necessary components of subject consent such as risks and benefits of a study and differentiated therapeutic from nontherapeutic research, among other points.

deductive reasoning Reasoning from the general to the specific, or from a general premise to a particular situation.

deductive thinking Thinking that begins with a theory or abstract principle that guides the selection of methods to gather data to support or refute the theory or principle.

degrees of freedom (df) Freedom of a score's value to vary given the other existing scores' values and the established sum of these scores: the number of values that are truly independent (formula varies according to statistical test).

de-identifying health data Removal of the 18 elements that could be used to identify an individual including relatives, employer, or household members. This term is part of the Health Insurance Portability and Accountability Act (HIPAA).

Delphi technique Method of measuring the judgments of a group of experts for assessing priorities or making forecasts.

demographic or attribute variables Specific variables such as age, gender, and ethnicity that are collected in a study to describe the sample.

denotative definition The literal meaning of a word.

dependent groups Groups in which the subjects or observations selected for data collection are in some way related to the selection of other subjects or observations. For example, if subjects serve as their own controls by using the pretest as a control, the observations (and therefore the groups) are dependent. Use of twins in a study or matching subjects on a selected variable, such as medical diagnosis or age, results in dependent groups.

dependent variable Response, behavior, or outcome that is predicted and measured in research. In interventional research, changes in the dependent variable are presumed to be caused by the independent variable.

description Involves identifying and understanding the nature and attributes of nursing phenomena and sometimes the relationships among these phenomena. This is one possible outcome of research.

descriptive design A design used to provide information about the prevalence of a variable or its characteristics in a data set, in quantitative research.

descriptive research Provides an accurate portrayal of what exists, determines the frequency with which something occurs, and categorizes information. Quantitative descriptive research generates statistics describing the prevalence of its variables, such as percentages, ratios, raw numbers, ranges, means and standard deviations. In qualitative research, refers to studies of various designs that investigate new areas of inquiry.

descriptive statistics Summary statistics that describe a sample's average and uniformity.

descriptive study designs Quantitative research designs that produce a statistical description of the phenomenon of interest.

design, research The researcher's choice of the best way in which to answer a research question, with respect to several considerations, including number of subject groups, timing of data collection, and researcher intervention, if any.

design validity Design-dependent truthfulness of a study: the degree to which an entity that the researcher believes is being performed, evaluated, measured, or represented is actually what is being performed, evaluated, measured, or represented. Its four components are construct validity, internal validity, external validity, and statistical conclusion validity.

deterministic relationship Causal statement of what always occurs in a particular situation, such as a scientific law.

deviation score Difference score, which is obtained by subtracting the mean from each score; indicates the extent to which a score deviates from the mean.

dialectic reasoning A type of reasoning that involves the holistic perspective, in which the whole is greater than the sum of the parts, and examining factors that are opposites and making sense of them by merging them into a single unit or idea that is greater than either alone.

diary A written record of personal experiences and reflections, maintained over time. In research, this refers to a research participant's record of experiences and reflections that may be used as data by a researcher. Use of diaries as data sources is more common in qualitative or mixed methods research than in quantitative.

difference score See *deviation score*.

diffusion of treatment Threat to internal validity in which experimental and control subjects interact and become aware of their group membership.

diminished autonomy Describes subjects with decreased ability to voluntarily give informed consent to participate in research, because of temporary or permanent inability to fully deliberate all aspects of the research consent process, or because of legal or mental incompetence.

direct costs The researcher's costs for materials and equipment to conduct a study that are identified in a proposal and included in the study's budget. Also, in outcomes research, refers to specific costs the patient incurs, for insurance payments and co-payments associated with health care.

direct measurement Used for quantification of a simple, concrete variable, such as a strategy that measures height, weight, or temperature.

direction of a relationship Refers to whether two variables are positively or negatively related. In a positive relationship, the two variables change in the same direction (increase or decrease together). In a negative relationship, the variables change in opposite directions (as one variable increases, the other decreases).

directional hypothesis A hypothesis that predicts the direction of the relationship between or among variables.

disproportionate sampling Selection of the sample for a study so that the number of subjects within identifiable strata are equal and do not reflect actual population proportions. Disproportionate sampling is used to eliminate bias introduced by stratum membership, such as gender, race, or area of residence.

dissemination of research findings Communication of research findings by means of presentations and publications.

dissertation An exhaustive and usually original research work, completed by a doctoral student under the supervision of faculty in the discipline. A dissertation is the final requirement for a doctoral degree.

distribution-free Term used to refer to statistical analyses that do not assume that data are normally distributed. Distribution-free analyses usually are non-parametric statistical techniques.

distribution In statistics, the relative frequency with which a variable assumes certain values.

divergent validity Type of measurement validity established by correlation of an instrument that measures a certain concept with another instrument that measures its opposite. Negative correlation supports the divergent validity of both instruments.

double-blinding A strategy in which neither subjects nor data-collectors are aware of subject assignment to group. Double-blinding avoids several threats to construct validity.

dummy variables Assignment of one or more numbers to categorical or dichotomous variables so that they can be included in a regression analysis.

duplicate publication bias Appearance of more research support for a finding than is accurate, because a study's findings have been published by the authors in more than one journal, without cross-referencing the other journal.

dwelling with the data Taking time to reflect on qualitative data before initiating analysis.

E

ebooks Books available in a digital or electronic format.

effect size Degree to which the phenomenon is present in the population or to which the null hypothesis is false. In examining relationships, it is the degree or size of the association between variables. Also refers to the effectiveness of an intervention in quasi-experimental and experimental research.

effectiveness The extent to which something produces a projected effect.

element Person (subject or participant), event, behavior, or any other single unit of a study.

eligibility criteria See *sampling criteria*.

embodied Heideggerian phenomenologist's belief that the person is a self within a body, and that events, perceptions, and feelings are experienced through the body and accompanied by physical sensations; thus, the person is referred to as *embodied*.

emergent concepts The ideas related to the phenomenon of interest that the researcher discovers during the processes of data collection and data analysis. Also referred to as *themes*, *essences*, *truths*, *factors*, and *factors of interest*, among other terms.

emic view In ethnographic research, a point of view that consists of studying the natives or insiders in a culture and reporting the results from their point of view.

empirical generalizations Inferences based on accumulated research evidence.

empirical literature Relevant studies published in journals, in books, and online, as well as unpublished studies, such as master's theses and doctoral dissertations.

empirical world The sum of reality experienced through our senses; the concrete portion of our existence.

endogenous variables Variables in a path analysis, or semantic equation model, whose values are influenced and possibly caused by exogenous variables and other endogenous variables.

environmental variable A variable that emanates from the research setting.

epistemology A point of view related to knowing and knowledge generation.

equivalence reliability A type of reliability that compares two versions of the same instrument or two observers measuring the same event.

error score Amount of random error in the measurement process, which is equal to the observed score minus the true score.

error in physiological measures Inaccuracy of physiological instruments related to environment, user, subject, equipment, and interpretation errors.

estimator Statistic that produces an approximate population value, based on the scores in a sample.

ethical principles Principles of respect for persons, beneficence, and justice.

ethnographic research Qualitative research methodology developed within the discipline of anthropology for investigating cultures. Ethnographic research is one of the principal qualitative strategies used in nursing research.

ethnographies The written reports of a culture from the perspective of insiders. These reports were initially the products of anthropologists who studied primitive, foreign, or remote cultures.

ethnography A word derived by combining the Greek roots of *ethno* (folk or people) and *graphos* (picture or portrait).

ethnonursing research A type of nursing research that focuses on nursing and health care within a culture. Ethnonursing research emerged from Leininger's theory of transcultural nursing.

etic approach Anthropological research approach of studying behavior from outside the culture and examining similarities and differences across cultures.

evaluation step of critical appraisal Determining the validity, credibility, significance, and meaning of the study by examining the links among the study process, study findings, and previous studies.

evidence-based practice (EBP) Conscientious integration of best research evidence with clinical expertise and patient values and needs in the delivery of quality, cost-effective health care.

evidence-based practice centers Universities and healthcare agencies identified by the Agency for Healthcare Research and Quality (AHRQ) as centers for the conduct, communication, and synthesis of research knowledge in selected areas to promote evidence-based health care.

evidence-based practice guidelines Rigorous, explicit clinical guidelines developed on the basis of the best research evidence available (such as findings from systematic reviews, meta-analyses, mixed-methods systematic reviews, meta-syntheses, and extensive clinical trials); supported by consensus from recognized national experts and affirmed by outcomes obtained by clinicians.

exclusion sampling criteria Descriptive criteria that eliminate some elements or subjects from inclusion in a research sample, for the purpose of eliminating sample characteristics that have the potential to introduce error.

exempt from review One of the three types of designations related to the extent of review required for study. Exempt from review status is reserved for studies that meet federally established criteria for exemption.

exogenous variables Variables in a path analysis, or semantic equation model, whose values influence the values of the other variables in the model but whose own causes are not explained within the model.

expedited IRB review One of the three types of designations related to the extent of review required for a study. In expedited review, risks posed to research subjects are determined to be no greater than those ordinarily encountered in daily life or during performance of routine physical or psychological examinations.

experimental group Subjects who are exposed to the experimental treatment or intervention.

experimental research Objective, systematic investigation that examines causality and is characterized by (1) researcher-controlled manipulation of the independent variable, (2) the presence of a distinct control group, and (3) random assignment of subjects to either the experimental or the control condition.

experimenter expectancies A threat to construct validity, characterized by a belief of the person collecting the data that may encourage certain responses from subjects, either in support of those beliefs or opposing them.

explanatory sequential design A mixed methods approach in which the researcher collects and analyzes quantitative data, and then collects and analyzes

qualitative data to explain the quantitative findings.

exploratory-descriptive qualitative research Qualitative research that lacks a clearly identified qualitative methodology (neither phenomenology, nor grounded theory, nor ethnography, nor historical research). In this text, a default term used for studies that the researchers have identified as being qualitative without indicating a specific approach or underlying philosophical basis.

exploratory factor analysis A subtype of factor analysis in which the researcher explores different solutions in choosing factors and their corresponding items. It is performed when the researcher has few prior expectations about the factor structure.

exploratory regression analysis Used when the researcher may not have sufficient information to determine which independent variables are effective predictors of the dependent variable; thus, many variables may be entered into the analysis simultaneously. This type is the most commonly used regression analysis strategy in nursing studies.

exploratory sequential design A mixed methods approach in which the collection and analysis of qualitative data precedes the collection of quantitative data.

exploratory studies Research designed to increase the knowledge of a field of study and not intended for generalization to large populations. Exploratory studies provide the basis for confirmatory studies.

external criticism Method of determining the validity of source materials in historical research that involves knowing where, when, why, and by whom a document was written.

external validity Extent to which study findings can be generalized beyond the sample included in the study.

extraneous variables Variables that are neither the independent nor the dependent variable, but that intrude upon the analysis and affect the strength of statistical measurements. Exist in all studies and can affect the measurement of study variables and the relationships among these variables.

F

F statistic Value or result obtained from conducting a type of analysis of variance.

fabrication in research Type of scientific misconduct that involves creating study results and recording or reporting them as true.

face validity A subjective assessment, usually by an expert, that verifies that a measurement instrument appears to measure the content it is purported to measure.

factor Hypothetical construct created by factor analysis that represents several separate factors or variables, and whose name reflects the focus of the variables with which it is associated.

factor analysis Statistical strategy in which variables or items in an instrument are evaluated for interrelationships, identifying those that are closely related. In explanatory factor analysis, the clusters or factors are then named, representing constructs or concepts of importance. The two types of factor analysis are exploratory and confirmatory.

factor loading In factor analysis, the magnitude of the correlation of a variable or item with one of the factors, ultimately the central concepts, of the data set.

factor scores The sum of the factor loadings for each variable for each study participant that is associated with one of the factors in a factor analysis. Thus, each subject will have a score for each factor in the instrument.

factorial design Experimental design in which two independent variables are tested for their effects upon one or more dependent variables, using four study groups. Its advantage is that it also provides results of the combined effect of both variables. Also called the *factorial experiment*.

fair treatment Ethical principle that promotes selection and treatment of subjects in a way that does not exclude some individuals or groups because of personal characteristics unrelated to the study.

false negative Result of a diagnostic or screening test that indicates a disease is not present when it is.

false positive Result of a diagnostic or screening test that indicates a disease is present when it is not.

falsification of research Type of research misconduct that involves either manipulating research materials, equipment, or processes, or changing or omitting data or results such that the research is not accurately represented in the research record.

feasibility of a study Whether or not resources are sufficient for study completion.

field notes Notes that a qualitative researcher makes during data collection.

field work Qualitative data collection that occurs in a naturalistic setting.

findings The researcher's explanation of the study results.

fishing and the error rate problem A threat to statistical conclusion validity that exists when a researcher conducts multiple statistical analyses of relationships or differences, "fishing" for statistically significant findings, when the analyses are not required by the study questions or hypotheses. Error is additive, so if hundreds of tests are performed it is likely that one or more will produce positive results, resulting in Type I error.

fixed-effect model A model in which the working assumption is that the effect size of an intervention or change is constant across studies and that observed differences are due to error.

focus groups Groups constituted with the purpose of collecting data on a specific topic from more than one research participant at the same time.

forced choice item A questionnaire item to which there is a response set that does not allow a written-in response. Also, a scale item with an even number of polar choices indicating opinion, at various levels of emphasis (agree strongly, agree somewhat, agree slightly, disagree slightly, etc.): there is no neutral position.

forest plots A graphical display of results of the individual studies examined in a quantitative meta-analysis or systematic review.

framework The abstract, logical structure of meaning that guides development of the study and enables the researcher to link the findings to the body of knowledge for nursing. A framework is a combination of concepts and the connections between them, used to explain relationships.

frequency distribution Statistical procedure that involves listing all possible values of a variable and tallying the number for each value in the data set.

Frequency distributions may be either ungrouped or grouped.

frequency table A visual display of the results of a frequency distribution, in which possible values appear in one column of a table and the frequency of each value in the other column.

funnel plot Used in a meta-analysis, a graphical display of effect sizes or odds ratios for a given intervention, in several studies.

G

gap In a research problem statement, an area that is unresearched or under-researched, and that consequently represents incomplete knowledge for theory or practice.

general proposition Highly abstract statement of the relationship between or among concepts that is found in a conceptual model.

generalization The act of applying the findings from a study to identical or similar people or situations.

geographical analyses Analysis of a variable, with respect to the co-variable of geography. Geographical analysis is a focus of spatial analysis in epidemiology and is used in healthcare to examine variations in health status, health services, patterns of care, or patterns of resource use. Sometimes referred to as *small area analyses*.

going native In ethnographic research, when the researcher becomes part of the culture and loses all objectivity. The concern is that the researcher cannot observe accurately and without bias.

gold standard The accepted benchmark for commodities, assessments, or analyses that serves as a basis of comparison with other commodities, assessments, or analyses. In medicine, the most accurate means of diagnosing a particular disease.

government report Document generated by a governmental agency, often quantitative and descriptive in nature. Government reports may be useful for providing information about incidence and status of a condition, disease, or social process, to be cited in the significance and background section of the problem statement of a research proposal or report.

grant Research funding from a private or public institution that supports the conduct of a study.

grantsmanship Expertise and skill in successfully developing proposals to obtain funding for selected studies.

grey literature Studies that have limited distribution, such as theses and dissertations, unpublished research reports, articles in obscure journals, some online journals, conference papers and abstracts, conference proceedings, research reports to funding agencies, and technical reports.

grounded theory research Qualitative, inductive research technique based on symbolic interaction theory that is conducted to investigate a human process within a sociological focus. Its result is the generation of conceptual categories, and sometimes theory.

grouped frequency distribution Visual presentation of a count of variable values, divided into subsets. For example, instead of providing numbers of subjects for all ages, the grouped frequency distribution provides numbers of subjects from ages 20 to 29, 30 to 39, and so forth.

Grove Model for Implementing Evidence-Based Guidelines in Practice Model developed by one of the textbook authors (Grove) to promote the use of national, standardized evidence-based guidelines in clinical practice.

H

Hawthorne effect A threat to construct validity, in which subjects alter their normal behaviors because they are being scrutinized. This is also referred to as *reactivity*. The Hawthorne effect can exist in both noninterventional and interventional studies.

hazard ratio (HR) The ratio of the likelihood of an event occurring, in the presence of a predictor variable, as compared with its likelihood in the absence of a predictor variable. Interpreted almost identically to an odds ratio (*OR*).

hazard risk In research, the risk or possibility of event occurrence.

heterogeneity Variety. In research, a heterogeneous sample is a varied sample, with respect to at least one characteristic. Use of a heterogeneous sample tends to reduce bias, but in interventional research may introduce potentially extraneous variables.

hierarchical statement set A set of three statements representing decreasing levels of abstraction, composed of a general proposition, a specific proposition, and a hypothesis or research question.

highly controlled setting A structured environment, artificially developed for the sole purpose of conducting research, such as a laboratory, experimental center, or medical research unit. Highly controlled settings are used for basic research studies and occasionally for applied research.

HIPAA Privacy Rule A United States set of standards federally implemented in 2003 that established the category of protected health information, limiting their use or disclosure by covered entities, such as healthcare providers and health plans, in order to protect an individual's health information. The HIPAA Privacy Rule pertains not only to the healthcare environment but also to the research conducted in that environment.

historical research Qualitative research method that includes a narrative description and analysis of past and ongoing events and processes.

history threat A threat to internal validity that exists when an event external to a study occurs and affects the value of the dependent variable.

homogeneity Sameness. In research, a homogeneous sample includes participants who are similar with respect to one or more characteristics. Use of a homogeneous sample eliminates potential extraneous variables but may produce results with limited generalizability, because the sample may be poorly representative of the target population.

homogeneity reliability Type of reliability testing used with multiple item scales that addresses the correlation of the items within an instrument to determine the consistency of the scale in measuring a study variable. Also referred to as *internal consistency reliability*.

homoscedastic Even dispersion of data on a scatter diagram, both above and below the regression line, which indicates that variance is similar throughout the range of values.

horizontal axis The *x*-axis of a graph. The horizontal axis is oriented in a left-right plane across the graph.

human rights Claims and demands related to legitimate expectations of safety, fairness, entitlement, and freedom that have been justified in the eyes of an individual or by the consensus of a group of individuals. Human rights are protected in research.

hypothesis Formal statement of a proposed relationship(s) between two or more variables. In research, a hypothesis is situated within a specified population.

hypothesis guessing within experimental conditions A threat to construct validity that occurs when subjects within a study guess the hypothesis of the researcher and modify their behavior so as to support or undermine that hypothesis.

hypothetical population A population that cannot be defined according to sampling theory rules, which require a list of all members of the population.

I

immersion in the data Initial phase of qualitative data analysis in which researchers become very familiar with the data by spending extensive time reading and rereading notes and transcripts, recalling observations and experiences, listening to audio tapes, and viewing videos.

imitation of treatment The threat to internal validity in which control group subjects self-administer the intervention intended only for the experimental group.

implications of research findings for nursing Meaning of research conclusions for the body of knowledge, theory, and practice in nursing, a term analogous to "usefulness."

inclusion sampling criteria Sampling requirements identified by the researcher that must be present for the element or subject to be included in the sample.

incomplete disclosure Failure to disclose to subjects the exact purpose of a study, based on the belief that subjects might alter their actions if they were made aware of the true purpose. After study completion, subjects must be debriefed about the complete purpose and the findings of the study.

independent groups Groups of subjects assigned to one or another condition, so that the assignment of one is totally unrelated to the assignment of others. An example is the random assignment of subjects to treatment versus control groups.

independent samples *t*-test Common parametric analysis technique used in nursing studies to test for significant differences between two groups unrelated to each other. Scores of one group are not linked to scores of the other group. *Compare to paired or dependent samples t-test.*

independent variable In interventional research, the treatment, intervention, or experimental activity that is manipulated or varied by the researcher to create an effect on the dependent variable. In correlational research, the variable or variables that predict the occurrence of the dependent variable. In the latter case, the predictive variables may or may not be found to be causative.

indirect costs The researcher's costs that are not specified in a grant proposal, such as use of space and some administrative costs. The amount of a grant may be increased to provide support to the institution to cover these costs. In outcomes research, the "hidden" costs the patient and family incur during hospitalization or treatment, such as loss of employment, lodging and meals away from home, and parking fees.

indirect measurement The strategy of quantification used with variables that cannot be measured directly but whose attributes can be quantified. Scales are examples of indirect measurement, such as the FACES Pain Rating Scale.

individually identifiable health information (IIHI) Any information collected from a person, including demographic information, that is created or received by healthcare providers, a health plan, or a healthcare clearinghouse, that is related to the past, present, or future physical or mental health or condition of an individual, and that identifies the person.

inductive reasoning Reasoning from the specific to the general in which particular instances are observed and then combined into a larger whole or general statement. It involves observing a connection or pattern and then attempting to derive a general explanation of that pattern.

inference Use of inductive reasoning to move from a specific case to a general truth. Inference is one basis of the qualitative analysis process. It is also the basis of inferential statistics used in quantitative research.

inferential statistics Statistics designed to allow inference from a sample statistic to a population parameter; commonly used to test hypotheses of similarities and differences in subsets of the sample under study.

informed consent Prospective subject's agreement to participate voluntarily in a study, which is reached after the subject assimilates essential information about the study.

institutional review Process of examining the design and methods of a proposed study for ethical considerations and also for overseeing studies in progress. Institutional review is undertaken by an independent committee of peers at an institution to determine the extent to which the proposed study protects the rights of subjects.

institutional review board (IRB) The committee of peers that reviews research to ensure that the investigator is conducting the research ethically. Universities, hospital corporations, and many managed care centers maintain IRBs, for the purpose of promoting the conduct of ethical research and protecting the rights of prospective subjects at their institutions.

instrumentation A component of measurement that involves the application of specific rules to develop a measurement device or instrument.

integration Making connections among ideas, theories, and experience.

intention to treat An analysis based on the principle that participant data are analyzed according to the groups into which they were randomly assigned regardless of what happens to them in the study.

interaction effects Threats to internal or external validity composed by the interaction of two separate threats. Examples are selection of subjects and treatment, setting and treatment, or history and treatment.

interaction of different treatments A threat to construct validity in which two independent variables are tested and the interaction between them is measured inadequately.

intercept In regression analysis, the point at which the regression line crosses (or intercepts) the y-axis. The intercept is represented by the letter a.

internal consistency reliability See *homogeneity reliability*.

internal criticism Involves examination of the authenticity of historical documents, with respect to their meaning. Internal criticism takes place after external criticism is complete.

internal validity The degree to which measured relationships among variables are truly due to their interaction, and the degree to which other intrusive variables might have accounted for the measured value.

interpretation of research outcomes The formal process by which a researcher considers the results of quantitative data analysis within contexts of previous research in the area, representativeness of the sample, usefulness within nursing, and state of the body of knowledge. The researcher's understanding of the meaning of the results of qualitative research and the research's usefulness in the context of existing knowledge.

interrater reliability Degree of consistency between two or more raters who independently assign ratings or interpretations to a variable, factor of interest, attribute, behavior, or other phenomenon being investigated.

interval data Numerical information that has equal distances between value points. Interval data are mutually exclusive and exhaustive, and they are artificial, in that they are obtained through artificial measurement instruments, such as scales, or devices with arbitrary values, such as a thermometer. Interval data are analyzed with parametric statistics.

interval estimate The researcher's approximation of the range of probable values of a population parameter.

interval level of measurement A measurement that exists at the interval level. See *interval data*.

intervening variable A variable whose existence explains the relationship between the independent variable and the dependent variable. An intervening variable, unlike a mediating variable, is often a psychological construct.

intervention fidelity Reliable and competent implementation of an experimental treatment that includes two core components: (1) adherence to the delivery of the prescribed treatment behaviors, session, or course, and (2) competence in the researcher or interventionalist's skill in delivery of the intervention.

interventional research Research that examines causation by means of an intervention delivered to the experimental subjects and a subsequent measure of its effects. Interventional research may be experimental or quasi-experimental.

interventions In research, treatments, therapies, procedures, or actions that are implemented to determine their outcomes. In healthcare practice, interventions are actions implemented by professionals to and with patients, in a particular situation, to promote beneficial health outcomes.

interview Structured or unstructured verbal communication between the researcher and subject during which information is obtained for a study.

introspection Process of turning one's attention inward, toward thoughts and feelings, to provide increased awareness and understanding of their flow and interplay.

intuition Insight or understanding of a situation or event as a whole that usually cannot be logically explained. It is reasoning-free knowledge, claimed to lack support from data.

invasion of privacy Ethical violation of an individual's right to privacy that occurs when private information is shared without that individual's knowledge or against his or her will.

investigator-initiated research proposal Research proposal in which the principal investigator identifies a significant problem, develops a study to examine it, and submits a proposal for the study to the appropriate federal funding agency.

inverse linear relationship A statistical finding in which as one variable or concept changes, the other variable or concept changes in the opposite direction, and both occur according to the standard regression formula of $y = ax + b$. It is also referred to as a *negative linear relationship*.

Iowa Model of Evidence-Based Practice Model developed in 1994 and revised in 2001 by Titler and colleagues to promote evidence-based practice in clinical agencies.

iteration A term used in mathematics and statistics, which refers to repeating sequential operations, using early solutions in subsequent calculations. In research, iteration refers to the ongoing process of revision of both design and methods while research is still in the planning stages, and to revision of interpretation during the latter phases of a study.

J

justice, principle of Ethical principle that states that human subjects should be treated fairly, as groups and as individuals.

K

key informants Participants in ethnographic studies whom the researcher purposely chooses for in-depth data collection, because they are both knowledgeable about the culture and articulate.

keywords Major concepts or variables that may be used in literature searches to find relevant references. Keywords or terms can be identified by determining the concepts in your study, the populations of particular interest in your study, interventions to be implemented, and measurement methods to be used in the study, or possible outcomes for the study.

knowledge Essential content or body of information for a discipline that is acquired through traditions, authority, borrowing, trial and error, personal experience, role-modeling and mentorship, intuition, reasoning, and research.

Kolmogorov-Smirnov two-sample test Nonparametric test used to determine whether two independent samples have been drawn from the same population.

kurtosis Degree of peakedness (platykurtic, mesokurtic, or leptokurtic) of the curve shape that is related to the spread or variance of scores.

L

landmark studies Published research that led to an important development or a turning point in a certain field of study. Landmark studies are well known by individuals in a specialty area, representing a change in conceptualization.

language bias Bias that may affect meta-analyses and reviews, when the search includes articles written in only one language, such as English, when important studies are written in other languages.

latent transition analyses (LTA) Projected probabilities or proportions of expected outcomes, which track movement over a series of outcomes. They are helpful in keeping perspective about a patient's recovery or progress during an attenuated treatment, providing an idea of how an individual patient responds to treatment. Because they are based on an average of actual patient progress within the population, they represent a quantification of the concept of outcome variance.

least-squares regression line A line drawn through a scatterplot that represents the smallest deviation of each value from the line.

legally authorized representative Individual or other body authorized under applicable law to consent on behalf of a prospective subject to the subject's participation in the procedures involved in the research.

leptokurtic Term used to describe an extremely peaked-shape distribution of a curve, which means that the scores in the distribution are similar and have limited variance.

level of significance See *alpha (α)*.

levels of measurement Scheme of hierarchical differentiation denoting the type of information inherent, and degree of precision, in a given measurement. The four levels, from low to high, are nominal (differentiation by names, not amounts), ordinal (differentiation by general magnitude), interval (differentiation by total number assigned by scale or by artificial numbering that uses whole numbers), and ratio (differentiation by the real number scale).

Likert scale Instrument designed to determine the opinion or attitude of a subject; it contains a number of declarative statements with a scale after each statement.

limitations Aspects of a study that decrease the generalizability of the findings and conclusions, or restrict the population to which findings can be generalized. Limitations are based on the design's validity. Construct validity-based limitations relate to faulty operational-ization of variables. Other limitations are embedded in the study's methods or design.

line graphs Graphical representations of point variable values joined by lines. A line graph may represent two different variables, or one variable over time, or one variable value and its frequency.

line of best fit The regression line drawn schematically that best fits all paired variable values. The line of best fit is represented by the regression equation.

linear relationship Numerical relationship between two variables, in which the formula $y = ax + b$ remains true for all variable values.

literature review See *relevant literature*.

location bias Bias that may affect meta-analyses and systematic reviews, in which the search includes only high-impact journals, or utilizes commonly-searched databases.

logic A branch of philosophy based on the study of valid reasoning. Also used to refer to valid reasoning and is inclusive of both abstract and concrete thinking.

logical positivism The branch of philosophy on which the scientific method is based. Logical positivists consider empirical discovery the only dependable source of knowledge. Quantitative research emerged from logical positivism.

longitudinal designs Noninterventional research in which data are collected on several occasions, in order to examine change in a variable over time, within a defined group.

low statistical power Power to detect relationships or differences that is below the acceptable standard power (0.8) needed to conduct a study. Low statistical power increases the likelihood of a Type II error.

M

manipulation The quantitative researcher's action of changing the value of the independent variable, in order to measure its effect on the dependent variable.

Mann-Whitney *U* test A statistical test conducted to determine whether two samples with nonparametric data are from the same population.

matching Technique by which subjects for a control or comparison group are purposively selected from a larger pool on the basis of their demographic similarity to the experimental group. This process results in dependent or related groups.

maturation The threat to internal validity in which normal changes that occur because of the passage of time affect the value of the dependent variable. An example of this might be measurements of improvement in gross motor task performance over a seven-hour testing period that do not take into consideration the subjects' fatigue or hunger.

mean Statistical measure of central tendency used with ratio-level and interval-level data. The mean value is obtained by summing all the values in a data set and dividing that total by the total number of data points in the set.

mean deviation Statistical measure of dispersion used with ratio-level and interval-level data. The mean deviation is the average magnitude of the difference between the mean and each individual score, using the absolute values.

mean difference A standard statistic that is calculated to determine the absolute difference between the means of two groups.

measurement Process of assigning values to objects, events, or situations in accord with some rule. The measurement method in quantitative research is determined by a concept's operational definition.

measurement error Difference between what exists in reality and what is measured by a research instrument.

measures of central tendency Statistical procedures (mode, median, and mean) calculated to determine the center of a distribution of scores.

measures of dispersion Statistical procedures (range, difference scores, sum of squares, variance, and standard deviation) conducted to determine the degree of distance between values in a set and their mean or median.

median Score at the exact center of an ungrouped frequency distribution. The median is the middle value; if the number of data points is even, the median value is the average of the two middle values.

mediating variables Variables that occur as intermediate links between independent and dependent variables. Often, they provide insight into the proposed relationship between cause and effect.

memo A reminder written by a qualitative researcher that contains insights or ideas related to data and pertinent to data analysis.

mentor Someone who serves as a teacher, sponsor, guide, exemplar, or counsellor for a novice or protégé. For example, an expert nurse serves as a guide or role model for a novice nurse or mentee.

mentorship Intense form of role-modeling in which a more experienced person works with a less experienced person to impart information about a new skill or way of being.

mesokurtic Term that describes a normal curve with an intermediate degree of kurtosis and intermediate variance of scores.

meta-analysis A technique that statistically pools data and results from several studies into a single quantitative analysis that provides one of the highest levels of evidence for practice. The studies all must share a similar design.

metasummary, qualitative Synthesis of findings across qualitative reports, performed in order to determine the current knowledge in an area.

meta-synthesis, qualitative Synthesis of qualitative studies that provides a fully integrated, novel description or explanation of a target event or experience versus a summary view of that event or experience. Meta-synthesis requires more complex, integrative thought than does metasummary, in developing a new perspective or theory based on the findings of previous qualitative studies.

method of least squares Procedure in regression analysis for developing the line of best fit.

methodological congruence The extent to which the methods of a qualitative study are consistent with the philosophical tradition and qualitative approach identified by the researchers.

methodological limitations Restrictions or weaknesses emanating from the design or methods of a quantitative study that limit the researcher's ability to interpret the study's results, draw conclusions, make generalizations, and suggest subsequent studies in the problem area.

methodology, research The general type of the research selected to answer the research question: quantitative research, qualitative research, outcomes research, or mixed methods research.

methods, research The specific ways in which the researcher chooses to conduct the study, within the chosen design. Methods include subject selection, choice of setting, attempts to limit factors that might introduce error, the manner in which a research intervention is strategized, ways in which data are collected, and choice of statistical tests.

metric ordinal scale Scale that has unequal intervals; its use in data collection yields ordinal-level data.

middle-range theories Theories that are less abstract than, and address more specific phenomena than do, grand theories; that are directly applicable to practice; and that focus on explanation and implementation. Also known as *practice theories*.

minimal risk Studies in which the potential for harm is not greater than what a person might encounter in everyday life or in routine healthcare.

mixed methods approach A research methodology in which two research designs are utilized in order to better represent truth. The vast majority of mixed methods studies use one quantitative design and one qualitative.

mixed methods systematic review A synthesis of studies having more than one methodology, conducted in order to determine the current knowledge in a problem area.

mixed results When more than one relationship or difference is examined, study results that are contradictory, such as opposite results of the effect of an independent variable.

mode Numerical value or score that occurs with the greatest frequency in a distribution. The mode does not necessarily indicate the center of the data set.

model-testing design Correlational research, such as structural equation modeling and path analysis, that measures proposed relationships within a theoretical model.

moderator A facilitator for a focus group, preferably one who reflects the age, gender, and race/ethnicity of the group members. The moderator, if not a member of the research team, must understand the purpose of the study and be trained in appropriate facilitation.

modifying variable Variable that alters the strength and occasionally the direction of the relationship between other variables.

monographs Books, booklets of conference proceedings, or pamphlets, which are written and published for a specific purpose and may be updated with a new edition, as needed.

monomethod bias A threat to construct validity in which the dependent variable is measured in several similar ways, for instance by use of three self-assessment instruments to measure life stress.

mono-operation bias A threat to construct validity, in which a given variable, especially a complex one like pain, is measured in only one way.

multiple causality The case in which two or more variables combine in causing an effect.

multicollinearity The case in which independent variables in a regression equation are strongly correlated with one another, making generalizability difficulty.

multidimensional scaling A measurement method that was developed to examine many aspects or elements of a concept or variable.

multilevel analysis The use of more than one way to analyze a data set. It is used in outcomes research, as well as epidemiology, to examine how variables, such as environmental factors and individual attributes or behavior, interact to influence outcomes.

multilevel synthesis In mixed methods research, independent synthesis of quantitative versus qualitative findings, followed by integration.

multimethod-multitrait technique An approach to validity in which the concepts in a study are measured in multiple ways to assess both the convergent and divergent validity of the testing methods.

multimodal A distribution of scores that has more than two modes or most frequently occurring scores.

multiple regression analysis A regression analysis of three of more variables and their interactions. Extension of simple linear regression with more than one independent variable entered into the analysis.

multistage cluster sampling Type of cluster sampling in which the random selection of the sample continues through several stages.

N

narrative analysis Qualitative approach that uses stories as its data. The narratives that comprise the data may originate from interviews, informal conversations, and field notes, as well as from tangible sources, such as journals and letters.

natural settings Naturalistic settings such as field settings, in which data are collected, without any attempts by the researcher to control for the effects of extraneous variables.

naturalistic inquiry encompasses research designed to study people and situations in their natural states.

necessary relationship One variable or concept must occur for a second variable or concept to occur.

negative likelihood ratio Ratio of true-negative results to false-negative results; is calculated as follows: Negative likelihood ratio = (100% − Sensitivity) ÷ Specificity.

negative linear relationship See *inverse linear relationship*.

negative results See *nonsignificant results*.

negatively skewed An asymmetry in a data set, in which instead of a bell curve shape, the resultant shape is more elongated on the left side. This means that the smaller values are further from the mean than the larger values, but the majority of data points are larger than the mean.

nested strategy Sometimes called a *nested design*, the nested strategy consists of randomly assigning clusters or "nests" of subjects instead of single subjects to group. Individual subjects are thus "nested" within a larger classification.

network sampling Nonprobability sampling method that includes a snowballing technique that takes advantage of social networks and the fact that friends tend to hold characteristics in common. Subjects meeting the sample criteria are asked to assist in locating others with similar characteristics. Network sampling is synonymous with *chain sampling* and *snowball sampling*.

networking Process of developing channels of communication among people with common interests.

nominal data Lowest level of data that can only be organized into categories that are exclusive and exhaustive, but the categories cannot be compared or rank-ordered. These data are analyzed using nonparametric statistical techniques.

nominal level of measurement Lowest level of measurement that is used when data can be organized into categories that are exclusive and exhaustive, but the categories cannot be compared or rank-ordered, such as gender, race, marital status, and diagnosis. See *nominal data*.

noncoercive disclaimer A statement included in a standard consent form that states that participation is voluntary and refusal to participate will involve no penalty or loss of benefits to which the subject would otherwise be entitled.

nondirectional hypothesis States that a relationship exists but does not predict the exact direction of the relationship, positive versus negative.

nonequivalent control group designs Interventional designs in which the control group is not selected by random means.

noninterventional research Studies in which researchers observe, measure, or test subjects, but do not enact experimental interventions. Within quantitative research, correlational studies and descriptive studies are noninterventional types of designs.

nonparametric statistical analysis Statistical techniques used when the first two assumptions of parametric statistics cannot be met: normal distribution and data that are at least at the interval level of measurement.

nonprobability sampling Nonrandom sampling technique in which not every element of the population has an opportunity for selection in the sample, such as convenience (accidental) sampling, quota sampling, purposive sampling, and network sampling.

nonsignificant results Research results not strong enough to reach statistical significance: the null hypothesis cannot be rejected. Nonsignificant results are synonymous with negative results.

nontherapeutic research Research conducted to generate knowledge for a discipline and in which the results from the study might benefit future patients but will probably not benefit those acting as research subjects.

normal curve A symmetrical, unimodal bell-shaped curve that is a theoretical distribution of all possible scores, but is rarely seen in real data sets. The normal curve is also called a *bell curve* because of its shape.

normally distributed Distribution of data points that follows the spread or distribution of a normal curve.

norm-referenced testing A type of evaluation that yields an estimate of the performance of the tested individual in comparison to the performance of a large set of other individuals, on whom the test was "normed."

null hypothesis A hypothesis that is the opposite of the research hypothesis, stating there is no significant difference between study groups, or no significant relationship among the variables. The null hypothesis is tested during data analysis and is used for interpreting statistical outcomes.

Nuremberg Code Ethical code of conduct developed in 1949, for the purpose of guiding investigators conducting research.

Nursing Care Report Card Evaluation of hospital nursing care developed in 1994 by the American Nurses Association and the American Academy of Nursing Expert Panel on Quality Health Care for the purpose of identifying and developing nursing-sensitive quality measures using 10 indicators (2 structure indicators, 2 process indicators, and 6 outcome indicators). This report card could facilitate benchmarking or setting a desired standard that would allow comparisons of hospitals in terms of their nursing care quality.

nursing interventions Deliberative cognitive, physical, or verbal activities performed with or on behalf of individuals and their families that are directed toward accomplishing particular therapeutic objectives relative to individuals' health and well-being. Nursing interventions are developed and revised through interventional research to promote EBP.

nursing research Formal inquiry through quantitative, qualitative, outcomes, or mixed methods research that validates and refines existing knowledge and generates new knowledge that directly and indirectly influences the delivery of evidence-based nursing practice.

nursing-sensitive patient outcomes Patient outcomes that are influenced by or associated with nursing care.

O

observation Collection of data through listening, smelling, touching, and seeing, with an emphasis on what is seen.

observational checklist A form used to collect observational data, on which a tally mark is used to count each occurrence of a listed behavior.

observational measurement Use of structured and unstructured observations to measure study variables.

observed level of significance The actual level of significance that is achieved or observed in a study.

observed score Actual score or value obtained for a subject on a measurement tool. Observed score = true score + random error.

odds ratio (*OR*) The ratio of the odds of an event occurring in one group, such as the treatment group, to the odds of it occurring in another group, such as the standard care or control group.

one-group pretest-posttest design A quasi-experimental design in which subjects act as their own controls, in a design that measures subjects both before and after intervention. Because it exerts almost no control over the effects of extraneous variables, interpretation of results is difficult.

one-tailed test of significance Analysis used with directional hypotheses in which extreme statistical values of interest are hypothesized to occur in a single tail of the distributional curve.

one-way chi-square A statistic that compares the distribution of a nominal-level variable with expected probability statistics for random occurrence.

operational definition Description of how concepts will be measured in a study, essentially converting them to variables.

operational reasoning Involves identification and discrimination among many alternatives or viewpoints and focuses on the process of debating alternatives.

operationalizing a variable or concept Establishment and description of the way in which a variable or concept shall be measured.

operator In a computer search, a set of directions that permits grouping of ideas, selection of places to search in a database record, and ways to show relationships within a database record, sentence, or paragraph. The most common operators are Boolean, locational, and positional.

operator, Boolean The three words AND, OR, and NOT are used with the researcher's identified concepts in conducting searches of databases.

operator, locational Search operator that identifies terms in specific areas or fields of a record, such as article title, author, and journal name.

operator, positional Search operator used to look for requested terms within certain distance of one another. Common positional operators are NEAR, WITH, and ADJ.

ordinal data Data that can be ranked, with intervals between the ranks that are not necessarily equal. Ordinal data are analyzed using nonparametric statistical techniques.

ordinal level measurement Measurement that yields ordinal or ranked data, such as levels of coping. See *ordinal data.*

outcome reporting bias Type of bias that occurs when study results are not reported clearly and with complete accuracy.

outcomes of care The dependent variables or clinical results of health care that are measured to determine quality. The outcomes from the Medical Outcomes Study Framework include clinical end points, functional status, general well-being, and satisfaction with care.

outcomes research Research that examines quality of care, as quantified by selected outcomes. It utilizes predominantly noninterventional quantitative designs from epidemiology, as well as other disciplines.

outliers Extreme scores or values in a set of data that are exceptions to the overall findings.

out-of-pocket costs Those expenses incurred by the patient, family, or both that are not reimbursed by the insurance company and might include non-covered expenses, co-payments, cost of travel to and from care, and the costs of buying supplies, dressings, selected medications, or special foods.

P

paired or dependent samples Samples that are related or matched in some way. See *dependent groups*.

paired or dependent samples *t*-test Parametric statistical test conducted to examine differences between dependent groups. The groups are dependent in repeated measures and case-control designs, and when participants in two groups are matched for relevant characteristics or variables.

paradigm A set of philosophical or theoretical concepts that characterize a particular way of viewing the world.

paradigm case In phenomenology, a quotation that best encapsulates a theme or an example that clearly depicts the study's findings.

parallel design In a mixed methods study, the quantitative and qualitative components are implemented concurrently. The components are equal in importance and convergence occurs during the interpretation phase.

parallel-forms reliability See *alternate-forms reliability*.

parallel synthesis Involves the separate synthesis of quantitative and qualitative studies, but the findings from the qualitative synthesis are used in interpreting the synthesized quantitative studies.

parameter Boundary or limit, usually used as a plural: the parameters of acceptable behavior. Also, the measure or numerical value of a characteristic of a population.

parametric statistical analyses Statistical techniques used when three assumptions are met: (1) the sample was drawn from a population for which the variance can be calculated, and the distribution is expected to be normal or approximately normal, (2) the level of measurement is interval or ratio, with an approximately normal distribution, and (3) the data can be treated as though they were obtained from random samples.

paraphrasing Restating an author's ideas in other words that capture the meaning. Paraphrasing implies understanding and, consequently, is preferred to direct quotation for theoretical content that is part of a scholarly paper.

partially controlled setting A naturalistic environment that the researcher modifies temporarily, in order to control for the effects of extraneous variables. Partially controlled settings are the most prevalent settings of experimental and quasi-experimental nursing research.

participant observation A form of observation used in qualitative research in which researchers either are already participants in a society or culture, or they become participants, in order to provide the insider view.

participants Individuals who participate in qualitative and quantitative research; also referred to as *subjects* in quantitative research. In ethnographic research, participants may also be called *informants*.

partitioning Strategy in which a researcher analyzes subjects according to a variable that can be regarded as dichotomous but actually has several different values. Partitioning provides more nuanced results than would be obtained from a dichotomously defined variable.

path analysis In a proposed model, the diagrammed relationships among pairs of variables, in which each is tested for its strength and direction, yielding a correlational value.

patient Someone who has already gained access to care in a given healthcare setting.

pattern A repeated word, phrase or occurrence. In qualitative data, a pattern may indicate similarities across participants and may be identified as a theme.

Pearson's product-moment correlation coefficient (*r*) Parametric statistical test conducted to determine the linear relationship between two variables.

percentage distribution Indicates the percentage of the sample with scores falling within a specific group or range.

percentage of variance Amount of variability explained by a linear relationship; the value is obtained by squaring Pearson's correlation coefficient (*r*). For example, if $r = 0.5$ in a study, the percentage of variance explained is $r^2 = 0.25$, or 25%.

periodicals Subset of serials with predictable publication dates, such as journals that are published over time and are numbered sequentially for the years published.

permission to participate in a study Agreement of parents or guardians that their child or ward of the state can be a subject in a study.

personal experience Gaining of knowledge by being individually or personally involved in an event, situation, or circumstance.

phenomenological research Inductive, descriptive qualitative methodology developed from phenomenological philosophy for the purpose of describing experiences as they are lived by the study participants and, often, the meaning of such experiences to the participants.

phenomenon (singular) Literally, a happening. In research, often means an idea or concept of interest (plural: phenomena).

phenomenon of interest The central topic of a quantitative, qualitative, outcomes, or mixed methods study. Also known as the *phenomenon*, the *study focus*, the *concept of interest*, and the *central issue*, among other terms.

philosophy Broad, global explanation of the world that gives meaning to nursing and provides a framework within which thinking, knowing, and doing occur. In nursing research, the overriding philosophical perspective that determines how reality is viewed, what is knowable, and how research is conducted.

Photovoice A qualitative research method that uses images taken by participants as data for analysis.

physiological measures Techniques and equipment used to measure physiological variables either directly or indirectly, such as techniques to measure heart rate or mean arterial pressure.

PICOS or PICO Format An acronym for Population or participants of interest; Intervention needed for practice; Comparisons of the intervention with control, placebo, standard care, variations of the same intervention, or different therapies; Outcomes needed for practice; and Study design. PICOS is one of the most common formats used to delimit a relevant clinical question.

pilot study Smaller-sample version of a proposed study conducted with the same research population, setting, intervention, and plans for data collection and analysis. The purpose of a pilot is to determine whether the proposed methods are effective in locating and consenting subjects, and in collecting useful data.

placebo In pharmacology, a substance without discernible effect, administered in research studies to the control group. Broadly, an intervention intended to have no effect.

plagiarism Type of research misconduct that involves the appropriation of another person's ideas, processes, results, or words without giving appropriate credit, including those obtained through confidential review of others' research proposals and manuscripts.

platykurtic Term that indicates a relatively flat curve, and a large variance for the set of scores.

population The particular group of elements (individuals, objects, events, or substances) that is the focus of a study.

population-based studies Cohort studies conducted so as to discover information about an entire population. In epidemiology and health fields, such studies often are conducted after an event that affects health occurs, such as a treatment, an outbreak, or an exposure. Also referred to as *population studies*.

population parameter A true but unknown numerical characteristic of a population. Parameters of the population are estimated with statistics.

position paper A formal essay, authored by an individual or group, and disseminated in order to present an opinion or viewpoint regarding an issue of debate or disagreement. Position papers often are disseminated by professional organizations and government agencies to represent that agency's position on an issue.

positive likelihood ratio Likelihood ratio calculated to determine the likelihood that a positive test result is a true positive. Positive Likelihood Ratio = Sensitivity ÷ (100% − Specificity).

positive linear relationship A numerical relationship between two variables, such that as one variable changes (value of the variable increases or decreases), the other variable will change in the same direction.

positively skewed An asymmetry in a data set, in which instead of a bell curve shape, the resultant shape is more elongated on the right side. This means that the larger values are further from the mean than the smaller values, but the majority of data points are smaller than the mean.

post hoc tests (Latin for *after this one*). Statistical tests developed specifically to determine the location of differences in studies with more than two groups and are performed after an initial test demonstrates a difference. When performed after an ANOVA to pinpoint location of differences, frequently used post hoc tests are Bonferroni's procedure, the Newman-Keuls test, the Tukey Honestly Significant Difference (HSD) test, the Scheffé test, and Dunnett's test. Also called *post hoc analyses*.

poster session A time during a professional conference when the results of selected studies are visually presented, usually on a two-dimensional surface, and including text, pictures, and illustrations. Other topics of general interest to conference attendees may also be presented in this way.

posttest-only control group design An experimental design in which there is no pre-intervention measurement of the value of the dependent variable in either the experimental group or the control group.

posttest-only design with comparison group Quasi-experimental design, referred to as pre-experimental by Campbell and Stanley, conducted to examine the difference between the experimental group that receives a treatment and the comparison group that does not. The design provides very poor control for threats to internal validity; however, with a very strong comparison group and concurrent data collection, the design can generate useful information about causation.

posttest-only design with comparison with norms A quasi-experimental design in which the results of an intervention in a single group are compared with average population values.

power Probability that a statistical test will detect a significant difference or relationship if one exists, which is the capacity to correctly reject a null hypothesis.

power analysis Statistical test conducted to determine the risk of Type II error so that the study can be modified to decrease the risk, if necessary. Conducting a power analysis uses alpha (level of significance), effect size, and standard power of 0.8 to determine the sample size for a study. Because effect size of an intervention varies from study to study, a power analysis often is conducted when nonsignificant results are obtained, to determine the actual power of the analysis.

practice pattern The pattern of *what* care is provided by a certain healthcare professional. Practice pattern is a term usually applied to physicians' practices, but it can refer to usual nursing care that is provided on a hospital unit or in a clinic setting.

practice pattern profiling Epidemiological technique used in outcomes research that focuses on patterns of care rather than individual occurrences of care. Practice pattern profiling was originally used to compare outcomes of physicians' practice patterns with one another, usually in the same type of practice and in the same region or specialty, and it may include patterns of referrals and resource utilization, as well. Practice pattern profiling now also includes comparisons among types of healthcare providers, such as advanced practice nurses and physician assistants.

practice style The pattern of *how* care is provided. This includes the skill of a practitioner in interpersonal relationships, in such aptitudes as communication skills. Practice style is part of the construct *processes of care* from Donabedian's theory of health care.

precision In general, a high degree of exactness with a small amount of variability. In statistics, accuracy with which the population parameters have been estimated within a study. Also used to describe the degree of consistency or reproducibility of measurements with physiological instruments.

prediction The offering of an opinion or guess about an unknown or future event, amount, outcome, or result. In statistics, a part of the process of inference.

prediction equation Outcome of regression analysis whereby a formula or equation is developed to predict a dependent variable.

predictive design Correlational design used to establish strength and direction of relationships between or among variables. Predictive correlational research is often the prelude to construction of a theoretical model.

predictive validity A type of criterion-related instrument validity, reflecting the extent to which an individual's score on a scale or instrument can be used to predict future performance or behavior on a criterion.

premise In research, a statement that identifies the proposed relationship between two or more variables or concepts. In a logical argument, a proposition from which a conclusion is drawn.

preproposal Short document (usually four to five pages plus appendices) written to explore the funding possibilities for a research project.

presentation A formal report of research findings, made at a professional meeting or conference either orally as a podium presentation or visually as a poster presentation.

pretest-posttest design with nonrandom control group A quantitative quasi-experimental design in which the intervention is applied to the experimental group, and both experimental and control groups are measured (tested) at the beginning of the process and again after the intervention occurs in the experimental group so that the effect of the intervention can be measured. This design is essentially the pretest-posttest control group design without random assignment to experimental/control group.

pretest-posttest control group design A quantitative experimental design in which, after random assignment to group, the intervention is applied to the experimental group, and both experimental and control groups are measured (tested) at the beginning of the process and again after intervention occurs in the experimental group so that the effect of the intervention can be measured. It is often called the *classic experimental design*.

primary source Source that is written by the person who originated or is responsible for generating the ideas published.

principal investigator (PI) The researcher who takes the major responsibility for the research proposal and design, and for the execution and the writing of the research report. When multiple authors' names appear in a published report, the first author is usually the principal investigator. In a research grant, the PI is the individual who will have primary responsibility for administering the grant and interacting with the funding agency. Also *primary investigator.*

privacy The freedom of an individual to determine the time, extent, and general circumstances under which private information will be shared with or withheld from others.

probability Likelihood. In statistics, probability refers to the percentage chance that the result of a certain statistical test performed with a sample actually represents the population from which the sample was drawn.

probability distributions Distributions of values for different statistical analysis techniques, such as tables of r values for Pearson Product Moment Correlation, t values for t-test, or F values for analysis of variance. Some common probability distribution tables are found in the appendices of this text.

probability sampling method Any random sampling technique in which each member (element) in the population has a greater than zero opportunity to be selected for the sample. The four types of probability sampling described in this text are simple random sampling, stratified random sampling, cluster sampling, and systematic sampling.

probability theory The branch of mathematics and statistics that addresses likelihood of occurrence and, in research, the likelihood that the findings or parameters of a sample are the same as the population parameters.

probing The act of posing secondary questions or questions during a qualitative interview so that the researcher can elicit contextual detail, clarification, and additional information.

problem statement The statement of the researcher at the end of the review of the literature that briefly synopsizes the state of the research and identifies the research gap. In clear language, the problem statement identifies the main concepts upon which the study will focus.

problematic reasoning Involves identifying a problem, selecting solutions to the problem, and resolving the problem.

process of care Construct that includes the actual care delivered by healthcare persons, both in a technical sense and in relation to patient-practitioner interactions with patients. Process of care is one of the three components (structure, process, and outcomes of care) of Donabedian's theory of quality of health care.

project grant proposal An application for a non-research grant to develop a new education program or implement an idea in clinical practice.

proportionate sampling A sampling strategy wherein subjects are selected from various strata so that their proportions are identical to those of the population.

proposal, research Written plan identifying the major elements of a study, such as the problem, purpose, and framework, and outlining the methods to conduct the study. The research proposal is written to request approval to conduct a study; it also must be submitted with requests for funding.

proposition Abstract, formal statement of the relationship between or among concepts.

prospective Looking forward in time. In data collection, refers to measurements made during the course of a study. Prospective is the opposite of retrospective.

prospective cohort study A study that uses a longitudinal design, either descriptive or correlational, in which a researcher identifies a group of persons at risk for a certain event, with data collection occurring at intervals. The prospective cohort study originated in the field of epidemiology.

protection from discomfort and harm A right of research participants based on the ethical principle of beneficence, which holds that one should do good and, above all, do no harm. The levels of discomfort and harm are (1) no anticipated effects, (2) temporary discomfort, (3) unusual levels of temporary discomfort, (4) risk of permanent damage, and (5) certainty of permanent damage.

providers of care Individuals responsible for delivering care, such as nurse practitioners and physicians, who are part of the structures of care of Donabedian's theory of health care.

publication bias Bias that occurs when studies with positive results are more likely to be published than studies with negative or inconclusive results.

published research Studies that are permanently recorded in hard copies of journals, monographs, conference proceedings, or books, or are posted online for readers to access.

purposive sampling Judgmental or selective sampling method that involves conscious selection by the researcher of certain subjects or elements to include in a study. Purposive sampling is a type of nonprobability or nonrandom sampling.

Q

Q-sort methodology Technique of comparative ratings in which a subject sorts cards with statements on them into designated piles (usually 7–10 piles in the distribution of a normal curve) that might range from best to worst. Q-sort methodology might be conducted to identify important items when developing a scale or for determining research priorities in specialty nursing areas.

qualitative research A scholarly and rigorous approach used to describe life experiences, cultures, and social processes from the perspectives of the persons involved.

qualitative research proposal A document developed by the researcher of a proposed qualitative study that often includes an introduction, a review of the literature, the philosophical foundation for the selected approach, and the method of inquiry.

qualitative research synthesis Process and product of systematically reviewing and formally integrating the findings from qualitative studies. Qualitative research synthesis produces either meta-summary or meta-synthesis.

qualitative research reports The written report of the results of qualitative inquiry, intended to describe the dynamic implementation of the research project and the unique, creative findings obtained. The report usually includes introduction, review of the literature, methods, results, and discussion sections.

quantitative research Formal, objective, systematic study process that counts or measures, in order to answer a research question. Its data are analyzed numerically.

quantitative research proposal A document developed by the researcher of a proposed quantitative study that often includes the introduction, review of the literature, framework, and methodology proposed for the study.

quantitative research report A written report that includes an introduction, review of the literature, methods, results, and a discussion of findings for a quantitative study.

quasi-experimental research Type of quantitative research conducted to test a cause-and-effect relationship, but which lacks one or more of the three essential elements of experimental research: (1) researcher-controlled manipulation of the independent variable, (2) the traditional type of control group, and (3) random assignment of subjects to groups.

query letter Letter sent to an editor of a journal to ask about the editor's interest in reviewing a manuscript.

questionnaire Self-report form designed to elicit information that can be obtained through the subject's selection from a list of predetermined options or through textual responses of the subject.

quota sampling Nonprobability convenience sampling technique in which the proportion of identified groups is predetermined by the researcher. Quota sampling may be used to ensure the inclusion of subject types likely to be underrepresented in the convenience sample, such as women, minority groups, and the undereducated, or to constitute the sample in order to achieve some sort of representativeness.

R

random assignment to groups Procedure used to assign subjects to treatment or comparison group, in which each subject has an equal opportunity to be assigned to either group.

random error Error that causes individuals' observed scores to vary haphazardly around the true score without a pattern.

random heterogeneity of respondents The threat to design validity that exists when subjects in a treatment or intervention group differ in ways that correlate with the dependent variable.

random sampling methods See *probability sampling method*.

random variation Normally-occurring and expected difference in values that occurs when one examines different subjects from the same sample.

randomization Term used in medical and biological research that is equivalent to random assignment.

randomized block design An experimental design in which the researcher assigns subjects to groups so that a potentially extraneous variable, whose values are known before intervention, is equally distributed among groups.

randomized controlled trial (RCT) A trial of an intervention using the pretest-posttest control group design, or another experimental design closely related to it, in order to produce definitive evidence for an intervention. An RCT may be single-site or multisite.

range Simplest measure of dispersion, obtained by subtracting the lowest score from the highest score ("range of 63") or by identifying the lowest and highest scores in a distribution of scores ("range from 118 to 181").

rating scales A method of measurement in which the rater assigns a value, sometimes numeric and sometimes not, from among an ordered set of predefined categories, in order to convey feelings, preferences, and other subjective perceptions. FACES Pain Rating Scale is a commonly used rating scale to measure pain in pediatric patients.

ratio data Numerical information based on the real number scale. Ratio data are mutually exclusive and mutually exhaustive, and they are real, in that they represent actual quanta and are capable of representing values between the numerals such as fractions and decimals. Ratio data are analyzed with parametric statistics.

ratio level of measurement Highest measurement form that meets all the rules of other forms of measure: mutually exclusive categories, exhaustive categories, rank ordering, equal spacing between intervals, and a continuum of values; also has an absolute zero, such as weight. A measurement that exists at the ratio level. See *ratio data*.

readability The degree of difficulty with which a text may be read and comprehended, often applied to a scale or survey instrument. Most available readability tools are based on the length of phrases or sentences, and number of syllables in words of the scale. The readability of a scale can influence its reliability and validity when used in a study.

repeated measures design A research design that repeatedly assesses or measures study variables in the same group of subjects.

reasoning Processing and organizing ideas to reach conclusions. Some types of reasoning described in this text are problematic, operational, dialectic, and logistical.

recommendations for further research An objective assessment of the state of the current research-generated body of knowledge in a discipline, based on the findings of the current study and a review of the literature, and the logical steps subsequent researchers might take in the future in order to expand that knowledge.

recruiting research participants The process of obtaining subjects or participants for a study that includes identifying potential subjects, approaching them to participate in the study, and gaining their agreement to participate.

refereed journal Publication that is peer-reviewed, using expert reviewers (referees) to determine whether a manuscript is suitable for publication in that particular journal.

reference group Group of individuals or other elements that constitutes the standard against which individual subjects' scores are compared.

referencing Comparing a subject's score against a standard, which is used in norm-referenced and criterion-referenced testing.

reflexivity A qualitative researcher's introspective self-awareness and critical examination of the interaction between self and the data during data collection and analysis. Reflexivity may lead the researcher to explore personal feelings and experiences that could introduce bias into the data analysis process.

refusal rate Percentage of potential subjects who decide not to participate in a study. The refusal rate is calculated by dividing the number refusing to participate by the number of potential subjects approached. For example, if 100 subjects are approached and 15 refuse to participate, the refusal rate is $(15 \div 100) \times 100\% = 0.15 \times 100\% = 15\%$.

regression analysis Analysis wherein the statistical relationship between or among variables is measured and characterized. The independent (predictor) variable or variables are analyzed to determine the influence upon variation or change in the value of the dependent variable.

regression coefficient (*R*) Statistic for multiple regression analysis.

regression line Line that best represents the linear relationship between two variables and may be depicted amidst the values of the raw scores plotted on a scatter diagram.

relational statement Declares that a relationship or link of some kind (positive or negative) exists between or among concepts. Within theories, relational statements also are called propositions and become the focus of testing in quantitative research.

relative risk A quantification of an occurrence, comparing two groups, sometimes comparing subjects in an experimental group and subjects in a control group. Relative risk is used most frequently to describe the risk associated with treated versus untreated conditions, with screening versus nonscreening, or with exposure versus nonexposure. Also referred to as *risk ratio*.

relevant literature Sources that are pertinent or highly important in providing the in-depth knowledge needed to synthesize the state of the body of knowledge within a problem area.

reliability Represents the consistency of the measure obtained. Also see *reliability testing*.

reliability testing Measure of the amount of random error in the measurement technique. Reliability testing of measurement methods focuses on the following three aspects of reliability: stability, equivalence, and internal consistency or homogeneity.

replication The act of reproducing or repeating a study in order to determine whether similar findings will be obtained, thus assessing the possibility of Type I or Type II error in the original study and sometimes allowing extension of findings to a larger population.

replication, approximate Operational replication that involves repeating the original study under similar conditions

and following the methods as closely as possible.

replication, concurrent A type of replication that involves collection of data for the original study and simultaneous replication of the data to provide a check of the reliability of the original study. Confirmation of the original study findings through replication is part of the original study's design.

replication, exact A type of replication that involves precise or exact duplication of the initial researcher's study to confirm the original findings. Exact replication is an ideal, not a reality.

replication, systematic Constructive replication that is done under distinctly new conditions in which the researchers conducting the replication follow the design but not the methods of the original researchers. The goal of such replication is to extend the findings of the original study to different settings, or to clients with different disease processes.

representativeness of the sample The degree to which the sample is like the population it purportedly represents.

request for applications (RFA) An opportunity for funding similar to the request for proposals (RFP), except that the government agency not only identifies the problem of concern but also describes what the goal of the research is. For example, an RFA may be released to discover the psychological characteristics of patients seeking bariatric surgery. Researchers design their own research and compete for this type of contract.

request for proposals (RFP) An opportunity for funding in which an agency within the federal government seeks proposals from researchers dealing with a specific clinical or system problem.

research Diligent, systematic inquiry or investigation to validate and refine existing knowledge and generate new knowledge.

research benefit Something of health-related, psychosocial, or other value to an individual research subject, or something that will contribute to the acquisition of generalizable knowledge. Assessing research benefits is part of the ethical process of balancing benefits and risks for a study.

research design See *design, research*.

research grant Funding awarded specifically for conducting a study.

research hypothesis Alternative hypothesis to the null hypothesis, stating that there is a relationship or a difference between two or more variables.

research methodology See *methodology, research*.

research methods See *methods, research*.

research misconduct Deliberate fabrication, falsification, or plagiarism in processing, performing, or reviewing research, or in reporting research results. Falsification does not include honest error or differences in opinion.

research objectives (or aims) The researcher's formal stated goal or goals of the study: its desired outcomes. If quantitative research has several articulated objectives or aims, each addresses the outcome of a specific statistical test or comparison.

research problem An area in which there is a gap in the knowledge base.

research proposal See *proposal, research*.

research purpose Concise, clear statement of the researcher's specific overriding focus or aim: the reason for conducting the study.

research questions Concise, interrogative statements developed to direct research studies.

research report The written description of a completed study designed to communicate study findings efficiently and effectively to nurses and other healthcare professionals.

research topics Concepts or broad problem areas that indicate the foci of essential research knowledge needed to provide evidence-based nursing practice. Research topics include numerous potential research problems.

research utilization Process of synthesizing, disseminating, and using research-generated knowledge to make an impact on or a change in a practice discipline.

research variable or concept A default term used to refer to a variable that is the focus of a quantitative study but that is not identified as an independent or a dependent variable.

research participants or informants See *subjects*.

researcher-participant relationships In qualitative research, the specific interactions between the researcher and the study participants that are initiated by the researcher and that establish

rapport, encouraging both information exchange and communication of the participants' perceptions, feelings, and opinions.

residual variable Term used in model-testing research that denotes a variable, either known or unknown, that is not included in a proposed model.

respect for persons, principle of Ethical principle that indicates that persons have the right to self-determination and the freedom to participate or not participate in research.

response set Parameters or possible answers within which a question or item is to be answered in a questionnaire. For example, a response set for a questionnaire might include a range of options between "strongly agree" and "strongly disagree."

results Outcomes from data analysis that are generated for each research objective, question, or hypothesis.

retaining research participants Keeping subjects participating in a study and preventing their attrition. A high retention rate provides a more representative sample and decreases the threats to design validity.

retention rate The number and percentage of subjects completing a study.

retrospective Looking backward in time. In data collection, refers to measurements made in the past that are retrieved by the research team from existent records, in the course of a study. Retrospective is the opposite of prospective.

retrospective study Literally a study that looks back. Retrospective research retrieves existent data and analyzes them.

right to self-determination See *self-determination, right to*.

rigor Literally, hardness or difficulty. In research, rigor is associated with paying attention to detail and exerting unflagging effort to adhere to scientific standards. In quantitative research, rigor implies a high degree of accuracy, consistency, and attention to all measurable aspects of the research. In qualitative research, rigor implies ensuring congruence between the philosophical foundation, qualitative approach, and methods with the goal of producing trustworthy findings.

risk ratio See *relative risk*.

rival hypothesis A second hypothesis that serves as an alternate explanation

for the study findings. Although the researcher may state a rival hypothesis in a research design, in nursing research, the rival hypothesis usually represents a dichotomy in interpretation introduced by an extraneous variable.

robustness The ability of a statistical analysis procedure to yield accurate results even when some of its assumptions are violated.

role-modeling Learning by imitating the behavior of an exemplar or role model.

S

sample Subset of the population that is selected for a study.

sample attrition See *attrition rate*.

sample characteristics Description of the research subjects who actually participate in a study, obtained by analyzing data acquired from the measurement of their demographic variables (e.g., age, gender, ethnicity, medical diagnosis).

sample size Number of subjects or participants who actually participate in at least the first phase of a study.

sampling Selecting groups of people, events, behaviors, or other elements with which to conduct a study.

sampling criteria List of the characteristics essential for membership in the target population. Sampling criteria consist of both inclusion and exclusion criteria. Sampling criteria are *not* the same as sample characteristics.

sampling error Difference between a sample statistic used to estimate a population parameter and the actual but unknown value of the parameter.

sampling frame A listing of every member of the population with membership defined by the sampling criteria.

sampling method The process of selecting a group of people, events, behaviors, or other elements that meet sampling criteria. Sampling methods may be random or nonrandom.

sampling plan A description of the strategies that will be used to obtain a sample for a study. The sampling plan may include either probability or nonprobability sampling methods.

scale Self-report form of measurement composed of several related items that are thought to measure the construct being studied. The subject responds to each item on the continuum or scale provided, such as a pain perception scale or state anxiety scale.

scatter diagrams or scatterplots   Graphs that provide a visual array of data points. Scatter diagrams provide a useful preliminary impression about the nature of the relationship between variables and the distribution of the data.

science   Coherent body of knowledge composed of research findings, tested theories, scientific principles, and laws for a discipline.

scientific method   All procedures that scientists have used, currently use, or may use in the future to pursue knowledge. "The scientific method," however, is a means of testing hypotheses, using deduction and hypothetical reasoning. It rests on the process of stating a hypothesis, testing it, and then either disproving it or testing it more fully.

scientific theory   Theory with valid and reliable methods of measuring each concept and relational statements that has been tested repeatedly through research and demonstrated to be valid.

secondary analysis   A strategy in which a researcher performs an analysis of data collected and originally analyzed by another researcher or agency. It may involve the use of administrative or research databases.

secondary source   Source that summarizes or quotes content from a primary source.

seeking approval to conduct a study   Process that involves submission of a research proposal to an authority or group for review.

selection   The process by which subjects are chosen to take part in a study.

selection threat   A threat to internal validity in which subject assignment to a group occurs in a nonrandom way. Selection threat occurs most frequently because of subject self-assignment to a group, or because experimental and control groups represent distinctly different populations.

selection-maturation   interaction   A threat to internal validity in a study with nonrandom group assignment, selection-maturation interaction occurs when the naturally occurring attributes in one group change due to the passage of time, independent of the study treatment.

self-determination, right to   A right that is based on the ethical principle of respect for persons, which states that because humans are capable of making their own decisions, they should be treated as autonomous agents who have the freedom to conduct their lives as they choose, without external controls.

seminal study   Study that prompted the initiation of a field of research.

sensitivity, physiological measure   The extent to which a physiologic measure can detect a small change. Higher sensitivity means more precision.

sensitivity of screening or diagnostic test   The accuracy of a screening or diagnostic test; the proportion of patients with the disease who have a true positive test result.

sequential relationship   Relationship in which one concept occurs later than the other.

serendipitous results   Research results that were not the primary focus of a study but that reveal new information that may prove useful.

serials   Literature published over time or in multiple volumes at one time. Serials do not necessarily have a predictable publication date.

setting, research   Location for conducting research. A research setting may be natural, partially controlled, or highly controlled.

sham   Something that appears to be something it is not: a deceit. A sham intervention may be used with a control group so that the subjects perceive that they have received an intervention, such as an intravenous medication. Use of a sham intervention prevents subjects from knowing their group assignment, avoiding potential threats to construct validity.

Shapiro-Wilk's *W* test   A statistical test of normality that assesses whether a variable's distribution is normal, versus skewed and/or kurtotic.

significance of a problem   Part of the research problem. In nursing, the significance statement expresses the importance of the problem to nursing and to the health of individuals, families, or communities.

significant results   Results of statistical analyses that are highly unlikely to have occurred by chance. Statistically significant results are those that are in keeping with the researcher's predictions, if predictions were made.

significant and not predicted results   Significant results that are the opposite of those predicted by the researcher. These also are referred to as *unexpected results.*

(simple) correlational design   Used to describe relationships between or among variables.

simple hypothesis   A statement of the posited relationship (associative or causal) between two variables.

simple linear regression   Parametric analysis technique that provides a means to estimate the value of a dependent variable based on the value of an independent variable.

simple random sampling   Selection of elements at random from a sampling frame for inclusion in a study. Each study element has a probability greater than zero of being selected for inclusion in the study.

situated   The time and place in which a person lives that shape his or her life experiences. Cultural, societal, relationship, and environmental factors create the unique context in which a person lives.

situated freedom   The amount of flexibility a person has to make certain choices based on his or her unique set of circumstances.

skewed   A curve that is asymmetrical (positively or negatively) because of an asymmetrical (non-normal) distribution of scores from a study.

skimming a source   Quickly reviewing a source to gain a broad overview of the content.

slope   The amount by which a line deviates from the horizontal. In statistics, the direction and angle of the regression line on a graph, represented by the letter *b*.

small area analyses   See *geographical analyses.*

snowball sampling   See *network sampling.*

Spearman rank-order correlation coefficient   Nonparametric analysis technique for ordinal data that is an adaptation of the Pearson's product-moment correlation used to examine relationships among variables in a study.

specific propositions   Statements found in theories that are at a moderate level of abstraction and provide the basis for the generation of hypotheses to guide a study.

specificity of a screening or diagnostic test   Proportion of patients without a disease who are actually identified as disease-free, as shown by negative test results.

split-half reliability   Process used to determine the homogeneity of an instrument's items. The instrument items are split in half, and a correlational procedure is performed, comparing the two halves for degree of similarity.

spurious correlations   Correlational tests found to be statistically significant when, in fact, the relationships they represent are not present. These represent a Type I error. Replication of the research usually results in statistically nonsignificant findings.

stability reliability   The degree to which a measurement instrument produces the same score on repeated administration.

standard deviation (*SD*)   A measure of the amount of dispersion from the mean that characterizes a data set.

standard of care   The norm on which quality of care is judged. Standards of care are based on research findings, in conjunction with current practice patterns. According to Donabedian, a standard of care is considered one of the processes of care.

standard scores   Used to express deviations from the mean (difference scores) in terms of standard deviation units, such as *z* scores, in which the mean is 0 and the standard deviation is 1.

standardized mean difference   Calculated in a meta-analysis when the same outcome, such as depression, is measured by different scales or methods.

statement synthesis   Combining information across theories and research findings about relationships among concepts to propose specific new or restated relationships among the concepts being studied. This step is a part of developing a framework for a study.

statistic   Numerical value obtained from a sample that is used to estimate a population parameter.

statistical conclusion validity   The degree to which the researcher makes decisions about proper use of statistics, so that the conclusions about relationships and differences drawn from the analyses are accurate reflections of reality.

statistical hypothesis   See *null hypothesis*.

statistical regression toward the mean   A threat to internal validity that is present when subjects display extreme scores of a variable. On remeasurement, the value tends to be closer to the population mean, so attribution of true cause is complicated.

statistical significance   The condition in which the value of the calculated statistic for a certain test exceeds the predetermined cut-off point. Statistical significance means that the null hypothesis is rejected.

Stetler Model of Research Utilization to Facilitate Evidence-Based Practice   Model developed by Stetler that provides a comprehensive framework to enhance the use of research findings by nurses to facilitate evidence-based practice.

stratification   A strategy used in one type of random sampling, in which the researcher predetermines the desired subject proportion of various levels (strata) of a characteristic of interest in the study population. Stratification may be used to create a sample proportionate to the population, or one that is intentionally disproportionate, depending on the study purpose and research question.

stratified random sampling   Used when the researcher knows some of the variables in the population that are critical to achieving representativeness. These identified variables are used to divide the sample into strata or groups.

strength of a relationship   Amount of variation explained by a relationship. A value of the statistic *r* that is close to 1 or to −1 represents a very strong relationship; a value of *r* close to 0 represents a very weak relationship.

structural equation modeling (SEM)   A complex analysis of theoretical interrelationships among variables displayed in a diagrammed model. Using multiple regression analysis, its complex calculations allow the researcher to identify the best model that explains interactions among variables, yielding the greatest explained variance.

structured interview   A set of interview questions in which questions are asked in the same order with all subjects. A quantitative structured interview's answer options are predefined and limited, while the answer options in qualitative structured interviews are flexible. Interviews in qualitative studies are more commonly semi-structured interviews.

structured observation   Clearly identifying what is to be observed and precisely defining how the observations are to be made, recorded, and coded.

structures of care   Set entities that affect quality of care in a healthcare environment. Some structures of care are the overall organization and administration of the healthcare agency, the essential equipment of care, educational preparation of qualified health personnel, staffing, and workforce size, as well as patient characteristics and the physical plant of the agency within its neighborhood.

study protocol   A step-by-step, detailed plan for implementing a study, beginning with recruitment and concluding with final data collection.

study validity   Measure of the truth or accuracy of research. It includes the degree to which measured variables represent what they are thought to represent.

study variables   Concepts at various levels of abstraction that are defined and measured during the course of a study.

subject attrition   See *attrition rate*.

subjects   Individuals participating in a study.

subject term   Frequently searched term included in a database thesaurus.

substantive theory   A theory that is contextual and that applies directly to practice. Synonymous with *middle-range theory*.

substitutable relationship   Relationship in which a similar concept can be substituted for the first concept and the second concept will occur.

substituted judgment standard   In the ethical conduct of research, a standard concerned with determining the course of action that incompetent individuals would take if they were capable of making their own decisions.

substruction, theoretical   The technique of diagramming a research study's constructs, concepts, variables, relationships, and measurement methods for easy review of logical consistency among levels.

sufficient relationship   States that when the first variable or concept occurs, the second will occur, regardless of the presence or absence of other factors.

sum of squares Mathematical manipulation involving summing the squares of the difference scores that is used as part of the analysis process for calculating the standard deviation.

summary statistics See *descriptive statistics.*

summated scales Scales in which various items are summed to obtain a single score.

survey Data collection technique in which questionnaires are used to gather data about an identified population.

symbolic meaning In symbolic interaction, the meaning attached to particular ideas or clusters of data. A shared symbol is one for which the meaning is the same for a group of persons or a society.

symmetrical curve A curve in which the left side is a mirror image of the right side.

symmetrical relationship A bi-directional relationship in which two variables are related, no matter which one occurs first. If A occurs (or changes), B will occur (or change); if B occurs (or changes), A will occur (or change).

synthesis of sources Clustering and interrelating ideas from several sources to promote a new understanding or provide a description of what is known and not known in an area.

systematic bias or variation Bias or variation obtained when subjects in a study share various characteristics, making the sample less representative than desired. Their resemblance to one another makes it more likely that demographics and measurements of effects of interventions will be quite similar for most of them.

systematic error Measurement error that is not random but occurs consistently, with the same magnitude and in the same direction, each time the measurement is applied.

systematic review Structured, comprehensive synthesis of quantitative studies in a particular healthcare area to determine the best research evidence available for expert clinicians to use to promote an evidence-based practice.

systematic sampling Conducted when an ordered list of all members of the population is available and involves selecting every *k*th individual on the list,

starting from a point that is selected randomly.

table Presentation of data, study results, or other information in columns and rows for easy review by the reader.

tails Extremes of the normal curve where significant statistical values can be found.

target population All elements (individuals, objects, events, or substances) that meet the sampling criteria for inclusion in a study, and to which the study findings will be generalized.

technical efficiency The degree to which there is waste-minimum utilization of precious resources, which are usually inadequate for serving an entire population and can be scarce.

tentative theory Theory that is newly proposed, has had minimal exposure to critical appraisal by the discipline, and has had little testing.

testable Study that contains variables that are measurable or can be manipulated in the real world.

test-retest reliability Determination of the stability or consistency of a measurement technique by correlating the scores obtained from repeated measures.

textbooks Monographs written to be used in formal educational programs.

themes See *emergent concepts.*

theoretical limitations Inability to conceptually define and operationalize study variables adequately, or inadequate connections among construct, concept, variable, and measurement. Theoretical limitations imply illogical or incomplete reasoning and substantially restrict abstract generalization of the findings.

theoretical literature Published concept analyses, conceptual maps, theories, and conceptual frameworks.

theoretical sampling A method of sampling often used in grounded theory research to advance the development of a theory throughout the research process. The researcher recruits eligible subjects on the basis of their ability to advance the emergent theory.

theory An integrated set of defined concepts, existence statements, and relational statements that are defined and interrelated to present a systematic view of a phenomenon.

therapeutic research Research that provides the patient an opportunity to receive an experimental treatment that might have beneficial results.

thesis Research project completed by a master's student as part of the requirements for a master's degree. A thesis is usually a culminating or capstone accomplishment.

threat to validity A factor or condition that decreases the validity of research results. The four threats to design validity are threats to construct validity, internal validity, external validity, and statistical conclusion validity.

threat to construct validity Design flaw in which the measurement of a variable is not suitable for the concept it represents. In most cases, this threat occurs because of the researcher's imprecise operational definition of the variable.

threat to external validity A limit to generalization based on differences between the conditions or participants of the study and the conditions or characteristics of persons or settings to which generalization is considered.

threat to internal validity In interventional research, a factor that causes changes in the dependent variable, so that these do not occur solely as a result of the action of the independent variable. In noninterventional research, a measurement that includes not only the concept of interest but other related concepts. In interventional research, two common reasons for these threats are that experimental and control groups are fundamentally dissimilar at the onset of the study or as the study progresses, and that groups are exposed in a dissimilar way to outside influences during the course of the study.

threat to statistical conclusion validity A factor that produces a false data analysis conclusion. Usually these threats occur because of inadequate sample size or inappropriate use of a statistical test.

time-lag bias A type of publication bias that occurs because studies with negative results are usually published later, sometimes 2 or 3 years later, than are studies with positive results.

time-dimensional designs Designs used extensively within the discipline of epidemiology to examine change over time, in relation to disease occurrence. In nursing, that change over time is often development, learning, personal growth, disease progression, exposure, aging, or deterioration.

time series designs One of a related set of quantitative quasi-experimental designs, in which data are collected repeatedly for a single group, both before and following an intervention.

time series design with comparison group Quasi-experimental design, in which simultaneous data are collected repeatedly for two groups. One of the groups reflects an intervention; the other does not.

time series design with repeated reversal Quasi-experimental design, in which data are collected repeated for a single group. An intervention is introduced and a measurement made; then the intervention is removed and another measurement made. This process of re-applying the intervention, with a measurement, and removing it, followed by another measurement, is repeated for at least two complete cycles. The design is also called the repeated-reversal design, and sometimes single subject research.

total variance The sum of the within-group variance and the between-group variance determined by conducting analysis of variance (ANOVA).

traditions Truths or beliefs that are based on customs and past trends and provide a way of acquiring knowledge.

translation/application Transforming from one language to another to facilitate understanding; in research, part of the process of interpreting quantitative research results, in which numerical results are translated into language and interpreted as findings. In qualitative research, theoretical and/or abstract results are translated into the language of daily life and clinical practice and interpreted as findings.

translational research An evolving concept that is defined by the National Institutes of Health as the translation of basic scientific discoveries into practical applications.

treatment Independent variable or intervention that is manipulated in a study to produce an effect on the dependent variable.

treatment fidelity The accuracy, consistency, and thoroughness in the manner in which an intervention is delivered, according to the specified protocol, treatment program, or intervention model.

trend designs Designs used to examine changes over time in the value of a variable, in an identified population.

trial and error An approach with unknown outcomes that is used in a situation of uncertainty when other sources of knowledge are unavailable.

triangulation The integration of data from two sources or sets of data. A metaphor taken from ship navigation and land surveying in which measurements are taken from two perspectives and the point of intersection is the location of a distant object.

truncated Shortened or cut off. In research, refers to an incomplete data set, in which the range of scores has been artificially compressed, by either eliminating outliers or representing values at the extremes as a small group such as "greater than 25."

true negative Result of a diagnostic or screening test that indicates accurately the absence of a disease/condition.

true positive Result of a diagnostic or screening test that indicates accurately the presence of a disease/condition.

true score Score that would be obtained if there were no error in measurement. Theoretically, some measurement error always occurs when a sample is used to estimate a population parameter.

t-test A parametric analysis technique used to determine significant differences between measures of two samples. See *independent samples* t-test and *paired samples* t-test.

two-tailed test of significance Type of analysis used for a nondirectional hypothesis in which the researcher assumes that an extreme score can occur in either tail.

two-way chi-square A nonparametric statistic that tests the association between two categorical variables.

Type I error Error that occurs when the researcher concludes that the samples tested are from different populations (the difference between groups is significant) when, in fact, the samples are from the same population (the difference between groups is not significant). The null hypothesis is rejected when it is, in fact, true.

Type II error Error that occurs when the researcher concludes that there is no significant difference between the samples examined when, in fact, a difference exists. The null hypothesis is regarded as true when it is, in fact, false. Type II error often occurs when a sample is of insufficient size to demonstrate a difference.

U

ungrouped frequency distribution A table or display listing all values of a variable and next to them the number of times in the set that the value was recorded.

unimodal Distribution of scores in a sample that displays one mode (most frequently occurring score).

unstructured interview Interview initiated with a broad question, after which subjects are encouraged to elaborate by telling their stories. The unstructured interview is a common data collection method used in qualitative research.

unstructured observations Spontaneously observing and recording what is seen with a minimum of planning. Unstructured observation is a common data collection method used in qualitative research.

V

validation phase Second phase of the Stetler Model, in which the research reports are critically appraised to determine their scientific soundness.

validity, instrument The extent to which an instrument actually reflects or is able to measure the construct being examined.

variables Concrete or abstract ideas that have been made measurable. In quantitative research, variables are studied in order to establish their incidence, the connections that may exist among them, or cause-and-effect relationships.

variance Measure of dispersion that is the mean or average of the sum of squares. Also, in a prediction model, the total amount of the dependent variable that is explained by the predictor variables.

variance analysis Outcomes research strategy that defines expected outcomes, and the approximate points at which they are expected to occur, and then tracks delay or non-achievement of these outcomes.

vary To be different. Numerical values associated with variables may vary or change, from one measurement to the next, or they may remain unchanged.

verbal presentation The communication of a research report at a professional conference or meeting.

vertical axis The *y*-axis in a graph of a regression line or scatterplot. The vertical axis is oriented in a top-to-bottom direction across the graph.

visual analog scale A line 100 mm in length with right-angle stops at each end on which subjects are asked to record their response to a study variable. Also referred to as *magnitude scale*.

volunteer sample Those willing to participate in the study. All samples with human subjects must be volunteer samples.

voluntary consent Indication that prospective subject has decided to take part in a study of his or her own volition without coercion or any undue influence.

W

wait-listed In experimental research, refers to a control group guaranteed to receive the treatment at the completion of the study. The strategy of wait-listing is sometimes used in the first tests of a new therapeutic medical intervention.

washout period The amount of time that is required for the effects of an intervention to dissipate, and the subject to return to baseline.

Wilcoxon matched-pairs test Nonparametric analysis technique conducted to examine changes that occur in pretest-posttest measures or matched-pairs measures.

within-group variance Variance that results when individual scores in a group vary from the group mean.

Y

y-intercept Point at which the regression line crosses (or intercepts) the *y*-axis. At this point on the regression line, $x = 0$.

Z

z scores Standardized scores developed from the normal curve.

Page numbers followed by "*f*" indicate figures, "*t*" indicate tables, and "*b*" indicate boxes.

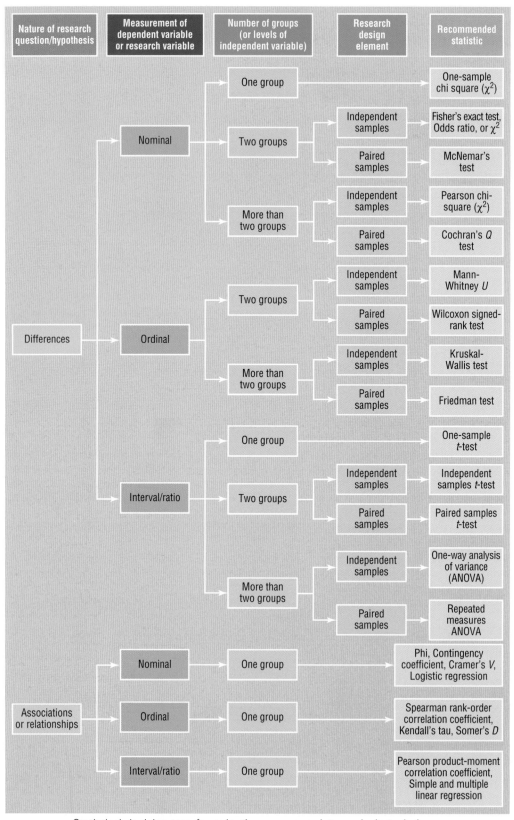

Statistical decision tree for selecting an appropriate analysis technique.